PSYCHO
DRUG
DIRECTORY
2010

THE PROFESSIONALS' POCKET HANDBOOK AND AIDE MEMOIRE

PSYCHOTROPIC
DRUG
DIRECTORY
2010

THE PROFESSIONALS' POCKET HANDBOOK AND AIDE MEMOIRE

STEPHEN BAZIRE

HEALTHCOMM UK Ltd

HealthComm UK Ltd, A Schofield Healthcare Media Company, Suite 3.1,
36 Upperkirkgate, Aberdeen AB10 1BA

British Library Cataloguing-in-Publication Data
A catalogue record is available for this book

ISBN-10   0-95555758-8-5
ISBN-13   978-0-9555758-8-4

Printed in Malta by Gutenberg Press Limited, Tarxien, Malta

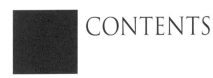

CONTENTS

CHAPTER 4: DRUG INTERACTIONS

CHAPTER 5: DRUG-INDUCED PSYCHIATRIC DISORDERS

CHAPTER 6: MANAGEMENT OF SIDE-EFFECTS

CHAPTER 7: PSYCHOTROPIC DRUGS

INDEX AND ABBREVIATIONS

INTRODUCTION

Why the *Psychotropic Drug Directory (PDD) 2010*? Well, the title tries to describe the contents, and how you should use them. The 'directory' part is because the book contains general principles, lists, issues, advice and references to help you make decisions but then directs you where to go to get the further information you might need, since it would be virtually impossible to convey all the subtleties of a research paper, case report or review in a couple of lines. I have, for instance, added well over 2000 new references to the text in this edition. If I spent a couple of hours thoroughly reading and analysing each and every paper, I'd never be able to finish the book and would have to give up the day job, before it gives up on me. So, you really should check papers before making important decisions. I would be hugely grateful for any advice or tips about papers that I may have taken at face value and inadvertently missed the errors, hidden bias or multiple publication.

It may be worth pointing out that this book is an entirely independent publication. There is no commercial sponsorship, support or influence on the content, which remains entirely my own work.

How to use the book...

The *PDD 2010* is arranged in a problem-solving way to aid optimum medication use:

- *Chapter 1*: select a mental health problem needing medication management and consider the pharmacological options from the BNF, combination and unlicensed lists.
- *Chapter 2* aids choosing a drug and dose, where a choice exists or is necessary.
- *Chapter 3* aids drug choice in a compromised patient.
- *Chapter 4* allows checking for drug–drug interactions.
- *Chapter 5* is an important check that the mental health problem is not drug-induced.
- *Chapter 6* helps to guide you where a drug works, but side-effects limit effectiveness.
- *Chapter 7* has got historical and other information I couldn't think where else to put.

A minimum level of knowledge is assumed and information given should be followed up in the appropriate sources when time allows. References, where quoted, are either of good recent review articles, or, of specific information.

Further information can be obtained by referring to the main paper or papers cited and also to the reference sections of those main papers. Lists and references are as comprehensive as viable but could never claim to be fully complete, nor could this book ever be as comprehensive as a MedLine search on a chosen topic. The listing of a drug use in this book does not in any way imply that it is licensed or safe for this use, and all information is presented in good faith. Throughout, I have tried to be as objective as possible. It must be up to the reader to make up his or her own mind on a topic, but I hope that the statements and references will have pointed you in the right direction and the time saved in looking papers up will allow more thought. It is inevitable that some papers are from specialist journals but, where possible, I have always quoted more accessible journals in preference. If the only paper published on the use of a drug is from an obscure or ancient source this may well indicate the status of the paper. Also, perhaps, I'll endeavour to remind readers of their ethical duty and responsibility (blindingly obvious statement) to include service-users' aspirations when choosing unlicensed and novel therapies.

Changes to this edition

Updates have been made to all chapters (marked with a *), including a full revision of *Chapter 5*, new sections in *Chapters 1, 2 and 6*.

Acknowledgements

Writing and continually updating a book such as this is a tremendous challenge and drain on my stamina and enthusiasm. Subsequently, the continued help, encouragement, constructive criticism and advice I have received from colleagues and correspondents throughout the world has always been utterly invaluable, not to mention very rewarding. It is wonderful to know that the book has helped improve the pharmaceutical care of many people with mental health needs. I would thus like to thank all the people I have thanked in previous editions, the many members of the College of Mental Health Pharmacy (formerly UKPPG) who have conveyed continued enthusiasm, encouragement and support, and all those people I have met at conferences and talks or who have written to me. Thanks as ever must go to my pharmacy staff and colleagues in the trust for continuing to tolerate and humour me, and special thanks to the University of East Anglia's fab School of Pharmacy for the honour. I also wish to thank the many people who have fed back on the book's contents and/or spotted ambiguities in the quarter of a million words, e.g. Laura Regan (for keeping the clozapine section up-to-date), Tanya Rimmer, Mojca Zvezdana, Paquita Bolton, Jackie Stark (Hull), Ben Browning and Dennis Liew. Thanks also to John Tams and Virgin Radio (especially The Geoff Show crew) for the company; to Ossi, Kadir, Shams, Muhrrem and Grandad Ossi at Grecco's (01603-624337) on Prince of Wales Road, Norwich for the world's best veggie pizzas (especially on a Monday night); to Jenny, Jill, Gail and Buz for being challenging; to my old mate Paul Woods; and of course, Binkie for being so good to work with; Judy in the library; Chris for keeping my computers running; my parents and my Godmother Kate Baxter for continuing to show interest; and Jill, Rosie and Chris for steering clear of me on Monday nights.

Stephen Bazire *BPharm, FRPharmS, DipPsychPharm, MCMHP*
Chief Pharmacist, Norfolk and Waveney Mental Health NHS Foundation Trust,
Hellesdon Hospital, Norwich NR6 5BE
Honorary Professor,
School Pharmacy,
University of East Anglia, Norwich
England
E-mail: steve.bazire@nwmhp.nhs.uk
Website for service users: www.nwmhp.nhs.uk/pharmacy
Website to aid service user choice of medication: www.choiceandmedication.org.uk
UKPPG website: www.ukppg.org.uk
Declaration of interests: www.ukppg.org.uk/committee.html

February, 2010

DRUG TREATMENT OPTIONS IN PSYCHIATRIC ILLNESS

This chapter lists medicines which are indicated for, or have been used in, the conditions listed and the author would welcome suggestions for further inclusions. References should be consulted for fuller details of non-approved uses. In some cases, drugs not available in the UK have been included as possible options if available, and for non-UK readers.

Drugs are classified as follows:

BNF listed

BNF listed drugs are listed in the *British National Formulary* and licensed in the UK for that condition, although there are a few drugs listed in the BNF for which no full licence has been granted. See the appropriate section in the BNF for a review of a drug's role in therapy and its prescribing details. Much information provided here is in addition to that in the standard texts.

+ Combinations

The combinations section includes some combinations that have been used, but carry the risks of additive side-effects and interactions.

● Unlicensed/some efficacy

This section includes drugs of some clinical efficacy (e.g. RCTs) or are strategies which can be used, but where no product licence exists.

■ Unlicensed/possible efficacy

This section includes drugs of minor or unproven importance or efficacy. No product licence exists.

◆ Others

This section includes drugs tried, but where no significant data exists since the original reports. The lack of positive follow-up data suggests a lack of efficacy although, if you know otherwise, the author would like to hear.

□ No efficacy

Drugs in this section are not thought to be of clinical use.

Information in these last four categories is given to provide help once all recognised and evidence-based treatments have been tried. These classifications are to some extent arbitrary, and the information is based on data presently available.

It is the prescriber's responsibility to ensure that all precautions are taken when prescribing a drug for an unlicensed use.

1.1 ACUTE PSYCHIATRIC EMERGENCY (APE) including RAPID TRANQUILLISATION
see Aggression (1.2), Mania and hypomania (1.10.2) and Psychosis and schizophrenia (1.23)

Violent patients (usually either schizophrenic, manic or substance abusers) present a risk to themselves and others. Swift, safe and effective treatment is often needed. Rapid tranquillisation (RT) is the term used to describe the procedure of giving varying amounts of antipsychotic medication, usually with benzodiazepines, over brief intervals of time to control agitated, threatening and potentially destructive patients.

Routes: IV administration is generally quicker-acting than IM, which is often little quicker than oral drugs (especially if concentrated liquids or melt-in-the-mouth tablets are used) and allows physical restraint to be removed more quickly. IV drug use does, however, carry additional dangers and the IM route should generally be the preferred choice except in exceptional circumstances. IM absorption will be more rapid in an active patient than a quiet one. Parenteral (IV/IM) doses generally have a higher potency than oral doses, so 'when required' or regular doses prescribed as 'IM/PO' are entirely inappropriate. All 'PRN' doses should be checked daily to ensure maximum doses are not being exceeded. Benzodiazepines are generally safe by (slow) injection, but antipsychotics can be fatal in moderate doses in drug-naïve people.

Doses: The need for high doses of antipsychotics is unnecessary, as violent patients respond to standard doses and higher doses may, in fact, be less effective, e.g. inducing akathisia. Use of concomitant benzodiazepines is safer and more effective than using high doses of antipsychotics as monotherapy.

Conditions: Manic patients may respond well to benzodiazepines, with antipsychotics as adjuncts. Schizophrenic patients usually respond best to antipsychotics, with benzodiazepines as adjuncts. In substance misuse, benzodiazepines and antipsychotics may be effective, but more studies are needed.

General principles of the management of acute psychiatric emergency (APE)

1. Obtain a drug history and carry out a physical examination if possible. Unless known previous exposure to psychotropics, use doses at the lower end of the ranges.
2. Antipsychotics in combination with benzodiazepines are preferred.
3. Parenteral administration is generally the quickest and most reliable route, but should be reserved **only** for when the patient cannot be persuaded to take drugs orally.
4. No anticholinergics should be used as this may confuse the clinical picture.
5. Switch to oral doses as soon as possible.
6. Check bp, pulse and temperature frequently.
7. Although APE can be carried out in the community, great care is needed and it is not recommended.

Potential complications of (particularly older) antipsychotics in APE:

1. Cardiovascular complications and sudden death — drugs causing QTc prolongation are contraindicated in patients with pre-existing cardiac problems, and care is needed in adrenaline-driven excited patients.
2. Respiratory depression.
3. Extrapyramidal symptoms, especially acute dystonia (may occur in 10–30% of patients within the first 24 hours and later in up to 50% of young males). Akathisia should be considered if agitation occurs, worsens or

recurs after antipsychotics have achieved adequate behavioural control, as it may be drug-induced and exacerbate the disturbed behaviour (see *Chapter 6.7*).
4. Acute hypotension (minimised if the patient can lie down) can occur, especially with phenothiazines and in the elderly.
5. Seizures, especially in non-compliant epileptics.
6. Mega-colon (rare), heatstroke, aspiration.
7. Neuroleptic malignant syndrome — see *Chapter 6.8* for risk factors. Close observation of temperature should be carried out, especially in early stages. Check CPK.
8. Local bruising, pain or extravasations (common, in up to 30% patients).
9. A depot given inadvertently into a vein may be rapidly fatal.
10. Disinhibition may occur with benzodiazepines, especially in people with poor impulse control or impulsivity, high-potency drugs, young or older age, developmental disabilities and/or pre-existing CNS damage. This remains controversial and probably over-rated (controlled study showing no effect: Rothschild *et al*, *J Clin Psychopharmacol* 2000;**20**:7–11; review by Paton, *Psychiatr Bull* 2002;**26**:460–2 noting the actual incidence may be lower than 1%).
11. In patients already taking antipsychotics, additional acute doses may reach toxic levels.

Reviews: Use of BDZs and antipsychotics in emergency departments (Rund *et al*, *J Emerg Med* 2006;**31**:317–24), reappraisal of current options (concludes that parenteral BDZs should now be the mainstay of treatment: McAllister-Williams and Ferrier, *Br J Psychiatry* 2002;**180**:485–9).

BNF listed *

Drugs in this section are licensed for emergency, short-term or adjunct therapy, of, e.g. acute psychosis, mania, anxiety or exacerbations of chronic psychosis, violent or impulsive behaviour, psychomotor agitation and excitement, or violent or dangerously impulsive behaviour. IM atypicals have a lower incidence of EPSE than IM haloperidol, unless the latter is combined with promethazine (n = 3425, Satterthwaite *et al*, *J Clin Psychiatry* 2008;**69**:1869–79).

ANTIPSYCHOTICS

Aripiprazole *

Aripiprazole is licensed for rapid control of agitation and disturbed behaviour in people with schizophrenia. The initial IM dose is 9.75 mg (range 5.25–15 mg). A second injection can be given after two hours, with no more than three doses in any 24 hours (maximum daily dose 30 mg, including all formulations). In acute psychotic agitation, aripiprazole (15–30 mg/d, n = 298) is as effective as olanzapine (20 mg/d, n = 306), with fewer side-effects (n = 604, RCT, d/b, 5/7, Kinon et al, J Clin Psychopharmacol 2008;28:601–7; MS, Lilly). In an earlier study, IM aripiprazole 9.5 mg was as effective as IM haloperidol 6.5 mg (but better tolerated) and superior to placebo in acute agitation in psychosis and schizophrenia (n = 448, RCT, d/b, p/c, Andrezina et al, Psychopharmacol [Berl] 2006;188:281–92). An analysis of three studies showed that aripiprazole IM can be used successfully to manage agitation, and may have a specific anti-agitation effect rather than just non-specific sedation (s = 3, Currier et al, J Psychiatr Pract 2007;13:159–69). Benzodiazepines can be given concomitantly but the patient must be monitored for excessive sedation and postural hypotension.

Chlorpromazine

Chlorpromazine is licensed for adjunctive short-term treatment of anxiety, agitation, violence or dangerously impulsive behaviour. The injection should be given by deep IM injection only, at 25–50 mg every 6–8 hours, with a lower dose (up to 25 mg eight-hourly) in the elderly. The IM injection is 2–4 times as potent, on a mg for mg basis, as oral chlorpromazine, and so prescriptions for '100 mg po/im' are entirely inappropriate and potentially dangerous. It can cause hypotension, has been associated with sudden death and is not recommended.

Haloperidol (see also combinations)

Haloperidol is licensed for adjunctive short-term treatment of moderate to severe agitation, violence or dangerously impulsive behaviour. It can be used at BNF doses, e.g. up to 30 mg/d orally or 18 mg/d by injection. Due to concerns about QTc prolongation (n = 596,

open, Reilly et al, Lancet 2000;355:1048–52) and reports of torsades de pointes, the SPC now recommends cardiac assessment and an ECG before starting treatment. The IV route in acutely disturbed patients should thus be avoided unless essential. Akathisia may exacerbate disturbed behaviour.

Olanzapine *

A number of studies (eg. n = 311 [c = 285]. RCT, d/b, p/c, Wright et al, Am J Psychiatry 2001;158:1149–51; n = 270, Wright et al, Schizophr Res 2001;49[Suppl 1]:250–1; n = 270, RCT, p/c, d/b, Breier et al, Arch Gen Psychiatry 2002;59:441–8) have shown olanzapine IM 10 mg to be at least as effective as haloperidol 7.5 mg IM in acute agitation in schizophrenia, with a possibly slightly quicker onset of action (e.g. at 30 minutes), no QT prolongation and significantly fewer EPS, including dystonia and akathisia (n = 311, RCT, p/c, Wright et al, Can J Psychiatry 2003;48:716–21, MS; review by Smith, EBMH 2003;6:27, noting that the response is in line with what would be expected from other antipsychotics). Other studies show olanzapine IM (n = 1294) to be more effective in APE after the first injection than zuclopenthixol IM or haloperidol IM (n = 2011, 7/7, Castle et al, World J Biol Psychiatry 2009;10:43–53), and orodispersible olanzapine was as effective as risperidone orodispersible in acute agitated psychosis, although olanzapine caused less tachycardia (n = 87, open, Hatta et al, Gen Hosp Psychiatry 2008;30:367–71). The following are Lilly's recommendations:

- Olanzapine IM can be used to rapidly control agitation and disturbed behaviours in patients with schizophrenia or manic episodes when oral is inappropriate.
- The maximum combined daily dose of oral and IM olanzapine is 20 mg.
- The initial dose of olanzapine IM should be 10 mg as a single injection (use lower doses in elderly patients and those with renal or hepatic impairment).
- A maximum of three injections of olanzapine IM may be administered in any 24 hours, and a minimum of two hours should elapse between each injection.
- Olanzapine IM is intended for short-term use, maximum of three consecutive days.

- Olanzapine 'Velotabs' produce a plasma level profile similar to oral tablets. IM peak plasma levels are five times higher than oral, peaking after a few minutes. Aggressive oral dosing strategies (e.g. up to 40mg/d) appear reasonably well tolerated and effective in controlling acutely agitated people with a variety of diagnoses (n = 148, RCT, p/c, 4/7, Baker et al, J Clin Psychopharmacol 2003;**23**:342–8, MS; comment by Citrome, EBMH 2004;**7**:12).
- There is no safety data on giving benzo-diazepines IM simultaneously with IM olanzapine. Benzodiazepines should not be given concomitantly (or within an hour) of olanzapine IM.
- Olanzapine pamoate should not be used for acute agitation or severe psychosis in people with schizophrenia (SPC).

Cochrane is critical of the supporting literature, noting the manufacturer's involvement, poor and incomplete reporting and the borderline ethical nature of the trials (s = 4, n = 769, Belgamwar and Fenton, Cochrane Database Syst Rev 2005; **2**:CD003729).

Review: use in acute agitation (Wagstaff et al, CNS Drugs 2005;**19**:147–64).

Quetiapine

Quetiapine is licensed for treatment of acute manic episodes, and 100–200mg stat may have some efficacy as a sedative in emergency settings, but with no clear dose-response pattern (n = 20, s/b, Currier et al, J Psychiatr Pract 2006;**12**:223–8).

Risperidone

Risperidone is licensed for acute mania (see combinations).

Trifluoperazine

Trifluoperazine is licensed as an adjunct therapy for acute anxiety and agitated states.

Zuclopenthixol acetate (Clopixol Acuphase®)

Clopixol Acuphase® (Lundbeck) can be given at a dose of 50–150mg stat, then repeated after 2–3 days (maximum every 1–2 days) after the first injection. The maximum cumulative dose is 400mg per 'course', i.e. four injections or over two weeks, whichever comes first. The onset of action is at about eight hours (peaking at about 36 hours; see psychosis 1.23), and so should only be used when initial control has been established with other agents. The maximum single dose in the elderly is 100mg. While zuclopenthixol acetate appears as effective as haloperidol in APE, sedation at four hours may be greater and there is an advantage of the need for fewer injections. Several reviews have suggested that more data is needed to prove an advantage over standard therapies (Gibson et al, Cochrane Database Syst Rev 2004;**3**:CD000525). Care is needed with Acuphase® to avoid it being given into a vein of a struggling or over-active patient.

BENZODIAZEPINES
(see also combinations)

Diazepam (see also combinations)

The recommended dose of diazepam is 10mg IV or IM, repeated after not less than four hours. IV infusion is possible, albeit difficult. IV diazepam is much more consistently absorbed than IM which, in turn, is little faster than oral and slower than the rectal route. If the IV route is used, it is strongly recommended to be into the large vein of the antecubital fossa with the patient, if possible, in a supine position to minimise the incidence of hypotension. The maximum IV dose is 5mg per minute. Mechanical ventilation and flumazenil should be available in case of respiratory depression, as hypoxic drive can be affected. Diazepam has a long half-life and active metabolites, and so accumulation and toxic delirium (especially in the elderly or hepatic impairment) must be avoided by use of decreased doses later on. A wide safety margin makes diazepam and lorazepam the drugs of choice.

Lorazepam (see also combinations)

Lorazepam is usually given by the IV route into a larger vein. IM absorption is as slow as oral administration, but more rapid in an active patient and IM generally carries less risk than IV. IM lorazepam alone was as effective as lorazepam IM plus either risperidone or haloperidol (both oral) in acute agitation and/

or psychosis, although the combination therapy was numerically superior (n = 30, RCT, d/b, d/b, Veser et al, J Psychiatr Pract 2006;**12**:103–8). Lorazepam injection may be diluted 50:50 with water or normal saline pre-injection. The dose in acute anxiety is 0.025–0.05 mg/kg (1.75–3.5 mg for a 70 kg person), repeated six-hourly. Some services use 0.5–2 mg PO/IM every 1–2 hours until symptoms are controlled, omitting doses when excessive sedation occurs. This can be a highly effective therapy. Caution is needed in renal and hepatic impairment and in the elderly, where lower doses may be needed. Lorazepam does not accumulate with repeated doses or in hepatic impairment; distinct advantages over diazepam.

● Unlicensed/some efficacy

Clomethiazole (chlormethiazole)
See SPC for doses for other indications.

Clonazepam
Clonazepam is licensed only for status epilepticus but can be used as an alternative to diazepam and lorazepam, albeit slower-acting. The dose is 1 mg (1 ml) by slow (1 mg per 30 seconds) IV injection, which is strongly recommended to be into the large vein of the antecubital fossa with the patient in a supine position, if possible, to minimise the incidence of hypotension. Care is needed in the elderly and caution in chronic pulmonary insufficiency.

+ Combinations

Combinations of antipsychotics and benzodiazepines are effective and allow lower doses of both to be used. Patients receiving monotherapy in APE at first are more likely to need second injections. A review concluded that combinations of a newer antipsychotic and a BDZ are optimal due to the lower incidence of EPS (s = 11, n = 701, Yildiz et al, Emerg Med J 2003;**20**:339–46).

Antipsychotic + benzodiazepine (see also separate drugs)
This combination is widely and strongly recommended, as the drugs act synergistically, reducing the amount of each drug (particularly the antipsychotic) required. The effect of the combination is rapid and predictable and the patient is less likely to require a second injection. **Lorazepam** is the most widely used benzodiazepine, with 2 mg IM plus haloperidol IM 5 mg being significantly better than lorazepam alone after 60–180 minutes in one APE study (n = 98, RCT, Battaglia et al, Am J Emerg Med 1997;**15**:335–40). Diazepam 10 mg IM/IV is a suitable alternative. In acute psychotic agitation, oral risperidone 2 mg plus lorazepam 2 mg was as effective and as well tolerated as haloperidol 5 mg IM plus lorazepam 2 mg IM over two hours (n = 83 + 79, RCT, s/b, Currier et al, J Clin Psychiatry 2004;**65**:386–94). The orodispersible risperidone tablets may be useful to ensure administration, although the peak plasma level occurs at 1.4–1.8 hours (the same as plain tablets) and can be as effective as an alternative to IM antipsychotics (n=191, open, Normann et al, Pharmacopsychiatry 2006;**39**:209–12). Risperidone liquid 2 mg plus oral lorazepam 2 mg was shown to be as effective in psychotic agitation as haloperidol 5 mg IM plus lorazepam 2 mg IM, but with less complications (n = 30, Currier and Simpson, J Clin Psychiatry 2001;**62**:153–7). In another trial, where patients were given a choice of oral risperidone (2 mg) plus oral lorazepam (2–2.5 mg) or standard IM antipsychotics, with or without lorazepam, most chose oral, which was more successful at two hours and significantly non-inferior with fewer side-effects (n=226, open, Lejeune et al, Int Clin Psychopharmacol 2004;**19**:259–69). Risperidone 2–6 mg/d was superior to oral zuclopenthixol (20–50 mg/d) when combined with lorazepam in acute psychosis (n = 75, open, 14/7, Hovens et al, J Psychopharmacol 2005;**19**:51–7).
Review: * general (Wilhelm et al, BMC Psychiatry 2008;**8**:61)

Haloperidol + promethazine (HAL-PRO) *
Three large trials have shown IM promethazine an effective adjunct to haloperidol, e.g. promethazine 25–50 mg plus haloperidol 10 mg IM was as effective as lorazepam IM 4 mg and 96% patients in each group were 'tranquil or asleep' after four hours, but 76% were asleep with the HAL-PRO combination compared with only 45% with lorazepam IM monotherapy (n = 200, RCT, Alexander et

al, *Br J Psychiatry* 2004;**185**:63–9; favourable comment by McAllister-Williams, *EBMH* 2005; **8**:7). In another study, haloperidol IM 5–10 mg plus promethazine IM up to 50 mg was more effective than haloperidol IM alone in acute agitation, with 10 cases of acute dystonia with haloperidol only (n = 316 [c = 311], open, Huf *et al*, *BMJ* 2007;**335**:839), and haloperidol IM plus promethazine IM was as effective as olanzapine IM alone in agitated and violent people with mental health problems. However, the combination required fewer additional medical interventions at four hours (n = 300 [c = 298], RCT, open, 2/52, Raveendran *et al*, *BMJ* 2007;**335**:865). Cochrane concludes that:

- 1% people given any haloperidol treatment experience a seizure.
- After 20 minutes, HAL-PRO was more tranquillising than haloperidol alone.
- After 15 minutes olanzapine was as tranquillising as HAL-PRO but did not have an enduring effect and more people needed additional treatment at 4 hours (s = 4, n = 1117, Huf *et al*, *Cochrane Database Syst Rev* 2009;**3**:CD005146; see also s = 4, Huf *et al*, *Rev Bras Psiquiatr* 2009;**31**:265–70).

■ Unlicensed/possible efficacy

Midazolam *

Midazolam may be useful for short-term sedation, with a quick onset and offset. IM can be used but IV is too dangerous in non-specialist mental health settings due to the potential for acute respiratory depression. Buccal midazolam, when used as an alternative to IM lorazepam, had an onset of action of 15 minutes, peaking at 30 minutes and lasting for at least an hour, with no serious adverse reactions or oversedation in a naturalistic study (n = 25, 115 doses, open, Taylor *et al*, *Int J Psychiatr Clin Pract* 2008;**12**:309–11). Midazolam 2.5–10 mg IM/IV may be rapidly effective (6–20 minutes) in controlling acute agitation, repeated every 20 minutes up to 20 mg per sedation event and monitored for at least four hours after the last dose. In a pragmatic real-world trial, with a simple end-point and only 1% drop-outs, IM midazolam was superior to haloperidol

plus promethazine at 20 and 40 minutes in aggressive or agitated emergency room patients, with few side-effects (n = 301, RCT, TREC-CG, *BMJ* 2003;**317**:708–13; comment by Waraich, *EBMH* 2004;**7**:42). Midazolam IM 5 mg was also as effective as, (and much quicker acting than) lorazepam IM 2 mg or haloperidol IM 5 mg in acute agitation, but the effects were shorter-lived (82 minutes vs 217 minutes vs 126 minutes respectively; n = 111, RCT, d/b, Nobay *et al*, *Acad Emerg Med* 2004;**11**:744–9).

Paraldehyde (now discontinued in UK)

Paraldehyde infusion should **only** be carried out in specialist centres, as it needs intensive care facilities.

Topiramate

A retrospective study suggested topiramate might have some efficacy for the control of aggression in psychosis (n = 45, Gobbi *et al*, *J Clin Psychopharmacol* 2006;**26**:467–73).

Valproate

While valproate loading may have an antimanic effect over 48–72 hours, it has no detectable effect when given IV over 120 minutes (n = 7, open, Phroloiv *et al*, *J Clin Psychiatry* 2004;**65**:68–70). See entry under mania (*1.10.2*).

Ziprasidone IM (not UK)

Ziprasidone IM is effective in doses of 10 mg IM every two hours or 20 mg IM every four hours. The maximum dose is 40 mg/day (n = 79, RCT, d/b, Daniel *et al*, *Psychopharmacol* 2001;**155**: 128–34). Although lorazepam may be given at the same time, the two must not be mixed in the same syringe due to compatibility issues.

1.2 AGGRESSION

see also Acute psychiatric emergency (*1.1*), Borderline personality disorder (*1.11*) and Self-injurious behaviour (*1.25*)

Aggression is defined as behaviour accompanied by verbal or physical threats which, if carried out, would cause harm to others, self or property. It can include situational (provoked), non-situational (unprovoked), passive, physical or interictal (especially in temporal lobe epilepsy). Aggression is not a diagnosis in itself, but as well as being potentially drug-induced (through either intoxication or withdrawal), can be a symptom of many conditions, including dementia, personality disorders, PTSD, PMS, trauma, etc, or as an expression of a variety of emotional or behavioural motivations. Low GABA and serotonin levels in various parts of the brain are associated with aggressive behaviour, and enhanced norepinephrine and dopamine levels in the brain are associated with increased aggression.

Role of drugs

Drugs may be useful in helping control some cases where suppression of aggression is considered important on safety grounds.

Reviews: * pharmacotherapy (Goedhard et al, J Clin Psychiatry 2006;**67**:1013–24; in brain injury, Fleminger et al, Cochrane Database Syst Rev 2006;**4**:CD003299), general (Volavka et al, Actas Esp Psiquiatr 2006;**34**:123–35), with anticonvulsants (Stanford et al, Curr Treat Options Neurol 2009;**11**:383–90), neurobiology (Siever, Am J Psychiatry 2008;**165**:429–42), in children (Parikh et al, J Child Adolesc Psychopharmacol 2008;**18**:157–78).

Lithium

Most studies with lithium have involved aggression in people with learning disabilities and a two-month trial at 0.6–1.0mmol/L may be justified in patients unmanageable by environmental factors. Lithium has been shown to reduce aggression and the frequency of episodes in learning disabilities (e.g. Langee, Am J Ment Retard 1990;**94**:448–52), reducing impulsive aggression with organic brain damage (n=2, 2 years, Bellus et al, Brain Inj 1996;**10**:849–60) and in children with aggression or conduct disorder, albeit poorly tolerated (e.g. n=86, RCT, d/b, p/c, Malone et al, Arch Gen Psychiatry 2000;**57**:649–54). Lithium may exert an effect via several mechanisms, e.g. enhancement of serotonin, but the potential adverse consequences of sudden discontinuation (accidental or deliberate) should be considered.

Antipsychotics *

Robust evidence for the efficacy of antipsychotics in aggression is lacking, as a clinical effect is difficult to quantify. It may be that raised dopamine levels are associated with aggression, in which case dopamine-blocking drugs may have some rationale. Use of higher doses of antipsychotics are generally considered to be effective only via a chemical strait-jacket or sedating effect. Indeed, in a trial in aggressive challenging behaviour in learning disabilities, aggression decreased substantially over 4/52 with haloperidol, risperidone and placebo, with no differences between the groups. The placebo group at no point showed a worse response than the antipsychotics and the authors concluded that antipsychotics should no longer be accepted routine therapy for aggressive behaviour in learning disabilities (n=86, RCT, d/b, p/c, 26/52, Tyrer et al, Lancet 2008;**371**:57–63).

However, they may still have a role if used carefully. An analysis of 19 studies suggested that **risperidone** is useful for treating aggression in a range of behavioural disorders, agitation and dementia (s=19, De Deyn and Buitelaar, Eur Psychiatry 2006;**21**:21–8), especially at lower dose, e.g. for severe, primary aggressive behaviour in adolescents with disruptive behaviours compounded by sub-average cognitive abilities (n=38, RCT, p/c, 6/52, Buitelaar et al, J Clin Psychiatry 2001;**62**:239–48; review by Young, EBMH 2002;**5**:11). **Clozapine** is not easy to use but reduced seclusion and restraint rates in aggressive, psychotic inpatients over 12 months have been shown, the effect not related to sedation (n=137, Chengappa et al, Schizophr Res 2002;**53**:1–6). Short-term use of clozapine for aggression in an adolescent with autistic disorder has been reported (n=1, Chen et al, J Clin Psychiatry 2001;**62**:479–80). **Quetiapine** may help at 25–300mg/d for aggression due to traumatic brain injury (n=7, open, 6/52, Kim and Bijlani, J Neuropsychiatry Clin Neurosci 2006;**18**:547–9). In **zuclopenthixol** responders (i.e. aggression reduced over 6/52 at 6–18mg/d) with learning disabilities, withdrawal produced an increase in aggression, so it either works and/or there is a rebound aggression on withdrawal (n = 49 [c = 39], RCT, d/b, p/c, 6/52, Haessler et al, Br J Psychiatry 2007;**190**:447–8). In aggression and SIB in learning disabilities, 80% improved on all measures with zuclopenthixol and discontinuation reversed the effect (n = 39, RCT, d/b, p/c, Hässler et al, Pharmacopsychiatry 2008;**41**:232–9).

Benzodiazepines

Benzodiazepines are reported to be effective in episodic behavioural disorders by aborting aggression in the prodromal stage. **Lorazepam** has been used in resistant aggression in dementia, with 1.5–3 mg/d effective orally over several years in some patients (n = 2, Fritz and Stewart, Am J Psychiatry 1990;**147**:1250), as has 1–2 mg lorazepam IV (d/b, Salzman et al, J Clin Psychiatry 1991;**52**:177–80). Use should normally be limited to only a few weeks to minimise the incidence of disinhibition or paradoxical reactions (review by Paton, Psychiatr Bull 2002;**26**:460–2, although the actual incidence may be lower than 1%).

Valproate *

Valproate may exert an effect by correcting any abnormally low GABA levels. Several small studies have shown a rapid effect, e.g. compared to quetiapine (n = 33, RCT, d/b, 28/7, Barzman et al, J Child Adolesc Psychopharmacol 2006;**16**:665–70) and oxcarbazepine (n = 31, MacMillan et al, J Psychiatr Pract 2006;**12**:214–22), but an earlier review was less than encouraging (s = 17, n = 164, Lindenmayer and Kotsaftis, J Clin Psychiatry 2000;**61**:123–8).

■ Unlicensed/possible efficacy

Aromatherapy

Lavender reduced agitation in Chinese patients with dementia (n = 70, RCT, c/o, 3 + 3/52, Lin et al, Int J Geriatr Psychiatry 2007;**22**:405–10).

Beta-blockers

Beta-blockers have been reported to help control aggression in learning disabilities (review, Am J Mental Retard 1990;**95**:110–9), autism, schizophrenia and in intermittent explosive disorders but have potential effects on bp and heart-rate (review by Haspel, Harv Rev Psychiatry 1995;**2**:274–81).

Buspirone

Several old studies and case reports have suggested some beneficial effect. A three-month trial at 30 mg/d seems necessary, and a transient worsening may occur initially (n = 20, 3/12, Stanislav et al, J Clin Psychopharmacol 1994;**14**:126–30). Buspirone 90 mg/d has been successful for reducing aggressive behaviour in an autistic woman with profound learning disabilities (n = 1, Brahm et al, Ann Pharmacother 2008;**42**:131–7).

Carbamazepine *

Evidence for carbamazepine in aggression is largely anecdotal, based on the proposed association between aggression and TLE or other EEG abnormalities. CBZ 600 mg/d may reduce aggressive behaviour in schizophrenia and has also been used in paroxysmal behaviour disorder and the elderly demented (n = 51, RCT, 6/52, Tariot et al, Am J Psychiatry 1998; **155**:54–61), 200 mg/d has been successful for BDZ-resistant impulsive aggression (n = 1, Nagata et al, Psychiatry Clin Neurosci 2007;**61**:695–7; n = 1, Pae, Psychiatry Clin Neurosci 2008;**62**:483). Beware of an interaction with antipsychotics.

Clonidine

Clonidine 150–400 mcg/d may reduce aggressiveness in destructive children (n = 17, open, Kemph et al, J Am Acad Child Adolesc Psychiatry 1993;**32**:577–81), possibly via increased CSF GABA levels.

Estrogens (estrogens)

See dementia (1.13).

Gabapentin

Gabapentin has been used in episodic agitation in severely mentally ill patients (n = 11, 6/12, Megna et al, Ann Pharmacother 2002;**36**:12–6). See also dementia (1.13).

Lamotrigine

See dementia (1.13).

Oxcarbazepine

Oxcarbazepine has improved a variety of measures of impulsive aggressiveness (n = 48 [c = 45], RCT, d/b, p/c, 4–10/52, Mattes, J Clin Psychopharmacol 2005;**25**:575–9).

Phenytoin
Phenytoin 300 mg/d may reduce impulsive aggressive acts but not premeditated attacks in prisoners (n = 60, d/b, p/c, Barratt et al, *J Clin Psychopharmacol* 1997;**17**:341–9).

SSRIs *
The use of SSRIs may be rational if low serotonin levels associated with aggression can be corrected. Aggression in learning disabilities may also be associated with unrecognised mood disorders, e.g. depression. **Citalopram** 20–60 mg/d has significantly reduced aggressive incidents with no deterioration or significant side-effects (n = 15, d/b, c/o, 24/52, Vartiainen, *Acta Psychiatr Scand* 1995;**91**:348–61), and up to 40 mg/d reduced impulsive aggression in children, adolescents (n = 12, open, 6/52, Armentos and Lewis, *J Am Acad Child Adolesc Psychiatry* 2002;**41**:522–9) and adults (n = 25, open, 8/52, Reist et al, *J Clin Psychiatry* 2003;**64**:81–5). A similar effect has been suggested with **sertraline** 50–200 mg/d (open, Kavoussi et al, *J Clin Psychiatry* 1994;**55**:137–41). **Fluoxetine** seems to have a clear anti-aggressive effect in IED (intermittent explosive disorder), although less than 50% achieve a full or partial remission (n = 100, RCT, d/b, p/c, Coccaro et al, *J Clin Psychiatry* 2009;**70**:653–62) and 20–60 mg/d was ineffective in reducing abuse and aggression by men against intimate-partners (n = 26, RCT, p/c, Lee et al, *Int Clin Psychopharmacol* 2008;**23**:337–41). SSRIs have been used successfully for dementia and chronic aggression after head injury (n = 3, Kim et al, *Pharmacother* 2001;**21**:498–501).

Vitamins
Nutritional supplements (containing vitamins, minerals and fatty acids) caused dramatic reductions in antisocial behaviour and violent incidents of young offenders within just two weeks (n = 231, RCT, p/c, Gesch et al, *Br J Psych- iatry* 2002;**181**:22–8; complimentary comment by Benton, *EBMH* 2003;**6**:41).

♦ Others

Other drugs tried include **cyproterone** 200 mg/d (e.g. Thibaut and Colonna, *Am J*

Psychiatry 1992;**149**:411; n = 1, Byrne et al, *Br J Psychiatry* 1992;**160**:282–3), **dexamfetamine** (Cherek et al, *Psychopharm* 1986;**88**:381–6), the synthetic progestogen **medroxy-progesterone** (n = 3, O'Connor and Baker, *Acta Psychiatr Scand* 1983;**67**:399–403) and **trazodone** (e.g. n = 1, Mashiko et al, *Psychiatry Clin Neurosci* 1996;**50**:133–6).

□ No efficacy

Levetiracetam *
Levetiracetam was of no efficacy for impulsive aggression in one study (n = 40 [c = 34], RCT, d/b, p/c, 10/52, Mattes, *J Clin Psychiatry* 2008;**69**:310–5).

1.3 AGORAPHOBIA
see also Anxiety disorder (*1.6*), Panic disorder (*1.21*) and Social anxiety (*1.27*)

Agoraphobia is an overwhelming and disabling anxiety provoked by being alone or in places where escape might be difficult or embarrassing and so these situations are avoided. Panic attacks may accompany the phobia and depression may be present in up to a half of patients. A link with serotonin deficiency has been shown.

Role of drugs *
Drug treatment may be effective in many patients, with psychotherapy being an essential component of the treatment package for many. A meta-analysis of 54 published studies has shown that symptoms are improved by tricyclics and high potency benzodiazepines and, although there may be a short-term deterioration, this usually turns to a longer-term improvement. The best long-term benefit is from exposure therapy, particularly combined with antidepressants. There is a weak but significant placebo response in drug trials. Adding a CBT package to SSRIs for panic (with or without agoraphobia) seems of little additional benefit, with SSRIs more effective than CBT alone (n = 150, 9/12, van Apeldoorn et al, *Acta Psychiatr Scand* 2008;**117**:260–70).

Reviews: * general (Perugi et al, *CNS Drugs* 2007;**21**:741–64), epidemiology (Goodwin et al, *Eur Neuropsychopharmacol* 2005;**15**:435–43).

BNF listed

Citalopram

Citalopram is licensed for the symptoms of panic disorder, with or without agoraphobia. The dose is 10mg/d for a week, increasing to 20–30mg/d, with a maximum of 60mg/d. The maximal effect may take three months to develop. See panic disorder (1.21).

Escitalopram

Escitalopram is licensed for the symptoms of panic disorder, with or without agoraphobia (see also 1.21). The dose is 5mg/d for the first week, then 10mg/d (maximum 20mg/d). Maximal effect may take three months to develop.

Paroxetine

Paroxetine is licensed for the symptoms and prevention of relapse of panic disorder, with or without agoraphobia. See panic disorder (1.21).

● Unlicensed/some efficacy

Benzodiazepines *

Alprazolam (n=69, 3.5 years, Kilic et al, Psychother Psychosom 1997;66:175–8) and diazepam have been used and shown to help, particularly with anxiety symptoms. Clonazepam 1–2mg/d has also shown significant efficacy (n=24, RCT, p/c, 6/52, Valenca et al, Arq Neuropsiquiatr 2000;58:1025–9). **Review:** Bruce et al, Am J Psychiatry 2003; 160:1432–8).

Tricyclics

While SSRIs are now first choice, up to 70% may respond to tricyclics, but with 30% dropping out due to side-effects. 20% may worsen, with an increase in panic attacks. Clomipramine, at doses up to 300mg/d, has been shown to be effective (n=108, d/b, p/c, 8/52, Johnson et al, Arch Gen Psychiatry 1988;45:453–9), with a continuous improvement shown over many weeks. See also panic (1.21).

■ Unlicensed/possible efficacy

Buspirone

Buspirone has been shown to be well tolerated

and enhance the effect of CBT in panic disorder with agoraphobia (n=41, d/b, 68/52, Cottraux et al, Br J Psychiatry 1995;167:635–41), although a subsequent naturalistic study was unable to replicate this long-term effect (open, p/c, Bouvard et al, Psychother Psychosom 1997;66:27–32).

◆ Others

Other drugs tried include MAOIs (Buigues and Vallejo, J Clin Psychiatry 1987;48:55–9), trazodone (n=11, Mavissakalian et al, Am J Psychiatry 1987;144:785–7) and valproate (Roy-Byrne et al, J Clin Psychiatry 1989;50[Suppl]:S44–S48).

1.4 ALCOHOL DEPENDENCE AND ABUSE

see also Alcohol withdrawal syndrome (1.5)

Symptoms

The main diagnostic symptoms of alcohol dependence are of a primacy of drinking over other activities, increased tolerance of alcohol, symptoms of repeated withdrawal, stereotyped pattern of drinking, compulsion to drink and relief drinking.

Risk factors *

Some risk factors for alcohol abuse or being an alcohol-dependent drinker include:

1. Occupation, e.g. brewers, reps, doctors.
2. Genetics (up to 30–40% influence).
3. Marital/social problems, e.g. work.
4. Personality, e.g. high anxiety levels.
5. Psychopaths and criminals, e.g. taking alcohol before criminal events.
6. Psychiatric illness, e.g. depression, phobia, etc.
7. Use for hypnotic or analgesic purposes.
8. Adverse childhood or adolescent experiences, e.g. prenatal alcohol exposure (n=433, Baer et al, Arch Gen Psychiatry 2003;60:377–85).
9. Parental misuse of alcohol (n=2427, Lieb et al, Psychol Med 2002;32:63–78).
10. Sweet taste preference (n=122, Kranzler et al, Am J Psychiatry 2001;158:813–5).
11. Following Norwich City FC and, indeed, now Ipswich Town FC too.

The body metabolises approximately one unit of alcohol per hour (varies between individuals but is the same regardless of the inital quantity) and peak levels occur one hour after the drink is consumed (absorption is more rapid with low volume drinks, eg. spirits and slower with higher volumes, e.g. beer. small amounts). One unit gives a man an alcohol blood level of about 15 mg/100 ml and a woman about 20 mg/100 ml. Alcohol consumption of 7.7–12.9 units per week is associated with the lowest mortality in men (White, J Clin Epidemiol 1999;52:967–75, review by Caan, EBMH 2000;3:61), a finding often quoted in bars throughout the world.

Role of drugs *

Pharmacological treatment can play its part in an overall plan. Any vitamin deficiency needs correcting (see AWS, 1.5). Other drugs may be useful to treat associated psychiatric morbidity, such as withdrawal, affective disorders, suicidal thoughts and hallucinations. A huge study (COMBINE) comparing naltrexone, acamprosate and Combined Behavioural Intervention (CBI) [9 arms:naltrexone 100 mg/d;acamprosate 3g/d;both; placebo; naltrexone + CBI; acamprosate + CBI; naltrexone + acamprosate + CBI; placebo + CBI; CBI only) concluded that acamprosate is ineffective but that naltrexone, CBI or both performed best (n = 1383, RCT, p/c, 16/52 and follow-up, Anton et al, JAMA 2006;295:2003–17). Other findings from COMBINE include that there is a significant placebo effect in large trial from pills, AA and seeing a healthcare professional (n = 1383 Weiss et al, J Stud Alcohol Drugs 2008;69:878–84) and CBI had little practical effect (Zweben et al, Alcohol Clin Exp Res 2008;32:1661–9).

In the longer term, disulfiram, naltrexone and acamprosate may have roles to play. Despite COMBINE acamprosate has a reasonable evidence base, is superior to placebo and is more effective in preventing a lapse, whereas naltrexone is better at preventing a lapse becoming a relapse (Rösner et al, J Psychopharmacol 2008;22:11–23; see also s = 42, Snyder and Bowers, Am J Drug Alcohol Abuse 2008;34:449–61), and so may be more useful for programmes aimed at controlled consumption. Disulfiram probably has limited efficacy. There is no real evidence for lithium or the SSRIs. Combinations of these drugs may be useful but the evidence base is not robust due to the difficulty of carrying out these types of study, e.g. high drop-out rates.

Reviews: * pharmacotherapy (Garbutt, J Subst Abuse Treat 2009;36:S15–23), genetics (Stacey et al, Curr Psychiatry Rep 2009;11:364–9), non-benzodiazepine GABAergic medicines (Leggio et al, Prog Neuropsychopharmacol Biol Psychiatry 2008;32:1106–17), opioid antagonists (Soyka and Rösner, Curr Drug Abuse Rev 2008;1:280–91), management of Korsakoff's (Kopelman et al, Alcohol Alcohol 2009;44:148–54).

BNF listed

Acamprosate *

Acamprosate is licensed in some countries for abstinence maintenance therapy for up to one year in motivated alcohol-dependent patients. It is a GABA analogue and may act to reduce the severity and frequency of relapse by enhancing GABA inhibitory neurotransmission and antagonising glutamate excitation by antagonising mGluR5 receptors (De Witte et al, CNS Drugs 2005;19:517–37; glutamate receptors increase in chronic alcohol dependency). This reduces intake via reduced reward, possibly restoring normal activity of glutaminergic neurons (which become overexcited by alcohol) and reducing craving (n = 29, p/c, 6/52, Weinstein et al, Addict Biol 2003;8:229–32). It takes about seven days to reach therapeutic levels and so can be started soon after detoxification (e.g. n = 296, RCT, d/b, p/c, 26/52, Gual and Legert, Alcohol Alcohol 2001;36:413–8) although this may have no particular advantage (n=40, RCT, d/b, p/c, 2/52 plus 10/52, Kampman et al, Addict Behav 2009;34:581–6). Continued alcohol consumption negates the therapeutic effect, but occasional lapses do not necessarily do this. Many RCTs have shown clinical effect and a large meta-analysis concluded that acamprosate has a significant beneficial effect in enhancing abstinence in recently detoxified alcohol-dependent individuals (s = 20, n = 4087, Mann et al, Alcohol Clin Exp Res 2004;28:51–63) and as part of a therapeutic approach targeted at achieving abstinence (s = 33, Carmen et al, Addiction 2004;99:811–28), although COMBINE was not too encouraging. There appear to be no predictors of the likelihood of efficacy (s = 7, n = 1485, RCT, p/c, Verheul et al,

Psychopharmacol [Berl] 2005;**178**:167–73) but may have no effect when craving is high (n=169, RCT, d/b, p/c, 12/52, Richardson *et al*, *Addiction* 2008;**103**:953–9). Its efficacy may be enhanced in combination with disulfiram, and may be effective as an adjunct to psychosocial and behavioural therapies including counselling (see combinations) for the maintenance of abstinence in detoxified patients. It should be combined with continued counselling.

Reviews: * general (Mann *et al*, *Alcohol Clin Exp Res* 2008;**32**:1105–10; Overman *et al*, *Ann Pharmacother* 2003;**37**:1090–9), mode of action (De Witte *et al*, *CNS Drugs* 2005;**19**:517–37; Zornoza *et al*, *CNS Drug Rev* 2003;**9**:359–74).

Disulfiram *

Disulfiram acts as a negative reinforcer for abstinence via the potential for the disulfiram-alcohol interaction, ie. an adversive/conditioning and maintenance therapy in alcoholics. It irreversibly inhibits ALDH (hepatic Aldehyde-NAD reductase) leading to accumulation of acetaldehyde from incomplete alcohol metabolism (Petersen, *Acta Psychiatr Scand* 1992;**369**[Suppl]:S7–S13, see also 4.7.1). Some published advice tends to underestimate doses needed, e.g. <250mg/d has only a minor interaction with alcohol (Malcolm *et al*, *Expert Opin Drug Saf* 2008;**7**:459–72), so it is suggested to start with a loading dose of 400mg/d, with 365mg/d the average dose used (n=33, retrospective, Mueser *et al*, *Am J Addict* 2003;**12**:242–52). Disulfiram seems superior to naltrexone in relapse prevention, although craving was lower with the naltrexone arm (n=100[c=97],

RCT, open, one year, De Sousa and De Sousa, *Alcohol Alcohol* 2004;**39**:528–31). 'Antabuse®' (Alpharma) tablets are dispersible and so can be given as a liquid in a supervised setting. It can also be given as a twice-a-week dose (i.e. daily dose × 7 divided by 2), as the enzyme inhibition is irreversible and the clinical effect lasts about 7–10 days.

Reviews: * general (Suh *et al*, *J Clin Psychopharmacol* 2006;**26**:290–302; Fuller and Gordis, *Addiction* 2004;**99**:21–4).

Vitamin B₁ (thiamine) *

Vitamin deficiency occurs after chronic alcohol abuse, and is due to inadequate diet, impaired absorption, increased metabolic demand and impaired utilisation. Thiamine (B_1) maintenance may be necessary to help reverse the mental confusion secondary to thiamine deficiency where 250mg IM for 3–5 days will minimise the risk of Wernicke's encephalopathy (Thompson and Marshall, *Alcohol Alcohol* 2006;**41**:159–67), but possibly only about 4.5mg is absorbed from each oral dose, via a saturable mechanism. Cochrane concludes that data to guide dose, frequency, route or duration is lacking (Day *et al*, *Cochrane Database Syst Rev* 2004;**1**:CD004033). See AWS 1.5.

Reviews: * general (Jackson and Teece, *Emerg Med J* 2004;**21**:501–2; Meier and Daeppen, *Rev Med Suisse* 2005;**1**:1740-4), thiamine utilisation (Singleton and Martin, *Curr Mol Med* 2001; **1**:197–207).

+ Combinations

The COMBINE study provides some guidance

Disulfiram test dose

A test dose is now considered dangerous due to the risks involved and because the mode of action is via a conditioning process. If considered necessary, wait five days after starting treatment for full enzyme block to occur.

1. Give 10–15ml of 95% alcohol (or 15–25ml spirits).
2. Reaction should start in 5–15 minutes.
3. Repeat in 30 minutes if no reaction. Reaction shows as flushed face, tachycardia, nausea, vomiting, fall in blood pressure. (Have crash box plus personnel available.)

Usual cause of no reaction is too low a dose of disulfiram. Bronchospasm has also been reported (Beri *et al*, *Br Med J* 1993;**306**:396). Noradrenaline has been effective in severe life-threatening hypotension with the disulfiram-alcohol reaction, when volume resuscitation and dopamine infusion failed (n=1, Ho *et al*, *Am J Med Sci* 2007;**333**:53–5).

but combining drugs with different modes of action may be useful.

Review: * general (Mattson and Litten, *J Stud Alcohol Suppl* 2005;**15**:8–16).

Acamprosate + disulfiram

In one study, alcoholics were randomised over one year to placebo or acamprosate, and could request additional disulfiram. Disulfiram improved the effectiveness of acamprosate, but a high drop-out did not allow full analysis (n = 118, RCT, Besson et al, *Alcohol Clin Exp Res* 1998;**22**:573–9).

Acamprosate + naltrexone *

Combined naltrexone and acamprosate were slightly superior to monotherapy and significantly superior to placebo for time to first drink and time to relapse (n = 160, RCT, d/b, p/c, 12/52, Kiefer et al, *Arch Gen Psychiatry* 2003;**60**:92–9).

Review: * Mason, *J Stud Alcohol Suppl* 2005;**15**:148–56).

Naltrexone + disulfiram

In a four-arm study, active medication produced lower craving and improved abstinence, but combining naltrexone and disulfiram had no advantage over either agent individually (n = 254, RCT, p/c, 12/52, Petrakis et al, *Biol Psychiatry* 2005;**57**:1128–37), but the combination may help alcohol dependence with comorbid PTSD (n = 93, RCT, d/b, p/c, 12/52, Petrakis et al, *Biol Psychiatry* 2006;**60**:777–83).

Naltrexone + ondansetron

Augmentation of naltrexone 50mg/d by ondansetron 0.5mg/d decreased alcohol craving (n = 90, RCT, d/b, p/c, 7/7, Myrick et al, *Arch Gen Psychiatry* 2007;**64**:466–75), supporting a previous small study (n = 20, RCT, d/b, 8/52, Ait-Daoud et al, *Alcohol Clin Exp Res* 2001;**25**:847–9).

● Unlicensed/some efficacy

Aripiprazole *

Aripiprazole 5–15mg/d was equivalent in efficacy to naltrexone 50mg/d (n = 57 [c = 43], RCT, d/b, 16/52, Martinotti et al, *J Psychopharmacol* 2009;**23**:123–9) and may reduce the reward and euphoria from alcohol and increase sedation (n = 18, RCT, 3/7, p/c, c/o, Kranzler et al, *Alcohol Clin Exp Res* 2008;**32**:573–9; see also n = 13, 16/52, Martinotti et al, *Am J Drug Alcohol Abuse* 2007;**33**:393–401).

Baclofen *

There is growing evidence for the use of baclofen. In alcohol-dependent people with cirrhosis of the liver, baclofen 30mg/d produces a well tolerated and highly significantly reduction in abstinence (71% vs 29% for placebo; n = 84, RCT, d/b, p/c, 12/52, Addolorato et al, *Lancet* 2007;**370**:1915–22). Baclofen doubles cumulative abstinence duration and other drinking measures (n = 148 [c = 129], RCT, p/c, 12/52, Gache and Hadengue, *J Hepatol* 2008; **49**:1083–5) and reduces craving, consumption and other measures of alcohol dependence (n = 39, RCT, d/b, p/c, 30/7, Addolorato et al, *Alcohol Alcohol* 2002;**37**:504–8). In case reports, baclofen 140mg/d produced dramatic reductions in craving and preoccupation with alcohol (n = 1, Bucknam, *Alcohol Alcohol* 2007;**42**:158–60) and 270mg/d (reduced to 120mg/d) allowed one person to become 'effortlessly' alcohol-free (n = 1, 9/12, Ameisen, *Alcohol Alcohol* 2005;**40**:147–50).

Review: * general (Addolorato et al, *Int J Clin Pract* 2006;**60**:1003–8).

Carbamazepine

A significant long-term effect has been shown on time to first drink and survival rates (n = 29, RCT, 12/12, Mueller et al, *Alcohol Clin Exp Res* 1997;**21**:86–92).

Gabapentin *

Gabapentin 600mg/d monotherapy post-detox significantly reduced alcohol consumption and craving, improving outcomes, and was very well tolerated and safe (n = 60, RCT, d/b, p/c, 4/52, Furieri et al, *J Clin Psychiatry* 2007;**68**:1691–1700). Gabapentin may have some use at night for reducing heavy drinking and improving insomnia (n = 21, RCT, d/b, p/c, 8/52, Brower et al, *Alcohol Clin Exp Res* 2008; **32**:1429–38; n = 55, Karam-Hage and Brower, *Psych Clin Neurosci* 2003;**57**:542–4).

Naltrexone *

Naltrexone has been well studied and may have significant efficacy in alcohol dependence. A systematic analysis has concluded that naltrexone is more useful in programmes geared to controlling consumption (s = 33, Carmen et al, Addiction 2004; **99**:811–28, see also COMBINE, n = 1383, RCT, p/c, 16/52 and follow-up, Anton et al, JAMA 2006;**295**:2003–17), possibly because it seems to have little effect on reducing alcohol sampling by abstinent alcoholics, but has a significant effect on reducing subsequent drinking by somehow blocking the craving for, and reward from, the next drink, especially when craving is high, unlike acamprosate (n = 169, RCT, d/b, p/c, 12/52, Richardson et al, Addiction 2008;**103**:953–9). This may be through blocking the pleasure (or 'high') caused by alcohol and reducing alcohol-seeking behaviour (n = 70, d/b, p/c, Volpicelli et al, Am J Psychiatry 1995;**152**:613–5), or reducing craving (n = 43, O'Malley et al, Am J Psychiatry 1996;**153**:281–3). The efficacy may be enhanced by limited psychosocial interventions (n = 111, RCT, p/c, 12/52, Morris et al, Addiction 2001;**96**:1565–73), CBT (n = 131, RCT, Anton et al, Am J Psychiatry 1999;**156**:1758–64; reviewed by Chick, EBMH 2000;**3**:75), medical advice (n = 107, RCT, d/b, p/c, 12/52, Latt et al, Med J Aust 2002;**176**:530–4) or by targetted naltrexone, i.e. prior to situations that might have a high risk of heavy drinking (n = 153, RCT, p/c, 8/52, Kranzler et al, J Clin Psychopharmacol 2003;**23**:294–304). However, naltrexone does not enhance the effect of cognitive behavioural coping skills therapy (CBCST) (n = 103, RCT, p/c, 12/52, O'Malley et al, Alcohol Clin Exp Res 2007;**31**:625–34). It may be more effective than monotherapy for improving alcohol-related outcomes if prescribed with an antidepressant (n = 627, Krystal et al, Alcohol Clin Exp Res 2008;**32**:85–91). Cochrane concludes that naltrexone 50 mg/d significantly decreases relapse in the short-term (NNT = 7), but that medium-term treatment gives no benefit (s = 27, RCTs, Srisurapanont and Jarusuraisin, Cochrane Database Syst Rev 2005;1:CD001867). Another extensive review concluded that the majority of double-blind trials support

that naltrexone reduces heavy alcohol drinking (s = 29, n = 5997, Pettinati et al, J Clin Psychopharmacol 2006;**26**:610–25), and a systematic review and meta-analysis concluded that naltrexone is safe and effective, reduces relapse rates, time to relapse and drinking frequency, suggesting a different application for each drug (s = 33, Bouza et al, Addiction 2004;**99**:811–28; comment by Feeney, EBMH 2005;**8**:14). One trial came to the reassuring conclusion that, while naltrexone is only moderately effective in reducing alcohol intake, its efficacy is far greater in people who actually take it (n = 97, p/c, Volpicelli et al, Arch Gen Psychiatry 1997;**54**:737–42).

Reviews: * general (Anton, N Engl J Med 2008; **359**:715-21; academic highlights, J Clin Psychiatry 2007;**68**:1117–28), depot injection (Mannelli et al, Expert Rev Neurother 2007;**7**:1265–77; Roozen et al, Eur Addict Res 2007;**13**:201–6; Comer et al, Expert Opin Investig Drugs 2007; **16**:1285–94).

Naltrexone depot injection
(UK license delayed)

A long-acting naltrexone injection (Vivitrex®, Alkermes; n = 315, RCT, p/c, DASNDSG, Alcohol Clin Exp Res 2004;**28**:1051–9) may help, e.g. 380 mg monthly significantly reduced heavy drinking days (n = 627 [c = 401], RCT, d/b, p/c, 6/12, Garbutt et al, JAMA 2005;**293**:1617–25; comment by Killeen, EBMH 2005;**8**:100). The monthly injection may be effective within two days and have a sustained action over at least 6/12 (n = 624, RCT, d/b, p/c, 24/52, Ciraulo et al, J Clin Psychiatry 2008;**69**:190–5).

Ondansetron (see also combinations)

Ondansetron, a 5-HT3 antagonist, at 8 mcg/kg/d was superior to placebo in increasing drink-free days, especially for early-onset (pre-25 years) alcoholism (n = 271, RCT, Johnson et al, JAMA 2000;**284**:963–71).

Topiramate *

Data is accumulating that topiramate may be a promising treatment, e.g. four studies show topiramate (around 300 mg/d) to be superior to placebo and at least as effective as naltrexone for reducing drinking (n = 102, RCT, 6/12, Flórez et al, Alcohol Clin Exp Res

2008;**32**:1251–9; n = 155, RCT, d/b, p/c, 12/52, Baltieri *et al, Addiction* 2008;**103**:2035–44; n = 150, RCT, p/c, d/b, 12/52, Johnson *et al, Arch Gen Psychiatry* 2004;**61**:905–12) and in reducing heavy drinking days and all other drinking outcomes in a large study (n = 371, RCT, d/b, p/c, 14/52, Johnson *et al, JAMA* 2007;**298**:1641–51). It may also reduce relapse (n = 155, RCT, d/b, p/c, 12/52, Baltieri *et al, Addiction* 2008;**103**:2035–44).

Review: * general (Olmsted and Kockler, *Ann Pharmacother* 2008;**42**:1475–80).

Valproate *

Valproate augmentation of TAU has decreased heavy drinking in people with bipolar I with comorbid alcohol dependence, an important finding (n = 59, RCT, d/b, p/c, 24/52, Salloum *et al, Arch Gen Psychiatry* 2005;**62**:37–45; enthusiastic review by Le Fauve, *EBMH* 2005;**8**:79; see also d/b, p/c, 12/52, Brady *et al, Drug Alcohol Depend* 2002;**67**:323–30), e.g. valproate 3 g/d has been used successfully to treat alcoholic hallucinosis (n = 40, RCT, d/b, 10/7, Aliyev and Aliyev, *Alcohol Alcohol* 2008;**43**:456–9).

■ Unlicensed/possible efficacy

Benzodiazepines

Although not recommended in alcoholics for the very real fear of addiction, benzodiazepines have been advocated if they are able to reduce alcohol dependence (as a 'lesser of two evils' strategy). Any use should be well-documented in the patient's notes.

Buspirone

Two trials in anxious alcoholics have shown reduced anxiety, alcohol consumption and drinking days (n = 61, 12/52, Kranzer *et al, Arch Gen Psychiatry* 1994;**51**:720–31), and a significant reduction in alcohol craving and consumption in motivated patients (n = 50, d/b, p/c, Bruno, *Psychopathology* 1989;**22**[Suppl 1]:S49–S59), but no effect on drinking or anxiety has been noted in two other studies (e.g. n = 156, RCT, Fawcett *et al, Alcohol Clin Exp Res* 2000;**24**:666–74). It may need four weeks at full therapeutic dose to achieve the effect and so a proper trial is necessary.

Levetiracetam *

In two pilot studies, levetiracetam 3 g/d reduced anxiety and alcohol consumption (n = 3, open, 8/52, Mariani and Levin, *Am J Drug Alcohol Abuse* 2008;**34**:683–91) and 2 g/d reduced alcohol consumption by 65% (n = 20, open, Sarid-Segal *et al, Am J Drug Alcohol Abuse* 2008;**34**:441–7).

Memantine *

There are two conflicting studies. Memantine 20–40 mg/d produced a dose-dependent attenuation of alcohol cue-induced craving (n = 38, RCT, 3/7, Krupitsky *et al, Am J Psychiatry* 2007;**164**:519–23) but up to 40 mg/d had no effect on any measures of alcohol use in treatment-seeking alcoholic-dependent patients (n = 34[c = 27], d/b, p/c, 16/52, Evans *et al, Alcohol Clin Exp Res* 2007;**31**:775–82). Finally, memantine 20 mg/d was as effective as escitalopram 20 mg/d for reducing drinking in depressed alcoholics, although it was more effective if abstinent at the start and there was no placebo arm (n = 80, d/b, 26/52, Muhonen *et al, Subst Abuse Treat Prev Policy* 2008;**3**:20).

Mirtazapine

There is a report of improvement in alcoholism with adjunctive mirtazapine for depression (n = 1, Crockford and White, *J Clin Psychiatry* 2005;**66**:540).

Oxcarbazepine

In a pilot study, oxcarbazepine was as effective as acamprosate in preventing alcohol relapse and as well tolerated (n = 30, RCT, open, 24/52, Croissant *et al, Alcohol Clin Exp Res* 2006;**30**:630–5; Croissant *et al, Pharmacopsychiatry* 2004;**37**:306–7; Martinotti *et al, Am J Addict* 2007;**16**:247–8).

Pregabalin *

Pregabalin 150–450 mg/d was as effective as naltrexone for drinking indices and craving scores but its effect may be more related to management of comorbid psychiatric symptoms (n = 71, RCT, d/b, Martinotti *et al, J Psychopharmacol* 2010;[in press]), although it may help prevent relapse (n = 20[c = 15], open, 16/52, Martinotti *et al, Adv Ther* 2008;**25**:608–18).

Quetiapine *

Quetiapine as monotherapy in dual diagnosis (alcohol and bipolar) markedly reduced alcohol consumption, craving and symptoms (n = 28, open, 16/52, Martinotti et al, Hum Psychopharmacol 2008;**23**:417–24; see also n = 9, case series, Croissant et al, Eur Psychiatry 2006;**21**:570–3).

SSRIs (see also SSRIs, no efficacy)

Citalopram has produced a modest (16–17%) but significant reduction in alcoholic drink intake and increase in drink-free days in studies of alcoholics, possibly by decreasing desire or reducing the reward (see also n = 62, d/b, p/c, Tiihonen et al, Pharmacopsychiatry 1996;**29**:27–9). Fluoxetine 60 mg/d reduced alcoholic and total drink intake compared to placebo and to fluoxetine 40 mg/d (n = 29, Naranjo et al, Clin Pharmacol Ther 1990; **47**:490–8), as has fluoxetine 20–40 mg/d in alcoholics with comorbid depression (RCT, n = 51, Cornelius et al, Arch Gen Psychiatry 1997; **54**:700–5; review by Haslam, EBMH 1998;**1**:41) but a larger study failed to reproduce these findings (n = 101, RCT, Kranzler et al, Am J Psychiatry 1995;**152**:391–7).
Review: (Naranjo and Knoke, J Clin Psychiatry 2001;**62**[Suppl 20]:S18–S25).

Tiagabine *

Tiagabine may have some role as adjunctive treatment in alcohol dependence (n = 120, open, 6/12, Paparrigopoulos et al, J Psychopharmacol 2010;[in press]) although it does not attenuate alcohol-induced activation of the human reward system (n = 20, Fehr et al, Psychopharmacol [Berl] 2007;**191**:975–83).

Zonisamide *

A pilot study showed a reduced urge to drink in risky drinkers (n = 10, d/b, p/c, Sarid-Segal et al, Am J Drug Alcohol Abuse 2010;[in press]).

◆ Others

Other drugs tried include imipramine (n = 60, Nunnes et al, Am J Psychiatry 1993;**150**:963–5), methylphenidate (p/c, c/o, 4/52, O'Donnell et al,

Clin Neuropharmacol 1986;**9**:65–70), trazodone (open, n = 25, Janiri et al, Alcohol Alcoholism 1998;**33**:362–5) and piracetam (Barnas et al, Psychopharmacology 1990;**100**:361–5).

□ No efficacy

Amisulpride

Low dose amisulpride 50 mg/d is ineffective in preventing relapse in primary alcohol dependence (n = 71, RCT, d/b, p/c, 6/12, Marra et al, Alcohol Clin Exp Res 2002;**26**:1545–52).

Donepezil

While donepezil was ineffective in one study in reversing Wernicke-Korsakoff's disease memory changes (n = 7, s/b, p/c, c/o, 30/7, Sahin et al, Clin Neuropharmacol 2002;**25**:16–20), high dose donepezil has been reported to help the memory deficits from Korsakoff's psychosis (n = 2, Codina et al, Rev Neurol 2002; **35**:341–5).

Flupentixol decanoate

After detoxification, flupentixol decanoate 10 mg 2/52 actually increased relapses compared to placebo (85% vs 65% for placebo), and so appears to have no role (n = 281, RCT, d/b, 12/12, Weisbeck et al, Alcohol Alcohol 2001;**36**:329–34).

Lithium

Three trials have shown no advantage over placebo (e.g. n = 156, RCT, 6/12, Fawcett et al, Alcohol Clin Exp Res 2000;**24**:666–74).

Olanzapine

Olanzapine was well tolerated but ineffective in reducing drinking outcomes (n = 60, RCT, b/d, 12/52, Guardia et al, Alcohol Clin Exp Res 2004;**28**:736–45).

SSRIs * (see also SSRIs, possible efficacy)

Fluvoxamine was worse than placebo on measures of abstinence and relapse (n = 493, RCT, d/b, p/c, 12/12, Chick et al, Drug Alcohol Depend 2004;**74**:61–70) and sertraline was ineffective on measures of drinking when used as an adjunct to naltrexone (n = 113, RCT, d/b, p/c, 10/52, Farren et al, Drug Alcohol Depend 2009;**99**:317–21).

1.5 ALCOHOL WITHDRAWAL SYNDROME (AWS)

see also Alcohol dependence and abuse (1.4)

Symptoms

The presentation of AWS includes psychological symptoms (e.g. anxiety, insomnia and restlessness), psychotic symptoms (e.g. hallucinations), tremor, sweating, tachycardia, gastrointestinal symptoms, GTC seizures, hallucinations and illusions, clouding of consciousness, delirium tremens (DT) and Wernicke's encephalopathy (WE). WE is the acute phase, lasting for about 48 hours after the last drink, and results from thiamine (B1) deficiency. If untreated it can lead on to the chronic form (Korsakoff psychosis, KP) characterised by severe short-term memory loss. Fits may first occur within 6–8 hours after cessation of alcohol use and peak at 12–24 hours (chronic alcohol consumption causes adaptation and downregulation of GABA receptors and upregulation of NMDA, so sudden withdrawal leads to hyperexcitability and hence seizures). In DT, seizures may occur (either primary or secondary to hypoglycaemia, hypomagnesaemia or hyponatraemia) as may suicidal ideation, gross disorientation, delusions, violence and marked tremor. DT peaks on the 3rd or 4th day, and physical complications are common, e.g. pulmonary infection and hepatic encephalopathy. Risk factors for alcohol withdrawal delirium include concurrent infection, tachycardia, symptoms of withdrawal with blood levels above 1 g/L, and a history of epileptic seizures or delirious episodes (n = 334, Palmstierna et al, Psychiatr Serv 2001;**52**:820–3).

Role of drugs

Seizures and psychiatric disturbances are serious problems and treatment of severe AWS is essential. Withdrawal symptoms in hospital may be underestimated and this may lead to undertreatment. A meta-analysis and practice guideline (Chang and Steinberg, Med Clin North Am 2001;**85**:1191–212) concludes that:

- benzodiazepines are suitable agents for AWS
- dosage should be individualised according to withdrawal severity, comorbidity and history of withdrawal seizures
- beta-blockers, clonidine, carbamazepine ameliorate withdrawal severity but evidence of

their effect on delirium and seizures is lacking
- phenothiazines ameliorate withdrawal but are less effective than benzodiazepines in reducing delirium or seizures
- thiamine (IM or IV) should be an additional first-line treatment.

Reviews: * general (McKeon et al, J Neurol Neurosurg Psychiatry 2008;**79**:854–62), Korsakoff psychosis (Smith and Hillman, Adv Psychiatr Treat 1999;**5**:271–8), seizures (Hughes, Epilepsy Behav 2009;**15**:92–7; Rathlev et al, J Emerg Med 2006;**31**:157–63), anticonvulsants in AWS (Hughes, Epilepsy Behav 2009;**15**:404–12), and in the elderly (Kraemer et al, Drugs Aging 1999;**14**:409–25).

BNF listed

Benzodiazepines *

Benzodiazepines are the drugs of choice for treating acute AWS (meta-analysis of 11 RCTs, n = 1286, Holbrook et al, Can Med Ass J 1999;**160**:649–55). Chlordiazepoxide (and diazepam) are the established treatments in the UK. Lorazepam (n = 186, p/c, D'Onofrio et al, N Engl J Med 1999;**340**:915–9; reviewed in EBMH 1999;**2**:107; Sosis et al, N Engl J Med 1999;**341**:609–10) has also been used, as it has an intermediate half-life and no active metabolites. Lorazepam starting at 8 mg/d was as effective as chlordiazepoxide 80 mg/d (both reducing over eight days) in alcohol withdrawal, and may be a suitable option at lower doses in people with impaired liver function (n = 100, RCT, d/b, 12/7, Kumar et al, J Stud Alcohol Drugs 2009;**70**:457–74). Doses may also be adjusted in a symptom-triggered way, with adequate monitoring of symptoms in patients with particular needs (e.g. chlordiazepoxide n = 108, Wiseman et al, J Clin Psychiatry 1998;**59**:289–93; and oxazepam, n = 117, RCT, Daeppen et al, Arch Intern Med 2002;**162**:1117–21). Higher doses of benzodiazepines may reduce the need for mechanical ventilation in acute-DTs (n = 54, Gold et al, Crit Care Med 2007;**35**:724–30). Beware of an extended metabolism in liver damage (see 3.6), and of respiratory depression.

Reviews: * general (Ntais et al, Cochrane Database Syst Rev 2005;**3**:CD005063), chlordiazepoxide withdrawal regimens

(Chick, *Adv Psychiatr Treat* 1996;**2**:249–57), chlordiazepoxide vs clomethiazole (Duncan and Taylor, *Psychiatr Bull* 1996;**20**:601–3), general (Peppers, *Pharmacotherapy* 1996;**16**:49–58).

Clomethiazole (chlormethiazole) *

Clomethiazole is regarded as a safe and effective treatment of AWS at up to 16 capsules/d, reducing over five to nine days. It has a low addictive potential, although dependence (mainly psychological) can be seen in some patients on longer-term therapy (Hession *et al*, *Lancet* 1979;**1**:953–4). Clomethiazole was as effective as carbamazepine for alcohol withdrawal, and was associated with less risk of premature discharge (n = 168, Hillemacher *et al*, *Pharmacopsychiatry* 2008;**41**:134–7). Clomethiazole may markedly suppress REM sleep in AWS (n = 20, RCT, p/c, d/b, 13/7, Gann *et al*, *Pharmacopsychiatry* 2004;**37**:228-35). The dangers of toxicity may have been exaggerated.

Reviews: Clomethiazole home detoxification schedules, and discussion that clomethiazole may not be as toxic as reputed (Sowerby and Hunter, *J Substance Misuse* 1997;**2**: 62–3; 114–7), general (Duncan and Taylor, *Psychiatr Bull* 1996; **20**: 6013).

Vitamin B supplementation

Classic signs of vitamin deficiency may only occur in extreme depletion and so are easily missed, being interpreted as intoxication. B vitamins act as co-enzymes for essential carbohydrate metabolism. Deficiency of nicotinamide, riboflavine (B_2) and pyridoxine (B_6) can cause neuropathies. Thiamine (B_1) supplementation must be primary and priority treatment to reverse the mental confusion secondary to thiamine deficiency (Wernicke's encephalopathy). Oral thiamine has a saturable absorption mechanism which allows only about 4.5 mg of a single dose to be absorbed. Thiamine 100 mg TDS allows about 13.5 mg to be absorbed, adequate only for mild deficiency. In chronic alcohol misusers, oral absorption can be reduced by 70%. Large oral doses are thus futile and adequate parenteral therapy should be routine, and is essential to treat or prevent KP (review, Thompson, *Alcohol Alcohol* 2000;**35**[Suppl 1]:S2–S7).

Indeed, only 16% patients with WE recovered when given low parenteral thiamine doses (50–100 mg/d) and 20% died (see Thompson *et al*, *Alcohol Alcohol* 2002;**37**:513–21). The parenteral dose necessary is about 500–1000 mg for three to five days (Thompson and Marshall, *Alcohol Alcohol* 2006;**41**:159–67). Although anaphylaxis has been reported with 'Parentrovite®' (Link) the incidence is about one report for every 5,000,000 IM ampoules used. It may be necessary to administer glucose after thiamine when administering thiamine to prevent Wernicke's encephalopathy (Chataway and Hardman, *Postgrad Med J* 1995;**71**:249–53).

Reviews: Thompson *et al*, *Alcohol Alcohol* 2002;**37**:513–21; McIntosh *et al*, *Psychiatr Bull* 2005;**29**:94–7.

+ Combinations

Carbamazepine + tiapride *

This combination was more effective than either drug separately for alcohol withdrawal (n = 56, RCT, open, Croissant *et al*, *Pharmacopsychiatry* 2009;**42**:175–81).

• Unlicensed/some efficacy

Baclofen *

Baclofen (30 mg/d, n = 15) was as effective as diazepam (n = 19) in uncomplicated AWS (n = 37, RCT, 10/7, Addolorato *et al*, *Am J Med* 2006;**119**:13–8; see also n = 42, Stallings and Schrader, *J Okla State Med Assoc* 2007; **100**:354–60).

Carbamazepine *

An effective and useful treatment, carbamazepine is probably active via an anti-kindling effect. It is non-addictive and its metabolism is generally little affected by liver dysfunction but may be inhibited by higher doses of alcohol. Carbamazepine may be as potent as clomethiazole in AWS (n = 37, RCT, s/b, Seifert *et al*, *Addict Biol* 2004;**9**:43–51), and it has also been used for outpatient detoxifications due to its safety and lack of abuse potential (n = 76 [c = 60], open, Collins *et al*, *Br J Psychiatry* 1990;**156**:871–4).

Review: * general (suggests limited evidence

of efficacy and cannot be recommended; s = 6, RCT, Prince and Turpin, *Am J Health Syst Pharm* 2008;**65**:1039–47).

Oxcarbazepine

A pilot study suggested that oxcarbazepine was more effective than carbamazepine in AWS, with less craving (n = 29, RCT, s/b, Schik et al, *Addict Biol* 2005;**10**:283–8).

■ Unlicensed/possible efficacy

Alcohol IV

In an acute setting, IV alcohol had no advantage over diazepam for acute AWS and the previously reported advantages were not evident (n = 50, RCT, 4/7, Weinberg et al, *J Trauma* 2008;**64**:99–104).

Antipsychotics

Decreased dopamine activity may occur in DT (*Postgrad Med J* 1990;**66**:1005–9) so care is needed with anti-dopaminergic drugs, as these may aggravate symptoms and lower the seizure threshold. NMS may also occur and not be recognised. Temperature regulation and liver function pose further difficulties.

Beta-blockers

Beta-blockers, such as atenolol and propranolol, have been used in treating some symptoms of mild to moderate AWS, e.g. tachycardia and tremor, and to reduce craving, but are generally not recommended (Neff and McQueen, *Drug Intell Clin Pharm* 1991;**25**:31–2). The variable kinetics of propranolol in cirrhosis and portal hypertension must be considered (Cales et al, *Br J Clin Pharmacol* 1989;**27**:763–70; comparison with diazepam, Worner, *Am J Drug Alcohol Abuse* 1994;**20**:115–24).

Gabapentin *

Gabapentin (1200 mg/d tapering down) may be as effective as lorazepam for AWS and more effective at reducing post-withdrawal drinking (n = 100, RCT, d/b, 12/7, Myrick et al, *Alcohol Clin Exp Res* 2009;**33**:1582–8). Reduction regimens have been used in outpatient detoxifications, with minimal abuse potential and lack of cognitive impairment (n = 3, open, 5/7, Bozikas et al, *Prog Neuropsychopharmacol Biol*

Psychiatry 2002;**26**:197–9). Augmentation of clomethiazole is well tolerated but ineffective (n = 61, RCT, d/b, 7/7, Bonnet et al, *J Clin Psychopharmacol* 2003;**23**:514–19).

Review: * general (suggests no evidence of efficacy and should not be used; s = 2, Prince and Turpin, *Am J Health Syst Pharm* 2008; **65**:1039–47).

Levetiracetam

An open-label pilot trial showed some efficacy (Krebs et al, *J Clin Psychopharmacol* 2006; **26**:347–9).

Lofexidine

Several studies have shown lofexidine (e.g. 0.4 mg qds for 2–3 days) to be superior to placebo in controlling AWS (e.g. n = 23, Cushman and Sowers, *Alcohol Clin Exp Res* 1989;**13**:361–4), but it appeared ineffective as an adjunct to chlordiazepoxide, with more withdrawal, hypotension, adverse effects and poorer retention with the combination compared to chlordiazepoxide alone (n = 72, RCT, Keaney et al, *Alcohol Alcohol* 2001;**36**:426–30).

Mirtazapine

Adjunctive mirtazapine 30–60 mg/d reduced anxiety and depressive symptoms during the detox process (n = 68, 4/52, Liappas et al, *J Psychopharmacol* 2004;**18**:88–93).

Phenobarbital *

Phenobarbital IV 65 mg with 130 mg 15 minutes later has been effective for BDZ-resistant DTs (n = 1, Hayner et al, *Pharmacotherapy* 2009; **29**:875–8). For those academically minded, the seizures had failed to respond to lorazepam at over 40 mg/hr IV, so that indisputably classifies as BDZ-resistant.

Propofol

Benzodiazepine refractory AWS has been successfully treated with propofol infusion (n = 4, McCowan and Marik, *Critical Care Med* 2000;**28**:1781–4; n = 1, Takeshita, *J Clin Psychiatry* 2004;**65**:134–5).

Tiapride

A retrospective and then open prospective study concluded that tiapride has potential efficacy (n = 60 + 80, Franz et al, Eur Arch Psychiatry Clin Neurosci 2001;**251**:185–92).

Trazodone

Severe AWS resistant to BDZs and clomethiazole responded to trazodone 600 mg/d (n = 1, Borras et al, Pharmacopsychiatry 2006; **39**:232).

Valproate

A review has concluded that only two of the six available studies show a significant effect for valproate and that it should not become a standard treatment (s = 6, Lum et al, Ann Pharmacother 2006;**40**:441–8), although adjunctive valproate (500 mg TDS) may help reduce benzodiazepine doses in AWS, particularly with more severe withdrawal symptoms (n = 36, RCT, 7/7, Reoux et al, Alcohol Clin Exp Res 2001;**25**:1324–9), and may also be a suitable alternative to BDZs due to its lack of abuse potential (n = 16, RCT, 6/52, Longo et al, J Addict Dis 2002;**21**:55–64).

◆ Others

Other drugs tried include **buprenorphine** (for abrupt withdrawal; Fudala et al, Clin Pharmacol Ther 1990;**47**:525–34), **clonidine** (for tremor, tachycardia and hypertension; J Stud Alcohol 1987;**48**:356–70), **dexamethasone** (as 4 mg injections; n = 110, Arch Int Med 1991;**114**:705–6), **flumazenil** (for AWS; n = 20, RCT, s/b, Gerra et al, Curr Ther Res 1991;**50**:62–6), **magnesium sulphate** (Ann Pharmacother 1992;**26**:650–2), **nitrous oxide** (rapid relief of AWS; n = 104, Br J Psychiatry 1991; **159**:672–5), and **phenytoin** (in pre-existing epilepsy; N Engl J Med 1988;**319**:715–6).

☐ No efficacy

Fluvoxamine

A trial of fluvoxamine in alcoholic Korsakoff syndrome showed no therapeutic role and included two apparently fluvoxamine-induced episodes of depression (n = 8, O'Carroll et al, Psychopharmacol 1994;**116**:85–8).

Nitrous oxide *

Although rapid relief of AWS has been reported (n = 104, Gillman and Lichtigfeld, Br J Psychiatry 1991;**159**:672–5), its use is not recommended (s = 6, Prince and Turpin, Am J Health Syst Pharm 2008;**65**:1039–47).

ALZHEIMER'S DISEASE
see Dementia (1.13)

ANOREXIA AND BULIMIA NERVOSA
see Eating disorders (1.16)

1.6 ANXIETY DISORDER
(generalised) — Generalised Anxiety disorder (GAD) includes also Panic disorder (1.21) with or without Agoraphobia (1.3), OCD (1.20) and Social phobia (1.27)

Symptoms

There are numerous symptoms of generalised anxiety disorder (although anxiety can in itself be a symptom of many conditions), but they can be classified into two main groups:

- **Psychological symptoms** include fearful apprehension, irritability, poor concentration, restlessness, being easily fatigued, sensitivity to noise, disturbed sleep (lying awake worrying, waking intermittently, unpleasant dreams, but not usually early morning waking) and poor memory (due to poor concentration).

- **Physical symptoms** are mainly due to overactivity of the sympathetic system or increased muscle tension, e.g. gastrointestinal (dry mouth, difficulty swallowing, wind, loose motions, etc), CNS (tinnitus, blurred vision, dizziness), respiratory (constricted chest, difficulty inhaling, overbreathing), cardiovascular (palpitations, heart pain, missed or ectopic beats, neck throbbing), genitourinary (increased micturition, lack of libido and impotence), muscular tension (tension headache, tremor) and panic attacks (sudden episodes of extreme anxiety or apprehension). Anxiety must be differentiated from depression, early schizophrenia, dementia, drugs/alcohol abuse including withdrawal and physical illness, e.g. thyroid dysfunction (n = 169, Simon et al, J Affect Disord 2002;**69**:209–17). The lifetime prevalence of anxiety disorders is about 17% in USA (Grant et al, Can J Psychiatry

2006;**51**:100–3; comment by Starcevic, *EBMH* 2006;**9**:115). GAD has a 90% lifetime comorbidity (Wittchen *et al, Arch Gen Psychiatry* 1994;**51**:355–64) and only about 25% of GAD cases present without any comorbidity (Maier *et al, Acta Psychiatr Scand* 2000;**101**:29–36).

Role of drugs

Anxiolytics such as benzodiazepines used as a 'first-line' measure are quite appropriate but it is difficult to assess the longer-term effectiveness of these drugs, as anxiety tends to fluctuate for reasons other than pharmacotherapy. The decision for longer-term treatment must be considered on an individual basis, with the risk:benefit analysis varying with the disability caused by the symptoms and the age of the person. Choice of therapy is not easy but an independent and thorough analysis concluded that the effect sizes were:

- 0.5 pregabalin
- 0.45 antihistamines (hydroxyzine)
- 0.42 SNRI (venlafaxine)
- 0.38 benzodiazepines
- 0.36 SSRIs
- 0.17 buspirone
- -0.31 complementary and alternative medicines (Kava kava and homeopathy).

Children and adolescents responded better to medication and Kava kava was worse than placebo (and has significant ADRs) (s = 21, d/b, p/c, Hidalgo *et al, J Psychopharmacol* 2007;**21**: 864–72), although another systematic review concluded that of the herbal remedies there was only sound evidence for Kava kava for anxiety and it is not free from risks (Ernst, *Adv Psych Treat* 2007;**13**:312–6).

The SSRIs and venlafaxine are effective across the range of anxiety disorders and are generally considered first-line treatment. Initial worsening and rare suicidal ideation can occur, so specific monitoring is needed early in treatment. BDZs are effective but use is not recommended by NICE and should only be used in the short-term unless anxiety is treatment-resistant. Low-dose trifluoperazine has been shown to be superior to placebo for GAD, but is about the only antipsychotic that has (review by Gao *et al, J Clin Psychiatry* 2006;**67**:1327–40). TCAs and anticonvulsants can be tried in resistant cases but need an individual risk-benefit assessment.

The role of pregabalin is yet to be established. Efficacy should be assessed at 12 weeks and, if successful, continued for six months (BAP evidence-based guidelines Baldwin *et al, J Psychopharmacol* 2005;**19**:567–96). Psychological interventions include explanations, reassurance, support and, in more persistent conditions, cognitive and behavioural therapy (Hoehn-Saric, *CNS Drugs* 1998;**9**:85–98).

Reviews: * evidence-base for drugs, review (Baldwin *et al, J Psychopharmacol* 2005;**19**:567–96; Baldwin and Polkinghorn, *Int J Neuropsychopharmacol* 2005;**8**:293–302), pharmacotherapy (Davidson, *J Clin Psychiatry* 2009;**70** Suppl 2:25–31; s = 48, Mitte *et al, J Clin Psychopharmacol* 2005;**25**:141–50; comment by Swinson, *EBMH* 2005;**8**:111), general (Gale and Davidson, *BMJ* 2007;**334**:579–81; Tyrer and Baldwin, *Lancet* 2006;**368**:2156–66).

BNF listed

BENZODIAZEPINES

Benzodiazepines may be extremely useful for chronic anxiety and should not be overlooked. A systematic review and meta-analysis of benzodiazepines showed robust evidence for efficacy if later, more rigorous, trials are favoured (s = 23, RCT, p/c, Martin *et al, J Psychopharmacol* 2007;**21**:774–82). Use of benzodiazepines can be restricted to short-term (up to four weeks) or intermittent courses. Prior benzodiazepine exposure does not predispose patients to more severe discontinuation symptoms in subsequent courses (review, Rickels and Freeman, *J Clin Psychiatry* 2000;**61**:409–13). Although the benzodiazepines have a relative lack of toxicity in overdose, there is some difference between

> Benzodiazepines are indicated for short-term relief of severe anxiety. Other treatment methods should then be started, e.g. relaxation, psychotherapy, treating any underlying depression, etc. Caution is advised for the use of benzodiazepines, e.g. use for short-term use, and avoid in depression and personality disorder.

different drugs, e.g. temazepam (with rapid absorption and high sedative effect) and possibly flurazepam have a greater toxicity in overdose than other benzodiazepines, e.g. diazepam, clonazepam, and oxazepam (303 overdose study by Buckley et al, Br Med J 1995;**310**:219–21). All are capable of being fatal in overdose (especially combined with alcohol) and should not be prescribed for patients at high risk of overdose. Users of benzodiazepines are also at greater risk of road-traffic accidents, especially if combined with alcohol (involved in accidents, n = 19 386 over three years, Barbone et al, Lancet 1998;**352**:1331–6). A retrospective review of hip fractures indicated that doses of > 3 mg/d diazepam (or equivalent) increased the risk of hip fractures by 50%, especially after initiation and after more than a month of treatment. Shorter half-life drugs did not appear to reduce the risk (n = 1 222 + 4 888, Wang et al, Am J Psychiatry 2001;**158**:892–8). Tremor in GAD is an enhanced physiological tremor and responds to propranolol and benzodiazepines (n = 120, open, c/o, Milanov, Electromyogr Clin Neurophysiol 2007;**47**:3–9).

Reviews: * general (Cloos and Ferreira, Curr Opin Psychiatry 2009;**22**:90–5), withdrawing BDZs (Lader et al, CNS Drugs 2009;**23**:19–34), guidelines for the clinical use of benzodiazepines (Nelson and Chouinard, Can J Clin Pharmacol 1999;**6**:69–83), advantages and disadvantages (Argyropoulos and Nutt, Prescriber 2001;**12**: 21–8).

Alprazolam

Alprazolam (review, Verster and Volkerts, CNS Drug Rev 2004;**10**:45–76) is a widely-used (except UK) BDZ. From 2063 BDZ overdoses, those with alprazolam (n = 131) were more likely to be admitted to ITUs than with other BDZs (n = 2063, Isbister et al, Br J Clin Pharmacol 2004;**58**:88–95).

Chlordiazepoxide

Chlordiazepoxide has a slower onset of action and many active metabolites.

Clobazam

Clobazam is licensed for the short-term (two to four weeks) treatment of anxiety. See entry under epilepsy (1.17.1).

Diazepam

Diazepam is the standard longer-acting benzodiazepine, with sedative, anxiolytic and muscle relaxant properties (among others). It has a long half-life and many active metabolites.

Lorazepam

Lorazepam is a shorter-acting benzodiazepine with potent receptor-binding properties. Despite previous media interest in alleged dependence it remains widely used.

Oxazepam

A shorter-acting benzodiazepine (the ultimate metabolite of diazepam and some other benzodiazepines) with no active metabolites.

There are many other benzodiazepines available commercially in the UK, e.g. **bromazepam**, **clorazepate**, and **ketazolam**.

Non-benzodiazepines

Beta-blockers

Propranolol at 20–60 mg/d may be useful for somatic anxiety symptoms such as tachycardia, sweating and tremor (n = 120, open, c/o, Milanov, Electromyogr Clin Neuophysiol 2007;**47**:3–9). Studies have shown propranolol to be less effective than diazepam (n = 26, d/b, p/c, c/o, Hallström et al, Br J Psychiatry 1981;**139**:417–21) and more effective than placebo (n = 57, p/c, Hudson, Br J Clin Pract 1988;**42**:419–26). The best response appears to be in doses sufficient to reduce resting pulse by 7 bpm (Hallström et al, Br J Psychiatry 1981;**139**:417–21), and in patients presenting with autonomic complaints, e.g. palpitations, shortness of breath, sweating, rapid ventilation, etc.

Buspirone

Buspirone is a non-benzodiazepine anxiolytic with negligible sedative, cognitive (n = 60, RCT, d/b, Chamberlain et al, J Psychopharmacol 2007; **21**:210–5), hypnotic, anticonvulsant and muscle relaxant properties. In general, it is considered as effective as the benzodiazepines in GAD, with a better side-effect profile, although it has been noted that early efficacy studies were not performed in patients diagnosed with GAD using current criteria. It has a slow onset of action and may be underused, as it needs four weeks at 10mg TDS for optimum efficacy. Buspirone possibly acts on 5-HT$_{1A}$ receptors and has no effect on withdrawal in benzodiazepine-dependent persons. Indeed, patients with GAD who have recently discontinued BDZs may suffer more ADRs and respond slower to buspirone than those who have neither had BDZs nor discontinued more than a month before (n = 735, DeMartinis et al, J Clin Psychiatry 2000;61:91–4). Buspirone does not significantly reduce anxiety symptoms in opioid-dependent individuals (n = 36, RCT, p/c, McRae et al, Am J Addict 2004;13:53–63), although it has a non-existent abuse potential and abrupt discontinuation has not been shown to produce withdrawal symptoms. Cochrane concludes that buspirone is superior to placebo but less effective than BDZs (s = 36, n = 5908, Chessick et al, Cochrane Database Syst Rev 2006;3:CD006115).

Reviews: general (Apter and Allen, J Clin Psychopharmacol 1999;19:86–93), clinical pharmacology and therapeutic applications (Fulton and Brogden, CNS Drugs 1997;7:68–88), pharmacokinetics (Mahmood and Sahajwalla, Clin Pharmacokinet 1999;36:277–87, 48 refs; Salazar et al, J Clin Pharmacol 2001;41:1351–8).

Duloxetine *

Duloxetine is licensed for GAD, with a starting dose of 30mg/d, increasing to 60mg/d if ineffective and with a maximum dose of 120mg/d. Data from three independent trials showed duloxetine 60–120mg/d to consistently improve functioning in GAD (s = 3, n = 1163, RCT, d/b, p/c, 9–10/52, Endicott et al, J Clin Psychiatry 2007;68:518–24) and 120mg/d is non-inferior to venlafaxine 75–225mg/d (56–58% response cf 40% with placebo) in adults with GAD (s = 2, n=984, RCT, d/b, p/c, 10/52, Allgulander et al, J Psychopharmacol 2008;22:417–25). In responders from an open active treatment phase, relapse with duloxetine 60–120mg/d was 14% vs 42% with placebo (n = 405, RCT, d/b, p/c, 26/52, Davidson et al, Eur Neuropsychopharmacol 2008;18:673–81).

Reviews: * general (s = 4, d/b, p/c, 9–10/52, Kornstein et al, Expert Rev Neurother 2009; 9:155–65 Khan and Macaluso, Neuropsychiatr

Dis Treat 2009;5:23–31; Norman and Olver, Neuropsychiatr Dis Treat 2008;4:1169–80).

Escitalopram *

Escitalopram is licensed for anxiety, with a 10mg/d starting dose and a 20mg/d maximum. There may be a significant improvement in GAD symptoms as early as the first week and the majority of patients respond by week eight with a significant improvement in functioning (n = 315, RCT, d/b, p/c, 8/52, Davidson et al, Depress Anxiety 2004;19:234–40). However, a trial should last at least four weeks before further intervention is considered (s = 40, Baldwin et al, Hum Psychopharmacol 2009;24:269–75). Several large studies have shown that escitalopram 10mg/d and 20mg/d are equally effective for GAD and superior to paroxetine (suggesting that perhaps not all SSRIs are the same in GAD) and placebo (n = 681, RCT, d/b, 12/52, Baldwin et al, Br J Psychiatry 2006;189:264–72; comment by Gale, EBMH 2007;10:45; n = 121, d/b, 24/52, Bielski et al, Ann Clin Psychiatry 2005;17:65–9; s = 3, RCT, p/c, Stein et al, Ann Clin Psychiatry 2005;17:71–5). Escitalopram also seems effective in the long-term (n = 526 [c = 299], open, 24/52, Davidson et al, J Clin Psychiatry 2005;66:1441–6). In older (>60) people with GAD, escitalopram was superior to placebo, but not significantly so (n = 177, RCT, d/b, p/c, 12/52, Lenze et al, JAMA 2009;301:295–303).

Hydroxyzine

Hydroxyzine is an antihistamine related to the phenothiazines, which may be mildly useful in some cases. Hydroxyzine 50mg/d may be as effective as bromazepam (but with less drowsiness) and both are more effective than placebo in GAD (n = 334, RCT, d/b, p/c, 3/52, Llorca et al, J Clin Psychiatry 2002;63:1020–7; comment by Akhondzadeh, EBMH 2003;6:91).

Paroxetine

Paroxetine is licensed in the UK for GAD, and a number of RCTs have shown 20–50mg/d to be rapidly effective (e.g. n = 324, RCT, p/c, Pollack et al, J Clin Psychiatry 2001;62:350–7). Paroxetine 20mg/d may be adequate (n = 384, RCT, d/b, p/c, Leibowitz et al, J Clin Psychiatry 2002;63:66–74; n = 278, RCT, d/b, p/c, 12/52,

Baldwin et al, Br J Psychiatry 2006;**189**:264–72) and 40 mg/d may be only slightly more effective than 20 mg/d (n=566, RCT, p/c, d/b, 8/52, Rickels et al, Am J Psychiatry 2003;**160**:749–56). Paroxetine may also be effective and well tolerated for long-term management of GAD and reduces relapse (n=652, d/b, p/c extension, 32/52, Stocchi et al, J Clin Psychiatry 2003;**64**:250–8; MS).

Reviews: overview of studies (s=4, n=1800, RCT, d/b, p/c, Rickels et al, J Clin Psychiatry 2006;**67**:41–7), use in anxiety (Snyderman et al, Expert Opin Pharmacother 2004;**5**:1799–806).

Pregabalin

Pregabalin is licensed for GAD and a recent review concluded that 200–450 mg/d is the optimal dose range, with 600 mg/d being no more effective (s=4, Bech, Pharmacopsychiatry 2007;**40**:163–8). Pregabalin 300 mg/d appears reasonably well tolerated, significantly superior to placebo, and equivalent to alprazolam (n=454, RCT, d/b, p/c, 4/52, Rickels et al, Arch Gen Psychiatry 2005;**62**:1022–30) and to venlafaxine (n=21, RCT, d/b, p/c, 6/52, Montgomery et al, J Clin Psychiatry 2006;**67**:771–82; MS). It may also be a quick-acting anxiolytic with few withdrawal symptoms (cf. lorazepam n=276, RCT, p/c, 6/52, Pande et al, Am J Psychiatry 2003;**160**:533–40). In responders, continuation therapy reduces relapse compared to placebo (42% vs 65%) and is reasonably well tolerated (n=624, open, 8/52; then n=338, RCT, p/c, d/b, 6/12, Feltner et al, Int Clin Psychopharmacol 2008;**23**:18–28, MS).

Reviews: general (Bendelow et al, Expert Rev Neurother 2007;**7**:769–81; Frampton and Foster, CNS Drugs 2006;**20**:685–95; Montgomery, Expert Opin Pharmacother 2006;**7**:2139–54).

Venlafaxine XL

Venlafaxine is licensed for GAD, with 75 mg/d considered the optimum dose (n=9, Melichar et al, J Psychopharmacol 2001;**15**:9–12). Venlafaxine 75 mg/d and pregabalin (400–600 mg/d) may be equipotent and superior to placebo for GAD, but venlafaxine was less well tolerated and pregabalin possibly had an earlier onset (n=426, RCT, d/b, 6/52, Montgomery et al, J Clin Psychiatry 2006;**67**:771–82; comment by Stein, EBMH 2007;**10**:23). For long-term treatment, 75 mg and 150 mg/d (but not 37.5 mg/d) have both been shown to be superior to placebo, showing a sustained effect (n=541, p/c, d/b, 24/52, Allgulander et al, Br J Psychiatry 2001;**179**:15–22, MS; n=377, RCT, 8/52, Rickels et al, Am J Psychiatry 2000;**157**:968–74). It is also effective for depression with anxiety, e.g. 75–225 mg/d was slightly more effective than fluoxetine (20–60 mg/d) in 92 patients with comorbid GAD and MDD (n=368, 12/52, Silverstone and Salinas, J Clin Psychiatry 2001;**62**:523–9). Higher doses are not routinely recommended but can be used, e.g. venlafaxine up to 225 mg/day was superior to placebo in non-depressed outpatients with generalised anxiety disorder (n=251, RCT, 6/52, Gelenberg et al, JAMA 2000;**283**:3082–8). In a pooled analysis, venlafaxine was found to be as well tolerated and effective in older adults for anxiety as in younger adults (s=5, n=1839, RCT, Katz et al, J Am Geriatr Soc 2002;**50**:18–25).

Review: general (Thase, Expert Rev Neurother 2006;**6**:269–82).

● Unlicensed/some efficacy

Agomelatine *

Agomelatine 25–50 mg/d has been shown to be effective and well-tolerated for pure GAD (n=121, RCT, d/b, p/c, 12/52, Stein et al, J Clin Psychopharmacol 2008;**28**:561–6).

Antipsychotics *

Antipsychotics have little proven efficacy in GAD and marked side-effects. **Trifluoperazine** 2–6 mg/d may be superior to placebo (n=415, d/b, p/c, 4/52, Mendels et al, J Clin Psychiatry 1986;**47**:170–4). Some newer antipsychotics have been used but the evidence for this currently makes it a costly strategy, e.g. **olanzapine** PRN is an expensive antihistamine. The use of PRN antipsychotics makes assessment of the underlying causes of agitation more difficult, especially as akathisia can be a side-effect. Antipsychotics should be used carefully and only for infrequent, sustained agitation (review by Druckenbrod et al, Ann Pharmacother 1993;**27**:645–8). A pilot study suggested **aripiprazole** may be useful as an adjunct in resistant GAD (n=13, open, 8/52,

Hoge et al, CNS Spectr 2008;**13**:522–7). Adjunctive low-dose **risperidone** (0.5–1.5mg/d) was superior (but not statistically) to placebo as add-on to existing anxiolytics (n = 40, RCT, d/b, p/c, 5/52, Brawman-Mintzer et al, J Clin Psychiatry 2005;**66**:1321–5), and up to 3mg/d may be useful in refractory anxiety disorders (n = 30[c = 21], open, 8/52, Simon et al, J Clin Psychiatry 2006;**67**:381–5), but was ineffective for anxiety comorbid within bipolar disorder (n = 111, RCT, d/b, p/c, 8/52, Sheehan et al, J Affect Disord 2009:**115**:376–85) and even low doses up to 2mg/d risk hyperprolactinaemia (n = 12, Kopecek et al, Neuro Endocrinol Lett 2006;**27**:803–6). **Quetiapine** (mean 386mg/d) may have some efficacy in resistant GAD as an adjunct to standard treatments (n = 40, open, 12/52, Katzman et al, J Anxiety Disord 2008; **22**:1480–6) and 150–300mg/d as monotherapy (n = 13[c = 10], open, 12/52, Schutters et al, J Clin Psychiatry 2005;**66**:540–2). Quetiapine 150mg/d seems the optimum dose for GAD, and as effective as paroxetine (n = 873, RCT, d/b, 8/52, Bandelow et al, Int J Neuropsychopharmacol 2009;**20**:1–16).

Reviews: * general (Gao et al, Expert Rev Neurother 2009;**9**:1147–58; Nemeroff, J Clin Psychiatry 2005;**66** Suppl 8:13–21).

Mirtazapine

Mirtazapine (15–45mg/d) may be effective within a week for the symptoms of GAD with comorbid depression (n = 10, open, 8/52, Goodnick et al, J Clin Psychiatry 1999;**60**:446–8) and 30mg produced response in 78% and remission in 36% in a pilot study (n = 44, open, 12/52, Gambi et al, J Psychopharmacol 2006;**20**:483–7).

SSRIs *
(see also paroxetine and escitalopram)

SSRIs have some efficacy in anxiety, with paroxetine and escitalopram licensed. Lower doses may be needed initially, as SSRIs may exacerbate symptoms over the first 1–2 weeks of treatment. **Citalopram** has been shown to be effective in 85% patients with GAD, including some who had failed with other SSRIs (n = 13, 12/52, Varia and Rauscher, Int Clin Psychopharmacol 2002;**17**:103–7), and also in children (n = 17, open, Prince et al,

Psychopharmacol Bull 2002;**36**:100–7). **Fluvoxamine** CR was superior to placebo for anxiety in adults, with few sexual side-effects (n = 300, RCT, d/b, p/c, 12/52, Westenberg et al, J Clin Psychopharmacol 2004;**24**:49–55) and it may be mildly effective for anxiety in children and adolescents (n = 128, RCT, 8/52, RUPPAS, N Engl J Med 2001;**344**:1279–85; critique by Hazell, EBMH 2001;**4**:116; review by Irons, Neuropsychiatr Dis Treat 2005;**1**:289–99). **Sertraline** 50–150mg/d was more effective than placebo for GAD (n = 370, RCT, d/b, p/c, 12/52, Allgulander et al, Am J Psychiatry 2004;**161**:1642–9), including acute treatment (n = 326, RCT, d/b, p/c, 10/52, Brawman-Mintzer et al, J Clin Psychiatry 2006;**67**:874–81).

Tricyclic antidepressants

Although not recommended by NICE, tricyclics may be useful for persistent or disabling anxiety that is not part of an adjustment/stress reaction. They may take several weeks to act but may be very potent, e.g. imipramine may be at least as effective as diazepam and trazodone (see also trazodone) (n = 230, d/b, p/c, 8/52, Rickels et al, Arch Gen Psychiatry 1993;**50**:884–95).

■ Unlicensed/possible efficacy

Gabapentin

In patients with a history of alcohol dependency or abuse, gabapentin 100–900mg/d may produce sustained clinical improvement in symptoms of anxiety (n = 4, Pollack et al, Am J Psychiatry 1998;**155**:992–3; review by Norton and Quarles, Hosp Pharm 2001;**36**:843–5, 12 refs). Gabapentin 800mg has reduced public-speaking provoked anxiety (n = 32, d/b, p/c, de-Paris et al, J Psychopharmacol 2003;**17**:184–8).

Galphimia glauca

Galphimia glauca is a traditional Mexican herbal medicine and was as effective and better tolerated than lorazepam 1mg/d in GAD (n = 152, RCT, d/b, 4/52, Herrera-Arellano et al, Planta Med 2007;**73**:713–7).

Kava kava

Kava kava has been reported to be as effective as sub-therapeutic buspirone and a drug

I've never heard of (opipramol), with a 75% response rate for all treatment arms which must say something about the illness severity in the trial (n = 129, RCT, 8/52, d/b, Boerner et al, *Phytomedicine* 2003;10[Suppl 4]:S38–S49). A meta-analysis showed it less than useful (see introduction).

Levetiracetam

Levetiracetam (mean 2 g/d) may have some efficacy for resistant GAD (n = 40, open, 9/52, Kinrys et al, *J Clin Psychiatry* 2007; 68:1010–3).

Passionflower (*Passiflora*)

Passionflower may have an anxiolytic effect, with a low incidence of drowsiness compared to oxazepam (n = 36, RCT, d/b, p/c, 4/52, Akhondzadeh et al, *J Clin Pharm Ther* 2001; 26:363–7), although Cochrane concludes that the data is too sparse to draw any conclusions (s = 2, n = 198, Miyasaka et al, *Cochrane Database Syst Rev* 2007: 1:CD004518).

Riluzole

Riluzole 100 mg/d was rapidly effective in 80%, producing remission in 53% over 2–3 weeks (n = 18 [c = 15], open, 8/52, Mathew et al, *Am J Psychiatry* 2005;162:2379–81).

Testosterone

Undiagnosed hypogonadism presenting as GAD has been treated successfully with testosterone injections (n = 1, Cooper and Ritchie, *Am J Psychiatry* 2000;157:1884).

Tiagabine *

An analysis of the three trials showed no significant advantage over placebo in adults with GAD (s = 3, RCT, p/c, d/b, 10/52, Pollack et al, *J Clin Psychopharmacol* 2008;28:308–16), although the two less robust studies suggested some efficacy at 8–20 mg/d (e.g. n = 40, open, RCT, 10/52, Rosenthal, *J Clin Psychiatry* 2003;64:1245–9; n = 18 [c = 17], open, 8/52, Schwartz et al, *Ann Clin Psychiatry* 2005;17:167–72).

Review: use in anxiety disorders (Schwartz and Nihalani, *Expert Opin Pharmacother* 2006; 7:1977–87).

Trazodone

Trazodone has been claimed to be equipotent with some benzodiazepines, e.g. trazodone may be at least as effective as diazepam and imipramine in GAD, although the antidepressants had more side-effects (n = 230, d/b, p/c, 8/52, Rickels et al, *Arch Gen Psychiatry* 1993;50:884–95).

Valproate

There has been some speculation that valproate may have anxiolytic actions (*Am J Psychiatry* 1990;147:950–1) via an effect of enhancing GABA.

◆ Others

Other drugs tried include **barbiturates** (such as amylobarbital), **mianserin** (n = 106, d/b, 6/52, Bjertnaes et al, *Acta Psychiatr Scand* 1982;66:199–207), **nabilone** (n = 8, RCT, Glass et al, *J Clin Pharmacol* 1981;21[Suppl 8–9]:S383–S96) and **St John's wort** (n = 100, d/b, 2/52, Panijel, *Therapiewoche* 1985;41:4659–68).

☐ No efficacy

Caffeine

Caffeine consumption should be calculated in GAD (*see Caffeinism 1.30*), as higher intakes can cause nervousness, anxiety, restlessness, irritability and palpitations, probably by an abnormal sensitivity to caffeine (n = 36, p/c, Bruce et al, *Arch Gen Psychiatry* 1992;49:867–9). One study, however, of chronic schizophrenic in-patients showed no change in anxiety when caffeine was removed from the diet (n = 26, Mayo et al, *Br J Psychiatry* 1993;162:543–5).

Review: * anxiogenic effects of caffeine (Broderick and Benjamin, *J Okla State Med Assoc* 2004;97:538–42).

Homeopathy

Classical homeopathy was no different in one study to placebo, although both groups had high response rates (n = 44, RCT, d/b, p/c, 10/52, Bonne et al, *J Clin Psychiatry* 2003;64:282–7).

Ondansetron

One study showed 4 mg/d to be no better than placebo, although placebo response was high (n=97, RCT, Romach et al, J Clin Psychopharmacol 1998;**18**:121–31).

Yohimbine

Yohimbine increases self-rated anxiety in anxiety-prone children (n=32, Sallee et al, Am J Psychiatry 2000;**157**:1236–42).

1.7 ATTENTION DEFICIT HYPER-ACTIVITY DISORDER (ADHD), including HYPERKINETIC DISORDER
1.7.1 ADHD IN CHILDREN AND ADOLESCENTS

Symptoms: *
Attention deficit hyperactivity disorder (ADHD) is characterised by a developmentally inappropriate degree of gross motor activity, impulsivity, inattention to detail and temper outbursts. Children with ADHD have extreme and persistent restlessness, sustained and prolonged motor activity and difficulty in organising and maintaining attention to work or play. They are also easily distracted, fidget, careless, reckless, prone to accidents, have learning difficulties (partly due to poor concentration), sleep problems (n=466, Gau and Chiang, Sleep 2009;**32**:671–9) and often have antisocial behaviour and a fluctuating mood. Onset is before seven years of age. Symptoms can fade by puberty but inattention and antisocial behaviour may persist into adult life and may, but not always, lead to poor achievement (see 1.7.2). ADHD is the most inheritable of all mental health conditions (up to 75%) and so there is a major genetic component. Studies implicate dysregulation of frontal-subcortical-cerebellar catecholamine circuits, including abnormal dopamine transport and impaired neurotransmission (Biederman and Faraone, Lancet 2005;**366**:237–48; Kuntsi et al, Neuromolecular Med 2006;**8**:461–84) especially in the nucleus accumbens and midbrain, areas that regulate reward and motivation (n=97, Volkow et al, JAMA 2009;**302**:1084–91).

Role of drugs *
Pharmacotherapy is an essential component for the treatment package for ADHD. Careful medication management is effective in reducing core ADHD symptoms, superior to behavioural therapy and with some limited evidence that

the combination is more effective than either alone (n=579, NTA-CG, Arch Gen Psychiatry 2000;**56**:1073–86; review by Sawyer and Graetz, EBMH 2000;**3**:82), although combining psychosocial treatment with methylphenidate may make no difference to response (n=103, RCT, 24/12, Abikoff et al, J Am Acad Child Adolesc Psychiatry 2004;**43**:802–11; comment by Scahill, EBMH 2005;**8**:9). A meta-analysis of methylphenidate and psychosocial treatments alone or together in adolescent ADHD showed that both were effective, but methylphenidate alone or in combination was superior to psychosocial treatments alone (s=26, RCTs, Van der Oord et al, Clin Psychol Rev 2008;**28**:783–800; comment by Jensen, EBMH 2009;**12**:18). The main pharmacotherapy strategy is the use of stimulants and a major meta-analysis has shown robust and consistent evidence that stimulants are more effective than placebo for improving overt and covert aggressive behaviours in ADHD (s=28, n=683, Connor et al, J Am Acad Child Adolesc Psych 2002;**41**:253–61; comment by Klein, EBMH 2002;**5**:108). Stimulants have an immediate effect compared to a delayed effect from noradrenergic agents, e.g. atomoxetine (Wilens et al, J Atten Disord 2002;**5**:189–202). Methylphenidate is clearly the first-line stimulant (s=62, n=2897, RCT, Schachter et al, CMAJ 2001;**165**:1475–88; review by Connor, EBMH 2002;**5**:50). There is a natural reluctance by many prescribers to use stimulants in younger children and so mild symptoms should be treated with environmental changes, but moderate to severe symptoms may require drug therapy. There is, however, no statistically significant association between stimulant treatment use between 6 and 17 years, and increased or decreased alcohol, drug or nicotine use in adult life (n=140 [c=112], 10-year follow-up, Biederman et al, Am J Psychiatry 2008;**165**:597–603).

Reviews: * general (Dopheide and Pliszka, Pharmacotherapy 2009;**29**:656–79, Shah, Pharm J 2008;**280**:191–4), treatment of comorbid ADHD and autism (Hazell, J Paediatr Child Health 2007;**43**:19–24), non-stimulant medications (Mohammadi and Akhondzadeh, Expert Rev Neurother 2007;**7**:195–201).

NB: Drug trials need to be interpreted carefully as different diagnostic criteria have been used in different studies.

BNF listed *

There are some comparisons between stimulants and atomoxetine. The most robust two show that atomoxetine is non-inferior to methylphenidate, and equally well tolerated, although atomoxetine had more TEAEs (n = 330, RCT, d/b, 8/52, Wang et al, Aust N Z J Psychiatry 2007;**41**:222–30). The other showed that methylphenidate was superior to atomoxetine and both were superior to placebo, buit that in non-responders to one, 42% then responded when switched to the other one (n=516, RCT, d/b, p/c, 6/52, Newcorn et al, Am J Psychiatry 2008;**165**:721–30).

Although there is still some concern about prescribing stimulants in adolescents, a long-term follow-up of methylphenidate in male children (6–12 years of age) with ADHD showed that an early age of initiation does not increase the risk for negative outcomes (e.g. substance misuse) and probably has the opposite effect (n = 354, Mannuzza et al, Am J Psychiatry 2008;**165**:604–9). There is no evidence for increased risk of sudden death with stimulants in ADHD (n = 18637, McCarthy et al, Drug Saf 2009;**32**:1089–96). For switching, see Chapter 2.

Review: atomoxetine vs stimulants (s = 5, Gibson et al, Ann Pharmacother 2006;**40**:1134–42).

Atomoxetine *

Atomoxetine is a noradrenaline reuptake inhibitor (NARI) with minimal effects on other transmitters, and is non-stimulant, with minimal abuse potential (comparison with methylphenidate, n = 16, d/b, p/c, Heil et al, Drug Alcohol Depend 2002;**67**:149–56) and no discontinuation syndrome (Wernicke et al, J Clin Psychopharmacol 2004;**24**:30–5, MS). The usual dose is 0.5 mg/kg up to 40 mg/d for the first week, increased up to 100 mg/d, although higher doses have been shown to have no advantages over standard doses (s = 2, n = 247, RCT, d/b, Kratochvil et al, J Am Acad Child Adolesc Psychiatry 2007;**46**:1128–37). Atomoxetine takes 3–4 weeks to work, so if switching from a stimulant continue the stimulant for several weeks while the atomoxetine kicks in. Efficacy in ADHD has been shown in a number of RCTs (e.g. s = 2, n = 291, RCT, d/b, p/c, 12/52, Spencer et al, J Clin Psychiatry 2002;**63**:1140–7). Once-daily dosing of atomoxetine seems equally effective and as

well tolerated as twice a day (n = 218, RCT, d/b, Adler et al, Ann Clin Psychiatry 2006;**18**:107–13; n = 153, RCT, p/c, 7/52, Weiss et al, J Am Acad Child Adolesc Psychiatry 2005;**44**:647–55, MS; comment by Barton, EBMH 2006;**9**:7) and may be effective throughout the day, including the next morning, unlike methylphenidate (n = 197, RCT, d/b, p/c, 8/52, Kelsey et al, Pediatrics 2004;**114**:1–8, MS). Long-term treatment seems effective (n = 272 [c = 97], 24/12, Kratochvil et al, J Am Acad Child Adolesc Psychiatry 2006;**45**:919–27; n = 125, 4 years, Adler et al, J Atten Disord 2008;**12**:248–53). A meta-analysis of long-term follow-up data, showed atomoxetine had only a minor effect on height, with none on those with the lowest height (n = 412, > 2 years, Spencer et al, Pediatrics 2005;**116**:74–80). Atomoxetine does not seem to make tics worse in ADHD with comorbid tic disorders (n = 148, RCT, d/b, p/c, < 18/52, Allen et al, Neurology 2005;**65**:1941–9; MS). While atomoxetine is effective for ADHD, it has no apparent efficacy for comorbid MDD (n = 142, d/b, 9/52, Atomoxetine ADHD-MDD study group, J Child Adolesc Psychopharmacol 2007;**17**:407–20, MS). In 2006, the UK MHRA issued guidance that people on atomoxetine should be monitored for signs of depression, suicidal thoughts or suicidal behaviour and referred for appropriate treatment if necessary, as increased suicidal thoughts or behaviour have been in association with atomoxetine (s = 12, n = 1357), although the incidence was only 0.4% and with no completed suicides.

Reviews: * general (Hammerness et al, Neuropsychiatr Dis Treat 2009;**5**:215–26; Vaughan et al, Expert Opin Pharmacother 2009;**10**:669–76; Barton, Arch Dis Child 2005;**90**(Suppl 1);26–9).

Dexamfetamine

Amfetamine is clearly superior to placebo on a variety of key measures, remaining effective over 15 months (n = 62, RCT, 15/12, Gillberg et al, Arch Gen Psychiatry 1997;**54**:857–64; review by Hall, EBMH 1998;**1**:86). A trial of dexamfetamine in adults with ADHD showed a significant effect in the short-term, with more data needed to justify long-term therapy (n = 68, RCT, Paterson et al, Aust N Z J Psychiatry 1999;**33**:494–502). Exacerbation of chronic tic disorder by methylphenidate or dexamfetamine has not been shown (n = 19, d/b, p/c, 1 yr; Nolan et al, *Pediatrics* 1999;**103**:730–7).

Methylphenidate *

At appropriate doses of methylphenidate (10–80 mg/d), a large proportion of children with ADHD obtain remission of symptoms. Methylphenidate's mode of action may be blockade of central dopamine transporters (Volkow et al, *Am J Psychiatry* 1998;**155**:1325–31), and may enhance the motivation to complete a task by increasing dopamine (n = 16, Volkow et al, *Am J Psychiatry* 2004;**161**:1173–80). Predictors of a positive response include demonstrable inattention, normal or near normal IQ, low anxiety (Buitelaar et al, *J Am Acad Child Adolesc Psychiatry* 1995;**34**:1025–32), high levels of hyperactivity at school and relatively low age (n = 36, RCT, Zeiner et al, *Acta Pediatr* 1999;**88**:298–303). However, a recent meta-analysis concluded that while methylphenidate is clearly superior to placebo, the effect size is smaller than expected (s = 16, Koesters et al, *J Psychopharmacol* 2009;**23**:733–44). The new SR preparations (eg. Concerta® XL, Janssen-Cilag, Equasym®, UCB Pharma, Medikinet®, Flynn) have made dosing much easier. The response to methylphenidate in ADHD does not appear to be moderated by comorbid anxiety (n = 91, RCT, 4/12, Diamond et al, *J Am Acad Child Adolesc Psychiatry* 1999;**38**:402–9; reviewed in *EBMH* 1999;**2**:108).

Methylphenidate formulations: plasma profiles

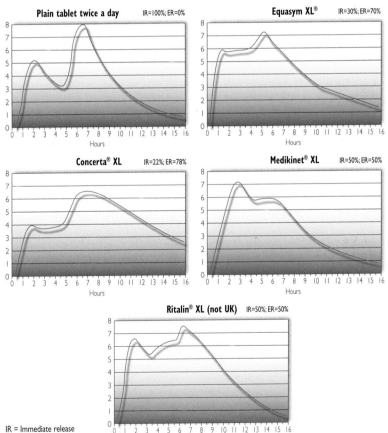

IR = Immediate release
ER = Extended release

Reviews: pharmacokinetics and efficacy (Kimko et al, *Clin Pharmacokinet* 1999;**37**:457–70, 75 refs), side-effects (review, Rappaport and Moffitt, *Clin Psychol Rev* 2002;**22**:1107–31).

+ Combinations

Review: general (Adler et al, *Curr Psychiatry Rep* 2006;**8**:409–15).

Antipsychotics (e.g. risperidone) + stimulants
See unlicensed/some efficacy.

Atomoxetine + methylphenidate
Adding methylphenidate to atomoxetine non-responders in previous stimulant non-responders seems a pointless exercise (n = 25, RCT, p/c, d/b, Carlson et al, *Child Adolesc Psychiatry Mental Health* 2007;**1**:10), although there is a case of successful use in a 10-year-old boy (n = 1, *J Child Adolesc Psychopharmacol* 2006;**16**:365–70).

• Unlicensed/some efficacy

Antipsychotics *
The 2008 NICE guidelines do not recommend use of antipsychotics in ADHD, as although they have been used for uncontrollable and explosive behaviour, their side-effect profile makes them unsatisfactory. This potential for long-term side-effects and worsening cognitive learning function usually outweighs their potential advantages. However, **risperidone** may be at least as effective as methylphenidate for ADHD in children and adolescents with moderate learning disabilities (n = 45, s/b, 4/52, Filho et al, *J Am Acad Child Adolesc Psychiatry* 2005;**44**:748–55) and risperidone (mean 1 mg/d) was very useful for treating aggression in ADHD (n = 25, RCT, p/c, 4/52, Armenteros et al, *J Am Acad Child Adolesc Psychiatry* 2007;**46**:558–65). In methylphenidate-resistant ADHD, addition of **quetiapine** produced significant improvement in 47% and was well tolerated (n = 30, open, 3 + 9/52, Kronenberger et al, *J Child Adolesc Psychopharmacol* 2007;**17**:334–47). **Aripiprazole** (mean 6.7 mg/d) reduced ADHD symptoms and improved overall functioning (n = 23, open, 6/52, Findling et al, *J Child Adolesc Psychopharmacol* 2008;**18**:347–54).

Bupropion

There is a growing body of evidence supporting the use of bupropion in ADHD. Bupropion XL up to 450 mg/d was effective (53% vs 31% for placebo) for ADHD, providing well tolerated and sustained benefit throughout the day (n = 162, RCT, d/b, p/c, 8/52, Wilens et al, *Biol Psychiatry* 2005;**57**:793–801). Bupropion (mean 3.3 mg/kg/d) and methylphenidate (mean 0.7 mg/kg/d) were equipotent in children with ADHD in one trial (n = 15, RCT, 6/52, Barrickman et al, *J Am Acad Child Adolesc Psychiatry* 1995;**34**:649–57) and provides another pharmacological alternative to stimulants in ADHD.

Clonidine *

Clonidine (an alpha-2 agonist) has been widely used for treatment-resistant ADHD. A recent study has shown 0.1–0.3 mg/d to be effective (but less so than methylphenidate) in ADHD (n = 122, RCT, d/b, p/c, 16/52, Palumbo et al, *J Am Acad Child Adolesc Psychiatry* 2008;**47**:180–8; see also s = 11, n = 150, Connor et al, *J Am Acad Child Adolesc Psychiatry* 1999;**38**:1551–9; reviewed by Greenhill, *EBMH* 2000;**3**:74). It may be useful as a well-tolerated (Daviss et al, *J Am Acad Child Adolesc Psychiatry* 2008;**47**:189–98) and cheaper alternative to methylphenidate (n = 50, RCT, d/b, Nair and Mahadevan, *J Trop Pediatr* 2009;**55**:116–21). Clonidine augmentation of psychostimulants can be used to improve conduct, but not hyperactivity, and may reduce stimulant adverse effects (n = 67, RCT, p/c, 6/52, Hazell and Stuart, *J Am Acad Child Adolesc Psychiatry* 2003;**42**:886–94).

Modafinil *

Modafinil appears to be promising in ADHD, e.g. once-daily modafinil (170–425 mg/d) was well tolerated and effective in children and adolescents on all rating systems (n = 246, RCT, d/b, p/c, 9/52, Biederman et al, *Pediatrics* 2005;**116**:777–84; positive comment by Barr and Clarke, *EBMH* 2006;**9**:68) and 200–300 mg/d was superior to placebo for ADHD (n = 46, RCT, d/b, p/c, 6/52, Kahbazi et al, *Psychiatry Res* 2009;**168**:237–7). The most recent review concludes that modafinil improves ADHD symptoms and behaviours compared to placebo (s = 3, n = 638, d/b, p/c, <9/52, Biederman and Pliszka, *J Pediatr* 2008;**152**:394–9), with no withdrawal symptoms on abrupt withdrawal (n = 190, RCT, d/b, p/c, 9/52, Swanson et al, *J Clin Psychiatry* 2006;**67**:137–47). Once-daily dosing is better tolerated than divided doses (n = 248 [c = 223], RCT, d/b, p/c, 4/52, Biederman et al, *J Clin Psychiatry* 2006;**67**:727–35).

Reboxetine *
Reboxetine is a NARI, like atomoxetine, and so logically it should be useful in ADHD. Reboxetine 4–6 mg/d was as effective as methylphenidate 20–50 mg/d (n = 33, d/b, 6/52, Arabgol et al, *Eur Child Adolesc Psychiatry* 2008; **18**:53–9) and 2–8 mg/d almost as effective as methylphenidate 10–20 mg/d (n = 27, open, 8/52, Cohen-Yavin et al, *Clin Neuropharmacol* 2009;**32**:179–82). Another pilot trial showed some efficacy in ADHD, seen within two weeks (n = 20, open, 6/52, Tehrani-Doost et al, *J Child Adolesc Psychopharmacol* 2008;**18**:179–84) and it may have some efficacy in stimulant-resistant ADHD (n = 31, RCT, open, 6/52, Ratner et al, *J Am Acad Child Adolesc Psychiatry* 2005;**44**:428–33).

Selegiline
In an active comparison, selegiline and methylphenidate were equally effective for child and adolescent ADHD (n = 40, RCT, 60/7, Mohammadi et al, *J Child Adolesc Psychopharmacol* 2004;**14**:418–25).

Tricyclics
Tricyclics are considered useful in patients non-responsive or intolerant of stimulants. Imipramine, clomipramine, nortriptyline and desipramine have been used in doses of 10–150 mg/d (mean 80 mg). In a retrospective, naturalistic study, tricyclics were shown to be effective at antidepressant doses (n = 37, Wilens et al, *J Nerv Ment Dis* 1995;**183**:48–9), although other authors have suggested that lower doses (e.g. 25–50 mg/d) are effective but sudden death, including cardiac arrest, has been reported with relatively low plasma levels (Riddle et al, *J Am Acad Child Adolesc Psychiatry* 1991;**30**:104–8) and so close monitoring is warranted.

■ Unlicensed/possible efficacy

Buspirone
A pilot study suggested buspirone may help hyperactive behaviour in ADHD (n = 8, Niederhofer, *Hum Psychopharmacol* 2003;**18**: 489–92).

Duloxetine *
Duloxetine has been used (n = 1, Niederhofer, *Eur Psychiatry* 2010;[in press]).

Gabapentin
A number of case reports exist, e.g. aggression, temper and violence responded almost completely ('a miracle') to gabapentin 900 mg/d in resistant ADHD (n = 1, Ryback and Ryback, *Am J Psychiatry* 1995;**152**:1399), and rapid and marked improvement with 200 mg/d as an adjunct to methylphenidate (n = 1, Hamrin and Bailey, *J Child Adolesc Psychopharmacol* 2001;**11**:301–9).

Ginkgo biloba *
GB has been shown to be less effective than methylphenidate in ADHD, but we do not know if it is better than placebo (n = 50, RCT, d/b, 6/52, Salehi et al, *Prog Neuropsychopharmacol Biol Psychiatry* 2010;34:76-80; see also n = 6, Niederhofer, *Phytother Res* 2010;**24**:26–7).

MAOIs
MAOIs are not considered as effective as stimulants but may help some non-responders, e.g. tranylcypromine has been considered as effective as stimulants but the dietary restrictions proved too difficult to manage.

Melatonin
Although melatonin advances circadian rhythms and enhances sleep time, there was no effect on behaviour, cognition or QoL (n = 105, RCT, d/b, p/c, 4/52, Van der Heijden et al, *J Am Acad Child Adolesc Psychiatry* 2007;**46**:233–41).

Memantine
A pilot study suggested a dose-dependent improvement in ADHD-IV and CGI-S with memantine 10–20 mg/d (n = 16, open, 8/52, Findling et al, *J Acad Adolesc Psychopharmacol* 2007;**17**:19–33).

Nicotine

Daily transdermal nicotine reduced hyper-activity and learning problems in a pilot study, but was poorly tolerated and so other methods of nicotinic receptor modulation may be worth investigating (n = 10, RCT, d/b, p/c, 2/52, Shytle et al, World J Biol Psychiatry 2002;**3**:150–5).

SSRIs

Serotonin function may be abnormal in ADHD (Fargason and Ford, South Med J 1994;**87**:302–9) and fluoxetine 20–60 mg/d may produce some statistical improvements in some rating scales (n = 22, open, Barrickman et al, J Am Acad Child Adolesc Psychiatry 1991;**30**:762–7).

Venlafaxine

There are case reports of use (e.g. Pleak and Gormly, Wilens et al, Am J Psychiatry 1995;**152**:1099–100).

Zinc

There is some evidence for zinc's efficacy (review by Arnold and DiSilvestro, J Child Adolesc Psychopharmacol 2005;**15**:619–27).

◆ Others

Other drugs tried include **thyroid** (n = 1, N Engl J Med 1993;**328**:997–1001).

☐ No efficacy

Barbiturates

These have been tried but excitation and agitation may be counter-productive.

Benzodiazepines

As for barbiturates.

Caffeine

Caffeine is ineffective as a minor stimulant (Dulcan, Pediatr Ann 1985;**14**:383–400) as tolerance develops too rapidly.

Donepezil

Adjunctive donepezil seems poorly tolerated and ineffectual for residual ADHD and cognitive symptoms (n = 13 [c = 7], open, 12/52, Wilens et al, J Child Adolesc Psychopharmacol 2005;**15**:947–55).

Homeopathy

There is no evidence for any efficacy for homeopathy in ADHD (s = 4, n = 168, Coulter and Dean, Cochrane Database Syst Rev 2007; **4**:CD005648).

Omega-3 fatty acids *

Recent trials of omega-3/6 only show limited response in a small sub-group of inattentive ADHD adolescents (n = 75, RCT, p/c, c/o, 6/12, Johnson et al, J Atten Disord 2009;**12**:394–401; n = 37 [c = 26], RCT, d/b, p/c, c/o, 16/52, Bélanger et al, Paediatr Child Health 2009;**14**:89–98) and a systematic review concluded that EFA supplements do not have an evidence base for routine use (Raz and Gabis, Dev Med Child Neurol 2009;**51**:580–92).

Selegiline

Selegiline may be mildly useful for the inattentive ADHD sub-type, but has little effect on impulsivity (n = 11, RCT, d/b, p/c, c/o, Rubenstein et al, J Child Adolesc Psychopharmacol 2006;**16**:404–15).

St John's wort *

SJW was ineffective in improving symptoms of ADHD (n = 54, RCT, d/b, p/c, 8/52, Weber et al, JAMA 2008;**299**:2633–41).

1.7.2 ADHD IN ADULTS see also ADHD in children and adolescents (1.7.1)

Incidence and importance *

Adult ADHD is widely under-recognised. Up to 65% adolescents with ADHD will have enduring symptoms, with around 3–4% adults affected, remarkably similar in different countries (n = 11422, Fayyad et al, Br J Psychiatry 2007;**190**:402–9; comment by Thome, EBMH 2008;**11**:31: n = 966, Faraone and Biederman, J Atten Disord 2005;**9**:384–91). Comorbidity is common (review by Barkley and Brown, CNS Spectr 2008;**13**:977–84), e.g. anxiety (n = 349, Karam et al, J Psychiatr Res 2009;**43**:697–701), BPD, SUD (Bukstein, Medscape J Med 2008;**10**:24), depression (McIntosh et al, Neuropsychiatr Dis Treat 2009;**5**:137–50), bipolar disorder (n = 159, Tamam et al, Eur Arch Psychiatry Clin Neurosci 2008;**258**:385–93), conduct disorders (Dowson, Acta Psychiatr Scand 2008;**117**:299–305, eating disorders (Nazar et al, Rev Bras Psiquiatr 2008;**30**:384–9) may overshadow ADHD. Indeed, around 20% adults with SUD have ADHD (11–35%, Kalbag and Levin, Subst Use Misuse 2005;**40**:1955–81;2043–8; review Wilens, J Clin Psychiatry 2007;**68**[Suppl 11]:4–8). Adults with ADHD may have lower educational achievement levels, but not because of low IQ (n=117, Antshel et al, Psychol Med 2009;**39**:1325–35). There is an 85% genetic link (adult ADHD having a greater inheritability), with some association with the D4 gene (Faraone, Psychiatr Clin North Am 2004;**27**:303–21).

Symptoms *

Adult ADHD (Hesslinger et al, Psychiatry Res 2003;**119**:217–23) may present as:

- Continuation of symptoms from adolescence
- Re-presentation after a treatment gap by young adults now realising they cannot cope
- First diagnosis, never diagnosed as children but with a history of symptoms
- Late-onset (as opposed to late diagnosis), which is controversial and relatively rare.

Adults with ADHD have problems with work, family and social activities. Driving is a particular problem, as they get fatigued quickly and are more likely to have accidents on motorways or open roads when attention lapses (Reimer et al, Traffic Inj Prev 2007;**8**:290–9), and have more tickets and offences, often as result of impulsivity (n=355, Thompson et al, J Pediatr Psychol 2007;**32**:745–59). Compared to ADHD in adolescents, hyperactivity diminishes, impulsivity is less but inattention persists. They are likely to have a lifetime history of sleep problems (n=2284, Gau et al, Sleep 2007;**30**:195–201).

Role of drugs *

Prescribing of ADHD treatments drops significantly from age 15–21, but at a greater rate than age-reported lessening of symptoms, suggesting prematurely stopped in some people who need treatment (McCarthy et al, Br J Psychiatry 2009;**194**:273–7). Stimulants are as effective in adults as in younger people, albeit currently unlicensed. Pharmacotherapy for ADHD is not compromised by psychiatric co-morbidity (Babock and Ornstein, Postgrad Med 2009;**121**:73–82). A systematic review and meta-analysis has concluded that the main evidence in adults is for immediate release methylphenidate, rather than the SR preparations (s=22, n=2203, Peterson et al, Psychopharmacology (Berl) 2008; **197**:1–11). Compliance is often good, and self-reported compliance correlates well with actual compliance (Safren et al, J Atten Disord 2007;**10**:257–60). Many will self-medicate, e.g. with amphetamines if sub-optimally treated. Although diversion is possible (reportedly 16–29%), it is less likely with SR preps (s=21, n=113,104, Wilens et al, J Am Acad Child Adolesc Psychiatry 2008;**47**:21–31). CBT in addition to medications can improve response (Rostain, Postgrad Med 2008;**120**:27–38).

Reviews: * general (Simon et al, Br J Psychiatry 2009;**194**:204–11; Feifel and MacDonald, Postgrad Med 2008;**120**:39–47; Tcheremissine and Salazar, Expert Opin Pharmacother 2008;**9**:1299–310. Rostain, Postgrad Med 2008; **120**:27–38; Thomsen and Damm, Igeskr Laeger 2008;**170**:3395–9; Asherson et al, Br J Psychiatry 2007;**190**:4–5, Cumyn et al, Expert Rev Neurother 2007;**7**:1375–90; Ohlmeier, Psychiatr Prax 2007; **34**[Suppl 3]:296–9), pharmacotherapy (Adler, J Clin Psychiatry 2009;**70**:e12; Mészáros et al, Int J Neuropsychopharmacol 2009;**12**:1137–47; Kolar et al, Neuropsychiatr Dis Treat 2008;**4**:107–21; systematic review, Mészáros et al, Psychiatr Hung 2007;**22**:259–70; non-stimulants, Newcorn, CNS Spectr 2008;**13**(9 Suppl 13):12–6; stimulants, Stein, CNS Spectr 2008;**13**(9 Suppl 13):8–11), antidepressants in adult ADHD (s=8, Verbeeck et al, Adv Ther 2009;**26**:170–84), managing adult ADHD and SUD (Upadhyaya, J Clin Psychiatry 2007;**68**[Suppl 11]:23–30), clinical guidelines (Gibbins and Weiss, Curr Psychiatry Rep 2007;**9**:420–6), BAP guidelines for adolescents in transition to adult services and in adults (Nutt et al, J Psychopharmacol 2007;**21**:10–41), neurobiological and genetics (Spencer, CNS Spectr 2008;**13**(9 Suppl 13):5–7; Cumyn et al, Expert Rev Neurother 2007;**7**:1375–90).

Unlicensed (but BNF listed for adolescents)

Atomoxetine *

Atomoxetine is not yet licensed for adult ADHD in UK (but is in e.g. USA) but has advantages in that the risk of diversion is minimal and it is not a controlled drug. A two-trial analysis showed discontinuations at under

10% in adult ADHD (s=2, n=536, RCT, d/b, p/c, 10/52, Michelson et al, Biol Psychiatry 2003;**53**:112–20). Atomoxetine 1.2 mg/kg/d has been shown to improve simulated driving performance (n=18, p/c, c/o, 3/52, Barkley et al, J Atten Disord 2007;**10**:306–16) and can help with comorbid social anxiety (n=442, RCT, d/b, p/c, 16/52, Adler et al, Depress Anxiety 2009;**26**:212–21). Analysis of four studies shows no discontinuation symptoms or rebound, and tapering is not required when stopped (s=4, 9–10/52, Wernicke et al, J Clin Psychopharmacol 2004;**24**:30–5, MS). Atomoxetine can be given once daily in adults, with an effect lasting into the evening, and for at least 6/12 (n=501, RCT, d/b, p/c, 6/12, Adler et al, J Clin Psychopharmacol 2009;**29**:44–50; see also s=2, n=421, open, 24/52, Wehmeier et al, Child Adolesc Psychiatry Ment Health 2009;**3**:5).

Reviews: * general (Vaughan et al, Expert Opin Pharmacother 2009;**10**:669–76; Durell et al, J Atten Disord 2010;**13**:401–6; SM).

Dexamfetamine

Dexamfetamine has been shown to be superior to placebo in adult ADHD (n=68 [c=67], RCT, d/b, p/c. Paterson et al, Aust N Z J Psychiatry 1999;**33**:494–502).

Methylphenidate *

Methylphenidate is not yet licensed for adult ADHD in the UK but has recently been approved in USA. A meta-analysis concluded that methylphenidate was well-tolerated and effective in adults, although it was associated with a modest rise in blood pressure and heart rate (s=26, n=811, Godfrey, J Psychopharmacol 2009;**23**:194–205). There remains some controversy about dosing. Large studies have suggested that 'robust' dosing (mean 1 mg/kg/d) may be highly effective (response 76% vs 19% placebo) compared to more traditional dosing (n=146, RCT, d/b, p/c, 6/52, Spencer et al, Biol Psychiatry 2005;**57**:456–63; n=45, RCT, d/b, p/c, c/o, Kooij et al, Psychol Med 2004;**34**:973–82). It seems that low dose methylphenidate has little efficacy for ADHD in substance misusers (n=25 [c=19], RCT, d/b, c/o, 8/52, Carpentier et al, Addiction 2005;**100**:1868–74), but other

studies show low to moderate doses (up to 60 mg/d) can have a sustained effect (n=359, RCT, d/b, p/c, 24/52, Rösler et al, Eur Arch Psychiatry Clin Neurosci 2009;**259**:120–9) and 18, 36 and 72 mg/d can be equally effective for adult ADHD, although 72 mg is slightly better (n=401, RCT, d/b, p/c, 5/52, Medori et al, Biol Psychiatry 2008;**63**:981–9, MS). There is a lower risk for diversion with SR preparations (n=50 [c=39], RCT, d/b, p/c, c/o, 2×5/52, Jain et al, J Clin Psychiatry 2007;**68**:268–77). Methylphenidate improves simulated driving performance in adult ADHD (n=53, RCT, d/b, p/c, c/o, Barkley et al, J Safety Res 2005;**36**:121–31; n=19 [c=18], RCT, d/b, p/c, c/o, 11/7, Verster et al, J Psychopharmacol 2008;**22**:230–7).

Review: * general (Nair and Moss, Neuropsychiatr Dis Treat 2009;**5**:421–32).

● Unlicensed/some efficacy

Bupropion

Bupropion has been investigated and it seems effective in adult ADHD, with a more rapid response than the significant placebo effect (n=162, RCT, p/c, d/b, 8/52, Wilens et al, Biol Psychiatry 2005;**57**:793–801). Bupropion was equivalent to methylphenidate and superior (but not statistically) to placebo in adult ADHD (n=30, RCT, d/b, p/c, 7/52, Kuperman et al, Ann Clin Psychiatry 2001;**13**:129–34) and up to 400 mg/d has been shown to be significantly superior to placebo (76% vs 37% improved) and, although the exclusion criteria were unclear, further trials are warranted (n=40 [c=38], RCT, d/b, 6/52, Wilens et al, Am J Psychiatry 2001;**158**:282–8; reviewed by Ferre and Nutt, EBMH 2001;**4**:92). Bupropion up to 400 mg/d may be effective in ADHD with comorbid SUD (n=14 [c=13], open, 6/12, Solhkhah et al, J Child Adolesc Psychopharmacol 2005;**15**:777–86). Usefully, in comorbid ADHD and bipolar, bupropion may be effective for ADHD without precipitating mania (n=36 [c=30], open, 6/52, Wilens et al, Biol Psychiatry 2003;**54**:9–16).

Clonidine

A license application for a CR product for adult ADHD has been submitted in USA.

Duloxetine *

There is a single case of efficacy in a 53-year-old male (n = 1, Tourjman and Bilodeau, *J Atten Disord* 2009;**13**:95–6).

Fish oils

High dose fish oil was better than flax oil or olive oil for correcting low serum phospholipid fatty acid levels in adults with ADHD (n = 30, RCT, 12/52, Young *et al*, *Reprod Nutr Dev* 2005; **45**:549–58).

Guanfacine *

This alpha-2 noradrenergic agonist (similar to clonidine) may have some potential (n = 17, d/b, p/c, c/o, Taylor and Russo, *J Clin Psychopharmacol* 2001;**21**:223–8).

Lithium

Lithium (up to 1200 mg/d) was equivalent to methylphenidate (up to 40 mg/d) on most outcome measures in one study (RCT, d/b, c/o, 2 × 8/52, Dorrego *et al*, *J Neuropsychiatry Clin Neurosci* 2002;**14**:289–95).

Milnacipran

There is a case of adult ADHD responding remarkably to milnacipran (n = 1, Kako *et al*, *Prog Neuropsychopharmacol Biol Psychiatry* 2007;**31**:772–5).

Moclobemide

There is a case of residual ADHD and co-morbid opiate dependence responding to moclobemide (n = 1, Vaiva *et al*, *Prog Neuro-psychopharmacol Biol Psychiatry* 2002;**26**:609–11).

Modafinil

Modafinil was comparable to dexamfetamine and superior to placebo in adult ADHD (n = 22 [c = 21], RCT, p/c, c/o, 3 × 3/52, Taylor and Russo, *J Child Adolesc Psychopharmacol* 2000;**10**:311–20).

Nicotine

This indirect dopamine agonist (smoked or transdermally) improves concentration in adult ADHD (s = 2, n = 17, d/b, c/o, Conners and Levin, *Psychopharmacol Bull* 1996;**32**:55–73).

Oxcarbazepine

A small study showed 300–1500 mg/d is effective in some people with adult ADHD (n = 9 [c = 8], open, 8/52, Davids *et al*, *Prog Neuropsychopharmacol Biol Psychiatry* 2006;**30**: 1033–8).

Tianeptine

Tianeptine might be 'a slightly effective beneficial and useful treatment for adult ADHD' according to the Medline abstract (n = 68, open, Niederhofer, *Neuropsychobiology* 2004;**49**:130–3).

Varenicline *

There is a case of a significant positive effect from varenicline 2 mg/d in an adult (n = 1, 6/52, Cocores and Gold, *J Neuropsychiatry Clin Neurosci* 2008;**20**:494–5).

Venlafaxine

Although 70% completers responded to venlafaxine 50–150 mg/d, it was poorly tolerated (n = 18 [c = 11], Hedges *et al*, *Psychopharmacol Bull* 1995;**31**:779–83). There has been one positive trial of 75 mg/d (n = 10 [= 9], open, 8/52, Findling *et al*, *J Clin Psychiatry* 1996;**57**:184–9).

☐ No efficacy

Anticholinesterases

A small open study of adjunctive **donepezil** showed it to be poorly tolerated and ineffective in adults (n = 6, open, 12/52, Wilens *et al*, *J Child Adolesc Psychopharmacol* 2005;**15**:947–55) and **galantamine** had no detectable effects (n = 36, RCT, d/b, p/c, 12/52, Biederman *et al*, *J Clin Psychopharmacol* 2006;**26**:163–6).

Homeopathy

There is no significant treatment effect on ADHD or related symptoms (s = 4, n = 168, Coulter and Dean, *Cochrane Database Syst Rev* 2007;**17**:CD005648).

Selegiline

Selegiline up to 60 mg/d was no more effective than placebo in adults and had significant ADRs (n = 24, RCT, d/b, p/c, 10/52, Ernst *et al*, *Psychopharmacol Bull* 1996;**32**:327–34) although it may have some efficacy in adolescents.

1.8 AUTISTIC DISORDER

Symptoms

Autism is a neurodevelopmental disorder, characterised by an excessive or morbid dislike of others or society, not responding with normal human emotions towards other people, a morbid self-centred attitude and with major impairments or abnormalities in language, communication, reciprocity, social interactions, imagination and behaviour. The main features include 'autistic aloneness', poor speech and language development, an obsessive desire for sameness, bizarre behaviour or mannerisms, a restricted repertoire of activities and interests, rituals and compulsive behaviour. Onset is not later than three years of age, the incidence four in 10 000, or up to 20 in 10 000 if including associated conditions (Gillberg and Wing, *Acta Psychiatr Scand* 1999;**99**:399–406). Up to 25% develop seizures in adolescence, 75% have an IQ in the retarded range, and up to 60% need long-term residential care. There is some evidence that dietary gluten could be implicated in autism, and that a gluten-free diet may ameliorate symptoms, particularly if implemented at a very early stage (review by Shattock and Whiteley, *Pharm J* 2001; **267**:17–9) although Cochrane concludes there is insufficient data (Millward *et al, Cochrane Database Syst Rev* 2008;**2**:CD003498).

Role of drugs

Drugs may be of limited use in treating some of the more severe behavioural symptoms. Self-injurious behaviour (SIB) is common (see *1.25*) and may be helped by low dose antipsychotics, to which autistic individuals seem very sensitive and so lower doses may be needed. Only risperidone and methylphenidate have more than one trial to show efficacy for aggressive symptoms in autism (s = 21, Parikh *et al, J Child Adolesc Psychopharmacol* 2008;**18**:157–78). A therapeutic window may exist, and higher doses may be counter-productive. Family support, education, skills training, behavioural therapy and social support can be significant aspects of the overall management.

Reviews: * general (Levy *et al, Lancet* 2009; **374**:1627–38; Moss and Howlin, *J Intellect Disabil Res* 2009;**53**:852–73), new treatments (Rossignol, *Ann Clin Psychiatry* 2009;**21**:213–36), drug therapy (s = 21, Parikh *et al, J Child Adolesc Psychopharmacol* 2008;**18**:157–78; Palermo and Curatolo, *J Child Neurol* 2004;**19**:155–64), genetics (Grigorenko, *Future Neurol* 2009;**4**:591–99; Kumar and Christian, *Curr Neurol Neurosci Rep* 2009;**9**:188–97), ADHD in autism (Hazell, *J Paediatr Child Health* 2007;**43**:19–24).

● Unlicensed/some efficacy

Antipsychotics *

Low-dose antipsychotics have a role to play. As adverse reactions can be significant, a 'start low and go slow' routine is recommended. **Risperidone** is now licensed in US for treatment of serious behavioural problems in children with autism and is the standard first-line antipsychotic in autism. Two reviews have concluded that although risperidone does not effect the core symptoms of autism, it has moderate efficacy in helping behavioural aspects, e.g. irritability, aggression, hyperactivity and stereotyping (s = 4, d/b, Canitano and Scandurra, *Neuropsychiatr Dis Treat* 2008;**4**:723–30), e.g. 0.5–3.5 mg/d had significant effects on overall non-specific behavioural symptoms (n = 101, RCT, d/b, p/c, 8/52, McDougle *et al, Am J Psychiatry* 2005;**162**:1142–8; comment by Fombonne, *EBMH* 2006;**9**:6), including in children aged 5–12 years (n = 55, RCT, d/b, p/c, 8/52, Pandina *et al, J Autism Dev Disord* 2007;**37**:367–73). Risperidone may also improve global functioning and social responsiveness while reducing hyperactivity and aggression (n = 40[c = 39], RCT, p/c, d/b, 18/12, Nagaraj *et al, J Child Neurol* 2006;**21**:450–5), and even Cochrane concludes that there is some evidence for the benefits of risperidone on irritability, repetition and social withdrawal in autism spectrum disorders (s = 3, Jesner *et al, Cochrane Database Syst Rev* 2007;**1**:CD005040). Long-term use seems safe and effective, e.g. for up to three years (n = 35, open, one year, Reyes *et al, Eur Child Adolesc Psychiatry* 2006;**15**:97–104) and a long-term discontinuation study suggested a significant relapse prevention efficacy, reducing disruptive behaviour in about half the children taking it (n = 36, d/b, 24/52, Troost *et al, J Am Acad Child Adolesc Psychiatry*

2005;**44**:1137–44), although this may disappear rapidly on discontinuation (n = 32, 6/12, d/b, Autism Network, *Am J Psychiatry* 2005;**162**:1361–9). It is well tolerated (n = 101, RCT, d/b, p/c, 8/52, Aman *et al*, *J Child Adolesc Psychopharmacol* 2005;**15**:844–5), although raised prolactin and weight gain are risks so monitor carefully (n = 20, 24/52, Gagliano *et al*, *J Child Adolesc Psychopharmacol* 2004;**14**:39–47). Although risperidone has the best evidence, other antipsychotics have been used. A review of 19 studies of atypicals concluded that risperidone (n = 133, s = 13) may be effective in reducing hyperactivity, aggression and repetitive behaviour (with low EPS), **olanzapine** (n = 11, s = 3; e.g. see n = 12, RCT, open, 6/52, Malone *et al*, *J Am Acad Child Adolesc Psychiatry* 2001;**40**:887–94) and **clozapine** (open, n = 3, Zuddas *et al*, *Am J Psychiatry* 1996;**153**:738) may also be effective, but there is little evidence that **amisulpride** (RCT, n = 9) or **quetiapine** (open, n = 6) are useful in this population (Barnard *et al*, *J Psychopharmacol* 2002;**16**:93–101). **Haloperidol** has been widely used, with 0.5–3 mg/d used to reduce behavioural symptoms (e.g. aggression and SIB) and improve learning (n = 60, 6/12, Perry *et al*, *J Am Acad Child Adolesc Psychiatry* 1989;**28**:87–92). **Ziprasidone** may have some promise in treating adolescents with autism (n = 12, open, 6/52, Malone *et al*, *J Child Adolesc Psychopharmacol* 2007;**17**:779–90). **Aripiprazole** at doses of 5, 10 and 15 mg/d all significantly improved aberrant behaviour and was well tolerated (n = 218, RCT, d/b, p/c, 8/52, Marcus *et al*, *J Am Acad Child Adolesc Psychiary* 2009;**48**:1110–9).

Reviews: * atypicals (McDougle *et al*, *J Clin Psychiatry* 2008;**69** (Suppl 4):15–20), general (Posey *et al*, *J Clin Invest* 2008;**118**:6–14; Malone and Waheed, *Drugs* 2009;**69**:535–48).

Methylphenidate

Methylphenidate has considerable negative effects on tantrums and moods but this may sometimes be outweighed by the positive effects on hyperactivity, attention and stereotype behaviour (e.g. n = 13, d/b, p/c, c/o, Handen *et al*, *J Autism Dev Disord* 2000;**30**:245–55; n = 72 [c = 66], RCT, RUPPAN, *Arch Gen Psychiatry* 2005;**62**:1266–74).

■ Unlicensed/possible efficacy

Antidepressants *

Serotonin reuptake inhibitors may have a role to play, particularly in adults with strong behavioural rigidity. Children and adolescents may be more sensitive to SSRIs and so, once again, 'start low and go slow' is the advice. A review of **SSRIs** in autism concludes that there are significant improvements in global functioning, anxiety and repetitive behaviour and they are well tolerated, but methodological weaknesses mean the findings are not robust (s = 3, RCT; s = 10, open; Kolevzon *et al*, *J Clin Psychiatry* 2006;**67**:407–14; review by Moore *et al*, *Ann Pharmacother* 2004;**38**:1515–9). **Fluoxetine** liquid (mean 10 mg/d) was superior to placebo for repetitive behaviours in autism (n = 45, RCT, d/b, p/c, c/o, 2 × 8/52, Hollander *et al*, *Neuropsychopharmacology* 2005;**30**:582–9). **Clomipramine** may be superior to placebo for autistic symptoms, anger and ritualism (n = 12, d/b, c/o, 10/52, *Arch Gen Psychiatry* 1993;**50**:441–7) and as an alternative to haloperidol for some symptoms (RCT, n = 36, p/c, 7/52, Remington *et al*, *J Clin Psychopharmacol* 2001;**1**:440–4). Low dose **venlafaxine** (18.75 mg/d) may help reduce SIB and ADHD-like symptoms in autism (n = 3, Carminati *et al*, *Prog Neuropsychopharmacol Biol Psychiatry* 2006; **30**:312–5). However, **citalopram** had no effect on repetitive behaviour in autistic spectrum disorders (n = 149, RCT, p/c, 12/52, King *et al*, *Arch Gen Psychiatry* 2009;**66**:583–90). **Mirtazapine** 15–30 mg/d had some efficacy (50% were very much improved) in reducing inappropriate sexual behaviours in autism (n = 10, open, 8/52, Coskun *et al*, *J Child Adolesc Psychopharmacol* 2009;**19**:203–6), but is only modestly effective in treating other autism-related symptoms (n = 26, open, Posey *et al*, *J Child Adolesc Psychopharmacol* 2001;**11**:267–77).

Atomoxetine

Atomoxetine has been used successfully for hyperactivity in autism spectrum disorders, so more trials are warranted (n = 16, RCT, p/c, c/o, 13/52, Arnold *et al*, *J Am Acad Child Adolesc Psychiatry* 2006;**45**:1196–205).

Buspirone

Buspirone 90 mg/d was successful for reducing aggressive behaviour in an autistic woman with profound learning disabilities (n = 1, Brahm et al, Ann Pharmacother 2008;**42**:131–7).

Cicloserin (D-cycloserine)

Cicloserin was well tolerated and improved CGI and ABC measures of social withdrawal (n = 12, 6/52, Posey et al, Am J Psychiatry 2004; **161**:2115–7).

Cyproheptadine

Cyproheptadine plus haloperidol was superior to haloperidol alone for ABC-C (aberrant behaviour) listed symptoms (RCT, d/b, p/c, 8/52, Akhondzadeh et al, J Clin Pharm Ther 2004;**29**:145–50).

Melatonin *

Melatonin 3–9 mg/d may be dramatically effective for severe circadian disturbances in adults with autism (n = 6, 6/52, Galli-Carminati et al, Swiss Med Wkly 2009;**139**:293–6), although long-term treatment may be needed as the effect may disappear on discontinuation (n = 25, open, 7/12, Giannotti et al, J Autism Dev Disord 2006;**36**:741–52).

Memantine

Memantine significantly improved language and social behaviour and appeared to have no serious side-effects (n = 151, open, 21/12, Chez et al, J Child Neurol 2007;**22**:574–9), and 10 mg/d has been used successfully for disruptive behaviour (n = 1, Erickson and Chambers, J Clin Psychiatry 2006;**67**:1000).

Naltrexone *

A recent review concluded that naltrexone was worth a try, especially if SIB occurs and other interventions have failed (s = 14, other reports =11, Elchaar et al, Ann Pharmacother 2006;**40**:1086–95). Naltrexone 1 mg/kg/d may reduce withdrawal, hyperactivity and SIB, with sedation being the only major side-effect (n = 10, Campbell et al, J Am Acad Child Adolesc Psychiatry 1989;**28**:200–6).

Pentoxifylline *

Pentoxifylline 600 mg/d added to risperidone may have some synergistic effects in treating behavioural problems in autism (n = 40, RCT, d/b, p/c, 10/52, Akhondzadeh et al, Prog Neuropsychopharmacol Biol Psychiatry 2010; **34**:32–6).

Propranolol *

Propranolol might help improve problem-solving in autistic spectrum disorders (see Beversdorf et al, Neurocase 2008;**14**:378–83).

Valproate

Two open trials have suggested some improvement in behavioural symptoms associated with autism, e.g. 91% who completed one trial showed sustained improvement in autistic spectrum symptoms, e.g. aggression and impulsivity, particularly if an EEG abnormality or seizure history was present (n = 14, open pilot, Hollander et al, J Clin Psychiatry 2001; **62**:530–4).

◆ Others

Other drugs tried include **buspirone** (e.g. n = 14, open, Ratey et al, J Clin Psychiatry 1989;**50**:382–4; n = 4, Realmuto et al, J Clin Psychopharmacol 1989;**9**:122–5), **carbamazepine** (eg. Gillberg, J Autism Dev Disord 1991;**21**:61–77), **clonidine** (n = 9, d/b, p/c, Fankhauser et al, J Clin Psychiatry 1992;**53**:77–82), **lithium** (e.g. n = 2, Kerbeshian et al, J Clin Psychopharmacol 1987;**7**:401–5) and high dose **pyridoxine**.

☐ No efficacy

Lamotrigine

Lamotrigine was ineffective on all measures in one study (n = 28, RCT, p/c, 18/52, Belsito et al, J Autism Dev Disord 2001;**31**:175–81).

Levetiracetam

Although levetiracetam may improve some symptoms (n = 10, open, Rugino and Samsock, J Dev Behav Pediatr 2002;**23**:225–30), the major study was unable to show an advantage for levetiracetam (mean 860 mg/d) over placebo (n = 20, p/c, d/b, 10/52, Wasserman et al, Int Clin Psychopharmacol 2006;**21**:363–7).

Omega-3 fatty acids *

A systematic review of small studies was unable to show evidence for efficacy in autistic spectrum disorder (s = 6, n = 94, Bent et al, J Autism Dev Disord 2009;**39**:1145–54) although individual cases exist, e.g. rapid response of anxiety and agitation (n = 1, Johnson and Hollander, J Clin Psychiatry 2003; **64**:848–9).

Secretin

Despite much interest, a complete lack of significant effect has been shown (Roberts et al, Pediatrics 2001;**107**:E71; reviewed by Levy, EBMH 2002;**5**:22; n = 56, RCT, p/c, 4/52, Owley et al, J Am Acad Child Adolesc Psychiatry 2001;**40**:1293–99) and thus remains an unproven therapy (review by Patel et al, Pharmacotherapy 2002:**22**:905–14).

St. John's wort *

SJW was essentially ineffective for measures of autistic behaviour in a small case series (n = 3, Niederhofer, Phytother Res 2009;**23**:1521–3).

1.9 BENZODIAZEPINE DEPENDENCE and WITHDRAWAL *

Although short-term benzodiazepine use at standard doses is usually without significant risk of toxicity and dependence, higher dose and longer-term use has potentially significant risks. The SDS (Severity of Dependence Scale) can be used to accurately detect the potential for BDZ dependence (de la Cuevas et al, Addiction 2000;**95**:245–50; reviewed by Law, EBMH 2000;**3**:119). In reviews of BDZ withdrawal strategies, minimal intervention (leaflet or group meeting) and clinician-led systematic discontinuation are both more effective than TAU (s = 29, Voshaar et al, Br J Psychiatry 2006;**189**:213–20; Parr et al, Addiction 2009;**104**:13–24), but psychotherapy during BDZ tapering may actually be detrimental to long-term outcomes (n = 180 [c = 170], RCT, 15/12, Oude Voshaar et al, Br J Psychiatry 2006;**188**:188–9). Predictors of poor long-term abstinence from BDZs includes more severe BDZ-dependence and continued alcohol intake, and this is independent of doses, personality and psychopathology (n = 180 [c = 174], Voshaar et al, Can J Psychiatry 2006;**51**:445–52). Craving is

also an independent risk factor for relapse after successful BDZ-discontinuation (n = 124, Mol et al, J Clin Psychiatry 2007;**68**:1894–900).

Reviews: * withdrawing BDZs in primary care (Lader et al, CNS Drugs 2009;**23**:19–34), treatment (Heberlein et al, Fortschr Neurol Psychiatr 2009;**77**:7–15), withdrawal syndrome (Petursson, Addiction 1994;**89**:11455–9), techniques and outcomes of BDZ detoxifications (Ferguson, Prescriber 2005;**16**:20–7; n = 82, Charney et al, J Clin Psychiatry 2000;**61**:190–5).

BNF listed

Antidepressants

Antidepressants may be useful for treating any concurrent depression and some are anxiolytics in their own right (see also introduction). **Mirtazapine** has been useful, particularly for sleep disturbance (n = 1, Chandrasekaran, Singapore Med J 2008;**49**:166–7).

Benzodiazepines

Transferring from the current benzodiazepine to diazepam (if necessary) is a common strategy, as diazepam is a longer-acting benzodiazepine and possibly easier from which to withdraw. If withdrawing chronic BDZs from old age in-patients, short-term (one week) substitution with a low-dose BDZ at night to help sleep may be effective (RCT, d/b, p/c, Petrovic et al, Eur J Clin Pharmacol 2002;**57**:759–64).

● Unlicensed/some efficacy

Buspirone

Caution is advised as buspirone has been reported to aggravate withdrawal symptoms (1.6). However, buspirone (38 mg/d) and imipramine (180 mg/d) have been used successfully in patients with GAD discontinuing long-term BDZs, introduced before a tapered discontinuation (n = 107, d/b, Rickels et al, Am J Psychiatry 2000;**157**:1973–9), and buspirone 15 mg/d may relieve lorazepam withdrawal symptoms, with no rebound anxiety on withdrawal (n = 44, RCT, Delle Chiaie et al, J Clin Psychopharmacol 1995;**15**:12–9). Buspirone may be helpful if established before BDZ withdrawal to manage underlying anxiety.

Carbamazepine *

Carbamazepine 600–800mg/d has been used as an alternative for benzodiazepine withdrawal in several studies (e.g. compared to tianeptine, Kornowski, *Psychiatr Pol* 2002;**36**(6 Suppl):311–8; Kaendler *et al*, *Nervenarzt* 1996; **67**:381–6). It reduces the chance of withdrawal convulsions and can minimise withdrawal symptoms (especially if withdrawal is abrupt) and reduces the incidence of relapse (n = 40, RCT, 12/52, Schweizer *et al*, *Arch Gen Psychiatry* 1991;**48**:448–52).

Oxcarbazepine *

Oxcarbazepine has been reported to enhance rapid BDZ withdrawal in as little as 11 days (n = 10, Croissant *et al*, *Am J Drug Alcohol Abuse* 2008;**34**:534–40).

Topiramate

Successful management of rapid BDZ-withdrawal with topiramate has been reported (n = 1, Cheseaux *et al*, *Hum Psychopharmacol* 2003;**18**:375–7), as has use of topiramate for alprazolam dependence (n = 1, Michopoulos *et*

■ **Unlicensed/possible efficacy**

Antihistamines

These may be useful as non-benzodiazepine hypnotics where insomnia is a problem.

Clonidine

This may be a helpful adjunct in withdrawal, especially at relatively high dose.

Flumazenil

IV flumazenil has been used to reduce BDZ craving, lower relapse rates and improve outcomes (n = 50, RCT, p/c, 6/52, Gerra *et al*, *Addict Biol* 2002;**7**:385–95). Caution is needed in BDZ dependence.

Melatonin

Controlled-release melatonin has been successfully used to facilitate discontinuation of benzodiazepines (n = 34, d/b, 6/52, Garfinkel *et al*, *Arch Intern Med* 1999;**159**:2456–60).

Characteristics of benzodiazepine users:

- Elderly maintained symptom-free by low and unchanging doses.
- Chronic physical disorders controlled by BDZs (e.g. epilepsy).
- Where quality of life is so improved by BDZs that long-term use, preferably with intermittent/variable doses, is justified (e.g. chronic or severe anxiety or insomnia and an inadequate personality, people who relapse to alcohol and other more dangerous substances when BDZ-free).

How to minimise the risks of dependence:

- Carefully select patients (e.g. avoid especially dependence-prone, lower education, multiple drug users, those with a criminal background).
- Keep the dose low.
- Stop where possible, e.g. use shorter courses.
- Use intermittent or variable doses.
- Use antidepressants if depression mixed with anxiety is present.
  (Darke *et al*, *Addiction* 1994;**89**:683–90)

Risk factors for poor withdrawal (need to seek specialist advice):

- Previously severe withdrawal (including history of seizures) or post-withdrawal reaction.
- Elderly or infirm.
- History of abuse of alcohol/other drugs.
- Concomitant severe medical or psychiatric illness (including personality problems).
- High dose/longer-term use (e.g. >30mg/d diazepam equivalent > 1 year).
- Cluster B personality/Borderline PD (n = 76, Vorma *et al*, *Subst Use Misuse* 2005;**40**:499–510).
- High neuroticism, higher behavioural inhibition and low social support (n = 41, 28/52, O'Connor *et al*, *Addict Behav* 2004;**29**:583–93).

al, World J Biol Psychiatry 2006;**7**:265–7).

Valproate

Valproate 150–1200mg/d may reduce the intensity of symptoms in protracted withdrawal (eg. n = 4, Apelt and Emrich, *Am J Psychiatry* 1994;**147**:1990), as well as acting as an anticonvulsant.

Patients where withdrawal should not be attempted:

- *Older medically ill or with spasticity or epilepsy:* Benzodiazepine usually prescribed by a non-psychiatrist. Seldom abused, doses not escalated, effective long-term. Care with subtle cognitive changes can occur.
- *Psychiatric patients with panic or agoraphobic disorders:* Seldom abused, doses not escalated, necessary long-term.
- *Psychiatric patients with recurrent dysphoria:* Long-term indications for use less clear. Abuse of other drugs often occurs.
- *Chronic sleep-disordered problems:* Drug may be active or preventing a rebound syndrome.

Withdrawal symptoms in the dependent patient:

- *Psychological:* Tension (to above pre-treatment levels), restlessness, agitation, panic attacks.
- *Physical:* Dry mouth, sweating, tremor, sleep disturbance, lethargy, headache, nausea, palpitations.
- *Mental:* Impaired memory and concentration, confusion.
- *Moderate:* Perceptual changes (i.e. hypersensitivity to light/sound), dysphoria, flu-like symptoms, anorexia, sore eyes, depersonalisation, depression, abnormal sensations of movement, rebound insomnia.
- *Severe:* (rare) Convulsions, psychoses (e.g. visual hallucinations, paranoia), delusions.

◆ Others

Other drugs tried include **phenobarbital** (*J Psychoact Drugs* 1983;**15**:85–95, 99–104) and **propranolol** (*Postgrad Med J* 1988; **64** [Suppl]:40–4).

□ No efficacy

Antipsychotics

Low dose anxiolytic use may be useful but may make withdrawal symptoms worse (Anon, *Lancet* 1987;**i**:78–9).

1.10 BIPOLAR MOOD DISORDER

1.10.1 PROPOPHYLAXIS AND MAINTENANCE
1.10.2 MANIA AND HYPOMANIA
1.10.3 BIPOLAR DEPRESSION
1.10.4 RAPID-CYCLING BIPOLAR DISORDER

Introduction

Bipolar mood disorder is a life-long illness with a variety of presentations, phases and sub-divisions. DSM-IV divides the condition into bipolar I (one or more manic or mixed episodes, wide mood swings), bipolar II (the most common form, one or more episodes of depression with at least one hypomanic but no manic episode) and bipolar III (pseudobipolar, often triggered by antidepressants, and which may present as a mixed state). There are many other classifications and sub-categories.

Diagnosis

Bipolar disorder is frequently unrecognised, misdiagnosed and inadequately treated. A survey of members of US bipolar association 'Chapters' showed that over 33% sought professional help within a year of the onset of symptoms. Of these, 69% were misdiagnosed (mostly as unipolar depression), there was an average of four physicians seen before getting an accurate diagnosis, and over 33% waited over 10 years before getting a diagnosis (n = 600, Hirschfeld *et al, J Clin Psychiatry* 2003;**64**:161–74), a finding stunningly similar to a previous survey (Lish *et al, J Affect Disord* 1994;**31**:281–94). The **average** time from the onset of symptoms to starting maintenance therapy is 8–10 years (e.g. n = 56, Goldberg and Ernst, *J Clin Psychiatry*

2002;**63**: 985–91), and may be even longer with women (n = 360, Viguera et al, Bipolar Disord 2001;**3**:245–52). Sadly, many suicide attempts are made during this latency period before lithium is started, the only mood stabiliser proven to reduce suicides. A longer delay also results in poorer social functioning over the last year, more annual hospitalisations and a higher likelihood of suicide attempts, regardless of the polarity of the first episode (n = 56, Goldberg and Ernst, J Clin Psychiatry 2002;**63**:985–91). A delay in starting mood stabilisers does not necessarily ultimately adversely influence the prophylactic outcome, but illness severity prior to prophylaxis does predict outcome, although those with a more severe illness were more likely to be treated early with better outcomes (n = 147, Baethge et al, Acta Psychiatr Scand 2003;**107**:260–7). Excess mortality has been shown in bipolar (n = 15 386) and unipolar (n = 39 182) disorder in Sweden, both in terms of suicides and from natural causes (population study, Osby et al, Arch Gen Psychiatry 2001;**58**:844–50); but suicide rates are significantly reduced by long-term medication with an antidepressant, neuroleptic, or lithium, or combinations thereof (n = 406, 22 years, Angst et al, J Affect Disord 2002;**68**:167–81).

Reviews: * general (Sie et al, Clin Pharmacist 2009;**1**:67–85), systematic (Ceron-Litvoc et al, Hum Psychopharmacol 2008;**24**:19–28).

1.10.1 PROPOPHYLAXIS AND MAINTENANCE

Role of drugs

The optimum outcomes in bipolar occur with the appropriate and consistent prescribing and concordance of mood stabilisers, training for the person to cope with stresses and risk factors, and family support. Lithium, valproate, some antipsychotics and carbamazepine are widely used for the prophylaxis of bipolar disorder, although the evidence for carbamazepine and perhaps valproate is not robust. It is clear that well-being and functioning are inversely proportional to the number of bipolar episodes, and so strategies to reduce relapse must be rigorously followed, especially minimising difficult-to-treat bipolar depression (see 1.10.3). Unfortunately, inappropriate use of antidepressants in un-diagnosed bipolar may lead to cycle worsening

in many (n = 85, naturalistic, Ghaemi et al, J Clin Psychiatry 2000;**61**:804–8). Regular compliance is important but be aware that impaired verbal learning and memory in bipolar could passively limit treatment adherence (n = 40, Cavanagh et al, Br J Psychiatry 2002;**180**:293–5, 320–6). There is some suggestion (from a small retrospective study) that lithium is not alone in producing rebound on discontinuation, as it may occur with CBZ, antipsychotics and valproate (n = 53, Franks et al, J Psychopharmacol 2008; **22**:452–6).

There is an overlap with ADHD, anxiety and personality disorder, e.g. labile effect, irritability, mood instability, stress, low mood/dysphoria, and many have warned of over-diagnosing PD and under-diagnosing bipolar disorder. CBT does not appear to reduce the overall episode recurrence in recurrent bipolar disorder (n = 253 [c = 200], RCT, s/b, 18/12, Scott et al, Br J Psychiatry 2006;**188**:313–20; comment by Lam, EBMH 2006;**9**:99; Beynon et al, Br J Psychiatry 2008;**192**:5–11), except perhaps in people with fewer episodes.

Reviews: * general (Vieta and Sanchez-Moreno, Dialogues Clin Neurosci 2008;**10**:165–79), BAP guidelines on bipolar disorder (Goodwin et al, J Psychopharmacol 2009;**23**:346–88), bipolar II and mixed depression (Benazzi, Lancet 2007;**369**:936–45), mood stabilisers and antipsychotics in maintenance bipolar disorder (Smith et al, Bipolar Disord 2007;**9**:394–412; Hellewell, J Psychopharmacol 2006;**20**(suppl 2):39–45), systematic review of relapse prevention (s = 34, Beynon et al, J Psychopharmacol 2009;**23**:574–91), complementary therapies (concludes SJW and SAMe [S-adenosyl-l-methionine] are both effective for depression but can cause mania; inconsistent evidence for acupuncture and omega-3-fatty acids; no data on massage, acupuncture, aromatherapy, yoga; Andreescu et al, J Affect Disord 2008;**110**:16–26).

BNF listed

Aripiprazole *

Aripiprazole is newly licensed for prevention of recurrence of manic episodes in bipolar I, in people who have responded acutely. The maintenance dose is the same as the acute dose. In supporting studies, 15–30mg/d was superior to placebo for reducing relapse in bipolar mania in those responding over 6/52 (n = 161, RCT, d/b, p/c, 6/12, Keck et al, J Clin Psychiatry 2006;**67**:626–37; two-year extension, n = 161, RCT, d/b, p/c, two years, Keck et al, Am J Psychiatry 2007;**164**:1480–91; see also n = 262, RCT, d/b, p/c, 3/52, Keck et al, Am J Psychiatry 2003;**160**:1651–8; observations by Jagadheesan and Muirhead, Am J Psychiatry 2004;**161**:1926–7).

Reviews: * Fountoulakis and Vieta, Ann Gen Psychiatry 2009;**8**:16; McIntyre et al, Expert Rev Neurother 2007;**7**:919–25).

Carbamazepine

Long-term therapy in affective disorders is licensed as an alternative to lithium although it is rapidly falling out of favour. Six studies of maintenance carbamazepine in bipolar disorder have shown equivocal results, e.g. incomplete protection, and so some uncertainty remains (reviewed by Keck et al, J Clin Psychiatry 1998;**59**[Suppl 6]:S74–S81, 114 refs). Indeed, one study showed that only 18% of carbamazepine-treated bipolars remained stable for 3–4 years, and another showed a 50% relapse rate (n = 24, open, four years, Post et al, J Clin Psychopharmacol 1990;**10**:318–27). A comparison of 10 studies of carbamazepine against lithium shows a roughly similar efficacy (n = 572, table in Davis et al, Acta Psychiatr Scand 1999;**100**:406–17). There has, however, been an increased interest in carbamazepine as a consequence of two studies of an SR preparation for use in mania and in a follow-on study as relapse prevention. Although 69% discontinued early, only 14% of the 77 completers relapsed (n = 92, open, 6/52, Ketter et al, J Clin Psychiatry 2004;**65**:668–73). There is little evidence for a rebound mania on discontinuation (e.g. n = 6, Macritchie and Hunt, J Psychopharmacol 2000;**14**:266–8). It has been suggested that the best thing you can do with carbamazepine in bipolar is to stop it and allow other drugs to reach therapeutic levels.

Lithium *

The use of lithium in bipolar was first published by Cade (Med J Aust 1949;**36**:49–52) and it is now widely used for the treatment and prophylaxis of bipolar illnesses and, with care, can be successful and safe. It is effective in bipolar I and II, by reducing relapses and increasing inter-episodic intervals.

Efficacy: Although the nine major placebo-controlled trials of lithium as prophylaxis of bipolar disorder have methodological flaws (e.g. most used an abrupt lithium-withdrawal control group shown to increase relapse in its own right), their findings are of great importance. Lithium clearly reduces the risk of relapse in bipolar disorder (61% with placebo, 33% with lithium), particularly for manic episodes (systematic review and meta-analysis, n = 770, Geddes et al, Am J Psychiatry 2004;**161**:217–22; review by Bauer, EBMH 2004;**7**:72). Bauer's review states it to be the first published, methodologically rigorous meta-analysis of RCT, d/b, p/c trials in relapse prevention, and concludes that lithium reduces the risk of relapse in affective relapse, especially manic, but that there is less evidence that it prevents depressive relapses. Response may be a familial trait (n = 146, Grof et al, J Clin Psychiatry 2002;**63**:942–7) and less likely with a high weight (Calkin et al, Bipolar Disord 2009;**11**:650–6).

Prophylaxis: Lithium appears highly effective as prophylactic therapy, provided it is taken and monitored regularly, and the dose and therapy reviewed regularly to minimise side-effects, especially those of weight gain and cognitive dulling. Commencing lithium within the first ten years of illness predicts better preventative outcomes than beginning prophylaxis later, both in major depression, recurrent and bipolar patients (n = 270, Franchini et al, Eur Arch Psychiatry Clin Neurosci 1999;**249**:227–30). The prophylactic efficacy is probably maintained for at least ten years (n = 86, mean 8.2 years, Berghofer et al, Acta Psychiatr Scand 1996;**93**:349–54). Data is accumulating that long-term lithium markedly reduces the excess mortality of people with recurrent affective disorders (retrospective study, n = 273, Müller-Oerlinghausen et al, Acta Psychiatr Scand 1996;**94**:344–7), probably at least in part by (see next section) reducing suicide (Gershon and Soares, Arch Gen Psychiatry 1997;**54**:16–20). Lithium maintenance yields striking long-term reductions of depressive as well as manic morbidity in both bipolar disorder subtypes, with greater overall benefits in bipolar II patients and with earlier treatment (n = 317, retrospective, Tondo et al, Am J Psychiatry 1998; **155**:638–45). Regular lithium use over five years has been shown to produce a drastic reduction in time in hospital as 'almost the rule', but irregular use leads to a much poorer outcome (n = 402, Maj et al, Am J Psychiatry 1998; **155**:30–5).

The main problems appear to be when therapy is given to carelessly selected patients given insufficient support (see compliance), education and supervision, illustrated by naturalistic studies which show a poorer outcome than controlled trials. Goodwin argues strongly that treatment with lithium should be for at least two years (and more probably three years at the minimum), and that up to two years it may have at best no beneficial effect (premature stopping resulting in premature recurrence of mania).

Suicide reduction: * Reduced suicide rate has been strongly associated with lithium, something unique in bipolar, e.g. a systematic review of RCTs showed that people with bipolar disorder taking lithium are less likely to die by suicide (2 vs 11, odds ratio = 0.26) and less likely to self-harm and with lower deaths overall (s = 32, n = 3458, Cipriani et al, Am J Psychiatry 2005; **162**:1805–19; see also Müller-Oerlinghausen et al, Arch Suicide Res 2005; **9**:307–19). In 18 municipalities in Oita in Japan where lithium is found in tapwater, lithium levels were significantly and negatively associated with SMR averages for 2002–2006, so maybe even very low levels of lithium may reduce the overall risk of suicide (Ohgami et al, B J Psychiatry 2009; **194**:464–5). Although suicide protection may be incomplete, it is seven-fold lower than in non-lithium treated patients (meta-analysis by Müller-Oerlinghausen, Eur Arch Psychiatry Clin Neurosci 2001; **251**[Suppl 2]:S72–S75), as are suicide attempts or successful suicide (2.7 times higher with valproate than lithium; n = 20 638, Goodwin et al, JAMA 2003; **290**:1467–73). Two publications present some caution (Coryell et al, Acta Psychiatr Scand 2001; **104**:193–7; editorial comment by Gelenberg, Acta Psychiatr Scand 2001; **104**:161–2; review by Burgess, EBMH 2002; **5**:52; n = 133, retrospective over

16 years, Brodersen et al, Br J Psychiatry 2000; **176**:429–33).

Mode of action: Lithium may exert its effect via many mechanisms, e.g. inositol monophosphatase enzyme inhibition, inhibiting secondary messenger systems, inhibition of Protein Kinase C activity (an action shared with valproate and tamoxifen), neuro-protection, regulating glycogen synthase kinase-3 (GSK-3) gene expression, increased human brain grey matter (Moore et al, Lancet 2000; **356**:1241–2), up-regulation of Bcl-2 (major neuroprotective protein, with speculated rebound reduction in Bcl-2 production on withdrawal: Manji et al, J Clin Psychiatry 2000; **61**[Suppl 9]:S82–S96), protection from glutamate apoptosis (programmed cell death) and serotonin regulation. Some of the long-term benefits of lithium may be mediated by neurotrophic effects.

Dosing: * Once-daily lithium reduces side-effects, simplifies dosage requirements and reduces renal damage (review Ljubicic et al, Can J Psychiatry 2008; **53**:323–31). Alternate daily lithium is not recommended (n = 50, d/b, Jensen et al, J Affect Disord 1996; **36**:89–93). There are several methods of predicting lithium dose and levels (e.g. n = 60, Abou-Auda et al, Bipolar Disord 2008; **10**:369–76).

Plasma levels: * Plasma levels of 0.4–0.8 mmol/L are generally considered safe and effective as prophylaxis, but below 0.4–0.6 mEq/L may be less protective against relapse. There was no difference in the protection against affective disorder relapse between high (0.8–1.0 mmol/L) and low (0.5–0.8 mmol/L) serum lithium levels (naturalistic, n = 91, Vestergaard et al, Acta Psychiatr Scand 1998; **98**:310–5), but only a third completed two years' lithium prophylaxis successfully, and alcohol or other medication abuse was associated with poor outcome. In the elderly, a third to half less lithium may be needed due to reduced clearance (n = 9, Hardy et al, J Clin Psychopharmacol 1987; **7**:153–8). Lower plasma levels of lithium may be better at preventing relapse of bipolar depression and higher levels better to prevent mania (n = 64, 18/12, Severus et al, J Affect Disord 2009; **115**:466–70).

Monitoring: * Plasma monitoring is often poor, with many litigation cases for poor monitoring, and the NPSA in the UK has recently (2009) set targets for adequate monitoring. Local databases may be a successful way to achieve this (Holmes and Bazire, *Bipolar Disorders* 2003;**5**[Suppl 1]:S53).

Compliance or concordance: The main reason for lithium failure is non-compliance (either complete or erratic), and the patient (and any partner or caregiver) should be aware of the long-term commitment needed. Specialised care, e.g. via lithium or mood clinics, may improve patient and professional compliance with lithium use (Guscott and Taylor, *Br J Psychiatry* 1994;**164**:741–6). For a general review of strategies to improve compliance, see Schou (*Acta Psychiatr Scand* 1997;**95**:361–3).

Discontinuation: Early (particularly manic) relapse following lithium discontinuation is now well recognised with several important studies showing a significant risk from rapid discontinuation. If stopped in under 14 days, the risk of relapse is much higher (median 50% risk of relapse within four months, 100% over 3.5 years) than with slower (15–30 days) withdrawal, with a significant excess over the first six months (n = 161, Baldessarini et al, *J Clin Psychiatry* 1996;**57**:441–8; n = 78, Baldessarini et al, *Am J Psychiatry* 1997; **154**:551–3). At seven-year follow-up, relapse was more common after acute lithium discontinuation, the excess morbidity being attributable to the first episode/relapse after discontinuation (n = 42, seven years, Cavanagh et al, *Acta Psychiatr Scand* 2004;**109**:91–5). Even controlled lithium discontinuation leads to a high relapse in people who have had a good response for at least five years, so be careful (n = 32, up to nine years, Yazici et al, *J Affect Disord* 2004;**80**:269–71). Since lithium has been shown to reduce mortality, discontinuation is also likely to be associated with increased mortality (review by MacQueen and Joffe, *Acta Psychiatr Scand* 2004;**109**:81–2).

Abrupt decrease: Decreasing lithium levels, (either through erratic compliance or major changes in dose) is also a powerful predictor of relapse (n = 94, Perlis et al, *Am J Psychiatry* 2002;**159**:1155–9). Indeed, the original paper that claims that > 0.8 mmol/L is superior to lower levels (n = 94, RCT, d/b, Gelenberg et al, *N Engl J Med* 1989;**321**:1489–93) notes that many in the lower level group had rapid reductions in levels which may have contributed to relapse.

Lithium refractoriness: Lithium discontinuation in stable patients, despite adequate lithium levels, has been reported to induce a refractory state. However, two studies of lithium maintenance treatment periods (mean four years) were unable to show this (n = 86, Tondo et al, *Am J Psychiatry* 1997;**154**:548–50; n = 28, Coryell et al, *Am J Psychiatry* 1998;**155**:895–8), although the latter study has been criticised as being underpowered (Maj, *Am J Psychiatry* 1999;**156**:1130; plus reply). In a longitudinal study of clinic-attending bipolars compliant with lithium for at least a year, and without comorbid substance misuse, retreatment showed a slightly reduced efficacy. There was no tendency for lesser responses later in treatment (n = 360, longitudinal, Tondo et al, *Br J Psychiatry* 2001;**178**[Suppl 41]:S184–S190).

Reviews: * general (Grandjean and Aubry, *CNS Drugs* 2009;**23**:225–40; Young and Newham, *J Psychopharmacol* 2006;**20**(suppl 2):17–22; Ferrier et al, *Adv Psychiatric Treat* 2006;**12**:256–64), metabolic adverse effects (Livingstone and Rampes, *J Psychopharmacol* 2006;**20**:347–55), in renal disease (Smith et al, *J Clin Psychiatry* 2005;**66**:396–9), history of lithium (Bech, *Psychother Psychosom* 2006; **75**:265–9).

Olanzapine *

Olanzapine is indicated for the prevention of recurrence in patients with bipolar disorder whose manic episode has responded to olanzapine, where maintenance olanzapine reduces relapse to subsequent mood disorder compared to placebo, although people with an index depressive episode in the open phase were excluded (n = 361, RCT, p/c, 48/52, Tohen et al, *Am J Psychiatry* 2006;**163**:247–56; MS; comment by Citrome, *EBMH* 2006;**9**:73). Two systematic reviews from Cipriani have summarised the data. One concludes that olanzapine helps prevent manic episodes, but only in people who have responded in an acute or mixed episode and have not responded to lithium or valproate (s = 5, RCT, Cipriani et al, *J Psychopharmacol* 2010;[in press]). Cochrane concludes that although the data is limited, olanzapine may prevent relapses in people responding during an index manic or mixed episode and who have previously not responded to lithium or valproate, although the evidence is stronger for lithium as a first-line maintenance treatment of bipolar disorder (s = 5, n = 1165, Cipriani et al, Cochrane Database Syst Rev 2009; 1:CD004367).

Risperidone (license anticipated 2010) *

Risperidone is licensed for acute mania or mixed episodes in bipolar mania and a license for adjunctive or maintenance treatment to prevent recurrence of bipolar 1, where relapse rates are significantly reduced (n = 124, RCT, d/b, p/c, 12/12, Macfadden et al, Bipolar Disord 2009;**11**:827–39), may be granted in 2010 (review, Kemp et al, Adv Ther 2009;**26**:588–99).

+ Combinations

There has been an increased use of poly-pharmacy in refractory bipolar disorder over recent decades.

Lithium + antipsychotics *

Lithium is frequently used with antipsychotics in maintenance therapy, although the evidence is poor, e.g. **flupentixol** was ineffective as an adjunct to lithium (n = 11, d/b, c/o, Esparon et al, Br J Psychiatry 1986;**148**:723–5). In patients stabilised on **quetiapine** and lithium, continued treatment reduced the risk of relapse (20% vs 52%) compared to placebo (n = 1953, open, <36/52; then n = 628, RCT, d/b, p/c, <104/52, Suppes et al, Am J Psychiatry 2009;**166**:476–88; see also RCT, d/b, p/c, <2 years, Vieta et al, J Affect Disord 2008;**109**:251–63). See also 'some efficacy' section.

Lithium + calcium-channel blockers

Although there are some reports of efficacy, potential drug interactions make this com-bination hazardous (reviewed by Freeman and Stoll, Am J Psychiatry 1998;**155**:12–21).

Lithium + carbamazepine/oxcarbazepine

Lithium plus carbamazepine has been widely used and can seem safe and effective, especially for rapid-cycling. Some old studies have shown a well tolerated and improved prophylactic effect compared to lithium monotherapy (e.g. n = 33, Small et al, Psychopharmacol Bull 1995;**31**:265–72), but in a pilot study, oxcarbazepine appeared more effective and better tolerated than carbamazepine as add-on to lithium for residual bipolar I and II symptoms (n = 52 [c = 52], RCT, d/b, 8/52, Juruena et al, Prog Neuropsychopharmacol Biol Psychiatry 2009;**33**:94–9).

Lithium + lamotrigine

A retrospective chart review showed the combination of lithium and lamotrigine was effective in reducing relapse of depression but not as good at preventing mania (n = 21, mean 55/52, Ghaemi et al, J Psychiatr Pract 2006;**12**:300–5).

Valproate + antipsychotics *

Many combinations are used, although there is little data to show a proven efficacy. In patients stabilised on **quetiapine** and valproate, continued treatment reduced the risk of relapse (20% vs 52%) compared to placebo (n = 1953, open, <36/52; then n = 628, RCT, d/b, p/c, <104/52, Suppes et al, Am J Psychiatry 2009;**166**:476–88; see also RCT, d/b, p/c, <2 years, Vieta et al, J Affect Disord 2008;**109**:251–63). There is also data that valproate may allow reduction in the doses of antipsychotics needed in bipolar disorder with psychosis, or even replace them (Reutens and Castle, Br J Psychiatry 1997;**170**:484–5). See also 'some efficacy'.

Valproate + carbamazepine

There have been several reports of efficacy, e.g. when valproate was added to carbamazepine non-responders, 69% responded (n = 29, Schaff et al, J Clin Psychiatry 1993;**54**:380–4).

Valproate + lamotrigine

An open study has indicated some efficacy (reviewed by Freeman and Stoll, Am J Psychiatry 1998;**155**:12–21), although the incidence of rash appears higher and valproate increases lamotrigine levels (see 4.5.5).

● Unlicensed/some efficacy

Antidepressants *

See bipolar depression (1.10.3) for use in bipolar disorder, with notes about the risk of inducing a switch to mania in bipolar depression. A meta-analysis has shown that long-term adjunctive antidepressants are not superior to mood-stabilisers alone, and with an unfavourable risk:benefit for antidepressants as long-term therapy in bipolar (s = 7, n = 350, Ghaemi *et al*, *Acta Psychiatr Scand* 2008;**118**:347–56).

Antipsychotics (see also aripiprazole, olanzapine and risperidone in BNF listed) *

The main roles of antipsychotics in bipolar disorder are:

1. Adjunctive to mood stabilisers for management of acute mania (see 1.10.2) or psychotic depression.
2. Adjunctive maintenance in treatment-resistance.

There is no compelling evidence that anti-psychotics, as such, are effective as mood stabilisers alone in bipolar disorder, although they may help prevent relapse of mania. Aripiprazole and olanzapine are licensed for relapse prevention in responders (see BNF section). Many other antipsychotics are licensed for bipolar mania and might thus have some relapse prevention efficacy. **Quetiapine** (see also combinations) is licensed in the short-term treatment of acute manic episodes and may have some applications as an alternative or adjunct in bipolar or schizoaffective disorders (n = 145, open, Zarate *et al*, *J Clin Psychiatry* 2000;**61**:185–9), and a pilot study in bipolar or schizoaffective patients poorly responsive to mood stabilisers, suggested that quetiapine (50–400 mg/d) may have some potential (n = 20, open, 12/52, Sajatovic *et al*, *J Clin Psychiatry* 2001;**62**:728–32). **Clozapine** may have some significant mood-stabilising effects in treatment-resistant bipolar or schizoaffective patients, e.g. as add-on therapy compared to placebo (n = 38, RCT, p/c, Suppes *et al*, *Am J Psychiatry* 1999;**156**:1164–9), and a longer trial showed some efficacy to improve symptoms in bipolar with psychotic features (n = 37, open, two years, Ciapparelli *et al*, *J Clin Psychiatry* 2003;**64**:451–8).

Reviews: atypicals in bipolar (Derry and Moore, *BMC Psychiatry* 2007;**7**:40; Gentile, *CNS Drugs* 2007;**21**:367–87; Perlis *et al*, *J Clin Psychiatry* 2006;**67**:509–16, comment by Jones, *EMBH* 2007;**10**:11).

Lamotrigine

Lamotrigine is licensed in the US (but not the UK) for the maintenance treatment of bipolar I depression and relapse prevention (see bipolar depression 1.10.3). The mode of action may be inhibiting excess glutamate release but it does not down-regulate PKC or MARCKS, so may be different to lithium and valproate (review by Hahn *et al*, *J Clin Psychiatry* 2004;**65**:791–804).

Review: use in bipolar (Bhagwagar and Goodwin, *Expert Opin Pharmacother* 2005;**476**: 1401–8).

Valproate

While valproate is licensed for mania, valproate salts are not actually licensed as mood stabilisers (and unlikely ever to be), albeit widely used for this purpose. The one-year study comparing divalproex, lithium and placebo (2:1:1) just failed to show divalproex to be superior to lithium or placebo in the time to any mood episode, but there was a noticeable trend for divalproex (40/52) over placebo (28/52) and lithium (24/52), and it was superior to placebo on nearly all secondary measures (n = 372, RCT, Bowden *et al*, *Arch Gen Psychiatry* 2000;**57**:481–9). Valproate may also reduce depressive symptoms compared to lithium (sub-analysis of Bowden study by Gyulai *et al*, *Neuropsychopharmacol* 2003;**28**:1374–82). Reduced suicide in bipolar has not been shown with valproate compared to lithium (n = 20 638, Goodwin *et al*, *JAMA* 2003;**290**:1467–73). See also entry under mania/hypomania (1.10.2).

■ Unlicensed/possible efficacy

Anticholinesterases *

While adjunctive **galantamine** improved some aspects of episodic memory in cognitive dysfunction, it had little overall positive effect (n = 30[c = 16], RCT, d/b, p/c, 3/12, Ghaemi *et al*, *J Clin Psychopharmacol* 2009;**29**:291–5). **Donepezil** 5–10 mg/d was not much use either for ADL or cognitive function in older people with bipolar (n = 12, 3/12, Gildengers et al, Int J Geriatr Psychiatry 2008;**23**:704–11).

Calcium-channel blockers

Verapamil 120–450mg/d and diltiazem (n = 8, open, 12/12, Silverstone and Birkett, J Psychiatry Neurosci 2000;**25**:276–80) have shown some promise as a mood stabiliser and may have some role as add-on therapy in resistant cases.

Cannabis

A review of cannabinoids in bipolar disorder concluded that there were no published studies of efficacy but much anecdotal evidence (Ashton et al, J Psychopharmacol 2005; **19**:293–300).

Gabapentin

See bipolar depression (1.10.3). Despite lacking efficacy in acute states, gabapentin added to a mood stabiliser (lithium, valproate or carbamazepine) may have some prophylactic effects (n = 25, RCT, d/b, p/c, 12/12, Vieta et al, J Clin Psychiatry 2006;**67**:473–7).

Omega-3 fatty acids

In a not very stringent four-month trial, omega-3 fatty acids produced a significantly longer remission than placebo, as well as scoring higher on most other outcome measures (n = 30, d/b, Stoll et al, Arch Gen Psychiatry 1999;**56**:407–12; general review by Greener, Prog Neurol Psychiatry 1999;**3**:26–7).

Oxcarbazepine (see also combinations)

There are case reports of success in bipolar II with comorbid substance abuse (n = 4, Nasr, Am J Psychiatry 2002;**159**:1793).

Tamoxifen

There is some interest in tamoxifen as a mood stabiliser in that it shares some intra-cellular properties with lithium, e.g. PKC inhibition (see lithium and tamoxifen in mania/hypomania; review by Zarate and Manji, CNS Drugs 2009; **23**:569–82).

Tiagabine

There are reports of tiagabine 4mg/d used successfully as adjunctive therapy in multiple drug-resistant bipolar disorder, continuing to be effective over several months (e.g. n = 2, Schaffer and Schaffer, Am J Psychiatry 1999; **156**:2014–15), although it was at best only modestly effective in refractory bipolar, with significant ADRs (n = 13, open, Suppes et al, Bipolar Disord 2002; **4**:283–9).

Topiramate

There is some evidence accumulating, but RCTs are awaited to confirm this. Several open studies suggest some efficacy, e.g. mild improvement was seen in 47% and marked-to-moderate in 13% bipolars treated with topiramate (mean 180mg/d), with a dose-related response and weight loss, as well as significant side-effects (n = 76, open, Ghaemi et al, Ann Clin Psychiatry 2001;**13**:185–9), in recurrent mania in bipolar I (n = 1, Letmaier et al, Int Clin Psychopharmacol 2001:**16**:295–8), as an adjunctive in treatment-resistant bipolar (n = 19, open, 12/52, Vieta et al, World J Biol Psychiatry 2003;**4**:172–6) and as add-on maintenance in bipolar, with low drop-outs and low relapses (n = 56, open, one year, Lykouras and Hatzimanolis, Curr Med Res Opin 2004;**20**:843–7).

Vitamins and minerals

A trial of 36 dietary nutrients has produced a 55–66% reduction in bipolar symptoms and a reduction in medication levels, leading to suggestions that bipolar disorder is an inborn error of metabolism, although the mechanism is unknown (n = 11, 6/12, Kaplan et al, J Clin Psychiatry 2001;**62**:936–44).

1.10.2 MANIA AND HYPOMANIA

Symptoms

Hypomania, the more common and less severe form of mania, includes an abnormal elation of mood, alternating with irritability, great energy, inability to concentrate, flight of ideas (rapid changing of the subject with some connections) and insomnia. Obsessive preoccupation with some idea, activity or desire may occur. The main presenting symptoms are a euphoric and labile mood (irritable, angry, grandiose), bright or untidy appearance, low sleep requirement, increased drive and energy, reduced insight, pressure of speech, flight of ideas, expansive thought and an overactive and intrusive manner.

Risk factors for chronicity of mania:
- Physical illness
- Substance misuse
- Positive family history
- Poor pre-morbid social functioning
- Depressed or mixed cycles
- Rapid-cycling
- Longer episodes and increased episodes

(review Tyrer, *J Psychopharmacol* 2006;**20**[suppl 2]:4–11).

Role of drugs

Hypomania or mania is a phase of a bipolar (or rarely a unipolar) illness. Both usually require specific long-term mood-stabiliser drug treatment for the bipolar component (i.e. lithium, valproate, atypicals, carbamazepine, etc), and non-specific shorter-term treatments (e.g. antipsychotics, benzodiazepines) for the insomnia, agitation and hyperactivity to calm the person and prevent exhaustion and harm. Systematic reviews have shown combining a second generation antipsychotic with a mood stabiliser (MS) is significantly more effective than a MS alone in acute mania (s = 24, n = 6187, Scherk et al, *Arch Gen Psychiatry* 2007;**64**:442–55; comment by Perlis, EBMH 2007;**10**:111; s = 8, n = 1124, RCT, Smith et al, *Acta Psychiatr Scand* 2007;**115**:12–20). A night of sleep deprivation is likely to escalate any manic patient to a higher degree of mania and so hypnotic/sedative use should be considered appropriate (n = 67, Wehr et al, *Arch Gen Psychiatry* 1982;**39**:559–65). Any comorbid substance misuse should be tackled at the same time, as recovery from mania is poorer in people with a history of substance abuse (retrospective review, n = 204, Goldberg et al, *J Clin Psychiatry* 1999;**60**:733–40). After recovery from a manic episode with an antipsychotic and a mood stabiliser, many people receive antipsychotics long-term. This may not always be the best thing to do, as one study showed that those continuing antipsychotics long-term had a quicker onset of depression, were more likely to discontinue, and have more EPS and dysphoria — a good collection of detrimental effects (n = 27, RCT, p/c, d/b, 6/12, Zarate and Tohen, *Am J Psychiatry* 2004;**161**:169–71). Most response to drugs occurs in the first few weeks and a meta-analysis of RCTs concludes that atypicals, lithium and haloperidol are equally effective

(and superior to placebo) in acute mania (s = 18, p/c, Perlis et al, *J Clin Psychiatry* 2006;**67**:509–16; comment by Jones, *EBMH* 2007;**10**:11). Lithium is an effective antimanic but difficult to use in the short and long-term. Evidence for an antimanic effect for valproate (particularly in mixed states) is better than carbamazepine.

Treatment goals for mania should be:

1. Discontinue any agents that may induce symptoms, including antidepressants and substances of misuse (see 5.7 for lists).
2. Stabilise any medical conditions.
3. Start non-specific calming medications, e.g. benzodiazepines, antipsychotics.
4. Start specific mood-stabilisers or relapse prevention agents (see 1.10.1) preferably when the patient is able to consent to longer-term therapy. For good reasons, in the real world patients presenting with mania are very different to those in clinical trials and inclusions, exclusions and differing assessments of severity (USA tends to rate the same presentation as more severe than UK) may have led to the over-estimating of anti-manic drug efficacy, as only about 16% of acute manic patients presenting in a routine mental hospital would seem to qualify for a standard placebo-controlled RCT (n = 74, Storosum et al, *Eur Neuropsychopharmacol* 2004;**14**:319–23). See bipolar mood disorder (1.10.1) for maintenance strategies.

Reviews: * pharmacological interventions (s = 13, n = 3089, Smith et al, *Bipolar Disord* 2007;**9**:551–60), anticonvulsants in mania (Cookson and Elliott, *J Psychopharmacol* 2006;**20**[Suppl]:23–30), evidence-based guidelines (Goodwin et al, *J Psychopharmacol* 2009;**23**:346–88), atypicals in mania (Cookson, *Adv Psych Treat* 2008; **14**:330–8).

BNF listed

Aripiprazole *

Aripiprazole is licensed for acute mania and relapse prevention. Initiate in mania at 15mg/d (range 5–20mg/d) if no other antipsychotics are involved (possibly with a lower dose if not urgent or caution is needed, e.g. Asian or black ethnic groups, which often have reduced 2D6 activity, and low BMI). Use adjunctive medications to manage agitation if necessary, e.g. benzodiazepines or promethazine. When switching from another antipsychotic, add aripiprazole 15mg/d (can be 5mg/d then 10mg/d first), then when stable (may be 5 half-lives of the previous drug) start tapering down the previous drug. Aripiprazole is at least as effective as haloperidol in acute mania, maintained for 12 weeks, with haloperidol having more side-effects (n = 485, RCT, d/b, p/c, 12/52, Young et al, Br J Psychiatry 2009; **194**:40–8; n = 272, RCT, d/b, p/c, 3/52, Sachs et al, J Psychopharmacol 2006; **20**:536–46; n = 347, RCT, d/b, 12/52, Vieta et al, Br J Psychiatry 2005; **187**:235–42; comment by Centorrino, EBMH 2006; **9**:41, noting that despite the relatively high haloperidol comparative dose and inclusion/ exclusion criteria, it is clear aripiprazole is effective and well tolerated in acute mania).

Reviews: * general (Muzina, Neuropsychiat Dis Treat 2009; **5**:279–88), consensus statement on use in mania (Aitchison et al, J Psychopharmacol 2009; **23**:231–40).

Asenapine (may be licensed 2010/11) *

In manic or mixed episodes, asenapine (mean 18.2mg/d) was rapidly effective, well tolerated and as effective as olanzapine (n = 488, RCT, d/b, p/c, 3/52, McIntyre et al, Bipolar Disord 2009; **11**:673–86).

Review: * general (Bishara and Taylor, Neuropsychiatr Dis Treat 2009; **5**:483–90).

Carbamazepine

There has been increased interest in carbamazepine with the launch of an MR preparation in USA. Carbamazepine MR up to 1600mg/d was effective in 41% (cf 22% for placebo) as monotherapy in acute bipolar mania (n = 204 [c = 96], RCT, d/b, p/c, 3/52, Weisler et al, J Clin Psychiatry 2004; **65**:478–84) and up to 1600mg/d was superior to placebo in acute mania (n = 239 [c = 144], RCT, d/b, p/c, 3/52, Weisler et al, J Clin Psychiatry 2005; **66**:323–30; pooled results analysis; n = 443 [c = 240], RCT, Weisler et al, CNS Drugs 2006; **20**:219–31). The previous five RCTs of carbamazepine in acute mania showed a response rate equivalent to lithium and chlorpromazine (review by Keck et al, J Clin Psychiatry 1998; **59**[Suppl 6]:S74–S81, 114 refs).

Reviews: acute mania (Owen, Drugs Today [Barc] 2006; **42**:283–9), CBZ for bipolar and mania (Stoner et al, Pharmacotherapy 2007; **27**: 68–88).

Lithium

Lithium is effective in acute mania/hypomania, although the onset of action may be delayed for five to seven days or longer (unless perhaps if loading doses are used). It is difficult to use in mania due to the need to monitor blood levels, problems with stopping later or prematurely, and the need for two to three years minimum treatment duration. Serum levels of 0.9–1.4mmol/L may be necessary in the short-term for a therapeutic effect and should be reduced once mood is normalised. Loading with lithium in mania is surprisingly poorly studied but has been tried with rapid success, many responding within 48 hours. The only recent study available showed that in 15 manic in-patients given 20mg/kg/d for up to 10 days, only five completed the trial (although seven drop-outs improved sufficiently to allow discharge and only two had ADRs). All had levels > 0.6mmol/L after the first day, which was generally well tolerated and showed a rapid improvement, although this needs confirming in a full study (n = 15, open, Keck et al, Bipolar Disord 2001; **3**:68–72). At least four previous depressive or 10–12 previous manic episodes are associated with reduced antimanic response to lithium (Swann et al, Acta Psychiatr Scand 2000; **101**:444–51; n = 154, Swann et al, Am J Psychiatry 1999; **156**:1264–6; n = 40, RCT, d/b, p/c, 4/52, Kafantaris et al, J Am Acad Child Adolesc Psychiatry 2004; **43**:984–93).

Review: efficacy and side-effects in mania (Bowden, J Clin Psychiatry 2000; **61**[Suppl 9]: S35–S40).

Olanzapine (see also combinations)

Olanzapine is licensed in many countries for acute mania. The starting dose is 15mg/d as monotherapy or 10mg/d in combination. Two Lilly RCTs have shown efficacy as monotherapy in mania, e.g. in acute mania, response to olanzapine (49%) was better than placebo (24%) (n = 139, RCT, 3/52, Tohen et al, Am J Psychiatry 1999; **156**:702–9, MS) and olanzapine (mean 17mg/d) produced a significantly greater improvement in mania scores and protocol-defined remission in acute mania than valproate (mean 1400 mg/d), with more weight gain, somnolence, dry mouth and increased appetite, but less nausea (n = 248, RCT, d/b, 3/52, Tohen et al, Am J Psychiatry 2002;**159**:1011–17, MS). It may be effective in bipolar mania in adolescents (13–17 years old) but had a significant side-effect burden (n = 161, RCT, d/b, p/c, 3/52, Tohen et al, Am J Psychiatry 2007;**164**:1547–56). Cochrane concludes that olanzapine is effective in mania, possibly more so than valproate, but with more weight gain and somnolence (n = 1422, s = 6, Rendell et al, Cochrane Database Syst Rev 2003;**3**:CD004040), although some feel valproate was underdosed (Lu, EBMH 2003;**6**:28). Olanzapine 'Velotabs' produce a plasma level profile similar to oral tablets but may be a suitable alternative to injections in some cases by assuring compliance.

Reviews: short-term management of bipolar I mania (Bhana and Perry, CNS Drugs 2001;**15**:871–904), evidence for relapse prevention following mania (Dando and Tohen, J Psychopharmacol 2006;**20**[suppl]:31–8).

Quetiapine * (see also combinations)

Quetiapine is licensed as monotherapy for the short-term treatment of acute manic episodes associated with bipolar I disorder. Two RCTs have shown efficacy, e.g. quetiapine was as effective as haloperidol in acute mania but better tolerated, with a final dose range of 400–800 mg/d (n = 302, RCT, d/b, p/c, 12/52, McIntyre et al, Eur Neuropsychopharmacol 2005;**15**:573–85) and up to 800 mg/d was as effective as lithium and both were superior to placebo in bipolar mania using YMRS (n = 302, RCT, d/b, p/c, 12/52, Bowden et al, J Clin Psychiatry 2005;**66**:111–21). Quetiapine was at least as effective as valproate in adolescent mania (n = 50, RCT, d/b, 28/7, DelBello et al, J Am Acad Child Adolesc Psychiatry 2006;**45**:305–13). Rapid dose escalation (300/600 mg/d on successive days) is generally tolerable and rapidly effective although additional bp monitoring would be prudent.

Risperidone (see also combinations)

Risperidone is licensed in the UK for monotherapy in bipolar mania. Two RCTs have shown efficacy, e.g. risperidone was more effective than placebo (42% vs 13% remission) in mania (n = 291, RCT, d/b, p/c, 3/52, Gopal et al, J Clin Psychiatry 2005;**66**:1016–20, MS; comment by Khanna, EBMH 2006;**9**:40) and in acute mania (YMRS > 20) risperidone 1–6 mg/d produced significant improvement in symptoms (n = 290, RCT, d/b, p/c, 3/52, Khanna et al, Br J Psychiatry 2005;**187**:229–34, MS). Although there is some controversy about this second study, the mania was severe and with low drop-outs, it shows that risperidone is also effective in very ill patients. Onset can be rapidly effective (within a week) as an adjunctive treatment to mood stabilisers in mania, especially if carbamazepine-treated patients are excluded (n = 151, RCT, d/b, p/c, 3/52, Yatham et al, Br J Psychiatry 2003;**182**:141–7; see 4.5.1 for reasons). In a further sub-analysis of this trial, it appears risperidone can be safely combined with valproate or lithium in acute mania (n = 79, 12/52, Yatham et al, Int Clin Psychopharmacol 2004;**19**:103–9). Cochrane concludes that risperidone is effective in mania as both monotherapy and adjunctive treatment (s = 6, n = 1343, Rendell et al, Cochrane Database Syst Rev 2006;**1**:CD004043).

Reviews: general (Nguyen and Guthrie, Ann Pharmacother 2006;**40**:674–82; Fenton and Scott, CNS Drugs 2005;**19**:429–44).

Valproate semisodium

Valproate semisodium (aka divalproex) is licensed in the UK as monotherapy for acute mania. Several RCTs have shown efficacy, e.g. a robust trial showed valproate to be as effective as lithium in acute mania, independently of a prior responsiveness to lithium (n = 174, RCT, p/c, 21/7, Bowden et al, JAMA 1994;**271**:918–24) and may be more effective than lithium and as effective as (but better tolerated than) olanzapine (n = 348, s = 3, RCT, d/b, Hirschfeld et al, J Clin Psychiatry 2003;**64**:841–6, MS; n = 120, RCT, d/b, 12/52, Zajecka et al, J Clin Psychiatry 2003;**63**:1148–55). A realistic study under realistic conditions, including more severely ill patients, suggests that prompt rapid stabilisation with valproate may allow transition to maintenance without antipsychotics (n = 136, RCT, d/b, p/c, 21/7, Müller-Oerlinghausen et al, J Clin Psychopharmacol 2000;**20**:195–203; review by Swann, *EBMH* 2000;**3**:113). Valproate augmentation of TAU decreased heavy drinking in bipolars with co-occurring alcohol dependence (n = 59, RCT, d/b, p/c, 24/52, Salloum et al, *Arch Gen Psychiatry* 2005; **62**:37–45). Cochrane concludes that there is consistent if limited evidence that valproate is effective in acute mania; it may be less effective than olanzapine but with less sedation and weight gain (s = 10, Macritchie et al, *Cochrane Database Syst Rev* 2003;**1**:CD004052). There appears to be a linear relationship between valproate serum concentration and response in acute mania, best response being above 94 mcg/ml, presumably as trough levels, although this is unclear in the paper (n = 374, s = 3, RCT, Allen et al, *Am J Psychiatry* 2006;**163**:272–5). Subsequently, oral loading doses of valproate are probably more rapidly effective in mania, e.g. 20 mg/kg/d may give a rapid response, often within three days (n = 36, RCT, 6/7, McElroy et al, *J Clin Psychiatry* 1996;**57**:142–6). Even more aggressive dosing (30 mg/kg/d on days one and two, then 20 mg/kg/d days 3–10) may produce more rapid therapeutic levels in acute mania, with no adverse effects (n = 59, RCT, Hirschfeld et al, *J Clin Psychiatry* 1999;**60**:815–18). High-dose IV valproate (20 mg/kg) over 30 minutes had no effect in acute mania (n = 7, Phrolov et al, *J Clin Psychiatry* 2004;**65**:68–70), but IV has been successfully used for adolescent mania (n = 5, Thakur et al, *Eur Child Adolesc Psychiatry* 2004;**13**:258–61). Valproate infusion (initially 125 mg over one hour) has been used and may also be rapidly effective (n = 1, Herbert and Nelson, *Am J Psychiatry* 2000;**157**:1023–4). The equivalent amount of valproic acid resulting from Depakote® 500 mg (Sanofi-Aventis), Epilim EC® 500 mg (Sanofi-Aventis) and Epilim Chrono® 500 mg (Sanofi-Aventis) are 500 mg, 433 mg and 433 mg respectively (MI).

Reviews: general (Bowden, *Bipolar Disord* 2003; **5**:189–202), loading dose strategies (Keck et al, *Bipolar Disord* 2000:**2**:42–6).

+ Combinations

In acute mania, combinations are rightfully commonly used. A review of all adjunctive treatment studies in acute mania notes that combinations are more effective than monotherapy and so lower doses can be used and tolerability is higher, improving longer-term retention in therapy (Sachs and Gardner-Schuster, *Acta Psychiatr Scand* Suppl 2007;**434**:27–34). A meta-analysis has concluded that adding an antipsychotic to an established mood stabliser is more effective than a mood stabliser alone (s = 8, n = 1124, RCT, Smith et al, *Acta Psychiatr Scand* 2007;**115**:12–20).

Review: * combining antipsychotics with another medicine (Goodwin et al, *Eur Neuropsychopharmacol* 2009;**19**:520–32).

Antipsychotics + benzodiazepines

See individual drugs or groups in this section (see also Acute Psychiatric Emergency 1.1).

Lithium + allopurinol *

Allopurinol 600 mg/d was significantly superior to placebo as an adjunct to lithium in mania and may provide an alternative to antipsychotics (n = 120, RCT, d/b, p/c, 4/52, Machado-Vieira et al, *J Clin Psychiatry* 2008;**69**:1237–45).

Lithium + antipsychotics

A review of these combinations concluded that the slow onset of action of lithium/valproate means that they are more adjuncts to antipsychotics initially, rather than vice versa (Cookson, *Br J Psychiatry* 2001;**178**[Suppl 41]:S148–S56). See also individual antipsychotics in BNF listed section. **Olanzapine** was superior to placebo as an add-on to valproate in manic and mixed bipolar episodes, although weight gain with olanzapine was significant (n = 344, RCT, d/b, 6/52, Tohen et al, *Arch Gen Psychiatry* 2002;**59**:62–9, MS; comment by Gardner, *EBMH* 2002;**5**:89). **Quetiapine** was also superior to placebo when added to lithium and well tolerated (n = 191[c = 105], RCT, 21/7, d/b, p/c, Sachs et al, *Bipolar Disord* 2004;**6**:213–23) and 500 mg/d (range 300–700 mg/d) was superior to placebo when combined with lithium or divalproex for bipolar mania, and was well tolerated (n = 402, RCT, d/b, p/c, 6/52, Yatham et al, *J Clin Psychopharmacol* 2004;**24**:599–606). **Risperidone** plus mood stabiliser (lithium or valproate) was as effective as haloperidol plus mood stabiliser and more effective than a mood stabiliser alone in acute mania (n = 156, RCT, d/b, p/c, 3/52, Sachs et al, Am J Psychiatry 2002;**159**:1146–54).

Lithium + carbamazepine

Carbamazepine can be used in resistant cases in combination with lithium (review of literature in Compr Psychiatry 1990;**31**:261–5). See 4.4 for neurotoxicity warning.

Olanzapine + carbamazepine

Olanzapine plus carbamazepine had no advantage (and had more side-effects) compared to carbamazepine alone in mania, (n = 118, RCT, d/b, p/c, 6 + 20/52, Tohen et al, Br J Psychiatry 2008;**192**:135–43; MS).

Valproate + antipsychotics *

Augmentation of valproate with amisulpride and haloperidol were equally effective but the former had fewer side-effects and was more tolerable (n = 123, RCT, open, 3/12, Thomas et al, Neuropsychiatr Dis Treat 2008;**4**:675–86). Olanzapine was superior to placebo as an add-on to valproate in manic and mixed bipolar episodes, although weight gain with olanzapine was significant (n = 344, RCT, d/b, 6/52, Tohen et al, Arch Gen Psychiatry 2002;**59**:62–9, MS; comment by Gardner, EBMH 2002;**5**:89). Quetiapine was also superior to placebo when added to valproate semisodium, and well tolerated (n = 191 [c = 105], RCT, 21/7, d/b, p/c, Sachs et al, Bipolar Disord 2004;**6**:213–23; n = 402, RCT, d/b, p/c, 6/52, Yatham et al, J Clin Psychopharmacol 2004;**24**:599–606). Risperidone plus mood stabiliser (lithium or valproate) was as effective as haloperidol plus mood stabiliser and more effective than a mood stabiliser alone in acute mania (n = 156, RCT, d/b, p/c, 3/52, Sachs et al, Am J Psychiatry 2002;**159**:1146–54).

Valproate + folic acid *

Folic acid added to valproate was superior to placebo as an adjuvant in acute mania, an astonishing finding (n=88, RCT, d/b, p/c, 3/52, Behzadi et al, Acta Psychiatr Scand 2009; 120:441–5).

Valproate + lithium

Valproate may successfully augment lithium in resistant rapid-cycling mania in elderly patients (n = 4, Schneider and Wilcox, J Affect Disord 1998;**47**:201–5) and in adults (n = 12, open, Reischies et al, Neuropsychobiol 2002;**46**[Suppl 1]:S22–S27).

● **Unlicensed/some efficacy**

Antipsychotics *
(see also aripiprazole, olanzapine, quetiapine and risperidone in BNF listed section) *

There is some evidence that hypomania has a hyperdopaminergic component (Cousins et al, Bipolar Disord 2009;**11**:787–806) and a review of 15 RCTs showed that antipsychotics produce a more rapid antimanic effect than lithium (predictably), but lithium is superior at three weeks (Keck et al, J Clin Psychiatry 1998;**59**[Suppl 6]:S74–S81). **Amisulpride** (about 700mg/d) was effective for mania in a pilot study (n = 20 [c = 14], open, 6/52, Vieta et al, J Clin Psychiatry 2005;**66**:575–8). Although obviously problematic, **clozapine** (mean 500mg/d) may be effective in 72% treatment-resistant manics or schizo-affectives (n = 25, open, Calabrese et al, Am J Psychiatry 1996;**153**:759–64) and compared to TAU in bipolar (n = 38, RCT, one year, Suppes et al, Am J Psychiatry 1999;**156**:1164–9). **Haloperidol** was superior to placebo at up to 8mg/d (n = 302, RCT, d/b, p/c, 12/52, McIntyre et al, Eur Neuropsychopharmacol 2005;**15**:573–85) and Cochrane concludes that haloperidol is superior to placebo and equivalent to other antimanic antipsychotics (but possibly inferior to aripiprazole), albeit poorly tolerated (s = 15, n = 2022, Cipriani et al, Cochrane Database Syst Rev 2006;**3**:CD004362). **Ziprasidone** is licensed in the USA for acute mania and 40–80mg BD produced a rapid (within two days) and sustained improvement in acute bipolar symptoms in one study (n = 210, RCT, p/c, d/b, 3/52, Keck et al, Am J Psychiatry 2003;**160**:741–8) A pilot study showed **zotepine** (mean 250mg/d) monotherapy is effective in severe mania (n = 12 [c = 10], open, 3/52, Amann et al, Bipolar Disord 2005;**7**:471–6).

Benzodiazepines

For a group of drugs routinely used in mania, there is remarkably little robust evidence for the efficacy of benzodiazepines, but use is supported by extensive clinical experience. Short-term medium or high doses of benzodiazepines can be used alone or as adjuncts to other therapies in acute phases of hypomania, e.g. diazepam by itself, lorazepam (Salzman et al, Psychosomatics 1986;**27**:17–21), or clonazepam at 4–16mg/d (n = 12, RCT, d/b, c/o, Chouinard et al, Biol Psychiatry 1983;**18**:451–66). For acute symptoms they have a rapid onset, are highly sedative and are well tolerated, with no EPSE side-effect risk, but have little or no long-term role. A meta-analysis concluded that the data supported the safe and effective use of clonazepam in mania, although there was not exactly a lot to meta-analyse (s = 7, n = 206, RCT, Curtin and Schulz, J Affect Disord 2004;**78**:201–8).

Phenytoin

Phenytoin augmentation of haloperidol in acute mania was more effective than haloperidol alone, and may indicate that blockade of voltage-activated sodium channels is a common therapeutic mechanism for anticonvulsants in acute mania (n = 39, RCT, 5/52, Mishory et al, Am J Psychiatry 2000;**157**:463–5).

Tamoxifen

Tamoxifen (a protein kinase C inhibitor) has, at last, an RCT confirming that it has significant antimanic activity and is remarkably well tolerated (n = 66 [c=50], RCT, d/b, p/c, 3/52, Yildiz et al, Arch Gen Psychiatry 2007;**64**:255–63). Tamoxifen 20–140mg/d was also significantly superior (63% response) to placebo (13% response) in bipolar mania, as early as day 5 (n = 16, d/b, p/c, 3/52, Zarate et al, Bipolar Disorders 2007;**9**:561–70).

■ Unlicensed/possible efficacy

Allopurinol

YMRS improved when allupurinol (300mg/d) was added to lithium and haloperidol in acute mania, albeit not quite statistically significant (n = 82, RCT, d/b, p/c, Akhondzadeh et al, Bipolar Disord 2006;**8**:485–9).

Levetiracetam

A pilot trial of adjunctive levetiracetam 500–2000mg/d showed some improvement in most manic patients, but was not wildly encouraging (n = 34, open, 8/52, Post et al, J Clin Psychiatry 2005;**66**:370–4). There is a well-documented case of acute mania responding to levetiracetam up to 2500mg/d (n = 1, Goldberg and Burdick, Am J Psychiatry 2002;**159**:148), and up to 4g/d appears to have some antimanic effect when used with haloperidol (n = 10, open, 28/7, Grunze et al, J Clin Psychiatry 2003;**64**:781–4).

Memantine *

Memantine may have some efficacy, and appears well tolerated (n = 33, open, Keck et al, Clin Neuropharmacol 2009;**32**:199–204).

Omega-3 fatty acids

Fish oils may have some efficacy (review by Maidment, Acta Psychiatr Scand 2000;**102**: 3–11).

Oxcarbazepine *

Oxcarbazepine has been used successfully in acute mania. Oxcarbazepine 1–2.4g/d was as effective as valproate in acute mania (n = 60, RCT, d/b, 12/52, Kakkar et al, Eur Psychiatry 2009;**24**:178–82), and 750–2000mg/d as an add-on to lithium was effective in 60%, and may be helpful long-term in some patients (n = 17, open, 8/52 + 12/12, Benedetti et al, J Affect Disord 2004;**79**:273–7). Oxcarbazepine was not significantly superior to placebo in youths (7–18 years) with bipolar mania (n = 116, RCT, d/b, p/c, 7/52, Wagner et al, Am J Psychiatry 2006;**163**:1179–86; comment by MacMillan and Heydrich, EBMH 2007;**10**:59).

Propofol

Propofol has been effective as an IV drip in multidrug resistant, severe, life-threatening mania (n = 1, Cluver and Hardesty, J Clin Psychiatry 2006; **67**:165–6).

Topiramate

Data on topiramate as an adjunct is mixed. Open trials have suggested modest efficacy in mania (n = 14, open, 4/52, Bozikas et al, Prog Neuropsychopharmacol Biol Psychiatry 2002;**26**:1203–6; 50% response, n = 10, open, 28/7, Calabrese et al, J Clin Psychopharmacol 2001;**21**:340–2), although a manufacturer's analysis concluded that there was no evidence to support routine use as monotherapy in mania (s = 4, RCT, Kushner et al, Bipolar Disord 2006;8:15–27). In the only RCT, topiramate had no effect as a mood stabiliser adjunct to lithium or valproate compared to placebo in bipolar I manic or mixed episodes, but at least people lost significant amounts of weight (n = 287, RCT, d/b, p/c, 12/52, Chengappa et al, J Clin Psychiatry 2006;67:1698–1706; MS). Topiramate and risperidone combined may be useful for short and long-term management of mania (n = 58[c = 41], open, 12/12, Vieta et al, J Clin Psychiatry 2003;64:834–9). Cochrane has concluded that there was, as yet, insufficient evidence for use as monotherapy or adjunctive for acute mania (Vasudev et al, Cochrane Database Syst Rev 2006;1:CD003384).

Tryptophan depletion

Acute tryptophan depletion may have an antimanic effect, albeit poorly tolerated (n = 23[c = 17], RCT, d/b, p/c, 7/7, Applebaum et al, Bipolar Disord 2007;9:884–7).

Verapamil *

Verapamil monotherapy appears to have no antimanic activity but may be highly effective in combination with lithium, possibly by enhancing pKC inhibition (n = 45, RCT, open, 9/52, Mallinger et al, Bipolar Disord 2008;10:856–66; n = 50[c = 50], RCT, d/b, 4/52, Singh, Int J Psychiatr Clin Pract 2008;12:303–8). An earlier naturalistic study in bipolar women suggested that verapamil was effective in mania with a response rate comparable to other mood stabilisers (n = 10437 women, open, Wisner et al, Biol Psychiatry 2002;5:745–52).

Zonisamide

Adjunctive zonisamide has improved mania and depression in many patients but mood deteriorated in 32% patients, although nearly all lost weight (n = 62[c=40], open, 8/52, McElroy et al, J Clin Psychiatry 2005;66:617–24).

◆ Others

Other drugs tried include **dexamfetamine** (Clower, Psychopharmacol Bull 1988;24:168), **clonidine** (in antipsychotic-resistant mania;

Jouvent et al, Br J Psychiatry 1988;152:293), **levothyroxine** (0.3–0.5 mg/d for rapid or 48-hour cycling mania; n = 7, Stancer and Persad, Arch Gen Psychiatry 1982;39:311–2), **methylene blue** (to reduce pathotoxic vanadium ion concentrations; Moody et al, Biol Psychiatry 1989; 26:850–2) and **spironolactone** (n = 1, Gillman and Lichtigfeld, Br Med J 1986;292:661–2).

□ No efficacy

Antidepressants

Antidepressants can either precipitate mania by provoking a mood switch, or exacerbate existing or developing mania (n = 1864, Lim et al, Bipolar Disord 2001;3:165–73).

Caffeine *

A high caffeine intake will risk disturbing sleep patterns and exacerbating mania, e.g. discontinuing heavy use has helped resolve treatment-resistant schizo-affective mania (n=1, Caykoylu et al, Prog Neuropsychopharmacol Biol Psychiatry 2008;32:1349–50).

Dipyridamole *

Dipyridamole 200mg/d was ineffective as an adjunct to lithium in bipolar mania (n = 120, RCT, d/b, p/c, 4/52, Machado-Vieira et al, J Clin Psychiatry 2008;69:1237–45; see also allopurinol, another purinergic agent).

Fosphenytoin

IV fosphenytoin appears ineffective in acute mania (n = 7, open, 1 hour, Applebaum et al, J Clin Psychiatry 2003;64:408–9).

Gabapentin

The only two controlled studies have failed to show any advantage as an adjunct over placebo in mania (e.g. n = 117, d/b, p/c, Pande, Gabapentin study group, Bipolar Disord 1999;1[Suppl 1]:S17; Pande et al, J Clin Psychopharmacol 1999;19:341–8), and the trend was towards a negative effect. However, a number of case reports and open studies (n = 25, up to 1440mg/d, Cabras et al, J Clin Psychiatry 1999;60:245–8) had suggested a potential effect in mania in some people, a good advert for evidence-based approaches to treatment.

Lamotrigine

Lamotrigine has no efficacy in acute mania and only delays the time to manic relapse in pooled data. It may be more effective in male bipolar patients with fewer prior medication trials (n = 45, Obrocea et al, Biol Psychiatry 2002;51:253–60).

Tiagabine

Tiagabine had no detectable anti-manic activity as monotherapy or adjunctive therapy compared to standard treatments (n = 8, open, 14/7, Grunze et al, J Clin Psychiatry 1999; 60:759–62).

1.10.3 BIPOLAR DEPRESSION *

Bipolar depression is longer-lasting than unipolar depression (up to 50% may still be depressed at one year; Hlastala et al, Depress Anxiety 1997;5:73–83), frequently misdiagnosed (a substantial proportion of antidepressant-refractory depression is probably undiagnosed bipolar; n = 6, Inoue et al, J Affect Disord 2006;95:61–7) and is more likely to have psychosis, diurnal variation, and hypersomnia during depressive episodes, and a greater number of shorter episodes (e.g. n = 1036, Forty et al, Br J Psychiatry 2008;192:388–9). It is clear that well-being and functioning are inversely proportional to the number of bipolar episodes and so strategies to reduce relapse must be rigorously followed, especially minimising difficult-to-treat bipolar depression. It can be potentiated by substance and alcohol misuse and is much more difficult to treat.

The general principles of management include:
1. **Avoid inducing mixed affective states** with antidepressants, particularly in bipolar III, where the risk of self-harm is high.
2. **Use mood stabilisers:** In the largest non-commercial study in acute phase bipolar depression, an antidepressant (paroxetine up to 40 mg/d or bupropion up to 375 mg/d) plus a mood stabiliser (lithium, valproate, carbamazepine or a licensed antimanic agent, e.g. olanzapine, risperidone, aripiprazole, quetiapine, ziprasidone) had a slightly poorer response (based on euthymia at 8/52) than people receiving just a mood stabiliser and placebo, indicating that longer-term adjunc-

tive antidepressants have no therapeutic advantage, but at least the antidepressant did not increase the risk of relapse, switch to mania or have greater ADRs (n = 366, RCT, d/b, p/c, 26/52, STEP-BD, Sachs et al, N Engl J Med 2007;356:1711–22; comment by Rao et al, EBMH 2007;10:109).
3. **Optimise antidepressants** (e.g. n = 2032, Moller et al, J Affect Disord 2001;67:141–6): Use with MS and start with lowest switch risk drugs, e.g. SSRIs, mirtazapine, bupropion or moclobemide, but avoid tricyclics, MAOIs and venlafaxine if possible (s = 12, n = 1088, RCTs, Gijsman et al, Am J Psychiatry 2004;161:1537–47; comment by Masand and Mago, EBMH 2005;8:35).
4. **Minimise antidepressant exposure** by attempting gradual taper after a continuation phase, provided the patient is genuinely euthymic. Consider, however, that premature discontinuing antidepressants within the first 3–6/12 of an episode (n = 25) has an up to three times higher relapse rate than those continuing for at least 8/12 (n = 19), with no increase in mania in the latter group (n = 44, retrospective, one year, Altshuler et al, J Clin Psychiatry 2001;62:612–6).
5. **Avoid switching to mania with anti-depressants** * — in bipolar depression this usually occurs within the first 12 weeks. The risk is highest in bipolar I and bipolar II then lowest with MDD (s = 13 [7 RCTs], Bond et al, J Clin Psychiatry 2008;69:1589–601; n = 184, 10/52, Altshuler et al, Am J Psychiatry 2006;163:313–5), and is lower if antidepressants are used with a mood stabiliser (n = 136, Mundo et al, J Affect Disord 2006;92:227–30). If depression develops, the best plan is to reduce the antidepressant dose immediately and allow the mood to settle for a month or so. Addition of an antidepressant to a mood stabiliser is probably more effective than adding a second mood stabiliser (paroxetine vs lithium or valproate; n = 27, RCT, d/b, 6/52, Young et al, Am J Psychiatry 2000;157:124–6), particularly in people unable to tolerate higher lithium doses (n = 117, d/b, p/c, 10/52, Nemeroff et al, Am J Psychiatry 2001;158:906–12). The switch rates in trials have been reported to be:

- placebo 7%
- sertraline 2%
- bupropion 4%.
- fluoxetine 0–16%
- venlafaxine 9%
- imipramine 9.5–28%
- tranylcypromine 24%.

A retrospective Polish study showed that antidepressant-induced switching from depression to mania was more common in women and with TCAs vs non-TCAs (36% vs. 17%), with amitriptyline (42%), imipramine (42%) and clomipramine (35%) being the highest risk (n=333, Koszewska and Rybakowski, *Neuropsychobiology* 2009; **59**:12–6).

References: n = 174, RCT, 10/52, Post *et al, Br J Psychiatry* 2006;**189**:124–31; n = 34, RCT, p/c, d/b, 8/52, Amsterdam and Shults, *J Affect Disord* 2005;**87**:121–30.

6. **Avoid sudden dose changes** or switches.
7. **Offer ECT** for patients at immediate risk of self-harm or unable to tolerate antidepressants (n = 6, Macedo-Soares *et al, J ECT* 2005;**21**:31–4). ECT may be better in older people.
8. **Check thyroid function** — poor response in bipolar depression may be related to low FTI and high TSH levels, even if in the alleged therapeutic range (n = 65, Cole *et al, Am J Psychiatry* 2002;**159**:116–21).

Reviews: * general (Goodnick, *Expert Opin Pharmacother* 2007;**8**:13–21; Azorin and Kaladjian, *Expert Opin Pharmacother* 2009;**10**:161–72; Malhi et al, *Bipolar Disorders* 2009;**11**(suppl 2):55–76; Vieta, *Acta Psychiatr Scand* 2008;**118**:335–6), ECNP consensus (Goodwin *et al, Eur Neuro-psychopharmacology* 2008;**18**:535–49), BAP guidelines (Goodwin *et al, J Psychopharmacol* 2009;**23**:346–88), newer antipsychotics (Cruz et al, *Int J Neuropsychopharmacol* 2009;[in press].

BNF listed

Quetiapine *

Quetiapine is now licensed for treatment of severe depressive episodes in bipolar disorder, but not for prevention of recurrence. A slower dose increase is recommended: (night-time, day 1 50mg; day 2 100mg; day 3 200mg; day 4 300mg). Monotherapy efficacy has been shown in two robust RCTs (BOLDER 1 and 2). BOLDER 1 showed response rates in bipolar I depression of 58.2% (600mg/d) and 57.6% (300mg/d), compared with 36% for placebo (remission was 52.9% vs 28.4%). Treatment for emergent mania was 3–4% for both groups (n = 542, RCT, d/b, p/c, 8/52, Calabrese et al, *Am J Psychiatry* 2005;**162**:1351–60). A secondary analysis showed an anxiolytic effect in bipolar I depression (n = 542, RCT, 8/52, p/c, Hirschfeld et al, *J Clin Psychiatry* 2006;**67**:355–62) and a post-hoc analysis showed an NNT = 5 for response and remission of bipolar depression (Cookson et al, *Int Clin Psychopharmacol* 2007;**22**:93–100). BOLDER 2 showed quetiapine 300mg and 600mg/d monotherapy were equally effective in bipolar I and II depression, with less switching than placebo and the effect visible from week 1 (n = 509 [c = 300], RCT, 8/52, d/b, p/c, Thase et al, *J Clin Psychopharmacol* 2006;**26**:600–9; s = 2, n = 694, RCT, d/b, p/c, 8/52, Weisler et al, *J Clin Psychiatry* 2008;**69**:769–82), replicated by the EMBOLDEN trials (e.g. n = 270, RCT, d/b, p/c, 8/52, Suppes et al, *J Affect Disord* 2010;**12**:106-15).

Reviews: * general (Thase, *Neuropsychiatr Dis Treat* 2008;**4**:11–21; s=5, RCT, d/b, p/c, Bogart and Chavez, *Ann Pharmacother* 2009; **43**:1848–56; Keating and Robinson, *Drugs* 2007;**67**:1077–95).

+ Combinations

Lithium + lamotrigine *

In the only augmentation study, significantly more people responded to lamotrigine augmentation of lithium than placebo in acute bipolar depression (n = 124, RCT, d/b, p/c, 8/52, van der Loos et al, *J Clin Psychiatry* 2009;**70**:223–31; see also n = 21, one year, Ghaemi et al, *J Psychiatr Pract* 2006;**12**:300–5).

Olanzapine + fluoxetine (OFC) *

The olanzapine-fluoxetine combination (OFC) is licensed for bipolar depression in the US as 'Symbyax' (6/25, 6/50, or 12/50 mg/day), and has been compared to olanzapine (5–20 mg/day), and placebo (n = 833, RCT, d/b, p/c, 8/52, Tohen et al, *Arch Gen Psychiatry* 2003;**60**:1079–88, MS; secondary analysis, n = 833, RCT, d/b, p/c, Shi et al, *Clin Ther* 2004;**26**:125–34, MS), although this study had no fluoxetine arm and so the combination's efficacy might be predominantly from fluoxetine and the effect may not be maintained if the fluoxetine is stopped (n = 114[c = 83], RCT, open, 7+12/52, Tamayo et al, J Clin Psychopharmacol 2009;**29**:358–61). OFC was more effective than lamotrigine 200mg/d for bipolar I depression but with more side-effects, although relapses were equivalent (n = 410, RCT, d/b, 25/52, Brown et al, Int J Neuropsychopharmacol 2009;**12**:773–82, MS; see also n = 410, RCT, d/b, 7/52, Brown et al, J Clin Psychiatry 2006;**67**:1025–33: MS; comment by Nirenberg, EBMH 2007;**10**:12, noting that the 5/52 titration period with lamotrigine would have left only 2/52 at full dose so it is surprising it did so well), and may have some efficacy in relapse prevention (n = 560, open, 76/52, Corya et al, J Clin Psychiatry 2003;**64**:1349–56; MS).

Reviews: * general (Deeks and Keating, CNS Drugs 2008;**22**:793–5; Owen, Drugs Today [Barc] 2006;**42**:185–92).

Lithium + fluoxetine

Fluoxetine-augmentation of lithium in bipolar mood disorder can help prevent breakthrough depression (n = 26, open, three-year, Tondo et al, Int J Psychiatry Clin Pract 1997;**1**:203–6).

● Unlicensed/some efficacy

Antidepressants *

Antidepressants can be effective in treating bipolar depression, but once mood has lifted there is the risk of inducing a switch to mania or rapid-cycling. In adults with bipolar depression, venlafaxine, bupropion and sertraline all produce similar acute responses (49–53%) and remission (34–41%), but the risk of switching to mania or hypomania is variable (see general principles, point 5). A recent review of antidepressants in bipolar depression (Licht et al, Acta Psychiatr Scand 2008;**118**:337–46) concludes:

- Switching occurs anyway
- Antidepressants seem safe when combined with a mood stabiliser
- Antidepressant monotherapy cannot be recommended, especially in bipolar I
- Perception of switching may be because

antidepressants shorten depressed phases
- If mania develops, stopping or reducing the antidepressant dose is advisable, although no guidance available
- Accelerated episode frequency is unproven but considered likely.

Fluoxetine may have a low switch rate in bipolar I and II (n = 34, RCT, p/c, d/b, 8/52, Amsterdam and Shults, J Affect Disord 2005;**87**:121–30). **Bupropion** has been used as an adjunct in resistant, bipolar depression (n = 13, open, Erfurth et al, Neuropsychobiology 2001;**45**[Suppl 1]:S33–S36). **Citalopram** has been shown to be effective in bipolar I and II depression, with a robust and sustained response rate and low ADRs (n = 45, open, 8/52, Kupfer et al, Clin Psych 2001;**62**:985–90). Citalopram and lamotrigine may be useful adjunctives in bipolar depression, with response rates rising considerably past the first six weeks (n = 20, RCT, d/b, 12/52, Schaffer et al, J Affect Disord 2006;**96**:95–9). **Escitalopram** may have some efficacy in bipolar depression (n = 20, open, 12/52, Fonseca et al, J Clin Psychiatry 2006;**67**:81–6). **Moclobemide** 450–750mg/d may be as effective as imipramine (150–250mg/d) in bipolar depression, with less side-effects and less switches to mania (2 vs 6) indicating a useful potential role (n = 156, RCT, 8/52, Silverstone et al, Acta Psychiatr Scand 2001;**104**:104–9). In the STEP-BD study, for bipolars developing a new-onset depressive episode there is no evidence that antidepressants were associated with new-onset suicidality, even in already high-risk populations (n = 425, Bauer et al, J Clin Psychiatry 2006;**67**:48–55). One study showed that continuing antidepressants after a depressive episode was **not** associated with an increased risk of manic episodes, but early discontinuation was associated with significantly increased depressive relapse (n = 84, one year, naturalistic, Altshuler et al, Am J Psychiatry 2003;**160**:1252–62). **Tricyclics** should be avoided unless covered with mood stabilisers (n = 136, Mundo et al, J Affect Disord 2006;**92**:227–30). In bipolar depression, response to **venlafaxine** reduces after repeated exposure (n=83, RCT, open, Amsterdam and Shults, J Aff Disorders 2009;**115**:234–40). **Tranylcypromine** appeared effective (62.5% responded) in refractory bipolar depression in an incomplete study (n = 19, RCT, open, Nolen et al, Acta Psychiatr Scand 2007;**115**:360–5).

Antipsychotics (see also quetiapine & OFC)*

The main roles of antipsychotics in bipolar depression are as adjunctives to mood stabilisers and as adjunctive maintenance in treatment-resistance. There is some preliminary data on the use of **aripiprazole**, e.g. mean 15mg/d was effective and reasonably well tolerated as add-on in resistant bipolar depression (n = 30[c = 16], open, Ketter et al, Ann Clin Psychiatry 2006;**18**:169–72) and aripiprazole as adjunctive (54%) or monotherapy (46%) was associated with some improvements (n = 85[c = 80], open, 16/52, Mazza et al, Expert Opin Pharmacother 2008;**9**:3145–9), supported by a chart review (n = 12, 8/52, Kemp et al, Prog Neuropsychopharmacol Biol Psychiatry 2007;**31**:574–7). Low-dose **ziprasidone** (mean 58mg/d) may have a potential for bipolar depression (n = 30, Liebowitz et al, J Affect Disord 2009;**118**:205–8).

Lamotrigine *

Lamotrigine is licensed in the US (but not UK) for the maintenance treatment of bipolar I depression and relapse prevention. A robust and independent meta-analysis of the five studies (three unpublished) showed a consistently beneficial effect in bipolar depression, greater in more severe depression (s = 5, n = 1072, RCT, d/b, p/c, Geddes et al, Br J Psychiatry 2009;**194**:4–9). In the key earlier study, lamotrigine 50–200mg/d monotherapy was significantly more effective than placebo in bipolar I depression, the effect being seen as early as the third week (n = 195[c = 136], RCT, d/b, p/c, 7/52, Calabrese et al, J Clin Psychiatry 1999;**60**:79–88). In patients with bipolar depression unresponsive to a mood stabiliser and at least one antidepressant, response to lamotrigine was 24% (cf. inositol 17% and risperidone 5%; n = 66, RCT, 16/52, open, Nierenberg et al, Am J Psychiatry 2006; **163**:210–6). Mode of action may be inhibition of sodium and calcium channels in presynaptic neurons, and subsequent neuronal membrane stabilisation. Increasing the dose slowly over 6/52 to 200mg/d minimises the incidence of serious rash, especially with valproate.

Reviews: * general (Thase, Neuropsychiatr Dis Treat 2008;**4**:11–21; Goldsmith et al, Drugs 2003;**63**:2029–50), mode of action in mood disorders (Ketter et al, J Clin Psychopharmacol 2003;**23**:484–95).

Omega-3 fatty acids

Ethyl-EPA (ethyl-eicopentaenoic acid) was effective in bipolar depression, with 1–2g/d superior to placebo (n = 75, RCT, d/b, p/c, 12/52, Frangou et al, Br J Psychiatry 2006;**188**:46–50), but in another study EPA 6g/d had no overall efficacy on any marker in bipolar depression (RCT, p/c, 4/12, Keck et al, Biol Psychiatry 2006;**60**:1020–3) so dose may be important (n = 12[c = 8], open, 6/12, Osher et al, J Clin Psychiatry 2005; **66**:726–9).

■ Unlicensed/possible efficacy

Gabapentin

While gabapentin has no antimanic activity (see 1.10.2), it may be useful as an adjunct in refractory and comorbid bipolar patients (review, s = 40, Carta et al, J Affect Disord 2003;**75**:83–91). Gabapentin augmentation was effective and well tolerated in mild-to-moderate bipolar depression (n = 22, open pilot, 12/52, Wang et al, Bipolar Disord 2002;**4**:296–301). However, in a trial against lamotrigine, gabapentin was no better than placebo (n = 45, RCT, p/c, d/b, c/o, 6/52, Obrocea et al, Biol Psychiatry 2002;**51**:253–60).

Inositol

Inositol may be useful in bipolar (as well as unipolar) depression, as shown in a trial where 50% responded to 12g/d inositol (cf 30% on placebo) (n = 24, RCT, 6/52, Chengappa et al, Bipolar Disord 2000;**2**:47–55) and in bipolar depression unresponsive to a mood stabiliser and at least one antidepressant, where response to inositol was 17% (cf lamotrigine 24% and risperidone 5%; n = 66, RCT, 16/52, open, Nierenberg et al, Am J Psychiatry 2006; **163**:210–6). However, inositol was numerically, but not statistically or clinically, superior to placebo as augmentation of lithium or valproate (n = 17, RCT, d/b, p/c, 6/52, Eden Evins et al, Bipolar Disord 2006;**8**:168–74).

Ketoconazole

Ketoconazole, 400 mg/d has been used as add-on therapy in resistant bipolar depression, with no increase in manic symptoms (n = 6, open, Brown et al, Bipolar Disord 2001;**3**:23–9).

Levetiracetam

A pilot trial of adjunctive levetiracetam 500–2000 mg/d showed a modest improvement in some depressed patients, but was not wildly encouraging (n = 34, open, 8/52, Post et al, J Clin Psychiatry 2005;**66**:370–4).

Melatonin

Melatonin secretion is altered in bipolar disorder and so melatonin may have some role (review by Srinivasan et al, World J Biol Psychiatry 2006;**7**:138–51).

Methylphenidate

In one study, methylphenidate was effective and tolerable in 78% depressed bipolars (n = 14, open, 12/52, El-Mallakh, Bipolar Disord 2000; **2**:56–9), and a retrospective chart analysis showed that methylphenidate (mean 14/12) could be effective for bipolar depression without apparent major problems, abuse or mood switching (n = 16, Lydon and El-Mallakh, J Clin Psychopharmacol 2006;**26**:516–8).

Modafinil

Modafinil 100–200 mg/d significantly improved depressive symptoms in bipolar depression, with no difference in treatment-emergent mania (n = 85, RCT, p/c, 6/52, Frye et al, Am J Psychiatry 2007;**164**:1242–9), and in remitted bipolar depression with hypersomnia, modafinil may be effective as an adjunct to mood stabilisers and antidepressants (n = 2, Fernandes and Petty, Ann Pharmacother 2003;**37**:1807–9). It does not seem to cause switching to mania when used for fatigue and sleepiness in bipolar depression (n = 39, Nasr et al, J Affect Disord 2006;**95**:111–4).

Oxcarbazepine

Oxcarbazepine as add-on to lithium in bipolar depression was effective in 60% and may be successful over the longer-term (n = 17, open,

8/52 + 12/12, Benedetti et al, J Affect Disord 2004;**79**:273–7).

Pramipexole

Pramipexole (a dopamine agonist) was clearly superior (60% response) to placebo (9%) in bipolar depression, when used as an adjunct to either lithium or valproate (n = 21, RCT, d/b, p/c, 6/52, Zarate et al, Biol Psychiatry 2004;**56**:54–60) and a mean 1.7 mg/d added to existing mood stabilisers produced a 67% response (cf 20% with placebo) in bipolar depression (n = 22, RCT, o/p, p/c, 6/52, Goldberg et al, Am J Psychiatry 2004;**161**:564–6).

Review: Whiskey and Taylor, Psychiatr Bull 2004;**28**:438–40).

Triiodothyronine *

Triiodothyronine (T3) (mean 90 mg/d) has been successful in treatment-resistant bipolar II (n = 159, retrospective, Kelly and Lieberman, J Affect Disord 2009;**116**:222–6) and low pretreatment thyroid function predicts slower response to antidepressants (n = 65, Cole et al, Am J Psychiatry 2002; **159**:116–21).

Valproate *

Two pilot studies have shown valproate superior to placebo for acute bipolar depression (n = 18, RCT, d/b, p/c, 6/52, Ghaemi et al, J Clin Psychiatry 2007;**68**:1840–4; n = 25, RCT, d/b, p/c, 8/52, Davis et al, J Affect Disord 2005;**85**:259–66; see also sub-analysis of Bowden study by Gyulai et al, Neuropsychopharmacol 2003;**28**:1374–82).

Zonisamide

Adjunctive zonisamide (mean 236 mg/d) may have modest effectiveness in bipolar depression in some patients, with low switching (e.g. Wilson and Findling, Expert Opin Pharmacother 2007;**8**:111–3) but relatively poor tolerability (n = 20 [c = 10], open, 8/52, Ghaemi et al, J Clin Psychopharmacol 2006;**26**:385–8), although up to 300 mg/d as add-on had significant effects in 50% of completers (n = 10 [c=8], open, 8/52, Anand et al, J Clin Psychiatry 2005;**66**:195–8).

1.10.4 RAPID-CYCLING BIPOLAR DISORDER

Introduction *

Rapid-cycling bipolar disorder is a variant of bipolar mood disorder, where four or more mood episodes occur in one year. Although it is relatively uncommon (e.g. one in six presenting with bipolar have a rapid-cycling pattern) and often a transient condition (about 80% will resolve in a year), the clinical significance of this sub-group is that it accounts for up to 80% of lithium non-responders, that antidepressant therapy of depressive phases can induce or worsen cycling and that rapid-cycling is a risk factor for suicide and suicide attempts (n = 345, mean 13 years, Coryell et al, Arch Gen Psychiatry 2003;**60**:914–20). Rapid-cycling is slightly more common in women and in bipolar II (n = 1742, STEP-BD, Schneck et al, Am J Psychiatry 2008;**165**:370–7). Risk factors include neurological damage, neuroendocrine factors (including hypothyrodism), psychotropic drugs (e.g. alcohol, antidepressants, stimulants) as well as some genetic factors (Sachs, in J Clin Psychiatry 2006;**67**:1140–51).

Role of drugs

There will probably always be a lack of robust data on the pharmacotherapy of rapid-cycling, as research is complicated by the unpredictable and spontaneously remitting nature of the condition. The initial strategies must be:

1. Reduce or stop any cycle-promoters, e.g. antidepressants.
2. Add/optimise anti-cycling mood stabilisers (start with lithium for treatment-naïve patients).
3. Add other drugs, e.g. lithium, antipsychotics, lamotrigine (especially for bipolar 2), perhaps valproate.
4. If ineffective, drugs may be used in combination. Levothyroxine and nimodipine may be effective in some patients not responsive to first-line drugs and may be worth a therapeutic trial.
4. Minimise ADRs to enhance compliance.
5. Recognise that full benefits may not be apparent for several months so do not abandon treatment too early.

References: n = 500, STEP-BD, Schneck et al, J Clin Psychiatry 2006;**67**[Suppl 11]:22–7; Coryell, CNS Drugs 2005;**19**:557–69.

Reviews: * definitions (Bauer et al, Bipolar Disord 2008;**10**:153–62), general (Mercer, Curr Psychiatr Rep 2007;**9**:53–62; Schneck, J Clin Psychiatry 2006; **67**(Suppl 22):22–7), evidence-based guidelines (Goodwin et al, J Psychopharmacol 2009;**23**:346–88).

BNF listed

Carbamazepine

The original carbamazepine study (n = 32, Kishimoto et al, Br J Psychiatry 1983;**143**:327–31) showed a particular effect in rapid-cycling and several studies (e.g. n = 18, open, 6/12, Joyce, Int Clin Psychopharmacol 1988;**3**:123–9) have shown a long-term response rate ranging from 20–70%. Doubt has, however, been raised about long-term efficacy as many people seem to lose the therapeutic response over several years (n = 24, open, four years, Post et al, J Clin Psychopharmacol 1990;**10**:318–27).

Lithium *

Around 20% of rapid-cyclers are lithium responders, probably by reducing the intensity of relapses rather than the actual number. Lithium response may be better if the sequence of relapse is mania, depression and then remission, rather than depression, then mania and remission (Grof et al, Prog Neuropsychopharmacol Biol Psychiatry 1987; **11**:199–203). Poor compliance with lithium, particularly if intermittent (e.g. frequent abrupt stopping), may complicate treatment by inducing relapse. Valproate seems as effective as lithium in preventing relapse in recently stabilised rapid-cyclers (n = 60[n = 254 in stabilisation phase], RCT, d/b, 20/12, Calabrese et al, Am J Psychiatry 2005;**162**:2152–61) and in patients stabilised for 6/12 on lithium plus valproate, the valproate had no additional effect over lithium alone (n = 31, RCT, d/b, 6/12, Kemp et al, J Clin Psychiatry 2009;**70**:113–21).

Review: * Muzina, Bipolar Disord 2009;**11**(Suppl 2):84–91.

+ Combinations

Carbamazepine + valproate

Synergy has been reported (n = 1 Ketter et al, J Clin Psychopharmacol 1992;**12**:276–81).

Lamotrigine + valproate

There is a case of successful use (n = 1, Woo et al, Psychiatry Clin Neurosci 2007; **61**:130–1).

Lithium + carbamazepine

The combination can be useful in rapid-cyclers non-responsive to the individual drugs (e.g. n = 16, retrospective, Di Costanzo and Schifano, Acta Psychiatr Scand 1991;**83**:456–9). See also interactions (4.5.1).

Lithium + levothyroxine

Low dose levothyroxine added to lithium has produced complete euthymia within seven days (n = 1, Bernstein, J Clin Psychopharmacol 1992;**12**:443–4).

Lithium + valproate

Open studies have included this combination in rapid-cyclers, and reported an additive or potentiating effect (mentioned by Sharma and Persad, Lithium 1994;**5**:117–25).

Thyroid + tricyclic

Sub-therapeutic doses of T_3 tri-iodothyronine 25–50 mcg/d (n = 1, Cooke, Am J Psychiatry 1990;**147**:255) or T_4 levothyroxine up to 0.1 mg/d have been used as augmentation to tricyclics and phenelzine (although care is needed with any use of antidepressants in rapid-cycling). See levothyroxine/liothyronine.

Topiramate + clozapine

There is one case of topiramate augmentation of clozapine retaining effectiveness for three years with no significant ADRs (n = 1, Chen et al, Clin Neuropharmacol 2005;**28**:136–8).

● **Unlicensed/some efficacy**

Lamotrigine (see also combinations)

In the largest and only prospective placebo-controlled study in rapid-cycling disorder, lamotrigine was well tolerated and appeared useful in some (n = 324, open + n = 182, d/b maintenance phase, Calabrese et al, J Clin Psychiatry 2000;**61**:841–50), with survival rates favouring lamotrigine (significantly so in bipolar II patients), and 41% stable without relapse at 6/12 (cf 26% placebo). Lamotrigine may be as effective as lithium in

a trial in refractory rapid-cycling (n = 14, RCT, open, one year, Walden et al, Bipolar Disorder 2000;**2**:336–9). The optimum dose appears to be 50–200 mg/d, although doses as high as 600 mg/d have been used.

Levothyroxine/liothyronine *

Levothyroxine has potential efficacy at 0.3–0.5 mg/d (or liothyronine 140–400 mcg/d) for rapid or 48-hour-cycling mania. Latent thyroid hypofunction may occur, revealed by a lithium challenge (n = 40, Gyulai et al, Biol Psychiatry 2003;**53**:899–905). Significant response was seen in a two-year study with high-dose levothyroxine (n = 6, open, Afflelou et al, Encephale 1997;**23**:209–17) and 0.25–0.3 mg/d, creating a slightly hyperthyroid state, was shown to be effective (via an unplanned dose reduction) in a lady with long-standing resistant rapid-cycling (n = 1, Extein, Am J Psychiatry 2000;**157**:1704–5).

Valproate (see also combinations)

Valproate seems as effective as lithium in preventing relapse in recently stabilised rapid-cyclers (n = 60 [n = 254 in stabilisation phase], RCT, d/b, 20/12, Calabrese et al, Am J Psychiatry 2005;**162**:2152–61).

■ **Unlicensed/possible efficacy**

Calcium-channel blockers

There are old reports of response to nimodipine (highly lipophilic, allowing adequate CNS concentrations and minimal peripheral effects) in rapid-cycling with a very marked response in some patients (n = 12 [c=9], RCT, d/b, p/c, Pazzaglia et al, Psychiatry Res 1993;**49**:257–72), with 90–180 mg/d optimal. Verapamil is poorly lipophilic with a low central effect.

Clonazepam

Clonazepam has been used as an adjunct to lithium in lithium-refractory bipolars (n = 5, open, Aronson et al, Am J Psychiatry 1989;**146**:77–80).

Clozapine

Clozapine may be effective in treatment-resistant rapid cycling (e.g. Suppes et al, Biol Psychiatry 1994;**36**:338–40).

Gabapentin

Some gabapentin studies in mania included some rapid-cycling patients and moderate efficacy was reported (Shelton and Calabrese, *Curr Psychiatry Reports* 2000;**2**:310–15).

Levetiracetam

There are cases of adjunctive treatment improving depression, interrupting rapid cycling (n = 2, Braünig and Krüger, *J Psychopharmacol* 2003;**17**:239–41) and in multiple drug-resistant rapid-cycling (n = 1, Kaufman, *Epilepsy Behav* 2004;**5**:1017–20).

Olanzapine

Ten rapid-cyclers were classified as responding to olanzapine during dysphoric mania (n = 13, open, 4/52, Gonzalez-Pinto et al, *J Clin Psychopharmacol* 2002;**22**:450–4).

Quetiapine *

Quetiapine 300 mg and 600 mg/d were more effective than placebo in treating depressive episodes in rapid-cycling bipolar I and II (n = 108, RCT, d/b, p/c, 8/52, Vieta et al, *Bipolar Disorder* 2007;**9**:413–25) and it may be more effective than valproate, albeit with more side-effects (n = 17, open, Langosch et al, *J Clin Psychopharmacol* 2008;**28**:555–60). Successful use with comorbid anxiety and social phobia has been reported (n = 1, Valerius et al, *Pharma-copsychiatry* 2005;**38**:225–6).

□ No efficacy

Antidepressants *

Antidepressants may induce rapid-cycling, especially in women prior to the first episode (but not in men, Yildiz and Sachs, *J Clin Psychiatry* 2003;**64**:814–18) and since up to 50% of cases may be antidepressant-induced, discontinuation has to be a first-line treatment. Antidepressants should only be used in rapid-cyclers in low dose and only in acute severe depression. Rates of TEM (Treatment Emergent Mania) are highest for fluoxetine (42%) and lowest for fluvoxamine and mirtazapine, but as a group there was no difference between SSRIs, bupropion and venlafaxine (n = 180, Gao et al, *Bipolar Disord* 2008;**10**:907–15), with one study showing

venlafaxine had no more chance of switching a rapid-cycler with depression into mania than a non-rapid-cycler (n = 83 [c = 50], RCT, open, 12/52, Amsterdam et al, *J Affect Disord* 2009;**112**:219–30).

1.11 BORDERLINE PERSONALITY DISORDER (BPD)
see also Aggression (*1.2*)

There are a large number of personality disorders, of which borderline personality disorder is but one. Treating personality disorders (and hence personality itself) is obviously somewhat controversial. Research is now often directed towards treating symptom clusters rather than the underlying personality disorder, e.g. anxiety, aggression and impulsiveness.

Symptoms

The main symptoms of BPD are of a deeply ingrained maladaptive pattern of behaviour, recognisable from adolescence and continuing through most of adult life. Such people show continued boredom, anger, unstable relationships, impulsive self-harmful behaviour (e.g. gambling, stealing, binge-eating or drinking), variable moods, recurrent suicide threats or behaviour, and uncertainty about their personal identity.

Role of drugs *

People with BPD may account for up to 7.5% of psychiatric admissions, with a raised incidence of psychiatric morbidity and mortality, and use a wide range of medication and services. Pharmacotherapy will not alter ingrained character traits or the effects of abuse, but they may produce modest benefits with the occasional striking result, and be more effective if combined with psychotherapy. Drug therapy, however, is fraught with problems. Side-effects may be grossly exaggerated to avoid treatment and patients may be actively antimedication. Cochrane concludes that current data for pharmacotherapy in BPD is poor, but that there may be a positive effect from antidepressants (Binks et al, *Cochrane Database Syst Rev* 2006;**1**:CD005653). Several meta-analyses of RCTs have concluded that the beneficial effects are as follows:

	Antipsychotics	Antidepressants	Mood stabilisers
Cognitive-perception	++	?	?
Anger	++/+++	+/++	++
Impulse-behaviour	+	o	++
Anxiety	?	+/++	+++
Depression	o	+	++
Global functioning	+	o	+

+++ Significant effect   + Minor effect
++ Moderate effect   o No effect

References: * s=21, Ingenhoven et al, J Clin Psychiatry 2010;[in press]; Mercer et al, J Pers Disord 2009;**23**:156–74; Dahl, Curr Opin Psychiatry 2008;**21**:78–83.

Reviews: * general (Bellion et al, CNS Drugs 2008; **22**:671–92; Diaz-Marsa et al, Actas Esp Psiquiatr 2008;**36**:39–49; Dahl, Curr Opin Psychiatry 2008; **21**:78–83), anticonvulsants (Díaz-Marsá et al, Actas Esp Psiquiatr 2008;**36**(Suppl 3):39–45), suicidality (Cardish, Can J Psychiatry 2007;**52**[suppl 1]:115S–127S).

● Unlicensed/some efficacy

Antipsychotics *

It has been generally accepted that people with DSM-IV borderline or schizotypical personality disorders may gain significant benefit from psychotherapy and small doses of antipsychotics. The first generation antipsychotics **haloperidol** and **trifluoperazine** have been used to improve anger, hostility and behavioural symptoms, but have been largely superseded, especially as two studies showed haloperidol to be no better than placebo (Soloff et al, Arch Gen Psychiatry 1993;**150**:377–85) and poorly tolerated (n=54, 16/52, Cornelius et al, Am J Psychiatry 1993;**150**:1843–8). **Aripiprazole** 15mg/d may improve many measures of BPD (n=52, RCT, d/b, p/c, 8/52, Nickel et al, Am J Psychiatry 2006;**163**:833–8; n=26[c=22], open, 18/12, Nickel, J Clin Psychiatry 2007;**68**:1815–6), including as an adjunct to sertraline (56% res-ponding to 10–15mg/d; n=21[c=16], open, 12/52, Bellion et al, Psychiatry Res 2008; **161**:206–12) and a low starting dose may

facilitate response (n=3, Mobascher et al, Pharmacopsychiatry 2006;**39**:111–2). Two small open trials of **clozapine** (25–100mg/d) in severe BPD produced a general improvement in one (n=12, Benedetti et al, J Clin Psychiatry 1998;**59**:13–107) and significantly reduced SIB, aggression, seclusion and violence in the other (n=7, Chengappa et al, J Clin Psychiatry 1999;**60**:477–84). **Olanzapine** may be effective against a range of psychopathological symptoms in females with BPD (weight gain being the only significant side-effect; n=28, d/b, p/c, 6/12, Zanarini and Frankenburg, J Clin Psychiatry 2001;**62**:849–54), with 5–10mg/d significantly superior to placebo for a mixed sample of BPD individuals (n=40, d/b, p/c, 12/52, Bogenschutz and Nurnberg, J Clin Psychiatry 2004;**65**:104–9, MS). IM may be effective over two hours for severe agitation in BPD in an emergency room observational study (n=25, Damsa et al, Gen Hosp Psychiatry 2007;**29**:51–3). **Quetiapine** (mean 250mg/d, range 175–400mg/d) may be well tolerated and significantly improve impulsivity and other symptoms in severe BPD (n=23, open, 12/52, Villeneuve and Lemelin, J Clin Psychiatry 2005;**66**:1298–303; see also n=14[c=11], open, 12/52, Bellion et al, J Clin Psychiatry 2006; **67**:1042–6) and a mean of 540mg/d may have an effect on hostility, suspiciousness and other rating scales in BPD (n=29[c=23], open, Perrella et al, Prog Neuropsychopharmacol Biol Psychiatry 2007; **31**:158–63; n=16[c=9], open, 8/52, Adityananjee et al, Ann Clin Psychiatry 2008;**20**:219–26). However, quetiapine 400mg/d was ineffective for impulsivity in BPD cluster B, although depressive symptoms might improve (n=15, open, 8/52, Roepke et al, Pharmacopsychiatry 2008;**41**:176–81). Low dose **risperidone** may be effective and well tolerated, e.g. risperidone (mean 3.3mg/d) helped as an add-on to existing therapies to improve BPD symptomatology, especially aggression and overall functioning (n=15, open, 8/52, Rocca et al, J Clin Psychiatry 2002; **63**:241–4). **Ziprasidone** does not seem to have a significant effect on BPD (n=60, RCT, d/b, p/c, 12/52, Pascual et al, J Clin Psychiatry 2008;**69**:603–8).

Review: general (Mobascher et al, Nervenarzt 2007;**78**:1003–13).

SSRIs

Some symptoms of BPD are shared with depression, e.g. self-condemnation, emptiness, hopelessness, boredom and somatic complaints, and so the use of antidepressants may have some logic. SSRIs may have a role, e.g. irritability and aggression improved in the 44% completers in a trial of **sertraline** 50–200 mg/d (n = 16, 8/52, Kavoussi et al, J Clin Psychiatry 1994;**55**:137–41). **Fluoxetine** 20–60 mg/d significantly reduced anger and distress, with a significant placebo effect detectable (n = 22, p/c, Selzman et al, J Clin Psychopharmacol 1995;**15**:23–9), and it was partially effective in reduced impulsive aggressive behaviour in another study, but with high drop-out rates (n = 40, RCT, Coccaro and Kavoussi, Arch Gen Psychiatry 1997;**54**:1081–8; review by Hawton, EBMH 1998;**1**:79). Combining with IPT may improve outcomes (n = 39 [c = 32], 6/12, Bellino et al, Can J Psychiatry 2006;**51**:453-60). **Fluvoxamine** may significantly improve rapid mood shifts in female BPDs, but not impulsivity and aggression (n = 38, RCT, d/b, p/c, c/o, 24/52 total, Rinne et al, Am J Psychiatry 2002;**159**:2048–54). Careful dose titration is needed to minimise agitation.

Topiramate

Two RCTs have shown topiramate to help to reduce anger in men (n = 42, RCT, d/b, p/c, 8/52, Nickel et al, Biol Psychiatry 2005;**57**:495–9) and women (n = 29, RCT, d/b, p/c, 8/52, Nickel et al, J Clin Psychiatry 2004;**65**:1515–9; IS), and in both studies participants lost weight. In another study, topiramate (up to 200 mg/d) reduced stress and some other symptoms, although SIB was not an outcome measure and the exclusion criteria included anyone suicidal or abusing drugs or alcohol, so the cohort was relatively limited (n = 56, RCT, d/b, 10/52, Loew et al, J Clin Psychopharmacol 2006;**26**:61–6; comment by Killaspy, EBMH 2006;**9**:74).

Valproate

Valproate significantly reduced irritability, anger, impulsiveness and relationship tempestuousness in women with comorbid bipolar II and BPD and was well tolerated (n = 20, RCT, p/c, d/b, 6/12, Frankenburg and Zanarini, J Clin Psychiatry 2002;**63**:442–6), supporting a previous study

in impulsive aggression in SSRI non-responders (e.g. n = 20 [c = 10], open, 12/52, Simeon et al, CNS Spectr 2007;**12**:439–43).

■ Unlicensed/possible efficacy

Carbamazepine

Carbamazepine may be useful for aggression and episodic dyscontrol and, although the latter is not epileptic, there are some common precipitating factors (e.g. prodromal symptoms, severe disturbance and post-episode relief of tension). Carbamazepine has been suggested as superior to placebo for behaviour control (n = 16, d/b, p/c, c/o, 6/52, Cowdry and Gardner, Arch Gen Psychiatry 1988;**45**:111–9) but an RCT failed to show any effects (n = 20, RCT, 30/7, de la Fuente and Lotstra, Eur Neuropsychopharmacol 1994;**4**:479–86).

Lamotrigine

Lamotrigine was relatively well tolerated and highly significantly effective for anger in women with BPD (n = 27, RCT, d/b, p/c, 8/52, Tritt et al, J Psychopharmacol 2005;**9**:287–91).

Lithium

Lithium has been reported to be useful for episodic dyscontrol and aggression, in BPD, emotionally unstable adolescents and in alcoholics with a BPD. Anecdotally, it produced a state of 'reflective delay', although the consequences of erratic compliance would be a significant disadvantage.

Methylphenidate

There is one case where methylphenidate was thought to have been effective in a patient with both ADHD and BPD (n = 1, Van Reekum and Links, Can J Psychiatry 1994;**39**:186–7), although this is open to debate (see amfetamines).

Oxcarbazepine

Oxcarbazepine 1.2–1.5 g BD may have a potential role (n = 17, open, Bellino et al, J Clin Psychiatry 2005;**66**:1111–5).

Tricyclics

Generally tricyclics are considered ineffective (or even detrimental) in depression associated with BPD.

□ No efficacy

Amfetamines

Dexamfetamine has been used but, with the exception of the occasional patient, has proved ineffective. It may be possible to test for amfetamine responsiveness (reviewed by Stein in *Br J Psychiatry* 1992;**161**:167–84).

Benzodiazepines

Benzodiazepines are considered to be contra-indicated in BPD due to their potential to disinhibit and induce rage reactions and dependence, e.g. **alprazolam** was significantly worse than placebo for behavioural control (n = 16, d/b, p/c, c/o, 6/52, Cowdry and Gardner, *Arch Gen Psychiatry* 1988;**45**:111–9), and the only major study showed **alprazolam** to be no better than placebo in children with anxious or avoidant disorders (n = 30, d/b, p/c, Simeon et al, *J Am Acad Child Adolesc Psychiatry* 1992;**31**:29–33). The occasional use of rapidly absorbed short-acting drugs (e.g. **lorazepam**) may have some limited use in patients with intermittent explosive disorders.

MAOIs

Two studies have shown phenelzine 60 mg/d to be no better than placebo (e.g. n = 108, RCT, d/b, p/c, 5/52, Soloff et al, *Arch Gen Psychiatry* 1993;**150**:377–85; n = 54, d/b, p/c, 21/52, Cornelius et al, *Am J Psychiatry* 1993;**150**: 1843–8).

Phenytoin

Two ancient studies showed an often negative effect (e.g. Rosenblatt et al, *Curr Ther Res* 1976; **19**:332–6).

Reboxetine

There is a case of worsening symptoms with reboxetine (n = 1, Anghelescu et al, *J Neuropsychiatry Clin Neurosci* 2005;**17**:559–60).

1.12: CATATONIA
see also Schizophrenia (*1.23*)

Symptoms

Catatonia is usually a rare and potentially lethal type of schizophrenia, dominated by psychosis, catalepsy, stupor, extreme negativism, resistant rigidity, hyperpyrexia, excitement (purposeless motor activity not influenced by external stimuli), echopraxia, grimacing or posturing. It may be associated with mixed (rather than pure) manic episodes in bipolars, and so may be misdiagnosed (n = 27, Krüger et al, *J Affect Disord* 2003;**74**:279–85). It may be linked to autism (Takaoka and Takata, *Psychol Rep* 2007;**101**:961–9) or even be a symptom of autism (Dhossche et al, *Int Rev Neurobiol* 2006;**72**:151–64).

Role of drugs

ECT is generally considered the treatment of choice for various forms of catatonia, e.g. organic, lethal and schizophrenic (n = 50, Hatta et al, *J ECT* 2007;**23**:233–5). Organic catatonia often responds to treatment of the underlying cause, e.g. withdrawal of the offending drug. Antipsychotic-induced catatonia is also potentially fatal and must be treated symptomatically. A careful history may elicit a drug-symptom association and the potentially offending drug(s) stopped. Antipsychotics are generally unhelpful.

Reviews: * drug-induced (Duggal and Singh, *Drugs Today* [Barc] 2005;**41**:599–607), clinical features, diagnosis, management and prognosis (Fink and Taylor, *Arch Gen Psychiatry* 2009;**66**:1173–7).

+ Combinations

Lorazepam + dexamfetamine
See separate drugs/groups.

Lorazepam + ECT
Concurrent or sequential use may be successful (n = 5, Petrides et al, *Biol Psychiatry* 1997;**42**, 375–81).

Olanzapine + amantadine
Dramatic reduction of symptoms has been reported with olanzapine and amantadine, weak NMDA receptor antagonists (n = 1, Babington and Spiegel, *Psychosomatics* 2007;**48**:534–6).

● Unlicensed/some efficacy

Amantadine
See memantine.

Benzodiazepines *
There are many case reports of successful

benzodiazepine use in catatonia, e.g. 1.5–2 mg IV **lorazepam** has improved antipsychotic-induced catatonia (n = 4, Fricchione et al, J Clin Psychopharmacol 1983;**3**:338–42) and lorazepam IM (or diazepam IV if lorazepam failed) showed a 100% success rate over 24 hours (n = 14, Huang, Psychiatry Clin Neurosci 2005;**59**:52–5). In an open study comparing lorazepam and ECT, 76% responded to lorazepam (IV and/or oral) within five days; most who failed responded promptly to ECT and a positive response to initial parenteral challenge with lorazepam predicted a positive outcome (n = 28, open, Bush et al, Acta Psychiatr Scand 1996;**93**:137–43). High-dose maintenance lorazepam has been effective long-term (Manjunatha et al, Aust NZ J Psychiatry 2007;**41**:625–7). Lorazepam IM or **diazepam** IV produced 100% resolution within a day in depressed people with catatonic features (n = 7, Hung and Huang, Clin Neuropharmacol 2006;**29**:144–7). **Clonazepam** at 2.5 mg/d orally or 1 mg IV (n = 3, Am J Psychiatry 1989; **146**:1230; n = 1, Kumar, Aust N Z J Psychiatry 2001;**35**:391) and **midazolam** (mentioned in Am J Psychiatry 1991;**148**:809) have also been used. However, Cochrane concludes that the evidence base for use is lacking (s = 0, n = 0, Gibson and Walcott, Cochrane Database Syst Rev 2008;**4**:CD006570).

Memantine

Amantadine and memantine may both have a role in improving symptoms of treatment-resistant catatonia (n = 25, Carroll et al, J Neuropsychiatry Clin Neurosci 2007;**19**:406–12) and there are case reports of rapid, significant response of catatonic schizophrenia to memantine 10–20 mg/d (n = 1, Carpenter et al, Ann Pharmacother 2006;**40**:344–6; n = 1, Thomas, Am J Psychiatry 2005;**162**:626; n = 1, Carroll et al, Ann Clin Psychiatry 2006;**18**: 133–4).

Zolpidem *

There have been a number of reports of dramatic improvement in catatonia with zolpidem (e.g. Mastain et al, Rev Neurol 1995; **151**:52–6), including a dramatic response when due to alcohol withdrawal (n = 1, Cottencin et al, Med Sci Monit 2009;**15**:129–31), to the

extent that it has been used as a diagnostic tool for catatonia, e.g. by inducing resolution in people thought to have schizophrenia and allowing interviews to take place (e.g. Thomas et al, Lancet 1997;**349**:702; Zaw and Bates, Lancet 1997;**349**:1914).

■ **Unlicensed/possible efficacy**

Antipsychotics *

Antipsychotics are generally considered unhelpful but there are cases of catatonic schizophrenia responsive to **amisulpride** (n = 1, French and Eastwood, Can J Psychiatry 2003;**48**:570), including a remarkable case of multi-resistant chronic catatonia responding to amisulpride 1200 mg/d over six months (n = 1, Srikanth and Baxter, Prog Neurol Psychiatry 2007;**11**:13–6), **aripiprazole** (Cummings and Noordsy, Schizophr Res 2009;**112**:194–5), **clozapine** (n = 2, Dursun et al, J Psychopharmacol 2005;**19**:432–3; n = 1, Sixt et al, Z Kinder Jugendosychiatr Psychother 2009;**37**:209–14) and **risperidone** (n = 2, Valevski et al, Clin Neuro-pharmacol 2001;**24**:228–31), including for periodic catatonia (Duggal and Gandotra, Can J Psychiatry 2005;**50**:241–2). Olanzapine has been used to successfully treat lethal catatonia (n = 1, Cassidy et al, J Psychopharmacol 2001;**15**:302–4; n = 1, Chang et al, Prog Neuropsychopharmacol Biol Psychiatry 2009;**33**:1559–60).

Carbamazepine

Carbamazepine may be an alternative in lorazepam-resistant patients (n = 9, Kritzinger and Jordaan, Int J Neuropsychopharmacol 2001; **4**:251–7).

Valproate

A very short review (entitled 'is there a role for valproic acid in the treatment of catatonia?') discussed the role, so the answer is 'probably not' (Bowers and Ajit, J Neuropsychiatry Clin Neurosci 2007;**19**:197–8), although a prophylactic effect may occur (n = 1, Yoshida et al, J Clin Psychopharmacol 2005;**25**:504–5).

Vitamin B12

There is a case of complete remission of catatonia with B12 replacement (n = 1, Berry et al, Acta Psychiatr Scand 2003;**108**:156–9).

◆ Others

Other drugs tried include **barbiturates** (thiopental and amobarbital; referred to by Masiar, *Am J Psychiatry* 1992;**149**:144–5), **bromocriptine** (n = 1, Mahmood, *Br J Psychiatry* 1991;**158**:437–8), IV **dantrolene** (n = 2, Pennati, *Am J Psychiatry* 1991; **148**:268), **dexamfetamine** (n = 1, Smith and Lebegue, *Am J Psychiatry* 1991;**148**:1265), and **lithium** (n = 1, Pheterson *et al*, *J Am Acad Child Adolesc Psychiatry* 1985;**24**:235–7).

1.13 DEMENTIA including:
1.13.1 Treatment of Alzheimer's disease
1.13.2 BPSD/BPSSD (behavioural and psychological [signs and] symptoms of dementia)
1.13.3 Vascular dementia
1.13.4 Prophylaxis and prevention

Symptoms

Dementia is an acquired progressive and irreversible reduction in the level of previously attained intellectual, memory and personality/ emotional functioning. The main clinical features include disturbed behaviour (disorganised, inappropriate, distracted, restless, antisocial), lack of insight, impaired thinking (slow, impoverished, incoherent, rigid), poverty of speech, low mood, poor cognitive function (forgetfulness, poor attention, disorientation in time and later place), and impaired memory. Some dementias can be treated, e.g. if caused by vitamin depletion (e.g. B_{12}, folic acid, thiamine), infections (encephalitis, neurosyphilis) or drug toxicity.

Alzheimer's disease (AD) * is a form of dementia characterised by amyloid plaques and neuro-fibrillary tangles, with reduced levels of acetylcholine and other transmitters in the brain. The amyloid hypothesis is that accumulation of the peptide amyloid beta, a toxic protein, precipitates the development of the sticky plaques that are common in Alzheimer's, although there are other theories. The degree of dementia is associated more with the degree of neurofibrillary pathology than with the amyloid plaque burden. It usually presents with an insidious onset and steady deterioration, forgetfulness, lack of spontaneity, disorientation, depressed mood, decline in self-care, poor sleep (waking disorientated and perplexed) and

intellectual impairment (dysphasia, dyspraxia, language decline). The incidence of comorbid cerebrovascular disease may be high, and ranges from 22% (n = 548, Feldman *et al*, *Int J Geriatr Psychiatry* 2008;**24**:479–88) to 89% (n = 232, Tabet *et al*, *Int J Clin Pract* 2009;**63**:338–45) depending on the threshold for identification.

Lewy body dementia* is a variant of Alzheimer's disease and is more common in men. The key features include early onset, persistent and well-formed visual hallucinations, and motor features of Parkinsonism. Patients may be extremely sensitive to antipsychotics and anticholinergics (Gold *et al*, *Front Neurol Neurosci* 2009;**24**:107–13), which may result in a sudden onset of EPSEs, profound confusion and deterioration, and can lead to death.

Vascular dementia is a variant of Alzheimer's (see separate section *1.13.3*).

Non-pharmacological interventions should include behavioural management, cognitive and multisensory stimulation, environmental design, physical activities, reality orientation and recreational activities.

Role of drugs

Currently there are six main classes of agents for dementia (management and prevention or delay):

- cholinesterase inhibitors
- NMDA receptor blockers (e.g. memantine)
- antioxidants (including gingko biloba)
- anti-inflammatory agents
- neurotrophic factors (including HRT)
- antiamyloid agents (including cholesterol-lowering drugs).

The use of cholinesterase inhibitors (ChEIs) will remain controversial in the UK, until the patents expire in 2012, when NICE will have to review their negative advice (based on cost-effectiveness). However, they clearly help many people, but the problem seems to be in identifying which ones. Drug trials have many exclusions, and extrapolation of the results to the general population is open to question, but even delaying admission to a nursing home by one month would pay for a year's drug. Unfortunately, the only extended trial failed to show an effect on time to institutionalisation or any other measure (n = 565, RCT, d/b, three years, Courtney et al, Lancet 2004;**363**:2105–15), concluding that donepezil was not cost-effective (although the trial has shortcomings, see correspondence in Lancet).

However, several independent reviews have concluded that the ChEIs are effective. A major systematic review and meta-analysis showed ChEIs to have a modest effect on neuropsychiatric and functional outcomes in Alzheimer's, but long-term outcomes, such as quality of life and caregiver burden, are unclear (s = 29, Trinh et al, JAMA 2003;**280**:210–16; comment by Lahiri and Farlow, EBMH 2003;**6**:94). Another review suggested the ChEIs result in a modest but significant therapeutic improvement, with an NNT of 7, and an NNH of 12 (s = 16, n = 5159 + 2795 controls, Lanctôt et al, CMAJ 2003;**169**:557–64).

Reviews: * general (Gifford and Jones, Prescriber 2009;**20**:45–9), mild-to-moderate dementia (Hogan et al, CMAJ 2008;**179**:1019–26), severe Alzheimer's disease (Herrmann and Gauthier, CMAJ 2008;**179**:1279–87;Voisin and Vellas, Drugs Aging 2009;**26**:135–44; Hsiung and Feldman, Expert Opin Pharmacother 2008; **9**:2575–8), vaccines (Foster et al, Mol Psychiatry 2009; **14**:239–51), medicines for inappropriate sexual behaviours in dementia (Guay, Am J Geriatr Pharmacother 2008;**6**:269–88), Alzheimer's and cerebrovascular disease (Gil et al, Clin Drug Investig 2008;**28**:429–37), Lewy body dementia (Borroni et al, Arch Gerentol Geriatr 2008; **46**:101–6), BAP guidelines (Burns et al, J Psychopharmacol 2006;**20**:732–55), genetics (Cacabelos, Eur Arch Psychiatry Clin Neurosci 2008;**258**[suppl 1]:28–47; Avramopoulos, Genome Med 2009;**27**:34), anticholinesterases and memantine (s = 59, Raina et al, Ann Intern Med 2008;**148**:379–97).

1.13.1 TREATMENT OF ALZHEIMER'S DISEASE

BNF listed

CHOLINESTERASE INHIBITORS (ChEIs)

Although there is little to clinically separate the three currently available ChEIs, there are slight differences between them. Donepezil inhibits AChE, rivastigmine inhibits AChE and BuChE (which gives more side-effects initially but may have advantages in later illness), and galantamine both inhibits AChE and enhances ACh's action on nicotinic receptors. ChEIs may offer continued benefit for up to two years in moderately-severe AD (n = 994[c = 575], RCT, d/b, two years, Bullock et al, Curr Med Res Opin 2005;**21**:1317–27) and in more severe AD (n = 145, RCT, p/c, 24/52, Feldman et al, Int J Geriatr Psychiatry 2005;**20**:559–69). All ChEIs may improve cognitive functioning in people with Lewy body dementia (s = 3, 12–20/52, Bhasin et al, Int J Ger Psychiatry 2007;**22**:890–5). Cochrane concludes that all three are effective, there is no evidence that they are **not** cost-effective, and that donepezil may be slightly better tolerated, although careful titration of galantamine and rivastigmine might overcome this (s = 13, RCT, d/b, p/c, Birks, Cochrane Database Syst Rev 2006;**1**:CD005593).

Reviews: * general (Musia et al, Curr Med Chem 2007;**14**:2654–79), systematic review and meta-analysis comparing anticholinesterases (s = 26, Hansen et al, Clin Interv Aging 2008;**3**:211–25).

Donepezil *

Donepezil is a piperidine-based reversible selective acetylcholinesterase inhibitor licensed for the symptomatic treatment of mild or moderate AD. The dose is 5mg/d for the first month, increasing to 10mg/d as tolerated. CYP2D6 ultrarapid metabolisers may have lower steady-state plasma levels than normals, and show no improvement as a consequence, a possible explanation of interindividual variation (n = 42, Varsaldi et al, Eur J Clin Pharmacol 2006;**62**:721–6). Withdrawal effects are rare (n = 2, Singh and Dudley, Int J Geriatr Psychiatry 2003;**18**:282–4), probably as its half-life is 70 hours. In the early stages of AD, donepezil 10mg/d may improve daily cognitive functioning (n = 153, RCT, d/b, p/c, 24/52, Seltzer et al, Arch Neurol 2004;**61**:1852–6) and may help preserve cognitive function in severe AD (n = 343, RCT, d/b, p/c, 24/52, Black et al, Neurology 2007;**69**:459–69). There is little data on who may respond to donepezil but poor visual-spatial motor abilities and lexical-semantic functioning may be predictive of good response (n = 30, open, 6/12, Saumier et al, Dement Geriatr Cogn Disord 2007;**24**:28–35). In moderate AD, a systematic review concluded donepezil was effective for cognitive and global function in AD for up to six months (s = 10, Whitehead et al, Int J Geriatr Psychiatry 2004;**19**:624–33; comment by Lanctôt, EBMH 2005;**8**:15, noting the AD-2000 trial was published too late to be included in the analysis). Donepezil maintains its effectiveness over one year while remaining well tolerated (n = 286, RCT, p/c, one year, Winblad et al, Neurology 2001;**57**:489–95; n = 431, p/c, Mohs et al, Neurology 2001;**57**:481–8; n = 423, Doody et al, Dement Geriatr Cogn Disord 2001;**12**:295–300), and even perhaps over two years, although the benefits are lost within six weeks of stopping (n = 763, open, two years, Doody et al, Arch Neurol 2001;**58**:427–33). In severe AD (MMSE 1–10), donepezil improved cognition and preserved function over an extended period (n = 248 [c = 194], RCT, d/b, p/c, 6/12, Winblad et al, Lancet 2006;**367**:1057–65; enthusiastic comment by Ringman, EBMH 2006;**9**:104). The AD-2000 trial concludes that donepezil does not delay the time to institutionalisation or progression of disability in AD, but this may be because of a number of design and practical reasons (n = 565, RCT, d/b, p/c, 60/52, AD2000 CG, Lancet 2004;**363**:2105–15; review by Standridge, EBMH 2004;**7**:112). Donepezil may be used in Lewy body dementia, but abrupt withdrawal can lead to acute cognitive and behavioural decline (n = 19, 20 + 6/52, Minett et al, Int J Geriatr Psychiatry 2003;**18**:988–93). In mild cognitive impairment, donepezil 10 mg/d (cf. placebo) may slow the progression to AD over the first year, but not over three years (n = 769, three years, RCT, p/c, d/b, Petersen et al, N Engl J Med 2005;**352**:2379–88). It might have some non-significant efficacy in mild cognitive impairment (n = 270, RCT, d/b, p/c, 24/52, Salloway et al, Neurology 2004;**63**:651–7), but it has no effect as a cognitive enhancer in healthy elderly volunteers (n = 26, RCT, 2/52, p/c, Beglinger et al, J Clin Psychopharmacol 2005;**25**:159–65). Cochrane concludes that donepezil produces modest improvements in cognitive function, ADL, and behaviour over one year (Birks et al, Cochrane Database Syst Rev 2006;**1**:CD001190).

Reviews: * general (Seltzer, Expert Opin Pharmacother 2007;**8**:1011–23; Tsuno, Expert Rev Neurother 2009;**9**:591–8; Winblad, Am J Alzheimer's Dis Other Demen 2009;**24**:185–92).

Galantamine *

Galantamine is a reversible competitive acetyl-cholinesterase inhibitor, but also stimulates pre- and post-synaptic nicotinic receptors and is indicated for mild-to-moderate AD. The sustained-release capsules (Galantamine XL) allow once a day dosing. A range of studies have shown effectiveness. Post-hoc analysis concludes the optimum dose is 16 mg/d for mild Alzheimer's and 24 mg/d for moderate Alzheimer's (n = 835, RCT, d/b, p/c, 5/12, Aronson et al, Drugs Aging 2009;**26**:231–9), with the benefit sustained over 12 months with the 24 mg/d dose (n = 636, RCT, 6/12 plus 6/12 extension, Raskind et al, Neurology 2000; **54**:2261–8; n = 182, RCT, s/b, 12/12, Wilcock et al, Drugs Aging 2003;**20**:777–89) or even longer (n = 194[c=119], RCT, d/b, p/c, 36/52, Raskind et al, Arch Neurol 2004;**61**:252–6). Galantamine (24 mg/d) is associated with a significant reduction in caregiver burden (n = 978, p/c, 21/52, Cummings et al, Am J Psychiatry 2004;**161**:532–8). In severe Alzheimer's it seems well-tolerated, safe and may improve cognitive function, but not ADL (n = 407 [c = 329], RCT, d/b, p/c, Lancet Neurol 2009;**8**:39–47; n = 407, RCT, d/b, p/c, 6/12, Burns et al, Lancet Neurology 2009;**8**:39–47). There appears to be no rebound from abrupt discontinuation. In Alzheimer's combined with cerebrovascular disease, galantamine showed improved cognitive function (n = 285 [c = 242], RCT, d/b, p/c, 6/12, Erkinjuntti et al, J Psychopharmacol 2008;**22**:761–8). Cochrane concludes that galantamine is effective at doses of 16–32 mg/d, with a consistent effect at 3–6 months (s = 10, Loy and Schneider, Cochrane Database Syst Rev 2006;**1**:CD001747).

Reviews: * general (Razay and Wilcock, Expert Rev Neurother 2008;**8**:9–17), pharmacology (Villarroya et al, Expert Opin Investig Drugs 2007;**16**:1987–98), kinetics (Farlow, Clin Pharmacokinet 2003;**42**:1383–92).

Rivastigmine *

Rivastigmine is a carbamate-derived 'pseudo-irreversible' acetylcholinesterase (preferentially the G1 sub-type) and butylcholinesterase inhibitor licensed for the treatment of mild-to-moderately severe AD and for mild-to-moderate dementia in patients with idiopathic Parkinson's disease. A number of trials have shown some efficacy. Rivastigmine 6–12 mg/d may also have a sustained effect in advanced moderate AD (n = 44, RCT, p/c, 12/12, Karaman et al, Dement Geriatr Cogn Disord 2005;**19**:51–6; see also s = 3, n = 117, RCTs, p/c, d/b, 6/12, Burns et al, Int J Geriatr Psychiatry 2004;**19**:243–9). Rivastigmine may be useful in people with rapidly progressing AD (s = 4, n = 517, 26/52, Farlow et al, Dement Geriatr Cogn Disord 2005;**20**:192–7). A sub-group analysis suggested that rivastigmine may be more effective and better tolerated than donepezil in Lewy body dementia (n = 49, RCT, d/b, Touchon et al, Curr Med Res Opin 2006;**22**:49–59), but with a return to pre-treatment levels of function 3/52 after discontinuation (n = 92 completers, RCT, d/b, p/c, 23/52, Wesnes et al, Dement Geriatr Cogn Disord 2002;**13**:183–92). Rivastigmine may also improve dementia in Parkinson's disease but increases nausea, vomiting and tremor (n = 541 [c = 410], RCT, d/b, 24/52, Emre et al, N Engl J Med 2004;**351**:2509–18; comment by Chow, EBMH 2005;**8**:41). Cochrane concludes that rivastigmine was beneficial at 6–12 mg/d in mild-to-moderate AD, with improvements in ADL and reduced rate of decline (s = 9, n = 4775, Birks et al, Cochrane Database Syst Rev 2009;**2**:CD001191).

Reviews: general (Onor et al, Clin Interv Aging 2007;**2**:17–32; Cummings et al, Neurology 2007;**69**[4 Suppl 1]:S10–3), patches (Winblad and Machado, Expert Opin Drug Deliv 2008; **5**:1377–86).

NON-ANTICHOLINESTERASES

Memantine *

Memantine is licensed in the UK and some European countries for moderate-to-severe dementia (not just mild-to-moderately severe), a unique indication. Memantine is a NMDA antagonist. It replaces the magnesium ion that blocks NMDA receptors, so acts as a voltage-dependent, non-competitive NMDA-antagonist, blocking the effect of excess glutamate release, thought to be responsible for many symptoms and for disease progression. It also appears to have a neuroprotective action (review, Jann, Expert Opin Investig Drugs 2000;**9**:1397–406). The dose is 5 mg/d for the first week, adding 5 mg/d each week up to a maximum of 20 mg/d as divided doses, although once and twice-daily dosing seems to be of equivalent efficacy and tolerability (n = 78, RCT, d/b, 12/52, Jones et al, Int J Geriatr Psychiatry 2007;**22**:258–62). Side-effects seem low compared to placebo (s = 6, n = 2311, d/b, p/c, >24/52, Farlow et al, Drug Saf 2008;**31**:577–85) but include hallucinations, confusion, dizziness, headache and tiredness. The NNTs are 3–6 for global outcomes, 7 for cognitive improvement and 3–6 for ADL improvements (s = 2, Livingston and Katona, Int J Geriatr Psychiatry 2004;**19**:19–25). In mild-to-moderate AD, memantine 20 mg/d showed statistically significant improvements at weeks 12 and 18, but not at 24 weeks due to an unexpectedly high placebo response (n = 470, RCT, d/b, p/c, 6/12, Bakchine and Loft, J Alzheimer's Dis 2007;**11**:471–9) and in another study memantine improved a wide range of cognitive measures without major drop-outs from ADRs (n = 403 [c = 332], RCT, d/b, p/c, 24/52, Peskind et al, Am J Geriatr Psychiatry 2006;**14**:704–15). Memantine has also, uniquely, been shown to reduce deterioration in moderate-to-severe AD (MMSE 3–14, mean 7.9) compared to placebo, based on CIBIC-plus and ADCS-ADLsev, and with low drop-outs (n = 252, RCT, p/c, 28/52, Reisberg et al, N Engl J Med 2003;**348**:1333–41) and to have a sustained effect (n = 175 [c = 136], open, 24/52, Reisberg et al, Arch Neurol 2006;**63**:49–54). Another study in moderate-to-severe Alzheimer's, 4% improved and 27% showed no deterioration over 6/12 (n = 451 [c = 412], 6/12, Clerici et al, Drugs Aging 2009;**26**:321–32). A pooled analysis of memantine in moderate-to-severe AD showed memantine was associated with reduced worsening of AD symptoms (s = 6, n = 1826, RCT, d/b, p/c, 6/12, Wilkinson and Andersen, Dement Geriatr Cogn Disord 2007;**24**:138–45). Memantine may also benefit language function (s = 4, n = 801, p/c,

Ferris et al, Alzheimer's Dement 2009;**5**:369–74). Memantine may be well-tolerated and useful in Lewy body dementia (n = 23, open, p/c, 16/52, Levin et al, Neurosci Behav Physiol 2009;**39**:597–604), and in dementia in Parkinson's disease or Lewy bodies (n = 72 [c = 56], RCT, d/b, p/c, 24/52, Aarsland et al, Lancet Neurol 2009;**8**:613–8). Cochrane concludes there is a beneficial effect at six months (McShane et al, Cochrane Database Syst Rev 2006;**2**:CD003154)

Reviews: * general (s = 7, van Marum, Neuropsychiatr Dis Treat 2009;**5**:237–47; Smith et al, Alzheimer Dis Assoc Disord 2006;**20**:133–7; McKeage, CNS Drugs 2009;**23**:881–97; Parsons et al, Neuropharmacology 2007;**53**:699–723), pharmacodynamics (Rammes et al, Curr Neuropharmacol 2008;**6**:55–78), cognitive functions (s = 6, n = 1826, Emre et al, J Alzheimer's Dis 2008;**14**:193–9).

+ Combinations

Memantine + ChEIs *

Memantine augmentation of **rivastigmine** may improve memory and executive function in mild-to-moderate AD (n = 90, open, 12/52, Riepe et al, Dement Geriatr Cogn Disord 2007; **23**:301–6) and had a sustained effect on slowing cognitive and functional decline in AD compared to anticholinesterase or no treatment (n = 382, 30/12, Atri et al, Alzheimer Dis Assoc Disord 2008;**22**:209–21). Rivastigmine and memantine appears tolerable but better with rivastigmine patches rather than capsules (n = 117, open, 26/52, Olin et al, Int J Geriatr Psychiatry 2010;[in press]). In an observational study of Alzheimer's, those patients taking memantine and an anticholinesterase (15%) had significantly delayed time to nursing home care compared to either as monotherapy (40% and 45% respectively) but made no change to time to death (n = 943, open, mean 3 years, Lopez et al, J Neurol Neurosurg Psychiatry 2009;**80**:600–7).

Reviews: memantine and galantamine (Grossberg et al, J Clin Pharmacol 2006;**46**[7 suppl 1]:17S–26S), memantine and donepezil (Xiong and Doraiswamy, Geriatrics 2005;**60**:13–4).

Sibutramine + ChEIs

Sibutramine had some efficacy in improving cognitive functioning in early and moderate AD

when used as an adjunct to donepezil (RCT, p/c, 3/12, Ollat et al, Encephale 2007;**33**:211–5).

● Unlicensed/some efficacy

Ginkgo biloba *

Ginkgo biloba (GB) 120mg/d stabilised and in some cases improved cognitive function for 6–12 months in patients with mild-to-moderate AD and multi-infarct dementia (n = 155) compared to placebo (n = 54), (RCT, Le Bars et al, JAMA 1997;**278**:1327–32). It must be given for at least 1–3 months before the full therapeutic effect is seen. In a trial of mild-to-severe AD, the placebo group showed a significant decline in all measures (ADAS-cog, GERRI and CGI), while the GB group were considered to have at least slightly improved on some scales (n = 309, d/b, p/c, 26/52, Le Bars et al, Dement Geriatr Cogn Disord 2000;**11**:230–7). GB (special extract EGb 761) has been shown to be equivalent to donepezil and superior to placebo on MMSE (RCT, d/b, p/c, 24/52, Mazza et al, Eur J Neurol 2006;**13**:981–5; n = 96, RCT, d/b, 22/52, Yancheva et al, Aging Ment Health 2009;**13**:183–90). However, it fails to boost memory in healthy older adults (n = 230, p/c, 6/52, Solomon et al, JAMA 2002;**288**:835–40) and GB 120mg/d had no detectable effect on mild-to-moderate dementia over 6/12 (n = 176, RCT, d/b, p/c, 6/12, McCarney et al, Int J Geriatr Psychiatry 2008;**23**:1222–30). Cochrane concludes that GB is safe, although evidence for efficacy is inconsistent and unreliable (s = 9, n = 2016, <6/12, Birks and Grimley Evans, Cochrane Database Syst Rev 2009;1:CD003120).

Review: Anon, Prescrire Int 2007;**16**:205–7.

SSRIs (see also sertraline in 'no efficacy')

Some studies have shown a potential effect from **citalopram**, e.g. improved confusion, mood, restlessness and irritability in AD, improved cognition and emotional functioning (review by Pollock et al, Consultant Pharm 1999;**14**:1251–8), and superiority over placebo (favourably with perphenazine) for behavioural disturbances associated with dementia (n = 85, RCT, d/b, 17/7, Pollock et al, Am J Psychiatry 2002;**159**:460–5). Fluvoxamine augmentation of perphenazine may be effective in reducing psychosis in Alzheimer's patients (n = 20, d/b, p/c, Levkovitz et al, J Nerv Ment Dis 2001;**189**:126–9).

Doxycycline and rifampicin
Significantly reduced decline has been shown with doxycycline 200 mg/d and rifampicin 300 mg/d for three months, which was well tolerated (n = 101, RCT, t/b, p/c, 12/12, Loeb et al, J Am Geriatr Soc 2004;**52**:381–7).

Folic acid *
Cochrane concludes that there is no consistent evidence one way or the other for the use of folic acid (with or without B12) to treat or prevent AD (s = 8, RCT, Malouf et al, Cochrane Database Syst Rev 2008;**4**:CD004514).

Insulin
Elevating insulin levels (with or without hyperglycaemia) improves memory in people with AD (n = 23 + 14 controls, Craft et al, Arch Gen Psychiatry 1999;**56**:1135–40).

Lamotrigine
A case exists of resistant frontal lobe dementia responding to lamotrigine 100 mg/d (n = 1, 6/12, Devarajan et al, Am J Psychiatry 2000; **157**:1178).

Levodopa
In people with dementia with Lewy bodies, levodopa produced 36% 'responders' for motor symptoms (n = 14 [c = 10], Molloy et al, J Neurol Neurosurg Psychiatry 2005; **76**:1200–3).

Methylphenidate *
Methylphenidate 10–20 mg/d has been used successfully for chronic apathy in dementia (n = 13, RCT, d/b, p/c, c/o, 5/52, Herrmann et al, J Clin Psychopharmacol 2008;**28**:296–301).

Naftidrofuryl
This is a cerebral vasodilator with some limited effect on cognitive and global functioning (e.g. n = 84, RCT, Emeriau et al, Clin Ther 2000;**22**:834–44).

Omega-3 fatty acids *
Reduced levels of DHAs have been related to dementia and so supplements may have some efficacy if started early (Cole et al, Prostaglandins Leukot Essent Fatty Acids 2009;**81**:213–21) and may help cognitive function in very mild AD (n = 204 [c = 174], RCT, d/b, p/c, Freund-Levi et al, Arch Neurol 2006;**63**:1402–8).

Piracetam
Piracetam stimulates ACh release. Mild effects may occur when used alone or with an ACh precursor, although Cochrane concludes that the evidence is too weak to prove an effect (Flicker and Grimley Evans, Cochrane Database Syst Rev 2001;**2**:1011).

Testosterone
Men with AD receiving weekly testosterone enanthante 100 mg performed clinically significantly better in spatial and memory tests, but with no change in aggression or unwanted behaviour (n = 32, RCT, p/c, 6/52, Cherrier et al, Neurology 2005;**64**:2063–8).

Vinpocetine *
Cochrane concludes that vinpocetine is well tolerated but has only a minor effect (s = 3, n = 583, p/c, Szatmari and Whitehouse, Cochrane Database Syst Rev 2003; **1**:CD003119).

Other drugs tried include **amantadine** (n = 33, Jibiki et al, Acta Therapeutica 1993;**19**:389–96) and **naltrexone** and **naloxone** (review in Ann Pharmacother 1993;**27**:447–80).

Cannabinoids *
Cochrane concludes that there is no evidence yet that cannabinoids are effective for dementia or BPSD (s = 1, Krishnan et al, Cochrane Database Syst Rev 2009;**2**:CD007204).

Cicloserin (D-cycloserine)
Cicloserin 5–50 mg/d (a partial agonist acting at the NMDA glycine receptor complex) has been shown to enhance implicit memory in Alzheimer's patients, supporting the development of NMDA receptor-mediated

glutamatergic interventions for the treatment of Alzheimer-related memory disorders (n= 108, p/c, d/b, 10/52, Schwartz et al, Neurology 1996;**46**:420–4). However, Cochrane concludes that it has no place in treatment (Laake and Oeksengaard, Cochrane Database Syst Rev 2002;**2**:CD003153).

Melatonin

There is no evidence that melatonin helps cognitive and non-cognitive symptoms of dementia (s = 3, Jansen et al, Cochrane Database Syst Rev 2006;**1**:CD003802).

Nicotine

Studies have shown reduced nicotinic cholinergic receptors in the frontal cortex. Nicotine may stimulate the release of acetylcholine in this area. Nicotine is known to improve attention, memory, vigilance and information processing in (so far) healthy humans, but transdermal nicotine (up to 21 mg/d) had no significant effect on cognitive functions in patients with AD (n = 18, p/c, d/b, c/o, Snaedal et al, Dementia 1996;**7**:47–52). Cochrane concludes that there is no reliable evidence for a beneficial effect (Lopez-Arrieta et al, Cochrane Database Syst Rev 2000;**2**:CD000149).

NSAIDs (see also prevention, 1.13.4)

Aspirin 75 mg e/c had no obvious effect on symptom progression in people (median age 75 years) already with diagnosed AD, and produced ADRs (n = 310, p/c, open, two years, AD2000 Group, Lancet Neurology 2008;**7**:41–9).

Prednisone

Prednisone 10–20 mg/d has been shown to be ineffective (n = 138, RCT, 56/52, Aisen et al, Neurology 2000;**54**:588–93), despite initial enthusiasm from a pilot study (n = 20, open, Aisen et al, Dementia 1996;**7**:201–6).

Procaine *

Despite some claims to the contrary, Cochrane concludes that procaine is detrimental in dementia and cognitive impairment (Szatmári and Bereczki, Cochrane Database Syst Rev 2008;**4**:CD005993).

Selegiline

Selegiline may improve MMSE scores, but with no apparent effect on brain lesions or degenerative changes in brain tissue (n = 17, Alafuzoff et al, Eur J Clin Pharmacol 2000;**55**:815–9), although one trial (with questionable methodology) of 10mg/d indicated some slowing of the disease (n = 341, RCT, Sano et al, N Engl J Med 1997;**336**:1216–22). Cochrane concludes that the evidence is poor, with no justification for use or any need for further studies (Birks and Flicker, Cochrane Database Syst Rev 2003;**1**:CD000442; see also n = 1073, Wilcock et al, Int J Geriatr Psychiatry 2002;**17**:175–83).

Sertraline

Sertraline augmentation of donepezil for BPSD in AD is ineffective, although, as they say, 'there may be a sub-group who respond' (n = 24 + 120, RCT, d/b, p/c, 12/52, Finkel et al, Int J Geriatr Psychiatry 2004;**19**:9–18).

Vitamins *

In mild-to-moderate AD in Taiwanese people, addition of multivitamins (including pyridoxine 5 mg, folic acid 1 mg and iron) had no effect on cognition or ADL functions (n = 89, RCT, d/b, p/c, 26/52, Sun et al, Clin Ther 2007;**29**:2204–14). Cochrane concludes that there is no evidence that vitamin E helps cognitive impairment in AD (Isaac et al, Cochrane Database Syst Rev 2008;**3**:CD002854)

1.13.2 BPSD/BPSSD (behavioural and psychological [signs and] symptoms of dementia) *

Behavioural and psychological (signs and) symptoms of dementia (BPSD/BPSSD) has a cluster of cognitive and non-cognitive symptoms (Petrovic et al, Acta Clin Belg 2007;**62**:426–32) and occurs in up to 90% of people with dementia (Robert et al, Eur Psychiatry 2005;**20**:490–6). BPSD likely to be an imbalance in a range of transmitters rather than one neurotransmitter abnormality (Kálmán et al, Neuropsychopharmacol Hung 2008;**10**:233–49). It includes aggression, agitation, anxiety, wandering, hoarding, sexual disinhibition, apathy and disruptive vocal activity.

Role of drugs

Symptoms of BPSD should be monitored for at least a month before treatment is considered, and non-drug approaches (e.g. environment, multisensory stimulation, etc) used first. Anticholinesterases and memantine have modest efficacy, antidepressants help depression (but more data is needed on agitation and aggression), carbamazepine may be effective (but has significant interactions) and use of valproate is not supported by current data (Herrmann and Lanctôt, *Can J Psychiatry* 2007;**52**:630–46). Antipsychotics may be helpful for severe BPSD but use low doses, time limit and document fully. They should not be used for mild-to-moderate symptoms.

Reviews: * general (Ballard *et al, Nat Rev Neurol* 2009;**5**:245–55; Hersch and Falzgraf, *Clin Interv Aging* 2007;**2**:611–21), symptoms (Chiu et al, *J Formos Med Assoc* 2006;**105**:556–62), psychopathology (Lanari *et al, Mech Ageing Dev* 2006;**127**:158–65), anticonvulsants (Pinheiro, *Encephale* 2008;**34**:409–15; Amann et al, *Clin Pract Epidemiol Ment Health* 2009;**5**:14), and genetics (Borroni *et al, Curr Alzheimer Res* 2010;[in press].

BNF listed

Anticholinesterases *

Anticholinesterases may help BPSD by slowing disease progression in AD, e.g. **donepezil** may significantly reduce delusions, disinhibition and other BPSD symptoms (n = 10, 24/52, Barak *et al, Arch Gerontol Geriatr* 2001;**33**:237–41; n = 28, open, Paleacu *et al, Clin Neuropharmacol* 2002;**25**:313–7) but not agitation (n = 272, RCT, p/c, 12/52, Howard *et al, N Engl J Med* 2007;**357**:1382–92; frustrated comment by Pelosi, *EBMH* 2008;**11**:84). A pooled analysis suggested **galantamine** might improve behavioural symptoms as well (s = 3, n = 2033, RCT, d/b, p/c, 3–6/12, Herrmann *et al, Am J Geriatr Psychiatry* 2005;**13**:527–34). A meta-analysis of studies of **rivastigmine** 6–12 mg/d shows it may be well tolerated and effective for BPSD (s = 3, p/c, 6/12, Finkel *et al, Clin Ther* 2004;**26**:980–90). A systematic review of all three anticholinesterases in BPSD concluded the evidence was limited but they were certainly an option (s = 14, median 24/52, Rodda *et al, Int Psychogeriatr* 2009;**21**:813–24).

Review: general (Miller, *Consult Pharm* 2007; **22**:754–62).

Memantine *

A systematic meta-analysis suggested that memantine decreases NPI (neuropsychiatric inventory) scores and may have a role in managing BPSD, although the effect size is relatively small (s = 5, n = 1750, RCT, d/b, p/c, Maidment *et al, Ann Pharmacother* 2008;**42**:32–8). In moderately severe to severe Alzheimer's disease, a pooled analysis of three studies showed memantine to have a significant effect on neuropsychiatric symptoms and disease progression (s = 3, RCT, p/c, 6/12, Wilcock *et al, J Clin Psychiatry* 2008;**69**:341–8).

Risperidone *

Due to SPC harmonisation across Europe, risperidone is now licensed for the short-term treatment (up to 6/52) of persistent aggression in people with moderate-to-severe Alzheimer's dementia unresponsive to non-pharmacological approaches and when there is a risk of harm to the self or others. A starting dose of 0.25 mg BD is recommended, increased to an optimum of 0.5 mg BD for most patients, although up to 1 mg BD can be used (n = 34, open, 8/52, Rainer *et al, J Clin Psychiatry* 2001;**62**:894–900). Risperidone (mean 1.5 mg/d) has been shown to be effective and well tolerated for BPSD, including sleep disturbances (n = 338 [c = 321], open, 12/52, Durán *et al, Int Psychogeriatr* 2005;**17**:591–604), aggression, agitation and psychosis (n = 337, RCT, p/c, 12/52, Brodaty *et al, J Clin Psychiatry* 2003;**64**:134–43). Additional care is needed in Lewy body dementia as, although psychotic and behavioural symptoms may respond well to low dose, severe EPSEs (especially rigidity) have occurred at 1 mg/d. Risperidone appears as effective as olanzapine (n = 39, d/b, 14/7, Fontaine *et al, J Clin Psychiatry* 2003;**64**:726–30), quetiapine (n = 72 [c = 69], RCT, s/b, 8/52, Rainer *et al, Eur Psychiatry* 2007;**22**:395–403) and superior to haloperidol (n = 114, RCT, d/b, c/o, 18/52, Suh *et al, Int J Geriatr Psychiatry* 2006;**21**:654–60).

+ Combinations

Donepezil + gabapentin (see also dementia)

Behavioural control from gabapentin may augment the cognitive improvement from donepezil (n = 2, Dallocchio et al, J Clin Psychiatry 2000;**61**:64).

Memantine + ChEIs

In patients stable on **donepezil**, addition of memantine may significantly improve BPSD in moderate-to-severe AD (n = 404 [c = 322], RCT, d/b, p/c, Tariot et al, JAMA 2004;**291**:317–24; review by McShane, EBMH 2004;**7**:76) and significantly lowered NPI scores by reducing agitation-related stress (d/b, p/c, 24/52, Cummings et al, Neurology 2006;**67**:57–63).

■ Unlicensed/probable efficacy

Antipsychotics (see also risperidone) *

Antipsychotics have been widely used for symptomatic management of BPSD, but this remains a high-profile and controversial subject. Antipsychotics should not be used as substitutes for poor standards of care, and can be adjuncts to other interventions, but must be monitored and reviewed regularly. Providing support and training for nursing staff to deliver enhanced psychosocial care can reduce antipsychotic use in nursing homes without an increase in agitation (n = 349, RCT, s/b, 12/12, Fossey et al, BMJ 2006;**332**:756–8; comment by Byrne, EBMH 2006;**9**:103). A one-year study showed that in patients with AD in residential care treated with antipsychotics, those that carried on had a survival probability of 70% compared to 77% in the switch-to-placebo group, clinically significant. In the follow-on study, the two-year survival was 46% vs 71%, and three-year was 30% vs 59%, even more marked (n = 128, RCT, p/c, 12/12, Ballard et al, Lancet Neurol 2009;**8**:151–7). In a comparison of olanzapine, risperidone and quetiapine in BPSD, olanzapine and risperidone showed greater improvement than placebo on anger, aggression and paranoia, but none improved functioning, care needs or quality of life (n = 421, RCT, p/c, <36/52, Sultzer et al, Am J Psychiatry 2008;**165**:844–54).

Stroke and cerebrovascular events: * In 2004, the UK CSM recommended that risperidone and olanzapine should not be used for behavioural problems in elderly people with dementia. Sadly, the options left are other newer antipsychotics (with no proof of safety data) or older typicals (from which we thought we had moved on). More recent data has shown that the risk of stroke per 1000 patient years in elderly adults (>65 years old) prescribed antipsychotics is higher with atypicals (47), butyrophenones (47), phenothiazines (72) and benzamides (25) than without (12), but the risk was higher with older antipsychotics than the atypicals (non-users n = 69 939 cf n = 4223 on antipsychotics; Sacchetti et al, J Psychopharmacol 2008;**22**:39–46). Cochrane concluded that risperidone and olanzapine reduce aggression in dementia, but the risk of severe CVA and EPSE means that they should not be used routinely unless there is marked distress (s = 16, RCT, p/c, Ballard and Waite, Cochrane Database Syst Rev 2006;**1**:CD003476).

Death: * On the positive side, an enormous Medicaid analysis was unable to show that atypicals (including risperidone) were more likely to cause CVEs than haloperidol or benzodiazepines (n = 8 million, Finkel et al, Int Psychogeriatr 2005;**17**:617–29) and a comparison of quetiapine, risperidone and olanzapine in the elderly for dementia or other indications showed no significant differences in CVA/TIA events, although dementia appeared to be an important risk factor (n = 18 236, 26/52, Layton et al, J Psychopharmacol 2006;**20**:473–82). However, a review concluded that antipsychotics are not particularly effective, there is most evidence for risperidone and olanzapine, but the effect is modest and increases the risk of stroke (s = 29, Sink et al, JAMA 2005;**293**:596–608). In older adults with dementia, antipsychotic use has been associated with an increased risk of death at 30 days compared to non-use, but conventional antipsychotics had a higher risk than atypicals (n = 27 259 pairs, Gill et al, Ann Intern Med 2007;**146**:775–86). Overall, ADRs from the atypicals may be the limiting factor and the modest benefits may be outweighed by the risks (n = 421, RCT, d/b, p/c, Schneider et al, N Engl J Med 2006;**355**:1525–38; comment by Ballard et al, EBMH 2007;**10**:58). In a fascinating recent report, the risk of cerebrovascular adverse events (CVAEs) appears significantly higher in the first nine weeks and then returns to baseline after three months, with chronic treatment no associated with CVAE (n = 26,157, Kleijer et al, J Psychopharmacol 2009;**23**:909–14).

The **haloperidol** SPC now states that elderly patients with dementia-related psychosis treated with antipsychotic drugs are at an increased risk of death (s = 17, p/c) being 1.6–1.7 times higher than placebo-treated patients, most appearing to be either cardiovascular (e.g. heart failure, sudden death) or infections (e.g. pneumonia) in nature.

Aripiprazole * has been suggested as a suitable alternative (Hamuro, Aust N Z J Psychiatry 2007; **41**:556) as 10mg/d appears safe and effective for psychosis associated with AD, improving psychosis, agitation and CGI (n = 487, RCT, d/b, p/c, 10/52, Mintzer et al, Am J Geriatr Psychiatry 2007;**15**:918–31). Aripiprazole IM was well-tolerated and superior to placebo for BPSD (n = 129, RCT, d/b, p/c, 24 hours, Rappaport et al, J Am Med Dir Assoc 2009;**10**:21–7), but aripiprazole (mean 9mg/d) was ineffective, albeit well tolerated, for psychotic symptoms in Alzheimer's disease (n = 256, RCT, d/b, p/c, 10/52, Streim et al, Am J Geriatr Psychiatry 2008; **16**:537–50).

Olanzapine at low dose, e.g. 5–10mg/d (but not 15mg/d) has been shown to be superior to placebo in treating BPSD and psychosis in patients with AD (n = 206, RCT, d/b, p/c, 6/52, Street et al, Arch Gen Psychiatry 2000;**57**:968–76) and 2.5mg/d seems a reasonable starting dose (n = 652, RCT, 10/52, d/b, p/c, De Deyn et al, Int J Geriatr Psychiatry 2004;**19**:115–26). It has also been used in Lewy body dementia, e.g. decreased psychotic symptoms but with no exacerbation of EPS (n = 29, RCT, Cummings et al, Dement Geriatr Cogn Disord 2002;**13**:67–73, sub-analysis), albeit not well tolerated (n = 8, open, Walker et al, Int J Geriatr Psychiatry 1999; **14**:459–66).

Quetiapine's * UK SPC has been updated with a warning that it is not approved for dementia-related psychosis due to a three-fold increased risk of CVA seen in RCTs with some atypical antipsychotics. However, despite lack of safety data, 25–150mg/d has become standard therapy for BPSD in dementia, e.g.

quetiapine (50–400mg/d) was as effective as risperidone (0.5–2mg/d) for BPSD with no cognitive impairment (n = 72 [c = 69], RCT, s/b, 8/52, Rainer et al, Eur Psychiatry 2007;**22**:395–403), and 200mg/d was superior to placebo for BPSD, but 100mg/d was not superior (n = 333 [c = 63–65%], RCT, d/b, p/c, 10/52, Zhong et al, Curr Alzheimer Res 2007;**4**:61–93). However, quetiapine (mean 200mg/d) did not improve psychosis or cause cognitive or motor deterioration, but reduced CGI-C scores compared to placebo (n = 40 [c = 27], RCT, d/b, p/c, 6/52, Paleacu et al, Int J Geriatr Psychiatry 2008;**23**:393–400). It has, however, been associated with significant cognitive decline (n = 80 [c = 71], RCT, p/c, d/b, 26/52, Ballard et al, Br Med J 2005;**330**:874).

Zotepine 12.5–150mg/d was well tolerated and effective on two measures of BPSD (n = 24, 8/52, open, Rainer et al, CNS Drugs 2004;**18**:49–55).

Review: * general (Liperoti et al, Curr Neuropharmacol 2008;**6**:117–24).

■ **Unlicensed/possible efficacy**

Antidepressants *

Antidepressants may have some use for comorbid depression. **Fluvoxamine** has been reported to be useful for BPSD (n = 3, Kurita et al, Fukushima J Med Sci 2006;**52**:143–8). Modest reductions of agitation in AD have been reported with **trazodone,** with fewer side-effects than placebo (e.g. n = 149, RCT, 16/52, Teri et al, Neurology 2000;**55**:1247–8). A small open study showed mirtazapine 15–30mg/d significantly reduced agitation in Alzheimer's, without significant ADRs or cognitive deterioration (n = 16 [c = 13], open, 12/52, Cakir and Kulaksizoglu, Neuropsychiatr Dis Treat 2008;**4**:963–6).

Aromatherapy *

Melissa, an essential balm oil, may reduce agitation in severe dementia (n = 71, d/b, p/c, Ballard et al, J Clin Psychiatry 2002;**63**:553–8) and lavender oil (two hours a day) produced a modest but significant reduction in agitation in dementia in a cunningly placebo-controlled trial (n = 15, p/c, Holmes et al, Int J Geriatr Psychiatry 2002;**17**:305–8). However, a review concludes that the evidence is scarce, incomplete, mixed and inconclusive (s = 11, Nguyen and Paton, *Int J Geriatr Psychiatry* 2008;**23**:337–46).

Review: Holmes and Ballard, *Adv Psychiatr Treat* 2004;**10**:296–300.

Buspirone

Buspirone has been used for vocal grunts, rocking and difficult behaviour (eg. n = 1, Hamner et al, *J Clin Psychopharmacol* 1996;**16**:261–2).

Carbamazepine

Carbamazepine proved useful in one trial for hostility and aggression in demented patients who had not responded to antipsychotics (n = 21, RCT, 6/52, Olin et al, *Am J Geriatr Psychiatry* 2001;**9**:400–5), but a literature review was less than enthusiastic about its efficacy (s = 7, Konovalov et al, *Int Psychogeriatr* 2008;**20**:293–308).

Cyproterone

Cyproterone was effective for aggression and impulsive behaviour but not aberrant motor behaviour in AD (n = 19, open, Caparros-Lefebvre and Dewailly, *Rev Neurol [Paris]* 2005;**161**:1071–8).

Gabapentin *

There is limited data in BPSD (Kim et al, *Drugs Aging* 2008;**25**:187–96) but it has been used for BPSD and sexual disinhibition in dementia (n = 3, Alkhalil et al, *Am J Ther* 2004;**11**:231–5; n = 24, Hawkins et al, *Am J Geriatr Psychiatry* 2000;**8**:221–5; review by Miller, *Ann Pharmacother* 2001;**35**:427–31). In a review of 11 case reports, three case series and one chart review, gabapentin was in most cases well tolerated and effective, but the data is incomplete (Kim et al, *Drugs Aging* 2008;**25**:187–96).

Prazosin *

Prazosin (mean 6 mg/d) was well tolerated and significantly useful for reducing BPSD (n = 22, RCT, d/b, p/c, 8/52, Wang et al, *Am J Geriatr Psychiatry* 2009;**17**:744–51).

Propranolol *

Propranolol has been used for agitation

in elderly demented patients (case study, Summers, *J Alzheimer's Dis* 2006;**9**:69–75).

Valproate *

Valproate may have some short-term efficacy but has tolerability issues (s = 4, p/c, Porsteinsson, *Drugs Aging* 2006;**23**:877–86), e.g. doses should generally be less than 1000 mg/d (n = 20, RCT, d/b, p/c, Profenno et al, *Curr Alzheimer Res* 2005;**2**:553–8). Positive studies include resistant patients (n = 39, open, 12/52, Sival et al, *Int J Geriatr Psychiatry* 2004;**19**:305–12) where it was generally well tolerated and moderately effective in decreasing physical agitation and aggression (n = 16, open, Herrmann, *Can J Psychiatry* 1998;**43**:69–72) with 86% response rates reported (n = 46, open, 6/52, Porteinsson et al, *Am J Geriatr Psychiatry* 2003;**11**:434–40). However, other trials showed no benefit in BPSD (n = 153 [c = 110], RCT, d/b, p/c, 6/52, Tariot et al, *Am J Geriatr Psychiatry* 2005;**13**:942–9; n = 14, RCT, d/b, p/c, c/o, Herrmann et al, *Dement Geriatr Cogn Disord* 2007;**23**:116–9). A literature review was less than enthusiastic about its efficacy (s = 7, Konovalov et al, *Int Psychogeriatr* 2008;**20**:293–308) and Cochrane concludes that valproate is ineffective in treating agitation in dementia, with unacceptable ADRs (s = 3, Lonergan and Luxenberg, *Cochrane Database Syst Rev* 2009; **3**:CD003945).

Yi-Gan San

Yi-Gan San (a traditional Chinese medicine) improved BPSD and ADL (n = 52 [c = 52], RCT, open, 4/52, Iwasaki et al, *J Clin Psychiatry* 2005;**66**:248–52; see also n = 5 [c = 5], open, 4/52, Shinno et al, *Prog Neuropsychopharmacol Biol Psychiatry* 2008;**32**:881–5).

Yokukansan *

Yokukansan, a traditional Japanese medicine, appeared effective and well tolerated in one study (n = 106, RCT, c/o, Mizukami et al [all 23 of them], *Int J Neuropsychopharmacol* 2009;**12**:191–9).

Zolpidem

This has been used for dementia-related insomnia and night-time wandering (Shelton and Hocking, *Ann Pharmacother* 1997;**31**:319–22).

☐ No efficacy

Cannabinoids *
Cochrane concludes there is no evidence that cannabinoids improve BPSD or other symptoms of dementia (s=1, Krishnan *et al, Cochrane Database Syst Rev* 2009;**2**:CD007204).

Estrogen
Short-term estrogen may increase disturbed and aggressive behaviour in dementia in the elderly (n=16, RCT, d/b, p/c, 4/52, Kyomen *et al, Am J Psychiatry* 2002;**159**:1225-7).

Melatonin *
Melatonin (1.5-8.5mg/d) at night had no effect on sleep, circadian rhythms or agitation in Alzheimer's, compared to placebo (n=41, RCT, p/c, d/b, 10/7, Gehrman *et al, Am J Geriatr Psychiatry* 2009;**17**;166-9).

Oxcarbazepine *
Oxcarbazepine appears to have no significant effect on BPSD in dementia (n=103, RCT, d/b, p/c, 8/52, Sommer *et al, Dement Geriatr Cogn Disord* 2009;**27**:155-63).

1.13.3 VASCULAR DEMENTIA *

Vascular dementia (VaD) is the second most common cause of dementia, affecting about 1-4% people over 65. It is a non-uniform disease due to a single strategic infarct, and can be comorbid with AD. A cholinergic deficiency has been postulated. VaD is characterised by executive dysfunction rather than memory impairment, usually with an acute onset of disorientation. The main symptoms are reading difficulties, loss in insight, apathy, impaired executive function and gait apraxia (n=219, Chan *et al, Dement Geriatr Cogn Disord* 2008;**26**:513-21). Neuroimaging shows cerebrovascular lesions (Murray *et al, Panminerva Med* 2007;**49**:197-207; Román, *J Neurol Sci* 2004;**226**:49-52).

Prevention (i.e. elimination of the main causes) may be the best option:
- hypertension (and lack of use of antihypertensives, probably the main factor)
- diabetes
- atherosclerosis
- cv disease (coronary artery disease, CHF, peripheral vascular disease)
- smoking
- atrial fibrillation
- lipid abnormalities
- hyperhomocystinemia
- sleep apnoea
- chronic infection
- elevation of C-reactive protein.

(McVeigh and Passmore, *Clin Interven Aging* 2006; **1**:229-35; Román, *Cerebrovasc Dis* 2005;**20**[suppl 2]:91-100).

Role of drugs
Anticholinesterases and memantine may produce small benefits but more data is needed (s=8, n=5183, RCT, 6/12, Kavirajan and Schneider, *Lancet Neurol* 2007; **6**:782-92), although a recent review concludes that there is insufficient evidence that anticholinesterases or memantine help (Zekry *et al, Front Neurol Neurosci* 2009;**24**:95-106).

Reviews: * general (Rojas-Fernandez and Moorhouse, *Ann Pharmacother* 2009;**43**:1310-23; Zekry, *Front Neurol Neurosci* 2009;**24**:95-106 Schneck, *Top Stroke Rehabil* 2008;**15**:22-6; Baskys and Hou, *Clin Interv Aging* 2007;**2**:327-35), symptoms (Stewart, *Am J Geriatr Cardiol* 2007;**16**:165-70), cholinergic dysfunction (Román, *Curr Psychiatry Rep* 2005;**7**:18-26), prevention and management (Kirschner, *Curr Neurol Neurosci Rep* 2009;**9**:437-42).

☐ BNF listed

Anticholinesterases *
Two large-scale studies show **donepezil** produces significant improvements in cognition and global functioning in VaD (n=616[c=491], RCT, p/c, 24/52, Wilkinson *et al, Neurology* 2003; **61**:479-86; n=603, RCT, p/c, 24/52, Black *et al, Stroke* 2003;**34**:2320-30; see also s=2, n=1219, 24/52, Malouf and Birks, *Cochrane Database Syst Rev* 2004;**1**:CD004395) and in an extension trial, donepezil appeared to improve cognition (s=2, n=885[c=707], RCT, 54/52, Wilkinson *et al, Int J Geriatr Psychiatry* 2009;**25**:305-13), memory and verbal recall (n=34[c=24], open, 24/52, Kwon *et al, Am J Alzheimer's Dis Other Demen* 2009;**24**:293-301). **Galantamine** may also be effective for patients with VaD or AD combined with cerebrovascular disease

(n = 396 + 196 controls, 6/12, Erkinjuntti et al, Lancet 2002;**359**:1283–90; MS). **Rivastigmine** does not provide any consistent response in probable VaD but some improvements may be seen, probably by improving Alzheimer's co-morbidity (n = 710, RCT, d/b, p/c, 24/52, Ballard et al, Curr Med Res Opin 2008;**24**:2561–74).

Aripiprazole *
Aripiprazole IM was well tolerated and superior to placebo for acute agitation in vascular dementia (n = 129, RCT, d/b, p/c, 24 hours, Rappaport et al, J Am Med Dir Assoc 2009;**10**:21–7).

Memantine
In mild-to-moderate vascular dementia, memantine improves cognition and is well tolerated (n = 579, RCT, d/b, p/c, 28/52, Wilcock et al, Int Clin Psychopharmacol 2002; **17**:297–305), and memantine 20 mg/d has improved ADAS-cog scores compared to placebo (where they declined) in the ITT analysis (n = 321 [c = 288], RCT, p/c, 28/52, Orgogozo et al, Stroke 2002;**33**:1834–9). Cochrane, however, concludes that there is a small beneficial effect at six months in AD, but no detectable effect in VaD (Areosa et al, Cochrane Database Syst Rev 2005;**2**:CD003154).

Reviews: vascular dementia (Smith et al, Alzheimer Dis Assoc Disord 2006;**20**:133–7; Mobius and Stoffler, Int Psychogeriatr 2003; **15**[suppl 1]:207–13)

■ Unlicensed/possible efficacy

Antihypertensives
Hypertension is a significant risk factor, and a persistent effect from calcium-channel blockers has been seen (NNT = 125: n = 2418, RCT, d/b, p/c, two years, Forette et al, Lancet 1998; **352**:1347–51; two-year follow-up, n = 2902, p/c, Forette et al, Arch Intern Med 2002;**162**:2046–52).

□ No efficacy

Cyproterone
Cyproterone was effective for aggression and impulsive behaviour but not aberrant motor behaviour in VaD (n = 19, open, Capparos-

Lefebvre and Dewailly, Rev Neurol [Paris] 2005;**161**:1071–8).

Huperzine A *
Cochrane concludes that there is no evidence that Huperzine A (a herbal medicine) has any efficacy in VaD (s = 1, n = 14, Hao et al, Cochrane Database Syst Rev 2009;**2**:CD007365).

SSRIs
Citalopram appears to have no efficacy in VaD (n = 98, RCT, d/b, 4/52, Nyth and Gottfries, Br J Psychiatry 1990;**157**:894–901).

1.13.4 PROPHYLAXIS AND PREVENTION OF DEMENTIA

This section may be useful in helping advise patients, carers, friends and relatives about possible strategies for reducing the risk of dementia, especially where a family history exists.

General measures (see also vascular dementia) include: *
* Alcohol — light to moderate alcohol consumption in later life is associated with a reduced risk of Alzheimer's and VaD (n = 36746, Anstey et al, Am J Geriatr Psychiatry 2009;**17**:542–55).
* Being overweight in midlife increases the risk of dementia (n = 1152, 40 years, Hassing et al, Int J Obes (Lond) 2009;**33**:893–8).
* Physical activity and exercise modestly improve cognition over two years (n = 170 [c = 138], RCT, two years, Lauten-schlager et al, JAMA 2008;**300**:1027–37).
* Hypertension (see antihypertensives); high and low bp is associated with faster cognitive decline in AD patients (n = 377, Razey et al, Dement Geriatr Cogn Disord 2009;**28**:70–4) and in hypertensive men, controlling blood pressure reduces the risk of AD (n = lots and lots, Peila et al, Stroke 2006;**37**:1165–70).
* Lower cholesterol (see statins)
* Fruit and vegetables — the risk of AD is reduced in people taking at least three fruit juices a week, but no effect was seen from vitamins E, C, or beta-carotene (n = 1836, mean eight years, Dai et al, Am J Med 2006;**119**:751–9). Higher folate helps (see vitamins)
* Not having diabetes (slower cognitive

decline in AD patients with diabetes; n = 154, Musicco et al, J Neurol 2009;**256**:1288–95).

- Drinking 3–5 cups of tea or coffee a day in midlife is associated with a 65% reduction in Alzheimer's. The effect most marked with tea but coffee as well (n = 1409, Eskelinen et al, J Alzheimers Dis 2009;**16**:85-91). See coffee.

Assessment of risk:

Score	Risk factor
1–2	Older age
2–4	Poor cognitive performance
2	BMI < 18.5
1	> 1 apolipoprotein E epsilon 4 alleles
1	MRI findings of white matter disease
1	Ventricular enlargement
1	Carotid artery thickening on ultrasound
1	History of bypass surgery
1	Slow physical performance
1	Lack of alcohol consumption

Range 0–15

Over six years, the percentage of people developing dementia were:
- 4% with low scores
- 23% with moderate scores
- 56% with high scores

(n = 3375, Barnes et al, Neurology 2009;**73**:173–9).

Reviews: * general (Sano et al, CNS Drugs 2008;**22**:887–902; Stephan and Brayne, Int Rev Psychiatry 2008;**20**:344–56; Szakely et al, Int Rev Psychiatry 2007;**19**:693–706), anti-amyloid disease modifying treatments (Christensen, Prim Care Companion J Clin Psychiatry 2007;**9**:32–41).

● **Unlicensed/some efficacy**

Anticholinesterases *

A systematic review concludes that these drugs do not delay the progression to AD or dementia when given to people with mild cognitive impairment (s = 8, RCT, 24/52–3 years, Raschetti et al, PLoS Medicine 2007;**4**:e338), but donepezil may delay the progression in the presence of depression (n = 756, d/b, p/c, three years, Lu et al, Neurology 2009;**72**:2115–21). Cochrane concludes that donepezil does not delay the onset of AD (s = 2, n = 782, RCT, d/b, p/c, Birks and Flicker, Cochrane Database Syst Rev 2006;**3**:CD006104).

NSAIDs *

NSAIDs may, or may not, reduce the risk of AD. **The case for:** A pooled analysis showed a significant effect on reducing the risk of AD but with no advantage for SALAs (e.g. diclofenac, flurbiprofen, ibuprofen) over non-SALAs (e.g. celecoxib, etodolac, mefenamic acid, nabumetone, naproxen) (s = 6, n = 13499, Szekely et al, Neurology 2008;**70**:2291–8). Duration may be an issue, e.g. taking NSAIDs for more than five years was protective against AD, with clearest evidence from ibuprofen (n = 246199, Vlad et al, Neurology 2008;**70**:1672–7; supported by n = 13211, s = 9, Etminan et al, Br Med J 2003;**327**:128–30). It may be that they reduce cognitive decline, but only if started in midlife (before 65 years) before cognitive decline starts, for a minimum of two years and if the person happens to have one or more predisposing APOE genotypes (n = 3383, Hayden et al, Neurology 2007;**69**:275–82), e.g. the APOE epsilon 4 allele (n = 3229, Szekely et al, Neurology 2008;**70**:17–24).

The case against: A five-year case-control study of postmortem brain tissue showed no significant differences in the amount of inflammatory glia, plaques, or tangles in either diagnostic group, and so, while long-term NSAIDs in people with AD may enhance cognitive performance, (n = 22, Halliday et al, Arch Neurol 2000;**57**:831–6; see also postmortem study, Mackenzie, Neurology 2000;**54**:732–5), they may not alleviate the progression in people with mild-to-moderate AD (n = 351, RCT, d/b, p/c, one year, Aisen et al, JAMA 2003;**289**:2819–26; comment by Jacoby, EBMH 2003;**6**:110). There have also been negative findings in older Catholic clergy (n = 1019, Arvanitakis et al, Neurol 2008;**70**:2219–25), from low-dose aspirin 75mg/d for two years (n = 310, RCT, open, mean three years, AD2000 Collaborative Group, Lancet Neurol 2008;**7**:41–9), over one year, from ibuprofen 800mg/d (n = 132[c = 97], RCT, d/b, p/c, 12/12, Pasqualetti et al, Aging Clin

Exp Res 2009;**21**:102–10) and from celecoxib and naproxen (n = 2528[c = 2117], RCT, d/b, p/c, mean two years, ADAPT Group, *Arch Neurol* 2008;**65**:896–905). Finally, in adults (mean 74 years of age), 13% had prior heavy NSAID use, and some became heavy users, but the heavy users actually had a higher AD incidence than non-users, although this could conceivably be because it delayed the onset until the trial (n = 2736, 10 years, Breitner *et al*, *Neurology* 2009;**22**:1899–905).

Review: * general (McGeer and McGeer, *Neurobiol Aging* 2007;**28**:639–47).

■ **Unlicensed/possible efficacy**

Antihypertensives * (see also introduction)

Cochrane concludes that there is no convincing evidence that lowering bp in later life prevents dementia or cognitive impairment in people with no apparent prior cerebrovascular disease, although the data is not robust (s = 4, n = 15936, McGuinness *et al*, *Cochrane Database Syst Rev* 2009;**4**: CD004034). However, cognition appears better preserved in elderly patients taking long-term antihypertensives (55% reduction in risk of dementia cf placebo, Forette *et al*, *Arch Intern Med* 2002;**162**:2046–52; n = 1900, Murray *et al*, *Arch Intern Med* 2002;**162**:2090–6), as blood pressure lowering may have a heterogeneous effect on cognitive function (s = 16, n = 19501, Birns *et al*, *J Hypertension* 2006;**24**:1907–14). ACE inhibitors do not seem as a class to affect cognitive decline, although there may be some differences between them, e.g. centrally active ACEI were associated with 65% less decline compared to a greater risk with non-centrally active ACEIs (n = 1054, six years, Sink *et al*, *Arch Intern Med* 2009;**169**:1195–202).

Beer

Beer contains silicon, which may reduce the bio-availability of aluminium (Gonzalez-Munoz *et al*, *Food Chem Toxicol* 2008;**46**:49–56). Well, it seems to be working for my Dad.

Coffee/caffeine/tea * (see also introduction)

A pooled analysis shows a clear protective effect for coffee on developing AD, although the evidence is not robust (s = 4, Barranco

Quintana *et al*, *Neurol Res* 2007;**29**:91–5), and may be from a neuroprotective effect from caffeine (Rosso *et al*, *Am J Alzheimers Dis Other Dement* 2008;**23**:417–22). However, coffee drinking did not appear to affect the risk of mild cognitive impairment of dementia in one study (n = 2606, mean follow-up 28 years, Laitala *et al*, *Am J Clin Nutr* 2009;**90**:640–6).

Estrogen (oestrogen) *

Estrogen is a potent chemical factor that prevents vascular disease and improves blood flow in diseased vessels, including blood flow in regions of the brain affected by AD. Estrogen also has direct effects on neuronal function that may play an important role in the preservation and repair of neurons and levels may decline in post-menopausal women in whom AD develops (n = 143, Manly *et al*, *Neurology* 2000;**54**:833–8). A number of trials have shown a potential effect. Long-term HRT may slow mental decline in older women, especially those over 85 (n = 2000, Carlson *et al*, *Neurology* 2001;**57**:2210–16), high-dose transdermal 17-beta-estradiol improved cognition in women with AD (n = 20, RCT, p/c, 8/52, Asthana *et al*, *Neurology* 2001;**57**:605–12) and estrogen HRT (oral or transdermal) enhanced verbal memory and performance in non-demented cognitively intact older women (n = 184, Maki *et al*, *Am J Psychiatry* 2001;**158**:227–33). However, some recent trials have failed to show a protective effect from, e.g. conjugated estrogens (n = 120, RCT, 12/12, Mulnard *et al*, *JAMA* 2000;**283**:1007–15; review by Hogervorst and McShane, *EBMH* 2000;**3**:83; n = 50, d/b, 12/52, Wang *et al*, *Neurology* 2000;**54**:2061–6) and from short-term estrogens (n = 42 women, RCT, 16/52, Henderson *et al*, *Neurology* 2000;**54**:295–302). Estrogen replacement therapy (ERT) did not appear to slow the decline in cognitive functioning in postmenopausal women (n = 2859, Alves de Moraes *et al*, *Am J Epidemiol* 2001;**154**:733–9) or reduce the risk of developing AD (n = 221406, case-control, Seshadri *et al*, *Arch Neurol* 2001;**58**:435–40) and actually increased the risk in another study (n = 4000, RCT, d/b, p/c, Shumaker *et al*, *JAMA* 2003;**289**:2651–62, 2663–72; comment by Sherwin and McGill, *EBMH* 2003;**6**:111).

Reviews: * general (Henderson, *Semin Reprod Med* 2009;**27**:283–93; Pike *et al*, *Front Neuroendocrinol* 2009;**30**:239–58; Zhao and Brinton, *BMC Neurosci* 2006;**7**:24).

Fish and n-3 fatty acids

People who eat fish at least once a week have 60% lower risk of developing AD compared with people who never, or seldom eat fish (n = 815, Morris *et al*, *Arch Neurol* 2003;**60**: 940–6). If you want to follow this, we can recommend 'Fishes' just across the road from our pharmacy. See also omega-3 fatty acids.

Folate *

A US study has shown that B6 and B12 levels are not related to AD onset but that higher folate intake decreases the risk of AD regardless of other factors and vitamin B levels (n = 965, mean six years, open, Luchsinger *et al*, *Arch Neurol* 2007;**64**:86–92). However, Cochrane concludes that there is no consistent evidence one way or the other for the use of folic acid (with or without B12) to treat or prevent AD (s = 8, RCT, Malouf *et al*, *Cochrane Database Syst Rev* 2008;**4**:CD004514).

Lithium *

The case for: There is some evidence that lithium could have a preventative role in AD, possibly by blocking accumulation of amyloid-beta peptides. Those with bipolar disorder have an increased risk of dementia compared to the general population (19% vs 7%), but in those who have had long-term lithium therapy it was 5% compared to 33% in non-lithium takers (n = 1423, Terao *et al*, *Prog Neuropsychopharmacol Biol Psychiatry* 2006; **30**:1125–8; n = 114, Nunes *et al*, *Br J Psychiatry* 2007;**190**:359–60; comment by Terao, *Br J Psychiatry* 2007;**190**:361–2).

The case against: A case-control study failed to show that lithium protects against the onset of dementia (Dunn *et al*, *Alzheimer Dis Assoc Disord* 2005;**19**:20–2). A short-term study showed no effect on GSK-3, which regulates the tau protein (n = 71, 10/52, Hampel *et al*, *J Clin Psychiatry* 2009;**70**:922–31), and lithium had no effect on MMSE in mild-to-moderate Alzheimer's disease (n = 22 [c = 8], open, < 12/12, *Int J Geriatr Psychiatry* 2008;**23**:704–11).

Reviews: * use in Alzheimer's disease (Zhong and Lee, *Expert Opin Drug Saf* 2007;**6**:375–83), possible mechanisms (Yeh and Tsai, *Med Hypotheses* 2008;**71**:948–51).

Melatonin *

Melatonin and its analogues have been proposed as potentially having some value (Srinivasan *et al*, *Behav Brain Funct* 2006;**2**:15).

Memantine *

A pilot study has suggested that memantine may effective cognitive function in some populations of postmenopausal women at risk of dementia (n = 22, open, 6/12, Wroolie *et al*, *Acta Neurol Scand* 2008;**119**:172–9).

Raloxifene

Raloxifene, a selective estrogen receptor modulator for osteoporosis, at 120 mg/d (but not 60 mg/d) may produce a 33% reduced risk of cognitive impairment in postmenopausal women (n = 5386, three years, Yaffe *et al*, *Am J Psychiatry* 2005;**62**:683–90).

Red wine *

Moderate consumption could help reduce or slow AD (Anon, *Health News* 2007;**13**:7–8). I thought you'd like to know.

Statins *

Raised midlife serum total cholesterol (even moderately) is associated with an increased risk of AD (n = 9844, 43 years, Solomon *et al*, *Dement Geriatr Cogn Disord* 2009;**28**:75–80), but it is unclear if statins help. Cochrane concludes that statins given in late life have no effect on preventing AD or VaD, but more studies would be needed to show an effect earlier in life (s = 2, n = 26340, McGuinness *et al*, *Cochrane Database Syst Rev* 2009; **2**:CD003160).

The case for: statins, e.g. lovastatin, pravastatin and atorvastatin 80 mg/d (n = 67 [c = 63], RCT, p/c, 3/12, Sparks *et al*, *Arch Neurol* 2005; **62**:753–7), have been reported to substantially lower the risk of developing dementias (n = 1364, Jick *et al*, *Lancet* 2000;**356**:1627–31; n = 60,000, Josefson, *Br Med J* 2000;**321**:1040). In cognitively normal people at enrolment, ongoing statin therapy has been associated at autopsy with reduced neurofibrillary tangle burden, so starting statins before the onset of AD is the important part (n = 110, Li et al, Neurology 2007;**69**:878–85). Non-statin cholesterol-lowering drugs do not show this effect (n = 6992, 15 years, Haag et al, J Neurol Neurosurg Psych 2009;**80**:13–7). Statins also seem to help people with increased risk, e.g. simvastatin 40mg/d improved selective measures of cognitive function (n = 57, RCT, d/b, p/c, 4/12, Carlsson et al, J Alzheimers Dis 2008;**13**:187–97) and in Down Syndrome (n = 123, mean five years, Zigman et al, Neurosci Lett 2007;**416**:279–84). Statin users about half as likely to develop dementia as those not taking them (n = 1674, five years, Cramer et al, Neurology 2008;**71**:344–50). In people with AD, use of statins and beta-blockers associated with delay in functional decline (n = 216, three years, Rosenberg et al, Am J Geriatr Psychiatry 2008;**16**:883–92).

The case against: in asymptomatic middle-aged adults at increased risk of AD, simvastatin improved some cognitive functions but did not affect cerebrospinal fluid biomarkers (n = 57, RCT, d/b, p/c, 4/12, Carlsson et al, J Alzheimers Dis 2008;**13**:187–97) and statin use over 4–5 years had no association with a lower incidence of dementia (n = 355 from n = 4895, Zandi et al, Arch Gen Psychiatry 2005; **62**:217–24; see also n = 2798, Rea et al, Arch Neurol 2005;**62**:1047–51).

Vitamins *

The case for: A study in Hawaii suggested that vitamin E and C supplements may protect against VaD and improve cognitive function in later life in men (n = 3385, Masaki et al, Neurology 2000;**54**:1265–72) and twice the risk if B12 or folate deficiency (n = 370, Wang et al, Neurology 2001;**56**:1188–94). Two large studies have shown that high dietary intake of vitamins C and E may lower the risk of AD (n = 5395, six years, Engelhart et al, JAMA 2002; **287**:3223–9), and that vitamin E from food (but not other antioxidants or supplements) may lower the risk of AD (n = 815, Morris et al, JAMA 2002;**287**:3230–7). Also, patients taking combined vitamin E (1000u/d) and donepezil 5mg/d declined at a slower rate than expected (n = 130, retrospective,

one year, Klatte et al, Alz Dis Assoc Disord 2003;**17**:113–6).

The case against: However, in patients with mild cognitive impairment, vitamin E 2000 IU (cf placebo) had no effect on impairment and did not slow the progression to AD (n = 769, three years, RCT, p/c, d/b, Petersen et al, N Engl J Med 2005;**352**:2379–88) and daily folate 5mg/d, vitamin B6 25mg and vitamin B12 1mg supplementation did not slow cognitive decline in people with mild-to-moderate AD (n = 409 [c = 340], RCT, d/b, p/c, 18/12, Aisen et al, JAMA 2008;**300**:1774–83). Cochrane concludes that there is no evidence for efficacy from vitamin E in either prevention or treatment of Alzheimer's disease (s = 2, Isaac et al, Cochrane Database Syst Rev 2008;**3**:CD002854).

□ No efficacy

Anticholinergics *

Older people taking a drug with an anticholinergic effect have an increased risk of cognitive decline and dementia (HR = 1.65) but discontinuing decreases the risk (n = 6912, four years, Carrière et al, Arch Intern Med 2009; **169**:1317–24).

Omega-3 fatty acids *

Two studies indicate that omega-3 fatty acids do not delay the rate of decline (n = 204 [c = 174], RCT, d/b, p/c, Freund-Levi et al, Arch Neurol 2006;**63**:1402–8), nor are they associated with reduced rates of dementia or Alzheimer's (n = 663, 11 years, Kröger et al, Am J Clin Nutr 2009;**90**:184–92). Another study showed no effect from omega-3 on reducing inflammatory or biomarkers for AD in CSF or plasma (n = 35, RCT, p/c, 6/12, Freund-Levi et al, Dement Geriatr Cogn Disord 2009;**27**:481–90). However, it has been suggested that they may be (more) effective if begun early or if used with an antioxidant (Cole et al, Prostaglandins Leukot Essent Fatty Acids 2009;**81**:213–21).

Gingko biloba *

GB 120mg BD had no effect on reducing the incidence rate of dementia (n = 3069, RCT, d/b, p/c, median six years, DeKosky et al, JAMA 2008;**300**:2253–62).

1.14 DEPRESSION

see also Bipolar mood disorder (*1.10*), Dysthymia (*1.15*), Rapid-cycling bipolar disorder (*1.10.4*) and Mania and hypomania (*1.10.2*)

Depression is a common illness, affecting up to 3% of the population per year, but remains underdiagnosed, undertreated (especially in men and in those under 30). Detection in primary care may be better than perceived by some (n = 18 414, Thompson et al, Br J Psychiatry 2001;**179**:317–23), although treatment may be adequate in fewer than 50% patients (n = 9090, Kessler et al, JAMA 2003;**289**:3095–105). The overall cost of depression (e.g. work, family, other illnesses) is high for this eminently treatable condition, although the UK press seems to have generally archaic views on this, with an apparent strong anti-pharmacotherapy bias.

Symptoms

Depression presents with a mixture of biological symptoms (insomnia or hypersomnia, diurnal variation in mood, low appetite, fatigue or loss of energy, constipation, loss of libido, weight loss or gain) and psychiatric symptoms (depressed mood, loss of interest or pleasure, poor memory, psychomotor agitation or retardation, recurrent thoughts of death or suicide, anxiety, feelings of worthlessness or guilt, including delusions, etc). Depression does not include the normal reaction to the death of a loved one. Atypical depression includes the symptoms of depression, plus two from hypersomnia, hyperphagia, rejection sensitivity and severe lethargy (n = 579, Posternak and Zimmerman, Arch Gen Psychiatry 2002; **59**:70–6).

Causes *

Risk factors can include prescribed or OTC drugs and substance misuse, genetic susceptibility, physical illness, menopause (n = 643 [c = 420], Cohen et al, Arch Gen Psychiatry 2006;**63**:385–90; comment by Woods, EBMH 2006;**9**:109), stress (e.g. bereavement, loss of job, birth of child, break-up of relationship, work stress), epilepsy (double risk, n = 130,880, Fuller-Thomson and Brennenstuhl, Epilepsia 2009;**50**:1051–8), poor social background and the time of year.

Role of drugs *

Although most depressions will resolve with time, antidepressants have a major role in hastening this recovery and reducing suffering. Antidepressants are effective, not addictive, and do not generally lose efficacy with prolonged use. Adequate doses are needed for clinical effect, and continuation for an appropriate period will minimise relapse.

The much publicised 2008 meta-analysis of short-term 4–8 weeks FDA licensing data for antidepressants pre-1999 (Kirsch et al, PLoS Med **5**:e45:0050045) concluded that antidepressants had no significant efficacy for anything except severe depression, once unpublished and inconvenient studies were excluded. This has been hotly disputed as e.g. an equally valid analysis of the same data comes up with different conclusions. There are a number of RCTs comparing CBT (cognitive behavioural therapy) with antidepressants over 12 weeks, and, overall, these show CBT is slightly less effective than antidepressants and even adding CBT to SSRIs in adolescent depression does not help (n = 208 [c = 193], RCT, s/b, 12 + 16/52, Goodyer et al, BMJ 2007;**335**:142–6; comment by Melvin, EBMH 2008;**11**:13) and adding CBT is also not more cost-effective than SSRIs alone (n = 208 [c = 193], RCT, s/b, 12 + 16/52, Byford et al, Br J Psychiatry 2007;**191**:521–7). So, what this analysis really shows is that short-term trials are not long enough and that the combination of SSRIs and CBT will, in many people, be the most effective treatment (critique of the evidence, or lack thereof, for psychotherapy; Nutt and Sharpe, J Psychopharmacol 2008;**22**:3–6; comment on Kirsch by McAllister-Williams, EBMH 2008;**11**:66–8), but that robust evidence for the efficacy of CBT is lacking and that adverse effects have not been properly investigated. CBT can reduce relapse, probably by tackling rumination, but only in people with four or more previous episodes (Conradi et al, Br J Psychiatry 2008;**193**:505–60) and, although there is some evidence for computerised CBT, there is a high drop-out rate and no measures for acceptability or adverse consequences (s = 4, Kaltenthaler et al, Br J Psychiatry 2008;**193**:181–4).

Treatment of depression

The general principles of the medicines

treatment of depression (with antidepressants) can be summed up by the six Ds:

- Diagnosis
- Drug-related
- Drug
- Dose
- Duration
- Discontinuation

1. **D**iagnosis: Making, or being able to make, a diagnosis helps. An obvious statement, but diagnosis does start with a D.

2. **D**rug-related causes eliminated: This might include excessive caffeine intake, other drugs liable to cause depression (see 5.5), and physical (e.g. low folate levels) and environmental causes.

3. **D**rug: All the main antidepressants appear to have broadly similar efficacy, although there may be some differences in efficacy and acceptability (see comparative section). As non-compliance or inadequate dosage are the main causes of drug failure, the choice of drug should consider these factors.

The Cipriani meta-analysis compared bupropion, citalopram, duloxetine, escitalopram, fluoxetine, fluvoxamine, milnacipran, mirtazapine, paroxetine, reboxetine, sertraline, and venlafaxine range for the acute treatment of unipolar major depression in adults. Cipriani concluded that:

- Escitalopram, mirtazapine, venlafaxine and sertraline were significantly more efficacious than duloxetine, fluoxetine, fluvoxamine, paroxetine and reboxetine (the latter significantly less efficacious than all the other antidepressants tested)
- Escitalopram and sertraline showed the best profile of acceptability, leading to significantly fewer discontinuations than duloxetine, fluvoxamine, paroxetine, reboxetine, and venlafaxine
- Clinically important differences exist, both in efficacy and acceptability, in favour of escitalopram and sertraline. Sertraline might be the best first choice because it has the most favourable balance between benefits, acceptability and acquisition cost, although escitalopram was not far behind (s = 117, n = 25,928, RCT, Cipriani *et al*, *Lancet* 2009;**373**:746–58).

Rankings of the top antidepressants for efficacy and cost-effectiveness (NICE, 2009) *

Efficacy	Cost-effectiveness	
	Moderate depression	Severe depression
1 Mirtazapine	1 Mirtazapine	1 Mirtazapine
2 Escitalopram	2 Sertraline	2 Sertraline
3 Venlafaxine	3 Escitalopram	3 Escitalopram
4 Sertraline	4 Citalopram	4 Citalopram
5 Citalopram	5 Venlafaxine	5 Venlafaxine
6 Paroxetine	6 Paroxetine	6 Paroxetine
7 Fluoxetine	7 Fluoxetine	7 Fluoxetine
8 Duloxetine	8 Fluvoxamine	8 Duloxetine
9 Fluvoxamine	9 Duloxetine	9 Fluvoxamine
10 Reboxetine	10 Reboxetine	10 Reboxetine

Onset of action: * Although commonly thought that antidepressants take four weeks to work, it is more accurate to say that 'time to substantial remission' (full statistical separation from placebo) may take four weeks in clinical trials (partly because trials are not powered to detect an earlier onset). The onset of action may actually be much quicker, with detectable positive effects after three hours (n = 26, RCT, d/b, Murphy *et al*, *Br J Psychiatry* 2009;**194**:535–40; n = 21 [c = 16], RCT, c/o, s/b, Bruhl *et al*, *Neuropsychopharmacology* 2010;**35**:521–33), separation from placebo by day 5 (review by Mitchell, *Br J Psychiatry* 2006; **188**:105–6), symptomatic improvement in a week (s = 28, n = 5872, RCT, Taylor *et al*, *Arch Gen Psychiatry* 2006;**63**:1217–23) and 57% differences apparent by week 2 (s = 47, n = 8500, d/b, p/c, Pasternak and Zimmerman, *J Clin Psychiatry* 2005; **66**:148–58). Early improvement within two weeks predicts subsequent positive outcome (s = 41, n = 6562, p/c, 4–8/52, Szegedi *et al*, *J Clin Psychiatry* 2009;**70**:344–53) and leads to better long-term compliance as recovery is associated with starting antidepressants. Telling people they take four weeks to work means any rapid improvement will be attributed to other reasons.

4. **D**ose: The therapeutic range of the newer antidepressants has been established through dose-finding studies but is less clear for the tricyclics (e.g. the need for tricyclic doses of 125–150 mg/d in 95% adults). Once-daily dosing is as effective as multiple daily doses, regardless of drug half-life (s = 22, Yyldyz, and Sachs, *J Affect Disord* 2001;**66**:199–206; review by Barbui, *EBMH* 2002;**5**:57).

5. **Duration:**

5a. Acute therapy — SSRIs are the standard first-line therapy, although starting at half the standard dose for a few days improves tolerability. The person must be monitored for akathisia, anxiety, agitation and suicidal ideation early in treatment. If depression remains completely unchanged at four weeks of therapeutic dosing, an alternate drug should be tried. Minimal improvement within the first four weeks should indicate a further two-week trial, then change to an alternate drug if there is no further response (n = 593, Quitkin et al, Arch Gen Psychiatry 1996;**53**:785–92). If there is no response by eight weeks, the trial should 'be declared a failure' (n = 840, 12/52, open, Quitkin et al, Am J Psychiatry 2003;**160**:734–40). These times should probably be doubled in the elderly and in chronic depression (review by Gelenberg and Chesen, J Clin Psychiatry 2000;**61**:712–21).

5b. Continuation therapy — proper treatment of depression requires relief not just of acute symptoms but continued treatment while the person remains vulnerable. Inadequate or no treatment for six months post-response in controlled trials has resulted in relapse rates as high as 50% (cf 20% with adequate treatment, although compliance was not certain in these cases). If a first episode of depression remits in 12 weeks, continued treatment for six months minimises the risk of relapse, but longer therapy may confer little additional benefit, except in people with additional relapse risk factors (n = 395, RCT, 52/52, Reimherr et al, Am J Psychiatry 1998;**155**:1247–53) and recurrent depression (s = 31, n = 4410, Geddes et al, Lancet 2003;**361**:653–61; comment by Donoghue, EBMH 2003;**6**:84). Continuation doses should be the **same or close to the therapeutic dose** (RCT, three years, Frank et al, J Affect Disord 1993;**27**:139–45). In the elderly, therapy for up to two years after recovery may be needed (Anon, Br J Psychiatry 1993;**162**:175–82). Patients should also be advised that antidepressants are not 'addictive' as such.

5c. Maintenance or relapse prevention * — relapse prevention has been shown for a number of antidepressants, e.g. imipramine over 3–5 years (n = 128, RCT, d/b, p/c, three years, Frank et al, Arch Gen Psychiatry 1990;**47**:1093–9; Kupfer et al, Arch Gen Psychiatry 1992;**49**:769–73), paroxetine in older adults (n = 116, RCT, d/b, p/c, two years, Reynolds et al, N Engl J Med 2006;**354**:1130–8;

comment by Shulman EBMH 2007;**9**:101 noting an NNT of only 4 and the lack of effect from IPT) and venlafaxine, but not sertraline (RCT, d/b, p/c, two years, Wilson et al, Br J Psychiatry 2003;**182**:492–7). Those likely to benefit from maintenance (Kasper and Eder in Winkler et al, Curr Opin Psychiatry 2002;**15**:63–8) include those with chronic depression, three episodes, or two episodes with risk factors (late or early onset, short interval between episodes, rapid onset, dysthymia, positive family history, comorbidity, incomplete response and low work adjustment). In a 10-year prospective study of multiple recurrences of major depression, the risk of recurrence increased by 16% with each successive episode, but the risk of recurrence progressively decreased as duration of recovery increased (n = 318, Solomon et al, Am J Psychiatry 2000;**157**:229–33), so keeping people well pays dividends.

General minimum treatment duration recommendations:

- First episode — six months post-recovery.
- Second episode — 2–3 years.
- Third episode — five years or longer.
- Fourth episode — you should need a very good reason to stop.

Pleasingly, the doubling in antidepressant prescribing in the UK over the last decade is apparently due to longer durations of treatment rather than a rise in depression (n = 189,851, Moore et al, BMJ 2009;**339**:b3999).

Reviews: maintenance (WFSBP Guidelines, Bauer et al, World J Biol Psychiatry 2002;**3**:69–86), relapse prevention (various artists, J Clin Psychiatry 2007;**68**:619–30).

6. **Discontinuation:** When discontinuing therapy is considered appropriate, slowly reduce doses over a minimum of four weeks. Discontinuation syndromes have been reported for nearly all antidepressants, but particularly paroxetine and venlafaxine. Discontinuation symptoms usually appear within 1–3 days of stopping treatment and they can improve within a week (although can last much longer), while recurrence of depression begins after three weeks and continues to worsen. See switching antidepressants in 2.2.2 for a further review, e.g. symptoms and management.

Treatment-resistant depression

True 'treatment-resistant' depression often needs a systematic approach to solve. Remember also that resistant depression may be undiagnosed bipolar (see *1.10.3*). Options include:

1. **Escalate antidepressant doses for an adequate duration:** This is appropriate for drugs with a dose-response curve, e.g. up to 300mg/d or more of a tricyclic or other drug (e.g. venlafaxine), or to tolerance (monitoring plasma levels carefully), remembering that a few people have multiple copies of, e.g. CYP2D6 and may rapidly metabolise tricyclics. Push SSRI doses to BNF maximum.

2. **Check blood levels:** to detect possible 2D6 ultrarapid metabolisers.

3. **Switch drugs:** Ensure all drug classes have been tried optimally, e.g. SSRIs, tricyclics, SNRIs, mirtazapine, agomelatine, moclobemide (at much higher doses than are currently recommended, e.g. over 600mg/d) and MAOIs (see *Chapter 2.2.6* for advice on switching antidepressants).

4. **Augment or combine:** Use logical combinations of antidepressants, (see later in this section), e.g. mirtazapine, lithium, carbamazepine (but not with tricyclics, where it reduces plasma levels, see *4.5.1*), valproate, or lithium/SSRI/tryptophan. SSRIs should not routinely be used with tricyclics, unless with regular blood level testing, or at all with MAOIs (see *4.3.4*).

5. **Assure compliance:** Around 42% people stop antidepressants within the first 30 days (mostly from ADRs), 30% in the next 60 days (mostly due to lack of efficacy), and only 28% carry on beyond three months (n = 829, Olfson *et al, Am J Psychiatry* 2006;**163**:101–8).

6. **Manage ADRs:** If response occurs but ADRs are limiting, see *Chapter 6* for strategies to manage, e.g. sexual dysfunction, sedation, etc.

7. **Check folate levels:** See adjunctive therapy.

8. **Consider individual CBT:** This should be considered in combination with antidepressants and may be effective, but requires a high level of expertise (n = 240, RCT, p/c, 16/52, DeRubeis *et al, Arch Gen Psychiatry* 2005;**62**:409–16).

Review: * drug treatments (Papakostas, *J Clin Psychiatry* 2009;**70**[Suppl 6]:16–25).

Bipolar depression

See separate section (*1.10.3*).

Loss of antidepressant efficacy (tachyphylaxis)

Loss of antidepressant efficacy (also termed 'operational tolerance', or more graphically as 'poop-out') has been reported during long-term maintenance treatment. An analysis of available studies estimates the incidence of relapse in people with a true drug response and continuing treatment is 7.4%, whereas in the relapse rate in placebo responders is 24%, so relapse in continuation treatment is most likely to be in people who were not true drug responders (s = 4, Zimmerman and Thongy, *J Clin Psychiatry* 2007;**68**:1271–6). There is, however, no sound data to support the view that antidepressants may actually worsen the course of depression (except perhaps bipolar depression). Possible mechanisms might include non-compliance, loss of initial placebo response, loss of true drug effect, pharmacological tolerance, accumulation of detrimental metabolites, change in illness pathology, unrecognised rapid-cycling, switching and cycle acceleration in bipolars, antidepressant-inducing paradoxical effects and a genuine lack of prophylactic efficacy (review by Fava, *J Clin Psychiatry* 2003;**64**:123–33).

Strategies to overcome loss of efficacy include:

1. **Increase** the dose.
2. **Decrease** the dose (this may work if the dose has exceeded any 'therapeutic window', but is poorly supported by published data).
3. **Addition** of dopamine agonists, e.g. bromocriptine.
4. **Augment** with, e.g. mood stabilisers, anticonvulsants, thyroid, another antidepressant.
5. **Drug holiday** (although this is poorly supported by the literature).
6. **Switch** to a different drug or class.
7. **Ensure compliance**.

Suicidality

The role of antidepressants in reducing or causing suicide or suicidal ideation remains controversial. The key issues are as follows (see also chapter 5.15 for more data, including reference to adolescents, etc):

- **Depression is a risk factor for suicide:** Suicide practically does not occur without the presence of mental health problems, most commonly depression, then alcoholism. Depressed individuals who have committed suicide have seldom been treated with antidepressants.
- **Antidepressants can cause a short-term increase in suicidal ideation but do**

not cause suicide: Antidepressants have been associated with the emergence of suicidal tendencies but an analysis of all FDA antidepressant trials was unable to find any link with increased suicide from any antidepressants compared to placebo (n = 49 277, Khan et al, Am J Psychiatry 2003;**160**:790–2). In other studies fluoxetine, paroxetine and dosulepin were associated with a slight increase in suicidal behaviour, especially days 1–9 (n = 159 810, Jick et al, JAMA 2004;**292**:338–43) and the suicide attempt risk with SSRI was 2.3 times higher than placebo and 1.9 times higher than other interventions (s = 702, n = 87 650, Fergusson et al, Br Med J 2005; **330**:396), although a five-fold increase in suicidal behaviour after discontinuation of antidepressants has been reported, suggesting a possible protective effect (n = 521, Yerevanian et al, Acta Psychiatr Scand 2004;**110**:452–8). Other negative studies include a meta-analysis of SSRIs, showing no increased risk of suicide in adults (s = 477, n = > 40 000, RCTs, p/c, Gunnell et al, Br Med J 2005;**330**:385; see also n = 146 095, Martinez et al, Br Med J 2005;**330**:389–93). To put this into perspective and add some balance, a thorough review of death/suicide and dependence concluded that while SSRIs have problems, they are less than the tricyclics or the depression (Nutt, J Psychopharmacol 2003;**17**:355–64).

- **Antidepressants reduce the incidence of suicide, especially in older adults:** The absolute risk of suicide during acute antidepressant treatment is about one in 3000, and serious suicide attempts is one in 1000, with no evidence of a statistically significant increase in suicide or ideation in the month after starting treatment with newer antidepressants (n = 65 103, Simon et al, Am J Psychiatry 2006;**163**:41–7). In Denmark, the suicide rate (1995–1999) dropped, particularly in people treated with SSRIs or older antidepressants (n = 438 625) compared to those not treated with antidepressants (n = 1 199 057) (four years, Søndergård et al, Acta Psychiatr Scand 2006;**114**:168–76). In Sweden,

an annual ongoing local educational programme (interactive seminars, 1995–2002) for GPs has led to antidepressant use being increased from 25% below national average to the same level, while suicide decreased to the national average (Henriksson and Isacsson, Acta Psychiatr Scand 2006;**114**:159–67). In Japan, for every extra DDD of antidepressant used per 1000 population, the suicide rate reduces by 6% (Nakagawa et al, J Clin Psychiatry 2007;**68**:908–16).

- **Antidepressants need to be treated with respect:** SSRIs and other newer agents have low toxicity in overdose but the tricyclics and some older antidepressants can be toxic in overdose.
- **Depressed patients with insomnia have significantly higher suicidal ideation** so do not forget hypnotics (n = 70, Chellappa and Araújo, Psychiatry Res 2007;**153**:131–6) and that SSRIs can disrupt sleep architecture so must be taken with breakfast.
- **Antidepressants do not cause an increase in suicide in depressed adolescents, although there may be an increase in suicidal ideation in under 25s:** A meta-analysis of RCTs indicated a small short-term risk of self-harm or suicidal events in children and adolescents with MDD treated with newer antidepressants (n = 2741, RCTs, Dubicka et al, Br J Psychiatry 2006;**189**:393–8). After the 2003 FDA and European regulators warning that antidepressants in younger people might increase suicide thoughts and attempts, there was a 22% reduction in SSRI use in < 19s in the Netherlands and a 30% reduction in SSRI use in < 19s in the USA. The result was a 49% *increase* in suicides in < 19s in the Netherlands (from 0.86 to 1.28 per 100 000 population) and a 14% increase in < 19s in the USA (from 2.83 to 3.23 per 100 000 population), the largest annual increase in US suicide rates and an abrupt reversal of 20-year trends (Gibbons et al, Am J Psychiatry 2007;**164**:1356–63).

Reviews: * BAP guidelines updated (Anderson et al, J Psychopharmacol 2008;**22**:343–96), pharmacotherapy (Reid and Cameron, Prescriber 2009;**20**:18–36; s = 104, Gartlehner et al,

Drug Saf 2008;**31**:851–65; Qaseem *et al, Ann Intern Med* 2008;**149**:725–33; Gartlehner *et al, Ann Intern Med* 2008;**149**:734–50), dopamine agonists (Clausius *et al, Neuropsychiatr* 2009; **23**:15–25), herbal remedies (Ernst, *Adv Psychiatr Treat* 2007;**13**:312–6), TDM of 15 antidepressants (Reis *et al, Ther Drug Monit* 2009;**31**:42–56), atypicals as augmentation (Shelton and Papakostas, *Acta Psychiatr Scand* 2008;**117**:253–9).

BNF listed

SELECTIVE SEROTONIN REUPTAKE INHIBITORS (SSRIs)

The SSRIs are now first choice drugs in depression in most patients due to their safety in overdose and better side-effect profile. Although chemically distinct from each other, the SSRIs are essentially more similar than different and are all effective antidepressants, but their ADR profiles and potential for interactions may show clinical differences, as well as efficacy and tolerability differences (see choice of drugs).

Citalopram

Citalopram is an established first-line anti-depressant and has been shown to be effective and well tolerated in studies against standard antidepressants. A review of 30 RCTs showed citalopram to be superior to placebo, of comparable efficacy to other antidepressants and well tolerated from 20–60 mg/d. STAR*D's phase I used an average of 42 mg/d for optimum effect. Relapse prevention has been shown over 15 months in adults (n = 427, RCT, 44–77/52, Hochstrasser *et al, Br J Psychiatry* 2001;**178**:304–10) and in the elderly (n = 121, RCT, 48/52, Klysner *et al, Br J Psychiatry* 2002; **181**:29–35; review by Appelberg, *EBMH* 2003: **6**:24).

Reviews: general (Pollock, *Expert Opin Pharmacother* 2001;**2**:681–98) and safety (Nemeroff, *Psychopharmacol Bull* 2003;**37**: 96–121).

Escitalopram *

Escitalopram is the pharmacologically active enantiomer of citalopram (a mix of R- and S-citalopram) and at least twice as potent on a mg for mg basis as citalopram (eg, n = 380, RCT, d/b, 8/52, Wade *et al, Int Clin Psychopharmacol* 2002;**17**:95–102). There is accumulating evidence that R-citalopram antagonises escitalopram at serotonin receptors (e.g. Storustovu *et al, Br J Pharmacol* 2004; **142**:172–80); escitalopram binds to the primary binding site **and** the allosteric site; whereas R-citalopram blocks the allosteric site in a dose-dependent manner, reducing the antidepressant effect on the primary site. R-citalopram has a greater affinity for the serotonin transporter than escitalopram (Sanchez, *Basic Clin Pharmacol Toxicol* 2006;**99**:91–5) and may also have a longer half-life (R-citalopram is metabolised slower than escitalopram), which might lead to an accumulating negative effect. The optimal dose in moderate MDD seems to be 10 mg/d with 20 mg/d the optimum in severe depression (p/c, 8/52, Bech *et al, Pharmacopsychiatry* 2006; **39**:128–34).

A series of meta-analyses have shown escitalopram superior to other antidepressants, e.g. the respected Cochrane review concludes that there are some consistent and significant advantages for escitalopram over other antidepressants for efficacy and acceptability (s = 14, Cipriani *et al, Cochrane Database Syst Rev* 2009;**2**:CD006532), e.g. there are 74% responders to escitalopram cf 63% for others (Montgomery and Møller, *Int Clin Psychopharmacol* 2009;**24**:111–8). Escitalopram was significantly more effective for response and remission of depression than other SSRIs [NNT = 25] and SNRIs [NNT = 15] (s = 16, n = 4549, Kennedy *et al, Curr Med Res Opin* 2009;**25**:161–75). While most antidepressants have greater efficacy with more severe depression, escitalopram appears to be effective across all grades of depression, especially severe (s = 15, n = 4301, Kilts *et al; Expert Opin Pharmacother* 2009;**10**:927–36). A trial should last at least four weeks before further intervention is considered (s = 40, Baldwin *et al, Hum Psychopharmacol* 2009;**24**:269–75). A long-term relapse prevention efficacy has been shown (n = 590 [c = 437], open, 12/12, Wade *et al, Ann Clin Psychiatry* 2006;**18**:83–9; n = 139, RCT, d/b, p/c, 52/52, Kornstein *et al, J Clin Psychiatry* 2006;**67**:1767–75; MS). Neither citalopram nor escitalopram had any effects on psychomotor performance and so have been recommended as suitable antidepressants for pilots (n = 24, d/b, p/c, c/o, 3×2/52, Paul et al, Aviat Space Environ Med 2007;**78**:693–7).

Reviews: general (Murdoch and Keam, Drugs 2005;**65**:2379–404; n > 4000, Baldwin et al, Ann Pharmacother 2007;**41**:1583–92), extensive (Dhillon et al, CNS Drugs 2006;**20**:763–90).

Fluoxetine

Fluoxetine is licensed across the world for depression, with or without anxiety. Although 20mg/d (n = 417, Beasley et al, J Clin Psychiatry 2000;**61**:722–8) is the standard dose (UK maximum 80mg/d), some resistant depressions may respond to 60–80mg/d. It has been shown to be clearly superior to placebo and slightly superior to tricyclics with significantly fewer drop-outs (rigorous meta-analysis, s = 30, n = 4120, Bech et al, Br J Psychiatry 2000;**176**:421–8)and evidence of relapse prevention (n = 140, RCT, 48/52, Gilaberte et al, J Clin Psychopharmacol 2001; **21**:417–24, MS). An interesting independent review suggesting inferior efficacy to other antidepressants (s = 131, Cipriani et al, J Clin Psychiatry 2006;**67**:850–64), and recently 60–80mg/d was shown not to be superior to venlafaxine nor placebo for MDD with melancholic features (n = 289, RCT, d/b, p/c, 6/52, Sheehan et al, Int Clin Psychopharmacol 2009;**24**:61–86). Cochrane calls for better trials with fluoxetine, a somewhat futile hope unless used as a comparator (Cipriani et al, Cochrane Database Syst Rev 2005;**19**:4185).

Review: safety and side-effects (Wernicke, Expert Opin Drug Saf 2004;**3**:495–504, MS).

Fluvoxamine *

Fluvoxamine is licensed in the UK for depression. The starting dose should be 100–150mg/d and lack of response at 6/52 accurately predicts non-response (n = 72, open, Morishita and Arita, Psychiatry Clin Neurosci 2003;**57**:177–81). A recent meta-analysis concludes there are no significant differences between fluvoxamine and other antidepressants (s = 53, n = 4000, Omori et al, J Psychopharmacol 2009;**23**:539–50). It may have a higher incidence of nausea and vomiting than other SSRIs.

Paroxetine *

Paroxetine is licensed for depression, including that accompanied by anxiety, with 20mg/d the optimum dose, although higher plasma levels are associated with early response in severely depressed patients so dose escalation might be effective (n = 84, 4-18/52, Gex-Fabry et al, Prog Neuropsychopharmacol Biol Psychiatry 2007;**31**:892–900). Relapse prevention has been shown with paroxetine in old age (n = 116, RCT, d/b, p/c, two years, Reynolds et al, N Engl J Med 2006;**354**:1130–8). Paroxetine's half-life increases from 10 to 21 hours on chronic dosing, but reduces when this is stopped, which may in part explain the many reports of discontinuation effects (see 2.2.2).

Reviews: * general (Marks et al, Expert Opin Drug Saf 2008;**7**:783–94; Tang and Helmeste, Expert Opin Pharmacother 2008;**9**:787–94).

> ### Switching or discontinuing antidepressants
>
> For a table on switching antidepressants and the gaps needed, or advice on the problems of discontinuing, see Chapter 2.2.7.

Sertraline *

The pharmacological profile of sertraline is similar to fluoxetine, but with a shorter half-life. The optimum dose may be 75 mg (n = 82, Morishita and Kinoshita, Hum Psychopharmacol 2008;**23**:647–51). A respected systematic review and meta-analysis shows a significant trend for sertraline over other antidepressants (s = 59, Cipriani et al, Cochrane Database Syst Rev 2009;**2**:CD006117). In recurrent depression (three or more episodes of MDD in four years), sertraline 50mg/d and 100mg/d were superior to placebo in preventing recurrences in people switched to sertraline for continuation treatment (n = 371, RCT, p/c, d/b, 18/12, Lépine et al, Am J Psychiatry 2004;**161**:836–42), but not in the elderly (n = 113 [c = 31], RCT, d/b, p/c, two years, Wilson et al, Br J Psychiatry 2003; **182**:492–7; MS).

Review: pharmacokinetic profile (DeVane et al, Clin Pharmacokinet 2002;**41**:1247–66).

TABLE 1.1: THE RATIONALE AND RISKS FOR COMBINATIONS OF ANTIDEPRESSANTS

Key:

SS	serotonin syndrome very possible
(SS)	serotonin syndrome possible or rarely reported
SSU	serotonin syndrome unlikely
LR	low rationale
SR	some rationale
HR	high rationale
UR	unknown rationale
LH	relatively low hazard or risk
MH	medium hazard or risk either known or predicted
HH	high hazard or risk of problems known or predicted so specialist monitoring required
UH	unknown or undocumented hazard
SM-LDT	specialist monitoring required and limit dose of tricyclic
VM	consider venlafaxine (>200mg/d) or mirtazapine instead for combined 5-HT and NA/NE reuptake blockade
CI	see Chapter 1 for data on positive use of combination
C4/5	see Chapters 4 or 5 for data on risk of interaction or adverse consequences

	Citalopram/ escitalopram	Fluoxetine	Fluvoxamine	Paroxetine	Sertraline	Tricyclics	MAOIs	Venlafaxine	Mirtazapine	Reboxetine	Trazodone	Duloxetine	Moclobemide	Agomelatine
Fluoxetine	SS LR-HH													
Fluvoxamine	SS LR-HH	SS LR-HH												
Paroxetine	SS LR-HH	SS LR-HH	SS LR-HR											
Sertraline	SS LR-HH	SS-C4/5/5 LR-HH	SS LR-HH	SS LR-HH										
Tricyclics	SS-C4/5 LR-HH-CI	SS-C4/5 LR-HH-CI SM-LDT	SS-C4/5 LR-HH-CI SM-LDT	SS-C4/5 LR-HH-CI SM-LDT	SS-C4/5 LR-HH-CI									
MAOIs	(SS)-C4/5 SR-HH	(SS)-C4/5 SR-HH	(SS)-C4/5 SR-HH	(SS)-C4/5 SR-HH	(SS)-C4/5 SR-HH	(SS) SR-HH-CI								
Venlafaxine	SS LR-HH	SS-C4/5 LR-HH	SS LR-HH	SS MR-HH-CI	SS LR-HH	SS LR-HH	SS-C4/5 SR-HH							
Mirtazapine	SSU LR-UH	(SS) LR-UH	SSU LR-UH	SSU C4/5 LR/UH	SSU C4/5 LR-UH	SSU C4/5 LR-UH	SSU C4/5 SR-MH	SSU HR-LH						
Reboxetine	SSU SR-UH VM	SSU SR-UH VM	SSU SR-UH VM	SSU SR-UH VM	SSU SR-UH VM	SSU LR-MH	SSU C4/5 LR-HH	SSU LR-UH	SSU MR-UH					
Trazodone	SS LR-UH	SS-C4/5 LR-MH	SS-C4/5 LR-UH	SS LR-UH	SS LR-UH	SSU C4/5 LR-LH	SSU C4/5 LR-HH	SS LR-HH	SSU SR-UH	SSU SR-UH VM				
Duloxetine	SS LR-HH	SS LR-MH	SS LR-HH	SS LR-HH	(SS) LR-HH	(SS)-C4 SR-HH	(SS)-C4 SR-HH	SS LR-HH	SSU SR-UH	SSU SR-UH VM	SS LR-HH			
Moclobemide	(SS)-C4/5 SR-MH	(SS)-C4/5 SR-LH	(SS)-C4/5 SR-MH	(SS)-C4/5 SR-MH	(SS) SR-MH	(SS) LR-HH	(SS) LR-HH	(SS)-C4/5 SR-HH	SSU SR-UH	SSU SR-UH	(SS) SR-UH	(SS) SR-HH		
Agomelatine	SSU HR-LH	SSU HR-LH	SSU HR-MH	SSU HR-LH	SSU HR-LH	SSU HR-LH	SSU HR-LH	SSU HR-LH	SSU HR-LH	SSU HR-LH	SSU HR-LH	SSU HR-LH	SSU HR-LH	
Tryptophan	(SS)-C4/5 UR-MH	(SS)-C4/5 UR-MH	(SS)-C4/5 UR-MH	(SS)-C4/5 UR-MH	(SS)-C4/5 UR-MH	(SS)-C4/5 UR-MH	(SS)-C4/5 UR-MH	(SS)-C4/5 UR-MH	SSU UR-LH	SSU UR-LH	(SS) UR-MH	(SS) UR-MH	SSU UR-MH	SSU UR-LH

TRICYCLICS

Doses of 125–150mg/d of tricyclics are effective in depression and clearly superior to placebo but due to cardiotoxicity, overdose toxicity (n = 2503, Shah et al, Psychol Med 2001;**31**:1203–10), sedation and anticholinergic effects are not recommended first-line, and in the UK, NICE recommends performing an ECG before prescribing tricyclics in depressed people at significant risk of cardiovascular disease. If using tricyclics, a therapeutic dose must be used before assessing the response.

Reviews: toxicity (Nutt, J Psychopharmacol 2005; **19**:123–4; pointing out the relative toxicity and sub-therapeutic dosing), cardiovascular toxicity from tricyclic poisoning (Thanacoody and Thomas, Toxicol Rev 2005;**24**:205–14).

Amitriptyline

Amitriptyline has long half-life (meta-analysis of amitriptyline vs the rest: Barbui and Hotopf, Br J Psychiatry 2001;**178**:129–44; reply by Thompson, Br J Psychiatry 2001;**178**:99–100) and Cochrane concludes that it is at least as effective as other antidepressants, but with a higher side-effect burden (s = 194, Guaiana et al, Cochrane Database Syst Rev 2007; **2**:CD004186).

Clomipramine

A potent tricyclic with an active metabolite, with a possible added advantage in treating depression with an obsessional component.

Dosulepin (dothiepin) *

Dosulepin is licensed in the UK, although in the UK NICE recommends that it is not used. Although often prescribed to aid sleep, both dosulepin and fluoxetine disrupt REM sleep and no sleep-promoting effects were seen from dosulepin (n = 12, RCT, 5/52, d/b, p/c, Wilson et al, J Psychopharmacol 2002;**16**:321–31).

Doxepin

Doxepin is a standard tricyclic with moderate sedation, which may have fewer anticholinergic and cardiac effects than older tricyclics.

Imipramine

Imipramine is a standard tricyclic. NICE states that women tolerate imipramine more poorly than men. Psychotic depression shows high response rate to imipramine (n = 52, Bruijn et al, J Affect Disord 2001;**66**:165–74). Stimulant side-effects may be troublesome as may the anticholinergic effects, especially in the elderly, and it may provoke fragmentation of motor activity during sleep (n = 52, Volkers et al, Eur Neuropsychopharm 2002;**12**:273–8).

Lofepramine

Lofepramine is an established UK tricyclic and NICE's tricyclic of choice. It may have relatively fewer side-effects than other tricyclics, e.g. it has minimal sedative effects and impairment of concentration and memory compared with dosulepin (Allen et al, J Psychopharmacol 1993;**7**:33–8). It is surprisingly safe in overdose, with lofepramine seeming to block the cardiotoxic effects of the main metabolite, desipramine (full review by Lancaster and Gonzalez, Drugs 1989;**37**:123–40).

Nortriptyline

Nortriptyline is a tricyclic with low cardio-toxic side-effects and suitable for once-daily administration. In treatment-resistant depression (failing 1–5 adequate trials), 40% may respond (12% remission) to nortriptyline, although 35% may not tolerate it (n = 92, open, 6/52, Nierenberg et al, J Clin Psychiatry 2003;**64**:35–9; n = 116, RCT, 12/52, Mulsant et al, Am J Geriatr Psychiatry 2001;**9**:406–14; n = 59, RCT, 18/12, Bump et al, Depress Anxiety 2001;**13**:38–44).

Trimipramine *

Structurally related to levomepromazine, trimipramine has significant sedative properties. High dose trimipramine (up to 400mg/d) has been shown to be at least as effective as amitriptyline and haloperidol for delusional depression (n = 94 [c = 57], RCT, d/b, p/c, 6/52, Künzel et al, J Psychiatr Res 2009;**43**:702–10).

OTHER ANTIDEPRESSANTS

Agomelatine *

Agomelatine is a 5HT2C and 5HT2B antagonist and a melatonin M1 and M2 agonist. In responders, the effective dose in 80% is

25 mg/d and 50 mg/d in the remaining 20% (n = 21, RCT, d/b, p/c, 6/52, Kennedy and Emsley, *Eur Neuropsychopharmacol* 2006;**16**:93–100. Agomelatine 25–50 mg/d was as effective as venlafaxine 75–150 mg/d, improving sleep quickly and with lower drop-outs (n = 332, RCT, d/b, 6/52, Lemoine et al, *J Clin Psychiatry* 2007;**68**:1723–32, MS). A pooled analysis shows efficacy also in severe depression (s = 3, n = 357, p/c, Montgomery and Kasper, *Int Clin Psychopharmacol* 2007;**22**:283–91) and being exceptionally well tolerated, appearing to have no sexual side-effects, no tolerability issues or discontinuation symptoms at a dose of 25 mg/d (n = 192, RCT, d/b, p/c, 2/52, Montgomery et al, *Int Clin Psychopharmacol* 2004;**19**:271–80). In a follow-on study of responders from an acute study, relapse over 6/12 was 21.7% for agomelatine and 46.6% for placebo, with no early relapse on discontinuation, suggesting no withdrawal or rebound effects (n = 239, RCT, d/b, p/c, 6/12, Goodwin et al, *J Clin Psychiatry* 2009;**70**:1128–37). Further data is accumulating showing a superior effect to other standard antidepressants.

Reviews: * general (Dolder et al, *Ann Pharmacother* 2008;**42**:1822–31; Le Strat and Gorwood, *J Psychopharmacol* 2008;**22**(Suppl):4–8; San and Arranz, *Eur Psychiatry* 2008;**23**:396–402; Ghosh and Hellewell, *Expert Opin Investig Drugs* 2007;**16**:1999–2004).

Duloxetine

Duloxetine is an SNRI that also weakly inhibits dopamine reuptake, but has no histamine, dopamine, cholinergic or adrenergic receptor affinity. The standard dose is 60 mg/d (but starting at a lower dose may improve tolerability; s = 6, n = 1619, d/b, p/c, Pritchett et al, *J Psychiatr Res* 2007;**41**:311–8), and, although there is no published evidence that 120 mg/d is more effective, some believe that to be the case. Efficacy has been shown in two major studies (n = 267, RCT, d/b, p/c, 9/52, Detke et al, *J Psychiatry Res* 2002;**36**:383–90; n = 245, RCT, d/b, p/c, 9/52, Detke et al, *J Clin Psychiatry* 2002;**63**:308–15). In other studies, duloxetine 40–120 mg/d was at least as effective as paroxetine 20 mg/d (RCT, d/b, p/c, Goldstein et al, *J Clin Psychopharmacol* 2004;**24**:389–99; MS; n = 392, RCT, d/b, p/c, 8/52, Perahia et al,

Eur Psychiatry 2006;**21**:367–78, MS), and non-inferior to escitalopram in depression, albeit slightly less well tolerated initially (n = 684, RCT, d/b, p/c, 8/52, Nierenberg et al, *Curr Med Res Opin* 2007;**23**:401–16). Follow-on studies show relapse prevention efficacy (e.g. n = 288, RCT, d/b, p/c, < 52/52, Perahia et al, *J Clin Psychiatry* 2009;**70**:706–16; MS). Duloxetine may be useful in older patients (n = 311, RCT, d/b, p/c, 8/52, Raskin et al, *Am J Psychiatry* 2007;**164**:900–9). A meta-analysis of published (and not fully reported) data on duloxetine's effect on painful physical symptoms in depression suggested the effect was very small and statistically non-significant (s = 5, Spielmans, *Psychother Psychosom* 2008;**77**:12–6).

Reviews: use in depression (Kirwin and Goren, *Pharmacother* 2005;**25**:396–410), general (Gupta et al, *Ann Clin Psychiatry* 2007; **19**: 125–32; Frampton and Plosker, *CNS Drugs* 2007; 21:581–609).

Switching or discontinuing antidepressants

For a table on switching antidepressants and the gaps needed, or advice on the problems of discontinuing, see *Chapter 2.2.7*.

Flupentixol *

The standard initial dosage is 1 mg as a single morning dose, which can be increased to 2 mg/d (maximum 3 mg/d) if there is inadequate clinical response.

Mianserin

Mianserin is a tetracyclic with prominent $5HT_{2A}$ and $5HT_{2C}$ antagonist properties, a good safety profile in overdose, low cardiotoxicity and marked sedative properties.

Mirtazapine *

Mirtazapine blocks presynaptic alpha-2 adreno-receptors (increasing norepinephrine transmission) and indirectly enhances serotonergic transmission, with additional $5\text{-}HT_2$ and $5\text{-}HT_3$ receptor blockade minimising the incidence of serotoninergic side-effects, e.g. nausea, headache and sexual dysfunction. The dose range is 15–45 mg/d and the optimum starting dose of 30 mg/d is well tolerated. Mirtazapine has been shown to be as effective as reference antidepressants (s = 10, n = 1904, RCT, d/b, Papakostas et al, J Psychopharmacol 2008;**22**:843–8). Mirtazapine may also be well tolerated and very effective as an adjunctive in antidepressant-resistant persistent MDD (n = 26, RCT, d/b, p/c, 4/52, Carpenter et al, Biol Psychiatry 2002;**51**:183–8). A meta-analysis of all three completed comparative studies of mirtazapine versus SSRIs (fluoxetine, paroxetine and citalopram) showed a similar AD profile, but hinted at superior efficacy and a robust faster onset of action, statistically significant in all three studies in the first few weeks (reviewed by Thompson, J Clin Psychiatry 1999,**60**[Suppl 17]:18–22; discussion 46–8; s = 3, n = 583, Quitkin et al, J Clin Psychiatry 2001;**62**:358–61; n = 212, RCT, d/b, 6/52, Szegedi et al, J Clin Psychiatry 2003;**64**:413–20 and n = 197, RCT, 24/52, Wade et al, Int Clin Psychopharmacol 2003;**18**:133–41). Relapse prevention is significantly superior to placebo (n = 156, RCT, d/b, 40/52, Thase et al, J Clin Psychiatry 2001;**62**:782–8). Mirtazapine started immediately after stroke may reduce the incidence of post-stroke depression (n = 70, RCT, open, one year, Niedermaier et al, J Clin Psychiatry 2005;**5**:1619–23; critical comment by Ween, EBMH 2005;**8**:74).

Reviews: * general (Croom et al, CNS Drugs 2009;**23**:427–52), kinetics (Timmer et al, Clin Pharmacokinet 2000;**38**:461–74, 56 refs).

Moclobemide

Moclobemide (a reversible inhibitor of mono-amine oxidase-A) inhibits only MAO-A and not MAO-B, so an excess of tyramine in the body will displace moclobemide from MAO-A, allowing tyramine metabolism to occur, MAO-B remaining free. This results in a 'cheese-reaction', usually only at amounts above 100–150 mg of tyramine (see 4.3.4), unlikely under normal conditions. A meta-analysis showed it to be about equipotent with imipramine or sedative tricyclic antidepressants in agitated-anxious depressive patients, and all were clearly superior to placebo (s = 38, n = 2416, d/b, Delini-Stula et al, J Affect Disord 1995;**35**:21–30). A review of moclobemide

overdose toxicity concludes that overdose is benign even with massive ingestions (only one death reported), but overdose in combination with other serotonergic agents can cause severe serotonin toxicity (n = 106, Isbister et al, Br J Clin Pharmacol 2003;**56**:441–50).

Review: Bonnet, CNS Drug Rev 2003;**9**:97–140.

Reboxetine

Reboxetine is a selective norepinephrine re-uptake inhibitor with no dopamine, histamine, adrenergic or serotonin effects at 8 mg/d, but a weak anticholinergic action. Analysis of four RCTs indicates reboxetine to be significantly more effective than placebo in severe depression (s = 4, RCT, d/b, p/c, 8/52, Montgomery et al, J Clin Psychopharmacol 2003;**23**:45–50). Relapse prevention has been shown against placebo (n = 283, d/b, p/c, 46/52, Versiani et al, J Clin Psychiatry 1999;**60**:400–6). Reboxetine may improve cognitive processing in depressed adults compared to paroxetine and placebo (n = 74, Ferguson et al, Int Clin Psychopharmacol 2003;**18**:9–14). There is no effect on reaction time (Hindmarsh, Eur Neuropsychopharmacol 1997;[Suppl 1]:S17–S21).

Reviews: general (Hajos et al, CNS Drug Rev 2004;**10**:23–44; Page, CNS Drug Rev 2003;**9**: 327–42).

Trazodone *

Trazodone increases NE and 5-HT turnover with low cardiotoxicity and anticholinergic side-effects, but a higher incidence of drowsiness and nausea, so it makes a good hypnotic as well. Trazodone SR 150–450 mg/d was as effective as sertraline 50–100 mg/d in MDD, and as well tolerated (n = 12, RCT, d/b, 6/52, Munizza et al, Curr Med Res Opin 2006;**22**:1703–13) and 300–350 mg/d was more effective than placebo (n = 412, RCT, d/b, p/c, 8/52, Sheehan et al, Psychiatry (Edgmont) 2009;**6**:20–33). It is best taken with food to reduce peak blood levels.

Venlafaxine *

Venlafaxine is an SNRI with 5-HT reuptake inhibition across the dosage range, NE reuptake inhibition becoming significant from 150 mg/d (n = 32, Harvey et al, Arch Gen Psychiatry 2000; **57**:503–9) and dopamine reuptake inhibition above 225 mg/d. A meta-analysis shows, as with other antidepressants, a greater effect on remission rates in more severe depression (s = 31, n = 6492, Schmitt et al, Eur Arch Psychiatry Clin Neurosci 2009;**259**:329–39). It is an effective antidepressant and there is evidence for a dose-response relationship (e.g. n = 147, RCT, Mehtonen et al, J Clin Psychiatry 2000;**61**:95–100), e.g. venlafaxine may be more effective at higher doses than certain SSRIs, with comparable tolerability (e.g. s = 32, Smith et al, Br J Psychiatry 2002;**180**:396–404). In SSRI-resistant MDD, venlafaxine (up to 150 mg/d) was effective, but higher doses (up to 375 mg/d) might be more effective (n = 96, retrospective, Vanoli et al, J Psychopharmacol 2008;**22**:434–40), but less well tolerated so is best reserved for people not responding to standard dose (n = 232, RCT, open, 12/52, Thase et al, J Clin Psychopharmacol 2006;**26**:250–8; comment by Dodd and Berk, EBMH 2007;**10**:17). Even higher doses, e.g. range 375–600 mg/d may be effective in severe depression but again have more side-effects albeit without higher drop-outs (n = 70, open, Harrison et al, J Psychopharmacol 2004;**18**:200–4). Relapse prevention has been shown in prior responders to venlafaxine over two years in the PREVENT studies (n = 258, RCT, d/b, p/c, 12/12, Kocsis et al, J Clin Psychiatry 2007;**68**:1014–23; n = 1096, RCT, d/b, two years, Keller et al, J Clin Psychiatry 2007;**68**:1246–56; review by Kornsten, Expert Rev Neurother 2008;**8**:737–42).

The UK MHRA have reduced their previous restrictions (comment by Taylor and Scott, J Psychopharmacol 2006;**20**:597–601) on venlafaxine:

- still to be reserved as 2nd line treatment
- shared care is only required for initiation in severely depressed people or in hospitalised patients who require doses of 300 mg daily, or above
- is only contraindicated in patients with an identified high risk of a serious cardiac ventricular arrhythmia or with uncontrolled hypertension. No baseline ECG is needed, but regular bp is recommended.

Although studies suggest a higher overdose toxicity with venlafaxine compared to SSRIs, this may be due to increased use in patients at higher risk factors for suicide (including severity

of depression), e.g. venlafaxine (n = 27096) patients were 4–6 times more likely to have been previously hospitalised for depression than fluoxetine (n = 134996) and citalopram (n = 52035), which might also explain the higher reported suicide rate with venlafaxine (n = 214127, Mines et al, Pharmacoepidemiol Drug Saf 2005;**14**:367–72, MS; Buckley and McManus, Br Med J 2002;**325**:1332–3). Discontinuation effects may be significant (see 2.2.6). Although the UK SPCs for XL and plain tablets have different maximum doses, this is just a licensing issue not a difference in absorption or safety. Venlafaxine is not recommended in children and adolescents under 18 years, due to lack of data on efficacy and an increase in the rate of harmful outcomes, including hostility, suicidal ideation and self-harm.

Review: general (Kienke and Rosenbaum, Depress Anxiety 2000;**12**[suppl 1]:50–4).

MONO-AMINE OXIDASE INHIBITORS (MAOIs)

Isocarboxazid

Isocarboxazid is a hydrazine derivative that irreversibly blocks the MAO enzyme (editorial by Shader and Greenblatt, J Clin Psychopharmacol 1999;**19**:105).

Phenelzine

Phenelzine is a hydrazine derivative that irreversibly blocks the MAO enzyme, and is NICE's MAOI of choice, although they recommend that it is only initiated by specialist mental health professionals (including GPs with a special interest in mental health). A comparison of tranylcypromine and phenelzine showed no significant difference between them, with a 52% response rate in severely depressed treatment-resistant patients (n = 77[c = 67], d/b, 5/52, Birkenhäger et al, J Clin Psychiatry 2004;**65**:1505–10).

Tranylcypromine *

Tranylcypromine is a non-hydrazine amfetamine-related MAOI with stimulant effects and a greater incidence of adverse drug interactions. Tranylcypromine did poorly in resistant depression in the STAR*D study (n = 109, open, McGrath et al, Am J Psychiatry

2006;**163**:1531–41), although the mean dose was only 37mg/d (doses towards 100mg/d or more may be much more effective, e.g. n=77, d/b, 5/52, Birkenhäger et al, J Clin Psychiatry 2004;**65**:1505–10; mean 52mg/d produced a 59% remission rate in treatment-resistant depression; n=32, Adli et al, Pharmacopsychiatry 2008;**41**:252–7), more patients were switched because of previous medication intolerance and the 2/52 washout/lead-in would have led to shorter duration of treatment. The use of concomitant amlodipine can attenuate hypertensive episodes with tranylcypromine, making MAOIs feasible in some resistant depressions (n=3, Taylor et al, J Clin Psychiatry 2005;**6**:657–8).

OTHER ANTIDEPRESSANTS

Lithium (see also combinations)
Use of lithium as monotherapy in the treatment and prophylaxis of unipolar (as well as bipolar) depression has been well-established, and associated with lower mortality, e.g. a meta-analysis of all available studies in MDD that had reported suicide or suicide attempts showed an 88% lower risk with vs without lithium, suggesting an anti-suicide effect in MDD as well as bipolar (s=8, n=329, Guzzetta et al, J Clin Psychiatry 2007;**68**:380–3). However, lithium is most effective as an adjunct to tricyclics and SSRIs (s=9, n=234, RCT, Bauer and Dopfmer, J Clin Psychopharmacol 1999;**19**:427–34; review by Lam, EBMH 2000;**3**:44; Bandolier 2000; **7**:4–5), where it may show a rapid effect over 1–2 weeks (e.g. in the elderly with unipolar MDD, a major protective effect: n=50, two years, Wilkinson et al, Int J Geriatr Psychiatry 2002;**17**:619–22, see also combinations later), although it may be of limited use in people resistant to multiple antidepressants (n=92, RCT, p/c, 12/52, Nierenberg et al, J Clin Psychopharmacol 2003;**23**:92–5). Some anti-depressant response to lithium is probably mood stabilisation in undiagnosed bipolar depression and so sudden withdrawal of lithium would be outright dangerous (Faedda et al, Am J Psychiatry 2001;**158**:1337–9). Cochrane concludes lithium is effective for relapse-prevention of long-term unipolar depression (s=8, n=475, Cipriani et al, Cochrane Database Syst Rev 2006;**4**:CD003492).

Reviews: lithium augmentation in refractory depression (Heit and Nemeroff, J Clin Psychiatry 1998;**59**[Suppl 6]:S28–S33, 36 refs), general review (Bauer and Dopfmer, J Clin Psychopharmacol 1999;**19**:427–34). See main entry under bipolar mood disorder (1.10) and bipolar depression (1.10.3).

Tryptophan
Tryptophan is a naturally occurring amino acid and precursor to serotonin, tryptophan is used in combination with other antidepressants. Tryptophan deficiency results in a rapid lowering of mood (review by Bell et al, Br J Psychiatry 2001;**178**:399–405) and tryptophan depletion reverses antidepressant-induced remission, so tryptophan might help if low tryptophan levels have occurred. Cochrane concludes that the trial data is limited and unreliable but suggests tryptophan may be superior to placebo (Shaw et al, Cochrane Database Syst Rev 2002;**1**:CD003198). Due to a previous association with eosinophilia-myalgia syndrome (EMS), it is now only licensed in the UK for resistant depression, by hospital specialists, in patients with severe depression continuously for more than two years, after adequate trials of standard drug treatments and as an adjunct to other treatments. These remain harsh restrictions for the low risk involved and possible antidepressant benefits.

+ Combinations (of antidepressants)

There is some evidence that combined NE and 5-HT reuptake blocking drugs can produce a quicker antidepressant effect, although it could be that combined drug use produces higher success rates by treating different depressive subgroups. It is better to combine mechanisms of action rather than simply adding drugs, aiming for synergy (de la Gándara et al, Acta Psychiatr Scand 2005;**112**[Suppl 428]:11–3).

Review: strategies for combination and augmentation for depression (DeBattista, J Psychopharmacol 2006;**20**[Suppl]:11–8).

Bupropion + SSRIs/SNRIs/MAOIs
Bupropion 200–300mg/d may be useful in

combination, e.g. 56% of **venlafaxine/SSRI**-resistant depressed patients responded when bupropion was added (n = 25, Spier et al, Depress Anxiety 1998; **7**:73–5). It may also counteract SSRI/venlafaxine-induced sexual dysfunction (n = 18, open, 8/52, Kennedy et al, J Clin Psychiatry 2002;**63**:181–6). A pilot study showed the combination of bupropion and **escitalopram** to be effective and well tolerated (n=51, open, 12/52, Leuchter et al, J Psychiatr Pract 2008;**14**:271–80). **Duloxetine** (mean 60 mg/d) combined with bupropion (mean 175 mg/d) was successful (remission 30%, response 60%) in non-responders to initial monotherapy with either drug (n = 10, open, Papakostas et al, Depress Anxiety 2006;**23**:178–81). Bupropion and **tranylcypromine** has been successful for multi-drug resistant depression (n = 1, Pierre and Gitlin, J Clin Psychiatry 2000; **61**:450–1).

Review: reduced side-effects (Zisook et al, Biol Psychiatry 2005;**59**:203–10).

Lithium + antidepressants *

There are many double-blind controlled trials of augmentation of tricyclics, sertraline, citalopram, venlafaxine and other antidepressants with lithium, with 10 studies reporting response rates averaging 52% (review by Fava, J Clin Psychiatry 2001;**62**[Suppl 18]:S4–S11). For SSRI augmentation, there is evidence of a substantial effect after 1–6 weeks, mostly within 1–2 weeks (review by Zullino and Baumann, Pharmacopsychiatry 2001;**34**:119–27), maintained for 6/12 (n = 30, RCT, d/b, p/c, 6/52, open 4/12 extension, Bauer et al, Am J Psychiatry 2000;**157**:1429–35). Lithium significantly augmented mirtazapine's onset of action compared to placebo, unlike carbamazepine (n=46, 5/52, open, Schule et al, World J Biol Psychiatry 2008;**25**:1–10). Adjunctive lithium may also reduce suicidal behaviour in unipolar depression (n = 167, Lauterbach et al, Acta Psychiatr Scand 2008;**118**:469–79). Adequate lithium levels (0.4 mmol/L or more) seem necessary. There is a view that many resistant depressions are part of unrecognised bipolar disorder and, hence, the use of lithium is logical (see also BNF section).

Review: lithium augmentation in refractory MDD (Bschor and Bauer, Curr Pharm Des 2006; **12**:2985–92).

Lithium + tryptophan + antidepressants (eg. clomipramine, SSRI or phenelzine)

Variously known as Triple Therapy or the MRC, Newcastle or London Cocktail, there have been reports of 55% remission rates in severe depression, eg. from:
- clomipramine (to 150 mg/d or to tolerance, e.g. 300–400 mg/d) plus
- tryptophan (2–4 g/d) plus
- lithium (standard levels).

Alternatives to clomipramine include phenelzine and the SSRIs (n = 20, RCT, Barker et al, Int Clin Psychopharmacol 1987;**2**:261–72). Tryptophan enhances the action of clomipramine on 5-HT sites and improves 5-HT absorption. Lithium also affects 5-HT and is an antidepressant in its own right.

Mirtazapine + venlafaxine/SSRIs

In persistent MDD, addition of mirtazapine 30 mg to existing therapy produced a response rate of 64% cf 20% with placebo (n = 26, RCT, d/b, p/c, 4/52, Carpenter et al, Biol Psychiatry 2002;**51**:183–88; short review in Fava, J Clin Psychiatry 2001;**62**[Suppl 18]:S4–S11). Mirtazapine has also been used with high-dose venlafaxine, the rationale being to use mirtazapine to block 5HT2 and 5HT3 receptors, reducing sexual and anxiety side-effects from venlafaxine, and allowing higher doses to be tolerated. The combination might have been under-rated in STAR*D phase 4 because the QIDS score was actually 23.5% vs only 12.1% for tranylcypromine. A retrospective study showed response rates of 50% at 8/52, and 56% at 6/12, with mirtazapine ADRs predominant (n = 32, Hannan et al, J Psychopharmacol 2007;**21**:161–4).

Reboxetine + duloxetine *

In duloxetine-resistant depression, a pilot study showed that addition of reboxetine produced an impressive 70% remission rate (n = 79, open, 12/52, Seguí et al, J Psychopharmacol 2010;[in press]).

Reboxetine + mirtazapine

Addition of reboxetine in mirtazapine-resistant depression may be a safe and effective strategy (n = 14, 12/52, Lopez-Munoz et al, Clin Neuropharmacol 2006;**29**:192–6).

Reboxetine + SSRIs

This logical combination has been used successfully with, e.g. citalopram in resistant depression (Devarajan and Dursun, *Can J Psychiatry* 2000;**45**:489–90). Reboxetine added to SSRI/mirtazapine/venlafaxine partial or non-responders produced a well tolerated improvement (n = 61, open, 6/52, Rubio et al, *J Affect Disord* 2004;**81**:67–72) and combined escitalopram and reboxetine may provide a rapid response (n = 3, Camarasa et al, *Prog Neuropsychopharmacol Biol Psychiatry* 2005;**29**: 165–8). In SSRI partial responders, addition of reboxetine produced 50% response and 34% remission rates, so RCTs would be useful to confirm this effect (n = 141, open, 12/52, López-Muñoz et al, *Pharmacopsychiatry* 2007;**40**:14–9).

SSRIs + SSRIs

Although there are anecdotal reports (e.g. Bondolfi et al, *Psychopharmacol* [Berl] 1996;**128**:421–5), the combination cannot be recommended and risks serotonin syndrome.

Tricyclics + MAOIs

Although extreme caution is advised, this combination is known to be effective in some resistant depressions, e.g. isocarboxazid plus amitriptyline (n = 25, open, Berlanga and Ortega-Soto, *J Affect Disord* 1995;**34**:187–92). Tranylcypromine plus clomipramine is known to be dangerous (at least two deaths) but other combinations can be used with care in an inpatient setting. Most problems occur when a tricyclic is added to an MAOI. Fewer adverse events have been reported with the reverse. It is best to take great care, e.g. separate the doses (e.g. MAOI in the morning, tricyclic in the evening), add one to the other in low dose and build up slowly or stop all antidepressants, wait a week, and then start both together at low dose and build up again.

Tricyclics + SSRIs

The only robust prospective study on the combination showed that high dose fluoxetine (60 mg/d) was, in fact, more effective in partial or non-responders to 20 mg/d than a fluoxetine/desipramine combination (n = 41, RCT, d/b, 4/52, Fava et al, *Am J Psychiatry*

1994;**151**:1372–4). Positive studies have not been robust (e.g. n = 30, open, Weilberg et al, *J Clin Psychiatry* 1989;**50**:447–9; n = 8, open, Seth et al, *Br J Psychiatry* 1992;**161**:562–5; disputed by Cowen and Power, *Br J Psychiatry* 1993; **162**:266–7). The combination should generally be avoided due to the high risk of an adverse interaction (*4.3.2*). Care is needed when prescribing the combination in potentially suicidal patients. (Cheeta et al, *Br J Psychiatry* 2004;**184**:41–7).

Venlafaxine + SSRIs

SSRIs have been used successfully to augment venlafaxine (n = 4, Gonul et al, *Prog Neuropsychopharmacol Biol Psychiatry* 2003; **27**:889–91), but the combination is not recommended.

+ Augmentation (of antidepressant drugs with no intrinsic antidepressant activity

Reviews: * general (DeBattista, *J Psychopharmacol* 2006;**20**[Suppl]:11–8), systematic review (s = 32, Fleurence et al, *Psychopharmacol Bull* 2009;**42**:57–90), atypical antipsychotics for treatment-resistant MDD (Papakostas and Shelton, *Curr Psychiatry Rep* 2008;**10**:481–6).

Anticholinesterases *

Donepezil augmentation of sertraline improved cognition in elderly people with depression and cognitive impairment (n= 23, RCT, d/b, p/c, 8/52, Pelton et al, *Int J Geriatr Psychiatry* 2008;**23**:670–6) but adding galantamine to venlafaxine or citalopram had no effect in MDD in 'older' (> 50) adults and with increased dropouts (n = 38, RCT, d/b, p/c, 24/52, Holtzheimer et al, *Int J Geriatr Psychiatry* 2008;**23**:625–31).

Antipsychotics *

A recent meta-analysis has concluded that second generation antipsychotics can successfully augment antidepressants in MDD but at increased risk of stopping due to side-effects (s = 16, n = 3480, p/c, Nelson and Papakostas, *Am J Psychiatry* 2009;**166**:980–91; see also s = 10, n = 1500, RCT, Papakostas et al, *J Clin Psychiatry* 2007;**68**:826–31; critical comment by Cipriani et al, *EBMH* 2008;**11**:14). They may have some role perhaps via 5HT$_{2A/2C}$

antagonism (review by Thase, J Clin Psychiatry 2002;**3**:95–103). Discontinuation after recovery can result in clear benefits (n = 55, case note review, Mortimer et al, J Clin Psychiatry 2003; **64**:668–72).

Amisulpride 50 mg/d monotherapy has been shown to have an antidepressant activity comparable with fluoxetine 20 mg/d, with a similar incidence of side-effects (n = 281, d/b, Smeraldi, J Affect Disord 1998;**48**:47–56), non-inferior to paroxetine 20 mg/d (n = 272, RCT, d/b, 56/7, Cassano et al, Int Clin Psychopharmacol 2002;**17**:27–32) and useful for psychotic depression in the elderly (n = 11, Politis et al, Prog Neuropsychopharmacol Biol Psychiatry 2008;**32**:1227–30).

Aripiprazole (s = 2, Weber et al, CNS Drugs 2008;**22**:807–13) has been approved in the US as adjunctive or add-on treatment to antidepressants for adults with MDD but a monotherapy license would require longer-term studies. In incomplete responders to an SSRI or venlafaxine, adjunctive aripiprazole (2–20 mg/d) improved MADRS scores and was well tolerated (n = 362, RCT, d/b, p/c, 8 + 6/52, Berman et al, J Clin Psychiatry 2007; **68**:843–53; critical review by Ciprani and Barbui, EBMH 2008;**11**:15) and adjunctive aripiprazole 2–20 mg/d was effective in 37% cf 19% with placebo (n = 349 [c = 297], RCT, d/b, p/c, 8/52, Berman et al, CNS Spect 2009;**14**:197–206; MS). A 50% response rate from adjunctive aripiprazole was seen in depression in older people (n = 24 [c = 19], open, 12/52, Sheffrin et al, J Clin Psychiatry 2009;**70**:208–13). It has also been useful as an adjunct to tranylcypromine (n = 1, Goforth and Carroll, J Clin Psychopharmacol 2007;**27**:216–7), bupropion (n = 4, 4/12, Sokolski, Ann Pharmacother 2008;**42**:1124–9) and escitalopram (n = 16 [c = 13], open, 7/52, Matthews et al, J Clin Psychopharmacol 2009; **29**:73–6). Even in people not responding to at least four antidepressants, aripiprazole (mean 11 mg/d) was moderately successful, although rates of akathisia were high at 25% (n = 381, RCT, d/b, 6/52, Marcus et al, J Clin Psychopharmacol 2008;**28**:156–65).

Clozapine has been used in refractory psychotic depression (n = 1, Dassa et al, Br J Psychiatry 1993;**163**:822–4).

Olanzapine-fluoxetine (OFC) is licensed in USA for treatment-resistant unipolar and bipolar depression. An analysis of Lilly data showed OFC to be superior to olanzapine or fluoxetine monotherapy (n = 1146, RCT, d/b, 6–8/52, Trivedi et al, J Clin Psychiatry 2009; **70**:387–96). However, OFC was no more effective than either drug alone or nortriptyline monotherapy in one trial (n = 500, RCT, d/b, 8/52, Shelton et al, J Clin Psychiatry 2005;**66**:1289–97, MS; comment by Dodd and Berk, EBMH 2006;**9**:42) and another trial showed that olanzapine plus sertraline improves psychotic depression better than olanzapine alone, suggesting that olanzapine monotherapy may not be a potent antidepressant (n = 259, RCT, d/b, p/c, 12/52, Meyers et al, Arch Gen Psychiatry 2009;**66**:838–47). A combined analysis of two RCTs in depression with psychotic features, showed olanzapine monotherapy to have no advantage over placebo, although OFC showed improvement in one of the less than convincing trials (s = 2, n = 249, RCT, 8/52, d/b, Rothschild et al, J Clin Psychopharmacol 2004;**24**:365–73).

Quetiapine (see also monotherapy) (n = 554, mean dose 318 mg/d) and risperidone (n = 175, mean dose 4.4 mg/d) produced improvements in HAM-D scores in psychotic depression, although quetiapine was superior to risperidone and better tolerated (n = 729, open, RCT, 4/12, Sajatovic et al, J Clin Psychiatry 2002;**63**:11 156–63). Quetiapine 50–750 mg/d (mean 300 mg/d) has been used with citalopram (n = 25, open, 6/52, Konstantinidis et al, Prog Neuropsychopharmacol Biol Psychiatry 2006;**32**:242–7). Quetiapine (mean 315 mg/d) may improve insomnia and other symptoms (n = 18 [c = 14], open, 20/52, Sagud et al, Psychopharmacol [Berl] 2006;**187**:511–4; n = 27, open, 4/52, Baune et al, Hum Psychopharmacol 2007;**22**:1–9). In treatment-resistant depression, augmentation with quetiapine 400 mg/d was at least as effective as lithium 600 mg/d (n = 20, open, Dorée et al, Curr Med Res Opin 2007;**23**:333–41). However, quetiapine 100 mg/d was ineffective as an adjunct to fluoxetine in unipolar depression, with no enhanced outcome nor speed the onset of action (n = 114, RCT, d/b, p/c, 8/52, Garakani et al, Int Clin Psychopharmacol 2008;**23**:269–75).

Risperidone 1–2 mg/d augmentation of sub-optimally effective antidepressants has increased response and remission (n = 274, RCT, d/b, p/c, 6/52, Mahmoud et al, Ann Intern Med 2007;147:593–602; comment by Barbee, EBMH 2008;11:77). In treatment-resistant non-psychotic, unipolar depression, risperidone 0.5–3 mg/d produced more rapid response and higher remission rates (n =97, RCT, d/b, p/c, 4/52, Keitner et al, J Psychiatr Res 2009;43:205–14). Perphenazine added to a tricyclic did not improve efficacy in late-life psychotic depression (n = 36, RCT, d/b, 4/52, Mulsant et al, J Clin Psychiatry 2001;62:597–604), although I personally object to late-life being defined as people aged 50 or older. Sulpiride 100 mg/d may accelerate the antidepressant effect of paroxetine 10–40 mg/d (n = 41 [c = 33], RCT, open, 12/52, Uchida et al, J Clin Psychopharmacol 2005;25:545–51). Ziprasidone has been used as augmentation in SSRI-resistance (n = 64, RCT, open, 6/52, Dunner et al, J Clin Psychiatry 2007;68:1071–7; MS).

Reviews: * olanzapine + fluoxetine (Bobo and Shelton, Expert Opin Pharmacother 2009; 10:2145–59; Bobo and Shelton, Neuropsychiatr Dis Treat 2009;5:369–83; Dodd and Berk, Expert Rev Neurother 2008;8:1299–306), aripiprazole as augmentation in MDD (Khan, Expert Rev Neurother 2008;8:1435–47), general (Selis and Peeters, Tijdschr Psychiatr 2008;50:213–22), atypicals as augmentation (Shelton and Papakostas, Acta Psychiatr Scand 2008;117:253–9).

Benzodiazepines *

Cochrane concludes that BDZ augmentation, e.g. clonazepam (optimum dose 2.5–6 mg/d, response takes 2–4 weeks; Morishita, Hum Psychopharmacol 2009;24:191–8), of anti-depressants leads to fewer drop-outs and less depression severity at 1–4 weeks, but the effect disappears at 6–8 weeks, so short-term use may be successful, possibly by minimising initial SSRI side-effects (e.g. anxiety), improving sleep or a direct action (s = 9, n = 679, Furukawa et al, Cochrane Database Syst Rev 2002;1:CD001026; comment by Gijsman, EBMH 2001;4:45). Predictors of response to clonazepam augmentation in protracted unipolar depression include negative family history of psychiatric illness, and doses

2.5–4 mg/d (n = 120, Morishita and Arita, Hum Psychopharmacol 2007;22:27–31).

Buspirone

Buspirone shares some pharmacodynamic properties with pindolol and augmentation of SSRIs may produce marked improvement in resistant depression (n = 30, 5/52, Dimitriou and Dimitriou, J Clin Psychopharmacol 1998; 18:465–9), e.g. adding 20–60 mg/d buspirone to SSRI non-responders produced significant reductions in MADRS scores at the end of week one compared to placebo, but both groups were equivalent at six weeks (n = 102, RCT, p/c, d/b, 6/52, Appelberg et al, J Clin Psychiatry 2001;62:448–52). However, an RCT failed to show any advantage of adding buspirone to an SSRI in treatment-resistant depression (n = 119, Landen et al, J Clin Psychiatry 1998;59:664–8), although the placebo (47%) and buspirone (51%) response rates were high. Another trial, suggested that buspirone actually slowed the onset of action of fluoxetine (n = 120, RCT, open, 12/52, Onder and Tural, J Affect Disord 2003;76:223–7), so great care is needed.

Carbamazepine (see also unlicensed) *

Carbamazepine augmentation may be useful in SSRI non-responders (n = 6, Steinacher et al, Eur Neuropsychopharmacol 2002;12:255–60), although beware of potential interactions, e.g. carbamazepine does not augment mirtazapine's onset of action compared to placebo, and reduces mirtazapine plasma levels (n = 46, 5/52, open, Schule et al, World J Biol Psychiatry 2008;25:1–10).

Celecoxib *

Celecoxib (400 mg/d) was more effective than placebo as an adjunct to fluoxetine in MDD (n = 40, RCT, p/c, 6/52, Akhondzadeh et al, Depress Anxiety 2009;26:607–11).

Estradiol/estrogen (see also unlicensed)

Estrogen supplementation of SSRIs may enhance their effectiveness (n = 5, Westlund et al, J Affect Disord 2003;77:87–92) in, e.g. postnatal depression (where sublingual estradiol produced clinical recovery in 83% at two weeks: n = 23, open, Ahokas et al, J Clin Psychiatry 2001;62:332–6) and the menopause (n = 145, Miller et al, J Am Geriatr Soc 2002;**50**:1826–30). Low-dose estrogen 0.625 mg/d as augmentation to partially effective SSRIs in perimenopausal depression significantly improved mood, but not memory (n = 17, RCT, d/b, p/c, 6/52, Morgan et al, J Clin Psychiatry 2005;**66**:774–80).

Folate

Low RBC folate levels have been linked to depression, persistent symptoms and a poor response to antidepressants (n = 127, RCT, p/c, 10/52, Coppen and Bailey, J Affect Disord 2000;**60**:121–30; comment by Goodwin, EBMH 2001;**4**:41), an easily rectified problem (e.g. n = 2948, Morris et al, Psychother Psychosom 2003;**72**:80–7). Folate 15 mg/d has significantly improved clinical response and recovery from acute psychiatric disorders (review by Reynolds, Br Med J 2002;**324**:1512–5, 32 refs) and oral supplementation with folic acid 800 mcg/d improves treatment outcomes (extensive review by Coppen and Bolander-Gouaille, J Psychopharmacol 2005;**19**:59–65, 63 refs, systematic review and meta-analysis by Taylor et al, J Psychopharmacol 2004;**18**:251–6). Leucovorin (metabolised to methylfolate) has a modest effect in SSRI non-response (n = 22, 8/52, Alpert et al, Ann Clin Psychiatry 2002; **14**:33–8).

Lamotrigine *

Lamotrigine's main role is in bipolar depression (see 1.10.3) but it may be useful as an adjunct for refractory unipolar depression, e.g. lamotrigine produced a rapid and robust resolution in symptoms (n = 14 [c = 12], open, 6/12, Gabriel, Depress Anxiety 2006;**23**:485–8) and 200 mg/d enhanced the onset of paroxetine (n = 40, p/c, d/b, 9/52, Normann et al, J Clin Psychiatry 2002;**63**:337–44), but 100 mg/d was not quite statistically superior to placebo as an adjunct to fluoxetine in MDD and bipolar II (n = 23, RCT, d/b, p/c, 6/52, Barbosa et al, J Clin Psychiatry 2003;**64**:403–7). Remember that even missing two days' doses means retitrating. However, in non-bipolar depression, lamotrigine augmentation of antidepressants was ineffective (n = 34, RCT, d/b, p/c, 8/52, Santos et al, Prim Care Companion J Clin Psychiatry 2008;**10**:187–90).

Levothyroxine (thyroxine, synthetic T4)

Low TSH and higher T4 levels are associated with current depressive syndrome in young adults (n = 6869, Forman-Hoffman et al, Acta Psychiatr Scand 2006;**114**:132–9), and augmentation with high-dose 150–300 mg/d levothyroxine had an antidepressant effect in more than 50% of the previously treatment-resistant patients with chronic depression and/or dysthymia (n = 9, open, 8/52, Rudas et al, Biol Psychiatry 1999;**15**:45, 229–33). Thyroid supplementation may accelerate the onset of tricyclic response in non-refractory depression (5/6 studies found T3 significantly superior to placebo, especially in women: meta-analysis, Altshuler et al, Am J Psychiatry 2001;**158**:1617–22).

Liothyronine (L-isomer of triiodothyronine, T3) *

A meta-analysis showed liothyronine augmentation to produce twice as many responses in refractory depression compared to controls, with moderately large improvements. T3 50 mcg/d was effective in 35% treatment-resistant depressives, especially for melancholic MDD (n = 20, open, 4/52, Iosifescu et al, J Clin Psychiatry 2005;**66**:1038–42) and 33% achieved full remission with T3 mean 90 mg/d after failing an average of 14 agents (n = 159, retrospective, Kelly and Lieberman, J Affect Disord 2009;**116**:222–6; see also n = 17, Kelly and Lieberman, J Affect Disord 2009;**115**:230–3). Augmentation of sertraline 100 mg/d by liothyronine 40–50 mcg/d improved ITT response rates from 57% to 70%, a significant effect (n = 124, RCT, d/b, p/c, 8/52, Cooper-Kazaz et al, Arch Gen Psychiatry 2007;**64**:679–88). Addition of liothyronine to paroxetine did not improve response (speed or total effect) and, in fact, more adverse reactions were seen (n = 106, RCT, d/b, p/c, 8/52, Appelhof et al, J Clin Endocrinol Metab 2004;**89**:6271–6). This may be effective, particularly in rapid-cycling bipolar disorder (1.10.4).

Reviews: * general (Cooper-Kazaz and Lerer, Int J Neuropsychopharmacol 2008;**11**:685–99), STAR*D (Nierenberg et al, Am J Psychiatry 2006;**163**:1519–30), HUNT study (Panicker et al, Clin Endocrinol (Oxf) 2009;**71**:574–80).

Metyrapone

Metyrapone 1 g/d accelerated the response to 'standard' antidepressants (nefazodone or fluvoxamine!) in MDD, possibly by counteracting stress hormones' inhibition of 5HT release in the forebrain (n=63, RCT, p/c, 5/52, Jahn et al, Arch Gen Psychiatry 2004;61:1235–44; comment by Young, EBMH 2005;8:72).

Methylphenidate *

Methylphenidate may be effective as augmentation where incomplete response has occurred with antidepressants, including the elderly, where apathy and withdrawal (but not hopelessness) are prominent features. Augmentation of citalopram may be rapidly successful and well tolerated in elderly depressed patients (n=16, RCT, d/b, p/c, 10/52, Lavretsky et al, Am J Geriatr Psychiatry 2006;14:181–5; n=9, open, 10/52, Lavretsky et al, J Clin Psychiatry 2003;64:1410–4; IS). Cochrane concludes that there is reasonable evidence for short-term psychostimulants (methylphenidate, dexamfetamine, modafinil) to reduce the symptoms of depression (s=24, RCT, Candy et al, Cochrane Database Syst Rev 2008;2:CD006722). However, adjunctive methylphenidate OROS 18–54 mg/d had no effect on depression ratings (MADRS) but improved apathy and fatigue (n=145, RCT, d/b, p/c, 5/52, Ravindran et al, J Clin Psychiatry 2008;69:87–94).

Modafinil

A review concluded that open studies show modafinil helps fatigue associated with depression but that RCTs have not been able to show this (Lam et al, Ann Pharmacother 2007;41:1005–12). Adjunctive modafinil to SSRIs at the start of treatment may enhance the onset of action in people with MDD and fatigue (n=29, open, 6/52, Ninan et al, J Clin Psychiatry 2004;65:414–20, MS). Adjunctive modafinil may help in patients with fatigue and sleepiness in MDD over the short-term, but the effect wears off over 6/52 (n=136 [c=118], RCT, d/b, p/c, 6/52, DeBattista et al, J Clin Psychiatry 2003;64:1057–64; n=245 [c=194], open, p/c, 12/52, Thase et al, CNS Spectr 2006;11:93–102; n=25 [c=21], open, 6/52, Konuk et al, Adv Ther 2006;23:646–54).

Nimodipine

Nimodipine augmentation of fluoxetine has been successful for 'vascular depression' (n=101, RCT, d/b, p/c, 8/52, Taragano et al, Int Psychogeriatr 2005;17:487–98).

Pergolide

The dopamine agonist pergolide has been tried with moderate success as an adjunct, e.g. 55% showed improvement within seven days, with doses of 0.5–1 mg/d (n=20, open, Bouckoms and Mangini, Psychopharmacol Bull 1993;29:207–11) and if added to tricyclics (n=20, open, Izumi et al, J Affect Disord 2000; 61:127–32).

Pindolol *

Antidepressants, e.g. SSRIs may act by inhibiting the 5-HT reuptake pump, increasing 5-HT but this also enhances 5-HT at 5-HT$_{1A}$ receptors situated on the cell body which operate a feedback loop, thus cancelling each other out. Over a period of weeks, however, the pre-synaptic 5-HT$_{1A}$ receptors become desensitised. Pindolol selectively blocks 5-HT$_{1A}$ receptors, and inhibits this initial feedback loop to increase the speed of onset of action (although not everyone agrees with this: Cremers et al, Biol Psychiatry 2001;50:13–21). In a very eloquent systematic review, Whale et al conclude that pindolol is clearly effective to enhance the onset of action of SSRIs, most clearly up to four weeks (s=11, Whale et al, J Psychopharmacol 2010;[in press]). In another interesting twist, reanalysis of an old study (n=11, RCT, Perez et al, Lancet 1997;349:1594–7) suggested that pindolol improves response (70% vs 40%) and speed of response (53 days vs 19 days) in first episode depression but not in recurrent patients (Portella et al, Eur Neuropsychopharmacol 2009;19:516–9).

Riluzole

Riluzole (mean 75 mg/d) is another dopamine agonist and may be useful as an adjunct to standard antidepressants, with a significant effect within the first week (n=10, open, 12/52, Sanacora et al, Biol Psychiatry 2007;61:822–5), and as monotherapy (mean 170 mg/d, n=19, open, 6/52, Zarate et al, Am J Psychiatry 2004;161:171–4).

Stimulants

See methylphenidate.

Topiramate

Adjunctive topiramate may be beneficial for some obese depressed females (n = 16, open, Carpenter et al, J Affect Disord 2002;**69**:251–5).

Valproate

A study of refractory depression indicated that valproate (750–1500 mg/d) augmentation of lithium (900–1500 mg/d) was effective in the eight patients who did not respond to lithium alone (n = 10, Sharma et al, Lithium 1994; **5**:99–103), and it may help reduce depressive agitation (n = 12 [c = 9], open, 4/52, DeBattista et al, J Clin Psychopharmacol 2005;**25**:476–9).

Vitamin B12 (cyanocobalamin)

Oral B12 1 mg/d supplementation has been recommended in treatment-resistant depression (Tiemeier et al, Am J Psychiatry 2002;**159**:2099–101; review by Coppen and Bolander-Gouaille, J Psychopharmacol 2005;**19**:59–65).

● Unlicensed/some efficacy (see also augmentation)

Bupropion *

Bupropion, a presynaptic dopamine and noradrenaline reuptake inhibitor, is licensed in the USA and other countries for the treatment of depression, as well as for smoking cessation. A meta-analysis of original data from seven studies comparing bupropion (n = 732) with SSRIs (n = 731) showed equivalent efficacy and tolerability, except bupropion caused no more sexual dysfunction than placebo (s = 7, RCT, d/b, Thase et al, J Clin Psychiatry 2005;**66**:974–81), less nausea, diarrhoea and somnolence, but higher cardiovascular, proconvulsive (at doses up to 450 mg/d: Pesola and Avasarala, J Emerg Med 2002;**22**:235–9) and overdose toxicity. Bupropion XR 300 mg/d was as effective as venlafaxine 150 mg/d and as well-tolerated, with dry mouth and insomnia the most reported ADRs (n = 571, RCT, d/b, p/c, 8/52, Hewett et al, J Psychopharmacol 2009;**23**:531–8), but there is no evidence for differential onset of action from SSRIs overall or escitalopram specifically (s = 7, n = 1672, RCT, d/b, 8/52, Papakostas et al, J Clin Psychiatry 2007;**68**:1907–12). Bupropion 300 mg/d (max 450 mg/d) helps MDD with decreased energy, pleasure, interest (n = 274, RCT, d/b, p/c, 8/52, Jefferson et al, J Clin Psychiatry 2006;**67**:865–73), sleepiness and fatigue (s = 6, n = 1317, RCT, d/b, Papakostas et al, Biol Psychiatry 2006;**60**:1350–5), anxiety symptoms in comorbid depression (s = 10, n = 2890, RCT, d/b, p/c, Papakostas et al, J Psychiatr Res 2008;**42**:134–40) and in fluoxetine-resistant depression (n = 29, 8/52, open, Fava et al, Ann Clin Psychiatry 2003;**15**:17–22). A relapse prevention effect has been shown (n = 423, RCT, d/b, p/c, 44/52, Weihs et al, Biol Psychiatry 2002;**51**:753–61). The maximum dosage of 450 mg/d should be adhered to since the risk of seizures is dose related (see 3.4).

Reviews: general (Koley et al, Expert Rev Neurol 2006;**6**:1249–65; Glayton, Expert Opin Pharmacother 2007;**8**:457–66), clinical profile and pharmacology (Dwoskin et al, CNS Drug Rev 2006;**12**:178–207).

Carbamazepine (see also augmentation)

Evidence for use as a pure antidepressant is poor (see augmentation) but, in one study, 44% of patients with resistant depression showed moderate or marked improvement with carbamazepine (n = 16, open, Cullen et al, J Clin Psychiatry 1991;**52**:472–6). See main entry under bipolar mood disorder (1.10.1).

Desvenlafaxine

Desvenlafaxine 100–200 mg/d was well tolerated but not superior to placebo for MDD in one study (n = 247, RCT, d/b, p/c, 8/52, Liebowitz et al, J Clin Psychiatry 2007;**68**:1663–72), although it is now licensed in some countries for depression.

Estradiol/estrogens (see also combinations) *

Estrogen receptors occur in the CNS and loss of estrogen has been shown to reduce serotonergic and other functioning. Estradiol (usually transdermal) has shown a striking improvement as monotherapy in severe postnatal depression (n = 37, d/b, p/c, Henderson et al, Lancet 1991;**338**:816–7; n = 61, d/b, p/c, Gregoire et al, Lancet 1996; **347**:930) and it improved depressive symptoms in postmenopausal women, albeit not cognition (n = 19, RCT, p/c, c/o, 24/52, Schiff et al, Psychoneuroendocrinology 2005;**30**:309–15). Conjugated estrogens 0.625 mg/d have significantly improved mood in perimenopausal women with MDD partially responding to antidepressants (n = 17, RCT, p/c, 6/52, Morgan et al, J Clin Psychiatry 2005;**66**:774–80), a progesterone derivative (chlormadinone) plus ethinylestradiol improved mood in women in an observational study (n = 50000, < 12/12, Huber et al, Clin Drug Invest 2008;**28**:783–91) and raloxifene, a partial estrogen receptor modulator, produced a remarkable improvement in fluvoxamine-intolerant and resistant MDD (n = 1, Sugiyama et al, J Clin Psychiatry 2007;**68**:636–7). However, a larger study showed transdermal estradiol did not improved depressive symptoms in postmenopausal women (n = 57, RCT, d/b, p/c, 8/52, Morrison et al, Biol Psychiatry 2004;**55**:406–12), nor enhance the effectiveness of sertraline in postmenopausal women with MDD, but it might have speeded the onset of response (n = 22, RCT, p/c, 10/52, Rasgon et al, J Psychiatr Res 2007;**41**:338–43). Cochrane concludes that estrogen may be of modest value for severe postpartum depression but that long-term efficacy has not been evaluated (s = 2, n = 229, Dennis et al, Cochrane Database Syst Rev 2008;**4**:CD001690).

Reviews: * general (Studd and Panay, Best Pract Res Clin Obstet Gynaecol 2009;**23**:63–71), mechanisms of action (Osterlund, Biochim Biophys Acta 2010;[in press]), transdermal estradiol (Moses-Kolko et al, Clin Obstet Gynecol 2009;**52**:516–29).

Methylphenidate (see also augmentation)

Methylphenidate can be used as monotherapy in acute depression (Klein and Wender, Arch Gen Psychiatry 1995;**52**:429–33), as it has the major advantage of a rapid action (often within 48 hours), although the effect tends to be transient and it may worsen anxiety and insomnia. The stimulant action of methylphenidate in the elderly may be grossly attenuated and so may not be appropriate in those reporting age-related cognitive decline (n = 60, RCT, p/c, d/b, Turner et al, Psychopharmacol [Berl] 2003;**168**:455–64).

Quetiapine (see also augmentation) *

In MDD, quetiapine 50–300 mg/d monotherapy seems effective, even from the fourth day (n = 723, RCT, d/b, p/c, 6/52, Weisler et al, CNS Spectr 2009;**14**:299–313), and 300mg/d XL was as effective as duloxetine for MDD (n = 612, RCT, d/b, p/c, 6/52, Cutler et al, J Clin Psychiatry 2009;**70**:526–39).

Review: Thase, Neuropsychiatr Dis Treat 2008;**4**: 11–21.

Selegiline

Transdermal selegiline (20 mg/d) is licensed in the USA and was surprisingly effective and well tolerated in one trial in MDD, as the transdermal route allows higher doses than possible orally, with no need for dietary restrictions (n = 177, RCT, p/c, 6/52, Bodkin and Amsterdam, Am J Psychiatry 2002;**159**:1869–75; comment by Benedictis, EBMH 2003;**6**:44; see also n = 289, d/b, p/c, 8/52, Amsterdam, J Clin Psychiatry 2003;**64**:208–14).

St John's wort (SJW) *

SJW is available over-the-counter in most European countries in a variety of preparations. The mode of action is uncertain but may include serotonin and/or norepinephrine reuptake inhibition, MAO-A and B inhibition and sigma receptor activity (review by Butterweck, CNS Drugs 2003;**17**:539–62). A variety of systematic reviews and meta-analyses conclude SJW has modest effects in major depression, but older smaller trials in a variety of depressions have shown a marked effect (e.g. s = 35, RCT, d/b, Linde et al, Br J Psychiatry 2005;**186**:99–107). The positive analyses of the varied quality literature on SJW include equivalent efficacy to the SSRIs but lower ADRs (s = 13, Rahimi et al, Prog Neuropsychopharmacol Biol Psychiatry 2009;**33**:118–27) and relapse prevention over 6/12 (n = 426, RCT, d/b, p/c, 26/52, Kasper et al, Eur Neuropsychopharmacol 2008;**18**:803–13). However, a major rigorous trial failed to show a significant antidepressant or anxiolytic effect in MDD (n = 200, RCT, p/c, 8/52, Shelton et al, JAMA 2001;**285**:1978–86; review by Hawley and Dale, EBMH 2002;**5**:24) and, in a second trial, neither sertraline nor SJW (generously dosed) were effective in moderately-severe depression (n = 340, RCT, d/b, p/c, 8/52,

Davidson et al, JAMA 2002;**287**:1807–14; review by Swann, EBMH 2002;**5**:111; vigorous discussion by Jonas et al, JAMA 2002;**288**:446–9). Most studies are short-term (up to 6/52), and many have high (up to 50%) drop-out rates, indicating that transient mild depression may be common in participants. Care is needed in adjunctive therapy (particularly if purchased OTC — see 4.3.3.9). Cochrane concludes that SJW is superior to placebo in MDD, equivalent to standard antidepressants and with fewer side-effects, although the source of SJW may be relevant (s = 29, n = 5489, Linde et al, Cochrane Database Syst Rev 2008;**4**:CD000448).

Reviews: general (Kelly, Hosp Med 2001;**62**: 274–6) and ADRs (s = 35, Knüppel and Linde, J Clin Psychiatry 2004;**5**:1470–9).

■ Unlicensed/possible efficacy

Antipsychotics
See augmentation.

Botox injections
One study showed that people with depression improved two months after botox injections (n = 10, Finzi and Wasserman, Dermatologic Surg 2006;**32**:645–50).

Buspirone (see also augmentation)
Buspirone may be more effective than placebo but less effective than imipramine as monotherapy in MDD in elderly patients (n = 177, RCT, Schweizer et al, J Clin Psychiatry 1998;**59**:175–83).

Chromium
Chromium picolinate may be an option in atypical depression, with a potential effect within two weeks (n = 15, 8/52, p/c, Davidson et al, Biol Psychiatry 2003;**53**:261–4).

Dexamethasone *
This synthetic glucocorticoid has shown a rapid and marked improvement, e.g. within a week when given 3–8 mg IV (n = 37, 4/7, Arana et al, Am J Psychiatry 1995;**152**:265–7; n = 7, Beale and Arana, Am J Psychiatry 1995;**152**:959–60), and up to 3 mg/d for four days (n = 10, Dinan et al, Acta Psychiatr Scand 1997;**95**:58–61), although probably only a minority of patients respond

(letter by Wolkowitz et al, Am J Psychiatry 1996; **153**:1112–3). This interesting effect may be via upregulation of glucocorticoid receptors, an effect shared with the SSRIs.

Reviews: * glucocorticoids (Pariente, Ann N Y Acad Sci 2009;**1179**:144–52; Kling et al, Depress Anxiety 2009;**26**:641–9; Yu et al, J Steroid Biochem Mol Biol 2008;**108**:300–9).

Dexamfetamine
Dexamfetamine may be rapidly effective for depression and fatigue, with one successful trial in men with HIV (n = 23, RCT, 2/52, Wagner and Rabkin, J Clin Psychiatry 2000;**61**:436–40).

DHEA (dehydroepiandrosterone)
DHEA (an adrenal androgen and neurosteroid) at 90–450 mg/d monotherapy was effective for mid-life depression (n = 18/52, RCT, d/b, p/c, c/o, 18/52, Schmidt et al, Arch Gen Psychiatry 2005;**62**:154–62), and in non-major depression in HIV/AIDS (n = 145 [c = 133], RCT, p/c, d/b, 8/52, Rabkin et al, Am J Psychiatry 2006;**163**:59–66), supporting earlier studies (n = 22, RCT, d/b, p/c, 6/52, Wolkowitz et al, Am J Psychiatry 1999;**156**:646–9), possibly by reducing the vulnerability to stress.

Donepezil
Donepezil may reduce REM latency in depressed patients (n = 16, c/o, Perlis et al, Biol Psychiatry 2002;**51**:457–62).

Glucocorticoid antagonists *
See hydrocortisone, ketoconazole, mifepristone and dexa-methasone.

Hydrocortisone
IV hydrocortisone produced a significantly greater and robust improvement in HAM-D scores than ovine CRH or placebo (n = 22, RCT, d/b, p/c, 2/7, DeBattista et al, Am J Psychiatry 2000;**157**:1334–7; comment by Watson and Young, Am J Psychiatry 2001;**158**:1536–7).

Hyoscine
A robust and rapid response occurred to short-term treatment with IV scopolamine in poor prognosis depression (n = 39 [c = 18], RCT, d/b, p/c, c/o, Furey and Drevets, Arch Gen Psychiatry 2006;**63**:1121–9).

Ketamine

There is a case of remarkable antidepressant response to inadvertent ketamine induction 'monotherapy' after seizure-free and hence failed ECT sessions (n = 1, Ostroff et al, Am J Psychiatry 2005;**162**:1385–6).

Ketoconazole

Ketoconazole inhibits cortisol secretion, lowering cortisol levels and may have a slow-onset antidepressant effect, particularly in hypercortisolemic (but not normal) patients (n = 20, RCT, d/b, p/c, 4/52, Wolkowitz et al, Biol Psychiatry 1999;**45**:1070–74). However, limited efficacy in treatment refractory MDD has been noted (n = 16, RCT, Malison et al, J Clin Psychopharmacol 1999;**19**:466–70).

Mifepristone

Mifepristone 600–1200 mg/d (another gluco-corticoid antagonist) may be an option for psychotic major depression (PMD), the theory being that 'the psychosis in PMD is caused by excessive activation of the HPA axis' (n = 30, open, 7/7, Belanoff et al, Biol Psychiatry 2002;**52**:386–92). A longer-term study showed that six days of mifepristone led to significant improvement in PMD even in the first week, maintained for four weeks, but probably not to eight weeks (n = 20, open, 8/52, Simpson et al, J Clin Psychiatry 2005;**66**:598–602).

Omega-3 fatty acids (PUFAs) *

There may be an association between PUFAs (polyunsaturated fatty acids) and depression, although a Finnish study showed low dietary intake of omega-3 fatty acids is **not** associated with low mood (n = 29 133, Hakkarainen et al, Am J Psychiatry 2004;**161**:567–9) and there has been a small negative study in perinatal depression (n = 26, RCT, d/b, p/c, 6/52, Rees et al, Aust N Z J Psychiatry 2008;**42**:199–205). A recent systematic review concludes that omega-3 fatty acids are a potential treatment for depression (s = 21, Kraguljac et al, Psychopharmacol Bull 2009;**42**:39–54), another review suggested an antidepressant effect superior to placebo (s = 3, n = 60, Osher and Belmaker, CNS Neurosci Ther 2009;**15**:128–33) and a pooled analysis showed significant antidepressant efficacy for omega-3 fatty acids, but noted significant heterogeneity and publication bias (s = 10, n = 329, d/b, p/c, > 4/52, Lin and Su, J Clin Psychiatry 2007;**68**:1056–61). Some beneficial effect has been reported with ethyl-EPA, e.g. with maintenance anti-depressants (n = 20, d/b, 4/52, Nemets et al, Am J Psychiatry 2002;**159**:477–9; n = 70, RCT, d/b, p/c,12/52, Peet and Horrobin, Arch Gen Psychiatry 2002;**59**:913–19), but EPA-E 1g/d was numerically but not statistically superior to placebo for MDD, albeit well-tolerated (n = 57 [c = 35],RCT,d/b,p/c,8/52,Mischoulon et al, J Clin Psychiatry 2009;**70**:1636–44). However, DHA (docosahexaenoic acid, an omega-3 fatty acid) was ineffective as monotherapy in major depression (n = 35, p/c, 6/52, Marangell et al, Am J Psychiatry 2003;**160**:996–8) and in people with CHD, augmentation of sertraline 50 mg/d with omega-3 fatty acids had no effects on depression (n = 122, RCT, d/b, 10/52, Carney et al, JAMA 2009;**302**:1651–7). However, intakes of fish and omega-3 fatty acids may be inversely associated with chronic depression, so supplementation may be helpful in people for whom fish is not an acceptable source (n = 3317, 20 years, Colangelo et al, Nutrition 2009;**25**:1011–9).

Opiates

Some anecdotal cases suggest that oxycodone or oxymorphone may produce a sustained effect in refractory and chronic depression, as well as reducing psychogenic pain and distress (n = 3, Stoll and Reuter, Am J Psychiatry 1999;**156**:2017) and buprenorphine may be useful in refractory, unipolar depression, with a striking response in four (n = 10, open, 6/52, Bodkin et al, J Clin Psychopharmacol 1995;**15**:49–57; see also Callaway, Biol Psychiatry 1996;**39**: 989–90). The potential for abuse limits their use.

Phenytoin

Phenytoin (up to 400 mg/d) was as effective as fluoxetine (up to 21 mg/d) for MDD (n = 33 [c = 28], RCT, d/b, Nemets et al, J Clin Psychiatry 2005;**66**:586–90).

Pramipexole

Pramipexole is a dopamine D2/D3 agonist licensed for Parkinson's disease and has been used with some success (n = 22, case series, Ostow, *Am J Psychiatry* 2002;**159**:320–1; n = 174, RCT, p/c, 8/52, Corrigan et al, *Depress Anxiety* 2000;**11**:58–65).

Pregabalin

There is a case of pregabalin 150–225 mg/d completely resolving resistant depression (n = 1, Showraki, *J Psychopharmacol* 2007; **21**:883–4).

Testosterone *

Low free testosterone levels are associated with a higher prevalence of depression, e.g. older men with low total or free testosterone levels are 1.5–2.7 times more likely to have depression (n = 3987, Almeida et al, *Arch Gen Psychiatry* 2008;**65**:283–9), and so supplementation might help (n = 3987, Almeida et al, *Arch Gen Psychiatry* 2007; **64**:283–9). Weekly testosterone cypionate 100–200 mg/d may be effective in some men with late-onset depression, but not earlier-onset depression (n = 15, RCT, 6/52, Perry et al, *J Clin Psychiatry* 2002;**63**:1096–101). Testosterone gel may be a non-parenteral route capable of producing an antidepressant effect in men with refractory depression and low testosterone (n = 22, RCT, p/c, 8/52, Pope et al, *Am J Psychiatry* 2003;**160**:105–11). However, the antidepressant effects of IM testosterone in hypogonadal men with MDD may only be equivalent to placebo (n = 30, RCT, d/b, p/c, 6/52, Seidmen et al, *J Clin Psychiatry* 2001;**62**:406–12).

Tramadol

Response of refractory MDD to tramadol (structurally similar to venlafaxine) 300–400 mg/d prescribed for pain has been reported (n = 1, Shapira et al, *J Clin Psychiatry* 2001;**62**:205–6).

Vardenafil

Vardenafil is effective for erectile dysfunction in milder MDD, and depressive symptoms may improve with treatment of one of the potential symptoms (n = 280, RCT, d/b, p/c, Rosen et al, *Am J Psychiatry* 2006;**163**:79–87).

Varenicline *

There is a case where a depressed tobacco-dependent patient became cigarette-free and euthymic with varenicline (n = 1, Grosshans et al, *Addiction* 2009;**104**:859–61).

◆ Others *

Other drugs tried include **ascorbic acid**, **captopril** 50–100 mg/d (n = 9, open, *J Clin Psychopharmacol* 1991;**11**:395–6), **bromocriptine** 10–60 mg/d (McGrath et al, *J Clin Psychopharmacol* 1995;**15**: 289–91), **cyproheptadine** (n = 6, RCT, Greenway et al, *Pharmacotherapy* 1995;**15**:357–60), **levo-dopa** (*J Psychopharmacol* 1990;**4**:152–67), **primidone** (n = 1, Brown et al, *Lancet* 1993; **342**:925), **tetracyclines** (minocycline; Pae et al, *Biomed Pharmacother* 2008;**62**:308–11, and demeclocycline; Levine et al, *Am J Psychiatry* 1996; **153**:582) and **thyrotropin-releasing hormone** (TRH, n = 5, Marangell et al, *Arch Gen Psychiatry* 1997;**54**:214–22).

□ No efficacy

Atomoxetine *

In SSRI-refractory depression, atomoxetine augmentation is of no benefit (n = 276, RCT, d/b, p/c, 8/52, Michelson et al, *J Clin Psychiatry* 2007;**68**:582–7; MS) and atomoxetine is in fact a failed antidepressant monotherapy (n = 15 [c = 11], open, 8/52, Carpenter et al, *J Clin Psychiatry* 2005;**66**:1234–8; see also n = 1, Pilhatsch et al, *Pharmacopsychiatry* 2006; **39**:79–80).

Benzodiazepines

Suggestions that **alprazolam** (n = 30, RCT, d/b, 6/52, Hubain et al, *J Affect Disord* 1990;**18**:67–73) and **diazepam** have some antidepressant activity were probably due to including measures of anxiety in the depression rating scales. The BNF states that BDZs should not be used to treat depression. Discontinuing drugs such as clonazepam prescribed for panic/anxiety control can often lead to improvement of depression (see 5.5). Short-term adjunctive use may have some role.

Caffeine

Some depressed people may have increased sensitivity to caffeine (Lee et al, *Am J Psychiatry* 1988;**145**:632–5).

Inositol *

Inositol is a precursor of an intracellular secondary messenger system for numerous neurotransmitters. The major trial showed no significant effect in SSRI augmentation (n = 27, RCT, p/c, Levine et al, Biol Psychiatry 1999;45:270–3) or in SSRI failures (RCT, d/b, Nemets et al, J Neural Transm 1999;106:795–8). Previous work had led to some enthusiasm (e.g. n = 28, p/c, Levine et al, Am J Psychiatry 1995;152:792–4).

Memantine

Memantine 5–20mg/d was ineffective for MDD (n = 32, RCT, d/b, p/c, Zarate et al, Am J Psychiatry 2006;163:153–5).

Pyridoxine (vitamin B6)

Low B6 levels have been associated with depression and supplementary B6 might be useful (n = 140, Hvas et al, Psychother Psychosom 2004;73:340–3), but a review (s = 10 including five RCTs) showed no apparent effect in men, although some minor effect in premenopausal women (Family Pract 2005;2:532–7).

1.15 DYSTHYMIA

see also Depression (1.14)

Symptoms

Dysthymia (literally 'ill-humored') is a low-grade chronic melancholic depression (often with anxiety) of insidious onset, chronic course (lasting at least two years with permanent or intermittent symptoms) and a high risk of relapse. It has few of the physical symptoms of depression and is compatible with stable social functioning. Almost all sufferers eventually develop super-imposed major depression (n = 86, three-year follow-up, Klein et al, Am J Psychiatry 2000;157:931–9). The life-time prevalence rate may be around 3–6%, and higher in the elderly. Dysthymia has been associated with low testosterone levels in men and hence a link made with HPG axis dysfunction (n = 220, open, Seidman et al, Am J Psychiatry 2002;159:456–9). It has been considered by some to be similar to depressive personality disorder or anxiety and, by others, as a way of medicalising (and hence ignoring) social problems, or as a way of giving someone a medical diagnosis to allow insurance claims.

Role of drugs

It is clear that antidepressants are effective in dysthymia, with no proven significant differences between classes but they should form part of an overall treatment strategy including, e.g. psychological therapies. A greater sensitivity to side-effects has been noted in dysthymics, with tricyclics the biggest culprits. SSRIs and moclobemide appear favoured. If one class does not work, switching to another may convey a 40–60% chance of response (Thase, Curr Opin Psychiatry 1998;11:77–83, 35 refs). A low (10–20%) placebo response is seen (Frances et al, Int Clin Psychopharmacol 1993;7:197–200). Cochrane concludes that drug therapy may be needed for several months (s = 15, Lima and Moncrieff, Cochrane Database Syst Rev 2000;4:CD001130) and might as well be chosen based on potential side-effects (s = 14, de Lima and Hotopf, Cochrane Database Syst Rev 2003;3:CD004047).

Reviews: diagnosis and treatment (de Lima and Hotopf, Drug Saf 2003;26:55–64), in the elderly (Bellino et al, Drugs Aging 2000;16:107–21).

● Unlicensed/some efficacy

ALCAR (acetyl-l-carnitine)

ALCAR may be as effective and tolerable as amisulpride (n = 204, RCT, d/b, 12/52, Zanardi and Smeraldi, Eur Neuropsychopharmacol 2006; 16:281–7).

Amisulpride

Amisulpride may have some efficacy in dysthymia, e.g. 50mg/d was as effective as sertraline 50–100mg/d, with a significantly faster onset of action (n = 313, RCT, d/b, 12/52, Amore et al, Int Clin Psychopharmacol 2001;16:317–24), and as effective as ALCAR (n = 204, RCT, d/b, 12/52, Zanardi and Smeraldi, Eur Neuropsychopharmacol 2006;16:281–7). It may also be effective for short-term treatment (n = 100, RCT, open, 8/52, Rocca et al, J Affect Disord 2002;70:313–7).

Review: substituted benzamides in dysthymia (Pani and Gessa, Mol Psychiatry 2002;7:247–53).

Bupropion

Bupropion SR up to 400mg/d was effective in 71% patients in one trial, with those having a history of substance misuse less likely to respond (n=21, open, 8/52, Hellerstein et al, J Clin Psychopharmacol 2001;**21**:325–9).

Moclobemide

Moclobemide (mean 675 mg/d) has been shown to be significantly more effective for dysthymia than imipramine (mean 220 mg/d), with fewer side-effects (n=315, RCT, Versiani et al, Int Clin Psychopharmacol 1997;**12**:183–93).

SSRIs

SSRIs are probably the treatment of choice for dysthymia. **Citalopram** (mean dose 39 mg/d) appeared effective in 73% of 'pure' dysthymics in one study (n=21, open, 12/52, Hellerstein et al, Int Clin Psychopharmacol 2004;**19**:143–8). **Fluoxetine** 20 mg/d may be more effective than placebo, with 50% of the non-responders at three months improving with a dose increase to 40 mg/d (n=140, RCT, Vanelle et al, Br J Psychiatry 1997;**170**:345–50), but may have limited efficacy in elderly patients (n=90 [c=71], RCT, d/b, p/c, 12/52, Devanand et al, Am J Geriatr Psychiatry 2005;**13**:59–68). **Fluvoxamine** may be well tolerated and effective in dysthymic adolescents (n=21, open, Rabe-Jablonska, J Child Adolesc Psychopharmacol 2000;**10**:9–18). **Paroxetine** was superior to psychotherapy and placebo in older dysthymics (n=415, RCT, 11/52, Williams et al, JAMA 2000;**284**:1519–26). In dysthymia without major depression, **sertraline** up to 200 mg/d may be effective over a wide range of efficacy and quality of life measures (n=310, RCT, p/c, 12/52, Ravindran et al, J Clin Psychiatry 2000;**61**:821–7), and may improve behaviour and personality in dysthymia (n=410, RCT, d/b, p/c, Hellerstein et al, Am J Psychiatry 2000;**157**:1436–44).

Tricyclics

Amitriptyline and desipramine (n=42, open, 8/52, Marin et al, Am J Psychiatry 1994; **151**:1079–80) have both been studied and found at doses of 150–300 mg/d to be 2–3 times more effective than placebo. 50–300 mg/d imipramine has been shown to be as effective (but with more drop-outs) as sertraline in long-standing dysthymia, and both were significantly better than placebo (n=416, RCT, 12/52, Kocsis et al, Am J Psychiatry 1997;**154**:390).

■ Unlicensed/possible efficacy

Chromium

Chromium (as the picolinate) provided a dramatic and complete resolution of dysthymia in a small trial (n=5, s/b, McLeod et al, J Clin Psychiatry 1999;**60**:237).

Duloxetine *

A pilot study has suggested some efficacy for duloxetine in dysthymia (n=24 [c=19], open, Koran et al, J Clin Psychiatry 2007;**68**:761–5).

Mirtazapine

Mirtazapine 15–45 mg/d was effective in 73% of patients with dysthymia in a small trial (n=15 [c=11], open, 10/52, Depress Anxiety 1999;**10**:68–72).

Sildenafil *

Sildenafil 25 mg/d has produced improvement in middle-aged male depression, the improvement not related to erectile function (n=20, open, 6/52, Orr et al, J Nerv Ment Dis 2008;**196**:496–500).

Testosterone *

In hypogonadal older men, testosterone gel may be effective for subsyndromal depression (n=33, RCT, d/b, p/c, 24/52, Shores et al, J Clin Psychiatry 2009;**70**:1009–16) and IM injections for middle-aged late-onset dysthymia in men (n=23, RCT, d/b, p/c, Seidman et al, J Clin Psychopharmacol 2009;**29**:216–21).

Venlafaxine

Several open studies suggest some efficacy, e.g. up to 225 mg/d was effective in 71% of completers (n=17 [c=14], 9/52, Dunner et al, J Clin Psychiatry 1997;**58**:528–31), and up to 300 mg/d may be reasonably effective and generally well tolerated for elderly patients (n=23 [c=18], open, 12/52, Devanand et al, J Geriatr Psychiatr Neurol 2004;**17**:219–24).

◆ Others

Other drugs tried include **lithium** (e.g. Akiskal et al, Arch Gen Psychiatry 1980;**37**:777–83), phenelzine and tranylcypromine (review, Anon, *Br J Psychiatry* 1995;**166**:174–83). and valproate (n = 1, Kemp, *Br J Psychiatry* 1992; **160**:121–3).

□ No efficacy

St John's wort
  People with dysthymia seem unresponsive to SJW, with placebo-level response, although non-dysthymics may improve (n = 150, RCT, d/b, p/c, 6/52, Randlov et al, *Phytomedicine* 2006; **13**:215–21).

1.16 EATING DISORDERS

1.16.1 Anorexia nervosa
1.16.2 Bulimia nervosa
1.16.3 Binge-eating disorder

DSM-IV includes three eating disorders; anorexia nervosa (AN), bulimia nervosa (BN) and eating disorders not otherwise specified (EDNOS), the latter including binge-eating disorder. Although sociocultural explanations are important and relevant, anorexia, bulimia and obesity may be heterogeneous disorders with a complex aetiology, including genetic factors and the environment (review by Collier and Treasure, *Br J Psychiatry* 2004;**185**:363–5).

Reviews: * general (Treasure et al, *Lancet* 2010;[in press]; Cooke and Sawyer, *Aust Fam Physician* 2004;**33**:27–31), anticonvulsants for eating disorders (McElroy et al, *CNS Drugs* 2009;**23**:139–56), pharmacotherapy (Powers and Bruty, *Child Adolesc Psychiatr Clin N Am* 2009;**18**:175–87; Pederson et al, *Expert Opin Pharmacother* 2003;**4**:1659–78), drug treatment of adolescent eating disorders (Couturier and Lock, *J Can Acad Child Adolesc Psychiatry* 2007;**16**:173–6; Pederson et al, *Expert Opin Pharmacother* 2003;**4**:1659–78), general and primary care (Pederson et al, *Expert Opin Pharmacother* 2003;**4**:1659–78).

1.16.1 ANOREXIA NERVOSA

Symptoms:
The main diagnostic symptoms of anorexia nervosa are:
1. Amenorrhoea in females (absence of three consecutive menstrual cycles).

2. Refusal to maintain body weight over the minimum normal for age and height.
3. Intense fear of gaining weight or becoming fat.
4. Disturbance in body perception, e.g. feeling fat even when emaciated.

Anorexia usually starts in the late teens, with distorted body image and relentless dieting. Patients may avoid carbohydrates, induce vomiting, abuse laxatives, take excess exercise, binge eat and suffer depression and social withdrawal. It may occur in up to 8–13 per 100 000 population, and 90% are female. Psychotherapy may be useful but with only a few small trials is unproven (s = 6, Hay et al, *Cochrane Database Syst Rev* 2003;**4**:CD003909).

Role of drugs
Drug therapy is generally most useful as a supportive measure to treat any concurrent conditions. In severely emaciated patients, enteral feeding or even TPN may be necessary.
Reviews: * overall management (Herpertz-Dahlmann and Salbach-Andrae, *Child Adolesc Psychiatr Clin N Am* 2009;**18**:131–45; Morris and Twaddle, *BMJ* 2007;**334**:894–8; Zandian et al, *Physiol Behav* 2007;**92**:283–90), systematic review (s = 32, Bulik et al, *Int J Eat Disord* 2007;**40**:310–20), use of SSRIs (Vaswani and Kalra, *Expert Opin Invest Drugs* 2004;**13**:349–57), genetics (Bulik et al, *Annu Rev Nutr* 2007;**27**:263–75), adolescent eating disorders: definitions, symptomatology, epidemiology and comorbidity (Herpertz-Dahlmann, *Child Adolesc Psychiatr Clin N Am* 2009; **18**:31–47).

+ Combinations

Olanzapine + mirtazapine
There is a report of successful use of olanzapine 10mg/d and mirtazapine 30mg/d (n = 1, 6/12, Wang et al, *Prog Neuropsychopharmacol Biol Psychiatry* 2006;**30**:306–9).

● Unlicensed/some efficacy

Nutritional feeding
TPN may be necessary in severely anorexic patients where a life-threatening weight loss has occurred, particularly if accompanied by low potassium levels and where conventional

therapies have failed. Weight gain can be significant in a relatively short period and TPN can help avert permanent damage or death. Great care is needed (review by Golden and Meyer, Int J Adolesc Med Health 2004; **16**:131–44) as patients are likely to interfere with the IV line with the possibility of infection in a compromised patient and of embolism. Supervised oral feeding with nutritional supplements can also be an effective acute treatment. Osteoporosis (Misra and Klibanski, Rev Endocr Metab Disord 2006; **7**:91–9) and osteopenia can be frequent and severe complications (Golden, Adolesc Med 2003; **14**:97–108) and vitamin D and calcium supplements are essential.

Reviews: * medical complications (Mitchell and Crow, Curr Opin Psychiatry 2006; **19**:438–43), nutrition (Golden and Meyer, Int J Adolesc Med Health 2004; **16**:131–44), tube feeding and nutrition (Rigaud et al, Presse Med 2009; **38**:1739–45; Rigaud et al, Clin Nutr 2007; **26**: 421–9).

Treatment of any PMS

This may help any premenstrual exacerbations.

■ Unlicensed/possible efficacy

Antipsychotics *

There are some reports that OCD and AN may respond to **olanzapine** 5 mg/d, with reduced fixed body perceptions and improved insight (e.g. n = 20, open, 10/52, Powers et al, Int J Eat Disord 2002; **32**:146–54; n = 1, Tateno et al, Psychiatry Clin Neurosci 2008; **62**:752) and although a review concludes that olanzapine 2.5–15 mg/d promotes weight gain and may have benefits on psychological symptoms, the reports are of limited scope with no RCTs (Dunican and DelDotto, Ann Pharmacother 2007; **41**:111–5). It has been used successfully in combination with psychotherapy for adoles-cent AN (n = 5, Dennis et al, Eat Weight Disord 2006; **11**:53–6; n = 1, Dadi-Hero et al, Psychiatr Danub 2009; **21**:122–5). **Risperidone** has been used (Newman-Toker, J Am Acad Child Adolesc Psychiatry 2000; **39**:941–2). **Aripiprazole** has been used to treat psychosis in AN where weight gain

from antipsychotics has been an issue (n = 1, Aragona, Eat Weight Disord 2007; **12**:54–7). Low-dose **haloperidol** has been suggested as an adjunct in severe AN (n = 13, open, 6/12, Cassano et al, Int J Eat Disord 2003; **33**:172–7). **Quetiapine** 150–300 mg/d has improved some general psychiatric symptoms in anorexia (n = 19 [c = 14], open, 10/52, Powers et al, Int J Eat Disord 2007; **40**:21–6).

Reviews: review (s = 4, Court et al, Eat Disord 2008; **16**:217–23), in children and adolescents (Mehler-Wex et al, Eur Eat Disord Rev 2008; **16**:100–8).

Antidepressants (see also fluoxetine)

There is some evidence that serotonergic control of the anterior pituitary function and impaired adrenal function occurs in AN (n = 12, Mondelli et al, Psychoneuroendocrinology 2006; **31**:1139–48). **Citalopram** 20 mg/d has been used successfully (e.g. n = 52, RCT, Fassino et al, Eur Neuropsychopharmacol 2002; **12**:453–9). There is a case of **mirtazapine** improving weight and treating underlying depression in a woman with AN over five months (n = 1, Jaafar et al, Aust N Z J Psychiatry 2007; **41**:768–9). A case has been reported of complete response to **sertraline** at 50 mg/d in a woman only partly responsive to fluoxetine (Roberts and Lydiard, Am J Psychiatry 1993; **150**:1753). **Tricyclics** have also been used.

Tramadol

Tramadol, which has significant MAOI activity and mu-opioid receptor antagonism, has been successful at 225 mg/d (n = 1, Mendelson, Am J Psychiatry 2001; **158**:963–94).

Zinc *

Zinc has virtually no side-effects. A four-week trial may help some people (e.g. Acta Psychiatr Scand 1990; **82**:14–7), and 100 mg/d produced an increase in BMI twice that of placebo (n = 35, RCT, Birmingham et al, Int J Eat Disord 1994; **15**:251–5). 14 mg/d for two months has been advocated as routine in all people with AN (Birmingham and Gritzner, Eat Weight Disord 2006; **11**:109–11; review by Su and Birmingham, Eat Weight Disord 2002; **7**:20–2).

◆ Others

Other drugs tried include **cyproheptadine** (n = 72, RCT, Halmi *et al, Arch Gen Psychiatry* 1986;**43**:177–81) and **lithium** (n = 16, d/b, 16/52, Gross, *J Clin Psychopharmacol* 1981; 1:376–81).

☐ No efficacy

Fluoxetine

In an important trial, fluoxetine had no advantage over placebo in anorexia following weight restoration (n = 93, RCT, d/b, p/c, < 1 year, Walsh *et al, JAMA* 2006;**295**:2605–12).

Topiramate

Topiramate caused relapse of anorexia in a patient when used for epilepsy (n = 1, Rosenow *et al, Am J Psychiatry* 2002;**159**:2112–3).

1.16.2 BULIMIA NERVOSA

Symptoms

The main diagnostic symptoms of bulimia nervosa are:

1. Recurrent binge eating, including lack of control.
2. An urge to overeat (including lack of control of eating during binges).
3. Regular self-induced vomiting, laxative abuse, strict dieting or fasting.
4. Persistent over-concern with body shape and weight.

There must be a minimum of two binge episodes per week for at least three months. Weight and menses are normal. The prevalence rates are about 1% for young women and 0.1% for young men. Mu-opioid receptor binding in bulimic women (n = 8) is lower than in healthy women (n = 8) in the left insular cortex, the area involved in processing taste, as well as the anticipation and reward of eating (n = 16, Bencherif *et al, J Nucl Med* 2005;**46**:1349–51).

Role of drugs

A meta-analysis of antidepressants vs placebo in bulimia showed that short-term remission was more likely with antidepressants, with equivalent drop-outs, but with no drug class better than any other (s = 16, RCTs, n = 1300, Bacaltchuk *et al, Aust N Z J Psychiatry* 2000;**34**:310–7). Cochrane concludes that all antidepressants appear equally effective compared to placebo, but with a high drop-out rate (Bacaltchuk and Hay, *Cochrane Database Syst Rev* 2003;**4**:CD003391; review by Morgan, *EBMH* 2002;**5**:75–6) and do not work as antidepressants. Adequate doses are needed, e.g. at least 150 mg/d equivalent of a tricyclic for adequate duration, e.g. at least four weeks. Side-effects (especially anticholinergic) can be severe and result in non-compliance. Drugs should be part of an individualised programme with nutrition and CBT the most effective interventions, although Cochrane concludes that the evidence for the efficacy of CBT in bulimia is small and of variable quality (s = 48, n = 3054, Hay *et al, Cochrane Database Syst Rev* 2009;**4**:CD000562).

Reviews: * general (Shapiro *et al, Int J Eat Disord* 2007;**40**:321–36; Mehler, *N Engl J Med* 2003; **28**:875–81; Brambilla, *CNS Drugs* 2001;**15**:119–36), systematic review (Bacaltchuk *et al, Aust N Z J Psychiatry* 2000;**34**:310–7), and binge-eating disorder (Dingemans *et al, Int J Obes* 2002; **26**:299–307).

BNF listed

Fluoxetine

Fluoxetine 60 mg/d has a significant effect on binge-eating and purging, eating attitudes, behaviour and food craving, and studies have confirmed this effect where psychological treatments have been inadequate, e.g. it was superior to placebo as maintenance therapy, albeit with a high drop-out rate (eg. n = 150, RCT, 12/12, Romano *et al, Am J Psychiatry* 2002;**159**:96–102; review by Palmer, *EBMH* 2002;**120**:120). Fluoxetine may also be effective in adolescent (12–18) bulimia (n = 10, open, 8/52, Kotler *et al, J Child Adolesc Psychopharmacol* 2003;**13**:329–35) but may have no benefit over a year once weight has been restored (n = 93, RCT, d/b, p/c, 12/12, Walsh *et al, JAMA* 2006;**295**:2605–12). It does not work purely as an antidepressant, as the improvement is independent of depression scores and needs higher doses. Its long half-life may help with missed doses.

+ Combinations

Naltrexone + fluoxetine

After a partial response to 60mg/d fluoxetine, addition of 100mg/d naltrexone has produced a 'robust' reduction in binge frequency and amount (n=1, Neumeister et al, Am J Psychiatry 1999;**156**:797).

● Unlicensed/some efficacy

SSRIs (see also fluoxetine above)

Citalopram may be useful for depressed patients for bulimia (n=37, RCT, s/b, Leombruni et al, Adv Ther 2006;**23**:481–94). Fluvoxamine 200mg/d may reduce binge-eating and purging and may be well tolerated (e.g. n=12, RCT, p/c, 12/52, Milano et al, Adv Ther 2005;**22**:178–83). Paroxetine has been reputed to have no beneficial effect in an unpublished study. Sertraline was significantly superior to placebo in most measures in two short studies (n=34, RCT, d/b, 6/52, McElroy et al, Am J Psychiatry 2000;**157**:1004–6; n=18, open, 8/52, Sloan et al, Int J Eat Dis 2004; **36**:48–54).

Topiramate *

There is growing interest in topiramate in bulimia. A systematic analysis has suggested topiramate is effective for the short-term treatment of BN but long-term use is unproven (s=5, Arbaizar et al, Gen Hosp Psych 2008;**30**:471–5). Two RCTs have shown that topiramate (median 100mg/d, range 25–400) may significantly improve binge and purge symptoms of BN (n=64, RCT, p/c, Hoopes et al, J Clin Psychiatry 2003;**64**:1335–41, ibid 1449–54; MS; n=60, RCT, d/b, p/c, 10/52, Nickel et al, Int J Eat Disord 2005;**38**:295–300). There have also been several published cases of dramatic response in drug-resistant bulimia (n=1, Knable, Am J Psychiatry 2001; **158**:322–3; n=1, Appolinario et al, Am J Psychiatry 2001;**158**:967–8; n=1, Felstrom and Blackshaw, Am J Psychiatry 2002;**159**:1246–7), and a case series, where topiramate was almost completely successful in stopping binging and purging in three patients with comorbid mood disorders, but was ineffective in two (n=5, Barbee, Int J Eat Disord 2003;**33**:469–72).

■ Unlicensed/possible efficacy

Buspirone

Buspirone may have similar efficacy to fluoxetine in short-term management of bulimic symptoms (n=57, open, 12/52, Rajewski and Rybakowski, Psychiatr Pol 2006;**40**:75–82).

Duloxetine

There are cases of treatment refractory bulimia responding to duloxetine, e.g. 120mg/d, effective over 2/52 and continuing over the next four months (n=1, Hazen and Fava, J Psychopharmacol 2006;**20**:723–4; n=1, Christensen and Averbuch, Psychiatry (Edgmont) 2009;**6**:27–8).

Flutamide

The testosterone receptor antagonist flutamide (250–500mg/d) produced a rapid and marked improvement in bulimic behaviour in two women (n=2, Bergman and Eriksson, Acta Psychiatr Scand 1996;**94**:137–9).

Lamotrigine *

Lamotrigine has been used to treat bulimia with comorbid bipolar (Rybakowski and Kaminska, Prog Neuropsychopharmacol 2008;**32**:2004–5).

MAOIs

MAOIs can be useful drugs if the dietary restrictions can be overcome.

Ondansetron

Ondansetron was reported to be effective in three small, short-term trials by one group of investigators, and may be an option after failure of conventional therapies (reviews by Fung and Ferrill, Ann Pharmacother 2001;**35**:1270–3; Generali and Cada, Hosp Pharm 2001;**36**:547–52;572). Decreased binge-eating and vomiting has been shown with ondansetron 24mg/d, possibly due to pharmacological decrease in vagal neuro-transmission (n=28, RCT, Faris et al, Lancet 2000;**355**:792–7; editorial by Kiss, Lancet 2000;**355**:769–70).

Oxcarbazepine

Oxcarbazepine has been used for self-mutilating bulimic patients (Cordas et al, Int J Neuropsychopharmacol 2006;**9**:769–71).

PMS treatments

Pyridoxine and progesterones may help to minimise the effects of premenstrual relapses.

Reboxetine

Reboxetine 4mg/d has produced a rapid response (50% decrease in bulimic behaviour) in 60% patients (n = 28, RCT, 3/12, Fassino et al, J Psychopharmacol 2004;**18**:423–8).

Stimulants

In women with comorbid ADHD and bulimia, complete response in binge eating has been reported with psychostimulants (n = 6, Dukarm, J Women's Health [Larchmt] 2005;**14**:345–50).

Tricyclics

Many tricyclics, e.g. amitriptyline (n = 32, d/b, p/c, Mitchell and Groat, J Clin Psychopharmacol 1984;**4**:186–93) have been used but are of arguable potency. Poor relapse rates suggest serious limitations with long-term efficacy (RCT, d/b, p/c, 6/12, Walsh et al, Am J Psychiatry 1991;**148**:1206–12).

◆ Others

Other drugs tried include **naltrexone** (n = 19, RCT, Marrazzi et al, Int Clin Psychopharmacol 1995;**10**:163–72), **trazodone** (n = 42, RCT, Pope et al, J Clin Psychopharmacol 1989;**9**:254–9), **valproate** (Tachibana et al, Jpn J Psychiatry Neurol 1989;**43**:77–84) and **zinc** (Safai-Kutti and Kutti, Ann Intern Med 1984;**100**:317–8).

□ No efficacy

Carbamazepine

No effect was seen in one study (n = 6, Safai-Kutti and Kutti, Am J Psychiatry 1983;**140**:1225–6).

Clozapine

There is a case of bulimia acutely worsening on clozapine 350mg/d (Brewerton and Shannon, Am J Psychiatry 1992;**149**:1408).

Cyproheptadine

Although potentially useful in anorexia, it appears to be detrimental in bulimia (n = 72, RCT, d/b, Halmi et al, Arch Gen Psychiatry 1986; **43**:177–81).

Lithium

Despite early enthusiasm, lithium appears no more effective than placebo (n = 91, Hsu et al, J Nerv Mental Dis 1991;**179**:351–5).

Mianserin

No effect was seen at 60mg/d (n = 50, 8/52, Sabine et al, Br J Clin Pharmacol 1983;**15**:S195–S202).

1.16.3 BINGE-EATING DISORDER (BED)

Symptoms

BED is characterised by binge-eating large amounts of food in discrete time periods, which is not then followed by compensatory behaviours such as purging or vomiting. BED is a chronic condition (mean duration 14 years, n = 888, Pope et al, Am J Psychiatry 2006;**163**:2181–3), with a longer duration than bulimia or anorexia. Many (but not all) patients are obese and may seek treatment for this. CBT is effective for behavioural and psychological features of BED but not for the obesity (n = 108 [c = 86], RCT, 16/52, d/b, p/c, Grilo et al, Biol Psychiatry 2005;**57**:301–9). Higher than expected rates of comorbid psychiatric conditions, especially depression, are seen. There is some controversy about its status and it is not mentioned in DSM-IV (Wilfley et al, Int J Eat Disord 2003;**34**[Suppl]:S96–S106).

Role of drugs *

A meta-analysis of p/c trials concluded that pharmacotherapy had a clinical advantage over placebo for achieving short-term remission and weight-loss from BED but there was no data for a long-term effect. Combining with psychotherapy does not enhance the effect (s = 33, p/c, Reas and Grilo, Obesity (Silver Spring) 2008;**16**:2024–38). Studies on desipramine, fluvoxamine, fluoxetine, sertraline, citalopram, dexfenfluramine, sibutra-mine and topiramate have shown some efficacy. An open trial of venlafaxine suggested a role.

Reviews: * general (Mathes et al, Appetite 2009; **52**:545–53; Yager, Am J Psychiatry 2008;**165**:4–6; Carter et al, Int J Eat Disord 2003;**34**[Suppl]:S74–S88; Appolinario and McElroy, Curr Drug Targets 2004;**5**:301–7).

● Unlicensed/some efficacy

Atomoxetine

Atomoxetine 40–120 mg/d was fairly well tolerated and significantly reduced binge-eating ratings (n = 40 [c = 36], RCT, d/b, p/c, 10/52, McElroy et al, J Clin Psychiatry 2007;**68**:390–8).

SSRIs * (see also 'no efficacy')

Citalopram may be effective in reducing binge-eating frequency, weight and severity (n = 38, RCT, d/b, p/c, 6/52, McElroy et al, J Clin Psychiatry 2003;**64**:807–13). Sertraline 100–200 mg/d and fluoxetine 40–80 mg/d were equally effective for measures of BED over an extended period (n = 42, RCT, d/b, 6/12, Leombruni et al, Prog Neuropsychopharmacol Biol Psychiatry 2008;**32**:1599–605). Fluoxetine (mean dose 71 mg/d) was well tolerated and effective in reducing binge-eating frequency, weight and illness severity (n = 60, RCT, d/b, 6/52, Arnold et al, J Clin Psychiatry 2002;**63**:1028–33), but had a low impact on BED symptoms compared to individualised CBT (n = 116, >2 years, Devlin et al, Obesity [Silver Spring] 2007;**15**:1702–9).

Lamotrigine *

Lamotrigine had a significant effect on all measures of BED in one study, but unfortunately so did placebo and this exceptionally high placebo response may have disguised any effect, or not, as the case may be (n = 51, RCT, d/b, p/c, 16/52, Guerdjikova et al, Int Clin Psychopharmacol 2009;**24**:150–8).

Lithium

In comorbid bipolar and BED, lithium has helped augment topiramate (n = 12, open, Kotwal et al, Hum Psychopharmacol 2006; **21**:425–31).

Memantine *

Memantine 5–20 mg/d may reduce binge-eating in BED but has little effect on BMI (n = 19 [c = 9], open, 12/52, Brennan et al, Int J Eat Disord 2008;**41**:520–6), and the effect may be complete within 24 hours, possibly blocking leptin response (n = 5, Hermanussen and Tresguerres, Econ Hum Biol 2005;**3**:329–37).

Reboxetine

A pilot study with reboxetine 8 mg/d produced a remarkable reduction in binge days per week, decreased BMI and improved other measures (n = 9 [c = 5], open, 12/52, Silveira et al, Eat Weight Disorder 2005;**10**;93–6).

Sibutramine

Two RCTs have shown sibutramine 15 mg/d to reduce binge episodes, weight and mental state (n = 60, RCT, d/b, p/c, 12/52, Appolinario et al, Arch Gen Psychiatry 2003;**60**:1109–16) and superior to placebo for reducing measures of BED (binges, weight, psychopathology) but with significant ADRs (n = 304, RCT, d/b, p/c, 24/52, Wilfley et al, Am J Psychiatry 2008;**165**:51–8).

Topiramate *

A systematic analysis has suggested that topiramate is effective for the short-term treatment of BED but long-term use is unproven (s = 5, Arbaizar et al, Gen Hosp Psychiatry 2008;**30**:471–5). Some of these studies included topiramate at up to 600 mg/d producing an enduring improvement in some patients with BED albeit poorly tolerated with a high drop-out rate (n = 61, 14 + 42/52, RCT, d/b, p/c, McElroy et al, J Clin Psychiatry 2004; **65**:1463–9; see also n = 61, RCT, d/b, p/c, 14/52, McElroy et al, Am J Psychiatry 2003;**160**:255–61). Adjunctive topiramate 200 mg/d improved the short-term efficacy of CBT (n = 73, RCT, d/b, p/c, 21/52, Claudino et al, J Clin Psychiatry 2007; **68**:1324–32) and topiramate has produced binge-eating remission in 58% (cf 29% on placebo) with 30% drop-out in both groups (n = 394, McElroy et al, Biol Psychiatry 2007; **61**:1039–48).

Review: Tata and Kockler, Ann Pharmacother 2006;**40**:1993–7.

Zonisamide

Zonisamide 100–600 mg/d may significantly reduce binge-eating frequency and other measures and controlled trials are now awaited (n = 15 [c = 8], open, 12/52, McElroy et al, J Clin Psychiatry 2004;**65**:50–6).

☐ No efficacy

Fluvoxamine (see also SSRIs)

Fluvoxamine was no better than placebo in

BED (n = 20, RCT, d/b, p/c, Pearlstein *et al, Arch Women Ment Health* 2003;**6**:147–51).

1.17 EPILEPSY
see also Status epilepticus (*1.17.1*)

The annual incidence of epilepsy is 50–70 cases per 100000 (excluding febrile seizure), with a point prevalence of 5–10 per 1000. The lifetime prevalence is 2–5% of the population.

Role of drugs
Drug therapy is probably the single most important aspect in managing seizures. Treatment after a first seizure probably halves the recurrence rate in the next 1–2 years but with no long-term remission in individuals with single or infrequent seizures (n = 1443, RCT, five years, Marson *et al, Lancet* 2005;**365**:2007–13).

Basic principles for the management of epilepsy are:
1. Choose the best drug for the seizure type and patient.
2. Start at a low dose.
3. Titrate slowly to allow tolerance to CNS ADRs.
4. Keep the regimen simple with OD or BD doses, even if polypharmacy.
5. Measure plasma concentrations if possible.
6. Try two monotherapies before polypharmacy.
7. If seizures persist, combine the best-tolerated first drug with one of the newer agents.
8. Aim to balance best seizure control with optimal quality of life

(Brodie *et al, Fast Facts: Epilepsy* 2005, Health Press).

Plasma level monitoring for anticonvulsants should be restricted to:
1. Patients on phenytoin or polytherapy where dosage adjustment is necessary due to poor seizure control or dose-related toxicity.
2. People with learning disabilities, where assessing toxicity is difficult.
3. Patients with renal or hepatic disease.
4. Pregnant women.
5. Where poor compliance is suspected.

Discontinuing anticonvulsants
Since all anticonvulsants have side-effects, especially when taken for long periods and even when optimum ranges are adhered to, they should be discontinued when no longer needed. Adults are not always given advice on anticonvulsant discontinuation, with many stopping on their own initiative. A concentration of seizures during or in the first few months after withdrawal suggest that at least some are provoked by drug withdrawal. Other withdrawal effects such as anxiety, agitation and insomnia are a problem, but only occur with the barbiturates and benzodiazepines. A prognostic index for recurrence of seizures, either on continued treatment or discontinuation, has been advised by the MRC Antiepileptic Drug Withdrawal Study Group (Chadwick *et al, Br Med J* 1993;**306**:1374–8). This important and accessible paper should be consulted in order to use this predictive model to its optimum. It should prove useful in counselling patients in the community who wish to withdraw from anticonvulsants. However, a recent randomised discontinuation study showed 15% relapses in the withdrawal group, and 7% in non-discontinuation, not significantly different (n=160, RCT, d/b, 12/12, Lossius *et al, Epilepsia* 2008;**49**:455–63). Unless, of course, you're one of the 8%.

Reviews: withdrawing anticonvulsants (Chadwick, *Epilepsia* 2006;**47**[Suppl 1]:58–61), comparative study (n = 1013, Chadwick, *Brain* 1999;**122**: 441–8).

Risk factors for relapse on discontinuing anticonvulsants:
- Polytherapy (four or more anticonvulsants).
- Active epilepsy.
- Age (50 years or older).
- Five weeks or less between reductions.
- Longer duration of treatment or illness (more than 30 months is a higher risk).
- Number of seizures before controlled (higher risk of relapse if more than 100 seizures occur before control).
- Interval seizure less than one month at onset of illness.
- Type of seizure: Complex partial seizures, tonic-clonic or combinations of seizures are more likely to relapse than simple partial seizures.

- Number of drugs required before seizure control (i.e. time taken to control seizures).
- Abnormal EEG .
- Adult/late onset seizures (after 10–12 years of age).
- Underlying cerebral disorder.
- Withdrawal in less than six months.

Review: practical (Crawford, *Prescriber* 2005;**16**: 43–7).

Favourable factors for discontinuing anticonvulsants:

- Primary generalised seizures.
- Childhood onset (after the age of one, better 5–12 years).
- Short duration of epilepsy.
- No cerebral disorder.
- Normal IQ.
- Normal EEG (or no gross abnormalities, underlying neurological disorder or learning disability), before and after discontinuation.
- Few seizures documented, especially juvenile myoclonic epilepsy.
- History of non-compliance/concordance without relapse.
- Medication below quoted therapeutic levels at time of discontinuation.
- More than two years since last seizure, especially in children.

Reviews: * pharmacotherapy (Johannessen Land-mark and Johannessen, *Drugs* 2008;**68**:1925–39), efficacy and tolerability (Kennedy and Lhatoo, *CNS Drugs* 2008;**22**:739–60), modes of action (Stahl, *J Clin Psychiatry* 2004;**65**:149–50), focal-onset seizures (Johannessen and Ben-Menachem, *Drugs* 2006;**66**:1701–25), catamenial epilepsy (Foldvary-Schaefer and Falcone, *Neurology* 2003;**61**[Suppl 2]:S2–S15), absence epilepsy (Manning *et al*, *Trends Pharmacol Sci* 2003; **24**:542–9), cognitive side-effects (Arif *et al*, *Epilepsy Behav* 2008;**14**:202–9).

BNF listed

FIRST-LINE/MONOTHERAPY DRUGS

Carbamazepine

Carbamazepine is a broad spectrum anti-convulsant, licensed for adjunctive or first-line therapy in tonic-clonic and partial seizures (excluding absences and myoclonic seizures). The sustained release tablets can be used as a once-a-day dosage, with careful monitoring if seizures continue, although lower trough concentrations mean some patients may need twice-daily dosing. Cochrane concludes carbamazepine and phenobarbital are equally effective, with phenobarbital possibly slightly better for partial onset seizures and carbamazepine for GTC seizures (Tudur Smith *et al*, *Cochrane Database Syst Rev* 2003; 1:CD001904).

Review: mode of action (Ambrosio *et al*, *Neurochem Res* 2002;**27**:121–30).

Lamotrigine

Lamotrigine is indicated for adjunctive or monotherapy in partial or generalised epilepsy, Lennox-Gastaut and juvenile myoclonic epilepsy. It is thought to stabilise pre-synaptic neuronal membranes by blockade of voltage-dependent sodium channels, with this secondarily inhibiting the release of excessive excitatory glutamate and aspartate. The 2–5% risk of rashes can be reduced in adults with a starting dose of 25 mg/d for two weeks, then 50 mg/d for two weeks, then increasing every 1–2 weeks, halved if added to valproate (where rash is also more likely to occur) or allergic to trimethoprim, and doubled if combined with concurrent enzyme-inducing drugs, e.g. phenytoin, carbamazepine, etc. The incidence of serious rash and Stevens-Johnson syndrome is relatively rare (higher if a history of previous AED-related rash; n = 988, Hirsch *et al*, *Epilepsia* 2006;**47**:318–22), but can be life-threatening and must be considered carefully (s = 2, n = 1955, Calabrese *et al*, *J Clin Psychiatry* 2002;**63**:1012–9). Cochrane con-cludes that while lamotrigine is much better tolerated than carbamazepine, the latter may be superior for seizure control (s = 5, n = 1384, Gamble *et al*, *Cochrane Database Syst Rev* 2006; 1:CD001031), but that it may be effective in drug-resistant partial epilepsy (n = 1243, s = 11, Ramaratnam *et al*, *Cochrane Database Syst Rev* 2001;**3**:CD001909).

Reviews: general (Malik *et al*, *Expert Rev Neurother* 2006;**6**:1609–27), kinetics, safety and toxicity (Biton, *Expert Opin Drug Metab Toxic* 2006;**2**:1009–18).

Levetiracetam

Levetiracetam is licensed as monotherapy for partial seizures, with or without secondary generalisation, in people aged 16 or over with newly-diagnosed epilepsy. Although structurally related to piracetam, it has a distinct pharmacological profile and the mode of action is unclear. The dose is 250mg BD, increasing to a maximum of 1500mg/d. It has been investigated at 1–3g/d for resistant partial seizures, where it has been effective and well tolerated as adjunctive and monotherapy. Levetiracetam seems to have long-term efficacy for partial seizures (n = 280, < 4 years, open follow-up, Abou-Khalil and Schaich, *Seizure* 2005;**14**:577–85). Cochrane concludes that levetiracetam is effective as an add-on in localised partial epilepsy (n = 1023, s = 4, 24/52, Chaisewikul *et al*, *Cochrane Database Syst Rev* 2001;**1**:CD001901) but that more data is needed. It has good bioavailability, rapidly achieves steady-state concentrations, has linear kinetics, minimal protein binding, and minimal metabolism, i.e. ideal pharmacokinetic properties although a BD dosage is needed due to its short half-life (review: Perucca and Johannessen, *Epileptic Disord* 2003;**5**[Suppl 1]: S17–S26).

Review: general (Carreno, *Drugs Today [Barc]* 2007;**43**:769–94).

Oxcarbazepine *

Oxcarbazepine is indicated for partial seizures with or without secondary generalised tonic-clonic seizures. Oxcarbazepine's mode of action mainly involves blocking sodium and calcium channels, but this may differ subtly from carbamazepine (review by Schmidt and Elger, *Epilepsy Behav* 2004;**5**:627–35). A consensus view suggested starting at 150mg/d, and increasing by 150mg/d on alternate days to 900–1200mg/d (Schmidt *et al*, *Acta Neurol Scand* 2001;**104**:167–70). Oxcarbazepine exerts its action primarily through its metabolite (the monohydroxy derivative, MHD). It can be used as monotherapy or adjunctive therapy in adults and children, with an average maintenance dose of 2400mg/day. About 25–30% of patients who have experienced hypersensitivity to carbamazepine may experience such reactions with oxcarbazepine, in which case oxcarbazepine should be immediately withdrawn. Hyponatraemia can occur and so regular sodium levels are advisable. If necessary, an abrupt switch from CBZ to oxcarbazepine on a 1:1.5 basis (or 1:1 for doses of CBZ > 800 mg/d followed by titration to tolerance if necessary) may be effective and well tolerated. Cochrane concludes that oxcarbazepine is better tolerated than phenytoin but that relative efficacy is unproven (Muller *et al, Cochrane Database Syst Rev* 2006;**2**:CD003615).

Reviews: * general (Bang and Goa, *CNS Drugs* 2004;**18**:57–61), TDM (probably unnecessary unless at extremes: Bring and Ensom, *Clin Pharmacokinet* 2008;**47**:767–78), clinical pharmacokinetics (May *et al, Clin Pharmacokinet* 2003; **42**:1023–42).

Phenytoin

Phenytoin is licensed for adjunctive or first-line therapy in partial or generalised epilepsy (excluding absence and myoclonus) and status epilepticus, and is believed to stabilise the seizure threshold. A wide range of side-effects and non-linear kinetics make it a difficult drug to use. A study of 45 patients aimed at establishing dosing rules to minimise toxic effects with phenytoin concluded the following:

1. Increase the dose by 100mg/d if the steady state plasma level is <7mcg/ml.
2. Increase the dose by 50mg/d if the steady state plasma level is 7–12mcg/ml.
3. Increase dose by 30mg/d when initial plasma levels are >12mcg/ml.

The 'optimal' range is only a guide and higher plasma levels may be needed, as interpatient and intrapatient variability in phenytoin protein binding mean serum concentration monitoring is unreliable (n = 48, 163 samples, Linh Banh *et al, Ther Drug Monit* 2002;**24**:379–85).

Topiramate

Topiramate is licensed as monotherapy for partial and generalised tonic-clonic seizures, with or without secondary generalisation. Topiramate is also licensed as adjunctive therapy in Lennox-Gastaut syndrome and partial seizures. There is a multiple mode of action, including sodium channel blockade, GABA enhancement, glutamate inhibition and weak carbonic anhydrase inhibition, which may explain its effect in resistant epilepsy and severity of side-effects, e.g. ataxia, dizziness and somnolence. The optimum dose now appears to be 100mg/d (as effective as 200mg/d but with less side-effects). Twice-daily dosing is appropriate and the recommended starting dose is now 25mg/d for the first week, increased by 25–50mg/d every one to two weeks to 200–400mg/d. Slow dose titration is important to minimise side-effects, which are the main reason for drop-outs (n=470, Bootsma et al, Epilepsy Behav 2004;5:380–7). Cochrane concludes that topiramate has efficacy as add-on therapy in partial epilepsy, but long-term and monotherapy were unproven (s=9, n=1049, RCT, Jette et al, Cochrane Database Syst Rev 2008;3:CD001417) and longer trials are needed.

Reviews: * general (Latini et al, Mini Rev Med Chem 2008;8:10–23; Lyseng-Williams and Yang, CNS Drugs 2008;22:171–4), in children (Ormrod and McClellan, Paediatr Drugs 2001; 3:293–319).

Valproate

Valproate is licensed for first-line or adjunctive therapy in partial, generalised or other epilepsies (excluding absence and myoclonus), including Lennox-Gastaut syndrome and juvenile myoclonic epilepsy. Valproate should not be used in women of child-bearing potential without a fully informed and documented discussion. The sustained release preparations overcome the short plasma half-life. There is little correlation between blood levels and therapeutic effect and so routine blood level monitoring is of limited use, although saturation protein-binding may occur above 100mg/L, requiring great care. Rapid IV loading of undiluted valproate 20–30mg/kg at 6–10mg/kg/min was well tolerated and produced no serious cardiac, neurological, hepatic or adverse effects (n=40, Limdi et al, Epilepsia 2007;48:478–83).

Reviews: mode of action in epilepsy (Johannsessen and Johannessen, CNS Drug Rev 2003;9:199–216), pharmacology (Owens and Nemeroff, Psychopharmacol Bull 2003; 37[Suppl 2]:S17–S24) and kinetics (DeVane, Psychopharmacol Bull 2003;37[Suppl 2]:S25–S42).

BENZODIAZEPINES *

Benzodiazepines are excellent anticonvulsants in the short-term, but tolerance limits their long-term use. They may also be useful for 'rescue' or special events, e.g. holidays and family events (review of pharmacology and pharmacokinetics; Riss et al, Acta Neurol Scand 2008;118:69–86).

Clobazam *

Clobazam is licensed as adjunctive therapy in partial or generalised epilepsy and as intermittent therapy. Tolerance can develop and so low doses (e.g. 10–20mg/d) and intermittent administration can help to minimise this. Sustained response is more likely in patients with a shorter duration of epilepsy and a known etiology. 11% of people with refractory epilepsy became seizure-free with addition of clobazam (n=251, Montenegro et al, Clin Neuropharmacol 2008;31:333–8). It may be effective for stimulus-provoked attacks, catamenial epilepsy (if given for one week in four), in intractable childhood epilepsy, as add-on in refractory epilepsy and as add-on for TLE with hippocampal sclerosis. Cochrane concludes clobazam is effective (particularly in partial onset seizures) but is unsure who would benefit most or the appropriate time-scales (s=4, n=196, Michael and Marson, Cochrane Database Syst Rev 2008; 2:CD004154)

Reviews: * general (Ng and Collins, Neurotherapeutics 2007;4:138–44), in Lennox-Gastaut syndrome (Conry et al, Epilepsia 2008;50: 1158–66).

Clonazepam

Clonazepam is licensed for adjunctive therapy in partial or generalised epilepsy (including absence and myoclonus), infantile spasms, status and Lennox-Gastaut syndrome. It has marked anticonvulsant properties but its usefulness is limited by tolerance (which may possibly be reversed with flumazenil 1.5mg IV) and sedation.

Diazepam

Diazepam is occasionally useful orally as an adjunct and in short-term therapy, although studies on it are limited. Use in status epilepticus is well-established.

BARBITURATES

Phenobarbital

Phenobarbital is licensed as adjunctive or monotherapy therapy in partial or generalised epilepsy (excluding absence and myoclonus). Concerns about cognitive and psychomotor impairment and dependence have rightly limited its use (Taylor et al, Cochrane Database Syst Rev 2001;**4**:CD002217). Cochrane concludes that carbamazepine and phenobarbital are equally effective (Tudur Smith et al, Cochrane Database Syst Rev 2003;**1**:CD001904).

Reviews: (Kale and Perucca, Br Med J 2004; **329**:1199–200; Kwan and Brodie, Epilepsia 2004;**45**:1141–9).

Primidone *

This obsolescent barbiturate is metabolised to phenobarbital and phenylethylmalonamide. It is probably less effective than valproate in carbamazepine-resistant epilepsy (n = 136, open, Sun et al, Seizure 2009;**18**:90–3).

ADD-ON OR ADJUNCT THERAPY/OTHERS

Acetazolamide *

Although this carbonic anhydrase inhibitor is a potent anticonvulsant, and is occasionally useful for absence and other seizures, rapid tolerance and long-term side-effects render it of limited use (review by Hoddevik, Tidsskr Nor Laegeforen 2000;**120**:1042–5; n = 1, Lyall, Can J Ophthalmol 2008;**43**:377).

Ethosuximide

Ethosuximide is primarily useful in absence seizures, but also as adjunctive therapy in GTC and other epilepsies. It is poorly studied and has largely now been replaced by valproate.

Gabapentin

Gabapentin is licensed as adjunctive therapy in refractory partial and secondary generalised epilepsy. There is a strong dose:response relationship, with much interpatient variability (requiring individual optimisation). A review concludes that gabapentin can be initiated at 900 mg/d and titrated (rapidly) to up to 3600 mg/d, with children treated with 23–78 mg/kg/d (McLean and Gidal, Clin

Ther 2003;**25**:1382–406). A TDS dosage is recommended, with no more than 12 hours between doses. It has a low order of toxicity, uncomplicated kinetics, no clinically important interactions, and plasma levels are not necessary. Cochrane concludes that gabapentin has efficacy as an add-on in drug-resistant epilepsy, but trials are short-term, with long-term efficacy and monotherapy unproven (Marson et al, Cochrane Database Syst Rev 2000;**3**:CD001415).

Review: general (n = 3100, PMSS, Wilton and Shakir, Epilepsia 2002;**43**:983–92).

Lacosamide *

Lacosamide is licensed for adjunctive therapy in partial onset seizures with or without secondary generalisation in patients with epilepsy aged 16 years or older. The starting dose is 50 mg BD up to a maximum of 200 mg BD. It selectively enhances slow inactivation of voltage-gated sodium channels and interacts with collapsin response mediator protein-2 (CRMP-2). Lacosamide produces a statistically significant reduction in seizure frequency at 400 mg and 600 mg/day versus placebo, with 400 mg/d better tolerated than 600 mg/d.

Reviews: * pharmacology (Beydoun et al, Expert Rev Neurother 2009;**9**:33–42) in partial seizures (Cross and Curran, Drugs 2009;**69**:449–59).

Piracetam

Piracetam is a GABA derivative, licensed in the UK for cortical myoclonus, in conjunction with other anti-myoclonic therapies. Up to 70% of patients may become seizure-free if they can swallow enough of it.

Pregabalin *

Pregabalin is licensed as an adjunctive therapy for adults with partial seizures, with or without secondary generalisation. It is a GABA analog that reduces excitatory neurotransmitter release by binding to alpha(2)-delta protein, modulating voltage-gated calcium channels (Warner and Figgitt, CNS Drugs 2005;**19**:265–72). The target dose is 600 mg/d in divided doses, starting at 150 mg/d, increasing to 300 mg/d after a week, and to a maximum of 600 mg/d after another week. Absorption is slightly reduced by food, and plasma level monitoring is unnecessary (review of serum concentrations, May et al, Ther Drug Monit 2007; **29**:789–94). It has a robust efficacy and good tolerability (s = 4, n = 1174, RCT, p/c, Gil-Nagel et al, Seizure 2009;**18**:184–92).

Rufinamide *

Rufinamide is a carboxamide derivative that modulates activity of sodium channels (prolonging their inactive state by membrane stabilising effects) and is licensed in UK as adjunctive therapy for seizures associated with Lennox-Gestaut syndrome in patients over three years old. It may also be effective in partial seizures. It should be dosed twice a day equally divided preferably with food (to slow absorption), starting at 200 mg/d increasing by 200 mg/d every two days at most, maximum recommended dose (600 mg/d) based on body weight (for patients weighing less than 30 kg halve these doses, e.g. start at 200 mg/d). If taking valproate start at a lower dose (see 4.5.12). Discontinuation at 25% every two days is recommended as the fastest. Cognitive effects are minimal in partial seizures compared to placebo (n = 189, 3/12, RCT, d/b, p/c, Aldenkamp and Alpherts, Epilepsia 2006; **47**:1153–9; see also n = 313, RCT, d/b, p/c, 21/52, Brodie et al, Epilepsia 2009;**50**:1899–90).
Reviews: * general (Herranz, Rev Neurol 2008; **47**:369–73; Kreutzkamp, Med Monatsschr Pharm 2007;**30**:358–61; Heaney and Walker, Drugs Today [Barc] 2007;**43**:455–60; Hakimian et al, Expert Opin Pharmacother 2007;**8**:1931–40).

Tiagabine

Tiagabine is licensed in the UK as adjunctive therapy for partial seizures, with or without secondary generalisation. It is a potent GABA reuptake inhibitor in neuronal and glial cells, increasing GABA-mediated inhibition of the CNS. Tiagabine has linear kinetics, a short half-life (requiring BD to QDS dosage), an inducible metabolism and a number of drug interactions (see 4.5.12). Cochrane concludes that tiagabine is effective as adjunctive therapy but is associated with many ADRs (Pereira et al, Cochrane Database Syst Rev 2002; **3**:CD001908).
Review: * general (Bauer and Cooper-Mahkorn, Neuropsychiatr Dis Treat 2008;**4**:731–6).

Vigabatrin

Vigabatrin is licensed as adjunctive therapy in refractory partial and secondary generalised epilepsy and as monotherapy for West's syndrome, but use is now limited by ocular changes (e.g. impaired contrast sensitivity and usually irreversible loss of field) in up to 50% of patients. Total vigabatrin exposure is the most significant factor in predicting visual field loss. It should only be used when there is no alternative, accompanied by a baseline and six-monthly peripheral field examination (Hardus et al, Epilepsia 2001;**42**:262–7; n = 17, Paul et al, Epilepsia 2001;**42**:525–30).
Reviews: general (Gidal et al, Ann Pharmacother 1999;**33**:1277–86), ocular problems (Newman et al, Eye 2002;**16**:567–71).

Zonisamide

Zonisamide is licensed for adjunctive therapy for adults with partial seizures, with or without secondary generalisation. Zonisamide may block voltage sensitive calcium channels and enhance the inhibitory effects, e.g. GABA. Its half-life is 60 hours, steady state is reached in 13 days, and accumulation occurs. The dose is 25 mg BD for a week, increasing by up to 100 mg a week to a maximum of 300–500 mg/d, with a dose-dependent effect. Cochrane concludes that zonisamide is effective as an add-on in drug-resistant partial epilepsy, but that the therapeutic dose is unclear and long-term studies are needed (s = 4, n = 850, RCT, p/c, Chadwick and Marson, Cochrane Database Syst Rev 2005;**4**:CD001416).
Reviews: * general (Arzimanoglou and Rahbani, Expert Rev Neurother 2006;**6**:1283–92; Frampton and Scott, CNS Drugs 2005;**19**: 347–67), long-term safety (Zaccara and Specchio, Neuropsychiatr Dis Treat 2009;**5**: 249–59).

+ Combinations

Numerous combinations are used but few have been, or can be, assessed systematically.

● Unlicensed/some efficacy

Calcium-channel blockers

Cochrane concludes the evidence for nifedipine and nimodipine is not convincing (s = 11, Chaisewikul et al, Cochrane Database Syst Rev 2001;**4**:CD002750).

Carnitine

Intractable epilepsy in a child with carnitine deficiency was treated successfully with L-carnitine 100mg TDS and valproate (n = 1, Shuper et al, Lancet 1999;**353**:1238; Campistol et al, Rev Neurol 2000;**30**[Suppl 1]:S105–9).

Fluoxetine

In patients with complex partial seizures, fluoxetine had a significant effect (n = 17, open, Favale et al, Neurology 1995;**45**:1926–7).

Goserelin

A reduction in the number of attacks in catamenial epilepsy has been shown, although long-term treatment would have problems (Reid and Gangar, Lancet 1992;**339**:253).

Melatonin

Adjunctive melatonin 6–9mg/d may be neuro-protective in children with epilepsy taking valproate (n = 31 [c = 29], RCT, d/b, p/c, Gupta et al, Br J Clin Pharmacol 2004;**58**:542–7).

Midazolam

Acute childhood seizures have been managed with intranasal midazolam (Smith and Carley, Emerg Med J 2005;**22**:436–7; Body and Ijaz, Emerg Med J 2005;**22**:364–5).

Nitrazepam

Nitrazepam has been used successfully in Lennox-Gestaut syndrome (n = 14, open, 12/12, Hosain et al, Pediatr Neurol 2003;**28**:16–9).

◆ Others

Other drugs used include **aromatherapy** (ylang ylang, chamomile and lavender: Anon, Pharm J 1993;**251**:798), **buspirone** (in progressive myoclonus epilepsy: Pranzatelli et al, J Neurol Neurosurg Psychiatry 1993;**56**:114–5), **magnesium** (Walker et al, Anesthesia 1995;**50**:130–5), **medroxyprogesterone** (in women: Epilepsia 1985;**26**:S40–S51), **progesterone** (especially catamenial exacerbations: n = 25, open, Herzog, Neurology 1995;**45**:1660–2).

□ No efficacy

Caffeine *

Caffeine may increase seizure frequency and so overall daily intake should be limited in epilepsy (Jankiewicz et al, Przegl Lek 2007;**64**:965–7).

Donepezil

Donepezil did not improve memory or cognitive functioning in epilepsy or exacerbate seizures (n = 23, RCT, s/b, p/c, c/o, 3 + 3/12, Hamberger et al, Epilepsia 2007;**48**:1283–91).

1.17.1 STATUS EPILEPTICUS

Status epilepticus is a state where multiple seizures occur without complete recovery between seizures, e.g. usually seizures longer than five minutes or two consecutive seizures without regaining consciousness. Mortality can be high, but rapid and aggressive management reduces this risk and any permanent neuronal damage.

Role of drugs

To prevent permanent brain damage, first-line therapy must be to support with oxygen and a glucose drip if possible. First-line drugs, e.g. benzodiazepines are usually successful to abort status epilepticus. Refractory seizures are frequently caused by acute neurological problems, e.g. encephalitis, CVA or trauma. Transfer to an ITU may be appropriate. The EFNS guidelines (Meierkord et al, Eur J Neurol 2006;**13**:445–50) recommend lorazepam 4mg IV or diazepam 10mg IV followed by 15–18mg/kg phenytoin (or fosphenytoin equivalents). If still fitting after 10 minutes, repeat lorazepam or diazepam. If refractory, use anaesthetic doses of midazolam, propofol or barbiturates with appropriate EEG monitoring. Isoflurane and desflurane adequately suppress refractory status epilepticus, albeit with complications (n = 7, Mirsattari et al, Arch Neurol 2004;**61**:1254–9).Cochrane concludes that lorazepam is superior to diazepam or phenytoin for cessation of seizures and carries a lower risk of continuation of status (Prasad et al, Cochrane Database Syst Rev 2005;**4**:CD003723).

Reviews: * general (Arif and Hirsch, Semin Neurol 2008;**28**:342–54; Wheless and Treiman, Epilepsia 2008;**49**(suppl 9):74–8; Selvitelli and Drislane, Curr Neurol Neurosci Rep 2007;**7**:529–

35; Treiman, *Int Rev Neurobiol* 2007;**81**:273–85), ICU management (Bleck, *Epilepsia* 2007;**48**[Suppl 8]:59–60), current developments (Selvitelli and Drislane, *Curr Neurol Neurosci Rep* 2007;**7**:529–35), anesthetics for refractory status (Rossetti, *Epilepsia* 2007;**48** Suppl 8:52–5).

BNF listed

Clonazepam

Clonazepam 0.5–1.5 mg by slow IV injection (possibly followed by an infusion) may be useful in refractory cases not responsive to diazepam. A prolonged effect may be seen.

Diazepam

Diazepam 0.15–0.25 mg/kg (i.e. around 10–30 mg) given as a slow IV injection over five minutes or rectally (e.g. rectal tubes) is first choice treatment in the UK. Rates above 5 mg/min IV are associated with respiratory depression. The speed of rectal absorption is second only to IV absorption (*Int J Pharmaceutics* 1980;**5**:127). It is also safe and effective when administered by paramedics in out-of-hospital situations (n = 205, RCT, p/c, Alldredge *et al, N Engl J Med* 2001;**345**:631–7).

Fosphenytoin

Fosphenytoin is a water soluble phosphate ester pro-drug converted to phenytoin. It is rapidly absorbed (therapeutic levels in 5–20 minutes) and is licensed for status and as a substitute for oral phenytoin. It is well tolerated at injection sites (open, Pryor *et al, Epilepsia* 2001;**42**:245–50) and has complete IM absorption. It can be given up to three times more rapidly IV than phenytoin and can be given IM, where cardiac monitoring is not necessary. Conversion to phenytoin takes about 7–15 minutes, with peak levels at about 30 minutes, and so fosphenytoin is less appropriate for the sole initial treatment of status epilepticus.
Review: general (Fischer *et al, Clin Pharmacokinet* 2003;**2**:33–58).

Lorazepam

Lorazepam may be preferable to diazepam, due to a longer duration of action (about two hours), shorter elimination half-life, no active metabolites and possibly less respiratory depression. In convulsive status epilepticus, lorazepam 4 mg IV was equivalent to diazepam 10 mg IV, but superior in terms of fewer recurrences (Cock and Schapira, *QJM* 2002;**95**:225–31).

Midazolam

Midazolam buccal (which can be with the injection liquid) and is licensed for status. Continuous IV infusion is unlicensed but can be rapidly successful in many patients with appropriate care. In refractory status, an IV bolus of midazolam followed by IV infusion was effective (mean 45 minutes) in 95% of ITU patients and appeared both safe and effective in this extreme situation (n = 19, open, Ulvi *et al, Neurol Sci* 2002;**23**:177–82). It has a rapid onset of action (30–90 seconds) but care is needed as it can cause potentially fatal respiratory depression, as midazolam's half-life prolongs significantly after sustained infusion (n = 2, Naritoku and Sinha, *Neurology* 2000;**54**:1366–8). Continuous midazolam infusion has been reported to be as effective as diazepam, although in one study recurrence and mortality were higher than with diazepam infusion (n = 40, RCT, open, Singhi *et al, J Child Neurol* 2002;**17**:106–10). Buccal midazolam was more effective than rectal diazepam in a multicentre emergency-room trial (n = 177, RCT, McIntyre *et al, Lancet* 2005;**366**:205–10) and more effective than rectal diazepam except for malaria-related seizures, where they were equally effective (n = 330, RCT, s/b, Mpimbaza *et al, Pediatrics* 2008;**121**:e58–64).
Review: general (Olkkola and Ahonen, *Handb Exp Pharmacol* 2008;**182**:335–60).

Paraldehyde *

Paraldehyde has been withdrawn in UK.

Phenobarbital sodium *

A parenteral loading dose of 10–20 mg/kg with a maintenance dose of 5–7 mg/kg/day can be used. Very high dose phenobarbital (mean 70 mg/kg/d) has been used successfully for refractory status (n = 10, Tiamkao *et al, J Med Assoc Thai* 2007;**90**:2597–600).

Phenytoin

Phenytoin (see also fosphenytoin) is a useful

second-line to the benzodiazepines, used as 10–20 mg/kg in 0.9% saline intravenously over 15 minutes (not exceeding 50 mg/minute) for recurrent or persistent seizures. It is effective from 20–30 minutes after injection but is not effective intramuscularly. It is not an easy drug to use due to the risk of hypotension and cardiac dysrhythmias.

Review: kinetics of phenytoin IV (Ogutu et al, Br J Clin Pharmacol 2003;**56**:112–9).

● **Unlicensed/some efficacy**

Propofol

Propofol has been used (review by Carley and Crawford, Emerg Med J 2002;**19**:143–4; see also Claassen et al, Epilepsia 2002;**43**:146–53), but two studies showed an increased risk of mortality (review by Niermeijer et al, J Neurol 2003;**250**:1237–40).

Thiamine

Thiamine may be indicated to prevent serious complications when glucose IV is given as supportive therapy in status, especially if due to alcoholic neuropathy (Koike and Sobue, Curr Opin Neurol 2006;**19**:481–6).

Thiopental (sodium thiopentone)

Induction of anaesthesia with a 2.5% solution (4–8 mg/kg) can be effective, continued with an infusion of 0.2% solution until seizure-free for 24 hours. Phenobarbital should be substituted once seizures stop, as thiopentone accumulates in fat and affects the myocardium.

Topiramate

In refractory status, loading doses of topiramate (10 mg/kg/d for two days then 5 mg/kg/d) may be effective, e.g. given by nasogastric tube over 2/7 in resistant status (n = 3, Kahriman et al, Epilepsia 2003;**44**:1353–6).

Valproate *

High-dose valproate IV can be successful (n = 97, Peters and Pohlmann-Eden, Seizure 2005;**14**:164–9) and may be at least as effective as diazepam infusion in refractory status, but without respiratory depression or hypotension (n = 40, RCT, open, Mehta et al, J

Child Neurol 2007;**22**:1191–7; n = 74, Gilad et al, Acta Neurol Scand 2008;**118**:296–300).

■ **Unlicensed/possible efficacy**

Chloral hydrate

Doses of up to 30 mg/kg at four-hourly intervals given orally or rectally may be effective in resistant status, although onset may be delayed (review in Ann Emerg Med 1990;**19**:674–7).

Etomidate

This non-barbiturate induction agent has some anticonvulsant activity. It has a length of action of about 6–10 minutes and doses of 0.2–0.3 mg/kg IV repeated after 20 minutes have been successful.

Flumazenil

Flumazenil IV may be effective in intractable epilepsy, although it may induce seizures (n = 67, Schulze-Bonhage and Elger, Epilepsia 2000;**41**:186–92).

Lidocaine

A 1% solution given as a 2–3 mg/kg bolus over two minutes can be rapidly effective (i.e. within minutes) in cases refractory to other drugs. The effect lasts about 30 minutes but due to the relatively short duration, a second dose is needed in about 50% of cases. It should be used only with caution if any form of heart block or sinus bradycardia exists, as it may induce ventricular arrhythmia or complete heart block.

□ **No efficacy**

Tiagabine

A retrospective chart analysis suggested tiagabine was more likely to increase NCSE than reduce it (n = 90, Koepp et al, Epilepsia 2005;**46**:1625–32).

GILLES DE LA TOURETTE
see Tourette's syndrome (*1.28*)

1.18 INSOMNIA

Insomnia, the difficulty in initiating or maintaining sleep, is generally a symptom of a condition, not an illness itself and should always be treated as such. Insomnia can be caused by a variety of external (e.g. environment) and internal stimuli (e.g. mental health problems, e.g. ADHD, stress, emotional conflict, physical illness and drugs, see 5.15), and can be transient, chronic, initial or with early morning wakening. The causes, where possible, should be determined and treated, as well as placing emphasis on sleep hygiene.

Principles of sleep hygiene:

1. Avoid excessive use of caffeine (particularly within 3–4 hours of going to bed), alcohol or nicotine. A hot milky drink may help.
2. Do not stay in bed for prolonged periods if not asleep. Go to another dimly lit room — watching TV can have an alerting effect.
3. Avoid daytime naps or long periods of inactivity.
4. A warm bath or exercise a few hours before bedtime may promote sleep.
5. Avoid engaging in strenuous exercise or mental activity near bedtime (although sex can aid sleep).
6. Make sure that the bed and bedroom are comfortable and avoid extremes of noise, temperature and humidity.
7. Establish a regular bedtime routine, e.g. going to bed at the same time and rising at the same time every morning, regardless of sleep duration.
8. Diet — carbohydrate (e.g. pasta, etc) helps sleep, but not eating a big meal within about two hours of going to bed. Sugar may inhibit sleep, as may some vitamin supplements.

Role of drugs

Assuming sleep hygiene is good, any hypnotics should always be used on a PRN basis, as tolerance may develop to the sedative effects within 2–3 weeks, especially with the benzodiazepines. Short-term use for short-term reasons is usually without problem and can be very useful and comforting for the patient. Longer-term use needs the risk:benefit analysis considered carefully. The principles of sleep hygiene should be discussed and any problems corrected before prescribing hypnotics. A meta-analysis of 22 RCTs of BDZs or zolpidem showed a consistent superiority over placebo for up to five weeks, but the evidence beyond five weeks is unclear (s = 22,

Nowell et al, JAMA 1997;**278**:2170–7, 86 refs). Anyone who had ever taken an hypnotic would know the differences between the Z hypnotics and the BDZs, but NICE failed to recognise this (see fervent rebuffs to NICE by Nutt, J Psychopharmacol 2005;**19**:125–7 and Alford and Verster, J Psychopharmacol 2005;**19**:129–32). About 30% older people prescribed BDZs or Zs may still be taking them two months later, but since they seem to be effective it may be that effort should go into avoiding long-term use, rather than stopping short-term for treatment of short-term anxiety and depression (n = 129, Simon and Ludman, Gen Hosp Psychiatry 2006; **28**:374–8).

Reviews: * general (Wilson and Nutt, Prescriber 2008;**19**:14–24; Passarella and Duong, Am J Health Syst Pharm 2008;**65**:927–34; Bhat et al, Expert Opin Pharmacother 2008;**9**:351–62), sleep disorders in elderly (Sivertsen et al, Br J Psychiatry 2007;**190**:285–6), maintenance therapies (Rosenberg, Ann Clin Psychiatry 2006;**18**:49–56), use antidepressants at low dose (Wiegand, Drugs 2008;**68**:2411–7), use of medicinal plants (Wheatley, J Psychopharmacol 2005;**19**:414–21), circadian rhythms and pharmacological management of insomnia (Richardson et al, Am J Manag Care 2007;**13**[5 Suppl]:S125–8), melatonin agonists modes of action (Srinivasan et al, Int J Neurosci 2009;**119**:821–46).

BNF listed

BENZODIAZEPINES

Benzodiazepines may be extremely useful in the short-term management of insomnia, helping to facilitate essential high-quality sleep. A meta-analysis indicated benzodiazepines are effective in improving sleep latency and duration but ADRs (e.g. drowsiness and dizziness) are common, although methodologically these studies are flawed (s = 45, n = 2672, RCTs, Holbrook et al, CMAJ 2000;**162**:225–33; reviewed by Furukawa, EBMH 2000;**3**:81). Users of benzodiazepines and zopiclone are also at greater risk of road-traffic accidents, especially if combined with alcohol (involved in accidents, n = 19386 over three years, Barbone et al, Lancet 1998;**352**:1331–6). Although relatively safe in over-dose, BDZs (especially flunitrazepam and nitrazepam) have been implicated in 39% of drug poisoning suicides in Sweden from 1992–1996, so care is needed (Carlsten et al, Scand J Public Health 2003;31:224–28). Withdrawal of long-term BDZ hypnotics may improve cognitive functioning in the elderly (n = 104, d/b, one year, Curran et al, Psychol Med 2003;33:1223–37; comment by Furukawa, EBMH 2004;7:46, noting a high drop-out rate).

Flunitrazepam

This longer-acting benzodiazepine may have an abuse potential (Woods and Winger, J Clin Psychopharmacol 1997;17[3 Suppl 2]:S1–S57; reviewed by Druid et al, Forensic Sci Int 2001; 122:136–41), including in combination with other drugs, and is probably under-rated in this respect, especially in forensic settings (Daderman and Edman, Psychiatry Res 2001; 103:27–42).

Flurazepam *

Flurazepam is a benzodiazepine with a short half-life but with longer-acting metabolites that can cause hangover in older people (n = 25, RCT, d/bb, p/c, c/o, Boyle et al, Hum Psychopharmacol 2009;24:61–71).

Loprazolam

Loprazolam is an intermediate-acting benzo-diazepine with a half-life of 7–15 hours.

Lormetazepam

Lormetazepam is an intermediate acting benzo-diazepine. Short-term use has no effect on daytime vigilance or motor task performance (n = 12, RCT, d/b, c/o, Iudice et al, Int J Clin Pharmacol Ther 2002;40:304–9), and it may produce minimal psychomotor impairment in younger adults (n = 18, RCT, d/b, p/c, Fabbrini et al, Clin Ther 2005;27:78–83).

Nitrazepam

Nitrazepam is a longer-acting benzodiazepine similar to diazepam, which has active meta-bolites. Stable plasma levels can be attained in five days, so avoid use in the elderly.

Temazepam

Temazepam is a shorter-acting benzodiazepine, whose abuse potential has been well

Predicting hypnotic dependence risk
(Tyrer, Br Med J 1993;306:706–8)

Factor	Score
Benzodiazepine hypnotic used	3
Dose higher than BNF mean	2
Duration of treatment > 3 months	2
Dependent personality	2
Short elimination half-life drug	2
Tolerance or dose escalation	2
Total	
No dependence, abrupt withdrawal	=0
Some dependence risk, withdraw over two weeks recommended	=1–4
Strong dependence risk, withdraw over 4–12 weeks	=5–8
High risk of dependence, withdraw gradually plus support programme	=8–13

recognised. 7.5 mg and 15 mg are equally effective (n = 131, RCT, d/b, Erman et al, Curr Med Res Opin 2004;20:441–9).

'Z' HYPNOTICS

The 'Z' hypnotics are now widely used and offer many benefits over the benzodiazepines. NICE in the UK concluded that there was nothing to chose between 'Z' hypnotics and the hypnotic benzodiazepines, a conclusion that has been hotly disputed (see introduction). Zolpidem is potent and quick-acting (often within 15 minutes) and ideal for initiating sleep and has many fans in the pharmaceutical and medical worlds. Zopiclone and the benzodiazepines have a slower onset but longer action. A large review concluded that the incidence of dependence with zopiclone and zolpidem is remarkably lower than hypnotic BDZs, and that they are relatively safe (n = 58, Hajak et al, Addiction 2003;98:1371–8).

Reviews: comparative tolerability of 'Z' hypnotics (Terzano et al, Drug Saf 2003;26:261–82), comprehensive (s = 24, n = 3909, Dundar et al, Hum Psychopharmacol 2004;19:305–22).

Zaleplon

Zaleplon is a pyrazolopyrimidine hypnotic, a selective full agonist at the omega-1 benzodiazepine receptor (Noguchi et al, Eur J Pharmacol 2002;**434**:21–8).

Zolpidem

Zolpidem is a imidazopyridine hypnotic which binds preferentially to the omega-1 benzodiazepine receptor. It decreases time to sleep and increases total sleep time and efficiency, but does not affect sleep architecture. It has a rapid onset of action and a short duration. It has been shown to be at least as effective as zopiclone, with less rebound on discontinuation and is better tolerated, e.g. no metallic taste (n=479, d/b, 14/7, Tsutsui et al, J Int Med Res 2001;**29**:163–77). In a comparison of zolpidem, zopiclone and lormetazepam in elderly patients, zolpidem caused least cognitive, memory and equilibrium adverse effects and should, thus, be the preferred hypnotic in the elderly (n=48, RCT, d/b, p/c, c/o, Allain et al, Eur J Clin Pharmacol 2003;**59**:179–88). In a fascinating study, zolpidem 10mg taken at night up to 3–5 times a week significantly improved overall sleep, which was sustained, with no evidence of rebound, dose escalation or withdrawal, showing that true PRN hypnotic use may be highly effective and safe (n=199, RCT, p/c, 12/52, Perlis et al, J Clin Psychiatry 2004;**65**:1128–37). It is so safe that it can even be taken by athletes the night before an event without adversely affecting performance (n=7, d/b, p/c, c/o, Ito et al, Neurosci Res 2007; **59**:309–13).

Reviews: general (Lee, CNS Drugs 2004; **18**[Suppl 1]:17–23, 43–5; Israel and Swainston-Harrison and Keating, CNS Drugs 2005;**19**:65–89).

Zopiclone

Zopiclone is an established and safe non-benzodiazepine hypnotic, albeit only licensed in the UK for up to 7.5mg/d for four weeks. Zopiclone is equivalent, but not superior, to BDZs (n=2672, meta-analysis, Holbrook et al, CMAJ 2000;**162**:225–33; reviewed by Furukawa, EBMH 2000;**3**:81). A New Zealand study concluded that the fatal toxicity for zopiclone was not significantly different to BDZs as a group, whereas alprazolam and clomethiazole had greater toxicity (Reith et al, J Toxicol Clin Toxicol 2003;**41**:975–80).

Zopiclone may impair memory storage during sleep (n=8, d/b, p/c, c/o, Silva et al, Neurosci Res 2003;**47**:241–3).

Review: extensive, including abuse potential (Cimolai, Can Fam Physician 2007;**53**:2124–9).

OTHER HYPNOTICS

Antihistamines

Antihistamines may be effective and are often used as OTC sleep aids. Promethazine has a relatively long half-life and a low abuse potential. Diphenhydramine may have an abuse potential and has been strongly linked to cognitive impairment and decline in older hospitalised patients and is best avoided in this patient group (n=426, Agostini et al, Arch Intern Med 2001;**161**:2091–7).

Barbiturates

Barbiturates should only be used for severe, intractable insomnia where there are compelling reasons, and only in patients already taking barbiturates. Toxicity in overdose can be high.

Chloral hydrate

Chloral hydrate has properties similar to the barbiturates and is relatively safe in the elderly as the half-life is not significantly lengthened. An abuse potential exists and it can be toxic in overdose (n=1, Frankland and Robinson, Can J Psychiatry 2001;**46**:763–4).

Clomethiazole (chlormethiazole)

Clomethiazole is a thiamine derivative with sedative-hypnotic and anticonvulsant properties. It has a rapid onset of action and short half-life even in the elderly, although they may be more sensitive to it. Dependence and abuse has been reported, but is not considered too important if the patient is not dependence prone (n=5, Hession et al, Lancet 1979;ii:953–4). It is unsafe in overdose.

Melatonin CR (Circadin PR®) *

Melatonin is an agonist at M1, M2 and M3 receptors. Circadin® is the only melatonin product to be licensed in the UK, as a monotherapy 21-day course for primary insomnia in people aged 55 and over. The dose is 2mg 1–2 hours before bedtime and after food (which slows absorption). The SR tablets contain a synthetic melatonin, which is released over several hours to match the normal human melatonin profile (increasing after dark, peaking at 2–4.00 AM, then diminishing), as elderly people with primary insomnia secrete significantly lower levels of melatonin than healthy elderly with good sleep quality. Pineal melatonin is synthesized and secreted in close association with the light/dark cycle (review, Srinivasan et al, Int J Neurosci 2009;**119**:821–46), and melatonin receptors may in fact only exist for a few hours. Efficacy has been shown in several major trials. In one study, PR-melatonin 2 mg significantly improved sleep quality, morning alertness, sleep onset and quality of life in primary insomnia (n = 354 [c = 334]. RCT, d/b, p/c, 5/52, Wade et al, Curr Med Res Opin 2007;**23**:2597–2605), a second study produced similar results with no withdrawal symptoms on discontinuation (n = 170 [c = 164], RCT, d/b, p/c, 7/52, Lemoine et al, J Sleep Res 2007;**16**:372–80) and a third showed that nightly treatment improved perceived quality of sleep (n=40, RCT, d/b, p/c, 6/52, Luthringer et al, Int Clin Psychopharmacol 2009;**24**:239–49). 5 mg 30 minutes before sleep helps shift workers fall off to sleep (n=86, RCT, d/b, p/c, c/o, Sadeghniiat-Haghighi et al, J Circadian Rhythms 2008;**6**:10), and adjunctive melatonin can also help older people discontinue conventional hypnotics (n=22, RCT, d/b, c/o, 4/12, Garzón et al, Aging Clin Exp Res 2009;**21**:38–42). Melatonin 5–10 mg PR may improve sleep in major depression as adjunct to fluoxetine (n=24 [c=19], d/b, p/c, 4/52, Dolberg et al, Am J Psychiatry 1998;**155**:1119–21), and 2–3 mg significantly improved sleep efficiency in chronic schizophrenics with poor sleep (n=40, RCT, d/b, p/c, 15/7, Kumar et al, J Clin Psychiatry 2007;**68**:237–41). Circadin® is well tolerated and safe, with low drop-outs in clinical trials, and is not associated with impairment of memory, vigilance, and driving performance as compared with placebo, has no discernible withdrawal symptoms and in older adults (>55) it causes no impaired function or cognitive performance, compared to zolpidem (n=16, RCT, d/b, p/c, c/o, Otmani et al, Hum Psychopharmacol 2008;**23**:693–705). It may have less efficacy in younger adults, as

the evidence for this group is mixed (s=32, n=97+427+651, RCT, Buscemi et al Br Med J 2006;**332**:385–93).

Review: * use for insomnia in over 55s (Wade and Downie, Expert Opin Investig Drugs 2008; **17**:1567–72).

Ramelteon (license delayed)

Ramelteon is a melatonin agonist, approved as a hypnotic in the US. A UK license is anticipated (see Chapter 7).

Triclofos *

Triclofos is a chloral-related drug with similar actions to chloral but with less gastric irritation and a more palatable taste. It is only available as a liquid in the UK and indicated for short-term treatment of severe insomnia which is interfering with normal daily life and where other therapies have failed (SPC).

● Unlicensed/some efficacy *

Other sedative drugs the patient may already be taking, especially antipsychotics and anti-depressants, may be prescribed as a single dose at night. In longer-term therapy most can be given this way. It is also important to avoid the use of 'stimulating' drugs at night, e.g. anticholinergics and MAOIs. Many sedative antidepressants are toxic in overdose and may disrupt REM sleep. If using antidepressants, a review suggests choosing sedating ones over activating ones, low anticholinergic effects, HT2A or 2C blockers over pure histamine blockers and use the lowest dose possible (e.g. doxepin 25 mg, mirtazapine 15 mg, trazodone 50 mg, trimipramine 25 mg; Wiegand, Drugs 2008;**68**:2411–7).

Doxepin *

Extraordinarily, doxepin 1 mg, 3 mg and 6 mg were superior to placebo for improving objective and subjective sleep measures in primary insomnia, with no apparent ADRs or residual effects (n=67, RCT, d/b, c/o, Roth et al, Sleep 2007;**30**:1555–61). Similarly, doxepin 25–50 mg has been shown to produce a mild-to-moderate but significant rapid and sustained improvement in insomnia, although rebound insomnia and side-effects were noted (n=47, p/c, Hajak et al, J Clin Psychiatry 2001;**62**:453–63).

Review: * (Goforth, *Expert Opin Pharmacother* 2009;**10**:1649–55).

Mirtazapine

Insomnia is reported by 90% depressed patients, but stimulation of 5-HT$_2$ receptors is thought to underlie the insomnia and adverse changes in sleep architecture seen with SSRIs/SNRIs. Mirtazapine blocks 5-HT$_2$ receptors and may improve sleep, e.g. 30mg increased sleep efficiency and decreased wakenings (and their duration), but with no effect on REM (n = 20, RCT, d/b, p/c, 3/7, Aslan et al, *Sleep* 2002;**25**:677–9). Mirtazapine may in fact help normalise abnormal REM sleep (n = 32, Schittecatte et al, *Psychiatry Res* 2002;**109**:1–8). It may also significantly improve objective sleep parameters compared to fluoxetine in people with MDD and insomnia (n = 19, RCT, d/b, 8/52, Winokur et al, *J Clin Psychiatry* 2003;**64**:1224–9).

Quetiapine *

Quetiapine 25–10mg has been shown to improve sleep, probably at least partly through its antihistaminic effects (n = 14, RCT, d/b, p/c, 17/7, Cohrs et al, *Psychopharmacology* 2004; **174**:421–9).
Review: * use in addictive conditions (Terán et al, *Subst Use Misuse* 2008;**43**:2169–71).

Trazodone

A review of trazodone as an hypnotic concluded that, except perhaps in depressed people, there is little or no data on efficacy or tolerability, and no dose-response data for sleep, so more research is needed before use can be considered of lower risk (Mendelson, *J Clin Psychiatry* 2005;**66**:469–76). More recently, 25–150mg has been shown to be effective (n = 28, open, 3/12, Wichniak et al, *Pol Merkur Lekarski* 2007;**23**:41–6).

■ Unlicensed/possible efficacy

Alcohol *

Alcohol causes sedation but increases slow-wave sleep, reduces and disrupts REM sleep, the diuretic effect may be counter-productive and overdose can have serious consequences. Rebound arousal can occur with higher doses when blood concentrations reach zero, leading to awakening. Alcohol is thus not recommended for routine medical use. It is, however, widely used as self-medication and is available in a number of highly palatable formulations, e.g. Farmer's, Chalk Hill and anything sold at the Ivy House, Stradbroke. Interestingly, ageing Scotch whisky upregulates GABA receptors more than younger or blended Scotch (regardless of ethanol concentration), and is better at calming and inducing sleep (Koda et al, *J Agriculture Food Chem* 2003;**51**:5238–44). Reasonable quantities of Spanish beer can also provide sufficient melatonin (and the more the alcohol, the more the melatonin) to increase the human body's antioxidant capacity (n = 1, b = 18, Maldonado et al, *Clin Nutr* 2009;**28**:188–91).

Donepezil

Anticholinesterases have been shown to improve REM sleep in younger adults and also in elderly healthy adults (n = 42, d/b, p/c, Schredl et al, *Pharmacopsychiatry* 2006;**39**:205–8).

Gabapentin

In alcoholics with persistent insomnia, gabapentin may improve sleep slightly more than trazodone (n = 55, open, 6/52, Karam-Hage and Brower, *Psych Clin Neurosci* 2003; **57**:542–4).

Herbal and OTC preparations

An extensive review of oral, non-prescription treatments for insomnia, e.g. herbals and others (Meolie et al, *J Clin Sleep Med* 2005;**1**:173–87) included passionflower, valerian, Jamaican dogwood, hops, Californian poppy, chamomile, lemon balm, St John's wort, kava kava, wild lettuce, skullcap, Patrina root, first-generation histamine-1-receptor antagonists, alcohol, calcium, vitamin A, nicotinamide, magnesium, vitamin B12, tryptophan, 5-hydroxytryptophan, dietary changes, Natrum muriaticum and Yoku-kan-san-ka-chimpi-hange. It concluded that the studies were small, of inadequate design and lacked statistical analysis. There was insufficient data to recommend any, except preliminary but conflicting data on valerian and H1-antagonists. There are significant potential risks for Jamaican dogwood, kava kava, alcohol and tryptophan.

Nicotine

Low concentrations of nicotine can cause mild sedation and relaxation and so a cigarette could help sleep in an anxious person. Higher levels cause arousal and agitation.

Paroxetine

Paroxetine 20mg/d may be an effective treatment for primary insomnia (n = 15, open, Nowell et al, J Clin Psychiatry 1999;**60**:89–95), although this might be a placebo response (Musa, J Clin Psychiatry 1999;**60**:795), and it was ineffective for treating primary insomnia in old age (n = 27, RCT, d/b, p/c, 6/52, Reynolds et al, Am J Geriatr Psychiatry 2006;**14**:803–7).

Tiagabine

Although tiagabine 4–6mg was effective in helping insomnia in the elderly (n = 24, RCT, d/b, p/c, Walsh et al, Sleep 2005;**28**:673–6), a second failed to show any effect (n = 207, RCT, d/b, p/c, Roth et al, Sleep 2006;**29**:335–41).

☐ No efficacy

Caffeine

Caffeine competes with the inhibitory neuro-transmitter adenosine, causing cortical arousal and decreased sleep. 150mg before retiring has a marked effect on sleep latency, reduces sleep efficacy and REM periods. Its half-life of five hours means any ingested near bedtime will effect sleep latency. See caffeinism (1.30).

MANIA AND HYPOMANIA
see Bipolar – Mania and hypomania (1.10.2)

1.19 NARCOLEPSY

Symptoms

Narcolepsy is a rare and often misdiagnosed disabling neurological disorder of excessive daytime sleepiness, sleep paralysis, hypnagogic hallucinations, cataplexy (sudden loss of muscle tone provoked by strong emotions, e.g. laughter) and abnormalities in REM sleep. There is a strong genetic linkage, and normally starts in the 20s or 30s. The incidence ranges from 1 in 1000 to 10000. Narcolepsy is probably caused by the loss of a relatively few neurons responsible for producing the neuropeptide hypocretin. Other specific symptoms include catalepsy (an abrupt, bilateral loss of skeletal muscle tone), hypnagogic hallucinations (vivid dreams while falling asleep or waking), sleep paralysis and automatic behaviour (unconscious functioning while asleep).

Role of drugs

The use of stimulants or modafinil is considered first-line treatment, with some antidepressants useful in some resistant cases. The risks of pharmacotherapy are usually outweighed by the risks to the patient of driving, work-place and other mishaps. The role of oxybate is as yet unclear. However, there is no robust evidence that antidepressants are effective for narcolepsy or improve quality of life (s = 2, Vignatelli et al, Cochrane Database Syst Rev 2005; **3**:CD003724).

Reviews: * general (Didato and Nobili, Expert Rev Neurother 2009;**9**:897–910; Mohsenin, Postgrad Med 2009;**121**:99–104; Bhat and El Solh, Expert Opin Pharmacother 2008;**9**:1721–33; Billiard, Neuropsychiatr Dis Treat 2008;**4**:557–8), EFNS management guidelines (Billiard et al, Eur J Neurol 2006;**13**:1035–48), narcolepsy-cataplexy (Mignot and Nishino, Sleep 2005;**28**:754–63), diagnosis (Hohsenin, Postgrad Med 2009;**121**:99–104).

BNF listed

Dexamfetamine

Dexamfetamine acts by enhancing release of noradrenaline, dopamine and serotonin, but the stimulant effect appears to be mainly via dopamine. Dexamfetamine 5–50mg/d can be highly effective, although doses of 40–60mg/d have been shown to be more effective than lower doses. If tolerance develops, drug holidays may be necessary. Although dexamfetamine is not immune from problems of chronic stimulant ingestion, many can take it for decades without apparent adverse consequences.

Modafinil

Modafinil is licensed for symptomatic relief of excessive sleepiness associated with narcolepsy, sleep apnoea and moderate-to-severe chronic shift work sleep disorder. Its precise mechanism of action is unknown, but it may activate the hippocampus which receives afferents from the hypothalamus, the centre of the sleep–

wake rhythm, promoting wakefulness (n = 8, Kim *et al, Neurosci Lett* 2007;**422**:91–6). It significantly increases daytime sleep latency but does not suppress cataplexy. Modafinil offers advantages because of its lack of rebound phenomena after treatment withdrawal and its low abuse potential. Modafinil 600 mg/d appears the maximum tolerated dose (n = 32, RCT, Wong *et al, J Clin Pharmacol* 1999;**39**:30–40). Splitting the doses, e.g. 200 mg BD may help promote wakefulness throughout a day compared to once-daily (s = 2, n = 56, RCT, d/b, Schwartz *et al, J Neuropsychiatry Clin Neurosci* 2005;**17**:405–12), with no tolerance or withdrawal in a 40-week follow-on (n = 271, RCT, 9/52, Modafinil study group, *Neurology* 2000;**54**:1166–75). It may also be useful for improving daytime wakefulness in people unresponsive to stimulants (n = 150, open, 6/52, Schwartz *et al, Sleep Med* 2003;**4**:43–9). Studies directly comparing modafinil to amfetamines and methylphenidate, currently the preferred therapies for narcolepsy are still not yet available. It should be withdrawn if rash or symptoms such as suicidal ideation, hallucinations, delusion, aggression, psychosis or mania (UK SPC) appear.

Reviews: general (Myrick *et al, Ann Clin Psychiatry* 2004;**16**:101–9), mode of action (Ballon and Feifel, *J Clin Psychiatry* 2006;**67**:554–66), pharmacokinetics (Robertson and Hellriegel, *Clin Pharmacokinet* 2003;**42**:123–37).

Sodium oxybate *

Sodium oxybate is licensed for cataplexy in adults with narcolepsy. Oxybate probably promotes slow (delta) wave sleep consolidating night-time sleep, increasing stage 3 and 4 sleep, reducing the onset of REM sleep. Nocturnal administration of oxybate shows a dose-related improvement in sleep and functional status in people with narcolepsy (n = 285, RCT, d/b, p/c, 4/52, Weaver and Cuellar, *Sleep* 2006;**29**:1189–94). The starting dose is 4.5 g/d, titrated slowly every two weeks (or longer) up to 9 g/d as a BD dose (bedtime and 2.5–4 hours later, due to its short half-life). If oxybate is stopped for more than 14 days it should be retitrated, although withdrawal symptoms with therapeutic doses are minimal (n = 55, Anon, *J Toxicol Clin Toxicol* 2003;**41**:131–5). Doses of 4.5, 6 and 9 g at night produce decreases in cataplexy attacks of 57%, 65% and 85% respectively (n = 228, RCT, d/b, p/c, 8/52, Xyrem ISG, *Sleep Med* 2005;**6**:415–21), and a discontinuation study suggested a long-term efficacy (n = 55, d/b, mean 21/12, US Xyrem MSG, *Sleep Med* 2004;**5**:119–23; see also n = 136, RCT, d/b, p/c, 4/52, Anon, *Sleep* 2002;**25**:42–9). Oxybate 9 g/d and modafinil 200–600 mg/d were both effective for excessive daytime sleepiness and produced additive effects when used together (n = 270, RCT, d/b, p/c, 10/52, Black and Houghton, *Sleep* 2006;**29**:939–46). Because of its abuse potential (it is the sodium salt of gamma-hydroxybutyrate [GHB]), prescribing is limited to physicians experienced in the treatment of sleep disorders. GHB is abused for its euphoric and weight loss effects, and its amnesic effect has led to it being used as a date-rape drug (Camacho *et al, Am J Drug Alcohol Abuse* 2005;**31**:601–7; Gonzalez and Nutt, *J Psychopharmacol* 2005;**19**:195–204). When switching to oxybate, gradual withdrawal of antidepressants can lead to a short-term increase in cataplexy, especially with TCAs (n = 57, Ristanovic *et al, Sleep Med* 2009;**10**:416–21).

Reviews: * general (Owen, *Drugs Today (Barc)* 2008;**44**:197–204; Scharf, *Expert Rev Neurother* 2006;**6**:1139–46; Robinson and Keating, *CNS Drugs* 2007;**21**:337–54; Lemon *et al, Ann Pharmacother* 2006;**40**:433–40), mode of action (Sills, *Curr Opin Pharmacol* 2006; **6**: 108–13).

+ Combinations

Modafinil + tranylcypromine

There is a report of successful use of tranylcypromine and modafinil for refractory narcolepsy (n = 1, Clemons *et al, Sleep Med* 2004;**5**:509–11).

● Unlicensed/some efficacy

Methylphenidate

Methylphenidate 2.5–5 mg BD (up to 60 mg/d) can be used (see also dexamfetamine above). Tolerance can be a problem, with drug holidays helpful. It has been considered as good as dexamfetamine and may have a better side-effect profile (reviewed by Challman and Lipsky, *Mayo Clin Proc* 2000;**75**:711–21).

Selegiline
Two trials have shown a potent and dose-related effect, at doses of at least 20mg/d (e.g. n = 30, RCT, d/b, p/c, 4/52, Mayer *et al*, *Clin Neuropharmacol* 1995;**18**:306–19), and may be useful in patients who get disturbing side-effects with stimulants.

■ Unlicensed/possible efficacy

Donepezil
Donepezil 10mg/d has been successfully used to improve narcolepsy (n = 1, 3/12, Niederhofer, *J Clin Sleep Med* 2006;**2**:71–2).

SSRIs
These are generally considered less effective than tricyclics but some positive results have been reported with, e.g. fluoxetine (Langdon *et al*, *Sleep* 1986;**9**:371–2).

Tricyclics *
Clomipramine and imipramine have been used for cataplexy and sleep paralysis, particularly in stimulant-resistant or intolerant patients. Tricyclic ADRs can be considerable and rebound cataplexy can occur with abrupt withdrawal (n = 57, 7/52, Ristanovic *et al*, *Sleep Med* 2009;**10**:416–21).

Venlafaxine *
Venlafaxine has been used for narcolepsy with cataplexy at 37.5–112.5mg/d in children (n = 6, Møller and Østergaard, *J Child Adolesc Psychopharmacol* 2009;**19**:197–201).

◆ Others

Other drugs used include benzodiazepines such as **clonazepam** (1–4mg/d; Thompson *et al*, *Ann Neurol* 1982;**12**:62–3), **clonidine** 150–300mcg/d (Salin-Pascual *et al*, *J Clin Psychiatry* 1985;**46**:528–31), **codeine** (n = 8, RCT, Fry *et al*, *Sleep* 1986;**9**:269–74), **levodopa** (n = 6, Boivin and Montplaisir, *Neurology* 1991;**41**:1267–9), **MAOIs** (e.g. tranylcypromine; n = 1, Gernaat *et al*, *Pharmacopsychiatry* 1995;**28**:98–100), **pentazocine** (n = 1, *Lancet* 1981; i:92), and **pro-**

pranolol (n = 48, 18/12, Meier-Ewart *et al*, *Sleep* 1985;**8**:95–104).

1.20 OBSESSIVE-COMPULSIVE DISORDERS (OCD)

Symptoms
OCD probably has a lifetime prevalence of 2–3%, an early onset (childhood or adolescence), and frequently becomes chronic and disabling if untreated. It is characterised by recurrent and intrusive thoughts of compulsive, stereotyped, repetitive behaviour, e.g. recurrent checking, hand-washing, etc. Functioning is impaired by obsessive thoughts and rituals. Resisting these thoughts causes heightened anxiety.

Role of drugs *
There is much evidence for the cause of OCD being related to a dysfunctional serotonin system, and SSRIs and clomipramine have been shown to be effective. The available data (meta-analyses/reviews by Ackerman and Greenland, *J Clin Psychopharmacol* 2002;**22**:309–17; Hollander and Kahn, *EBMH* 2003;**6**:23; s = 9, n = 278, RCT, b/d, Bloch *et al*, *Mol Psychiatry* 2006: **11**:622–32) concludes that:

1. **Drug:** Only antidepressants affecting the serotonin system are effective:
   - the SSRIs as a class are similarly effective to clomipramine and both are superior to non-serotonergic drugs
   - clomipramine is perhaps slightly more effective than SSRIs
   - tricyclics (other than clomipramine) and mirtazapine seem ineffective
   - concomitant depression does not seem necessary for improvement in obsessive-compulsive symptoms.

2. **Dose:** The daily dose usually needs to be high, e.g. 250–300mg clomipramine, or 60–80mg fluoxetine or paroxetine. A meta-analysis has concluded that higher doses of SSRIs are less well tolerated but are clearly associated with improved efficacy (s = 9, n = 2268, RCT, d/b, p/c, Bloch *et al*, *Mol Psychiatry* 2010;[in press]).

3. **Duration:** Response is slow and may not occur for many weeks so continue with the maximum tolerated dose of an SSRI for **three months** (25% respond given adequate

dose and duration). A minimum of 1–2 years pharmacotherapy is recommended, as relapse is common on discontinuation and the risks of long-term therapy may be outweighed by the risks of relapse and its consequences.

4. **Treatment resistance:** Switching from an SSRI (paroxetine) to venlafaxine or vice versa if no response may be an effective strategy (n = 150, RCT, d/b, Denys et al, J Clin Psychiatry 2004;**65**:37–43; review by Bhui, EBMH 2004;**7**:114). Add an antipsychotic (best evidence is for risperidone and haloperidol), although only 30% will show a meaningful response.

5. **Discontinuation:** Very gradual discontinuation over several months is widely recommended.

In the UK, NICE has produced guidance on OCD and uses a stepped care approach. However, this did not emphasise the need to use higher doses for prolonged periods of time. Drugs may only reduce symptomatology by 30–60%, but many patients consider this a significant benefit. The effects of SSRIs may be enhanced by CBT (n = 48 [c = 43], O'Connor et al, Acta Psychiatr Scand 2006;**113**:408–19; 17 sessions, n = 108, RCT, Simpson et al, Am J Psychiatry 2008;**165**:621–30), especially if the CBT is added immediately after drug response (n = 96 [c = 59], RCT, s/b, 12/52, Tenneij et al, J Clin Psychiatry 2005;**66**:1169–75; comment by Cottraux, EBMH 2006;**9**:53).

Reviews: * general (Abramowitz et al, Lancet 2009;**374**:491–9; Fontenelle et al, Expert Opin Pharmacother 2007;**8**:563–83; Ravindran et al, Can J Psychiatry 2009;**54**:331–43), WCA guidelines (Greist et al, CNS Spectr 2003;[Suppl 1]:S7–S16), British Association of Psychopharmacology evidence-based guidelines (Baldwin et al, J Psychopharmacol 2005;**19**:567–96), antipsychotics in OCD (Fineberg et al, J Psychopharmacol 2006; **20**:97–103).

BNF listed

Clomipramine

Clomipramine is superior to placebo and non-serotonergic drugs (e.g. n = 122, RCT, d/b, p/c, 12/52, Foa et al, Am J Psychiatry 2005;**162**:151–61; see also review of meta-analyses in

introduction). IV clomipramine may be effective in patients intolerant or non-responsive to oral clomipramine (n = 54, RCT, Fallon et al, Arch Gen Psychiatry 1998;**55**:918–24).

Escitalopram

Escitalopram is licensed for the treatment of OCD at a dose of 10–20 mg/d. Escitalopram 10 mg/d was as effective as (and better tolerated than) paroxetine 40 mg/d, and escitalopram 20 mg/d was effective as early as six weeks (n = 466, RCT, d/b, p/c, 24/52, Stein et al, Curr Med Res Opin 2007;**23**:701–11). High-dose escitalopram (up to 50 mg/d, mean 34 mg/d) may be needed and is well tolerated and effective in resistant OCD (n = 67 [c = 64], open, 16/52, Rabinowitz et al, Int Clin Psychopharmacol 2008;**23**:49–53). Long-term efficacy has also been shown in an open 16-week study, followed by a discontinuation phase in the 320 responders, where escitalopram had a relapse rate of 23% compared to 52% in the placebo group (n = 468, RCT, d/b, 24/52, Fineberg et al, Eur Neuropsychopharmacol 2007;**17**:480–9).

Fluoxetine *

Fluoxetine has shown a significant clinical effect at 20–60 mg/d, developing over 13 weeks, and continuing to be effective for at least nine months with few side-effects (e.g. n = 130, RCT, p/c, 12/12, Romano et al, J Clin Psychopharmacol 2001;**21**:46–52) and may be more effective in washers and with obsessive thoughts rather than checkers (n = 265, Farnam et al, Arch Iran Med 2008;**11**:522–5).

Fluvoxamine

Fluvoxamine has been shown to be partially or very effective in several trials and it may be equivalent to clomipramine but better tolerated (n = 227, RCT, d/b, 10/52, Mundo et al, Hum Psychopharmacol 2001;**16**:461–8).

Paroxetine *

Paroxetine is licensed for the symptoms of OCD and for relapse prevention at doses of 40–60 mg (reviews by Owen, Drugs Today (Barc) 2008;**44**:887–93 and Kamijima and Aoki, Expert Rev Neurother 2006;**6**:945–56). Higher doses are necessary, particularly in acute OCD, as 20 mg/d is not effective (n = 348, RCT, d/b, p/c, 12/52, Hollander *et al*, *J Clin Psychiatry* 2003;**64**:1113–21).

Sertraline

Sertraline is licensed for OCD in adults and also in children and adolescents (dose: 6–12 years, 25–50 mg/d; for 13–17 years, use the adult dose but with no dose increases after less than a week, and a lower body weight may require lower doses). Sertraline has been shown to be effective in many studies, e.g. slightly more effective than fluoxetine but as well tolerated (n = 150, RCT, d/b, 6/12, Bergeron *et al*, *J Clin Psychopharmacol* 2002;**22**:148–54). Rapid titration to 150 mg/d over five days may give a faster onset of action in acute OCD, with similar tolerability to slower (15 days) titration (n = 32, s/b, 12/52, Bogetto *et al*, *Eur Neuropsychopharm* 2002;**12**:181–6). Relapse prevention has been shown, with lack of prominent discontinuation symptoms (n = 649[c=223], RCT, 6/12, Koran *et al*, *Am J Psychiatry* 2002;**159**:88–95; review by Soomro, *EBMH* 2002;**5**:115). High-dose sertraline (up to 400 mg/d) may be effective in refractory OCD (n = 66, RCT, d/b, 12/52, Ninan *et al*, *J Clin Psychiatry* 2006;**67**:15–22).

+ Combinations of SSRIs/clomipramine

Review: combination and augmentation therapies (Walsh and McDougle, *Expert Opin Pharmacother* 2004;**5**:2059–67).

Antipsychotics + SSRIs/clomipramine *

A meta-analysis of RCTs supports the use of antipsychotics as an augmentation strategy (s = 10,n = 305,RCT,Skapinakis *et al*,*Eur Neuropsychopharmacol* 2007;**17**:79–93), supporting a previous systematic review and meta-analysis,which concluded that risperidone and haloperidol (but not olanzapine) significantly improve response in at least a third of people who have tried (but not responded to) an SSRI monotherapy at full dose for at least 12 weeks (but have no effect if given earlier than 12/52), particularly in people with comorbid tic disorder (s = 9, n = 278, < 16/52, RCT, Bloch *et al*, *Mol Psychiatry* 2006;**11**:622–32; comment by Dell'Osso, *EBMH* 2007;**10**:24). If successful, they should probably continue

for at least several months, as relapse on discontinuation is high. **Risperidone** has been shown to be effective as SSRI augmentation at 3 mg/d (e.g. n = 70, RCT, 12/52, McDougle *et al*, *Arch Gen Psychiatry* 2000;**57**:794–801; comment by Ramasubbu, *Arch Gen Psychiatry* 2002;**59**:472–3) and even at really low-dose, adjunctive risperidone (0.5 mg/d) may be effective (n = 45, RCT, d/b, p/c, 6/52, Erzeovesi *et al*, *Eur Neuropsychopharmacol* 2005;**15**:69–74). Smaller studies have suggested some efficacy for **olanzapine** 5 mg/d in SSRI-resistant OCD (n = 26, open, two years, Marazziti *et al*, *J Psychopharmacol* 2005;**19**:392–4), but the only RCT showed no additional advantage of adding olanzapine in fluoxetine-refractory OCD patients (n = 44, RCT, p/c, 6/52, Shapira *et al*, *Biol Psychiatry* 2004;**55**:553–5). A small pilot study suggested **aripiprazole** may have some efficacy as SSRI augmentation (n = 8, open, 8/52, Connor *et al*, *J Clin Psychiatry* 2005;**66**:49–51; n = 1, 16/52, Friedman *et al*, *J Clin Psychiatry* 2007;**68**:972–3). A meta-analysis showed **quetiapine** up to 400 mg/d had some efficacy as an adjunct to SSRIs in resistant OCD (s = 3, n = 102, RCT, d/b, p/c, Fineberg *et al*, *Int Clin Psychopharmacol* 2006; **21**:337–43). More recently, when used in non-refractory OCD, quetiapine 300–450 mg/d augmentation of citalopram 60 mg/d from the start significantly enhanced the number of responses (n = 76 [c = 66], RCT, d/b, p/c, 10/52, Vulink *et al*, *J Clin Psychiatry* 2009;**70**:1001–8), although quetiapine 400–600 mg/d was ineffective as an adjunct to an SSRI in resistant OCD (n = 40, RCT, d/b, p/c, 12/52, Kordon *et al*, *J Clin Psychopharmacol* 2008;**28**:550–4).

Buspirone + SSRIs

There are case reports with, e.g. **sertraline** (e.g. n = 2, Menkes, *Br J Psychiatry* 1995;**167**:823–4) and **fluoxetine** (Alessi and Bos, *Am J Psychiatry* 1991;**148**:1605) but not **fluvoxamine** (n = 33, RCT, p/c, McDougle, *Am J Psychiatry* 1993;**150**:647–9; 819–21).

Carbamazepine + clomipramine

Carbamazepine has been used as augmentation in refractory OCD (n = 1, Iwata *et al*, *J Clin Psychiatry* 2000;**161**:528–9).

Clomipramine + SSRIs *

Citalopram plus clomipramine was markedly more effective than clomipramine in treatment-resistant OCD (n = 16, open, 3/12, Pallanti et al, Eur Psychiatry 1999;**14**:101–6) and around 50% people taking clomipramine (after failing at least two SSRIs previously) responded after addition of citalopram up to 60mg/d (n = 20, 11/12, Marazziti et al, CNS Spectr 2008;**13**:971–6).

Dexamfetamine and caffeine + SSRIs *

In partial response to SNRIs or SSRIs, augmentation with d-amphetamine (30mg/d) and caffeine (300mg/d) were equally effective in improving residual symptoms, although this book's author would think there are quite a few people who have 300mg/d caffeine without an augmentation strategy (n = 24, RCT, d/b, 5/52, Koran et al, J Clin Psychiatry 2009;70:1530-5).

Gabapentin + SSRIs

Gabapentin up to 3600mg/d has been used in patients only partially responsive to fluoxetine 30–100mg/d (n = 5, open, 6/52, Cora-Locatelli et al, J Clin Psychiatry 1998;**59**:480–1).

Inositol + SSRIs

Inositol 18g/d may significantly reduce Y-BOCS rating scale scores (n = 13, d/b, c/o, 6/52, Fux et al, Am J Psychiatry 1996;**153**:1219–21; n = 10, open, Seedat and Stein, Int Clin Psychopharmacol 1999;**14**:353–6), but the only RCT has shown no effect on symptoms (n = 10, RCT, d/b, p/c, c/o, 6/52, Fux et al, Int J Neuropsychopharmacol 1999;**2**:193–5).

Lithium + SSRIs

Lithium augmentation of fluvoxamine in OCD appears ineffective (n = 30, d/b, p/c, McDougle et al, J Clin Psychopharmacol 1991;**11**:175–84).

Memantine + SSRIs/clomipramine *

Memantine 20mg/d has been used as augmentation to SSRI-non-responsive OCD, producing a meaningful improvement in 43% completers (n = 15 [c = 14], 12/52, Aboujaoude et al, J Clin Psychopharmacol 2009;**29**:51–5) and 20mg/d produced a response over 3/52 as an adjunct to clomipramine 300mg/d and sulpiride 400mg/d, maintained over 3/12 (n = 1, Poyurovsky et al, Am J Psychiatry 2005;

162:2191–2; see also n = 2, Pasquini and Biondi, Prog Neuropsychopharmacol Biol Psychiatry 2006;**30**:1173–5).

Mirtazapine + citalopram

Mirtazapine 15–30mg/d may speed the response to citalopram by four weeks, but with similar response rates from week 8, which could be significant in severe OCD, although a robust study would be needed to confirm this (n = 49, s/b, 12/52, Pallanti et al, J Clin Psychiatry 2004;**65**:1394–9; comment by Schüle and Laakmann, EBMH 2005;**8**:42). In mirtazapine-responders, discontinuation led to relapse suggesting a prophylactic effect (n = 30, d/b, p/c, 8/52, Koran et al, J Clin Psychiatry 2005;**66**:515–20).

Naltrexone + SSRIs/clomipramine

Naltrexone augmentation in SSRI-resistant OCD was ineffective (n = 10, RCT, d/b, p/c, c/o, 5/52, Amiaz et al, Eur Neuropsychopharmacol 2008;**18**:455–61).

Pindolol + SSRIs

Pindolol 7.5mg/d may possibly improve the response to paroxetine in multiple SSRI-resistant OCD (n = 14, d/b, p/c, 6/52, Dannon et al, Eur Neuropsychopharmacol 2000;**10**:165–9).

Pregabalin + SSRI *

There is a case of pregabalin 600mg/d used as a successful adjunct to a sertraline-risperidone combination (n = 1, Oulis et al, Prim Care Companion J Clin Psychiatry 2008;**10**:249).

Riluzole + SSRIs

Riluzole 100mg/d appeared to have some activity as an adjunct in a treatment-resistant OCD (n = 13, open, Coric et al, Biol Psychiatry 2005;**58**:424–8).

Topiramate + SSRIs *

Topiramate (mean 250mg/d) may be useful as an adjunct to SSRIs in resistant OCD (n = 16, < 13/52, Van Ameringen et al, Depress Anxiety 2006;**23**:1–5; n = 1, Vinkers et al, Tijdschr Psychiatr 2008;**50**:747–50).

Tricyclics + clomipramine

Addition of nortriptyline 50mg/d to clomipramine 150mg/d produced a more rapid onset of action than clomipramine alone (n = 30, d/b, p/c, RCT, Noorbala et al, J Clin Pharm Ther 1998;**23**:155–9).

• Unlicensed/some efficacy

Citalopram
Citalopram has been shown to be as effective as fluvoxamine and paroxetine and predictors of response include longer duration of more severe illness, no previous SSRI and an adequate dose for adequate duration (RCT, Stein et al, Int Clin Psychopharmacol 2001;**16**:357–61). Very high dose citalopram (160mg/d) may be effective in severe, resistant OCD (n = 1, Bejerot and Bodlund, Acta Psychiatr Scand 1998; **98**:423–4).

Venlafaxine
Venlafaxine has been shown to be as effective as paroxetine but not superior (n = 150, RCT, d/b, Denys et al, J Clin Psychopharmacol 2003; **23**:568–75). In one trial, venlafaxine (n = 26; 225–350mg/d) was almost as effective as clomipramine (n = 47; 150–225mg/d) but better tolerated (n = 73, RCT, s/b, 12/52, Albert et al, J Clin Psychiatry 2002;**63**:1004–9).
Reviews: SNRIs in OCD (Phelps and Cates, Ann Pharmacother 2005;**39**:136–40; Dell'Osso et al, J Clin Psychiatry 2006;**67**:600–10).

■ Unlicensed/possible efficacy

Cycloserine
Cycloserine 100mg given before behavioural therapy improves OCD and depressive symptoms (n = 23, RCT, d/b, p/c, 5/52, Wilhelm et al, Am J Psychiatry 2008;**165**:335–41), and when used before exposure therapy (d/b, p/c, Kushner et al, Biol Psychiatry 2007;**62**:835–8).

Glycine *
Glycine 60g/d appears poorly tolerated but may work well in some people, with some significant sustained responses in a pilot study (n = 24[c = 14], RCT, d/b, p/c, 12/52, Greenberg et al, J Psychiatr Res 2009;**43**:664–70).

Mirtazapine *
Mirtazapine 60mg/d showed advantage over

placebo (n = 30[c = 26], open, 12/52 followed by d/b, p/c discontinuation, 8/52, Koran et al, J Clin Psychiatry 2005;**66**:515–20).

Morphine
Rather bizarrely, once-weekly oral morphine was effective in some treatment-resistant OCD patients, unlike lorazepam or placebo (n = 23, RCT, d/b, c/o, p/c, 6/52, Koran et al, J Clin Psychiatry 2005;**66**:353–9).

Nicotine
Nicotine chewing gum 4mg has improved treatment-resistant OCD (n = 1, Pasquini et al, Prog Neuropsychopharmacol Biol Psychiatry 2005;**29**:157–9).

Ondansetron
Ondansetron 3mg/d was effective in some OCD patients (n = 8[c = 6], open, 8/52, Hewlett et al, J Clin Psychiatry 2003;**64**:1025–30).

Oxcarbazepine
There is a case of successful use of oxcarbazepine for OCD (n = 1, McMeekin, J S C Med Assoc 2002;**98**:316–20).

Paliperidone *
Paliperidone has been used successfully in resistant OCD (n = 1, Angelucci et al, Prog Neuropsychopharmacol Biol Psychiatry 2009; **33**:1277–8).

Phenelzine
Phenelzine 60mg/d was shown to be inferior to fluoxetine (80mg/d) except in patients with asymmetry/other atypical obsession, and no preferential response was detected in patients with high anxiety levels (n = 60, RCT, Jenike et al, Am J Psychiatry 1997;**154**:1261–4).

Psilocybin
Psilocybin reduced acute OCD symptoms in some patients in a carefully controlled situation (n = 9, Moreno et al, J Clin Psychiatry 2006; **67**:1735–40).

Tramadol
There is a report of rapid reduction in OCD symptoms with 100mg/d tramadol, allowing fluoxetine to be introduced as the long-

term treatment (n=1, Goldsmith *et al*, *Am J Psychiatry* 1999;**156**:660–1).

◆ Others

Other drugs tried include **diphenhydramine** up to 250mg/d (n=28, d/b, c/o, 6/52, Hewlett *et al*, *J Clin Psychopharmacol* 1992;**12**:420–30).

□ No efficacy

Bupropion *
Bupropion had no significant effect in OCD (n=12, open, 8/52, Vulink *et al*, *J Clin Psychiatry* 2005;**66**:228–30).

Clonazepam
Clonazepam seems ineffective as monotherapy in treating OCD, although it may be helpful for specific sub-groups with comorbid anxiety (n=27, d/b, p/c, 10/52, Hollander *et al*, *World J Biol Psychiatry* 2003;**4**:30–4) and as augmentation of sertraline (n=37, RCT, d/b, p/c, 12/52, Crockett *et al*, *Ann Clin Psychiatry* 2004;**16**:127–32).

Clozapine
Clozapine has been used for OCD symptoms in schizophrenia (n=15, open, Reznik *et al*, *Pharmacopsychiatry* 2004;**37**:52–6), but has been shown to be ineffective (n=10, McDougle *et al*, *Am J Psychiatry* 1995;**152**:1812–4) or even detrimental (eg. Baker *et al*, *J Clin Psychiatry* 1992;**53**:439–42).

Flutamide
The anti-androgen flutamide was ineffective in one trial (n=8, Altemus *et al*, *J Clin Psychiatry* 1999;**60**:442–5).

Naltrexone *
Naltrexone appears to have no beneficial effect (n=10, RCT, d/b, p/c, c/o, 2/12, Amiaz *et al*, *Eur Neuropsychopharmacol* 2008;**18**:455–61).

Oxytocin
Initial enthusiasm was not confirmed in a study of intranasal administration (n=3, Salzberg and Swedo, *Am J Psychiatry* 1992;**149**:713–4).

Trazodone
A study showed trazodone up to 300mg/d to be equipotent with placebo (n=21, d/b, c/o, 10/52, Pigott *et al*, *J Clin Psychopharmacol* 1992;**12**:156–62).

Tricyclics (except clomipramine)
Imipramine (Volavka *et al*, *Psychiatry Res* 1985;**14**:85–93), amitriptyline and nortriptyline have been shown to be ineffective.

1.20.1 BODY DYSMORPHIC DISORDER (BDD)

Symptoms *
Body dysmorphic disorder (BDD) is characterised by a disabling preoccupation with an imagined or minor defect in appearance (especially skin, hair and nose), with time-consuming behaviours such as mirror gazing, excessive camouflaging and need for reassurance. The adult incidence is thought to be around 0.5–1% (Bohne *et al*, *Psychosomatics* 2002;**43**:486–90), although it may be as high as 2.4% (Koran *et al*, *CNS Spectr* 2008;**13**:316–22). It has a fluctuating or episodic course, often lifelong, with a higher risk/comorbidity in people with depression, social phobia, SUDs, OCD and eating disorders. There is a high risk of suicide (around a quarter may have attempted suicide sometime during their life, 2.6% per year and 0.3% succeed, Phillips and Menard, *Am J Psychiatry* 2006;**163**:1280–2), which is 45 times higher than the general population and 2–3 times more than depression and bipolar.

Role of drugs *
There are few trials or RCTs in BDD. NICE says use either an SSRI or more intensive targeted CBT for moderate BDD. The onset of action of SSRIs (as in OCD) may be delayed for up to 12/52. The best evidence is available for fluoxetine; clomipramine monotherapy is a second line; with buspirone as an adjunct in resistant cases. Treatment duration should be 12 months if effective to prevent relapse and allow further improvement. TCAs (other than clomipramine), SNRIs, MAOIs, anxiolytics (except short-term) or antipsychotic monotherapy are not recommended. Cochrane concludes that SSRIs/clomipramine are superior

to placebo and to desipramine (s = 2, n = 96) and CBT may be effective (s = 3, n = 83), mostly in women (s = 5, n = 179, Ipser et al, *Cochrane Syst Database Rev* 2009; **1**:CD005332).

Reviews: * pharmacological therapies (Phillips, *CNS Spectr* 2002;**7**:453–60), general (Phillips et al, *Am J Psychiatry* 2008;**165**:1111–8; Fiori and Giannetti, *Neuropsychiatr Dis Treat* 2009;**5**:477–81), relationship to eating disorders (Phillips and Kaye, *CNS Spectr* 2007;**12**:347–58) and OC spectrum (Ravindran et al, *Can J Psychiatry* 2009; **54**:331–43).

● Unlicensed/some efficacy

Buspirone *
A small open study showed a 46% response with buspirone as augmentation of SSRIs (n = 13, open, Phillips, *Psychopharmacol Bull* 1996;**32**:175–80).

Bupropion *
There are some cases reports of response (Nardi et al, *Aust N Z J Psychiatry* 2005;**39**:112).

Citalopram *
An open study showed a 73% response rate in BDD (n = 15, open, 12/52, Phillips and Najjar, *J Clin Psychiatry* 2003;**64**:715–20).

Clomipramine *
Clomipramine was clearly superior to desipramine in BDD even if delusions were prominent (n = 29, RCT, d/b, c/o, 16/52, Hollander et al, *Arch Gen Psychiatry* 1999;**56**:1033–9).

Escitalopram *
A small study showed some well-tolerated efficacy (47% were much improved) in BDD (n = 15[c = 11], open, Phillips, *Int Clin Psychopharmacol* 2006;**21**:177–9).

Fluoxetine *
A 53% response rate (cf 18% with placebo) has been seen (NNT = 2.7, n = 67, RCT, d/b, p/c, 12/52, Phillips et al, *Arch Gen Psychiatry* 2002;**59**:381–8). There is no evidence that fluoxetine increases suicidality in BDD and, in fact, appears to have a protective effect (n = 67, RCT, d/b, p/c, 12/52, Phillips and Kelly, *Int Clin Psychopharmacol* 2009;**24**:26–8).

Fluvoxamine *
In an open study, fluvoxamine had a 63% response rate using BDD-YBOCS (n = 30, open, 16/52, Phillips et al, *J Clin Psychiatry* 2001; **62**:87–91; n = 1, Khan and Decker, *J Child Adoles Psychopharmacol* 2001;**11**:105–7).

Review: Irons, *Neuropsychiatr Dis Treat* 2005; **1**:289–99.

Levetiracetam *
A pilot study suggested that levetiracetam (mean 2000 mg/d) can improve many measures of BDD (n = 17, open, 12/52, Phillips and Menard, *CNS Spectr* 2009;**14**:252–60).

Olanzapine *
Olanzapine (up to 15 mg/d) augmentation of fluoxetine was effective in 33%, but 67% remained unchanged (n = 6, d/b, p/c, 8/52, Phillips, *Am J Psychiatry* 2005;**162**:1022–3). It has been used to augment paroxetine (n = 1, Nakaaki et al, *Psychiatry Clin Neurosci* 2008; **62**:370) and as monotherapy (n = 1, Grant, *J Clin Psychiatry* 2001;**62**:297–8).

Venlafaxine *
Venlafaxine (minimum 150 mg/d) may improve global severity and specific symptoms (n = 17 [c = 11], open, 12–16/52, Allen et al, *CNS Spectr* 2008;**13**:138–44).

□ No efficacy

Desipramine *
Desipramine was not considered effective in a comparison with clomipramine (n = 29, RCT, d/b, c/o, 16/52, Hollander et al, *Arch Gen Psychiatry* 1999;**56**:1033–9).

Pimozide *
Pimozide was ineffective as an adjunct to fluoxetine (n = 28, d/b, p/c, 8/52, Phillips, *Am J Psychiatry* 2005;**162**:377–9).

1.21 PANIC DISORDER
see also Anxiety disorder (1.6)

Symptoms
Panic disorder is usually characterised by sudden attacks of anxiety, where physical symptoms predominate, peaking within 10 minutes and with

an associated fear of serious consequences, e.g. heart attack. These attacks need to include four of the following: palpitations, abdominal distress/nausea, numbness/tingling, inability to breathe or shortness of breath, choking, sweating, chest pains, dizziness, depersonalisation (common), flushes/chills, fear of dying and trembling/shaking. The lifetime prevalence of panic disorder is about 5% in the USA (Grant et al, J Clin Psychiatry 2006;**67**:363–74; comment by Bienvenu, EBMH 2006;**9**:114), with a point prevalence of 1.5% (males) and 2.8% (females). There is frequently a family history and it can be a presenting feature of depression.

Role of drugs *

In general, short-term benefits may be gained with drug therapy. The main principle is to start low and go slow (to minimise initial jitteriness), and accept that response may take some time to occur, e.g. SSRIs are effective long-term with a slow onset of action, initial worsening (meta-analysis, 34 RCTs, nine open, n = 2367; Bakker et al, Acta Psychiatr Scand 2002;**106**:163–7; although efficacy may have been overestimated: s = 12, Otto et al, Am J Psychiatry 2001;**158**:1989–92) and some exacerbation may occur on discontinuation. After a standard dose SSRI for 6/52, there is little evidence for the efficacy of increasing the dose (n = 39, Simon et al, J Clin Psychiatry 2009;**70**:1563–70). Benzodiazepines have a quicker onset of action but obvious potential problems, e.g. the dependence potential and tolerance, and NICE concludes that they have a poor long-term outcome. Placebo responders tend to show an early and temporary remission. Combining CBT and antidepressants increases the response compared to either therapy alone (meta-analysis, s = 21, n = 1709, RCTs, Furukawa et al, Br J Psychiatry 2006;**188**:305–12; comment by Mitte, EBMH 2006;**9**:98; CBT vs imipramine, a poorly-tolerated and less serotonergic agent; n = 326, RCT,12/12, Barlow et al, JAMA 2000; **283**:2529–36). Relapse rates at 6–12 months can be as high as 75% on discontinuation of psychotropics, and so continued treatment and support is necessary in most patients over at least a year (Scott et al, Adv Psychiatr Treat 2001;**7**:275–82). CBT has an unproven role, e.g. CBT plus SSRI was superior to SSRI monotherapy, in turn superior to CBT alone for panic disorder (n = 150, 9/12, van Apeldoorn

et al, Acta Psychiatr Scand 2008;**117**:260–70). Adding a CBT package to SSRIs seems of little additional benefit, with SSRIs more effective than CBT alone (n = 150, 9/12, van Apeldoorn et al, Acta Psychiatr Scand 2008;**117**:260–70). Cochrane concludes that there is no evidence for psychotherapy as an adjunct for BDZs in panic (s = 3, n = 243, Watanabe et al, Cochrane Database Syst Rev 2009;**2**:CD005335).

Reviews: diagnosis (Perugi et al, CNS Drugs 2007;**21**:741–64), general (Katon, N Engl J Med 2006;**354**:2360–7; Taylor, BMJ 2006;**332**:951–5; Roy-Byrne et al, Lancet 2006;**368**:1023–32; Kumar and Oakley-Browne, Clin Evid 2006;**15**:1438–52; Katon, N Engl J Med 2006;**354**:2360–7), BAP evidence-based guidelines (Baldwin et al, J Psychopharmacol 2005;**19**:567–96); refractory panic (Bandelow and Ruther, CNS Spectr 2004, **9**:725–39), epidemiology (Batelaan et al, Tijdschr Psychiatr 2006;**48**:195–205).

BNF listed

Benzodiazepines

Benzodiazepines are rapidly effective and useful in people needing immediate relief (review by Kasper and Resinger, Eur Neuropsychopharmacol 2001;**11**:307–21). Many benzodiazepines have been studied, e.g. **clonazepam** is longer-acting, with 1–2mg/d the best balance between benefit and tolerability (n = 413, RCT, p/c, 13/52, Rosenbaum et al, J Clin Psychopharmacol 1997;**17**:390–400) and it may have a sustained effect (n = 67, three years, open, Nardi et al, Psychiatry Res 2005;**137**:61–70). Early co-administration of clonazepam with sertraline may facilitate early improvement in panic symptoms (n = 50, RCT, d/b, Goddard et al, Arch Gen Psychiatry 2001;**58**:681–86). The main problem is discontinuation, where relapse may be more common with shorter-acting benzodiazepines so transferring to an SSRI is advisable.

Citalopram

Citalopram is licensed in the UK for panic disorder, with or without agoraphobia. The starting dose in panic disorder is 10mg/d for one week, increasing to 20–30mg/d as the optimum dose to a maximum of 60mg/d and 20–60mg/d appears to be effective and well tolerated over one year (n = 279, RCT, d/b, 8/52,

Lepola et al, J Clin Psychiatry 1998;**59**:528–34). Citalopram may also control phobic symptoms in panic, especially at 20–30mg/d (n = 475, RCT, 8/52, Leinonen et al, J Psychiatry Neurosci 2000;**25**:25–32). It may be quicker acting than paroxetine, but equipotent (n = 58, RCT, s/b, 60/7, Perna et al, Pharmacopsychiatry 2001; **34**:85–90). Escitalopram and citalopram appear equally effective in panic disorder (n = 366, RCT, d/b, p/c, 10/52, Stahl et al, J Clin Psychiatry 2003;**64**:1322–7, MS).

Escitalopram

Escitalopram is licensed in the UK for panic disorder, with or without agoraphobia. The initial dose is 5mg/d for the first week, then 10mg/d, increasing to a maximum of 20mg/d. Escitalopram and citalopram appear equally effective in panic disorder (n = 366, RCT, d/b, p/c, 10/52, Stahl et al, J Clin Psychiatry 2003;**64**: 1322–7, MS).

Paroxetine

Paroxetine is licensed for panic and agoraphobia. A 10mg/d starting dose is recommended. Several studies have shown a significant effect, e.g. as effective as citalopram (n = 58, RCT, s/b, 60/7, Perna et al, Pharmacopsychiatry 2001;**34**:85–90) and as effective as clomipramine, but with a more rapid onset of action and less side-effects (e.g. n = 367, d/b, p/c, 12/52, Lecrubier et al, Acta Psychiatr Scand 1997;**95**:145–52). The optimum effective dose is 40mg/d (n = 278, d/b, p/c, Ballenger et al, Am J Psychiatry 1998;**155**:36–42). After 12 months treatment, a further year of paroxetine did not reduce relapse rates compared to discontinuation in panic disorder (with or without agoraphobia) (n = 143, open, three years, Dannon et al, BMC Psychiatry 2004;**11**:16). Combining with CBT is significantly more effective than placebo plus CBT (n = 120, RCT, p/c, 12/52, Oehrberg et al, Br J Psychiatry 1995;**167**:374–9).

Tricyclics

Tricyclics are effective in panic disorder. They may take four weeks to start to work and 12 weeks for maximal effect. Initial jitteriness is a common problem and so it is usually necessary to start at a low dose (10–25mg/d). **Clomipramine** is as effective as paroxetine in panic disorder,

but with a slower onset of action and more side-effects (n = 176, RCT, Lecrubier et al, Acta Psychiatr Scand 1997;**95**:153–60), and may have a biphasic response, symptoms worsening over 12 weeks before improving. **Imipramine** is effective (vs placebo) in all studies using doses above 150mg/d and with a substantial prophylactic efficacy (n = 18, RCT, Mavissakalian and Perel, Ann Clin Psychiatry 2001;**13**:63–7). A modest dose of **trimipramine** 50mg/d proved effective in multi-drug resistant panic disorder (n = 1, Cerra, Am J Psychiatry 2006;**163**:548). Long-term maintenance is needed for most patients, especially with a high baseline BDI and who need higher doses to reach remission (n = 51, RCT, Lotufo-Neto et al, J Clin Psychopharmacol 2001;**15**:13–7). Weight gain is a specific and significant adverse effect, as are dry mouth, sweating and increased heart rate, and sexual dysfunction (n = 51, RCT, p/c, d/b, 12/12, Mavissakalian et al, J Clin Psychopharmacol 2002;**22**:155–61). Early detection of relapse may be a viable alternative to long-term therapy (n = 51, RCT, d/b, 12/12, Mavissakalian and Perel, J Clin Psychopharmacol 2002;**22**:294–9).

+ Combinations

Clonazepam + SSRI

Use of clonazepam, slowly tapered after four weeks, as an initial adjunct to paroxetine was as affective as continued clonazepam, facilitating longer-term monotherapy (n = 60, RCT, p/c, 12/52, Pollack et al, J Psychopharmacol 2003;**17**:276–82).

Olanzapine + SSRI

There is a case of complete remission when olanzapine was added to paroxetine (n = 1, Chao, Pharmacopsychiatry 2004; **37**:239–40).

● Unlicensed/some efficacy

Fluoxetine

Fluoxetine is effective when initial doses are kept very low (2.5–5 mg/d) then increased, as higher doses produce side-effects such as anxiety and over-stimulation, possibly due to serotonergic supersensitivity. Fluoxetine 20mg/d is clearly superior to placebo over a range of symptoms in panic disorder (n=165[c=145], RCT, p/c, 24/52, Michelson et al, Br J Psychiatry 1999;**174**:213–8).If there is no response by 6/52, it may benefit from an increase up to 60mg/d (n=180[c=153],12/52, RCT, Michelson et al, Br J Psychiatry 2001;**179**:514–8).

Fluvoxamine
Fluvoxamine has been compared favourably with placebo and cognitive therapy (n=55, RCT, p/c, 8/52, Black et al, Arch Gen Psychiatry 1993;**50**:44–50), but not all placebo trials have shown efficacy.

Gabapentin
Gabapentin 600–3600mg/d may have anxiolytic effects in severe panic disorder (n=103, RCT, d/b, p/c, 8/52, Pande et al, J Clin Psychopharmacol 2000;**20**:467–71).

Sertraline *
Pooled data indicates that sertraline is an effective treatment for panic disorder, even in people with risk factors for poor response (s=4, n=664, d/b, Pollack et al, J Clin Psychiatry 2000;**61**:922–7) and prevents relapse (n=240, RCT, d/b, p/c, 8/52, Kamijima et al, Int Clin Psychopharmacol 2005;**20**:265–73). Early response predicts final remission, a useful aid to decision-making (n=544, p/c, Pollack et al, J Psychiatr Res 2002;**36**:229–36). Sertraline 50–150mg/d is equivalent in efficacy to paroxetine (40–60mg/d) but better tolerated and easier to stop (n=225, RCT, d/b, 12/52, Bandelow et al, J Clin Psychiatry 2004;**65**:405–13; MS).
Review: * Hobgood and Clayton, Drugs Today (Barc) 2009;**45**:351–61.

■ **Unlicensed/possible efficacy**

Aripiprazole *
A pilot study suggested aripiprazole may be useful as an adjunct in resistant panic disorder (n=10, open, 8/52, Hoge et al, CNS Spectr 2008;**13**:522–7). Adjunctive aripiprazole has been used successfully (n=1, Harada et al, J Clin Psychopharmacol 2009;**29**:301–2).

Bupropion *
There is a single case of panic improving markedly when bupropion was used for

MDD in a patient with comorbid Parkinson's Disease (n=1, Gebhardt et al, J Clin Pharm Ther 2008;**33**:575–7).

Cicloserin (D-cycloserine) *
D-cycloserine may have a role in enhancing the response to CBT for panic (n=31, RCT, d/b, p/c, Otto et al, Biol Psychiatry 2010;**67**:365–70).

Duloxetine *
A pilot study suggests duloxetine 60–120mg/d may have some efficacy in panic disorder (n=15, open, 6/52, Simon et al, CNS Neurosci Ther 2009;**15**:19–23).

Inositol
In one trial, inositol 12g/d improved panic symptoms, whereas lorazepam did not (n=25, d/b, p/c, c/o, 4/52, Benjamin et al, Am J Psychiatry 1995;**152**:1084–6) and was superior to fluvoxamine 150mg/d (n=20, RCT, c/o, 8/52, Palatnik et al, J Clin Psychopharmacol 2001;**21**:335–9).

Levetiracetam
Levetiracetam was effective in 84% completers in a pilot study (n=18[c=13], open, 12/52, Papp, J Clin Psychiatry 2006;**67**:1573–6).

MAOIs
Phenelzine at 45–90mg/d may be effective, e.g. in multi-drug-resistant severe panic attacks (n=1, Buch and Wagner, J Clin Psychiatry 2007; **68**:335–6) and in atypical depression with panic attacks. MAOIs have fallen out of use but may be useful in resistant cases.

Mirtazapine
Mirtazapine may be a rapidly effective alternative to SSRIs (n=28, RCT, open, 12/52, Boshuisen et al, Int Clin Psychopharmacol 2001;**16**:363–8; n=45, open, 3/12, Sarchiapone et al, Int Clin Psychopharmacol 2003;**8**:35–8). Mirtazapine was similar in efficacy and tolerability to fluoxetine in another trial (n=27, RCT, 8/52, Ribeiro et al, Braz J Med Biol Res 2001;**34**:1303–7).

Moclobemide
Moclobemide was ineffective as monotherapy (n=55, RCT, 8/52, Loerch et al, Br J Psychiatry

1999;**174**:205–12), but comparisons with clomipramine (n = 135, RCT, 8/52, Kruger and Dahl, *Eur Arch Psych Clin Neurosci* 1999; **249**[Suppl 1]:S7–S10) and fluoxetine (RCT, d/b, 8/52, Tiller *et al*, *Eur Arch Psych Clin Neurosci* 1999;**249**[Suppl 1]:S19–S24) show similar efficacy, although the comparator drugs may have been at sub-therapeutic doses.

Olanzapine

Olanzapine (mean 12.3 mg/d) was remarkably effective in reducing refractory panic attacks, with 50% even being panic-free at the trial end (n = 10, open, 8/52, Hollifield *et al*, *Depress Anx* 2005;**21**:33–40).

Pramipexole

Successful augmentation of SSRIs with pramipexole up to 1.5 mg/d has been reported (n = 2, Marazziti *et al*, *Am J Psychiatry* 2001;**158**: 498–9).

Reboxetine

Reboxetine is less effective than citalopram (n = 19, RCT, s/b, c/o, 18/52, Seedat *et al*, *Int Clin Psychopharmacol* 2003;**18**:279–84) and paroxetine (n = 68, RCT, s/b, Bertani *et al*, *Pharmacopsychiatry* 2004;**37**:206–10).

Valproate

Valproate 300–1500 mg/d may be useful for resistant panic disorder (e.g. n = 13[c = 10], open, 8/52, Baetz and Bowen, *Can J Psychiatry* 1998;**43**:73–7).

Venlafaxine

Venlafaxine (75–225 mg/d) was superior to placebo for panic disorder, higher doses being most effective (n = 624, RCT, p/c, 12/52, Pollack *et al*, *Psychopharmacol* [Berl] 2007;**194**:233–42), although a previous study was negative (n = 361, RCT, d/b, p/c, 10/52, Bradwejn *et al*, *Br J Psychiatry* 2005;**187**:352–9).

◆ **Others**

Other drugs tried include **carbamazepine** (review by Keck *et al*, *J Clin Psychopharmacol* 1992;**12**[Suppl]:S36–S41), **clonidine** (review by Puzantian and Hart, *Ann Pharmacother* 1993;**2**:1351–3), **ondansetron** (Schneier *et al*,

Anxiety 1996;**2**:199–202), **oxcarbazepine** (n = 1, Windhaber *et al*, *J Clin Psychiatry* 1997;**58**:404–5) and **pindolol** (see Mathew *et al*, *Psychopharmacol Bull* 2001;**35**:97–110).

□ **No efficacy**

Buspirone

Buspirone is not superior to placebo (d/b, c/o, *J Clin Psychiatry* 1988;**49**[8, Suppl]:S30–S36), or in combination with CBT (n = 77, RCT, Bouvard *et al*, *Psychother Psychosom* 1997;**66**:7–32).

Caffeine *

Caffeine is anxiogenic and panic patients seem to be more sensitive to its effects. Challenge doses of 480 mg have been shown to provoke panic attacks (n = 98, RCT, d/b, 1/52, Nardi *et al*, *Psychiatry Res* 2009;**169**:149–53).

1.22 POST-TRAUMATIC STRESS DISORDER (PTSD)

Symptoms

PTSD is an anxiety disorder resulting from an extreme stressful event, e.g. serious threat to life or involvement of a loved one in a catastrophic event, and where a personal vulnerability exists. The person then re-experiences the event recurrently through dreams and feelings. PTSD may be quite common yet often unrecognised and may lead to significant morbidity and mortality. The lifetime prevalence may be 1–9%. Severe trauma can produce long-lasting neurobiological changes and only drugs with a significant effect on the serotonin system seem to work.

Role of drugs

Drug treatment is still relatively poorly studied but from current data it seems that 'positive' symptoms (e.g. nightmares, etc) respond better, whereas 'negative' symptoms of avoidance (e.g. social withdrawal, etc) are less responsive to drugs. There is an almost total lack of response to placebo in chronic PTSD. SSRIs (e.g. sertraline and paroxetine) have been shown to be effective in short-term studies (6–12/52), and for relapse prevention over 6–12/12. Higher doses of serotonergic drugs for longer periods (at least five weeks) seem necessary. Extended treatment is needed, as there is a great risk of relapse and symptom recurrence if discontinued (s = 3, RCT, d/b, p/c, < 14/52, Davis et al, CNS Drugs 2006;**20**:465–76). Long-term atypicals, non-SSRIs and AEDs may also be effective (s = 9, Davis et al, CNS Drugs 2006;**20**:465–76). BDZs are probably ineffective (review by Asnis et al, Drugs 2004;**64**:383–404). Some, but not all, psychological treatments help PTSD (Bisson and Andrew, Cochrane Database Syst Rev 2007;**3**:CD003388).

Reviews: * general (Mellman and Lydiard, J Clin Psychiatry 2008;**69**:e2; Bisson, Adv Psych Treat 2007;**13**:119–26; Zohar et al, Curr Opin Psychiatry 2008;**21**:74–7), BAP evidence-based guidelines (Baldwin et al, J Psychopharmacol 2005;**19**:567–96), pharmacotherapy (Mohamed and Rosenheck, J Clin Psychiatry 2008;**69**:959–65), alternatives to antidepressants (Berger et al, Prog Neuropsychopharmacol Biol Psychiatry 2009; **33**:169–80), AEDs in PTSD (Berlin, Curr Psychiatry Rep 2007;**9**:291–300).

Paroxetine

Paroxetine is licensed for PTSD, with a standard dose of 20mg/d, increasing gradually to 50mg/d if needed. Doses of 20–40mg/d have been shown to be effective and well tolerated in adults (both male and female) with chronic PTSD (n = 551, RCT, p/c, 12/52, Marshall et al, Am J Psychiatry 2001;**158**:1982–8; n = 307, d/b, p/c, 12/52, Tucker et al, J Clin Psychiatry 2001;**62**:960–8). It has also been used successfully for post-traumatic grief (n = 15, open, Zygmont et al, J Clin Psychiatry 1998; **59**:241–5), non-combat-related chronic PTSD (n = 17, open, 12/52, Marshall et al, J Clin Psychopharmacol 1998;**18**:10–8), dissociation in chronic PTSD in adults (n = 52, RCT, d/b, p/c, 10/52, Marshall et al, Depress Anxiety 2007;**24**:77–84) and in chronic PTSD (n = 30, open, 6/12, Kucukali et al, Bosn J Basic Med Sci 2008;**8**:76–9; n=52[c=25], 12/12, open, Kim et al, Psychiatry Clin Neurosci 2008;**62**:646–52).

Sertraline

Sertraline is licensed for PTSD in women, but may not be effective in men. Two RCTs in PTSD have shown sertraline (mean dose 150mg/d) to be superior to placebo in measures of global and functional outcomes and symptom severity (n = 187, RCT, 12/52, Brady et al, JAMA 2000;**283**:1837–44; critical review by Bisson, EBMH 2000;**3**:109) and at 50–200mg/d to produce a 60% response rate cf 38% with placebo (n = 208, RCT, p/c, 12/52, Davidson et al, Arch Gen Psychiatry 2001;**58**:485–92). Sertraline seems particularly effective in treating psychological symptoms of PTSD, e.g. anger, anhedonia, detachment and numbing as opposed to somatic symptoms, e.g. insomnia and exaggerated startle response (n = 400, 12/52, Davidson et al, Psychol Med 2002;**32**:661–70), and for PTSD caused by either interpersonal trauma or childhood abuse (n = 395, RCT, d/b, p/c, 12/52, Stein et al, Ann Clin Psychiatry 2006;**18**:243–9), but was not effective for PTSD in a VA clinic setting (n = 169, RCT, d/b, p/c, 12/52, Friedman et al, J Clin Psychiatry 2007;**68**:711–20; MS). A prophylactic effect has been suggested (n = 96, open, 24/52, Davidson et al, Am J Psychiatry 2001;**158**:1974–81; review by Bisson, EBMH 2002;**5**:110, which noted that although there are major methodology concerns, it is good data and suggests at least one year's treatment with sertraline should be effective; see also n = 128, open 24/52, Londberg et al, J Clin Psychiatry 2001;**62**:325–31).

Review: Schwartz and Rothbaum, Expert Opin Pharmacother 2002;**3**:1489–99.

SSRIs (paroxetine and sertraline licensed)

Fluoxetine (up to 60mg/d) was shown to be superior to placebo in civilians with PTSD, with a very low placebo response rate (eg. n = 131, RCT, p/c, d/b, 6/12, Martenyi et al, Br J Psychiatry 2002;**181**:315–20; comment by Butterfield, EBMH 2003;**6**:51; strong criticism by Agell, Br J Psychiatry 2003;**182**:366–7 and defence by Eli Lilly; Br J Psychiatry 2003;**182**:367–8). Fluoxetine was more effective for relapse prevention than placebo (50% vs 22%) in responders over 6/12 (n = 123[c = 114], open, 6/12, Davidson et al, J Clin Psychopharmacol 2005;**25**:166–9). Care may be needed initially with use in patients with comorbid panic attacks, as fluoxetine may increase panic and anxiety so start low and go slow. **Citalopram** was partly effective in two cases (n = 2, Khouzam et al, Mil Med 2001;**166**:921–3). **Escitalopram** (up to 20 mg/d) was effective in 45% patients (n = 25 [c = 24], open, 12/52, Robert et al, J Clin Psychiatry 2006;**67**:1522–6). **Fluvoxamine** 100–300 mg/d (mean 150 mg) appeared to improve combat-related PTSD but not depressive symptoms (n = 15, open, 14/52, Escalona et al, Depress Anxiety 2002;**15**:29–33).

Venlafaxine

Venlafaxine 37.5–300 mg/d (mean 222 mg/d) was significantly more effective than placebo for enduring PTSD (n = 329, RCT, d/b, p/c, 6/12, Davidson et al, Arch Gen Psychiatry 2006; **63**:1158–65; review, Pae et al, Expert Rev Neurosci 2007;**7**:603–15).

■ Unlicensed/possible efficacy

Antipsychotics *

Antipsychotics are generally considered to be relatively poorly effective (e.g. n = 15, RCT, d/b, p/c, 10/52, Butterfield et al, Int Clin Psychopharmacol 2001;**16**:197–203) but a meta-analysis of studies shows that **olanzapine** and **risperidone** were superior to placebo for PTSD symptoms, particularly 'intrusion' symptoms (s = 7, n = 192, RCT, d/b, p/c, Pae et al, Int Clin Psychopharmacol 2008;**23**:1–8). **Aripiprazole** has been studied in a series of open studies in PTSD, e.g. it was effective in about 60% of those who tolerated the drug, starting at a low dose, i.e. 5 mg/d rather than 10 mg/d, to aid tolerability (n = 22 [c = 14], open, 12/52, Villarreal et al, Psychopharmacol Bull 2007;**40**:6–18; n = 32 [c = 23], open, 16/52, Mello et al, Rev Bras Psiquiatr 2008;**30**:358–61) and adjunctive aripiprazole (mean 13 mg/d) produced a 53% response rate with PTSD, and again treatment-emergent ADRs were improved with a low starting dose (5 mg) and slower titration (n = 17 [c = 8], open, 12/52, Robert et al, Psychopharmacol Bull 2009;**42**:69–80). It may help sleep disturbances and hyperarousal (n = 5, Lambert, Int Clin Psychopharmacol 2006;**21**:185–7). **Clozapine** has been used successfully in comorbid psychosis and PTSD

(n = 1, Hamner, Am J Psychiatry 1996;**153**:841) and in treatment-resistant, abused adolescents with psychosis and PTSD (n = 6, Wheatley et al, J Clin Psychopharmacol 2004;**24**:167–73). **Levomepromazine** may help reduce sleep problems in PTSD (Aukst-Margetic et al, Eur Psychiatry 2004;**19**:235–6). **Olanzapine** augmentation of SSRIs may be useful (e.g. n = 5, open, Jakovljevic et al, Acta Psychiatr Scand 2003;**107**:394–6; n = 19, d/b, p/c, 8/52, Stein et al, Am J Psychiatry 2002;**159**:1777–9). **Quetiapine** (mean 200–250 mg/d) may also be an option as augmentation of SSRIs (Sokolski et al, Mil Med 2003;**168**:486–9) and encouraging outcomes were seen in small pilot studies as adjunctive treatment in resistant PTSD (n = 20 [c = 18], open, 6/52, Hamner et al, J Clin Psychopharmacol 2003;**23**:5–20; n = 15, open, 8/52, Ahearn et al, Int Clin Psychopharmacol 2006;**21**:29–33). Adjunctive **risperidone** in resistant combat PTSD was well tolerated and produced a modest improvement in one study (n = 40, RCT, d/b, p/c, 5/52, Hamner et al, Int Clin Psychopharmacol 2003;**18**:1–8) and 2–4 mg/d has helped decrease some psychotic and PTSD symptoms in antidepressant-resistant patients (n = 26, open, 6/52, Kozaric-Kovacic et al, J Clin Psychiatry 2005;**66**:922–7). However, in sertraline part-response, addition of risperidone is of limited value (n = 45 [c = 34], Rothbaum et al, J Clin Psychiatry 2008;**69**:520–5). **Ziprasidone** has been used successfully (n = 2, Siddiqui et al, J Psychiatry Neurosci 2005;**30**:430–1).

Benzodiazepines

Although generally considered ineffective, potential anti-arousal effects can be useful and beneficial effects have been seen with **clonazepam** at 4–5 mg/d (n = 13, open, 6/12, Gelpin et al, J Clin Psychiatry 1996;**57**:390–4), but it was largely ineffective in improving sleep disturbances and nightmares in combat-related PTSD (n = 6, 2 + 2/52, p/c, c/o, s/b, Cates et al, Ann Pharmacother 2004;**38**:1395–9). Care is needed with possible abuse, induction of depression, the potential for the release of impulsive or antisocial behaviour and severe withdrawal reactions (n = 8, Risse et al, J Clin Psychiatry 1990;**51**:206–9).

Beta-blockers *

Propranolol may reduce the consolidation of emotional memory and is a potential, albeit controversial treatment for minimisation of PTSD (Henry et al, Am J Bioeth 2007;**7**:12–20; Rosenberg, Am J Bioeth 2007;**7**:27–8), e.g. propranolol 40mg TDS for seven days immediately post-trauma (n = 11) has shown lower levels of PTSD symptoms than in those refusing (n = 8) propranolol (n = 19, open, Vaiva et al, Biol Psychiatry 2003;**54**:947–9). However, propranolol was ineffective in preventing PTSD in soldiers experiencing burns in conflict (n = 65, McGee et al, J Burn Care Res 2009;**30**:92–7).

DHEA (dehydroepiandrosterone)

7-keto DHEA has been used successfully in treatment-resistant PTSD (n = 5, Sageman and Brown, J Clin Psychiatry 2006;**67**:493–6).

Gabapentin

Successful use has been reported (e.g. n = 30, Hamner et al, Ann Clin Psychiatry 2001;**13**:141–6; n = 1, Malek-Ahmadi, Ann Pharmacother 2003; **37**:664–6).

Levetiracetam

Levetiracetam (mean 2000mg/d) may be useful as antidepressant augmentation in refractory PTSD (n = 23, retrospective, mean 10/52, Kinrys et al, J Clin Psychiatry 2006;**67**:211–4).

Liothyronine/triiodothyronine

Triiodothyronine 25mcg/d has been used successfully to augment ineffective SSRI (fluoxetine or paroxetine 40mg/d) mono-therapy (n = 5, 8/52, Agid et al, J Clin Psychiatry 2001;**62**:169–73).

MAOIs

Phenelzine may exert a notable effect on intrusive and avoidance symptoms (n = 60, RCT, d/b, 8/52, Kosten et al, J Nerv Ment Dis 1991;**179**:366–70). The strong inhibitory effect on REM sleep may be contributory.

Memantine

Memantine showed consistent positive results in a case series (n = 4, open, 12/52, Battista et al, Psychiatry 2007;**70**:167–74).

Mirtazapine

A number of studies have suggested an effect in some symptoms at 45mg/d (64% response vs 20% for placebo; n = 29, RCT, d/b, p/c, 8/52, Davidson et al, Biol Psychiatry 2003;**53**:188–91). It was effective and well tolerated in PTSD in Korea (n = 15, open, 8/52, Bahk et al, Hum Psychopharmacol 2002;**17**:341–4) and in Korean veterans (n = 100, RCT, open, 6/52, Chung et al, Hum Psychopharmacol 2004; **19**:489–94). For PTSD nightmares, mirtazapine may have some significant effects, perhaps by an effect on sleep (n = > 300, open, Lewis, Am J Psychiatry 2002;**159**:1948–9). A continuation study showed a modest enduring effect for six months (n = 15 [c = 12], 24/52, Kim et al, Psychiatry Clin Neurosci 2005;**59**:743–7).

Oxcarbazepine

Oxcarbazepine has been used for PTSD (n = 1, Berigan, Can J Psychiatry 2002; **7**:973–4).

Phenytoin

Phenytoin may have some use at anticonvulsant doses and may be associated with changes in brain structure (n = 9, open, 3/12, Bremner et al, J Clin Psychiatry 2004;**65**:1559–64; Bremner et al, J Psychopharmacol 2005;**19**:159–65).

Prazosin *

Prazosin (mean dose 9.5mg/d) may reduce nightmares in veterans with chronic PTSD if taken for at least eight weeks (n = 59, retrospective chart analysis, Raskind et al, J Clin Psychiatry 2002;**63**:565–8), and is well tolerated and superior to placebo on primary outcome measures in PTSD if taken at night (n = 40 [c = 34], RCT, d/b, p/c, 8/52, Raskind et al, Biol Psychiatry 2007;**61**:928–34).

Reviews: general (Taylor et al, Am J Health Syst Pharm 2008;**65**:716–22; Miller, Pharmacother 2008;**28**:656–66).

Pregabalin *

A small pilot study suggested pregabalin may be useful for accident-related PTSD (n = 9, 6/52, Pae et al, Int Clin Psychopharmacol 2009; **24**:29–33; Strawn et al, J Clin Psychopharmacol 2008;**28**:596–7).

Quetiapine

Quetiapine 25–400 mg/d monotherapy has reduced psychotic and PTSD symptoms (n = 53, open, 8/52, Kozaric-Kovacic and Pivac, *Int J Neuropsychopharmacol* 2007;**10**:253–61).

Tiagabine

Tiagabine 8 mg/d (range 4–12 mg/d) may be worth investigating in PTSD (n = 7, open, 8/52, Taylor, *J Clin Psychiatry* 2003;**64**:1421–5; UG) and a discontinuation study in responders suggested some relapse prevention efficacy (n = 29[c = 19], open, 12/52, Connor *et al*, *Psychopharmacol* [Berl] 2006;**184**:21–5).

Topiramate *

Topiramate (up to 400 mg/d) has shown a significant effect on re-experiencing symptoms and treatment outcome scales in civilian PTSD (e.g. n = 38, RCT, d/b, p/c, Tucker *et al*, *J Clin Psychiatry* 2007;**68**:201–6; n = 43[c = 29], open, 8/52, Alderman *et al*, *Ann Pharmacother* 2009;**43**:635–41).

Tricyclics

Amitriptyline (n = 46, p/c, 8/52, Davidson *et al*, *Arch Gen Psychiatry* 1990;**4**:259–69) and imipramine (n = 60, RCT, p/c, 8/52, Kosten *et al*, *J Nerv Ment Dis* 1991;**179**:366–70) have been shown to produce a modest and clinically meaningful effect. However, doses of 300 mg/d for at least eight weeks may be needed.

Valproate

Intrusion, hyperarousal and depressive symptoms may respond to valproate (n = 16, 8/52, Clark *et al*, *J Trauma Stress* 1999;**12**:395–401; n = 16, open, Fesler, *J Clin Psychiatry* 1991;**52**:361–4) and in civilians with non-combat-related PTSD (open, Otte *et al*, *J Clin Psychopharmacol* 2004;**24**:106–8).

◆ Others

Other drugs tried include **buspirone** (e.g. Hamner *et al*, *Depress Anxiety* 1997;**5**:137–9), **carbamazepine** (e.g. Wolf *et al*, *Biol Psychiatry* 1988;**23**:642–4), **clonidine** (n = 9, Kinzie and Leung, *J Nerv Ment Dis* 1989;**177**:546–50), **cyproheptadine** for nightmares (e.g. Brophy, *Mil Med* 1991;**156**:100–1), **lithium** (Kitchner and Greenstein, *Mil Med* 1985;**150**:378–81), and **trazodone** (n = 6, open, Hertzberg *et al*, *J Clin Psychopharmacol* 1996;**1**:294–8).

□ No efficacy

Bupropion *

Bupropion may improve depression but appears ineffective for PTSD (n = 30, d/b, p/c, 8/52, Becker *et al*, *J Clin Psychopharmacol* 2007;**27**:193–7).

Flumazenil

Two studies have shown no effects (e.g. Coupland *et al*, *Biol Psychiatry* 1997;**41**:988–90).

Guanfacine

Guanfacine had no effect on any PTSD symptoms (n = 63, RCT, d/b, p/c, 8/52, Neylan *et al*, *Am J Psychiatry* 2006;**163**:2186–8).

Naltrexone

Only non-significant improvements were seen in a small, short trial (n = 8, open, 2/52, Lubin *et al*, *Hum Psychopharmacol* 2002;**17**:181–5).

PSYCHIATRIC EMERGENCY, ACUTE

see Acute psychiatric emergency (*1.1*)

1.23 PSYCHOSIS AND SCHIZOPHRENIA

1.23.1. Psychosis and schizophrenia
1.23.2. First episode (early intervention)
1.23.3. Cognitive impairment
see also Catatonia (*1.12*)

Symptoms

Schizophrenia is an enduring and fluctuating mental health problem with a high chance of relapse. Schneider's 'First rank symptoms' are often used as the main diagnostic features. They include hearing thoughts spoken aloud, 'third person' hallucinations, hallucinations in the form of a commentary, somatic hallucinations, thought withdrawal or insertion, thought broadcasting, delusional perceptions and feelings, or actions experienced as being made or influenced by external agents. The most frequent symptoms are a lack of insight, auditory hallucinations, ideas of reference, suspiciousness, flat affect, voices speaking to them, delusional mood, delusions of persecution and thoughts spoken aloud.

Possible causes of schizophrenia *

The dopamine hypothesis, i.e. excess dopamine activity in the mesolimbic remains the most enduring explanation for the main symptoms (Toda and Abi-Dargham, *Curr Psychiatry Rep* 2007; **9**:329–36) but is clearly not the whole story and there are many other theories, e.g. hypofunction of the glutamate systems, particularly at the NMDA sub-type of glutamate receptor (Harrison, *Br J Psychiatry* 2008; **192**:86–7), combined dopamine hyperfunction and glutamate hypofunction (Paz et al, *Eur Neuropsychopharmacol* 2008; **18**:773–86) and 5-HT$_2$ hyperfunction (Di Pietro and Seamans, *Pharmacopsychiatry* 2007; **40**(Suppl 1):S27–33). The balance between D$_2$ and 5-HT$_2$ may be important. Abnormal connections between nerves involving amino acid neurotransmitters may be a consequence of developmentally reduced synaptic connectivity (during perinatal and adolescent periods), rather than loss of neuronal or glial cells. Antipsychotics are thought to exert a significant part of their clinical effect via blockade of mesolimbic (Strange, *Trends Pharmacol Sci* 2008; **29**:314–21) D$_2$ receptors.

Role of drugs in schizophrenia

Antipsychotics have a major role in the management of the symptoms of schizophrenia but the actual choice of drug is difficult. In nearly all RCTs using haloperidol as the comparator, haloperidol doses were higher than recommended even for severely ill patients, so it is not surprising some of the newer drugs appear better tolerated (s = 49, Hugenholtz et al, *J Clin Psychiatry* 2006; **67**:897–903).

1. Choice of antipsychotic *

There have only been two major independent comparisons.

The **CATIE** study compared olanzapine (7.5–30 mg/d), risperidone (1.5–6 mg/d), perphenazine (8–32 mg/d), quetiapine (200–800 mg/d) and ziprasidone (40–160 mg/d). Among the many findings, 74% patients discontinued their first antipsychotic within 18 months, olanzapine had the lowest drop-

out rate (but had its known side-effects), and perphenazine was as effective as the others (n = 1493, RCT, < 18/12, Lieberman et al, *N Engl J Med* 2005; **353**:1209–23). Those who did not respond to a second generation antipsychotic, clozapine was more effective than switching to another atypical (n = 99, CATIE, McEvoy et al, *Am J Psychiatry* 2006; **163**:600–10). Switching to risperidone or olanzapine was more effective than quetiapine or ziprasidone, based on time to discontinuation (n = 444, RCT, d/b, CATIE, Stroup et al, *Am J Psychiatry* 2006; **163**:611–22). **CUtLASS** compared switching to either first or second generation antipsychotics in people who needed a change and showed striking consistency over all drugs for quality of life scores (n = 227, RCT, open-s/b, 12/12, Jones et al, *Arch Gen Psychiatry* 2006; **63**:1079–87). The choice of antipsychotic in the acute phase thus remains an individual decision. A meta-analysis of 2nd generation vs 1st generation antipsychotic trials has confirmed that 2nd generations are not a homogenous class (s = 150, n = 21,533, d/b, Leucht et al, *Lancet* 2009; **373**:31–41).

2. Early-onset and limitation of progression

Evidence is accumulating that antipsychotics started after the symptoms first appear, or even in a prodromal stage, may prevent or delay the progression of schizophrenia. See section 1.23.2.

3. Acute phase *

Many antipsychotics have an immediate calming effect (useful in relieving distress in the acute stage) and then reduce the intensity of psychotic symptoms. There is little proven advantage of using higher doses of some drugs, e.g. above about 12–15 mg/d of high-potency antipsychotics (e.g. haloperidol), and higher doses potentially give the recipient an adverse experience. A pooled-data analysis has shown that if there was no improvement after two weeks, the person is unlikely to respond at week 4 and so may benefit from an earlier change (s = 7, n = 1708, RCT, Leucht et al, *J Clin Psychiatry* 2007; **68**:352–60). Most response is likely within 3–4 weeks, so objective rating scales may be a useful, time-effective and cost-effective tool in decision-making.

4. Relapse prevention

Relapse of schizophrenia occurs in around 80% of untreated schizophrenics and so maintenance therapy, which reduces relapse rates significantly, is usually an important component of the management. If antipsychotics are stopped, relapse may be delayed for 2–6 months, with the individual often feeling better (due to a reduced side-effect burden) before the relapse. Intermittent therapy (prodrome-based or crisis intervention) is generally accepted as ineffective (n = 363, RCT, Gaebel et al, Schizophr Res 2002;**53**:145–59) and risks sudden relapse. Side-effects, particularly the under-rated akathisia, weight gain and dysphoria, tend to reduce compliance.

Although long-term antipsychotics are the most important relapse-prevention strategy, it is difficult to motivate people to continue while relatively asymptomatic. While compliance and adherence are terms used, 'concordance' implies an agreement between the prescriber and patient as to the degree of medicine-taking acceptable to both. In patients, this will balance the positive effects of the drug (e.g. symptom suppression) and the negative effects (e.g. side-effects) and finding a good reason not to relapse, e.g. family, friends or job, may aid effective maintenance therapy.

Long-term medication is obviously of major concern due to the potential for adverse consequences. To address this, an 11-year follow-up study of mortality in people with schizophrenia concluded that there was no evidence of an increase in deaths and that the gap in life expectancy between people with schizophrenia and the general population is reducing, e.g. there was a lower mortality in people with schizophrenia taking antipsychotics (for 7–11 years during study period) than not, (n = 66881 schizophrenics from national register cf 5.2m in general population, 11 years, Tiihonen et al, Lancet 2009;**374**:620–7).

Year	Life expectancy		Difference
	Schizophrenia	General population	
1996	32.5 years	57.5 years	25 years
2006	37.4 years	59.9 years	22.5 years

In people taking antipsychotics, the highest mortality was with quetiapine (OR 1.41), the lowest with clozapine (OR 0.74).

5. Discontinuation *

Many people with schizophrenia are on long-term antipsychotics (depot or oral) at the dose they received when acutely ill. With depression 'the dose that got you well keeps you well' is probably true, but there is abundant evidence that this may not be necessary in schizophrenia as continuous antipsychotic intake is 'topping-up' D2 blockade as significant D2 blockade can persist for 16 weeks after discontinuing depots (Pani et al, Eur Psychiatry 2207;**22**:267–75). Reducing doses from their acute levels may actually improve outcomes and symptoms but (and it is a big but) some people appear to need higher doses long-term. This does not mean you should not try reducing doses but that care is needed to prevent unnecessary and potentially catastrophic relapses.

Reducing doses or stopping antipsychotics in someone on a high dose long-term

- Check the history carefully to see if there is clear evidence of previous illness. If so, proceed only with great caution (especially if any evidence of a forensic potential) and document carefully. A history of non-compliance without relapse is a good sign, but not to be taken as confirmation that antipsychotics are not needed.
- Make only small changes each time.
- Remember that the peak for relapse may be at about 3–6 months post-dose reduction or discontinuation. So, leave for six months to assess the outcome of each change.
- Have a robust system in place for detecting early signs of relapse.
- Have a robust plan for increasing or reintroducing doses when early signs of relapse occur to restabilise the patient.
- Remember that some people need higher doses and there is much to gain by reducing doses but, probably more to lose should the person relapse and not be able to return to their previous levels of functioning.
- Consider the consequences of relapse, damage to the individual and others, and previous events.

The use of high dose antipsychotic medication (Thompson, *Br J Psychiatry* 1994;**164**:448–58; revised by Royal College of Psychiatrists, 2006)

The upper end of the dose ranges of older antipsychotics is often not clearly established and usually defined by limits of safety and the SPCs. Doses above these limits should only be used 'with caution and under specialist supervision'. 'Chlorpromazine equivalents' have been used to compare drugs or calculate total doses of multiple drugs, but maximum doses vary between drugs, and dosage equivalents are of only limited use (see 2.2.1). The evidence and scientific rationale for the effectiveness of high doses is very limited.

Main dangers of high dose antipsychotics:

1. Sudden cardiac-related death, e.g. QT prolongation, torsades de pointes.
2. CNS toxicity, e.g. CNS and respiratory depression, hypoxia, seizures.

Main uses of antipsychotics above BNF limits:

1. **Psychiatric emergency:** see 'Acute psychiatric emergency' (*Chapter 1.1*).
2. **Acute treatment:** i.e. after the emergency, but before the antipsychotic takes full effect. Doses should be reduced as soon as possible once the patient has responded.
3. **Long-term treatment:** e.g. in treatment-resistant schizophrenia where residual symptoms impair living or rehabilitation:
   - **as polypharmacy:** the prescribing of multiple antipsychotics is 'not recommended' as it 'may constitute a hazard' and side-effects are not minimised
   - **poor resources:** inadequate resources/environment often result in the need for more medication at higher doses.

Factors to be considered before prescribing high-dose antipsychotics:

- The diagnosis is fully confirmed and documented.
- Plasma levels are therapeutic and compliance with regimen is assured.
- Treatment duration has been fully adequate.
- Reduced doses for a trial period have been tried to rule out, e.g. akathisia.
- Adverse social and psychological factors have been minimised.
- Alternative antipsychotic therapies tried.

If exceeding standard BNF antipsychotic doses, the following should be routine and documented:

- Multidisciplinary team and patient (or advocate) discussion, obtaining valid consent if possible, making a thorough record of the decision and reasoning, including target signs and symptoms, and outcome evaluation.
- Consideration of any contraindications, e.g. cardiac, age, renal, hepatic, weight, and smoking, and any interactions, e.g. with tricyclics, carbamazepine, etc.
- ECG pre-treatment to exclude QTc prolongation, repeated every 1–3 months, especially with haloperidol.
- Doses increased only slowly.
- Regular checks carried out on pulse, bp temperature and hydration.
- Prescription reviewed regularly and reduced after three months if no improvement.

Risk factors for relapse

Medication risk factors include:

- **Drug used,** e.g. rehospitalisation rates for schizophrenics discharged on olanzapine (n=313) or risperidone (n=268) were similar (31% and 33% respectively) but considerably lower than those (n=458) discharged on conventional antipsychotics (48%) (2yrs, Rabinowitz et al, Am J Psychiatry 2001;**58**:266–9), confirmed by CATIE.
- **Doses:** there are some ethnic trends in drug responses, and doses may need to be lower in some racial groups (n=192, 6/52, Emsley et al, J Clin Psychiatry 2002;**63**:9–14). Higher long-term doses lead to extra ADRs and a higher risk of non-compliance.
- **Duration of untreated psychosis (DUP):** DUP is a good predictor of outcome.
- **Unmanaged substance misuse:** this reduces antipsychotic effects in dual diagnosis, with sooner and longer readmissions, especially in those non-compliant (n=99, four years, Hunt et al, Schizophr Res 2002; **54**:253–64).
- **Non-compliance/concordance.**

Review: optimal duration of prophylactic antipsychotics in schizophrenia (Bosveld-van Haandel et al, Acta Psychiatr Scand 2001;**103**:335–46).

Suicide prevention

Around 5% of schizophrenics will commit suicide, usually near illness onset (n=22598, Palmer et al, Arch Gen Psychiatry 2005;**62**:247–53). A five-year retrospective study suggested both risperidone and olanzapine gave some protection from suicidality compared to other (excluding clozapine) antipsychotics (n=756, Barak et al, Psychopharmacol [Berl] 2004;**175**: 215–9). Clozapine has a clear anti-suicide effect.

Reviews: * metabolic syndrome review (Thakore, Br J Psychiatry 2005;**186**:455–6), metabolic side-effects of atypicals in children (Fedorowicz and Fombonne, J Psychopharmacol 2006;**20**:533–50), systematic review and meta-analysis of second generation antipsychotics vs low-potency first generation (s=150,n=21,533, d/b, Leucht et al, Lancet 2009;**373**:31–41), long-term efficacy of atypicals (Martin and Stewart, J Psychopharmacol 2006;**20**[suppl]:S20–S37), plasma levels of atypicals (Mauri et al, Clin Pharmacokinet 2007;**46**:359–88).

1.23.1 PSYCHOSIS AND SCHIZOPHRENIA

BNF listed

PHENOTHIAZINES

Chlorpromazine *

Chlorpromazine can be used for a wide range of psychotic conditions but use in the elderly is problematic. Cochrane concludes that chlorpromazine remains a global 'benchmark' for schizophrenia, as a well-established, effective but imperfect treatment (Adams et al, Cochrane Database Syst Rev 2007;**2**:CD000284) with a relapse prevention efficacy (s=10, n=1042, Almerie et al, Cochrane Database Syst Rev 2007; **1**:CD006329) and remains one of the three listed drugs for psychosis and is on the WHO Essential Drug List (WHO 2009). Cochrane also concludes that, based on available studies (all 1968-78) that the optimum dose of chlorpromazine is in the 400-800mg/d range, with no advantages for lower or higher doses (s=4, n=1012, RCT, Liu and De Haan, Cochrane Syst Database Rev 2009;**2**:CD007778). IV use is not recommended unless the injection is diluted and the patient is in a supine position.

Fluphenazine (see also depots)

The oral preparation has been discontinued in the UK. Cochrane concluded that oral fluphenazine was effective 'but imperfect' (s=7, Mataer and Almerie, Cochrane Database Syst Rev 2007;**1**:CD006352).

Levomepromazine (methotrimeprazine)

Levomepromazine (600–1000mg/d, mean 710mg/d) may be more effective than chlorpromazine in TRS (n=38, RCT, open/d/b, 30/52, Lal et al, J Psychiatry Neurosci 2006; **31**: 271–9). It has significant sedative effects.

Pericyazine

Pericyazine is a piperidine phenothiazine similar to thioridazine, with marked sedative and hypotensive side-effects. Use as a low-dose anxiolytic-sedative has increased with the fall of thioridazine. Little is published about the drug.

Perphenazine

Perphenazine is a piperazine phenothiazine with a relatively short half-life (8–12 hours). Chosen as a 'typical' comparator, the CATIE study has shown perphenazine to be as effective as olanzapine, risperidone, quetiapine and ziprasidone (n = 1493, RCT, < 18/12, Lieberman et al, N Engl J Med 2005; **353**:1209–23; see also Rosenheck; Kane et al, J Clin Psychiatry 2007;**68**:1812–4).

Prochlorperazine

Prochlorperazine is a piperazine phenothiazine better known for its use as an antiemetic and in Ménières disease, but also licensed for schizophrenia and acute mania.

Promazine

Promazine is similar to chlorpromazine and retains a minor role as a non-dependence-prone hypnotic, although the potential for side-effects should not be ignored.

Trifluoperazine

Trifluoperazine is a piperazine phenothiazine widely used as an antipsychotic and sometimes claimed to have 'activating' effects at low doses. Cochrane concludes that trifluoperazine is of similar efficacy to other antipsychotics (s = 13, n = 1162, Marques et al, Cochrane Database Syst Rev 2004;**1**:CD003545).

BUTYROPHENONES

Benperidol

Benperidol is a potent D2 blocker marketed originally as specific for antisocial sexual behaviour, with uncontrolled studies and reports claiming beneficial effects. Cochrane concludes that there is insufficient evidence to assess the drug's effectiveness, with a single poor RCT, where it was inferior to perphenazine (Leucht and Hartung, Cochrane Database Syst Rev 2005;**2**:CD003083). See 1.26.

Haloperidol (see also depots) *

Haloperidol is the prototype and standard reference butyrophenone used for the treatment of acute and chronic psychosis, both orally and as an injection (aqueous and depot), although in the CUtLASS study few patients remained on haloperidol long-term. The BNF oral limit is 30mg/d, but there is no additional antipsychotic advantage from doses higher than 12mg/d in psychosis and acute mania and 4mg/d may be as effective as 10mg/d and 40mg/d (n = 24, RCT, d/b, 2/52, Stone et al, Am J Psychiatry 1995;**152**:1210–2). Even ultra-low doses (1–2mg/d) may be effective and well tolerated in first-episode psychosis (n = 35, open, Oosthuizen et al, J Psychopharmacol 2001;**15**:251–5), although reported to cause as much TD as standard dose typicals (n = 57, 12/12, Oosthuizen et al, J Clin Psychiatry 2003; **64**:1075–80). Cochrane concludes that doses above 7.5 mg/d should only be prescribed with caution (s = 16, n = 426, Waraich et al, Cochrane Database Syst Rev 2002;**3**:CD001951). The elimination half-life in brain tissue is about 6–8 days, with significant amounts still detectable after two weeks. Thus, residual side-effects may continue for many weeks or months after stopping the drug, due to persistence of active CNS levels (Kornhuber et al, Am J Psychiatry 1999;**156**:885–90). Cochrane concludes that haloperidol is superior to placebo but that its ADRs are such that alternative antipsychotics should be prescribed (Joy et al, Cochrane Database Syst Rev 2006;**4**:CD003082). The UK SPC now recommends an ECG before treatment due to the risk of a dose-related increase in QT-interval (n = 596, Reilly et al, Lancet 2000;**355**:1048–52), especially if given by the IV, rather than IM route.

Review: Pharmacokinetics (Kudo and Ishizaki, Clin Pharmacokinetics 1999;**37**:435–56).

THIOXANTHENES

Flupentixol (see also depots)

Oral flupentixol is usually used in low dose for anxiety and depression. Flupentixol 5–20mg/d was as effective as olanzapine 5–20mg/d with more EPS but less weight gain (n = 28, RCT, d/b, 4/52, Gattaz et al, Pharmacopsychiatry 2004;**37**:279–85) and 4–12mg/d was as effective as risperidone 2–6mg/d for negative, affective and cognitive symptoms (n = 144, RCT, d/b, 25/52, Ruhrmann et al, Prog Neuropsychopharmacol Biol Psychiatry 2007; **31**:1012–22).

Zuclopenthixol (see also depots)

Zuclopenthixol is a relatively long-acting oral antipsychotic, and in a trial of oral vs depot zuclopenthixol in people with violence and schizophrenia, violence was inversely proportional to compliance, and much lower in the depot group (n = 46, RCT, s/b, one year, Arango et al, Eur Psychiatry 2006;**21**:34–40). Cochrane concludes that oral zuclopenthixol is a viable option but needs routine anticholinergics (s = 18, n = 1578, Kumar and Strech, Cochrane Database Syst Rev 2005;**4**:CD005474).

DIPHENYLBUTYLPIPERIDINES

Fluspirilene

See depots.

Pimozide

Pimozide is licensed for chronic schizophrenia and other psychoses, especially paranoid and monosymptomatic hypochondriacal psychoses, e.g. parasitosis. It is effective against a wide range of positive symptoms (s = 35, n = 1348, Rathbone and McMonagle, Cochrane Database Syst Rev 2007;**3**:CD001949), but with potential cardiotoxic effects (see 3.2). Any use in delusional disorders is based almost entirely on case reports (Gray, EBMH 2000;**3**:117).

BENZAMIDES, substituted

Review: consensus statement on substituted benzamides in psychiatry (Racagni et al, Neuro-psychobiol 2004;**50**:134–43).

Amisulpride

Low dose amisulpride (related to sulpiride) blocks pre-synaptic D2 and D3 autoreceptors, higher doses blocking post-synaptic receptors, with little effect on other receptors. It is often classified as 'atypical' (or even an 'atypical' atypical: Lecrubier, Int Clin Psychopharmacol 2000;**15**[Suppl 4]:S21–S26). A meta-analysis showed some effect at 50–100mg/d for predominantly negative symptoms and lower use of anticholinergic drugs (s = 18, n = 2214, RCT, Leucht et al, Am J Psychiatry 2002;**159**:180–90; caution expressed by Remington and Kapur, EBMH 2002;**5**:85). Another meta-analysis suggests negative symptoms may respond to low-dose amisulpride at the dose necessary for positive symptom response (when it becomes a D2/D3 blocker), its effect is essentially that of a 'typical' agent (s = 4, Storosum et al, Schizo Bull 2002;**28**;193–201). Amisulpride has been compared with risperidone (n = 309, RCT, d/b, 6/12, Sechter et al, Neuropsychopharmacol 2002;**27**;1071–81) and at 200–800mg/d is equivalent to olanzapine 5–20mg/d but with less weight gain (n = 377, RCT, d/b, 6/12, Martin et al, Curr Med Res Opin 2002;**18**:355–62) and dose-dependent hyperprolactinaemia (RCT, d/b, 6/12, Mortimer et al, Int Clin Psychopharmacol 2004;**19**:63–9). Cochrane concludes that amisulpride has a good general profile, may improve global and negative symptoms and might be more acceptable and more tolerable than high-potency, conventional antipsychotics (s = 19, n = 2443, RCTs, Mota et al, Cochrane Database Syst Rev 2002;**2**:CD001357).

Reviews: * general (Mortimer, Neuropsychiatr Dis Treat 2009;**5**:267–77; Pani et al, Clin Drug Invest 2008;**28**:465–77), TDM (Sparshatt et al, Acta Psychiatr Scand 2009;**120**:416–28).

Sulpiride *

Sulpiride is a specific dopamine (D2, plus some D3 and D4) receptor blocker, well-established in the UK. Cochrane concludes that sulpiride may be effective but the evidence is extremely limited (s = 2, n = 113, Omori and Wang, Cochrane Database Syst Rev 2009;**2**:CD007811). It was the most commonly chosen first generation antipsychotic in the CUtLASS study (n = 227, RCT, open-s/b, 12/12, Jones et al, Arch Gen Psychiatry 2006;**63**:1079–87).

SECOND GENERATION (OR ATYPICAL) ANTIPSYCHOTICS *

'Atypical' has been a widely-used term to describe a diverse group of antipsychotics with specific characteristics, e.g. minimal EPS, lack of sedation or a fast dissociation from D2 receptors. It may be better to either consider antipsychotics on a spectrum from typical (e.g. chlorpromazine) at one end to atypical (e.g. clozapine) at the other, or to base it upon a particular definition of atypicality, e.g. serotonin-dopamine antagonism (SDA), limbic specificity or a structural grouping (Grunder et al, Nat Rev Drug Discov 2009;**8**:197–

202).The CATIE and CUtLASS studies have shown similar efficacy but different ADRs. CATIE, CUtLASS and the Leucht meta-analysis have shown similar efficacy but different ADRs.

Reviews of atypicals: dosing (Cutler et al, CNS Spectr 2008;**13**[Suppl 9]:1–16), TDM (Hiemke et al, Ther Drug Monit 2004;**26**:156–60), doses (Kinon et al, CNS Drugs 2004;**18**:597–616) and mechanisms of action (Horacek et al, CNS Drugs 2006;**20**:389–409).

Aripiprazole *

Aripiprazole is a dopamine D2 and $5HT_{1A}$ receptor partial agonist, and a $5HT_{2A}$ receptor antagonist. It stimulates dopamine receptors but to a lower level than dopamine, while blocking endogenous dopamine (100% D2 occupancy by aripiprazole reduces dopaminergic activity to about 30%). There is only a minimal effect on alpha-1, H_1 and $5HT_{2C}$ receptors. The starting dose should be 5 mg/d if the patient is switching from another antipsychotic, increasing to 10 mg/d, and then 15 mg/d as tolerated. Time to steady state takes one to two and maybe four weeks so rapid dose escalation may not be advisable (Uzun et al, Psychiatr Danub 2005;**17**:67–75). A thorough analysis has concluded that the optimum dose of aripiprazole is 10 mg/d, with doses above 20 mg/d providing no additional benefit (s=5, Mace and Taylor, CNS Drugs 2009;**23**:773–80), although higher doses have been used, albeit with variable success (35–60 mg/d, n=4, Crossman and Lindenmayer, J Clin Psychiatry 2006;**67**:1158–9; 75 mg/d n=1, Duggan and Mendhekar, J Clin Psychiatry 2006;**67**:674–5). A rather critical systematic review and meta-analysis has concluded that aripiprazole is superior to placebo with less raised prolactin than other antipsychotics, although study attrition rates were large and poorly reported (s=10, El-Sayeh et al, Br J Psychiatry 2006;**189**:102–8; biting and justified criticism by Mortimer, EBMH 2007;**10**:14). Long-term efficacy equivalent to olanzapine has been shown in a one-year extension trial to a 6/12 RCT (n=214, one year, Chrzanowski et al, Psychopharmacology [Berl] 2006;**189**:259–66), where 15 mg/d seems well tolerated and effective (n=310, RCT, p/c, d/b, 6/12, Pigott et al, J Clin Psychiatry 2003;**64**:1048–56; comment

by Mortimer, EBMH 2004;**7**:41 noting placebo level side-effects, no dose titration, simple dosing, that 30% of stable people relapsed over 6/12 when switched, and a lack of symptom reduction in more severely ill patients). In olanzapine or risperidone non-responders, switching to either aripiprazole (15–30 mg/d) or perphenazine (8–64 mg/d), resulting in 27% and 25% respectively responding, with aripiprazole better tolerated and with higher QoL scores (n=300, RCT, d/b, 6/52, Kane et al, J Clin Psychiatry 2007;**68**:213–23; MS). Aripiprazole 9.75 mg IM is rapidly effective and well tolerated for agitation in schizophrenia (n=357, RCT, p/c, Tran-Johnson et al, J Clin Psychiatry 2007;**68**:111–9; MS). Cochrane concludes that aripiprazole is effective, with a lower risk of akathisia, raised prolactin and QTc prolongation than other atypicals (El-Sayeh and Morganti, Cochrane Database Syst Rev 2006**2**:CD004578), efficacy is similar to typicals but with superior tolerability (s=9, n=3122, Bhattacharjee and El-Sayeh, Cochrane Database Syst Rev 2008;**3**:CD006617) but somewhat less effective than olanzapine, albeit better tolerated for metabolic effects and sedation (s=4, n=1404, Komossa et al, Cochrane Database Syst Rev 2009;**4**:CD006569; see also n=703, RCT, d/b, 46/52, Fleischacker et al, Biol Psychiatry 2009;**65**:510–7).

Reviews: * consensus statement (Sullivan et al, Curr Med Res Opin 2007;**23**:1733–44), safety and tolerability (Pae, Expert Opin Drug Saf 2009;**8**:373–86), use in children and adolescents (Greenaway and Elbe, J Can Acad Child Adolesc Psychiatry 2009;**18**:250–60), oral vs IM kinetics (Boulton et al, Clin Pharmacokinet 2008;**47**:475–85).

Asenapine * (UK license planned 2010/11)

Asenapine is licensed in USA for acute schizophrenia and acute mania or mixed episodes in bipolar I with or without psychotic features. It has a high affinity for 5HT1A/1B/2A/2B/2C/5/6/7, D1/2/3/4, alpha 1 and 2, H1 and H2 but not cholinergic receptors (Citrome, Int J Clin Pract 2009;**63**:1762–84). Asenapine 10 mg/d was as effective as risperidone and superior to placebo in acute schizophrenia, and as well-tolerated as placebo (n=174, RCT, p/c, 6/52, Potkin et *al, J Clin Psychiatry* 2007;**68**:1492–1500; MS), and 10mg/d was superior to risperidone 6mg/d and placebo in acute schizophrenia (n = 174, RCT, p/c, d/b, 6/52, Potkin *et al, J Clin Psychiatry* 2007;**68**:1492–1500). It is available as an oral melt formulation of 'fragile wafer'. It is 35% bioavailable orally, but less than 2% if swallowed, so no drinking or eating for 10 minutes after a dose is recommended. Food just before a dose decreases absorption by 20% and by 10% up to four hours afterwards. The US PI for asenapine recommends gradual discontinuation and minimising overlap with other antipsychotics.

Reviews: * in schizophrenia (Bishara and Taylor, *Neuropsychiatr Dis Treat* 2009;**5**:483–90), general (Shahid *et al, J Psychopharmacol* 2008; **23**:65–73; Weber and McCormack, *CNS Drugs* 2009;**23**:781–92).

Clozapine (see also *Tables 1.2–1.5*) *

Clozapine is indicated for treatment-resistant schizophrenia (TRS) and unresponsive psychotic disorders in Parkinson's disease. Before starting, patients should have a physical examination and any cardiac disease excluded.

Efficacy: Clozapine is probably effective in up to 30–50% of treatment-resistant schizophrenics (n = 268, RCT, d/b, p/c, 6/52, Kane *et al, Arch Gen Psychiatry* 1988;**45**:789–96). This may rise to 60% if adequate doses are given for up to 12 months, e.g. a one-year study in TRS showed that 50–76% responded to clozapine over 52 weeks, the peak response occurring at 12–24 weeks (n = 84, open, Lieberman *et al, Am J Psychiatry* 1994;**151**:1744–52). There is probably little clinical gain in prolonging exposure to clozapine beyond eight weeks at any particular dose if no response is seen (n = 50, open, Conley *et al, Am J Psychiatry* 1997;**154**:1243–7). Cochrane concludes that the benefit of clozapine over typicals is not significant, although this included all studies, not just in TRS where it is clearly superior and has a differential efficacy (s = 42, n = 3950, Essali *et al, Cochrane Database Syst Rev* 2009; 1:CD000059).

Mode of action: Clozapine's mode of action remains unclear, e.g. it has a low occupancy of D_2 receptors (30–60%) and thus may act via D_1, $5-HT_{2}$, ACh, $5-HT_6$ and $5-HT_7$ receptors and

inhibition of pre-synaptic alpha-2 autoreceptors. Some D_2 limbic specificity has been shown. Adjunctive aripiprazole (with potent D2 affinity) does not diminish clozapine's efficacy, suggesting its efficacy is not predominantly D2 blockade.

Blood levels: Plasma levels may be useful in optimising therapy if poor response occurs. ADRs can be far higher than spontaneously reported, and plasma level related (n = 103, Yusufi *et al, Int Clin Psychopharmacol* 2007; **22**:238–43). Plasma clozapine levels of 200–450ng/ml have been shown to be superior to levels of 150ng/ml and below (n = 56, VanderZwaag *et al, Am J Psychiatry* 1996; **153**:1579–84). Levels over 350ng/ml should only be reached with extreme care and blood levels may not necessarily be related to therapeutic efficacy (n = 41, Kurz *et al, Br J Psychiatry* 1998;**173**:341–4). Low plasma levels may occur in CYP1A2 ultra-rapid metabolisers (review by Greenwood-Smith *et al, J Psychopharmacol* 2003;**17**:234–8) and may account for some non-responders.

Blood dyscrasias: Clozapine can cause a usually reversible neutropenia in 3–4% of patients, which may lead on to agranulocytosis in 0.8% of patients over one year, with a non-dose-related higher risk in older people and those with lower base-line wbc counts (n = 11555, Alvir *et al, N Engl J Med* 1993;**329**:162–7). The onset peaks at around 8–10 weeks (range 0.5–24+ weeks), lasts between 12 and 20 days and treatment is thus restricted (see *Table 1.2*), although the incidence after three years is minimal. The UK CPMS database study indicated that agranulocytosis is 2.4-fold higher in Asians compared to Caucasians, and there is an age-related increase in risk of 53% per decade, but no dose-relationship (n = 12760, Munro *et al, Br J Psychiatry* 1999;**175**:576–80). Clozapine is also able to induce transient granulocytopenia without the usual rise in granulocyte colony stimulating factor (G-CSF) levels. The use of clozapine in people with a low wbc count due to benign ethnic neutropenia (BEN) may be allowed with haematologist advice. Of 53 patients rechallenged after clozapine-induced leucopenia or neutropenia, 38% had a further dyscrasia and, in most of these, it was more severe, longer-lasting

Clozapine UK prescribing and monitoring summary

Clozapine is indicated in the UK for treatment-resistant schizophrenia and psychosis in Parkinson's disease, ie. patients 'non-responsive' or 'intolerant' of conventional antipsychotics (*Table 1.2*). It can be dispensed on a weekly, fortnightly or four-weekly basis (*Table 1.3*), but only following a satisfactory blood result (*Table 1.4*).

TABLE 1.2: SUMMARY OF UK CLOZAPINE PRESCRIBING RESTRICTIONS

'Non-responsive'	Lack of satisfactory clinical improvements despite the use of at least two marketed antipsychotics prescribed at adequate dose for an adequate duration
'Intolerant'	The impossibility of achieving clinical benefit with conventional antipsychotics because of severe or untreatable neurological or other adverse reactions, eg. extrapyramidal or tardive dyskinesia
Patient requirements	Hospital-based originally. Normal white blood cell and differential blood counts. Enrolled with clozapine non-rechallenge database (CNRD)
Prescriber and dispensing requirements	Consultant must be registered with CNRD (clozapine non-rechallenge database). Hospital or nominated community pharmacy must be registered with CNRD

TABLE 1.3: SUMMARY OF UK CLOZAPINE MINIMUM BLOOD TEST REQUIREMENTS *

Blood tests	Required frequency	Validity
Pre-treatment	Single blood screen	10 days, if satisfactory (green)
First 18 weeks of treatment First sample at three days	Weekly (usually Monday or Tuesday)	11 days (not including day of sample) if satisfactory (green)
Weeks 19–52	Every two weeks if blood results have been satisfactory	21 days (not including day of sample) if satisfactory (green)
Weeks 53 onwards	Every four weeks, if 'stable haematological profile'	42 days (not including day of sample) if satisfactory (green)
Discontinuation (temporary or permanent)	Weekly (up to 18 weeks), or fortnightly (19 weeks onwards) for four weeks after completely stopping clozapine	In total one month's follow-up is required at previous monitoring frequency e.g. 4x1/52, 2x2/52 or 1x4/52.. If test result has not been, or does not go, red clozapine may be restarted. See *Table 1.5*

TABLE 1.4: SUMMARY OF UK TEST RESULTS

Results	Meaning	Action
Green	Satisfactory	Routine tests
Amber	wbc or neutrophil counts below accepted levels	Repeat test twice a week until either red or green
Red	wbc below 3000/mm^3 and/or absolute neutrophils below 1500/mm^3	Immediate cessation of therapy. Sample blood daily until patient recovered. No further prescribing allowed unless an error has occurred or Consultant takes full responsibility.

TABLE 1.5: SUMMARY OF TEMPORARY BREAKS IN CLOZAPINE THERAPY ADVICE *

1. Dose		
Dose on discontinuation	Break	Dose on restart (contact your supplying pharmacy for advice)
Any	<48 hours	Restart on previous dose
Any	>48 hours	Restart at 12.5–25 mg and build up gradually to previous dose to minimise dose-related side-effects
2. Sampling frequency		
Previous monitoring frequency	Break	Monitoring on restart
Weekly	<1 week	Weekly, no need to restart 18-week period
Weekly	>1 week	Weekly, **must** restart 18-week period
After 18 weeks *		
Fortnightly	≤3 days	Fortnightly
Fortnightly	≥3 days	Weekly for six weeks, then fortnightly
Four-weekly	≤3 days	Four-weekly
Four-weekly	>3 days	Weekly for six weeks, then four-weekly
Fortnightly or four-weekly	>4 weeks	Requires full re-registration and monitoring again fully as if commencing for the first time.

and occurred more quickly than the original episode, but 55% were rechallenged successfully and remained in treatment (n = 53, Dunk et al, Br J Psychiatry 2006;**188**:255–63). G-CSF or GM-CSF stimulates cell production and shortens the period of clozapine-induced agranulocytosis by about a half, at which point it can be discontinued (e.g. n = 1, Schuld et al, Acta Psychiatr Scand 2000;**102**:153–5; n = 1, Sperner-Unterweger et al, Br J Psychiatry 1998; **173**:82–4).

Reviews: * restarting clozapine after neutropenia (Whiskey and Taylor, CNS Drugs 2007; **21**:25–35), genetics of clozapine-induced agranulocytosis (Opgen-Rhein and Dettling, Pharmacogenomics 2008;**9**:1101–11).

Suicide reduction: It is now reasonably well-established that clozapine reduces suicide rates in schizophrenia, which can be as high as 10%, a startling comparison with the risk of one in 50 for reversible agranulocytosis. The InterSePT study (n = 980, RCT, d/b, two years, Meltzer et al, Arch Gen Psychiatry 2003;**60**:82–91; comment by Volavka, EBMH 2003;**6**:93) has shown a 25% reduction in suicide events compared to olanzapine (a drug itself with possible antisuicide effects) which appears to be due to clozapine's intrinsic action (e.g. reducing impulsiveness and aggression, n = 44, open, 6/12, prospective, Spivak et al, J Clin Psychiatry 2003;**64**:755–60) not from concomitant medication (Glick et al, J Clin Psychiatry 2004;**65**:679–85), making a contribution to the risk:benefit analysis of clozapine. However, one study failed to show a reduced completed suicide rate with clozapine (9.2–10.5% in each group over four years), as the reduced death rate was entirely due to reduced respiratory disorders (n = 1514 plus 2830 matched-controls, four years, Sernyak et al, Am J Psychiatry 2001;**158**:931–7; disputed by Ertugrul and Meltzer, Am J Psychiatry 2002; **159**:323–5; comment by Reinstein et al, Clin Drug Investig 2002;**22**:341–6).

Reviews: * combination therapies (Mouaffak et al, Clin Neuropharmacol 2006;**29**:28–33), in children (Gogtay and Rapoport, Expert Opin Pharmacother 2008;**9**:459–65), ADRs (Flanagan, Curr Drug Saf 2008;**3**:115-22), clozapine vs typicals (s = 42, n = 3950, Essali et al, Cochrane Database Syst Rev 2009;**1**:CD000059).

Olanzapine *

Olanzapine is licensed for the treatment of schizophrenia and relapse prevention. It blocks a wide variety of receptors, e.g. $5-HT_{2A/C}$, $5-HT_3$, $5-HT_6$, D_{1-5}, M_{1-5}, alpha-one and H1, with some mesolimbic dopamine selectivity. The starting and main therapeutic dose is 10mg/d (range 5–20mg/d, mean 15–18mg/d). Many studies have shown a clinical effect, e.g. where olanzapine (mean dose 15mg/d) was more effective than haloperidol (10–20mg/d) on negative symptoms (n = 335, RCT, d/b, 12/12, Tollefson and Sanger, Am J Psychiatry 1997;**154**:466–74), superior to haloperidol for all symptoms of schizophrenia, with fewer side-effects, including EPS and prolactin levels (n = 1996, d/b, 6/52, Tollefson et al, Am J Psychiatry 1997;**154**:457–65) and superior to risperidone for primary negative symptoms and with less side-effects (n = 339, d/b, 28/52, Tran et al, J Clin Psychopharmacol 1997;**17**:407–18, MS; review by Cunningham Owens, EBMH 1998;**1**:55). An independent study in TRS suggested that switching from an atypical/haloperidol to olanzapine may improve cognitive function but improve psychopathology in only 9% (n = 45, Lindenmayer et al, J Clin Psychiatry 2002;**63**:931–5). Olanzapine appeared highly effective in a relapse prevention study (n = 583, RCT, d/b, one year, Beasley et al, J Clin Psychopharmacol 2003;**23**:582–94, MS).

Higher doses: Use of higher doses may be increasing, and there is some evidence for efficacy (Citrome and Kantrowitz, Expert Rev Neurother 2009;**9**:1045–58), although high dose olanzapine (10mg vs 20mg vs 40mg/d) had no advantage over lower doses in TRS (n = 599, RCT, d/b, 8/52, Kinon et al, J Clin Psychopharmacol 2008;**28**:392–400; MS). In a comparison of high-dose olanzapine mean 34mg/d (vs clozapine mean 564mg/d) showed similar efficacy in TRS (n = 40, RCT, d/b, 6/12, Meltzer et al, J Clin Psychiatry 2008;**69**:274–85; comment by Roth, J Clin Psychiatry 2008;**69**:176–7). Higher dose olanzapine (30–40mg/d) has similar kinetics as 20mg/d but akathisia is more common (n = 37, RCT, d/b, Mitchell et al, Clin Ther 2006;**28**:881–92). Olanzapine levels may be useful to optimise doses and assess the influence of gender, smoking and interactions (n = 194, Skogh et al, Ther Drug Monit 2002;**24**:518–26). Cochrane concludes that olanzapine may be effective, with low EPS and greater weight gain, but that the high drop-outs and unfamiliar rating scales make firm conclusions difficult to draw (Duggan et al, Cochrane Database Syst Rev 2005;**2**:CD001329).

Reviews: * TDM/plasma levels, dosing and interactions (n = 71, Bergemann et al, Pharmacopsychiatry 2004;**37**:63–8), safety (Kantrowitz and Citrome, Expert Opin Drug Saf 2008;**7**:761–9).

Paliperidone *

Paliperidone, the 9-hydroxy metabolite of risperidone, has a starting and standard dose of 6 mg/d, which has placebo level EPS, and no need for dose titration. The oral form uses the OROS sustained release system giving a once-daily dosage and steady plasma levels. Paliperidone is also an antagonist at alpha-1 and alpha-2 adrenergic receptors and H1 histaminergic receptors but no affinity for cholinergic muscarinic or beta-1 or beta-2 adrenergic receptors. It has been shown to be effective at 6–12 mg/d in acute schizophrenia (s = 3, n = 1326, RCT, d/b, p/c, 6/52, Meltzer et al, J Clin Psychiatry 2008;**69**:817–29), quicker-acting and more effective than quetiapine in acute schizophrenia (n = 397 [c = 281], RCT, d/b, p/c, 6/52, Canuso et al, Am J Psychiatry 2009;**166**:691–701, MS) and in relapse prevention studies (s = 3, n = 1083, 52/52, open extension, Emsley et al, Int Clin Psychopharmacol 2008;**23**:343–56). Paliperidone seems to be effective regardless of the presence of negative symptoms (s = 3, n = 1193, d/b, p/c, 6/52, Canuso et al, Schizophr Res 2009;**113**:56–64). In older adults (mean 70 years) paliperidone was generally well tolerated (n = 114, RCT, d/b, p/c, 6/52 + 24/52 open extension, Tzimos et al, Am J Geriatr Psychiatry 2008;**16**:31–43). Paliperidone 9 mg/d improved sleep architecture and continuity in schizophrenia with concomitant insomnia (n = 36, RCT, d/b, p/c, 2/52, Luthringer et al, Int Clin Psychopharmacol 2007;**22**:299-308). Administration with high fat high caloric meal increases peak concentration 60% and the AUC 54% compared with administration under fasting conditions. Cochrane concludes paliperidone is effective (s = 5, n = 3067, RCT,

p/c, Nussbaum and Stroup, Cochrane Database Syst Rev 2008;**2**:CD006369; comment by Dolder, EBMH 2008;**11**:114).

Reviews: * general (Marino and Caballero, Pharmacopsychiatry 2008;**28**:1283–98; Dolder et al, Am J Health Syst Pharm 2008;**65**:403–13; Spina and Cavallaro, Expert Opin Drug Saf 2007;**6**:651–62; Dlugosz and Nasrallah, Expert Opin Pharmacother 2007;**8**:2307–13; Spina and Cavallaro, Expert Opin Drug Saf 2007;**6**:651–62; Yang and Plosker, CNS Drugs 2007;**21**:417–25).

Quetiapine *

Quetiapine is an established antipsychotic with effects on many receptors, e.g. it shows transiently high D2 occupancy which drops rapidly over 12–14 hours, which may explain the low EPS and low prolactin elevation (n = 12, Kapur et al, Arch Gen Psychiatry 2000;**57**:553–9). The target dose of 600 mg/d (range 150–750 mg/d) is probably the most effective, with once-daily dosing viable with the new XL preparation, although a few may experience worsening symptoms or orthostatic hypotension (n = 21, RCT, d/b, c/o, 4 + 4/52, Chengappa et al, Can J Psychiatry 2003;**48**:187–94). Doses need to be increased gradually over several days initially to reduce the incidence of postural hypotension. Many double-blind randomised trials indicate that the drug is as effective in schizophrenia as reference drugs (e.g. n = 448, RCT, 6/52, Copolov et al, Psychol Med 2000;**30**:95–105). In schizophrenics only partially responsive to typicals, significantly more responded to quetiapine 600 mg/d than haloperidol 20 mg/d, and quetiapine was better tolerated (n = 288, d/b, 8/52, Emsley et al, Int Clin Psychopharmacol 2000;**15**:121–31). Quetiapine XL was as effective as plain tablets, but with less ADRs (n = 58, RCT, d/b, c/o, Datto et al, Clin Ther 2009 **31**:492–502). Quetiapine may improve cognitive functioning (n = 58, RCT, Velligan et al, Schizophr Res 2002;**53**:239–48) and negative symptoms (s = 4, n = 1106, Tandon, Hum Psychopharmacol 2004;**19**:559–63). An analysis has shown that the onset of action of quetiapine is significant by the end of week one (SANS and BPRS), sooner than usually expected (s = 3, n = 620, RCT, d/b, Small et al, *Curr Med Res Opin* 2004;**20**:1017–23). A review of high-dose quetiapine concluding that there is little or no evidence for use of supra-BNF doses (Sparshatt *et al, CNS Drugs* 2008;**22**:49–72). Cochrane concludes that although quetiapine is more effective than placebo, no difference could be detected against traditional antipsychotics, and drop-outs due to adverse effects were lower with quetiapine but still high (Srisurapanont *et al, Cochrane Database Syst Rev* 2004;**2**:CD000967).

Reviews: general (Miodownik and Lerner, *Expert Rev Neurother* 2006;**6**:983–92; Miodownik and Lerner, *Expert Rev Neurother* 2006;**6**:983–92), dosing strategies (Citrome *et al, J Clin Psychiatry* 2005;**66**:1512–6).

Risperidone *

Risperidone is licensed for acute and chronic psychosis and has D_2 and $5-HT_2$ blocking actions.

Dose: An extensive literature analysis concluded that risperidone's optimum dose is 4mg/d, lower doses being consistently less effective and > 6mg/d having more side-effects, and with less efficacy at >10mg/d (Ezewuzie and Taylor, *J Psychopharmacol* 2006;**20**:86–90). Cochrane agrees that generally the optimal dose is 4–6mg/d, with 2–4mg/d of value in first episode and doses above 10mg/d have no advantage (Li *et al, Cochrane Database Syst Rev* 2009;**4**:CD007474). Titration to 6mg/d over three days is standard practice, but a slower titration has been recommended (over weeks rather than days, stabilising on 2–4mg/d initially before proceeding to higher doses), particularly in drug-naive first-episode schizophrenics and in the elderly. Slow titration markedly reduces the final doses needed, EPS and reduces non-compliance (n = 17, Kontaxakis *et al, Am J Psychiatry* 2000;**157**:1178–9), and may lead to better outcomes. Even very low dose (1–2mg/d) can produce dramatic improvements in prodromal phase or first episode schizophrenia (see *1.23.2*).

Efficacy: Risperidone has shown efficacy across a wide range of symptoms of psychosis and schizophrenia. Comparisons with olanzapine have been favourable, e.g. more effective with comparable side-effects (n = 42, open, 6/12,

Ho *et al, J Clin Psychiatry* 1999;**60**:658–63), or lower weight gain (n = 377, RCT, Conley and Mahmoud, *Am J Psychiatry* 2001;**158**:765–74). Relapse prevention has been shown over one year (n = 397, average follow-up one-year, Csernansky *et al, N Engl J Med* 2002;**346**:16–22; comment by McIntosh, *EBMH* 2002;**5**:77). Risperidone (4–6mg/d, n = 153) was superior to placebo (n = 73) and quetiapine (600–800mg/d, n = 156) in acute exacerbations of schizophrenia requiring hospitalisation (n = 382, RCT, d/b, p/c, 6/52, Potkin *et al, Schzophr Res* 2006;**85**:254–65).

Review: TDM (therapeutic range of 25–150microg/L, n = 50, Odou *et al, Clin Drug Invest* 2000;**19**:283–92).

Sertindole *

Sertindole is now only available on a named-patient basis in the UK and Lundbeck will not be applying for a full license. Cochrane concluded that sertindole is effective and as tolerable as placebo at 20mg/d (s = 3, n = 1104, Lewis *et al, Cochrane Database Syst Rev* 2005;**3**:CD001715) but with little evidence of superiority over other atypicals (Komossa *et al, Cochrane Database Syst Rev* 2009;**2**:CD006752).

Review: general (Murdoch and Keating, *CNS Drugs* 2006;**20**:233–55).

Zotepine

Zotepine is a tricyclic dibenzothiepine licensed for schizophrenia in some countries. Both zotepine and its active metabolite norzotepine have a high affinity for a range of dopamine and serotonin receptor sub-types, and have some NARI activity. To minimise hypotension, the dose should be titrated from 25mg TDS every four days to a maximum of 300mg/d (as a TDS dose). It has been compared to haloperidol, low dose chlorpromazine and higher dose chlorpromazine 300–600mg/d (less EPSE and greater improvement in BPRS, n = 158, RCT, 8/52, Cooper *et al, Acta Psychiatr Scand* 2000;**101**:218–25). Relapse prevention has been shown (n = 121, d/b, p/c, 6/12, Cooper *et al, Psychopharmacol* [Berl] 2000;**150**:237–43). The risk of seizures is dose-related and rises above 300mg/d. An ECG is recommended pre-treatment in people with CHD, at risk of hypokalaemia or taking other drugs known to prolong QTc. Cochrane concludes that zotepine is as effective as other antipsychotics and superior to placebo, although most studies were less than 12/52 duration (s = 141, n = 966, Fenton et al, Cochrane Database Syst Rev 2006; 4:CD001948).

Review: * Green, Expert Opin Drug Metab Toxicol 2009;**5**:181–6).

Ziprasidone (not available in the UK) *

Ziprasidone is licensed in the USA and some European countries for schizophrenia, and is effective in the treatment of positive, negative and depressive symptoms of schizophrenia and schizoaffective disorder. Ziprasidone 5–20 mg has been shown to be effective in acute psychosis, and better tolerated than haloperidol IM (n = 132, 3/7, Brook et al, J Clin Psychiatry 2000;**61**:933–41), superior to placebo on PANSS with placebo level EPS (n = 278, RCT, d/b, p/c, one year, Arato et al, Int Clin Psychopharmacol 2002;**17**:207–15) and effective for relapse prevention (n = 301, RCT, d/b, 28/52, Hirsch et al, J Clin Psychiatry 2002;**63**:516–23; n = 168, d/b, 196/52, Potkin et al, Int J Neuropsychopharmacol 2009;**12**:1233–48). Ziprasidone has been compared with clozapine in TRS, where it showed efficacy, but with less metabolic ADRs than clozapine (n = 147, RCT, d/b, p/c, 18/52, Sacchetti et al, Schizophr Res 2009;**110**:80–9). Cochrane concludes that ziprasidone is slightly less effective than amisulpride, olanzapine and risperidone but with low weight gain (s = 9, n = 3361, Komossa et al, Cochrane Database Syst Rev 2009;**4**:CD006627).

DEPOT AND LONG-ACTING INJECTIONS

The major advantage of depots is assured compliance and steady plasma levels, with associated and proven reduction in relapses, rehospitalisation and severity of relapse. There may also be some reduction in bioavailability problems (some people metabolise anti-psychotics extensively via the first-pass effect). Used properly, depots can lead to reduced relapses, stable therapeutic effects and better downward titration of doses to reduce the incidence of side-effects (Adams et al, Br J Psychiatry 2001;**179**:290–9; reviewed by McGorry, EBMH 2002;**5**:42). With CATIE's low retention rates, long-acting injections may help improve retention and reduce relapse, readmissions, brain tissue loss, and deterioration (Nasrallah, Acta Psychiatr Scand 2007;**115**:260–7). The major disadvantages include the impossibility of altering a dose if side-effects develop (e.g. dystonia, NMS), patients seeing depot administration as 'being controlled', having no control over or involvement in their treatment or, worse still, as being a punishment. Many users and carers are insufficiently educated about the pros and cons of depot administration. It is not enough just to prevent relapse with a depot.

Depot injections do, of course, also hurt, the pain declining over 10 days and this has a negative effect on patient attitude towards medication (n = 34, Bloch et al, J Clin Psychiatry 2001;**62**:855–9), although there is some evidence to the contrary (Walburn et al, Br J Psychiatry 2001;**179**:300–7). There is need for a meticulous (Z-tracking) injection technique (Cocoman and Murray, J Psychiatr Ment Health Nurs 2008;**15**:424–34).

Licensed UK depot/long-acting injection sites:*

Depot/LAI	Licensed IM routes
Flupentixol decanoate	Gluteal, lateral thigh
Fluphenazine decanoate	Gluteal
Fluspirilene	Gluteal, lateral thigh
Haloperidol decanoate	Gluteal
Olanzapine pamoate	Gluteal
Pipothiazine palmitate	Gluteal
Risperidone	Gluteal, deltoid
Zuclopentixol decanoate	Gluteal, lateral thigh

Reviews: overviews (Altamura et al, Drugs 2003;**3**:493–512; Kennedy and Mikhail, Lancet 2000;**356**:594).

Pharmacokinetics

The tables on pages 161–163 show the plasma levels for each depot as single doses (although these have been difficult to obtain and are not reliable), and as computer-generated profiles for multiple doses (based on single-dose profiles).

Depot and longer-acting injection pharmacokinetics

These graphs show the known plasma levels of the available longer-acting antipsychotic injections in the UK. The single dose kinetics are reasonably well-established for many of these preparations. The multiple-dose graphs are computer-generated as little or no data exists on long-term kinetics, with downward arrows indicating when injections are given. These graphs will, however, give *some* indication of the time to steady state, and the length of time before plasma levels fall to zero after a depot has been stopped, although half-lives tend to lengthen with chronic use. The 'y' axis units are not established for any of the multiple dose graphs, and there will of course be some inter-individual variation.

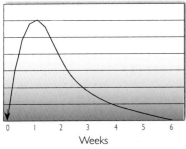

Flupentixol decanoate single dose

Weeks

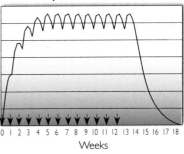

Flupentixol decanoate 1/52

Weeks

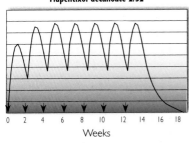

Flupentixol decanoate 2/52

Weeks

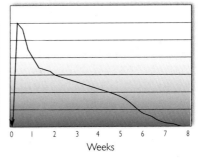

Fluphenazine decanoate single dose

Weeks

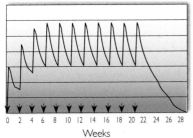

Fluphenazine decanoate 2/52

Weeks

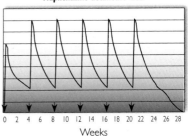

Fluphenazine decanoate 4/52

Weeks

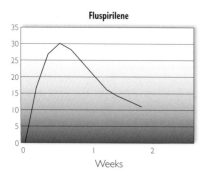

Fluspirilene

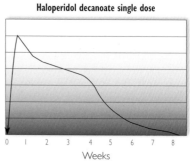

Haloperidol decanoate single dose

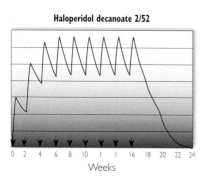

Haloperidol decanoate 2/52

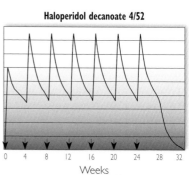

Haloperidol decanoate 4/52

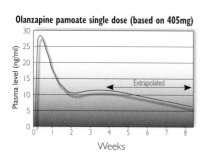

Olanzapine pamoate single dose (based on 405mg)

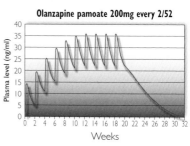

Olanzapine pamoate 200mg every 2/52

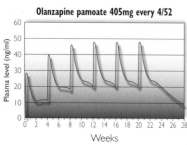

Olanzapine pamoate 405mg every 4/52

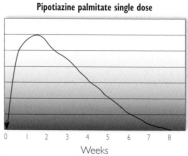

Pipotiazine palmitate single dose

Pipotiazine palmitate 2/52

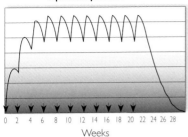

Weeks

Pipotiazine palmitate 4/52

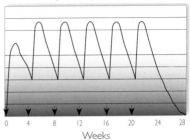

Weeks

Risperidone Consta single dose

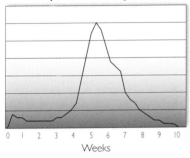

Weeks

Risperdal Consta 2/52

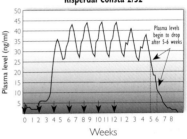

Plasma level (ng/ml)

Plasma levels begin to drop after 5-6 weeks

Weeks

Zuclopenthixol decanoate single dose

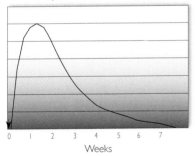

Weeks

Zuclopenthixol decanoate 1/52

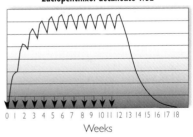

Weeks

Zuclopenthixol decanoate 2/52

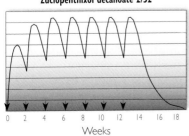

Weeks

Zuclopenthixol acetate single dose

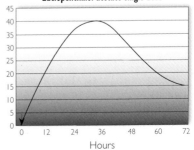

Hours

Flupentixol decanoate *
(e.g. Depixol®, Lundbeck)

Flupentixol is a dopamine specific thioxanthene antipsychotic (Kuhn et al, Fortschr Neurol Psychiatr 2000;**68**[Suppl 1]: S38–S41). It is contraindicated in people with circulatory collapse or depressed consciousness due to any cause (e.g. intoxication with alcohol or opiates)
- Duration of action = 3–4 weeks.
- Peak = 7–10 days.
- Rate limiting half-life = eight days (single dose), 17 days (multiple doses).
- Time to steady state = 10–12 weeks.

Fluphenazine decanoate
(e.g. Modecate®, Sanofi-Synthelabo)

Fluphenazine decanoate is a longer-acting phenothiazine and a four-week interval between injections is possible. The efficacy data is very limited, showing little difference between depots and orals (s = 70, n = 1892, RCT, David et al, Cochrane Database Syst Rev 2005;1:CD000307). Responders have been shown to have greatest improvement with fluphenazine levels above 1.0 ng/ml and doses above 0.2–0.25 mg/kg/d (n = 72, RCT, d/b, 4/52, Levinson et al, Am J Psychiatry 1995;**152**:765–71). Fluphenazine 25 mg every two or six weeks produces similar side-effects, efficacy and relapse rates, but with reduced drug exposure using the longer dosage interval (n = 50, RCT, 54/52, Carpenter et al, Am J Psychiatry 1999;**156**:412–8).
- Duration of action = 1–3 weeks.
- Peak = 6–48 hours.
- Rate-limiting half-life = 6–10 days (single doses), 14–100 days (multiple doses).
- Time to steady state = 6–12 weeks.

Fluspirilene
(e.g. Redeptin®, SmithKline French)

Fluspirilene is only available in the UK as an import, as a water-based weekly micro-crystalline injection. Cochrane concludes that it has no advantage over orals or other depots, albeit with limited data (s = 12, RCT, Abhijnhan et al, Cochrane Database Syst Rev 2007;1:CD001718).
- Duration of action = 1.5 weeks.
- Peak within two days.
- Rate limiting half-life = 7–9 days.

- Time to steady state = 5–6 weeks.

Haloperidol decanoate
(Haldol Decanoate ®, Janssen-Cilag)

Haloperidol decanoate is longer-acting and a four-week interval between injections is possible. An analysis suggests a maximal effect at 50 mg/4 weeks, with no evidence that doses above 100 mg/4 weeks have any additional effects (s = 13, Taylor, Psychiatr Bull 2005;**29**:104–7), e.g. rates of deterioration with 50–100 mg/month were not significantly greater in one study compared to 25 mg/month, and ADRs were possibly higher (n = 105, RCT, d/b, Kane et al, Am J Psychiatry 2002;**4**:554–60; review by Marois and Roy, EBMH 2002;**5**:113). It is best reserved for chronic relapsing schizophrenics responsive to haloperidol.
- Duration of action = six weeks.
- Peak = 3–9 days.
- Rate limiting half-life = 18–21 days (single + chronic).
- Time to steady state = 10–12 weeks at monthly dosing.

Olanzapine pamoate (Zypadhera®, Zyprexa Relprevv®, Lilly) *

Olanzapine pamoate is licensed long-acting formulation for deep IM gluteal injection in people who have previously received oral doses. Olanzapine pamoate releases olanzapine slowly over approximately 6–8 weeks after each injection, so care needed is after discontinuation. Oral supplementation is not recommended, e.g. in acute TRS, olanzapine pamoate every two or four weeks was more effective than placebo, despite no use of additional oral supplementation (RCT, d/b, p/c, 8/52, Lauriello et al, J Clin Psychiatry 2008;**69**:790–9). However, if supplementation is used, it should be the equivalent of a maximum of 20 mg/d (all preparations) and the 'loading dose' should be reduced after two months (n = 9, Mamo et al, Neuropsychopharmacology 2008;**33**:298–304). Doses should be as per the chart for the first two months, then reduced.
- Duration of action = 6 weeks?
- Peak = 4 days
- Half-life = 30 days.
- Time to steady state = 3 months.

Dose conversion:

Oral dose	Starting dose (initial 2/12)	Maintenance dose (after 2/12)
10 mg/d	210 mg 2/52 or 405 mg 4/52	150 mg 2/52 or 300 mg 4/52
15 mg/d	300 mg 2/52	210 mg 2/52 or 405 mg 4/52
20 mg/d	300 mg 2/52	300 mg 2/52

Post-injection syndrome: There have been reports of unpredictable (around one in 1500 injections and in around 1.4% patients) and idiosyncratic excessive sedation, resembling olanzapine overdose (Citrome, *Int J Clin Pract* 2009; **63**:140-50) 1–6 hours post-injection (usually one hour) with full recovery within 24–72 hours. To avoid adverse consequences, after injection the patient must be observed in a healthcare facility by appropriately qualified personnel for at least three hours for signs and symptoms of apparent overdose, e.g. sedation (mild to coma), delirium, EPSE, dysarthria, ataxia, aggression and convulsions.

Review: * general (Citrome, *Int J Clin Pract* 2009;**62**:140–50).

Paliperidone palmitate (Invega Sustenna®)*
Paliperidone palmitate (n = 1795, Samtani et al, *Clin Pharmacokinet* 2009;**48**:585–600)is licensed in USA for schizophrenia and a UK license may be granted in 2010–11.

Pipothiazine palmitate
(Piportil®, Sanofi-Aventis)
Pipothiazine is a piperidine phenothiazine marketed in the UK as the palmitate. Cochrane concludes that although better data is needed, pipothiazine is a viable antipsychotic choice (Dinesh et al, *Cochrane Database Syst Rev* 2004; **4**:CD001720).

- Duration of action = 4–6 weeks.
- Peak = 9–10 days.
- Rate limiting half-life = 14–21 days.
- Time to steady state = 8–12 weeks.

Risperidone
(Risperdal Consta®, Janssen-Cilag) *
This novel, long-acting injection uses risperidone molecules in a synthetic and absorbable polymer microsphere base suspended in water. It is licensed for schizophrenic and other psychoses. Release: The initial dose is 25–37.5 mg fortnightly, with a maximum of 50 mg every two weeks. Plasma levels are stable after 3–4 injections and maintained for 4–5 weeks after the last injection, then decline rapidly. D2 receptor studies show risperidone 25, 50 and 75 mg fortnightly are in the range found in patients effectively treated with 2–6 mg/d oral risperidone (n = 13, Gefvert et al, *Int J Neuropsychopharmacol* 2005;**8**:27–36; see also Love and Conley, *Am J Health Syst Pharm* 2004; **61**:1792–800), although 75 mg had higher side-effects (n = 400, RCT, d/b, p/c, 12/52, Kane et al, *Am J Psychiatry* 2003;**160**:1125–32). Where possible, patients should be pre-treated with risperidone orally for at least a few days before the injection is commenced to rule out any severe EPS, hypotensive or other idiosyncratic reactions. Oral cover may be needed for the first 3–4 weeks, then tapered during weeks 4–5. Since steady state occurs about 6–8 weeks after each dose change, some have recommended dose increases only every eight weeks (Knox and Stimmel, *Clin Ther* 2004; **26**:1994–2002). There may be a small release of risperidone in the first few days from the surface of the granules and transient EPSE may occur after one day (n = 3, Adamou and Hale, *Am J Psychiatry* 2004;**161**:576–7). Elimination is complete 7–8 weeks after the last injection. The vials must be stored at 2–8°C, although can be kept at < 25°C for up to seven days, no longer, or be put back in a fridge again. The injection can now be given in the deltoid muscle, with a specific needle.

Efficacy: There have been several published reviews of Consta outcomes (e.g. n = 541 [c = 298], 12/12, Lindenmayer et al, *Eur Neuropsychopharmacol* 2007;**17**:138–44). Risperidone injection 25–50 mg every 2/52 was as effective as olanzapine oral 5–20 mg/d (n = 377, RCT, open, one year; Keks et al, *Br J Psychiatry* 2007; **191**:131–9; MS) and more effective than zuclopenthixol depot (n = 115, RCT, open, 6/12, Rubio et al, *Can J Psychiatry* 2006;**51**:531–9). Of 65% of patients completing one year on Consta, 5% dropped out because of ADRs, and 25% suffered ADRs (n = 615, open, 12/12, Fleischacker et al, *J Clin Psychiatry* 2003;**64**:1250–7; see also n = 347[c = 243], open, 12/12, Rossi *et al*, *Hum Psychopharmacol* 2009;**24**:574–83). In a retrospective case note review, a mirror-image analysis of Consta use showed it resulted in a 58% retention in treatment at one year, and roughly halved readmission rates and stays (n = 67, three years, Niaz and Haddad, *Acta Psychiatr Scand* 2007;**116**:36–46), and in clinically stable patients, Consta 25 mg and 50 mg were effective, produced modest improvements and relapse and readmission rates were low for 25 mg (21.6% and 10% respectively) and 50 mg (14.9% and 6%) (n = 324, RCT, d/b, one year, Simpson *et al*, *J Clin Psychiatry* 2006;**67**:1194–1203). Optimum efficacy may take many months, e.g. half of those with a good outcome at 6/12 had not yet improved by 3/12 and oral doses may be needed longer than the first 3/52 (n = 50, naturalistic follow-up, Paton and Okocha, *Psychiatr Bull* 2004;**28**:12–4, IS). There may be a significant effect on negative symptoms when used for prolonged period of time (n = 842[c = 631], 6/12, Curtis *et al*, *J Psychopharmacol* 2008;**22**:254–61).

Factors predicting response: There have been many attempts to identify those likely to respond better. These include previous poor concordance and older people (n = 250, 6/12, Taylor *et al*, *Int J Neuropsychopharmacol* 2006; **9**:685–94).

Dose and switching: Switching to Consta can be done by abrupt switch from other depots without oral transition (open, 12/52, Turner *et al*, *Int Clin Psychopharmacol* 2004;**19**:241–9). Risperidone levels may be lower with Consta than oral, but there is also a lower 9-OH risperidone:risperidone ratio with Consta, which may indicate higher depot doses are needed (n = 78+82, Nesväg *et al*, *Acta Psychiatr Scand* 2006;**114**:21–6) and 25 mg/fortnight may be insufficient since it provides low plasma levels and possibly sub-therapeutic in vivo D2 occupancies (editorial by Taylor, *Acta Psychiatr Scand* 2006;**114**:1–2).

A careful switching study concluded:
- oral dose < 3 mg/d = Consta 25 mg 2/52
- oral 3–5 mg/d = Consta 37.5 mg 2/52
- oral > 5 mg/d = Consta 50 mg 2/52

(n = 50[c = 45], RCT, s/b, 48/52, Bai *et al*, *J Clin Psychiatry* 2007;**68**:1218–25).

Reviews: general (Rainer, *Neuropsychiatr Dis Treat* 2008;**4**:919–27; Möller, *Drugs* 2007;**67**: 1541–66; Niaz and Haddad, *Acta Psychiatr Scand* 2007;**116**:36–46; Ehter and Fuller, *Ann Pharmacother* 2004;**38**:2122–7).

Zuclopenthixol acetate
(Clopixol Acuphase®, Lundbeck)

Zuclopenthixol acetate is available as 'Clopixol Acuphase' in the UK. 50–150 mg as a single dose provides reduction in psychotic symptoms over about 78 hours. The maximum cumulative dose is 400 mg over two weeks, with no more than four injections. Cochrane concludes that there is inadequate data on Acuphase and no convincing evidence either way in APE compared to IM haloperidol (Fenton *et al*, *Cochrane Database Syst Rev* 2004;**2**:CD00525). See also 1.1.

- Duration of action = 2–3 days.
- Peak = 24–40 hours.
- Rate limiting half-life = 32 hours +/- 7.

Zuclopenthixol decanoate
(Clopixol®, Lundbeck)

This is an established antipsychotic which has also been used in high dose in aggression, particularly in learning disabilities and forensic patients but is not indicated for this.

- Duration of action = 2–4 weeks.
- Peak = 4–9 days.
- Rate limiting half-life = 17–21 days (multiple doses).
- Time to steady state = 10–12 weeks.

+ Combinations

Polypharmacy with antipsychotics falls into three main categories:

- two or more drugs of the same class
- multiclass (two drugs in different classes at full dose)
- adjunctive and augmentation (low dose of one with a standard dose of another).

Appropriate reasons for the use of antipsychotic combinations include:

- Failure to respond to clozapine.
- Poor clozapine tolerance, with a second drug as augmentation of a low clozapine dose.

- As augmentation in clozapine partial response.
- Patients unwilling to stop an old drug or refusing to try clozapine.
- During a switch from one antipsychotic to another.
- When discontinuing a depot poses an unacceptable risk, e.g. forensic patients.
- As a temporary measure during an acute exacerbation of illness.

Inappropriate reasons for the use of antipsychotic combinations include:

- Confusing a sedative effect with an antipsychotic effect.
- Not waiting long enough for an antipsychotic to work (i.e. at least six weeks) before making changes.
- As a substitute for failing to plan and communicate a switch, which is then never fully completed.
- Where clinical improvement occurs before a switch is completed, and the clinician 'quits while ahead' rather than risking completing the change.
- Using high doses to make up for inadequate resources and environment.

Despite widespread use of combinations (with increased ADRs and possibly reduced outcomes; n = 1043, McCue et al, J Clin Psychiatry 2003; 64:984–9), there are only a very few RCTs of combination antipsychotics in schizophrenia and in a retrospective case-control study, multiple antipsychotics were associated with a major increase in drug exposure, adverse events and time in hospital, but with no apparent clinical gain compared to monotherapy (n = 70 pairs, Centorrino et al, Am J Psychiatry 2004; 161:700–6). A critical review concludes there is some evidence for sulpiride, lamotrigine and E-EPA as clozapine augmentation (s = 11, n = 270, Kontaxakis et al, Eur Psychiatry 2005; 20:409–15). Combinations should thus only be used once standard monotherapies have been found inadequate, and then with carefully monitored outcomes (clinical and adverse) and discontinued if no clear advantage is seen.
Review: * editorial review of the lack of evidence and trials of combinations (Stahl et al, Acta Psychiatr Scand 2004; 110:241–2; Zink et al, Curr Opin Psychiatry 2010; 23:103–11).

Clozapine combinations & augmentation *

A recent meta-analysis was unable to show any short-term benefit from clozapine augmentation over 16 weeks, but longer-term trials are needed (s = 10, n = 522, Taylor and Smith, Acta Psychiatr Scand 2009; 119:419–25), but Cochrane concludes that there is insufficient data to conclude anything (s = 3, Cipriani et al, Cochrane Database Syst Rev 2009; 3:CD006324).
Reviews: * thorough (Chan and Sweeting, J Psychopharmacol 2007; 21:657–64; Barbui et al, Schizophr Bull 2008; 35:458–68).

Clozapine + aripiprazole

Although there have been many case reports and series of aripiprazole combined with clozapine (e.g. n = 11[c = 11], open, 3/12, Ziegenbein et al, Clin Drug Invest 2006; 26:117–24), a recent RCT showed aripiprazole augmentation of clozapine to slightly improve negative symptoms but did not lead to significant improvement in total symptoms of schizophrenia (n = 62, RCT, d/b, p/c, Chang et al, J Clin Psychiatry 2008; 69:720-31), but interestingly did not lead to deterioration either. Other open studies include aripiprazole 15 mg/d augmentation of clozapine significantly improving all symptom measures (except PANSS positive) with no increase in ADRs (n = 27[c = 23], open, 16/52, Mitsonis et al, Prog Neuropsychopharmacol Biol Psychiatry 2007; 31:373–7) and weight loss, reduction in clozapine dosage and improved symptoms (n = 26, Karunakaran et al, J Psychopharmacol 2007; 21:453–56).
Review: * Englisch and Zink, Prog Neuropsychopharmacol Biol Psychiatry 2008; 32:1386–92.

Clozapine + amisulpride (see also sulpiride)

Combining a specific D2-blocker with clozapine is a well-known strategy. There are some open studies (but no RCT yet), e.g. amisulpride significantly improved response to clozapine without significant additional side-effects (n = 33[c = 28], open, 6/12, Munro et al, Acta Psychiatr Scand 2004; 110:292–8) and 80% improved with amisulpride 700 mg/d (range 520–980 mg/d) as adjunctive therapy (n = 56[c = 50], s/b, 8/52, Genç et al, Adv Ther 2007; 24:1–13).

Clozapine + anticholinesterases

See 1.23.3 for the effect on cognition.

Clozapine + gingko biloba *

In TRS, addition of Gingko biloba to clozapine had some beneficial effects on negative symptoms, but not positive or overall symptoms (n=42, p/c, 12/52, Doruk et al, Int Clin Psychopharmacol 2008;**23**:223–7).

Clozapine + lamotrigine *

A meta-analysis of lamotrigine augmentation of clozapine concluded lamotrigine was superior to placebo on primary and secondary outcome measures with a clinically meaningful benefit (s=5, n=161, RCT, p/c, 10–24/52, Tiihonen et al, Schizophr Res 2009;**109**:10–4).

Clozapine + mirtazapine

Mirtazapine augmentation of clozapine has improved negative symptoms (especially apathy and anhedonia) and BPRS scores (n= 24, RCT, d/b, p/c, 8/52, Zoccali et al, Int Clin Psychopharmacol 2004;**19**:71–6).

Clozapine + olanzapine

One patient responded to clozapine 100mg/d and olanzapine 10mg/d when individually neither were satisfactory (n=1, Rhoads, J Clin Psychiatry 2000;**61**:678–80).

Clozapine + quetiapine

Although quetiapine has some effect as augmentation of clozapine, it may be less effective than amisulpride (n=56[c=50], s/b, 8/52, Genç et al, Adv Ther 2007;**24**:1–13). Weight loss has been reported when 25% of the clozapine dose was converted to quetiapine (1 mg clozapine:2 mg quetiapine) (n=65, open, 10/12, Reinstein et al, Clin Drug Invest 1999;**18**:99–104).

Clozapine + risperidone *

An RCT has shown risperidone 4–6mg/d to improve sub-optimal clozapine response (n=40, RCT, d/b, p/c, 12/52, Josiassen et al, Am J Psychiatry 2005;**162**:130–6), although a moderate (four-fold) rise in prolactin levels can occur (n=40, open, Henderson et al, J Clin Psychiatry 2001;**62**:605–8). However,

addition of risperidone 3mg/d to clozapine had no significant effect in symptoms of severe schizophrenia (n=68, RCT, p/c, d/b, 8+18/52, Honer et al, N Engl J Med 2006;**354**:472–82), and up to 6mg/d made no difference to psychopathology or quality of life compared to placebo (n=30, RCT, p/c, d/b, 6/52, Yagcioglu et al, J Clin Psychiatry 2005;**66**:63–72). A critical review concludes the evidence is encouraging, with the best response with lower risperidone dose and longer duration (s=15[2=RCT], n=86, Kontaxakis et al, Eur Arch Psychiatry Clin Neurosci 2006;**256**:350–5).

Clozapine + sulpiride

In the first RCT of combined antipsychotics, clozapine and sulpiride produced a substantially greater improvement than clozapine alone in TRS (n=24, RCT, Shiloh et al, Br J Psychiatry 1997;**171**:569–73), although the two study groups had some initial differences.

Clozapine + ziprasidone *

In TRS, clozapine augmentation by ziprasidone or risperidone was equally effective and well-tolerated, with slight QT prolongation with ziprasidone and prolactin rise with risperidone (n=24, open, RCT, 6/52, Zink et al, J Psychopharmacol 2009;**23**:305–14).

Other antipsychotic combinations and augmentation

Amisulpride + aripiprazole *

There is a case of worsening psychosis when aripiprazole was added to amisulpride (n=1, Adan-Manes and Garcia-Parajua, J Clin Pharm Ther 2009;**34**:245–6).

Amisulpride + risperidone or ziprasidone

In a small trial, 80% improved on the combination with amisulpride at a mean dose of 693mg/d (n=15, open, Lerner et al, Clin Neuropharmacol 2005;**28**:66–71).

Olanzapine + quetiapine

This combination was completely successful in a patient with raised prolactin intolerant of clozapine, with no elevation of prolactin (n=1, Dunkley and Reveley, J Psychopharmacol 2005;**19**:97–101).

Olanzapine + sulpiride

Sulpiride 600 mg/d augmentation of partially effective olanzapine had no effect on PANSS but significantly improved depressive symptoms (n = 17, RCT, 8/52, Kotler *et al*, *Int Clin Psychopharmacol* 2004;**19**:23–6).

Risperidone + olanzapine *

Risperidone plus olanzapine was successful in TRS resistant to sequential olanzapine, quetiapine and risperidone monotherapy, and was well tolerated albeit with increased side-effects (e.g. n = 17 [c = 17], open, 8/52, Suzuki *et al*, *Hum Psychopharmacol* 2008; **23**:455–63).

● **Augmentation** (with drugs with no intrinsic antipsychotic activity)

Anticholinesterases

See *1.23.3*.

Benzodiazepines

Short-term use may reduce anxiety, tension and insomnia and high doses may have some tranquillising effects. They may also allow lower doses of antipsychotics to be used, as high doses of antipsychotics are often used for their additional sedative properties, e.g. in psychotic agitation. Cochrane concludes that there is little or no evidence that BDZs are useful as monotherapy or even adjunctive therapy in schizophrenia, although widely used to augment antipsychotics in acute states (s = 31, n = 2000, Volz *et al*, *Cochrane Database Syst Rev* 2007;**1**:CD006391). See also 'Acute psychiatric emergency' (*1.1*).

Carbamazepine

Carbamazepine has been used in addition to antipsychotics to improve behaviour in over-active or aggressive schizophrenics but Cochrane could not recommend carbamazepine for routine use, either as monotherapy, augmentation or maintenance (s = 10, n = 258, RCT, Leucht *et al*, *Cochrane Database Syst Rev* 2007;**3**:CD001258). A related systematic review and meta-analysis of carbamazepine augmentation in schizophrenia failed to show any clinically significant positive effect (s = 10, n = 283,

Leucht *et al*, *J Clin Psychiatry* 2002;**63**:218–24). Remember that carbamazepine will induce CYP3A4 and reduce the plasma levels of many antipsychotics.

Chinese herbal medicines

A systematic review and meta-analysis suggested that monotherapy was not effective but that adjunctive use might help some outcomes (s = 7, RCTs, Rathbone *et al*, *Br J Psychiatry* 2007;**190**:379–84; probably an inappropriate conclusion, comment by Werneke, *EBMH* 2008;**11**:19).

Cicloserin (D-cycloserine)

Cicloserin is a partial agonist of a glutamate receptor sub-type and addition of 50 mg/d to typicals, risperidone and olanzapine produced a significant reduction in negative symptoms (n = 24, d/b, p/c, c/o, 6/52, Heresco-Levy *et al*, *Am J Psychiatry* 2002;**159**:480–2), supporting the view that glutamate function may be important in schizophrenia. However, not all data is positive (e.g. n = 10, Goff *et al*, *Am J Psychiatry* 1996;**153**:1628–30).

Cox-2 inhibitors

Celecoxib 400 mg/d added to risperidone in resistant schizophrenia may produce a significant reduction in PANSS compared to risperidone monotherapy (n = 50, RCT, d/b, p/c, 5/52, Muller *et al*, *Eur Arch Psychiatry Clin Neurosci* 2004;**254**:14–22) and reduce EPSEs (n = 60, RCT, d/b, p/c, 8/52, Akhondzadeh *et al*, *Schizophr Res* 2007;**90**:179–85).

Cyproheptadine

Adding cyproheptadine 24 mg/d to haloperidol 30 mg/d has significantly reduced negative symptoms (n = 30, RCT, Akhondzadeh *et al*, *J Clin Pharm Ther* 1999;**24**:49).

DHEA (dehydroepiandrosterone)

DHEA 100 mg/d produced significant improvements as adjunctive therapy in negative, depressive and anxiety symptoms of schizophrenia, although Cochrane concludes that the available studies are inconclusive and unconvincing (s = 3, n = 126, Elias and Kumar, *Cochrane Database Syst Rev* 2007;**3**:CD006197).

Dipyridamole

Dipyridamole (75 mg/d) and haloperidol (16–20 mg/d) was superior to haloperidol alone in schizophrenia, possibly via an effect on the interaction between the adenosine and dopamine systems (n = 30, RCT, Akhondzadeh et al, J Clin Pharm Ther 2000; **25**:131–8).

ECT

ECT plus antipsychotics combination may be beneficial for positive (but not negative) symptoms of schizophrenia, with a 55% response rate and has a possible role early in an acute exacerbation of chronic schizophrenia (n = 160, Chanpattana and Chakrabhand, Psychiatry Res 2001;**105**:107–15).

Folate *

Although there have been some reports, a review suggests that the data is inadequate, inconsistent and unconvincing (s = 7, n = 325 + 560, Muntjewerff and Blom, Prog Neuropsychopharmacol Biol Psychiatry 2005;**29**: 1133–9), although low folate levels have been reported in schizophrenia (n = 91, Goff et al, Am J Psychiatry 2004; **161**:1705–8).

Ginkgo biloba (see also clozapine)

Ginkgo biloba has enhanced the effectiveness of haloperidol and reduced EPS compared to placebo (n = 109, RCT, d/b, p/c, 12/52, Zhang et al, J Clin Psychiatry 2001;**62**:878–83; comment by Knable, EBMH 2002;**5**:90).

Glycine

High-dose glycine (0.8 g/kg/d) as add-on to olanzapine or risperidone significantly reduced negative symptoms by 23% and improved cognitive function (n = 17, RCT, d/b, p/c, c/o, 6/52, Heresco-Levy et al, Biol Psychiatry 2004; **15**:165–71), particularly in people with low pre-treatment plasma glycine levels. High-dose glycine added to antipsychotics was effective with no increase in antipsychotic levels (n = 12, RCT, Javitt et al, Int J Neuropsychopharmacol 2001;**4**:385–91), although some studies are negative (n = 30, d/b, p/c, Evins et al, Am J Psychiatry 2000;**157**:826–8).

Lamotrigine (see clozapine augmentation) *

Evidence for augmentation (especially of

clozapine) is considered reasonable, but monotherapy lacking. Cochrane concludes that the available data on lamotrigine for schizophrenia is poor and no global response is detectable (s = 5, n = 537, Premkumar and Pick, Cochrane Database Syst Rev 2006;**4**: CD005962).

Reviews: concise (Thomas et al, Int J Neuropsychopharmacol 2005;**8**:1–3), mode of action (Large et al, Psychopharmacology [Berl] 2005; **6**:1–22).

Mirtazapine *

Mirtazapine was clearly and robustly superior to placebo on almost all measures of improvement as an adjunct to antipsychotics in TRS (n = 39, RCT, d/b, 6/52, Joffe et al, Schizophr Res 2009;**108**:245–51), but had no efficacy on PANSS scores as an adjunct to atypicals (n = 40, RCT, d/b, p/c, 6/52, Berk et al, Hum Psychopharmacol 2009;**24**:233–8). Visual hallucinations have ceased with mirtazapine (n = 1, Koethe et al, Pharmacopsychiatry 2007; **40**:82–3).

Ondansetron *

There are now two RCTs showing efficacy as an adjunctive therapy. Ondansetron 8 mg/d significantly improved negative symptoms and general symptoms as an adjunct to risperidone (n = 30, RCT, d/b, p/c, >8/52, Akhondzadeh et al, Schizophr Res 2009;**107**:206–12) and 8 mg/d improved PANSS and reduced EPSE in people with TRS on haloperidol 4–30 mg/d, (n = 121, RCT, d/b, p/c, 12/52, Zhang et al, Schizophr Res 2006;**88**:102–10).

Oxcarbazepine

Oxcarbazepine has been used as an adjunctive treatment in acute schizophrenia (n = 6, open, Leweke et al, Am J Psychiatry 2004;**161**:1130–1).

Pergolide

Pergolide as an adjunct to partially effective amisulpride has improved negative and depressive symptoms without affecting positive symptoms or increasing ADRs (n = 1, Roesch-Ely et al, Pharmacopsychiatry 2006;**39**:115–6).

Selegiline

Low-dose oral selegiline as antipsychotic

augmentation may improve negative symptoms of schizophrenia (n = 67, d/b, p/c, 12/52, Bodkin et al, Am J Psychiatry 2005;**162**:388–90).

D-serine

D-serine is a full agonist at glycine NMDA receptors and, when used at 30 mg/kg/d as adjunct to olanzapine or risperidone, significantly improved PANSS, 20% reduction in BRS in 35% of patients, with no detrimental adverse effects (n = 39, RCT, d/b, p/c, c/o, 6/52, Heresco-Levy et al, Biol Psychiatry 2005;**15**:577–85).

SSRIs

The largest meta-analysis of trials of SSRIs as add-on therapy for negative symptoms of schizophrenia concluded that there was no evidence to support this strategy, although there may be a modest effect in 'chronic patients' (s = 11, n = 667, Sepehry et al, J Clin Psychiatry 2007;**68**:604–10; comment by Lecrubier, EBMH 2007;**10**:113). Citalopram has been trialled successfully for the depressive/anxiety symptoms of PANSS (RCT, Taiminen et al, Int Clin Psychopharmacol 1997;**12**:31–5) and improving subjective well-being, but addition of citalopram 40 mg/d to atypicals had no effect on any clinical or cognition measures (n = 19, RCT, p/c, c/o, 24/52, Friedman et al, J Clin Psychopharmacol 2005;**25**:237–42). Fluoxetine 20 mg/d significantly improved PANSS in open studies of TRS (e.g. n = 9, open, 6/52, Goff et al, Am J Psychiatry 1990;**147**:492–4), but may increase EPS and was ineffective as an adjunct to clozapine (n = 33, open, p/c, 8/52, Buchanan et al, Am J Psychiatry 1996;**153**:1625–7). Fluvoxamine was ineffective as augmentation of risperidone-resistant schizophrenia (n = 30, open, 12/52, Takashi et al, Hum Psychopharmacol 2002;**17**:95–8) and must only be used with clozapine with extreme care (see 4.2.3). Paroxetine (n = 8, open, 30/12, Jockers-Scherubl et al, J Clin Psychiatry 2001;**62**:573) and sertraline (n = 26, d/b, p/c, 8/52, Mulholland et al, J Psychopharmacol 2003;**17**:107–12) may improve negative or depressive symptoms.

Topiramate *

Topiramate 300 mg/d as antipsychotic adjuncts in TRS has reduced PANSS scores in some (n = 26, RCT, d/b, p/c, c/o, 2×12/52, Tiihonen et al, J Clin Psychiatry 2005;**66**:1012–5, IS), particularly for negative symptoms and reducing weight gain (n = 32, RCT, d/b, p/c, Afshar et al, J Psychopharmacol 2009;**23**:157–62). However, topiramate had no effect on BPRS when added to clozapine, risperidone, olanzapine or flupentixol (n = 9, open, Dursun and Deakin, J Psychopharmacol 2001;**15**:297–301), and significant deterioration has been reported so it should not be used with clozapine as anticonvulsant cover (n = 5, open, Millson et al, Am J Psychiatry 2002;**159**:675; n = 1, Hofer et al, J Clin Psychiatry 2003;**64**:1267–8).

Valproate

Reviews have concluded that there is no proven advantage for valproate augmentation in schizophrenia. Some studies show inconsistent benefit but that it may be useful in acute management (Basan et al, Schizophr Res 2004;**70**:33–7; Basan and Leucht, Cochrane Database Syst Rev 2004;1:4028; see also Citrome, Psychopharmacol Bull 2003;**37**[Suppl 2]:S74–S88). Valproate as an adjunct to risperidone or olanzapine for acute exacerbation of schizophrenia has resulted in an earlier response of psychotic symptoms (n = 249, RCT, d/b, Casey et al, Neuropsychopharmacol 2003;**28**:182–92). Cochrane concludes that there is no data to support or refute the use of valproate as monotherapy in schizophrenia (s = 7, n = 519, Schwarz et al, Cochrane Database Syst Rev 2008;**3**:CD004028).

● Unlicensed/some efficacy

Estradiol/estrogen *

Estrogen may have specific antipsychotic-like effects in schizophrenic women (n = 125, Bergemann et al, Psychol Med 2007;**37**:1427–36), e.g. 100 mcg estradiol significantly reduced positive and general psychopathology, suggesting a possible role (n = 102, RCT, p/c, 28/7, Kulkarni et al, Arch Gen Psychiatry 2008; **65**:955–60), e.g. estrogen as an adjunct to haloperidol significantly reduced positive and general symptoms in women of child-bearing age with chronic schizophrenia (n = 32, RCT, d/b, p/c, 8/52, Akhondzadeh et al, Prog Neuropsychopharmacol Biol Psychiatry 2003;**27**:1007–12). Transdermal estrogen was, however, unable to prevent relapse of postnatal affective psychosis when started within 48 hours of delivery (n=29, open, 12/7, Kumar et al, *J Clin Psychiatry* 2003;**64**:112–8).

■ Unlicensed/possible efficacy

Bromocriptine

It has been speculated that increasing some dopaminergic function may improve negative symptoms of schizophrenia. Bromocriptine (n=6, open, Levi-Minzi et al, *Compr Psychiatry* 1991;**32**:210–6) may decrease negative symptoms, at least in some patient sub-groups.

Betel nut

Male high-consumption betel nut (an anti-muscarinic) chewers with schizophrenia have significantly milder positive symptoms than low users (n=65, Sullivan et al, *Am J Psychiatry* 2007;**164**:670).

Flunarizine *

Flunarizine has some dopamine-blocking properties, and has been shown to be as effective as haloperidol and, with a half-life of 2–7 weeks, could have a potential role as a long-acting oral antipsychotic (n=70, RCT, d/b, 12/52, Bisol et al, *J Clin Psychiatry* 2008; **69**:1572–9).

Lithium

Lithium-responsive psychosis can occur and may be familial and is perhaps genetically distinct from the bulk of schizophrenias. A meta-analysis has concluded that although a few studies show some efficacy of lithium in schizophrenia, the overall results are inconclusive (n=611, s=20, Leucht et al, *J Clin Psychiatry* 2004;**65**:177–86) and Cochrane agrees that lithium is ineffective as a sole agent, but may potentially be useful in a few patients (n=611, s=20, Leucht et al, *Cochrane Database Syst Rev* 2003;**3**:CD003834; review by Bender and Dittmann-Balcar, *EBMH* 2004;**7**:104). Lithium augmentation of clozapine may provide additional clinical benefit in schizoaffective but not schizophrenic patients (n=20, p/c, 4/52, Small et al, *J Clin Psychopharmacol* 2003; **23**:223–8).

Melatonin

Melatonin 3 mg/d may be useful as a hypnotic in schizophrenia (see insomnia, n=40, RCT, d/b, p/c, 15/7, Kumar et al, *J Clin Psychiatry* 2007;**68**:237–41), but not in those with better sleep efficiency (n=19, RCT, c/o, p/c, Shamir et al, *J Clin Psychiatry* 2000;**61**:373–7).

Minocycline

There are cases of acute schizophrenia with predominantly catatonic symptoms responding to minocycline (n=2, Miyaoka et al, *Prog Neuropsychopharmacol Biol Psychiatry* 2007;**31**:304–7).

Omega-3 fatty acids

There is some evidence for abnormal phospholipid metabolism in schizophrenia, and trials with PUVAs have produced inconsistent but usually favourable findings. There may be a bell-shaped response curve, with 2 g the optimum dose and 4 g and higher possibly counter-productive (Horrobin, *Am J Psychiatry* 2003;**160**:188–9). E-EPA (ethyl-eicosapentaenoic acid) may be effective as adjunctive therapy for persistent psychotic symptoms (n=40, RCT, 12/52, Emsley et al, *Am J Psychiatry* 2002;**159**:1696–8), e.g. patients with schizophrenia may be able to improve their general symptoms by taking a supplement that combines essential polyunsaturated fatty acids (EPUFAs) with antioxidants (n=73, 4/12, Arvindaksham et al, *Schizophr Res* 2003;**62**:195–204). A small open study of adjunctive omega-3 fatty acids and vitamins E and C to haloperidol suggested significantly improved symptoms on all rating scales, particularly on reduced akathisia (n=17, open, Sivrioglu et al, *Prog Neuropsychopharmacol Biol Psychiatry* 2007; **31**:1493–9). However, omega-3 fatty acids have been shown to be ineffective in treating residual symptoms of schizophrenia (n=87, RCT, 16/52, Fenton et al, *Am J Psychiatry* 2001; **158**:2071–4).

Tetrabenazine

Tetrabenazine has been used for the treatment of psychoses and psychoneuroses but the high incidence of side-effects makes this a relatively unsuitable drug.

◆ Others

Other drugs that have been tried include azathioprine (n = 1, Levine, *Lancet* 1994; **344**:59–60), high dose beta-blockers (propranolol: *Lancet* 1980;ii:627–8; nadolol up to 120mg/d; *Clin Pharm* 1989;**8**:132–5), clonidine as augmentation (*Br J Psychiatry* 1988;**152**:293), calcium-channel blockers (*Am J Psychiatry* 1992;**149**:1615; *Drug Intell Clin Pharm* 1990;**24**:838–40), dexamfetamine (van Kammen and Bornow, *Int Clin Psychopharmacol* 1988;**3**:111–21), famotidine (review by Martinez, *Ann Pharmacother* 1999;**33**:742–7), levodopa (*Am J Psychiatry* 1988;**145**:1180), naltrexone/naloxone (Welch and Thompson, *J Clin Pharm Ther* 1994;**19**:279–83) and prednisone (n = 1, Cohen et al, *Lancet* 1996; **347**:1228).

□ No efficacy

Ayurvedic medicine

Ayurvedic medicine may have some effects but there is inadequate data to draw any conclusions (s = 3, n = 250, Agarwal et al, *Cochrane Database Syst Rev* 2007;**4**:CD006867).

Buspirone

Buspirone has various receptor activities, e.g. 5-HT$_{1A}$ partial antagonism and dopamine antagonism but exacerbation of psychosis has been reported.

Caffeine

Excess caffeine consumption can present as psychosis, increasing arousal and may have a psychotogenic effect, but moderate use probably has little effect on anxiety, depression and psychosis (e.g. n = 26, RCT, d/b, c/o, Mayo et al, *Br J Psychiatry* 1993;**162**:543–5).

Cannabidiol

In a small case series in TRS, only one showed mild improvement with cannabidiol, the others showing none (n = 3, 35/7, Zuardi et al, *J Psychopharmacol* 2006;**20**:683–6).

Cannabis *

Cochrane concludes that there is insufficient evidence to support or refute the use of cannabis to treat schizophrenia (s = 1, RCT, Rathbone et al, *Cochrane Database Syst Rev* 2008;**3**:CD004837).

Creatine

Adjunctive creatine 5g/d had no effect on cognitive function or symptoms (n = 12, RCT, d/b, p/c, c/o, 3/12, Kaptsan et al, *J Clin Psychiatry* 2007;**68**:881–4).

Hypnosis

There is no evidence for the efficacy of hypnosis in schizophrenia, although it is apparently as tolerable as Sibelius after four weeks. I felt you ought to know (Izquierdo et al, *Cochrane Database Syst Rev* 2007;**4**:CD004160).

Methylphenidate

Bolus IV methylphenidate has been used to induce an exacerbation of symptoms in an attempt to predict those people most likely to relapse when antipsychotics are discontinued (mentioned in Klein and Wender, *Arch Gen Psychiatry* 1995;**52**:429–33).

Memantine *

Memantine 20mg/d was ineffective on all primary and secondary measures as an adjunct to antipsychotics in schizophrenia (n = 138, RCT, d/b, p/c, 8/52, Lieberman et al, *Neuropsychopharmacology* 2009;**34**:1322–9).

Nifedipine *

Adjunctive nifedipine is of little efficacy although it had a numerical advantage in negative PANSS scores (n = 62, open, 10/52, Dzhuga and Kozlovski, *Zh Nevrol Psikhiatr Im S S Korsakova* 2009;**109**:32–5).

Tricyclics

Tricyclics are at best ineffective for acute psychotic episodes (n = 58, RCT, d/b, p/c, 4/52, Kramer et al, *Arch Gen Psychiatry* 1989; **46**:922–8).

Vitamin B6

No difference in PANSS scores was detectable with B$_6$ supplementation in stable chronic schizophrenics (n = 15, d/b, p/c, c/o, 9/52, Lerner et al, *J Clin Psychiatry* 2002;**63**:54–8).

1.23.2 FIRST EPISODE (EARLY INTERVENTION) *

Early intervention can include both treating a first episode quickly, and treating people at high risk before symptoms actually appear. Social decline, associated with neurocognitive deficits, often occurs in the prodromal phase or in the early course of schizophrenia and so management of this is vital.

A longer duration of untreated psychosis (DUP) shows a consistent but modest relationship (s = 26, n = 4490, Marshall et al, Arch Gen Psychiatry 2005;**62**:975–83; comment by Perkins, EBMH 2006;**9**:36; n = 157, Wunderink et al, Acta Psychiatr Scand 2006;**113**:332–9) with:

- worse symptoms, poor social functioning independent of symptoms (n=98, one year, Barnes et al, Br J Psychiatry 2008;**193**:203–9)
- less chance of remission, and reduced improvement in after one year (n = 49, Fusar-Poli et al, Br J Psychiatry 2009;**194**:181–2)
- impaired verbal IQ, verbal learning and working memory (n = 273, Lappin et al, Schizophr Res 2007;**95**:103–10).

However, delay in starting antipsychotics in first-episode psychosis is not necessarily neurotoxic for the brain or leads to reduced hippocampal volumes (n = 105, Ho et al, Am J Psychiatry 2005;**162**:1527–9). Structured early intervention programmes improve overall functioning and adherence but not necessarily symptoms (n = 144, RCT, 18/12, Garety et al, Br J Psychiatry 2006;**188**:37–45; comment by van Meijl, EBMH 2006;**9**:69). Substance misuse early in the illness has been linked with increased severity of illness (n = 232, Bühler et al, Schizophr Res 2002;**54**:234–51), and so should also be managed. Cochrane concludes that there is insufficient data to draw conclusions for use in children with onset prior to 13 years (Kennedy et al, Cochrane Database Syst Rev 2007;**3**:CD004027). Addition of CBT, family therapy and other inputs to optimal pharmacotherapy and case management may improve symptoms and outcomes, although psychotic symptoms and readmissions may be unchanged (n = 50, RCT, two years, Grawe et al, Acta Psychiatr Scand 2006;**114**:328–36).

Role of antipsychotics in first episodes *

- Minimise deterioration (or even perhaps prevent the illness developing, although this remains unproven; s = 7, n = 941, Marshall and Rathbone, Cochrane Database Syst Rev 2006;**4**:CD004718).
- Reduce stigma from symptoms, aiming for complete, not incomplete, remission.
- Increase engagement by minimising adverse experience with medication through use of minimum effective doses.

Antipsychotic therapy is usually considered essential treatment, and is definitely more effective if taken regularly. Improving concordance (and effectiveness) in a first episode has a number of principles:

1. Optimal drug dose:

- Slow titration is needed, both starting and stopping. The mean time to response is nine weeks (n = 118, Robinson et al, Am J Psychiatry 1999;**156**:544–9) but may be longer (n = 522, RCT, median 30/52, Emsley et al, Am J Psychiatry 2006; **163**:743–45).

2. Patient choice considered a high priority:

- Consider what the patient prefers (weight gain is the most unpopular side-effect and its impact on the user must not be trivialised). Antipsychotic-induced weight gain 3–4 times more common in younger, first-episode patients compared to older, chronic patients. The increase is consistent by drug but idiosyncratic by individual, with oanzapine>risperidone>haloperidol (s = 51, n = 14769, Alvarez-Jiménez et al, CNS Drugs 2008;**22**:547–62).
- Explain that there is no clear way of treating prodromal symptoms without the high risk of treating 'false positives' (Larsen et al, Acta Psychiatr Scand 2001;**103**:323–4).
- Minimise 'obvious' ADRs that might make patients look different, and which reduces compliance and engagement (n = 42, Amminger et al, Schizophr Res 2002;**54**:223–30).

3. Adequate duration of treatment: the relapse rate over five years is high with diagnosed but untreated schizophrenia.

- On discontinuation, up to 78% may experience an exacerbation or relapse within one year, and 96% may do so within two years (n = 53, RCT, open, 18/12, Gitlin et al, Am J Psychiatry 2001;**158**:1835–42). In a recent study in remitted first-episode psychosis patients stable for 6/12, maintenance with low-dose antipsychotics was compared to gradual discontinuation, with an 18/12 follow-up. Twice as many relapses occurred in the discontinuation group compared to maintenance (43% vs 21%), with 30% requiring restarting antipsychotics and only 20% successfully discontinuing. The authors concluded that although more work is needed on risk factors, the risk from low doses appears low compared to the risk of relapse and subsequent potential deterioration (n = 131, RCT, open, 18/12, Wunderink et al, J Clin Psychiatry 2007;**68**:654–61).

- Patients should be advised that not taking antipsychotics for several years will almost inevitably lead to relapse and rehospitalisation (n = 104, Robinson et al, Arch Gen Psychiatry 1999;**56**:241–7). The optimum duration of therapy is as yet unclear.

4. Treatment is monitored:

- Older drugs have high incidence of EPS (even with low dose haloperidol; n = 57, 12/12, Oosterhuizen et al, J Clin Psychiatry 2003;**64**:1075–80), raised prolactin and adverse cognitive effects.
- Newer drugs have higher incidence of weight gain (which should be dealt with early) and diabetes, which needs to be screened for, monitored and managed.

Reviews: * the case for early intervention (McGorry, BMJ 2008;**337**:a695), the case against (Pelosi, BMJ 2008;**337**:a710), general (Salimi et al, CNS Drugs 2009;**23**:837–55; Crespo-Facorro et al, Curr Psychiatry Rep 2008;**10**:202–9; Rotgé et al, Encephale 2008;**34**:194–204), efficacy and tolerability (Kumra et al, Schizophrenia Bull 2008; **34**:60–71).

BNF listed

Few antipsychotic trials are carried out in first episode patients (Remington, Br J Psychiatry 2005; **187**[Suppl 48]:S77–S84) so optimum doses are unclear, e.g. relatively low doses of risperidone 4 mg/d, olanzapine 15.3 mg/d, haloperidol 5.4 mg/d were equally effective for first episode psychosis, with haloperidol worst for EPSE and olanzapine worst for weight gain (n = 172, RCT, open, 6/52, Crespo-Facorro

et al, J Clin Psychiatry 2006;**67**:1511–21; IS, comment by Barbui et al, EBMH 2007;**10**:54). In a pragmatic naturalistic comparison of haloperidol 1–4 mg/d, amisulpride 200–800 mg/d, olanzapine 5–20 mg/d, quetiapine 200–750 mg/d and ziprasidone 40–160 mg/d, symptom reduction remained virtually the same for all groups, but clinically meaningful in those completing, suggesting that at least a year's treatment can be achieved (n = 498 [c = 291], open, RCT, 12/12, Kahn et al, Lancet 2008;**371**: 1085–97).

Amisulpride

Amisulpride (mean 250 mg/d) is licensed from age 15 years upwards and may have some efficacy for primary negative symptoms in first-episode psychosis (n = 14 [c = 12], open, 6/52, Murphy et al, Hum Psychopharmacol 2006; **21**:511–7).

Aripiprazole *

Aripiprazole is licensed in the UK for schizophrenia in adolescents aged 15 years or older (US 13–17 years). In first episode patients, aripiprazole had a responder rate of 79% and was well tolerated (n = 45 [c = 42], open, 12/52, Takahashi et al, Clin Neuropharmacol 2009;**32**:149–50) and a chart review suggested some efficacy as an adjunct (n = 15, Bachmann et al, Pharmacopsychiatry 2009;**42**:153–7).

Clozapine

Clozapine is licensed from age 16 upwards. There was a 15% decrease in the odds of achieving remission for every year of untreated psychoses. Early use of clozapine (after as few as 25 weeks in people failing two other antipsychotics) has been associated with significant and meaningful reductions in symptoms (n = 13, Agid et al, J Clin Psycho-pharmacol 2007;**27**:369–73; see also n = 54, d/b or open, Sporn et al, J Am Acad Child Adolesc Psychiatry 2007;**46**:1349–56), but it has more ADRs and toxicity (n = 25, RCT, d/b, 8/52 + open two-year follow-up, Shaw et al, Arch Gen Psychiatry 2006;**63**:721–30).

Haloperidol

Haloperidol is licensed for childhood behavioural disorders and schizophrenia with no age limit. Haloperidol 2 mg/d is much better tolerated than 8 mg/d and as effective, shown by PANSS scores (n=40, RCT, d/b, 6/52, Oosthuizen et al, Int J Neuropsychopharmacol 2004;**7**:125–31) and has equivalent efficacy to olanzapine, although drop-out rates were high and this trial excluded more severely ill people (n=263[c=83], RCT, d/b, one year; Strakowski et al, Schizophr Res 2005;**78**:161–9; comment by Awad, EBMH 2006;**9**:47). Unlike olanzapine, haloperidol is associated with reduced grey matter volume in first episode, either due to haloperidol-induced toxicity or superior olanzapine efficacy (n=263, RCT, d/b, volunteer controlled, 24/12, Lieberman et al, Arch Gen Psychiatry 2005;**62**:361–70). Haloperidol and risperidone (both 2–4 mg/d) were equally effective in relapse prevention in first-episode schizophrenia, with similar ADRs and drop-outs (n=151, RCT, d/b, one year; Gaebel et al, J Clin Psychiatry 2007;**68**:1763–74).

Olanzapine *

Olanzapine is only licensed in UK from age 18 years upwards. Low dose olanzapine is preferable to haloperidol in first-episode psychosis, with superior efficacy, lower discontinuations, greater retention in treatment and reduced side-effects (n=158, open, Bobes et al, Prog Neuropsychopharmacol Biol Psychiatry 2003;**27**:473–81; n=107, RCT, d/b, p/c, 6/52, Kryzhanovskaya et al, J Am Acad Child Adolesc Psychiatry 2009;**48**:60–70), although weight gain is a significant adverse effect (mean 15.4 kg) in first-episode psychosis (n=263, open, two years, Zipursky et al, Br J Psychiatry 2005;**187**:537–43; comment by Lambert, EBMH 2006;**9**:72). Olanzapine (2.5–20 mg/d) and risperidone (1–6 mg/d) have been shown to be equipotent in first-episode schizophrenia (n=112, RCT, open, 4/12, Robinson et al, Am J Psychiatry 2006;**163**:2096–102; n=100[c=77], RCT, open, 6/12, Cuesta et al, Br J Psychiatry 2009;**194**:439–45) and as effective as quetiapine (n=50[c=32], open, 6/12, Arango et al, Eur Child Adolesc Psychiatry 2009;**18**:418–28), but weight gain was greater with olanzapine.

Quetiapine *

Quetiapine is licensed for schizophrenia in adults. Low EPS, weight gain and prolactin effects make quetiapine a suitable antipsychotic. It seems to be as effective as olanzapine but with less weight gain (n=50[c=32], open, 6/12, Arango et al, Eur Child Adolesc Psychiatry 2009;**18**:418–28).

Risperidone *

Risperidone is licensed from age 15 years upwards and is now the standard first choice. Risperidone needs a low but adequate dose, e.g. 1.5–6 mg/d is more effective than really low-dose (0.15–0.6) (n=257, RCT, d/b, 87/52, Haas et al, Br J Psychiatry 2009;**194**:158–64) but 2 mg/d was as effective as 4 mg/d with fewer side-effects and, although 4 mg/d (especially with slow titration; Williams, J Clin Psychiatry 2001;**62**:282–9; n=183, RCT, 6/52, Emsley, Schizophr Bull 1999;**25**:721–9) was slightly better at 4/52, the two were similar at 8/52, so it makes little pharmacological sense in escalating doses at an early stage (n=49, d/b, 8/52, Merlo et al, J Clin Psychiatry 2002;**63**:885–91). In the 75% who initially clinically improved, relapses were delayed longer with risperidone (mean 3.3 mg/d; median 466 days) than haloperidol (mean 2.9 mg/d; median 205 days) (n=555, RCT, d/b, <5 years, median 30/52, Schooler et al, Am J Psychiatry 2005;**162**:947–53). Risperidone 1–6 mg/d was equipotent with olanzapine (2.5–20 mg/d) in first-episode schizophrenia, but patients may be more stable with risperidone (n=112, RCT, open, 4/12, Robinson et al, Am J Psychiatry 2006;**163**:2096–102; see also n=25, RCT, open, 12/52, Mozes et al, J Child Adolesc Psychopharmacol 2006;**16**:393–403). Use of RLAI improves compliance and reduces relapse rate (n=50[c=32], open, two years, Emsley et al, Int Clin Psychopharmacol 2008;**23**:325–31) in first episode schizophrenia compared to oral risperidone (n=50, Kim et al, Prog Neuropsychopharmacol Biol Psychiatry 2008;**32**:1231–5).

☐ No efficacy

Omega-3 fatty acids (E-EPA)

There were no significant effects from E-EPA as augmentation of antipsychotics in first-episode psychosis, although there was perhaps a slightly quicker onset of action (n=69, RCT, d/b, p/c, 12/52, Berger et al, J Clin Psychiatry 2007;**68**:1867–75).

1.23.3 COGNITIVE IMPAIRMENT

Cognitive impairment is a known complication of schizophrenia and antipsychotics, and so methods to improve cognitive function are needed. Some antipsychotics may have a better cognitive profile than others, e.g. risperidone over haloperidol, (n = 533 [c = 359], RCT, 3/12 follow-up, Harvey et al, Am J Psychiatry 2005;**162**:1888–95) and olanzapine (mean 9.6 mg/d) over haloperidol mean 4.6 mg/d (n = 167, RCT, d/b, 12/52, Keefe et al, Am J Psychiatry 2004;**161**:985–95).
Reviews: * general (Galletly, Psychopharmacol [Berl] 2009;**202**:259–73), pharmacological treatment of cognition in schizophrenia (Harvey and Cornblatt, Am J Psychiatry 2008;**165**:163–5).

Anticholinesterases + antipsychotics *
A review concluded that a meta-analysis was difficult to carry out and did not reveal clear evidence for efficacy for anticholinesterases for memory dysfunction in schizophrenia (s = 8, Stip et al, Clin Neuropharmacol 2007;**30**:218–29). Of the available drugs, **donepezil** 5–10 mg/d appears to have little effect on cognitive deficits in schizophrenia (e.g. n = 36, RCT, d/b, p/c, 8/52, Freudenrich et al, Psychopharmacol [Berl] 2005;**181**:358–63; n = 26, RCT, d/b, p/c, 16/52, Kohler et al, Cognit Neuropsychiatry 2007;**12**:412–21). However, some mild improvements have been shown (n = 24, RCT, d/b, p/c, 12/52, Lee et al, J Psychopharmacol 2007;**21**:421–7 n=28, open, 12/52, Chung et al World J Biol Psychiatry 2009;**10**:156–62) and 10 mg/d as an adjunct to risperidone significantly improved negative symptoms in chronic schizophrenia with cognitive impairments (n = 30, RCT, d/b, p/c, 12/52, Akhondzadeh et al, Prog Neuropsychopharmacol Biol Psychiatry 2008;**32**:1810–5). Improvement in refractory negative symptoms and cognition has been reported with adjunctive **galantamine**, e.g. improved processing speed, WAIS-III and verbal memory, although it interfered with practice effects in attention tasks (n = 86, RCT, d/b, p/c, 12/52, Buchanan et al, Am J Psychiatry 2008;**165**:82–9), but 24 mg/d had no apparent effect on cognitive function or negative

symptoms in stable schizophrenia with low baseline functioning (n = 83 [c = 73], RCT, d/b, p/c, 12/52, Conley et al, Clin Neuropharmacol 2009;**32**:69–74). **Rivastigmine** up to 9 mg/d had no effect on cognitive function in schizophrenics with significant impairment (n = 20, RCT, c/o, 6/12, Chouinard et al, Curr Med Res Opin 2007;**23**:575–83) and adjunctive use had no detectable effect on cognitive function when added to stable antipsychotic therapy in schizophrenia (n = 40 [c = 21], RCT, d/b, p/c, 24/52, Sharma et al, Schizophr Res 2006;**85**:73–83), although up to 16 mg BD has significantly improved quality of life and cognitive functioning with few ADRs (n = 16, 12/12, Lenzi et al, Clin Neuropharmacol 2003; **26**:317–21).

Clozapine + mirtazapine
In stabilised clozapine patients, addition of mirtazapine produced a significant improvement in cognitive performance (n = 15, 8/52, open, Delle Chiaie et al, Exp Clin Psychopharmacol 2007;**15**:563–8).

Clozapine + risperidone
The combination did not significantly improve cognitive function cf clozapine alone (n = 30, RCT, d/b, p/c, 6/52, Akdede et al, J Clin Psychiatry 2006;**67**:1912–9).

Buspirone
Buspirone augmentation has improved attention in schizophrenia but not statistically (n = 73, RCT, d/b, p/c, 6/12, Sumiyoshi et al, Schizophr Res 2007;**95**:158–68).

Modafinil
Modafinil 200 mg/d has produced improvements in cognitive functioning in schizophrenia (n = 20, RCT, d/b, p/c, c/o, Turner et al, Neuropsychopharmacol 2004;**29**:1363–73) and 100-200 mg/d may improve fatigue and cognitive functioning in schizophrenia (n = 11, open, 4/52, Rosenthal and Bryant, Clin Neuropharmacol 2004;**27**:38–43). However, modafinil had no effect on negative symptoms of schizophrenia, but some global improvements were seen (n = 20, RCT, d/b, p/c, 8/52, Pierre et al, J Clin

Psychiatry 2007;**68**:705–10) and single doses did not improve cognitive control in schizophrenics with prominent negative symptoms but had some effect in patients with suboptimal baseline function (n = 12, d/b, c/o, Hunter et al, *Am J Psychiatry* 2006;**163**:2184–6).

Pregnenolone *

A pilot study of the neurosteroid pregnenolone (which enhances cognition in rats and modulates NMDA receptors) as an adjunct to antipsychotics showed significantly improved SANS scores (n = 21 [c = 18], RCT, d/b, p/c, 8/52, Marx et al, *Neuropsychopharmacology* 2009;**34**:1885–903).

☐ No efficacy

Atomoxetine *

Adjunctive atomoxetine was ineffective for improving cognitive impairment in schizophrenia (n = 32, RCT, d/b, p/c, 8/52, Kelly et al, *J Clin Psychiatry* 2009;**70**:518–25).

Cicloserin (D-cycloserine)

In severe negative symptoms and cognitive impairment (without marked positive, depressive or EP symptoms) there was no improvement when either glycine or cicloserin were added (n = 157, RCT, d/b, p/c, 12/52, Buchanan et al, *Am J Psychiatry* 2007;**164**:1593–602).

Glycine

See cicloserine above.

RAPID-CYCLING BIPOLAR DISORDER

see Rapid-cycling bipolar disorder (*1.10.4*)

1.24 SEASONAL AFFECTIVE DISORDER (SAD)

see Depression (*1.14*), Mania and hypomania (*1.10.2*) and Bipolar mood disorder (*1.10*)

SAD is a recurrent affective disorder, pre-dominantly major depression, but can include mania or hypomania. It has a characteristic seasonal relationship, usually autumn or winter (s = 20, Magnusson, *Acta Psychiatr Scand* 2000: **101**:176–84), for at least two or three years,

with full remission at a characteristic time of the year and outnumbering any non-seasonal episodes. The incidence may be around 1–10% (e.g. 2.4% in North Wales) and peaks in winter. Atypical depressive features include hypersomnia, increased appetite and weight and carbohydrate cravings. Theories for the cause include excess melatonin secretion, delayed or reduced amplitude circadian rhythms, and serotonergic dysfunction. It is often undiagnosed and half of sufferers are given other depressive diagnoses and antidepressants (n = 1999, Michalak et al, *Br J Psychiatry* 2001;**179**:31–4). Light therapy is first choice for SAD (n = 96, RCT, Lam et al, *Am J Psychiatry* 2006;**163**:805–12; comment by Gaynes, *EBMH* 2007;**10**:26) and, although better tolerated than fluoxetine, it is not without risk, with side-effects including jumpiness (9%), headache (8%), and nausea (16%).

Role of drugs

While phototherapy is well established, pre-liminary data from controlled trials indicates that drug treatment may also be effective, with bupropion and sertraline suggested as effective. Seasonal major depression can be prevented by starting an antidepressant early in the season while patient is still well (e.g. with bupropion 150–300 mg/d; s = 3, n = 1042, RCT, p/c, Modell et al, *Biol Psychiatry* 2005;**58**:658–67).

Reviews: * general (*DTB* 2009;**47**:128–32;Westrin and Lam, *Ann Clin Psychiatry* 2007;**19**:239–46; Pjrek et al, *CNS Spectr* 2005;**10**:664–9), long-term treatment (Westrin and Lam, *CNS Drugs* 2007;**21**:901–9), light therapy (Golden et al, *Am J Psychiatry* 2005;**162**:656–62; Terman, *EBMH* 2006;**9**:21).

● Unlicensed/some efficacy

Bupropion

Bupropion XL is licensed in the USA for SAD, using 150–300 mg/d where treatment was started in the autumn while the patients were still well (s = 3, n = 1042, RCT, p/c, d/b, Modell et al, *Biol Psychiatry* 2005;**58**:658–67).

Sertraline

Sertraline (50–200 mg/d) was significantly superior to placebo in winter pattern SAD in one study (n = 187, RCT, d/b, p/c, O/P, 8/52,

Moscovitch et al, Psychopharmacol [Berl] 2004; 171:390–7).

■ Unlicensed/possible efficacy

Agomelatine
A pilot study suggested that seasonal depression may respond to agomelatine (n = 37, open, 14/52, Pjrek et al, Psychopharmacology [Berl] 2007;190:575–9).

Beta-blockers
Propranolol 60 mg/d administered pre-sunrise (5.30–6.00 AM) may produce response in winter depression possibly via short-term, short-acting beta-blocker-induced truncation of nocturnal melatonin secretion early morning but not in the evening (n = 33, d/b, p/c, Schlager, Am J Psychiatry 1994;151:1383–5). Atenolol appears less effective (n = 19, d/b, p/c, c/o, Rosenthal et al, Am J Psychiatry 1988;145:52–6).

Duloxetine *
Duloxetine may be useful for SAD (n = 26, open, 8/52, Pjrek et al, Pharmacopsychiatry 2008;41:100–5).

Melatonin
Melatonin secretion is altered in SAD and melatonin may have some role (review by Srinivasan et al, World J Biol Psychiatry 2006;7:138–51).

Mirtazapine
A pilot study has shown a rapid and well tolerated effect in SAD (n = 8, open, 4/52, Hesselmann et al, Hum Psychopharmacol Clin Exp 1999;14:59–62).

Modafinil
A pilot study suggested modafinil significantly reduces fatigue and sleepiness (n = 13 [c = 9], open, 8/52, Lundt, J Affect Disord 2004; 81:173–8).

Reboxetine
A study indicated a rapid and significant effect in 65% of patients, including atypical symptoms in the first week (n = 16, open, 6/52, Hilger et al, Eur Neuropsychopharmacol 2001;11:1–5).

SSRIs
Light therapy has an early onset of action and, in responders, **citalopram** significantly reduces relapse in the continuation phase (n = 282, p/c, 15/52, Martiny et al, Acta Psychiatr Scand 2004;109:230–4). **Escitalopram** 10–20 mg/d appears effective and very well tolerated (n = 20, open, 8/52, Pjrek et al, Pharmacopsychiatry 2007;40:20–4) and **fluoxetine** 20 mg/d was superior to placebo (59–34%), but was not quite statistically significant (n = 68, p/c, 5/52, Lam et al, Am J Psychiatry 1995;152:1765–70).

◆ Others ◆

Other drugs used include **moclobemide** (n = 581, RCT, d/b, 6/52, Partonen and Lonnqvist, J Affect Disord 1996;41:93–9), **St John's wort** (s/b, Kasper, Pharmacopsychiatry 1997;30[Suppl 2]: S89–S93) and **tranylcypromine** (n = 14, open, Dilsaver and Jaeckle, J Clin Psychiatry 1990; 51:326–9).

□ No efficacy

Ginkgo biloba
One study was unable to show an effect from 'Bio-Biloba' in preventing winter depression (n = 27, RCT, 10/52, Lingaerde et al, Acta Psychiatr Scand 1999;100:62–6).

1.25 SELF-INJURIOUS BEHAVIOUR (SIB)

SIB is a self-destructive behaviour resulting in significant tissue damage, but without lethal intent. It can occur in learning disabilities (e.g. Lesch-Nyhan syndrome), as well as in OCD, sadomasochism, schizophrenia and borderline personality disorder. There seems to be a variety of causes, e.g. relief of dysphoria, poor impulse control and dissociation.

Role of drugs
Opiate antagonists may be useful where a reward mechanism seems to exist. There is some evidence of a serotonergic involvement. Antipsychotics seem to work mainly via a non-specific sedating mechanism.
Review: psychopharmacology of severe SIB associated with learning disabilities (Clarke, Br J Psychiatry 1998;172:389–94).

+ Combinations

Clozapine + clomipramine

This combination was successful in treating compulsive self-mutilation in a drug-resistant mild learning disability patient (n = 1, Holzer et al, Am J Psychiatry 1996;**153**:133).

Lamotrigine + fluoxetine

These have been used in compulsive sexual behaviour (n = 1, Schupak, Prog Neuropsychopharmacol Biol Psychiatry 2007;**31**: 1337–8).

● Unlicensed/some efficacy

Antipsychotics

Antipsychotics are frequently prescribed but evidence for their efficacy is suggestive rather than conclusive. **Risperidone** was shown to be effective for up to 52 months in 75% of developmentally disabled inpatients (retrospective chart analysis, Brahm et al, Pharmacotherapy 2001;**21**:382). Low-dose **olanzapine** (5 mg/d) has been used successfully for SIB (n = 2, Hough, J Clin Psychiatry 2001; **62**:96–7) and **clozapine** 200 mg/d has been effective in a few cases (n = 2, Hammock et al, J Autism Dev Disord 2001;**31**:109–13).
Review: Janowsky et al, J Clin Psychopharmacol 2005;**25**:19–25.

Buspirone

In a trial of developmentally disabled individuals with self-injury and anxiety, 64% responded to doses of 20–45 mg/d with a maximal response seen more than three weeks later (n = 14, open, Ratey et al, J Clin Psychiatry 1989;**50**:382).

Lithium

Some old studies have suggested that lithium is effective in both aggression and SIB, e.g. response was seen in 2–8 weeks with a lithium serum concentration of 0.7–1.0 mEq/L (n = 42, d/b, p/c, 4/12, Craft et al, Br J Psychiatry 1987; **150**:685–9).

Naltrexone/naloxone

There is conflicting data about the efficacy of naltrexone in SIB. Some studies show some efficacy when used in adequate dose for adequate duration, e.g. 25–100 mg/d orally (n = 4, Sandman et al, Am J Ment Retard 1990;**95**:93–102), although lower doses (e.g. 10–50 mg/d) may also be effective and it undoubtedly helps some patients (e.g. n = 1, 32/52, Griengl et al, Acta Psychiatr Scand 2001;**103**:234–6; n = 1 plus review, White and Schultz, Am J Psychiatry 2000;**157**:1574–82). Some trials have, however, shown a lack of efficacy (n = 33, d/b, p/c, c/o, Willemsen-Swinkels et al, Arch Gen Psychiatry 1995;**52**:766–73). SIB may get worse over the first few weeks of naltrexone but then improve and so short studies could miss the effect. There is some evidence of raised opioid peptide activity in autism, Fragile-X syndrome and other mental handicaps.
Review: Symons et al, Ment Retard Dev Disabil Res Rev 2004;**10**:193–200.

■ Unlicensed/possible efficacy

Anticholinesterases

These have been successful for an elderly demented woman with sexual aggression (n = 1, Alagiakrishnan et al, J Am Geriatr Soc 2003;**51**:1326).

Omega-3 fatty acids

Omega-3 fatty acid supplements reduced suicidal markers and improved well-being in recurrent self-harmers, but had no effect on impulsivity, aggression and hostility (n = 49, RCT, d/b, p/c, 12/52, Hallahan et al, Br J Psychiatry 2007;**190**:118–22) compared to placebo (Goff van Essa, Self Inj Behav 2009;**12**:45).

Oxcarbazepine

Oxcarbazepine has been used for self-mutilating bulimic patients (Cordas et al, Int J Neuropsychopharmacol 2006;**9**:769–71).

Topiramate

Topiramate 200 mg/d was observed to produce remission of SIB in a patient with BPD (n = 1, Cassano et al, Bipolar Disorders 2001;**3**:161).

◆ Others *

Other drugs used include **clomipramine** (n = 11, open, Garber et al, J Am Acad Child Adolesc Psych

1992;**31**:1157–60), **dextromethorphan** (n = 1, Welch and Sovner, *Br J Psychiatry* 1992;**161**:118–20), **fluoxetine** (n = 4, Ricketts *et al*, *J Am Acad Child Adolesc Psychiatry* 1993;**32**:865–9) and **propranolol** (review; Ruedrich *et al*, *Am J Ment Retard* 1990;**95**:110–9).

1.26 SEXUAL DEVIANCY DISORDERS

Sexual deviancy disorders are abnormalities of a basic biological drive and are recognised as psychiatric syndromes. They include exhibitionism, fetishism, sexual masochism or sadism, paedophilia and voyeurism, but not rape (considered a sexual expression of aggression rather than an aggressive expression of sexuality). The main characteristic is of intense, recurrent sexual arousal and fantasies, particularly connected with inanimate objects, children, non-consenting adults or the self.

Role of drugs
Drug therapy is controversial but may sometimes be a useful adjunct to other therapies, due to the chronic nature of the disease and its high and unpredictable relapse rates. One review (Bradford, *J Sex Res* 2000;**37**:248–57) suggested a treatment hierarchy of CBT, SSRIs, low-dose antiandrogens, higher dose antiandrogens, then very high dose antiandrogens. Deviant sexual behaviour is rare in women and so drug therapy is usually aimed at reducing sexual drive in men. The success of any form of treatment is highly dependent on detailed evaluations and diagnosis. Placebo-controlled studies have huge ethical complications.
Reviews: * general (Guay, *Am J Geriatr Pharmacother* 2008;**6**:269–88), sexual functioning (Meston and Frohlich, *Arch Gen Psychiatry* 2000;**57**:1012–30), treatment protocols for cyproterone, medroxyprogesterone, etc (Reilly *et al*, *Can J Psychiatry* 2000;**45**:559–63).

BNF listed

Benperidol
Benperidol is a standard butyrophenone which, although used for the control of deviant antisocial sexual behaviour, has no proven use other than as an antipsychotic. The only double-blind study published showed a slight reduction in sexual thoughts, but not in behaviour (*Drug Ther Bull* 1974;**12**:2).

Cyproterone (acetate)
Cyproterone is available in many countries to treat severe hypersexuality and sexual deviation in men. It has both antiandrogenic and antigonadotropic actions and probably acts by disrupting the receptors' response to androgens. It can reduce sexual interest, drive and arousal, as well as deviant fantasies and behaviour, and significantly reduces some sexual behaviours in paraphilias and paedophilia (n = 19, RCT, d/b, p/c, c/o, Bradford *et al*, *Arch Sex Behav* 1993;**22**:383–402). The onset of action may be delayed for 2–3 weeks and is reversible within 3–6 weeks of stopping. An adequate trial of four months is usually recommended. A depot injection is available on a named patient basis and a syrup can be made.

• Unlicensed/some efficacy

LHRH antagonists
Luteinising hormone-releasing hormone (gonadorelin, LHRH) antagonists can produce complete chemical castration and thus have a potent effect on sexual deviancy. A thorough review concluded that LHRH antagonists offer a treatment option for severe paraphilia, with little or no relapse if the patient remains under treatment (s = 13, n = 118, Briken *et al*, *J Clin Psychiatry* 2003;**64**:890–7). **Nafarelin** has been used and **flutamide**, a pure antiandrogen similar to cyproterone, has been used in conjunction with nafarelin (n = 1, Rousseau *et al*, *Can J Psychiatry* 1990;**35**:338–41). **Leuprolide** acetate is an alternative and a depot leuprolide significantly suppressed self-reported deviant sexual interests and behaviour and was well tolerated, although bone demineralisation occurred in 25% (n = 12, open, Krueger and Kaplan, *Arch Sex Behav* 2001;**30**:409–22). **Triptorelin** has also been used (n = 6, Thibaut *et al*, *Acta Psychiatr Scand* 1993;**87**:445–50), where depot triptorelin palmoate 3.75 mg/month plus psychotherapy was effective for reducing episodes of deviant sexual behaviours over 3–12 months in all men with severe paraphilia (n = 30, open, Rosler and Witztum, *N Engl J Med* 1998;**338**:416–22).

Medroxyprogesterone (acetate)

Medroxyprogesterone has indirect anti-androgenic activity by preventing testosterone release from the testicles (review by Cooper, *Can J Psychiatry* 1986;**31**:73–9) and increasing the metabolic clearance of testosterone, resulting in suppression of sexual arousal and libido. Adverse effects include weight gain, diabetes and DVTs, although feminisation has not been reported. Few proper trials have been carried out but there is a case series where it was successful for inappropriate sexual behaviour in elderly men with dementia (n = 5, case series, Light and Holroyd, *J Psychiatry Neurosci* 2006;**31**:132–4). Due to a possible central tranquillising effect, care is needed on ethical grounds (Berlin, *Bull Am Acad Psychiatry Law* 1989;**17**:233–9).

SSRIs *

Reduced daily frequency and duration of paraphilia and related disorders has been shown (n = 26, open case series, Kafka and Hennen, *J Clin Psychiatry* 2000;**61**:664–70; n = 1, Mania et al, *Prim Care Companion J Clin Psychiatry* 2006;**8**:106). Citalopram has been used successfully for hypersexuality in early Alzheimer's disease (n = 1, Tosto et al, *Neurol Sci* 2008;**29**:269–70). SSRI-induced anorgasmia may be a contributory factor to this effect.

■ Unlicensed/possible efficacy

Carbamazepine *

Carbamazepine has been used to treat sexual disinhibition in dementia (n = 1, Freymann et al, *Pharmacopsychiatry* 2005;**38**:144–5) and in hypersexuality in Parkinson's disease (n = 1, Bach et al, *Mov Disord* 2009;**24**:1241–2).

Gabapentin

Gabapentin has been used to treat sexual disinhibition in dementia (n = 3, Alkhalil et al, *Am J Ther* 2004;**11**:231–5).

Imipramine

Some improvements in paraphilic and non-paraphilic sexual addictions and depressive symptoms were noted in 90% of patients treated with imipramine, fluoxetine or lithium (n = 10, Kafka, *J Clin Psychiatry* 1991;**52**:60–5).

Lithium

See imipramine.

Methylphenidate

Methylphenidate may be used cautiously to augment the effect of SSRIs in paraphilias and related disorders (n = 26, Kafka and Hennen, *J Clin Psychiatry* 2000;**61**:664–70).

Mirtazapine *

Mirtazapine 15–30 mg/d had some efficacy (50% were very much improved) in reducing inappropriate sexual behaviours in people with autism (n = 10, open, 8/52, Coskun et al, *J Child Adolesc Psychopharmacol* 2009;**19**:203–6).

Naltrexone

Compulsive sexual behaviour has been treated with naltrexone and SSRIs (n = 2, Raymond et al, *Int Clin Psychopharmacol* 2002;**17**:201–5), and naltrexone was reported to have a positive response in 15 adolescent sexual offenders, with a therapeutic window of 50–200 mg/d. Of the six non-responders, five responded to leuprolide (n = 21, open, Ryback, *J Clin Psychiatry* 2004;**65**:982–6).

Quetiapine *

There is a case of inappropriate sexual behaviour improving rapidly with quetiapine (n = 1, Prakash et al, *Am J Alzheimer's Dis Other Demen* 2009;**24**:136–40).

Topiramate

Topiramate 50 mg/d reduced compulsive non-paraphilic sexual behaviours strongly triggered by environmental cues in one patient (n = 1, Khazaal and Zullion, *BMC Psychiatry* 2006; **6**:22).

Valproate

Valproate has been a useful adjunct in bipolar sex offenders, but only for mood, not for paraphilic symptoms (open, retrospective, Nelson et al, *J Affect Disord* 2001;**64**:249–55).

1.27 SOCIAL ANXIETY DISORDER (SOCIAL PHOBIA DISORDER)
see also Anxiety disorder (*1.6*)

Social anxiety is the second most common phobia (incidence in USA is 5%; n = 43 093,

Grant et al, J Clin Psychiatry 2005;**66**:1351–61; comment by Manfro, EBMH 2006;**9**:88) where the sufferers fear public ridicule, scrutiny and negative evaluation, with fear of embarrassment, criticism or making a public mistake. Feared situations include public speaking, social gatherings, writing under supervision or eating and drinking in public. Anticipatory anxiety leads to impaired performance. Two sub-divisions include general and specific social phobia. This is a serious, disabling anxiety disorder associated with reduction in quality of life (s = 3, n = 829, RCTs, p/c, Stein and Kean, Am J Psychiatry 2000;**157**:1606–13), but is underdiagnosed with less than 5% of sufferers receiving a diagnosis (n = 3862, Katzelnick et al, Am J Psychiatry 2001; **158**:1999–2007). Early diagnosis and treatment may be vital (Kahalid-Khan et al, Paediatr Drugs 2007;**9**:227–37).

Role of drugs *
Drugs and behavioural approaches are commonly used. A meta-analysis of effect sizes (including all six UK SSRIs) concluded that SSRIs are more effective than placebo, with improvements also in social and occupational functioning (s = 15, n = 3527, RCT, d/b, p/c, 10–24/52, Hansen et al, Int Clin Psychopharmacol 2008;**23**:170–9; see also s = 15, RCT, d/b, p/c, Hedges et al, J Psychopharmacol 2007;**21**:102–11). Venlafaxine XL may be second-line, with moclobemide, MAOIs and benzodiazepines third choice. The only predictor of response is length of treatment, which should be at least 12 weeks (Stein et al, J Clin Psychiatry 2002;**63**:152–5). Cochrane concludes that SSRIs have the strongest evidence for short-term and probably the long-term (s = 36, n = 4268, RCT, Stein et al, Cochrane Database Syst Rev 2004;**4**:CD001206). The placebo response may be moderately large (15 p/c studies, Oosterbaan et al, J Psychopharmacol 2001;**15**:199–203). CBT alone is probably more effective than fluoxetine and placebo (n = 60, RCT, d/b, 12/12, Clark et al, J Consult Clin Psychol 2003;**71**:1058–67; review Taylor EBMH 2004;**7**:75) but compared to clonazepam alone, combined psychodynamic group therapy (PGT) and clonazepam improved global functioning, but not any secondary measures (n = 57, RCT, 12/52, Knijnik et al, Eur Psychiatry 2008;**23**:567–74).
Reviews: * general (Westenberg, CNS Spectr

2009;**14**(2 Suppl 3):24–33; Schneier, N Engl J Med 2006;**355**:1029–36; Nash, Prescriber 2005; **16**:7–24), BAP evidence-based guidelines (Baldwin et al, J Psychopharmacol 2005;**19**:567–96).

BNF listed

Escitalopram *
Escitalopram is licensed in the UK for social anxiety (although citalopram is not licensed). The starting dose is 10mg/d, increased to a maximum of 20mg/d or reduced to 5mg/d, depending upon the individual's response, and any trial should last at least four weeks before further intervention is considered (s = 40, Baldwin et al, Hum Psychopharmacol 2009;**24**:269–75). Efficacy has been shown in a number of major trials. Escitalopram 10–20mg/d was superior to placebo (54% vs 39% response) using the LSAS total score (n = 358, RCT, p/c, d/b, 12/52, Kasper et al, Br J Psychiatry 2005;**186**:222–6; MS) and appeared effective and well tolerated in the long-term (n = 517, RCT, d/b, p/c, 24/52, Montgomery et al, J Clin Psychiatry 2005;**66**:1270–8; comment by Stein, EBMH 2006;**9**:52). A sub-analysis of pooled data showed efficacy against all symptom dimensions (s = 2, RCT, p/c, 12/52, Stein et al, Depress Anxiety 2004;**20**:175–81).

Paroxetine
Several studies show paroxetine to be superior to placebo, e.g. at 20–50mg/d reducing symptoms and avoidance, with 40mg/d the optimum dose (n = 384, d/b, 12/52, Liebowitz et al, J Clin Psychiatry 2002;**63**:66–74). Paroxetine 10–50mg/d is also effective and well tolerated for social anxiety in children and adolescents (8–17) (n = 322, RCT, p/c, d/b, 16/52, Wagner et al, Arch Gen Psychiatry 2004;**61**:1153–62). Lack of response at eight weeks does not necessarily predict long-term lack of response and so a minimum of 12 weeks treatment is necessary (review, s = 3, Stein et al, J Clin Psychiatry 2002;**63**:152–5). It may be effective for relapse prevention (n = 323[c = 257], RCT, p/c, Stein et al, Arch Gen Psychiatry 2002; **59**:1111–8).

Venlafaxine
Venlafaxine XL is now licensed for moderate-to-severe generalised social anxiety disorder

(n = 279 [c = 173], RCT, d/b, p/c, 12/52, Liebowitz et al, J Clin Psychiatry 2005;66:238-47). The standard dose of 75 mg/d is as effective and well tolerated as paroxetine 20–50 mg/d (n = 413 [c = 318], RCT, p/c, d/b, 12/52, Liebowitz et al, Arch Gen Psychiatry 2005;62:190–8), although 150–225 mg/d has been used (n = 386, d/b, p/c, 6/12, Stein et al, Psychopharmacol [Berl] 2004;177:280–8). Lower doses may be useful in children and adolescents (n = 293, RCT, p/c, 16/52, March et al, Biol Psychiatry 2007;62:1149–54).

Combinations

Paroxetine + clonazepam

Unlike panic disorder, combining a BDZ with paroxetine did not lead to a quicker response (n = 28 [c = 19], d/b, p/c, 10/52, Seedat and Stein, J Clin Psychiatry 2004;65:244–8).

● Unlicensed/some efficacy

Benzodiazepines

Benzodiazepines have a rapid onset, good tolerability and flexible dosing, but cause sedation, lack of coordination and long-term use has some potential risks. **Diazepam** may be ineffective but **alprazolam** (n = 65, 12/52, Gelernter et al, Arch Gen Psychiatry 1991;48:938–45) is equivalent to other treatments and **clonazepam** has been widely studied (review by Jefferson, J Clin Psychiatry 2001;62[Suppl 1]:S50–S53) and appears safe and effective.

Gabapentin *

Gabapentin (900–3600 mg/d) was well tolerated and significantly reduced symptoms in one trial (n = 69, RCT, d/b, p/c, 14/52, Pande et al, J Clin Psychopharmacol 1999;19:341–8) and 1800 mg/d was as effective as tiagabine for reducing symptoms of social anxiety (n = 8, RCT, d/b, c/o, 2x4/52, Urbano et al, Prim Care Companion J Clin Psychiatry 2009;11:123).

MAOIs

Phenelzine (mean dose 66 mg/d) was effective in 85% patients with refractory social anxiety (n = 7, open, Aarre, Nord J Psychiatry 2003;57:313–5) and in a complex trial, phenelzine was slightly superior to group CBT,

and both were superior to placebo (n = 133, 12/52, Heimberg et al, Arch Gen Psychiatry 1998;55:1113–4; reviewed by Thyer, EBMH 1999;2:80).

Mirtazapine

Mirtazapine seemed effective and well tolerated in women with social anxiety but not comorbid psychiatric illness (n = 66 [c = 60], RCT, d/b, p/c, 10/52, Muehlbacher et al, J Clin Psychopharmacol 2005;25:580–3; comment by Mörtberg, EBMH 2006;9:75), supporting an earlier pilot study with a 41% response rate (n = 14, open, 12/52, van Veen et al, Int Clin Psychopharmacol 2002;17:315–7).

Moclobemide

In a comparison of moclobemide, CBT and the combination, moclobemide was better for subjective general anxiety, CBT for avoidant behaviour (and best overall) and the combination most rapidly effective (n = 81 [c = 66], RCT, p/c, 6/12 + 24/12, Prasko et al, Neuro Endocrinol Lett 2006;27:473–81). Moclobemide has been compared favourably with phenelzine (n = 78, RCT, d/b, 24/52, Versani et al, Br J Psychiatry 1992;161:353–60).

Pregabalin

Pregabalin 600 mg/d was effective and well tolerated in social anxiety, whereas 150 mg/d and placebo were ineffective (n = 135, RCT, d/b, p/c, 10/52, Pande et al, J Clin Psychopharmacol 2004;24:141–9, MS). In a comparative study, it was as effective as lorazepam 6 mg/d (n = 271, RCT, d/b, p/c, 4/52, Feltner et al, J Clin Psychopharmacol 2003;23:240–9, MS; see also Pary, EBMH 2004;7:17).

SSRIs (paroxetine, escitalopram and venlafaxine are licensed)

Citalopram 40 mg/d appears well tolerated and as effective (75% response) as moclobemide (n = 71, RCT, s/b, 8/52, Atmaca et al, Hum Psychopharmacol 2002;17:401–5), supported by additional reports (e.g. Varia et al, Prog Neuropsychopharmacol Biol Psychiatry 2002;26:205–8). Improvement in social anxiety symptoms may lag behind depression resolution, and may need more than 12 weeks for full response (n = 21, open, 12/52, Schneier et al, Depress Anxiety 2003;**17**:191–6). **Fluvoxamine** may have some role, e.g. 200 mg/d (mean dose) was superior to placebo in one study (n = 92, RCT, Stein et al, Am J Psychiatry 1999;**156**:756–60), the CR version was superior to placebo in another (n = 279, RCT, p/c, 12/52, Davidson et al, J Clin Psychopharmacol 2004;**24**:118–25). It may be useful long-term if the person has responded to short-term treatment (n = 112, 24/52 extension, Stein et al, Int J Neuropsychopharmacol 2003;**6**:317–23). **Sertraline** is licensed in several countries for social anxiety and at up to 200 mg/d was more effective than placebo in one well-designed flexible-dose trial, although the exclusion criteria were unclear (n = 204, RCT, 20/52, van Ameringen et al, Am J Psychiatry 2001;**158**:275–81; review by Pieters, EBMH 2001;**4**:91; see also n = 415, RCT, d/b, p/c, 12/52, Liebowitz et al, J Clin Psychiatry 2003;**64**:785–92). Its efficacy may be enhanced by combination with exposure therapy (n = 387, RCT, d/b, 24/52, Blomhoff et al, Br J Psychiatry 2001;**179**:23–30). Sertraline may be effective long-term, but relapse may occur on discontinuation (n = 375, RCT, p/c, d/b, one year, Haug et al, Br J Psychiatry 2003;**182**:312–8). However, a large pilot study failed to show that **fluoxetine** up to 60 mg/d was superior to placebo, although the latter had an unusually high response rate (n = 60, RCT, d/b, 14/52, Kobak et al, J Clin Psychopharmacol 2002; **22**:257–62).

■ Unlicensed/possible efficacy

Botulinum toxin
Severe axillary hyperhydrosis has been treated with botulinum toxin, significantly improving overall disability (n = 40, RCT, p/c, 8/52, Connor et al, J Clin Psychiatry 2006;**67**:30–6).

Levetiracetam
Levetiracetam had a significant effect on symptoms at up to 3 g/d (n = 20, open, 8/52, Simon et al, J Clin Psychiatry 2004;**65**:1219–22) but 500–3000 mg/d was not statistically superior to placebo (n = 16, RCT, d/b, p/c, 7/52, Zhang et al, J Psychopharmacol 2006;**20**:551–3).

Quetiapine *
One study has shown a slight positive effect as monotherapy (n = 15, RCT, p/c, Vaishnavi et al, Prog Neuropsychopharmacol Biol Psychiatry 2007;**31**:1464–9), but single doses of 25 mg were ineffective for social anxiety, and cause drowsiness (n = 20, RCT, d/b, p/c, c/o, Donahue et al, J Anxiety Disord 2008; **23**:362–8).

◆ Others

Other drugs used include **bupropion** (n = 10, open, 12/52, Emmanuel et al, Depress Anxiety 2000; **12**:111–3) and **tricyclics** (n = 15, open, 8/52, Simpson et al, J Clin Psychopharmacol 1998; **18**:132–5)

□ No efficacy

Beta-blockers
There is no evidence for efficacy, except perhaps in people where management of tremor is essential, e.g. musicians (e.g. nadolol; n = 31, d/b, c/o, s/b, James and Savage, Am Heart J 1984;**108**:1150–5). Pindolol 15 mg/d was no more effective than placebo in augmenting SSRI treatment of generalised social phobia (n = 14, d/b, p/c, c/o, 4/52, Stein et al, Am J Psychiatry 2001;**158**:1725–7). However, illicit self-medication with propranolol (up to 320 mg/d) has been reported (n = 1, Fontanella, Rev Bras Psiquiatr 2003;**25**:228–30), with symptoms manageable with adjunctive paroxetine, so maybe it does work, but at higher doses.

Caffeine *
Caffeine induces more severe performance anxiety suggesting a hyperreactivity to caffeine (n = 28 + 26, RCT, d/b, c/o, Nardi et al, Psychiatry Res 2009;**169**:149–53).

St John's wort
SJW was not superior to placebo in one trial (n = 40, RCT, p/c, 12/52, Kobak et al, J Clin Psychopharmacol 2005;**25**:51–8).

Valproate
A small study showed complete ineffectiveness of valproate at up to 1500 mg/d (n = 16, mentioned by Jefferson, J Clin Psychiatry 2001; **62**[Suppl 1]:S50–S53).

1.28 TOURETTE'S SYNDROME (GILLES DE LA TOURETTE)
see also OCD (*1.20*) and SIB (*1.25*)

The main diagnostic symptoms of this hereditary disorder include multiple tics, vocal tics (grunts, snarls and obscenities), stereotyped movements (jumping and dancing), overactivity, learning difficulties and emotional problems. the incidence is 1–5 per 10000 and is more common in males. It has an onset at 5–6 years, beginning with respiratory or vocal tics with grunting or barking noises. Psychiatric comorbidity is common, e.g. OCD, anxiety, depression and ADHD.

Role of drugs
If the condition is affecting the person's abilities to function, drug therapy may be useful. Low starting doses, gradual increases and adequate trials are necessary.
Reviews: pharmacological options (Silay and Jankovic, *Expert Opin Emerg Drugs* 2005;**10**:365–80; Jimenez-Jimenez and Garcia-Ruiz, *Drugs* 2001;**61**:2207–20).

BNF listed

Haloperidol
Haloperidol 0.5–40mg/d was the licensed drug of choice and remains a treatment option. Side-effects may be limiting and its efficacy has been questioned (n = 22, p/c, d/b, Sallee et al, *Am J Psychiatry* 1997;**154**:1057–62). See also pimozide and nicotine chewing gum.

Pimozide *
Pimozide 1–20mg/d may be as effective as, or superior to, haloperidol (eg. n = 22, p/c, d/b, Sallee et al, *Am J Psychiatry* 1997;**154**:1057–62), with less side-effects. Cochrane concludes that pimozide is effective, although the data is limited (s = 6, n = 162, RCT, Pringsheim and Marras, *Cochrane Database Syst Rev* 2009;**2**:CD006996). An ECG is essential monitoring (see *3.2.1*).

+ Combinations

Naltrexone + codeine
Sequential use of naltrexone (100–300mg/d) and codeine phosphate (15–120mg/d) has proved effective (n = 2, McConville et al, *Lancet* 1994;**343**:601). See also naltrexone/opiate antagonists.

● Unlicensed/some efficacy

Antipsychotics (see also BNF Listed) *
There are now a number of studies showing a significant effect from **risperidone**, eg. a mean dose of 2.5mg/d was clearly superior to placebo on global assessment of Tourette symptoms (n = 48, RCT, d/b, p/c, Dion et al, *J Clin Psychopharmacol* 2002;**22**:31–9), and a mean dose of 3.8mg/d was at least as effective as pimozide (mean 2.9mg/d), but was much better tolerated (n = 50, d/b, 12/52, Bruggeman et al, *J Clin Psychiatry* 2001;**62**:50–6). Risperidone (mean 2.5mg/d) may also be useful for the short-term management of tics in Tourette's (n = 34, RCT, d/b, p/c, 8/52, Scahill et al, *Neurology* 2003;**60**:1130–5) and may have similar efficacy to clonidine over a wide range of symptoms (n = 21, RCT, d/b, 8/52, Gaffney et al, *J Am Acad Child Adolesc Psychiatry* 2002;**41**:330–6). **Sulpiride** 200–400mg/d has been used, as has **amisulpride** (n = 1, Fountoulakis et al, *Ann Pharmacother* 2004;**38**:901). **Aripiprazole** (mean 12mg/d) reduced tics and explosive outbursts in 100% and 96% completers respectively (n = 37 [c = 29], open, retrospective, Budman et al, *J Child Adolesc Psychopharmacol* 2008;**18**:509–15), with low-doses seeming effective for Tourette's and tics (n = 15, open, 12/52, Seo et al, *J Child Adolesc Psychopharmacol* 2008;**18**:197–205; Kastrup et al, *J Clin Psychopharmacol* 2005;**25**:94–6). 10–20mg/d has been dramatically and rapidly effective in some patients (n = 11, Davies et al, *Hum Psychopharmacol* 2006;**21**:447–53; Bubl et al, *World J Biol Psychiatry* 2006;**7**:123–5), including late-onset Tourette's (n = 1, Ikenouchi-Sugita et al, *World J Biol Psychiatry* 2009;**10**:977–80; for review see Kawohl et al, *World J Biol Psychiatry* 2008;**10**:827–31). In a small study, **olanzapine** (mean 14.5mg/d) improved aggression and tics in Tourette's, albeit with significant weight gain (n = 10, RCT, s/b, 10/52, Stephens et al, *J Child Adolesc Psychopharmacol* 2004;**14**:255–66; n = 12, open, 6/12, McCracken et al, *J Child*

Adolesc Psychopharmacol 2008;**18**:501–8) and it may be superior to pimozide (n = 4, d/b, c/o, 12/12, Onofrj et al, *J Neurol* 2000;**247**:443–6). **Quetiapine** (mean 175 mg/d) may have some efficacy in Tourette's syndrome (n = 12, retrospective, 8/52, Copur et al, *Clin Drug Invest* 2007;**27**:123–30). and 200 mg/d had a significant effect on tics, but was not well tolerated (n = 12 [c = 9], open, 8–12/52, de Jonge et al, *J Clin Psychiatry* 2007; **68**:1148–50).

Clonidine *

Clonidine 0.1–0.6 mg/d may be as effective as haloperidol. Clonidine or methylphenidate alone or in combination are effective for ADHD with comorbid tics (n = 16, RCT, p/c, 16/52, TSSG, *Neurology* 2002;**58**:527–36; review by Goldberg, *EBMH* 2002;**5**:122), and clonidine 0.1 mg/d was effective in a trial vs levetiracetam (n = 12 [c = 10], RCT, d/b, c/o, 15/52, Hedderick et al, *Pediatr Neurol* 2009; **40**:420–5).

Lorazepam

Lorazepam 1.5–10 mg/d may be useful as adjuvant therapy.

Topiramate *

Topiramate has been used with some success (n = 29 [c = 20], RCT, d/b, p/c, 10/52, Jankovic et al, *J Neurol Neurosurg Psychiatry* 2010;**81**:70–3; see also n = 2, Abuzzhab and Brown, *Am J Psychiatry* 2001;**158**:968).

■ Unlicensed/possible efficacy

Cannabinoids

In a survey of people with Tourette's who had tried marijuana, 82% reported a reduction or complete remission in motor and vocal tics, urges and OCD symptoms (n = 17, Muller-Vahl et al, *Acta Psychiatr Scand* 1998;**98**:502–6), and an RCT showed that THC doses of up to 10 mg/d showed significant trends in favour of THC on a variety of measures, with no reported adverse effects (n = 24, RCT, d/b, 6/52, Muller-Vahl et al, *J Clin Psychiatry* 2003;**64**:459–65).

Donepezil

Successful use has been proposed (Niederhofer, *Mov Disord* 2006;**21**:2027).

Finasteride

Finasteride 5 mg/d has been used successfully in a resistant case (n = 1, Bortolato et al, *Am J Psychiatry* 2007;**164**:1914–5).

Fluoxetine

81% patients with OCD in Tourette's syndrome had improved symptoms on fluoxetine (n = 32, open, *Neurology* 1991;**41**:872–4). A potential effect has been suggested in children with OCD symptoms in Tourette's (n = 11, Kyrlan et al, *Clin Neuropharmacol* 1993; **16**:167–72).

Methylphenidate

Methylphenidate can aggravate tics or be associated with their appearance (Klein and Wender, *Arch Gen Psychiatry* 1995;**52**:429–33), but some tics may be significantly worse, although generally these are not to the extent of contraindicating a trial, e.g. in ADHD with Tourette's (Gadow et al, *Arch Gen Psychiatry* 1995;**52**:444–55). See also clonidine.

Nicotine

Transdermal nicotine (7 mg/d) has been shown to be superior to placebo as an adjunct to haloperidol (eg. n = 70 [c = 56], d/b, p/c, Silver et al, *J Clin Psychiatry* 2001;**62**:707–14). Nicotine chewing gum is an alternative that enhances the symptomatic effects of haloperidol (n = 10, open, McConville et al, *Am J Psychiatry* 1991;**148**:793–4) and PRN usage may have a low risk and help to minimise this.

Ondansetron

In haloperidol-resistant Tourette's, ondansetron 24 mg/d significantly improved tic severity on one rating scale but not on others (n = 30, RCT, d/b, p/c, 3/52, Toren et al, *J Clin Psychiatry* 2005;**66**:499–503).

Pergolide

Pergolide (up to 300 mcg/d) may be safe and effective in children with Tourette's disorder, chronic motor or vocal tic disorder (n = 245, RCT, 6/52, Gilbert et al, *Neurology* 2000;**54**:1310–6).

Tetrabenazine *

For a review of use see Porta et al, *Clin Drug Investig* 2008;**28**:443–59.

◆ Others *

Other drugs used include **buspirone** 30mg/d (n=1, Dursun et al, Lancet 1995;**345**:1366–7), **calcium-channel blockers** (verapamil and nifedipine, but not diltiazem; n=2, Walsh et al, Am J Psychiatry 1986;**143**:1467–68), methadone 110mg/d (n=1, Meuldijk and Colon, Am J Psychiatry 1992;**149**:139–40), **nifedipine** (Berg, Acta Psychiatr Scand 1985;**72**:400–1),**paroxetine** (n=45, open, 8/52, Bruun and Budman, J Clin Psychiatry 1998;**59**:581–4), pentazocine (Clin Pharm 1985; **4**:494), and **selegiline** (n=24, d/b, p/c, c/o, Feigin et al, Neurology 1996;**46**:965–8).

□ No efficacy

**Levetiracetam *

In a small but perfectly formed trial, levetiracetam (10mg/kg/d) was completely ineffective (n=12 [c=10],RCT,d/b,c/o,15/52,Hedderick et al, Pediatr Neurol 2009;**40**:420–5).

1.29 TRICHOTILLOMANIA
see also OCD (1.20)

Symptoms
Trichotillomania presents as impulsive pulling out of a person's own hair (scalp, eyebrows, and eyelashes, pubic, chest, etc), resulting in hair loss. It is associated with OCD, and can occur in the presence of learning disability, anxiety, depression, schizophrenia and borderline personality disorder. It may result in relief of tension, can be episodic or chronic, and is more common in females.

Role of drugs *
A range of psychological and behaviour therapies are used and may be most effective when combined with pharmacotherapy. A significant review has concluded that clomipramine is effective, but that SSRIs are not (s=7, Bloch et al, Biol Psychiatry 2007;**62**:839–46), and trials need to be of at least 8–10 weeks duration to prove or disprove an effect in an individual case. HRT (habit reversal training) combined with sertraline is more effective than either approach alone (n=24, RCT, d/b, Dougherty et al, J Clin Psychiatry 2006;**67**:1086–92). Dermatological help is beneficial.
Reviews: general (Papadopulos et al, Int J

Dermatol 2003;**42**:330–4; Nuss et al, Cutis 2003;**72**:191–6; Hautmann et al, J Am Acad Dermatol 2002;**46**:807–21).

+ Combinations

Antipsychotics + SSRI
Symptom improvement has been reported when **olanzapine** 10mg/d was added to **fluoxetine** 40mg/d (n=1, Potenza et al, Am J Psychiatry 1998;**155**:1329–30). Olanzapine 1.25–7.5mg/d has been used with some success as augmentation of citalopram in refractory cases (n=4, Ashton, Am J Psychiatry 2001;**158**:1929–30). Resistant trichotillomania has responded to **risperidone** augmentation of **fluvoxamine** (n=1, Gabriel, Can J Psychiatry 2001;**46**:285–6).

● Unlicensed/some efficacy

Clomipramine
Several studies (s=7, Bloch et al, Biol Psychiatry 2007;**62**:839–46) have shown clomipramine in doses of around 180mg/d to be effective in some patients with trichotillomania.

■ Unlicensed/possible efficacy

Bupropion
Bupropion 300mg/d (but not 150mg/d) has produced almost complete resolution of symptoms in one treatment-resistant case (n=1, Bhanji and Margolese, J Clin Psychiatry 2004;**65**:1283).

SSRIs
A major review concluded that SSRIs lack significant clinical effect (s=7, Bloch et al, Biol Psychiatry 2007;**62**:839–46), although there are some positive reports. **Citalopram** may be safe in trichotillomania, with modest but significant effects (n=14, open, 12/52, Stein et al, Eur Arch Psychiatry Clin Neurosci 1997;**247**:234–6). **Escitalopram** 10mg/d produced complete remission in a 10-year-old boy (n=1, Bhatia and Sapra, Eur Psychiatry 2004;**19**:239–40). **Fluoxetine** appears minimally effective (e.g. Winchel et al, J Clin Psychiatry 1992;**53**:304–8; n=21, RCT, d/b, c/o, 18/52, Christenson, Am J Psychiatry 1991;**148**:1566–71), the doses

required are high (up to 80mg/d) and if response occurs, relapse is not uncommon and was no better than placebo in two studies (n=43, RCT, 12/52, van Minnen et al, Arch Gen Psychiatry 2003;**60**:517–22; n=23, d/b, c/o, 31/52, Streichenwein and Thornby, Am J Psychiatry 1995;**152**:1192–6). Potential use has been reported from **fluvoxamine** in reducing distress, but not hair pulling (n=21, open, 12/52, Stanley et al, J Clin Psychopharmacol 1997;**17**:278–83).

Haloperidol
Haloperidol has been used successfully as SSRI augmentation (n=9, open, Van Ameringen et al, J Affect Disord 1999; **56**:219–26).

Inositol
Inositol, a glucose isomer with notable effects on serotonin, was well tolerated and effective in reducing hair pulling in patients unwilling to take, or who are intolerant of SSRIs (n=3, Seedat et al, J Clin Psychiatry 2001;**62**:60–1).

Lithium *
80% patients tried on lithium showed reduced hair pulling and some hair regrowth, possibly via an effect on aggressive behaviour (n=10, open, 14/12, Christenson et al, J Clin Psychiatry 1991;**52**:116–20; see also Sharma and Corpse, Arch Women's Ment Health 2008;**11**:305–6).

Olanzapine
Olanzapine monotherapy up to 10mg/d has produced a significant reduction in hair pulling and anxiety, with 22% achieving full remission (n=18, open, 3/12, Stewart and Nejtek, J Clin Psychiatry 2003;**64**:49–52), and it has been successfully used to augment fluoxetine (n=2, Srivastava et al, Aust NZ J Psychiatry 2005; **39**:112–3).

Quetiapine
There is one case report of response (n=1, Khouzam et al, Psychiatry 2002;**65**:261–70).

Valproate *
Higher-dose valproate has produced a sustained improvement in a 10-year-old girl (n=1, Adewuya et al, J Child Adolesc Psychopharmacol 2008;**18**:533–6).

■ Others

Other drugs include **paroxetine** (n=1, Reid, Am J Psychiatry 1994;**151**:290), **pimozide** (e.g. J Clin Psychiatry 1992;**53**:123–6) and **trazodone** (e.g. Sunkureddi and Markovitz, Am J Psychiatry 1993;**150**:523–4).

1.30 CAFFEINISM

Caffeine is an antagonist at adenosine receptors. Reducing adenosine activity increases dopamine activity, leading to increased activity. Tolerance develops very quickly to the stimulant effect, e.g. complete tolerance to sleep disruption from 400mg/d occurs in seven days. Caffeine consumption at 250–500mg/d is regarded as moderate use. Caffeinism is estimated to start at a consumption of between 600mg and 750mg/d, with above 1000mg/d well into the toxic range. Caffeine dependence displays features of a typical psychoactive substance dependence, i.e. withdrawal, continued use despite caffeine-induced problems, tolerance and persistent desire or unsuccessful attempts to cut down or control use (n=16, Strain et al, JAMA 1994;**272**:1043–8).

Caffeine withdrawal *
Caffeine withdrawal is a DSM-IV diagnosis and thus should be taken seriously. The 14 main withdrawal symptoms fall into three groups (Ozsungur et al, Psychopharmacology [Berl] 2009; **201**:541–8):

1. Fatigue and headache (52%) – more likely with high habitual use
2. Dysphoric mood, rebound drowsiness – more likely with high habitual use
3. Flu-like, somatic – no more likely with high habitual use than low use

(review by Dews et al, Food Chem Toxicol 2002; **40**:1257–61).

Symptoms of caffeinism (acute or chronic) *
Adverse effects of low-to-moderate doses: Diuresis, increased gastric secretion, fine tremor, increased skeletal muscle stamina, mild anxiety, negative mood, palpitations and nervousness. Adverse effects of high doses: Chronic insomnia, persistent anxiety, restlessness, tension, irritability, tremulousness, panic, poor con-

centration, confusion, disorientation, paranoia, delirium, tremor, muscle twitching, convulsions, vertigo, dizziness, tinnitus, auditory and visual hallucinations, facial flushing, hyperthermia, nausea, vomiting, abdominal discomfort and tachypnoea. High caffeine use is also associated with high daily cigarette use, and aggression, conduct disorder, ADHD and social problems in adolescents (n = 132, Martin et al, Scientific World Journal 2008;**8**:512–6).

Adverse consequences: There is some contradictory evidence about the effect of caffeine on people with mental health problems. Clearly, high doses can cause significant effects. Acute high doses (10mg/kg) significantly increase arousal and have a psychotogenic effect in schizophrenics (n = 13, d/b, Lucas et al, Biol Psychiatry 1990;**28**:35–40). Schizophrenics often have higher caffeine intakes and average intake should be routinely monitored (Rihs et al, Eur Arch Psychiatry Clin Neurosci 1996;**246**:83–92). Caffeinism can precipitate or exacerbate psychoses and make these more resistant (n = 2, Zaslove et al, Br J Psychiatry 1991;**159**:565–7) to drug treatment, especially antipsychotics. The clinical signs of affective diseases can be modified. Caffeine 150mg at bedtime has a marked effect on sleep latency, total sleep time and reduced sleep efficacy and REM periods. Consumption may be influenced by some genetic factors (n = 1934 twin study, Kendler and Prescott, Am J Psychiatry 1999;**156**:223–8). Conversely, there are reports of lack of correlation between caffeine consumption and anxiety and depression.

Methods of caffeine reduction
1. Recognition of the problems of excess caffeine consumption (>750mg/d) and the likely benefits of reduction.
2. Identification of all current caffeine sources and the pattern of consumption.
3. Implement a planned gradual reduction, e.g. making weaker drinks, taken less often, increasing use of caffeine-free equivalent drinks (particularly at 'usual' drinking times of the day), using half-caffeine coffee, or mixing caffeine and decaffeinated coffee to give a lower strength.
4. Use of analgesia (caffeine-free, of course) for withdrawal headaches.

5. Setting a target for consumption, which will not need to be complete abstinence, e.g. caffeine drinks only at set times in the day, e.g. on rising, etc.

Calculating caffeine intake:

Source	Caffeine content	
	per 100ml	per container
Brewed coffee*	55–85mg	140–210mg/cup
Instant coffee	35–45mg	85–110mg/cup
Decaf. coffee	2mg	5mg/cup
Cocoa	3mg	7mg/cup
Brewed tea*	25–55mg	55–140mg/cup
Coca-cola	11mg	36mg/can
Pepsi cola	7mg	22mg/can
Milk chocolate		22mg/100g
Hedex seltzer		60mg/sachet
A cup is taken as being 250ml		

Reviews: general (Smith, Food Chem Toxicol 2002;**40**:1243–55), caffeine craving questionnaire (West and Roderique-Davies, J Psychopharmacol 2008;**22**:80–91), withdrawal (Juliano and Griffiths, Psychopharmacology [Berl] 2004;**176**:1–29).

1.31 ELECTROCONVULSIVE THERAPY (ECT)

ECT was first used in its current form in 1938 (Linington and Harris, Br Med J 1988;**297**:1354–5). It is effective for rapid and short-term improvement in severe depression where other treatments have proven ineffective or life is threatened. The risks are higher in pregnancy, older people and in children. It is also used in mania (especially manic delirium), more rarely catatonia and drug-resistant Parkinsonism. ECT is probably superior to, or at least as effective as, antidepressants and tends to be quicker-acting in severely depressed patients, although there remains some dispute about this. ECT may be better than antidepressants for the short-term treatment of acute depression (n = 256, s = 6, UK ECT Group, Lancet 2003;**361**:799–808; comment by Bauer, EBMH 2003;**6**:83). Combining maintenance ECT with antidepressants has been suggested as improving outcomes in patients who have responded to acute treatment with ECT, compared to antidepressants only (n = 58, retrospective chart review, Gagné et al, Am J Psychiatry 2000;**157**:1960–5).

High-risk patients: These include those with severe cardiovascular disease, arrhythmias, pacemakers, obstructive pulmonary disease, asthma, pregnancy, osteoporosis, cerebral tumours, hydrocephalus and multiple sclerosis. If the patient has hypertension, sublingual nifedipine 20 minutes prior to ECT attenuates the hypertensive response (n = 5, Wells et al, Anaesth Intensive Care 1989;**17**:31–3).

Premedication: Atropine or glycopyrrolate can be used as antimuscarinics, mainly in patients with cardiovascular risks (n = 19, Bouckoms et al, Convulsive Therapy 1989;**5**:48–55).

Muscle relaxants: Suxamethonium is used to prevent fractures that can occur during the procedure secondary to the tonic-clonic muscular contractions (n = 52, d/b, Konarzewski et al, Anaesthesia 1988;**43**:474–6).

Induction agents: * **Propofol** is now widely used as it is well tolerated and short-acting with a quick recovery. It shortens seizure length by up to 30% but seemingly without significant effect on the clinical outcome (n = 62, RCT, Bauer et al, J ECT 2009;**25**:85–90; n = 20, d/b, Fear et al, Br J Psychiatry 1994;**165**:506–9), although ECT courses may be prolonged. It may be associated with bradycardia and hypotension. **Etomidate** is short-acting, has a rapid recovery, less hypotension than propofol and may lengthen seizure duration compared to methohexital and propofol (Ilivicky et al, Am J Psychiatry 1995;**152**:957–8) but is painful at the injection site, has a high incidence of extraneous muscle movements, and rarely causes adrenocortical dysfunction with repeated doses (a major concern which limits use with longer courses), although it can be successful (n = 3, Benbow et al, Psychiatr Bull 2002;**26**:351–3). Inhaled **sevoflurane** has been used successfully as an induction agent for ECT (n = 5, Palmer et al, Psychiatr Bull 2004;**28**:326–8) and is equivalent to thiopental for induction, and significantly better for postictal orientation 20 minutes after treatment (n = 31, RCT, d/b, Rasmussen et al, J ECT 2007;**23**:236–8).

Maintenance: * ECT has been used at two-, three- and then four-weekly intervals for six months to prevent relapse, with variable success rates (reviews; n = 201, RCT, 6/12, Kellner et al, Arch Gen Psychiatry 2006;**63**:1337–44; van Beusekom et al, J ECT 2007;**23**:17–20; n = 43, Russell et al, J ECT 2003;**19**:4–9; Gupta et al, J ECT 2008;**24**:191–4).

Post-ECT memory loss and agitation: * High anticholinergic drug levels have been associated with a greater risk of post-ECT confusion (n = 20, Mondimore et al, Am J Psychiatry 1983; **140**:930–1). Oral thiamine 50–200mg/d may lead to rapid resolution (3–5 days) of post-ECT confusion and memory loss, and so thiamine deficiency is implicated in post-ECT confusional state (n = 3, Linton et al, Int J Geriatr Psychiatry 2002;**7**:189–92). **Promethazine** 25–50mg orally 1–2 hours before ECT has been used successfully for severe post-ECT agitation (n = 8, Vishne et al, J ECT 2005;**21**:118–21). **Piracetam** appears to have no effect in reducing post-ECT cognitive impairment either in short (n = 18, d/b, c/o, 3/7, Mindus et al, Acta Psychiatr Scand 1975; **51**:319–26) or longer courses (given during and after an ECT course), although it might slightly enhance ECT's clinical effect (n = 38, RCT, d/b, p/c, >2/52, Tang et al, J ECT 2002;**18**:130–7). In recurrent post-ECT aggression, 5mg IV immediately after the seizure each time resolved the recovery without incident (n = 1, Labbate and Miller, Am J Psychiatry 1995;**152**:472–3). Propofol has been used to help manage postictal agitation after ECT (n = 10, O'Reardon et al, J ECT 2006;**22**:247–52). **Donepezil** has been used successfully for cognitive deficits associated with maintenance ECT (see donepezil).

Reviews: * comprehensive reviews (Lisanby, N Engl J Med 2007;**357**:1939–45; Scott, Adv Psychiatr Treat 2005;**11**:150–6), in the elderly (Flint and Gagnon, Can J Psychiatry 2002;**47**:734–41).

Drug considerations

There are no RCTs of ECT given with concurrent anticonvulsants and one thorough review suggests that there is no evidence that ECT and anticonvulsants cannot be used together (Sienaert and Peuskens, J ECT 2007;**23**:120–3).

Agomelatine

There is no experience on the use of agomelatine with ECT, but no pro- or anticonvulsant effects have been shown (MI).

Antipsychotics * (see also clozapine)

Antipsychotics lower the seizure threshold and would be expected to lead to seizures at lower ECT doses. A review of ECT with antipsychotics in schizophrenia concluded that the combination appeared to be safe and effective (review by Braga and Petrides, *J ECT* 2005;**21**:75–83). ECT and risperidone Consta have been used successfully together (n = 1, Sengul et al, *J ECT* 2009;**25**:282–3). Weekly ECT followed by maintenance as indicated as an adjunct to sulpiride (n = 17), risperidone (n = 26) and olanzapine (n = 27) showed long-term safety and some efficacy (especially with olanzapine), albeit with a high drop-out rate (n = 70 [c = 32], two years, Ravani et al, *Psychiatr Danub* 2009;**21**:179–86). There were also no apparent problems with ECT in a patient taking olanzapine and duloxetine (n = 1, Hanretta and Malek-Ahmadi, *J ECT* 2006;**22**:139–41). There were no significant adverse effects when ECT was used with aripiprazole (n = 4, Masdrakis et al, *J ECT* 2008;**24**:236–8).

Benzodiazepines

Benzodiazepines may lessen the improvement with unilateral ECT (n = 124, Jha and Stein, *Acta Psychiatr Scand* 1996;**94**:101–4). They may reduce the effectiveness of ECT, even several months after treatment is stopped, probably by raising the seizure threshold, having an effect on seizure duration, the number of sub-maximal seizures or by increasing the number of treatments needed.

Bupropion

Use with ECT has been reported (n = 2, Kellner et al, *J Clin Psychopharmacol* 1994;**14**:215–6), as has prolonged seizures when used with lithium and venlafaxine (n = 1, Conway and Nelson, *J ECT* 2001;**17**:216–8).

Caffeine

Caffeine 240 mg IV has been used to augment seizure duration (reported by the ideally named Coffey et al, *Am J Psychiatry* 1990;**147**:579–85) or 300–1000 mg orally (n = 30, Ancill and Carlyle, *Am J Psychiatry* 1992;**149**:137), as has 125 mg IV during treatment (Jaffe and Dubin, *Am J Psychiatry* 1992;**149**:1610). A small study showed a complex effect which deserves a full study to determine the optimum dose and timing (Francis et al, *Am J Psychiatry* 1994;**151**:1524–6). Cases of cardiac dysrhythmia have been reported.

Carbamazepine

Logic would dictate that since carbamazepine is an anticonvulsant it would have an effect on reducing seizures (as for benzodiazepines). A small retrospective study showed that in seven patients taking either valproate or carbamazepine, seizure durations were slightly shorter but that this appeared to have no dramatic effect on either the efficacy or side-effects of ECT (n = 7, Zarate et al, *Ann Clin Psychiatry* 1997;**9**:19–25).

Ciprofloxacin

There is a case of prolonged seizures related to concurrent ciprofloxacin 1 g/d (n = 1, Kisa et al, *J ECT* 2005;**21**:43–4).

Clozapine *

The UK SPCs recommend suspending clozapine for 24 hours pre-ECT to reduce the risk of unwanted seizures. However, there have been four case series that may help. One showed that 2–20 sessions of ECT with clozapine (mean 518 mg/d, range 200–900 mg/d) to probably be safe and with short-term efficacy (72% showing marked initial improvement but only in 23% beyond 4/12) in resistant cases (n = 22, Havaki-Kontaxaki et al, *Clin Neuropharmacol* 2006;**29**:52–6). An active comparison, combined ECT and clozapine improved TRS more than either alone (PANSS scores reductions 71% combination, 46% clozapine and 40% placebo) and there were no significant adverse effects with the combination (n = 18, p/c, Masoudzadeh and Khalilian, *Pak J Biol Sci* 2007;**10**:4287–90). Finally, the combination appeared particularly effective in schizoaffective patients (n = 43, Gazdag et al, *Ideggyogy Sz* 2006;**59**:261–7; see also n = 36, Kupchik et al, *Clin Neuropharmacol* 2000;**23**:14–16). Prolonged seizures (n = 1, Bloch et al, *Br J Psychiatry* 1996;**169**:253–4) and supra-ventricular tachycardia (Beale et al, *Convul Ther* 1994;**10**:228–31) have been reported. Apart from mild cognitive disturbances, there were no negative consequences from 24 ECTs in someone taking high-dose clozapine (1600 mg/d), although there were no positive consequences either (n = 1, Keller et al, *J ECT* 2009;**25**:280–1). However, not omitting doses is, however, a risky strategy, especially with higher doses of clozapine where the seizure threshold may be significantly lower.

Donepezil *

Donepezil has been used successfully for treating cognitive deficits from maintenance ECT (n=1, Rao et al, J ECT 2009;**25**:216-8). Donepezil 5mg given from before ECT until three days after ECT finishes improves post-ECT cognitive function recovery time compared to placebo (n=45, RCT, t/b, p/c, Prakash et al, J ECT 2006;**22**:163–8; n=1, Logan and Stewart, J ECT 2007;**23**:28–9).

Duloxetine

There were no apparent problems with ECT in a patient taking olanzapine and duloxetine (n=1, Hanretta and Malek-Ahmadi, J ECT 2006;**22**:139–41).

Escitalopram *

There is a report of ECT being well-tolerated with escitalopram 20mg/d (n=3, Masdrakis et al, J ECT 2008;**24**:289–91).

Flumazenil

Effective ECT was only possible in a benzodiazepine-dependent depressed woman when the anticonvulsant effect of clonazepam was reversed by flumazenil 0.1mg (n=1, Berigan et al, Am J Psychiatry 1995;**152**:957).

Ibuprofen

Ibuprofen 600mg/d 90 minutes before ECT may reduce the frequency and severity of post-ECT headache (n=34, RCT, p/c, d/b, Leung et al, J Clin Psychiatry 2003;**64**:551–3), although Kessler thinks their data shows that it might actually increase seizure duration (Kessler, J Clin Psychiatry 2004;**65**:442).

Ketamine

Enhanced ECT seizure duration has been reported (mentioned in review by Weiner et al, 1991;**14**:857–67).

Lamotrigine

Lamotrigine (mean 100mg/d) had no adverse effect on concurrent ECT in bipolar depression, with no rashes, no worsening cognitive function and clinically adequate ECT

seizures (n=9, Penland and Ostroff, J ECT 2006;**22**:142–7).

Lithium

The use of lithium with ECT has been reported to cause severe memory loss, neurological abnormalities and a reduced antidepressant effect, although a retrospective study showed no increase in side-effects or other problems (e.g. n=12 and review, Dolenc and Rasmussen, J ECT 2005;**21**:165–70). There are reports of prolonged seizure, serotonin syndrome and focal seizure with ECT and lithium at sub-therapeutic levels (n=3, Sartorius et al, World J Biol Psychiatry 2005;**6**:121–4). It has been suggested that ECT facilitates lithium toxicity, possibly by releasing lithium from cells, producing a pure toxicity. Elderly patients may be more susceptible to this combination. Some sources recommend discontinuing lithium 48 hours before ECT to prevent this neurotoxicity and not re-starting for several days after the last treatment (Ferrier et al, Adv Psychiatr Treat 1995;**1**:102–10). A review of the pros and cons of the use of lithium in ECT (Lippmann and El-Mallakh, Lithium 1994;**5**:205–9) concluded that there must be clear indications for concurrent use of both treatments. However, discontinuing lithium would risk discontinuation effects and be potentially dangerous (see lithium in 1.10).

MAOIs

MAOIs are normally contraindicated with surgery as they can interact with opiates. However, a review has concluded that there is no dangerous interaction between MAOIs and ECT (n=4, Dolenc et al, J ECT 2004;**20**:258–61).

Moxifloxacin

Moxifloxacin has been associated with prolonged seizures (n=1, Reti and Davydow, J ECT 2007;**23**:289–90).

Mirtazapine

An open study indicated that there were no problems with mirtazapine, either started before or during a course of ECT (n=19, Söderström, poster, WCP, 1999, Germany). There are cases of successful and uneventful use (n=2, Farah, Convul Ther 1997;**13**:116–7).

Moclobemide
The SPC recommends suspending moclobemide for 24 hours pre-ECT, although there is no data on its use with ECT.

Naloxone
Naloxone has no detectable effect (Rasmussen et al, Convuls Ther 1997;**13**: 44–6).

Rivastigmine
There is a case of eight ECTs being successful with the person taking rivastigmine throughout (n = 1, Zink et al, J ECT 2002;**18**:162–4).

SSRIs
A small study showed a significantly longer seizure duration in patients taking SSRIs compared to other antidepressants (n = 13, Potokar et al, Int J Psychiatr Clin Pract 1997;**1**:277–80), although an earlier review did not support the theory that **fluoxetine** causes prolonged seizures (n = 12, Gutierrez-Esteinou and Pope, Convul Ther 1989;**5**:344–8). There are reports of prolonged seizures with ECT and **paroxetine** and in a rater-blinded comparison seizure length was twice as long in those taking paroxetine (n = 14, Curran, Acta Psychiatr Scand 1995;**92**:239–40). Prolonged seizures may occur with **fluvoxamine** and ECT and the SPC recommends a four-day interval between stopping fluvoxamine and giving ECT. There is only limited experience with ECT and **sertraline** or **citalopram**.

Steroids *
In chronic steroid users, additional 'stress doses' are sometimes given before general anaesthesia, but this appears unnecessary for prednisolone and ECT (n = 27, Rasmussen et al, J ECT 2008;**24**:128–30).

Sumatriptan
Sumatriptan may prevent post-ECT headaches (White et al, Headache 2006;**46**:692).

Theophylline
Theophylline (related to caffeine) at 100–400 mg IV has been reported to facilitate ECT seizures in previously resistant patients (n = 7,

Leentjens et al, Convuls Ther 1996;**12**:232–7). There are, however, reports of status epilepticus and increase in seizure duration with concomitant ECT.

Trazodone
A prolonged seizure duration has been reported (n = 1, Lanes and Ravaris, Am J Psychiatry 1993;**150**:525), although low-dose use did not produce any problems in one retrospective study (n = 100, Krahn et al, J Clin Psychiatry 2001;**62**:108–10).

Tricyclics *
Combined tricyclic and ECT therapy is often used and seems to present no routine problems. Indeed, nortriptyline enhances the effect of ECT and reduces cognitive adverse effects (n < 319, RCT, Sackeim et al, Arch Gen Psychiatry 2009;**66**:729–37). The use of anaesthetics could enhance the risk of cardiac arrhythmias and hypotension.

Valproate
A small retrospective study showed that in patients taking either valproate or carbamazepine, seizure durations were slightly shorter but that this appeared to have no dramatic effect on the efficacy, or side-effects of ECT (n = 7, Zarate et al, Ann Clin Psychiatry 1997;**9**:19–25).

Venlafaxine *
Venlafaxine seems to reduce the effect of ECT and tends to worsen cognitive adverse effects (n < 319, RCT, Sackeim et al, Arch Gen Psychiatry 2009;**66**:729–37; n = 1, Jha and Tomar, Int J Geriatr Psychiatry 2002;**17**:979–80). Venlafaxine at doses of up to 300 mg/d seems safe if propofol is the anaesthetic but the possibility of asystole cannot be excluded (n = 13, Gonzalez-Pinto et al, J Neuropsychiatry Clin Neurosci 2002; **14**:206–9).

Zopiclone
Reduced seizure length has been reported with 7.5–15 mg of zopiclone the previous night (n = 2, Tobiansky, J Psychopharmacol 1991; **5**:268–9) and so is best avoided.

SELECTING DRUGS, DOSES AND PREPARATIONS

TABLE 2.1.1: HYPNOTICS — RELATIVE SIDE-EFFECTS

Class	Drug	Usual night dose mg/d	Adult max dose mg/d	Elderly max dose mg/d	Elimination half-life (hours) adult	Elimination half-life (hours) elderly	G/I upset	Hang-over	Dependence potential
Shorter-acting benzodiazepines									
1a	Loprazolam	1	2	7	10	24	O	●	●
1a	Lormetazepam	1	1.5+	<Ad	10	14	O	●	●
1a	Temazepam	10–20	40	20	5–11	14+	O	●	●●
Longer-acting benzodiazepines									
1b	Flunitrazepam	1	2	1	35	35	O	●●	●
1b	Flurazepam	15	30	15+	47–95	?	O	●●●	●●
1b	Nitrazepam	5	10	5	18–36	40+	O	●●●	●
Chloral and derivatives									
2	Chloral betane	707	5 tabs	<Ad?	7–10	Same	●●●	●	●
2	Triclofos	1 g	2 g	1 g	?	?	●	?	?
Other hypnotics									
3	Clomethiazole#	N/A#	2 caps#	Same	4–5	Same	O	●	●●
4	Promethazine	25	50	–	10–19	10–19	O	O	O
5	Zaleplon	10	10	5	2	3	O	O	O
6	Zopiclone	7.5	7.5	<Ad	3.5–6	8	●	●	●
7	Zolpidem	5	(10)	10	2(2–3)	Longer	O	O	O
8	Melatonin	2	2 for 3/52	2	3.5–4	3.5-4	O	O	O
9	Ramelteon (U)	8	8	8	1–2	1–2	O	O	O

Classes
1a = Shorter-acting or minimally-accumulating benzodiazepines
1b = Longer-acting or accumulating benzodiazepines
2 = Chloral and derivative
3 = Clomethiazole (chormethiazole)
4 = Antihistamine
5 = Pyrazolopyrimidine
6 = Imidazopyridine
7 = Cyclopyrrone
8 = Melatonin
9 = Melatonin receptor agonist

Side-effects
●●● = Marked effect
●● = Moderate effect
● = Mild effect
O = Little or nothing reported
? = No information available

Other abbreviations
Usual night dose = Suggested usual dose for an adult in the UK SPC
Adult max dose = Suggested maximum adult hypnotic dose in the UK SPC
Elderly max dose = Suggested maximum elderly hypnotic dose in the UK SPC
# = 1 capsule is therapeutically equivalent to 5 ml syrup. Indicated for severe insomnia in the elderly only.
U = Unlicensed in UK at time of writing

TABLE 2.1.2: ANTIDEPRESSANTS — RELATIVE SIDE-EFFECTS *

Drug	Adult max dose mg/d	Elderly max dose mg/d	Relative side-effects (most will be dose-related)						
			Anti-cholinergic	Cardiac	Nausea ‡	Sedation	Overdose §	Pro-convulsant	Sexual dysfunction
Tricyclics									
Amitriptyline	200	75	●●●	●●●	●●	●●●	●●●	●●	●●
Clomipramine	250	75	●●●	●●	●●	●●	●	●●	●●●
Dosulepin (dothiepin)	150	75	●●	●●	○	●●●	●●●		●●
Doxepin	300	<Ad	●	●●	●	●●	●●		●●
Imipramine	300	50	●●	●●	●●	●	●●●		●●
Lofepramine	210	<Ad	●●	●	●●	●	○	○	●●
Nortriptyline	150	50	●●	●	●●	●	●●	●	●●●
Trimipramine	300	<Ad	●●●	●●	●	●●	●●	●	●●
SSRIs									
Citalopram	60	40	○	○	●●●	○	●	○	●●
Escitalopram	20	<20	○	○	●●	○	○	○	●●
Fluoxetine	(20)	(80)	○	○	●●	○	○	○	●●
Fluvoxamine	300	300	●	○	●●●	●	○	○	●
Paroxetine	50	40	○	○	●●	○	○	○	●●●
Sertraline	200	200	○	○	●●	○	○	○	●●
MAOIs									
Isocarboxazid	60	<Ad	●●	●●	●●	○	●●	○	●
Phenelzine	90	(90)	●●	●	●●	●	●●●	○	●●
Tranylcypromine	CA30	(30)	●	●	●●	●	●●●	○	●

TABLE 2.1.2: ANTIDEPRESSANTS — RELATIVE SIDE-EFFECTS (CONT) *

Drug	Adult max dose mg/d	Elderly max dose mg/d	Relative side-effects (most will be dose-related)						
			Anti-cholinergic	Cardiac	Nausea ‡	Sedation	Overdose §	Pro-convulsant	Sexual dysfunction
Others									
Agomelatine	50	50?	○	○	○	○	○	○	○
Bupropion/amfebutamone (U)	–	–	●	○	●	○	●●	●●	○
Duloxetine	120	Caution	○	○	●●	●	?	?	●●
Flupentixol	3	2	●●	○	○	●	●	?	●
Mianserin	90+	<Ad	●	○	○	●●●	○	○	●
Mirtazapine	45	45	○	○	○	●●	○	●●	●●
Moclobemide	600	600	●	○	●	○	○	?	●
Reboxetine	12	NR	●	●	●	○	○	○	○
Trazodone	600	+300	○	○	●●●	●●	●	○	●●
Tryptophan	6g	6g	○	○	●●	●●	●	○	○
Venlafaxine	Plain 375 XL ≥225	Same	○	●●	●●	○	●●	●	●●

Side-effects

●●● = Marked effect
●● = Moderate effect
● = Mild effect
○ = Little or minimal effect
? = No information or little reported
U = Unlicensed in UK for depression

Other abbreviations

‡ = Typical serotonergic side-effect
Adult max dose = Maximum adult oral antidepressant dose in UK SPC
Elderly max dose = Maximum elderly oral antidepressant dose as stated in UK SPC. Most state that half the adult dose may be sufficient
Overdose § = Based on UK Fatal Toxicity Index (Henry et al, Br J Med 1995;**310**:221–48). For review of epidemiology and relative toxicity of antidepressant drugs in overdose see Henry (Drug Safety 1997;**16**:374–90, 92 refs)

TABLE 2.1.3: ANTIDEPRESSANTS — PHARMACOKINETICS AND RECEPTOR EFFECTS *

Drug	Major active metabolites	Half-life (hours)	Peak plasma conc (hours)	Transmitter reuptake inhibition 5-HT	NA/NE	DA
Tricyclics						
Amitriptyline		8–24	6	+++	++++	+
	Nortriptyline	18–96	(4–5)	+	++++	+
Clomipramine		17–28	2.5	+++	+	–
	Desmethylclomipramine	>36	4–24	+	+++	–
Dosulepin (dothiepin)		14–40	3	+	+	+
	Desmethyldothiepin	22–60	2			–
Doxepin		8–24	4	+	+	–
	Desmethyldoxepin	30–72	–			–
Imipramine		4–18	2	+++	+	–
	Desipramine	12–24	(4–5)	+	++++	–
Lofepramine		1.6	1–2	+	++++	–
	Desipramine	12–24	(4–5)	+	++++	–
Nortriptyline		18–96	(4–5)	+	+++	–
Trimipramine	(Desmethyltrimipramine)	7–23	3	+	+	+
Selective serotonin reuptake inhibitors (SSRIs)						
Citalopram		33	2–4	++++	–	–
Escitalopram		30	2–4	++++	–	–
Fluoxetine		24–140	6–8	++++	–	+
	Norfluoxetine	168–216	–	+	–	–
Fluvoxamine	None	13–22	2–8	+++	–	–
Paroxetine	None	24	6	++++	+	–
Sertraline		25–36	4–10	+++	–	–
	Desmethylsertraline	66–109	8–12	+	–	–

TABLE 2.1.3: ANTIDEPRESSANTS — PHARMACOKINETICS AND RECEPTOR EFFECTS (CONT) *

Drug	Major active metabolites	Half-life (hours)	Peak plasma conc (hours)	Transmitter reuptake inhibition		
				5-HT	NA/NE	DA
Monoamine oxidase inhibitors						
Isocarboxazid	NK	N/K	2-3	↑	↑	↑
Phenelzine	NK	1.5	2-3	↑	↑	↑
Tranylcypromine	NK	2.5	2–3	↑	↑	↑
Others						
Agomelatine	None	1-2	1-2	5HT2C antagonist	O	O
Bupropion (U)	Hydroxybupropion	3-16 (highly variable) 12-38	4	-	+	++
Duloxetine	NK	8-17	6	+++	+++	-
Flupentixol	NK	35	3-8	-	-	-
Mianserin	Desmethyl-8-hydroxy	12-29	1-3	O	O	+
Mirtazapine	None	20-40	1-3	+++ ←	←	←
Moclobemide	None	1-2	1	O	O	O
Reboxetine	NK	13	2	O	+++	O
Trazodone	mCPP	½-2	½-2	++# PPSA	O	O
Venlafaxine §	Desmethylvenlafaxine	1-2	5(2-7) 10(8-13)	+++§	+++§	+§

Abbreviations

+++ = Marked potency ++ = Minor potency
+++ = Moderate potency + = Minimal
                        O = Nil

↑ = Cytoplasm levels increase
5-HT = 5-hydroxytryptamine or serotonin
= Also potent central 5HT antagonist

Other abbreviations

§ = Dose-dependent reuptake inhibiton (see CI)
PPSA = Potent postsynaptic 5-HT agonist
NA/NE = Noradrenaline or norepinephrine

TABLE 2.1.4: ANTIPSYCHOTICS — RELATIVE SIDE-EFFECTS *

Drug	Adult max dose mg/d	Elderly max dose mg/d	Relative side-effects (most will be dose related)								
			Anti-cholinergic	Cardiac	EPSE	Hypo-tension	Sedation	Minor O/D	Weight gain	Prolactin	Procon-vulsant
Phenothiazines											
Chlorpromazine	1000	<Ad	●●●	●●●	●●	●●●	●●●	●●●	●●	●●●?	●●●
Levomepromazine (methotrimeprazine)	1000	NR	●●●	●●●	●●?	●●●	●●●	●●●	?	●●●?	●●?
Promazine	800	<Ad	●●	●●	●●	●●●	●●●	●●●	?	●●●?	●●?
Pericyazine	(300)	<Ad	●	●●	●●	●●●	●●●	●●●	?	●●●?	●●?
Thioridazine	600	<Ad	●●	●●●	●	●●	●●	●●	●	●●●?	●●
Fluphenazine	CA20	CA10	●●	●●	●●●	●	●●	●	●●	●●●?	●
Perphenazine	24	<Ad	●	●●	●●●	●	●●	●●	●●●	●●●?	●●?
Trifluoperazine	–	<Ad	○	●●	●●	●	●	●	?	●●●?	●
Others											
Benperidol	1.5	<Ad	?	?	?	●	●●	?	?	●●●	●?
Haloperidol	30	30	●●	●●	●●●	●	●	●	●	●●●?	●?
Flupentixol	18	<Ad	●●	○	●●●	○	●	●	●	●●?	●
Zuclopenthixol	150	<Ad	●	●	●●●	●	●	●●	?	●●?	○?
Pimozide	20	<Ad	●	●●●	●	●●	●	●	○	●●●?	●
Amisulpride	1200	1200	○	○	●	○	○	○	●	●●	●?
Sulpiride	2400	2400	●	○	●	○	●	●	●	●●	○?
Depot and long-acting injections ◆											
Fluphenazine decanoate	100–2/52	<Ad	●●	●●	●●●	●	●	●	●	●●●?	●
Pipotiazine palmitate	200–4/52	<Ad	●●	●●	●●	●	●	?	?	●●●?	●●?
Haloperidol decanoate	300–4/52	<Ad	●	●	●●●	●	●	●	●	●●	●
Flupentixol decanoate	400–1/52	<Ad	●●	○	●●	○	●	●	?	●●?	●?
Zuclopentixol decanoate	600–1/52	<Ad	●●	●	●●	●	●●	●●	?	●●?	○?

TABLE 2.1.4: ANTIPSYCHOTICS — RELATIVE SIDE-EFFECTS (CONT) *

Drug	Adult max dose mg/d	Elderly max dose mg/d ?	Relative side-effects (most will be dose related)								
			Anti-cholinergic	Cardiac	EPSE	Hypo-tension	Sedation	Minor O/D	Weight gain	Prolactin	Procon-vulsant
Depot and long-acting injections ◆											
Fluspirilene	20–1/52	<Ad	●	●	●●●	●●	●●	?	?	●●?	●
Risperidone Consta	50–2/52	25–2/52	○	○	●●	●●	?	?	●	●●	○
Olanzapine pamoate	300–2/52	See SPC	●	○	○	○	●●	○	●●	●	●●
Second generation/atypicals											
Aripiprazole	30	30	○	●	○	○	●	?	●	○	○
Asenapine (U,TBC)	(10)	(20)	○?	?	●?	●?	●●?	?	●?	?	?
Clozapine	900	(900)	●●	●●	○	●	●●●	?	●●●	○	●●●
Olanzapine	20	20	●	○	○	○	●●	○	●●●	●	●●
Paliperidone	12	12	○	○	●	●	●	○	●	●●	●
Quetiapine	800	<Ad	●	●	○	●●	●●	●	●	●	○
Risperidone	(16)	4	○	○	●	●	?	?	●	●●●	○
Sertindole	(20)	(20)	○	●●	○	●●	○	○	●	○	●●
Zotepine	300	150	●●	●●	●	●●	●●	?	●●?	●●?	●●●
Ziprasidone (U)	–	–	○	●●	○	○	○	?	○	○	○

201

Side-effects

●●● = Marked effect
●● = Moderate effect
● = Mild/transient effect

○ = Little or minimal effect
? = No information or little reported
U = Unlicensed in UK at time of writing

Other abbreviations

Adult max dose = Maximum adult oral antipsychotic dose as stated in UK SPC or BNF. May be different for other indications

Elderly max dose = Maximum oral antipsychotic dose in the elderly as stated in UK SPC or BNF Most state that a starting dose of half to a quarter of the adult dose should be adequate, with smaller dose increments

◆ = 100–2/52 means 100mg every two weeks; 400–1/52 means 400mg every week, etc

TABLE 2.1.5: ANTIPSYCHOTICS — PHARMACOKINETICS AND RECEPTOR EFFECTS

Drug/group	Receptor blockade (5)										5HT₂ₐ:D₂ affinity ratio	Half-life (hours)	Time to peak (oral) (2) hours	Main metabolite(s)
	D_1	D_2	D_3	D_4	$5HT_{1A}$	$5HT_{2A}$	M_1	α-1	α-2	H_1				
Phenothiazines														
Chlorpromazine	++	+	++	+		+++	++	+++	+	++	10:1	6(2–119)	3(IM 1–4, IV 2–4)	Many
Fluphenazine HCl	++	+++	+++	++		++	+	++	O	+	1:2	FHCl 33 FD 14–27/7	FHCl 3	Some, unclear if active
Fluphenazine decanoate														
Levomepromazine	++	++	+++	?		+++	+++	+++	O	+++	5:1	15–30	1–3	Some, unclear if active
Pericyazine (3)	++?	+?	++?	+?		+++?	+++?			++?		NK	NK	NK
Perphenazine	++	++	NK	?		+++	+	++	++	+++	2:1	10(8–12)	4–8	Some, unclear if active
Thioridazine	++	+	++	+		+++	+++	+++	+	+	5:1	21–24	NK	Mesoridazine
Trifluoperazine	++	++	NK	+	+	+++	+	+++	+	+	2:1	24	2–4	Several
Others														
Benperidol	+?	+++	+?	+?		+?	O?	+?	+?	++?	NK	8	2	1% unchanged in urine
Haloperidol HCl	++	+++	+++	+++		++	+	++	+	+	1:25	HHCl 21(9–38) HD 21/7	2–6	Hydroxy-haloperidol
Haloperidol decanoate														
Flupentixol HCl												FHCl 22–36 FD 3–7/7(1)	FHCl 3–6 FD 3–10/7	Inactive
Flupentixol decanoate														
Zuclopenthixol HCl	++	+++	+	NK		+++	++	++	NK	++	1:3	20	ZHCl 3–4 ZD 5–7 days ZA 24–48	Inactive
Zuclopenthixol decanoate														
Zuclopenthixol acetate														
Sulpiride	O	+++	+	O		O	O	O	O	O	1:50	6–8	2–6	Nil
Amisulpride	O	+++	+++	O		O	O	O	O	O		12–17	1–4	Nil
Pimozide	+	+++	+++	+		+++	+	+++	+	O	1:5	53–55	6–8	Some, unclear if active
Fluspirilene	NK	NK	NK	NK	NK	NK	NK	NK	NK	NK	NK	32–>300	1–48	Inactive

TABLE 2.1.5: ANTIPSYCHOTICS — PHARMACOKINETICS AND RECEPTOR EFFECTS (CONT) *

Drug/group	Receptor blockade (5)										$5HT_{2a}:D_2$ affinity ratio	Half-life (hours)	Time to peak (oral) (2) hours	Main metabolite(s)
	D_1	D_2	D_3	D_4	$5HT_{1A}$	$5HT_{2A}$	M_1	α-1	α-2	H_1				
Second generation/Atypicals														
Aripiprazole	O	++++	O	O	PAg	AAnt	O	O	O	O	N/A	75(31–146)	3–7	None known
Asenapine (TBC)	++	+++	++	++	+++	+++	O	++	++	++	20:1?	6 [8]	0.5-1.5	Minor
Clozapine	++	++4	++	++	++	+++	+++	+++	++	+++	20-30:1	4-12	2-3	Norclozapine
Olanzapine	++	++4	++	++	+	+++	++	++	+	+++	50:1	30(21-54)	3-6	Inactive
Paliperidone	+	+++	+++	++	+	+++	O	+++	++	++		23	23-29	None known
Quetiapine	O	++	+	+	++	++	O	++	O	+	1:1	7	1.5, XL 5-6hrs	N-desalkylquetiapine (t1/2 12hrs)
Risperidone	+	+++	++	++	++	+++	O	+++	+++	++	8-11:1	20-30	1-2 (7)	Hydroxyrisperidone
Sertindole	+	++++4	++	++	+	+++	O	+++	O	+	100:1	55-90	10	Dehydrosertindole
Ziprasidone	+	+++	++	+	+++	+++	O	++	+	O	3:1	7	4-5	Many
Zotepine	++	+++	+++	++	++	+++	+	+++	++	+++	4:1	14-24	1 and 10-12	Norzotepine (inactive)

Receptor binding: +++ = High affinity; ++ = Moderate; + = Low; O = Very low; NK = Not known; ? = Possible; PAg = Partial agonist with very high affinity; AAnt = Antagonist.

Additional ref: Siloh, Nutt and Weizman (2000) *Atlas of Psychiatric Pharmacotherapy*, Martin Dunitz, London (very colourful and useful)

1. Flupentixol decanoate's half-life is longer (up to 17 days) on continuous administration
2. Time to oral peak may vary with food
3. Receptor-binding studies for pericyazine have not been published, but it has been reported to have some differences to chlorpromazine
4. Sertindole, olanzapine and clozapine appear to have some D2 limbic selectivity
5. Inclusion of a receptor may give some guide to therapeutic action and adverse effects
6. There is a considerable degree of variation between published sources, depending upon how the results are presented, whether they are single studies or averages, the receptor sources, assay type, etc. These figures should be taken only as a guide, eg there is little, or nothing published about fluspirilene or pericyazine
7. All oral preparations, including tablets, orodispersable and liquid
8. Biphasic half-life: 6hrs for the first 18hrs, then terminal half-life is 23hrs.

TABLE 2.1.6: ANXIOLYTICS — RELATIVE SIDE-EFFECTS

Class	Drug	Usual dose mg/d	Adult max dose mg/d	Elderly max dose mg/d	Half-life (hours) adult (+ range)	elderly	Hang-over	Depen-dence po-tential
Shorter-acting benzodiazepines								
1a	Clonazepam	2	20	1	35 (20–60)	Same	●●	●●
1a	Loprazolam	1	3	0.75	14 (6–20)	L	●	●
1a	Lorazepam	4	4	<Ad	12 (8–25)	Same	●●●	●●●
1a	Oxazepam	30	120	80	8 (5–15)	Same	●●●	●●
Longer-acting benzodiazepines								
1b	Chlordiazepoxide	30	100	<50	12 (6–30)	L	●●●	●●
1b	Clobazam	30	60	20	18 (9–77)	L	●	●●
1b	Clorazepate	15	15?	<Ad	PD	L	●●●	●●
1b	Diazepam	6	30	15	32 (21–50)	L	●●●	●●
Beta-blockers								
2	Oxprenolol	80	80	80	4# (3–6)	Same	●	○
2	Propranolol	80	120	–	2# (1–2)	Same	●	○
Other anxiolytics								
3	Buspirone	30	45	45	7 (2–11)	Same	○	○
4	Pregabalin	300	600	<600	6	L	○	○
5	Duloxetine	30	120	120	8-17	Same?	○	○
5	Venlafaxine	75	75	75	1-2	Same	○	○

Classes
1a = Shorter-acting or minimally-accumulating benzodiazepines
1b = Longer-acting or accumulating benzodiazepines. These also have metabolites which enhance their
      length of action
2 = Beta-blockers
3 = Azapirone (Azaspirodecanedione)
4 = Anticonvulsant
5 = SNRI

Side-effects
●●● = Marked effect   ○ = Little or nothing reported
●● = Moderate effect   ? = No information available
● = Mild effect

Other abbreviations

Adult max dose   = Suggested maximum oral dose in the UK SPC. Most recommend
                        treatment for up to four weeks
Elderly max dose   = Suggested maximum oral dose in the elderly in the UK SPC. Most state that half
                        the adult dose should be adequate
# = Pharmacological action longer than half-life suggests
L = Longer
The data on this and the previous pages is based on a large number of papers. Note was taken of presentation of data, equivalence of dose used, etc. When non-comparable papers are excluded, there is a surprisingly high level of consistency on reported relative side-effects. Individuals response may, of course, vary widely. Many effects may be dose-related.

2.2 SWITCHING OR DISCONTINUING PSYCHOTROPICS

Switching psychotropics can be achieved using a variety of methods, varying in rate, overlap, gap and complexity. The main types are summarised in the graphs and comments. The remarks below specifically relating to antipsychotics are marked with #.

Switch 1: Drug-free interval

(Discontinue first drug, leave drug-free interval, introduce second drug.)

Advantages:
1. Minimises combined ADRs.
2. Relapse risk not too high, if the patient is relatively stable and the gap is not prolonged.
3. Minimal interaction potential.
4. Side-effects from the second drug are less likely to be confused with discontinuation effects from the first drug.
5. Anticholinergic drug doses can be titrated as needed. #
6. Ideal (but often impractical) for switches to clozapine to reduce additive myelosuppressive potential. #
7. Lowest medication error potential.

Disadvantages:
1. Takes time, which delays the desired relief of symptoms or side-effects. #
2. Potential for relapse or deterioration during the gap and changeover.
3. Early relapse before reaching a therapeutic dose might be interpreted as lack of efficacy of the second drug.

Switch 2: No interval

(Stop first drug, start second immediately.)

Advantages:
1. Straightforward.
2. Low medication error potential.
3. Appropriate for inpatient settings with better supervision.
4. Appropriate where an acute severe reaction to a drug has occurred, e.g. statutory abrupt withdrawal of clozapine due to a blood dyscrasia. #
5. Sometimes acceptable for high-risk switches to clozapine to reduce additive myelosuppressive potential, but retaining antipsychotic cover. #

TABLE 2.2.1: SWITCHING PSYCHOTROPICS

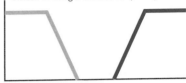

Switch 1: Drug-free interval (safest)

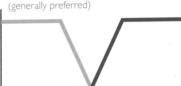

Switch 2: No interval (generally preferred)

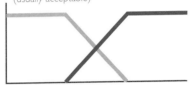

Switch 3: Partial overlap (usually acceptable)

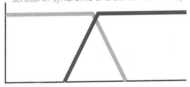

Switch 4a: Full overlap (risks NMS, serotonin syndrome and combined ADRs)

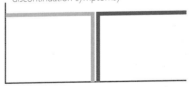

Switch 4b: Abrupt switch (risks discontinuation symptoms)

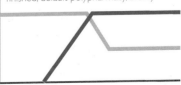

Switch 5: Incomplete (switch never finished, default polypharmacy, avoid)

Disadvantages:

1. May raise unrealistic expectations from the patient and family of a rapid improvement on the second drug.
2. Combined ADRs, albeit short-lived.
4. Potential for drug interactions if the first drug has a long half-life, e.g. fluoxetine.
5. Rapid discontinuation of the first drug may produce higher relapse rates, e.g. antipsychotics.
6. Discontinuation effects from the first drug might be interpreted as side-effects of the second, e.g. some antipsychotics.

Switch 3: Partial overlap

(Add new drug, either at standard dose or quickly titrated upwards, while slowly tapering the first drug.)

Advantages:

1. Appropriate when symptom or side-effect relief is needed but there is a high risk or relapse or deterioration
2. No sudden changes occur (which might destabilise the patient).
3. This switch may be unavoidable for depot to oral switches, where plasma levels of depot will decline slowly. #
4. Useful for switches from a high potency antipsychotic to a newer or lower potency drug where cholinergic rebound may occur. Either way, anticholinergic cover can be retained for several weeks. #

Disadvantages:

1. If the taper is too quick, two drugs may be given at sub-therapeutic doses.
2. Combined ADRs may occur.
3. Potential for drug interactions, especially with antidepressants.
4. Potential for medication errors if not planned fully in advance — involve carers and patient if patient is at home.
5. High potential for polypharmacy if the switch is never completed (see Switch 5). #

Switch 4: Full overlap *

(Add new drug to therapeutic dose and then slowly taper previous drug.)

Advantages:

1. Safest if relapse prevention is of greatest concern.
2. Most appropriate if the patient has recently

(e.g. < 3 months) recovered from acute relapse with the first drug.
3. Low risk of discontinuation effects of the first drug.
4. If depot to oral antipsychotic switch, this may be the lowest risk opportunity to assess compliance with oral drugs. #
5. Slow taper is possible and is better for drugs with a high anticholinergic activity.
6. Probably the safest switch for aripiprazole.

Disadvantages:

1. Combined ADRs may occur (but not necessarily with antipsychotics, Gardner et al, Can J Psychiatry 1997;**42**:430–1).
2. Potential severe reactions, e.g. NMS or serotonin syndrome.
3. Potential for drug interactions.
4. Potential for medication errors if not planned and completed fully.
5. High potential for polypharmacy if switch never completed (see switch 5 below)

Switch 5: Incomplete

(Add new drug to therapeutic dose and then never stop previous drug).

This can happen if the switch is started but the treatment plan is not passed on or the patient improves and there is a reluctance to discontinue the first drug and possibly destabilise the patient#. 'Default polypharmacy' should be avoided. The advantages of long-term monotherapy include that it is easier to judge the effectiveness of any given drug accurately, and medication regimens are simple and not confused by polypharmacy (extensive review, Weiden et al, J Clin Psychiatry 1998;**59**[Suppl 19]:36–49). Monotherapy should thus always be tried first and if at some time later a rational, planned and assessed polypharmacy is tried then that is reasonable. See *1.23* for a discussion on combined antipsychotics.

2.2.1 SWITCHING OR DISCONTINUING ANTIPSYCHOTICS

Reviews: * strategies (Lambert, *J Clin Psychiatry* 2007;**68**(Suppl 6):10–3), general (Remington et al, *Schizophr Res* 2005;**76**:267–72), discontinuing antipsychotics (Tranter and Healy, *J Psychopharmacol* 1998;**12**:401–6), general (Buckley and Correll, *J Clin Psychiatry* 2008;**69**(Suppl 1):4–17).

2.2.1.1 GENERAL ADVICE ON SWITCHING ANTIPSYCHOTICS

Reasons for switching antipsychotics include (Weiden et al, J Clin Psychiatry 1997;**58**[Suppl 10]: S63–S72):

1. Persistent positive (distressing and disruptive) symptoms.
2. Persistent negative (restrictive and burdening) symptoms.
3. Relapse despite compliance.
4. Persistent distressing adverse effects such as EPS, akathisia, hyperprolactinaemia, poor self-image and sexual dysfunction.
5. Oral to depot or other formulation change.

Risks of discontinuing (or switching) anti-psychotics * (review and guidance, Keks et al, CNS Drugs 1995;**4**:351–6):

1. Cholinergic rebound (e.g. nausea, vomiting, restlessness, anxiety, insomnia, fatigue, malaise, myalgia, diaphoresis, rhinitis, paraesthesia, GI distress, headaches, nightmares) may occur on discontinuation, particularly if a second drug has less anticholinergic effect or if anticholinergics are withdrawn too soon. It can be severe but brief and predictable.
2. Withdrawal dyskinesias, e.g. extrapyramidal symptoms, rebound akathisia (may be confused with anxiety or psychosis), rebound dystonia and worsening tardive dyskinesia. These may partly be related to cholinergic rebound, and have been reported in mentally 'healthy' people taking metoclopramide as an antiemetic (Tranter and Healy, J Psychopharmacol 1998;**12**:401–6), and can be minimised by slow tapering.
3. Other discontinuation symptoms, e.g. NMS (Spivak et al, Acta Psychiatr Scand 1990; **81**:168–9).
4. Relapse or destabilisation * — this may present an unacceptable risk to the patient. Relapse rates of up to 50% at six months after abrupt discontinuation have been reported (n = 1210, Viguera et al, Arch Gen Psychiatry 1997;**54**:49–55) and people with schizophrenia who switch antipsychotics have poorer outcomes, e.g. are more likely to use in-patient and crisis services (n = 651, open, 12/12, Faries et al, BMC Psychiatry 2009;**9**:54). Gradual

discontinuation reduces this risk (reviewed by Tranter and Healy, J Psychopharmacol 1998;**12**:401–6). True relapses tend to occur from 1–6 months after abrupt withdrawal of oral drugs and 3–6 months with depots, probably due to persistence of the drug at receptor level. There may be a particular problem with clozapine, where relapse or rebound psychosis can be more severe (e.g. Baldessarini et al, Arch Gen Psychiatry 1995; **52**:1071–2, see also 2.2.1.4).
5. Anxiety or stress from the switch causing symptom flare-up.
6. Medication errors.
7. The replacement drug being less effective than the former, or having different but still unacceptable side-effects, resulting in premature abandonment and an inadequate trial of the new drug.

General principles for switching antipsychotics:

1. Ensure the optimum effect is obtained from the first drug (see CATIE study in C1.23)
2. Ensure a treatment target is set and measured (take care that the key aims of a switch are not easier and less risky to achieve by, e.g. dose or timing adjustment of the first drug).
3. Avoid switches:
   - coinciding with major life stress events
   - after a change in treatment team - allow full assimilation into the new team first
   - from a drug which was successfully used to treat a major relapse within the last 3–6/12
   - in patients previously non-compliant with oral drugs now stable for under a year on a depot (Weiden et al, J Clin Psychiatry 1997;**58**[Suppl 10]:63–72).
4. If possible, slowly taper the first antipsychotic, probably over at least eight weeks, as this reduces the risk of relapse and emergent extrapyramidal and psychotic symptoms.
5. Slowly taper any anticholinergic, which may also be allowed to continue for a time after the drug has been discontinued. Reintroduce if necessary for any emergent symptoms.
6. Monitor mental and physical state regularly (particularly during the first month).

Before switching to a newer antipsychotic:

1. Warn about possible ADRs (e.g. weight gain,

short-term sedation, diabetes, implications of reduced prolactin inhibition).

2. Discuss the need for an adequate trial and the need to complete the switch.
3. Agree how to define success or failure, and the chances thereof.
4. Warn that the new drug is not perfect — that one is swapping one set of side-effects for another.

2.2.1.2 SPECIFIC DRUG SWITCHES
NMS has been reported during many antipsychotic switches.

1. Phenothiazine to phenothiazine

Get the dose equivalent right, then switches 2 or 3 are probably reasonable.

2. Phenothiazine to D2-blocker

Get the optimum dose equivalent, then switches 2 or 3 are reasonable, but beware of cholinergic rebound (nausea, vomiting, restlessness, anxiety, insomnia, fatigue, GI distress) and stronger D2-blockade leading to additional EPSE.

3. Switching to a typical depot

Studies have shown that this is usually relatively straightforward if done carefully, remembering that typical depots peak plasma levels may vary (see Table 2.2.2) and so reduce doses accordingly. Beware of additive EPSEs.

3a. Oral antipsychotic to typical depot:
Anecdotal evidence shows that the change can usually be made uneventfully (e.g. review in

TABLE 2.2.2: SWITCHING ANTIPSYCHOTICS *

From \ To	Pheno-thiazines	D2 blockers	Typical depots	Aripiprazole[15]	Asenapine[15]	Clozapine[15]	Olanzapine[15]	Olanzapine pamoate[15]	Risperidone	Risperidone consta	Quetiapine[15]
Phenothiazines	RT (1)	RT (2)	RT (3)	RT (4)	RT (12)	Care (5,)	NOP (6)	NOP (13)	RT (7)	RT (8a)	RT (9a)
D2 blockers	RT (10)	RT (11)	RT (3)	RT (4)	RT (12)	Care (5)	NOP (6)	NOP (13)	RT (7)	RT (8a)	RT (9b)
Typical depots	RT (3)	RT (3)	RT (3)	RT (3,4)	RT (3,12)	Care (3,5)	RT (3,6)	NOP (3,13)	RT (3,7)	RT (3,8c)	RT (3,9c)
Aripiprazole[15]	RT (4)	RT (4)	RT (3,4)	-	RT (12)	Care (4,5)	RT (4,6)	NOP (13)	RT (4,7)	RT (4,8a)	NOP (4,9d)
Asenapine[15]	RT (12)	RT (12)	RT (3,12)	RT (4,12)	-	NOP (5,12)	RT (6,12)	NOP (12,13)	RT (7,12)	RT (8a,12)	RT (9,12)
Clozapine[15]	Care (5)	Care (5)	Care (3,5)	RT (4,5)	NOP (5,12)	-	Care (5,6c)	NOP (5,13)	RT (5,7)	RT (5,8a)	RT (5,9e)
Olanzapine[15]	NOP (6)	NOP (6)	NOP (3,13)	RT (4,6)	RT (6,12)	Care (5,6)	-	NOP (6,13)	RT (6,7)	RT (6,8a)	NOP (6,9f)
Olanzapine pamoate[15]	RT (13)	RT (13)	RT (3,13e)	RT (4,13)	RT (13,12)	RT (5,13)	RT (6,13)	-	RT (7,13)	RT (8,13)	RT (9,13)
Risperidone	RT (14)	RT (14)	RT (3,14)	RT (4,14)	RT (14,12)	Care (5,14)	NOP (6a,14)	NOP (13,14)	-	RT (8d,14)	NOP (9g,14)
Risperidone Consta	RT (8e)	RT (8e)	RT (3,8)	RT (4,8e,16)	RT (8e,12)	Care (5,8e)	RT (6,8,16)	NOP (8a,13)	RT (7,8e)	-	RT (8e,9)
Quetiapine[15]	NOP (9,14)	NOP (9,14)	NOP (3,14)	RT (4,9,14)	RT (9,12,14)	Care (5,9,14)	NOP (6,9,14)	NOP (9,13,14)	RT (7,9,14)	RT (8a9,14)	-
Stopping	RT (16)	RT (16)	RT (16)	RT (16)	RT (16)	RT (16)	RT (16)	RT (16)	RT (16)	RT (16)	RT (16)

NOP = No obvious problems, although there is the definite risk of NMS with **all** switches
RT = Read text
Care = Great care needed, also read text

Clin Pharmacokinet 1985;**10**:315–33), although there are no formal studies. Converting to the same drug as a depot should present no great problems if doses are chosen carefully (e.g. switch 3, see also *2.2.1.4*).

3b. Changing from one typical depot to another typical depot:
No significant problems are usually experienced (Soni *et al*, *Acta Psychiatr Scand* 1992;**85**:354–9) and a direct exchange from one depot to another can often be made uneventfully (e.g. switch 3).

3c. Combined oral antipsychotic plus depot to depot alone:
This can be an unusually difficult procedure and relapses may occur more frequently with this change when compared to other changes. Relapses can occur, particularly in the first 3–4 months, when antipsychotic levels can be inadvertently sub-therapeutic (Soni *et al*, *Acta Psychiatr Scand* 1992;**85**:354–9). If the risk of relapse is high, any change should probably be done verging on the side of caution, e.g. increasing the depot dose, then reducing oral doses later.

3d. Oral fluphenazine to depot fluphenazine:
If transferring from oral fluphenazine, multiply the total daily oral dose by 1.2 and administer as fluphenazine decanoate IM every one to two weeks. Accumulation occurs and so the dosing interval may be increased to every three weeks or so after four to six weeks of therapy (review, Ereshefsky *et al*, *J Clin Psychiatry* 1984;**45**:50–9). Concomitant oral therapy should be limited to the initial period or during times of decompensation.

3e. Oral haloperidol to depot haloperidol:
If transferring from stabilised oral haloperidol to haloperidol depot, multiply the total daily oral dose by 15–20, to a maximum of 300 mg monthly, preferably much lower. Accumulation occurs and so the decanoate dose should be decreased by 25% a month until the minimum effective dose is achieved. The average maintenance dose appears to be about 100 mg every four weeks. Elderly patients or those stabilised on less than 10 mg/d oral haloperidol should receive haloperidol decanoate in an IM dose that is 10–15 times the oral dose every four weeks. Concomitant oral therapy should be limited to the initial period or during times of decompensation.

3f. Altering the frequency of a typical depot: *
Such a change should present no great problems, provided antipsychotic levels do not drop too low or rise too high. Computer modelling suggests that:

- If switching from weekly to fortnightly, add 25-40% to the last weekly dose, then go to fortnightly with double the weekly dose, e.g. 100 mg/wk to 200 mg/fortnight:

Week	1	2	3	4	5	6	7
Dose	100	100	125-140	-	200	-	200

- If switching from fortnightly to 4-weekly, add 50% to the last fortnightly dose then go to 4-weekly with double the weekly dose, e.g. 100 mg/fortnight to 200 mg/monthly:

Week	1	3	5	7	9	11	13
Dose	100	100	150	-	200		200

3g. Depot typicals to others: *
Stop the depot and introduce the next antipsychotic when the next depot dose would have been due, remembering that a slow decay in depot plasma levels may occur so beware of adding the new drug too quickly, e.g. 33% of people stopping fluphenazine decanoate had notable plasma levels 12/52 after last dose (Gitlin *et al*, *J Clin Psychopharmacol* 1988;**8**:53–6). Depots are occasionally given more often than strictly necessary.

3h. Typical depot to typical depot:
This is not usually a problem, with a direct switch often possible.

4. Switching to aripiprazole *

For most antipsychotics it would seem that abrupt switching to aripiprazole can often be poorly tolerated. Aripiprazole strongly binds to dopamine receptors, with a long half-life, displacing almost every other antipsychotic and stimulating receptors to about 30% activity. This abrupt change from minimal dopamine activity to 30% within hours can be acutely distressing and adversive. A cross-taper is most likely to be successful, starting aripiprazole at 5 mg/d (SPC mentions 10 mg/d) then increasing stepwise to 15 mg/d, and reducing the previous antipsychotic by 25% twice a week (n = 53 [c = 48], RCT, open, 14/52, Takeuchi *et al*, *J Clin Psychopharmacol* 2008; **28**:540–3; n = 77, RCT, open, 12/52, Pae *et al*,

Eur Neuropsychopharmacol 2009;**19**:562–70). In a switching study, although all 3 switches from risperidone (n=105) or olanzapine (n=164) to aripiprazole (abrupt; immediate aripiprazole start with tapered reduction of first drug; or a 14-day cross-taper) were reportedly well tolerated (n=269, 8/52, Byerly *et al, Schizophr Res* 2009;**107**:218–22), the data is inconsistent (e.g. 12/52, Ryckmans *et al, Pharmacopsychiatry* 2009; **42**:114–21):

- Switching from FGAs/D2 specific antipsychotics may have a lower success rate than SGAs and may be more difficult than thought, possibly because of higher receptor affinity with FGAs.
- Olanzapine and quetiapine may need a smoother switching process with a longer cross-taper (n=45[c=31], 12/52, Lin *et al, Chang Gung Med J* 2009;**32**:409–16).

Also, warn women about the possible normalisation of prolactin (see 15).

5. Switching to/from clozapine *

5a. Switching to clozapine: Care would be needed with the increased risk of dyscrasias with phenothiazines and delayed clearance of depots (especially Risperdal Consta®, Janssen-Cilag and olanzapine pamoate). Ideally, a previous drug should be completely withdrawn before clozapine is started, including depots (e.g. switch 1), but this is rarely practical. Clozapine is markedly sedative and hypotensive, so care is needed with additive effects and start with the usual gradual dose titration but monitor carefully. Warn women about possible normalisation of prolactin and the need for adequate oral contraception if necessary. Pharmacokinetic interactions are unlikely (see *4.2.2*).

5b. Switching from clozapine (see also 16. discontinuing antipsychotics)
Converting clozapine to other antipsychotics seems particularly problematic (n=30, RCT, Shiovitz *et al, Schizophr Bull* 1996;**22**:591–5). Relapse after clozapine discontinuation seems to be of a higher incidence, may be more rapid and withdrawal symptoms may be more severe than with other drugs (see 16). For gradual discontinuation of clozapine, it is best to simultaneously introduce and escalate the doses of another antipsychotic.

6. Switching to/from oral olanzapine

There are no apparent problems with stopping olanzapine suddenly, so any switch from olanzapine should be possible. When switching to olanzapine, additive EPSE, hypotension and drug interactions are unlikely to occur and so switch 3 is usually suitable with care. Due to a lesser effect on prolactin, unexpected pregnancies have been reported a couple of months after a switch from typicals to olanzapine, despite no contraceptive use for 4–5 years (n=2, Neumann and Frasch, *Nervenarzt* 2001;**72**:876–8).

6a. Risperidone to oral olanzapine: In a comparison of four different typical/risperidone to olanzapine switches in partially remitted, stable schizophrenic out-patients, the most successful method was starting 10mg olanzapine then gradually discontinuing the original drug. The next most successful was gradual introduction/gradual discontinuation; and probably best for elderly/frail patients. Most drop-outs (usually sleep-related)

TABLE 2.2.3: SUMMARY OF ANTIPSYCHOTIC INJECTIONS *

Drug	Peak (days)	Usual frequency	Main duration	Depot half-life	Time to steady state from first dose
Flupentixol	7–10	2/52	2–4/52	7/7	10–12/52
Fluphenazine	1–2	2–4/52	3–4/52	14/7	6–12/52
Fluspirilene	1–2	1/52	1/52	?	5–6/52
Haloperidol	3–9	4/52	4/52	21–28/7	10–12/52
Pipothiazine	9–10	4/52	4/52	21–28/7	8–12/52
Zuclopenthixol	4–9	2/52	2–4/52	7/7	10–12/52
Risperidone	35	2/52	2–3/52	?	12/52
Olanzapine	2–4	2/52 or 4/52	4–6/52?	30 (13–42)/7	12/52

were with abrupt discontinuation (switch 2) and gradual olanzapine introduction (n = 209, 82% completed, open, Kinon et al, J Clin Psychiatry 2000;**61**:833–40). In first-episode schizophrenics with residual symptoms from risperidone, a switch to **olanzapine** was effective in 30%, although 47% gained significant weight from baseline (n = 58[c = 51], open, 12/52, Takahashi et al, J Clin Psychiatry 2006;**67**:1577–82; IS).

6b. Depots to oral olanzapine: There has been a three-month trial (which may have been of inadequate duration) of switching of clinically stable schizophrenics on depots, either continuing the depot or transferred to olanzapine over 4/52. After 3/12 those transferring to olanzapine were clinically improved and all preferred olanzapine, so a four-week switch is clinically viable (n = 26, RCT, open, 3/12, Godleski et al, J Clin Psychiatry 2003;**64**:119–22).

6c. Clozapine to oral olanzapine: An open study of a clozapine to olanzapine switch by patients wishing to avoid blood monitoring, eight of 19 successfully completed the switch (using switch 4) and the others required restabilising on clozapine (n = 19, Henderson et al, J Clin Psychiatry 1998;**59**:585–8). In patients responsive to clozapine but suffering adverse effects, a slow cross-titration over at least two weeks to olanzapine may be successful in about 90% patients (n = 20, open, 24/52, Littrell et al, J Clin Psychiatry 2000;**61**:912–5; Lilly part-funded).

6d. Others to olanzapine: One study showed that in resistant schizophrenia, switching to olanzapine may be successful (n = 25, open, five years, Karagianis et al, Curr Med Res Opin 2003;**6**:47–80), with both a direct switch (2) and tapered switch (3), over 2/52, having equivalent outcomes, both therapeutic (67–74% successful) and for adverse effects (n = 108, RCT, open, 6/52, Lee et al, J Clin Psychiatry 2002;**63**:569–76).

7. Switching to/from oral risperidone

Hypotension may occur, so gradual dose titration over at least 3/7 (or longer if possible) to 4 mg/d is recommended. Additive hypotension with low potency drugs may occur during a switch. A sudden switch (along with gradual withdrawal of anticholinergics) may be successful in about 60% patients, but a more gradual switch and dose escalation is preferable (n = 36, Kirov et al, Acta

Psychiatr Scand 1997;**95**:439–43). A review of switching to risperidone recommended reducing the existing antipsychotic dose, then overlapping risperidone with the existing therapy, rather than making an abrupt switch (Borison et al, Clin Ther 1996;**18**:592–607). Risperidone may be a suitable replacement if introduced before slow clozapine withdrawal, i.e. switch 4 (Zimbroff, Am J Psychiatry 1995;**152**:1102). There are few obvious other problems with stopping or switching risperidone (e.g. interactions), except the standard potential for NMS, prolactin altered and additive EPS if switching to a phenothiazine or D2-blocker. Switches 2 or 3 should be possible.

8. Switching to/from Risperdal Consta®(LAI)*

8a. Switching to risperidone LAI: It is important to understand the release kinetics of Consta before deciding a switch strategy, i.e. therapeutic levels are not reached until week 4 (i.e. just before the third injection) but only reach optimum in weeks 5–6 (i.e. after the third injection). Assessment of the response to oral risperidone is strongly recommended before giving the first injection, then giving oral for 3–4 weeks, or more. Consta may have the best chance of success if the person has been shown to respond to oral risperidone first.

8b. Oral antipsychotics to risperidone LAI Continue for three weeks after starting Consta, then discontinue step-wise during week 4 (preferably through time-limited prescriptions to avoid polypharmacy). There has been a study of three **olanzapine** to risperidone switches:

1. Olanzapine stopped abruptly, risperidone started immediately and increased as usual
2. Gradual 1; week 1 olanzapine reduced by 50% for a week and risperidone started; week 2 olanzapine stopped
3. Gradual 2; week 1 olanzapine full dose, risperidone started, week 2 olanzapine 50%, week 3 olanzapine stopped.

Gradual 2 had the least drop-outs and the best outcomes (n = 123[c = 97], RCT, open, 6/52, Ganguli et al, BMC Med 2008;**6**:17).

8c. Typical depot to risperidone LAI: JC recommend starting Consta one week before the last fortnightly injection, with an oral drug available if the risk of relapse is high. Alternatively, switch on the depot due date, supplementing with oral risperidone for 3–4 weeks.

8d. Oral risperidone to risperidone LAI: Continue risperidone for three weeks, then gradually discontinue in week 4.

8e. Risperidone LAI to others: The last dose of Consta will finally stop releasing risperidone about six weeks later, so wait until then and introduce the new drug gradually from about day 42.

9. Switching to/from quetiapine *

Quetiapine has a short receptor half-life so warn women about a possible normalisation of prolactin and the need for adequate oral contraception if necessary. A switching study to quetiapine XL from other antipsychotics (mostly conventionals and risperidone) used:

Day 1:   300mg plus 75% previous antipsychotic

Day 2:   600mg plus 50% previous;

Day 3:   400–800mg/d plus 25% of previous, then stop

Day 4:   400–800mg over four days

63% of the completers achieved clinical benefit and tolerated the switch (n = 477 [c = 370], open, 12/52, Ganesan et al, Curr Med Res Opin 2008; 24:21–32; MS).

9a. Phenothiazine to quetiapine: Switch 3 may be reasonable, but be aware of additional initial postural hypotension, so a slightly slower dose titration or additional monitoring might be prudent.

9b. D2-blocker to quetiapine: Switch 2 or 3 should be tolerable, as receptor blockade with quetiapine is quite different to that of standard D2-blockers.

9c. Typical depot to quetiapine: Switch 2 should be tolerable, starting quetiapine when the next depot dose is due.

9d. Aripiprazole to quetiapine: Quetiapine will not displace aripiprazole from receptors so the onset of quetiapine's action will be dependent upon the rate at which aripiprazole dissociates from dopamine and serotonin receptors.

9e. Clozapine to quetiapine: Switches 2, 3 or 4 should be tolerable, depending on the reason for the switch.

9f. Olanzapine to quetiapine: Any switch should be acceptable.

9g. Risperidone to quetiapine: Switches 2 or 3 should be tolerable. An abrupt switch from risperidone (mean 1.4mg/d) to quetiapine (mean 87mg/d) in elderly people (mean 82-year-old) with BPSD was well tolerated, with only three discontinuing (n = 67, open, Madhusoodanan and Bogunovic, Am J Alzheimer's Dis Other Demen 2006; 21:169–74).

9h. Switching from quetiapine: * There are few obvious problems with stopping or switching from quetiapine (except perhaps NMS), so switches 2 or 3 should be OK (for review see Weiden, J Psychopharmacol 2006; 20:104–18).

10. Switching D2-blockers to phenothiazines

Switches 2 or 3 should be considered first.

11. Switching D2-blocker to D2 blocker

Consider switches 1–3 first, bearing in mind the potential for NMS and additional EPSE. For a general, waffly review on switching to or from amisulpride, see Peuskens (Curr Med Res Opin 2002; 18[Suppl 3]:S23–S28).

12. Switching to/from asenapine *

The US PI for asenapine recommends gradual discontinuation and minimising overlap with other antipsychotics.

13. Switching to/from olanzapine pamoate *

There is no published information on switching to or from olanzapine pamoate. Switching to it should present few problems as olanzapine pamoate takes 12 weeks to reach steady state, so some crossover, e.g. switches 2–4 would be viable. As with Consta, switching from olanzapine pamoate requires a gradual switch as olanzapine levels can persist for several months after discontinuation.

14. Switching to/from ziprasidone *

14a. Haloperidol to ziprasidone: This has good completion rate with, surprisingly, some weight increase (n = 99 [c = 67, 68%], open, 12/52, Alptekin et al, Int Clin Psychopharmacol 2009; 24:229–38).

14b. Olanzapine to ziprasidone: Again this

has a good completion rate, with some weight reduction (n=82[c=71, 86%], open, 12/52, Alptekin et al, Int Clin Psychopharmacol 2009;**24**:229–38).

14c. Risperidone to ziprasidone: This has an average completion rate, with some weight reduction (n=104[c=62, 60%], open, 12/52, Alptekin et al, Int Clin Psychopharmacol 2009;**24**:229–38).

15. Prolactin warning

Warn women about the possibility of currently raised prolactin (particularly with D2-blockers) causing amenorrhoea, and normalisation of prolactin with the new drug and, if necessary, the need for adequate oral contraception.

16. Discontinuing antipsychotics *

Stopping an antipsychotic has three main risks; discontinuation symptoms, withdrawal/rebound psychosis, and relapse. Discontinuing gradually is the ideal and has the lowest incidence of these adverse outcomes. See individual drugs for their specific reports:

16a. Withdrawal symptoms *
Cholinergic rebound (Lieberman, Psychosomatics 1981;**22**:253–4) from abrupt withdrawal of phenothiazine and other low-potency or antipsychotics can include headache, restlessness, nausea, emesis, anorexia, diarrhoea, rhinorrhea, diaphoresis, myalgia, paraesthesia, anxiety (Dilsaver and Alessi, Acta Psychiatr Scand 1988; **77**:241–6) and rebound insomnia (n=3, van Sweden, Pharmacopsychiatry 1987;**20**:116–9). When switching to high-potency antipsychotics, 85% suffer insomnia, anxiety and tensional restlessness (akathisia), again probably from cholinergic rebound (n=26, Chouinard et al, J Clin Psychiatry 1984;**45**:500–2). Dramatic withdrawal-emergent cachexia (loss of weight, appetite, muscle atrophy, wasting) has also been reported in learning disabilities (n=10, Mikkelsen et al, N Engl J Med 1988;**318**:929).

16b. Withdrawal psychosis *
Rapid-onset psychosis (so-called 'supersensitivity psychosis') has been reported with antipsychotic withdrawal (incidence possibly 12–20%, peak 24–48 hours), but is less common with gradual compared to abrupt withdrawal (n=2, Ekblom

et al, Psychopharmacology [Berl] 1984;**83**:293–4), can occur even in bipolar patients (n=1, Witschy et al, Am J Psychiatry 1984;**141**:105–6) and usually disappears rapidly on reinstitution. It may occur more with clozapine, possibly because of its short half-life (Baldessarini et al, Arch Gen Psychiatry 1995;**52**:1071–2).

16c. Relapse *
Obviously, if an antipsychotic has been effective, discontinuation risks relapse. Relapse after gradual withdrawal may be heralded by anxiety, agitation, restlessness and insomnia (Dilsaver and Alessi, Acta Psychiatr Scand 1988;**77**:241–6). A number of studies and analyses (e.g. Moncrieff, Acta Psychiatr Scand 2006;**114**:3–13; 57 refs; n=17, Zander et al, Psychopharmacology [Berl] 1981;**73**:43–7) have concluded that:

- About 25–50% relapse within 10–12 weeks (s=66, n=4365), 50% after 6/12 (s=13, n=1210)
- The relapse rate with slow discontinuation (32%) is half that of rapid discontinuation (65%)
- People who remain stable after 6/12 tend to remain relapse-free without medication (n=1210, retrospective, Viguera et al, Arch Gen Psychiatry 1997;**54**:49–55)

16d. Discontinuing aripiprazole *
Supersensitivity psychosis has been reported after tapering aripiprazole (n=1, Chang et al, Prog Neuropsychopharmacol Biol Psychiatry 2009; **33**:388–9).

16e. Discontinuing clozapine *
Sudden discontinuation of clozapine due to a blood dyscrasia is sometimes necessary and can lead to more difficult to treat psychosis in TRS, e.g. in a retrospective comparison, doses needed to be 43% higher on re-treatment (n=43), compared to 12.5% lower if the person (n=12) had stayed on clozapine (n=55, Miodowniok et al, J Clin Psychiatry 2006;**67**:1204-8). After sudden withdrawal of 200mg/d clozapine taken for 4/52 (in schizophrenia in remission),

- 39% (11/28) had no withdrawal symptoms
- 43% (12/28) had mild symptoms (agitation, headache, nausea)
- 14% (4/28) had moderate symptoms (nausea, vomiting, diarrhoea)
- 4% (1/28) had rebound psychosis requiring hospitalisation for manic episodes.

Most symptoms occurred within 24–36 hours and

resolved over 3–7 days (n = 30 [c = 28], 7/7, open, Shiovitz *et al, Schizophr Bull* 1996;**22**:591–5).

16f. Withdrawal symptoms *

A major mechanism of clozapine withdrawal symptoms is cholinergic rebound, within 24–48 hours of stopping, with reports of limb and neck dystonias, choreoform movements, dyskinesias lasting 5–14 days (n = 4, Ahmed *et al, J Clin Psychiatry* 1998;**59**:472–7), delirium (n = 3, Stanillla *et al, J Clin Psychiatry* 1997;**58**:252–5), and oculogyric crisis (n = 1, Mendhekar and Duggal, *J Neuropsychiatry Clin Neurosci* 2006;**18**:424–3). Other withdrawal symptoms reported include *de novo* OCD (n = 2, Poyurovsky *et al, Clin Neuropharmacol* 1998;**21**:97–100), Tourette-like tics (n = 1, Poyurovsky *et al, Clin Neuropharmacol* 1998;**21**:97–100), catatonia (after abrupt withdrawal, n = 1, Yeh *et al, Clin Neuropharmacol* 2004;**27**:216–8), rebound insomnia (n = 1, Staedt *et al, Eur Arch Psychiatry Clin Neurosci* 1996;**246**:79–82), severe akathisia with suicidal and autoaggressive behaviour (n = 1, Poyurovsky *et al, Int Clin Psychopharmacol* 1996;**11**:283-6) and NMS (n = 1, Margeti and Aukst-Margeti, *Prog Neuropsychopharmacol Biol Psychiatry*2005;**29**:14507). Most dramatically resolve on recommencement or use of anticholinergics (De Leon *et al, J Clin Psychiatry* 1994; **55**:119–20). They may occur in 25% clozapine patients (< 300 mg/d) but this is reduced significantly if switching to olanzapine (n = 106, RCT, d/b, p/c, Tollefson *et al, J Clin Psychopharmacol* 1999;**19**:435–43).

16g. Discontinuing haloperidol *

Rebound psychosis (n = 1, Kahne, *Can J Psychiatry* 1989;**34**:227–9) and dyskinesia (n = 1, Sexson and Barak, *J Perinatol* 1989;**9**:170–2; n = 5, Riker *et al, Chest* 1997;**111**:1778–81) have been reported with haloperidol.

16h. Discontinuing olanzapine *

Supersensitivity psychosis 48 hours after sudden olanzapine discontinuation has been reported (n = 3, Llorca *et al, Can J Psychiatry* 2001;**46**:87–8), as has myoclonus (as part of a possible serotonin syndrome caused by serotonin rebound) after a six-month course (n = 1, Nayudu and Scheftner, *J Clin Psychopharmacol* 2000;**20**:489–90).

16i. Discontinuing quetiapine *

Acute withdrawal symptoms such as nausea, vomiting, insomnia, headache, diarrhoea, dizziness, chorea (Jiménez-Caballero *et al, Rev Neurol* 2004;**38**:1094) and irritability have been reported with acute cessation of high doses. In one case, these occurred within 24 hours of a dose reduction, where a very slow taper or ondansetron did not help, but prochlorperazine did (n = 1, Kim and Staab, *Am J Psychiatry* 2005; **162**:1020). The SPC recommends withdraw over at least 1–2 weeks.

16j. Discontinuing risperidone *

Risperidone discontinuation symptoms have included tics (Rowan and Malone, *J Am Acad Child Adolesc Psychiatry* 1997;**36**:162–3), dyskinesia during dose reduction (n = 1, Anand and Dewan, *Ann Clin Psychiatry* 1996;**8**:179–82), or abrupt discontinuation, (n = 1, Miller, *Ann Pharmacother* 2000;**34**:269), respiratory dyskinesia, e.g. involuntary movements of respiratory muscles, and grunting (n = 1, Ehrt *et al, J Clin Psychopharmacol* 2005;**25**:609) and akathisia (n = 2, Bertolín Guillén *et al, Actas Esp Psiquiatr* 2002;**30**:195–7).

Reviews:* neuroleptic discontinuation syndromes (Tranter and Healy, *J Psychopharmacol* 1998;**12**:401–6; Baldessarini and Viguera, *Arch Gen Psychiatry* 1995;**52**:189–92; Moncrieff, *Acta Psychiatr Scand* 2006;**114**:3–13).

Median and near maximal daily dose		
Drug	ED 50	ED 85–95
Oral:		
Chlorpromazine	150 mg	400–450 mg
Fluphenazine	–	< 6.9 mg
Haloperidol	0.5–2 mg	3.5–10 mg
Trifluoperazine	–	10–15 mg/d
Amisulpride	50 mg	200 mg
Aripiprazole	< 1.5	10 mg/d
Clozapine		> 400 mg
Olanzapine	9 mg	> 16 mg
Quetiapine	80–215 mg	150–600 mg
Risperidone	2 mg	4 mg
Sertindole	10 mg	12–20 mg
Depots		
Fluphenazine dec	–	25 mg/fortnight
Risperidone		
Consta	15 mg/mon	50 mg/mon

TABLE 2.2.4: ANTIPSYCHOTIC DOSE EQUIVALENTS *

Oral	mg/d (+ range)
Chlorpromazine	100 mg (25–50 mg IM or 250 mg rectally)
Fluphenazine	2 mg (1.25–5 mg)
Levomepromazine	NK
Pericyazine	24 mg
Perphenazine	8 mg (7–15 mg)
Promazine	100 mg (50–200 mg)
Thioridazine	100 mg (75–104 mg)
Trifluoperazine	5 mg (2–8 mg)
Benperidol	2 mg
Haloperidol	3 mg (1–5 mg), or 1.5 mg IM/IV for doses up to 20 mg
Flupentixol	2 mg
Zuclopenthixol	25 mg (25–60 mg) up to 150 mg/d
Pimozide	2 mg (25–60 mg) up to 150 mg/d
Amisulpride	100 mg (40–150 mg)
Sulpiride	200 mg (200–333 mg)
Clozapine	100 mg (30–150 mg)
Olanzapine	NE
Quetiapine	NE
Zotepine	NE
Paliperidone	NE
Risperidone	0.5–1 mg (0.5–3 mg)
Depots and LAIs *	**mg/week**
Fluphenazine decanoate	5–10 mg (1–12.5 mg)
Pipothiazine palmitate	10 mg (5–12.5 mg)
Haloperidol decanoate	15 mg (5–25 mg)
Flupentixol decanoate	10 mg (8–20 mg)
Zuclopenthixol decanoate	100 mg (40–100 mg)
Fluspirilene	2 mg (NE)
Risperidone Consta LAI	12.5 mg (25 mg/fortnight)
Olanzapine pamoate *	Should only be used for people responding to oral olanzapine. See *Chapter 1* for oral to depot dose equivalent..

Bioavailability from oral haloperidol is about 50% of IM, with IV approximately equivalent to IM.

Key:

NE   = Not fully established

90 mg (75–100) = Recommended average dose + ranges quoted in the literature. The wider the range, the greater the uncertainty about the exact equivalent

> **The actual dose of a new drug required =**
>
> $$\frac{\text{Current total daily (oral) or weekly (depot) dose of the existing drug}}{\text{Equivalent dose stated for the existing drug in that form}} \quad \times \quad \text{equivalent dose of the new drug as stated in that table}$$

2.2.1.3 ANTIPSYCHOTIC DOSE EQUIVALENTS

The antipsychotic dose(s) of each drug within each heading of this section are approximately equivalent to others under the same heading (e.g. perphenazine 24mg/d is equivalent to chlorpromazine 300mg/d and to flupentixol 60mg 2/52), based on the references indicated. There is, however, a genuine lack of agreement about antipsychotic equivalents. This is mainly because the five methods of assessing anti-psychotic equivalence (clinical studies, non-clinical/receptor binding studies, median effective doses and manufacturers' information) can produce up to a five-fold difference in the equivalents calculated, particularly true in the case of high-potency antipsychotics. Ranges quoted here are thus unweighted for individual variation and are valid, but imprecise. The five methods are:

1. **Clinical studies** — there aren't any.

2. **Receptor binding** — antipsychotics displace ligands from dopamine receptors (particularly D2) at a rate that to some extent correlates with their antipsychotic potency and so roughly equivalent antipsychotic doses can be calculated. However, some dose relationships, e.g. haloperidol, are unlikely to be linear and sedation and anxiety may not be directly related to dopamine blockade. High-potency drugs, e.g. haloperidol and fluphenazine, have the highest quoted variance, over 1000% in some cases, which may lead to prescribing in higher doses than necessary (Dewan and Koss, *Acta Psychiatr Scand* 1995;**91**:229–32). Additionally, higher doses of antipsychotics tend to be used to control disruptive behaviour rather than just to control psychotic symptoms (Peralta et al, *Acta Psychiatr Scand* 1994;**90**:354–7).

3. **Median effective doses** — median effective doses (ED50) and near maximal effective doses (ED85 to ED95) can be used (systematic review and meta-analysis, Davis and Chen, *J Clin Psychopharmacol* 2004;**24**:192–208; review by Woods, *EBMH* 2004;**7**:106).

4. **Percentage of maximum dose** — this has been proposed as an alternative, but is also imprecise, as maximum doses may not be equivalent, e.g. is flupentixol decanoate 400mg a week really equivalent to 50mg a week of fluphenazine decanoate? Defined daily doses (DDDs) are an alternative to CPZ equivalents, but do not really match up as they

assume optimum doses are being used, which is not always the case (Rikcken et al, *J Clin Psychopharmacol* 2003;**23**:657–9).

Antipsychotic equivalence is specifically quoted here and the doses are as accurate as data allows, but to avoid any confusion you must consider the following:

1. Antipsychotic equivalence must not be confused with sedation, e.g. there may be no extra antipsychotic effect from haloperidol above 8–12mg/d (see *1.10.4*). If using a sedating 'broad-spectrum' drug (e.g. a phenothiazine) and converting to a D2 receptor selective drug (e.g. flupentixol, sulpiride, etc), the use of conversion tables may not thus be appropriate and may result in enhanced side-effects or over-dosage.

2. With some drugs there may not be a linear relationship between the dose and antipsychotic effect.

3. Dose frequency with depots may be important as the first pass effect may reduce the effective doses of oral preparations.

4. Differing half-lives may complicate the calculations and final dose recommendation.

5. These equivalent doses are not necessarily equivalent in terms of maximum doses.

6. For the newer antipsychotics, therapeutic doses are better defined and so no equivalent doses are appropriate.

You should always check your answer against the SPC to ensure an inappropriately high dose is not inadvertently considered (review, Atkins et al, *Psychiatr Bull* 1997;**21**:224–6).

Review: general (Remington et al, *Am J Psychiatry* 1998;**155**:1301–2).

2.2.1.4 POST-SWITCHING ANTIPSYCHOTIC ISSUES

(Based on an extensive review by Weiden et al, *J Clin Psychiatry* 1998;**59**[Suppl 19]:36–49.)

Assessing response:

1. For all drugs, aim for a minimum of three months at full therapeutic dosage.

2. Be cautious of any significant gains (e.g. reduced side-effects) within 6/52 of the last drug stopping, as drug concentrations at receptor level may outlast plasma levels (see haloperidol, *1.27*).

3. Even if gains occur, make sure a full therapeutic trial is achieved, as discontinuation of the previous drug will lead to a gradual loss of its side-effects (including cognitive impairment), which may be interpreted as improvement.
4. If therapeutic gains occur, it has been suggested to delay discontinuing any anticholinergic and/or antiakathisia drugs until during the second month.
5. Raised prolactin levels may take over 3/12 to resolve, so women need to be warned about this, and to ensure that they have adequate contraceptive cover.
6. If positive changes occur, caution the patient not to risk relapse by 'over-doing it'.

Managing a sub-optimum response to a switch:
1. No improvement by 6/52 — exclude non-compliance with the switch, substance misuse and inadequate dosage. Try to work towards 12/52 at full dose.
2. Some response by 6/52 — do not get too excited, continue to 12/52.
3. Partial response between 6/52 and 12/52 — consider an increase in dose, and try to go for a 6/12 trial.
4. Initial response followed by worsening of positive symptoms — check worsening is not actually improvement (e.g. previous positive symptoms hidden by the patient now surfacing), try to restabilise and aim for 12/52 at full dose.

Long-term issues:
1. With improvements in insight, increased psychosocial support and monitoring will be needed to reduce the risk of post-psychotic depression and self-harm.

2.2.2 SWITCHING BENZODIAZEPINES

Switching benzodiazepines may be advantageous for a variety of reasons, eg. to a drug with a longer half-life prior to discontinuation. While there is broad agreement in the literature about equivalent doses, clonazepam has a wide variety of reported equivalences and particular care is needed with this drug. Inter-patient variability and differing half-lives means the figures can never be exact and should be interpreted using your own pharmaceutical knowledge.

2.2.3 SWITCHING ANTICHOLINERGICS

See 6.7 about the overall indications for the use of anticholinergics. Equivalent doses are:

Biperiden	2 mg
Orphenadrine	50 mg
Procyclidine	2 mg
Trihexyphenidyl (benzhexol)	2 mg

(Saklad, personal communication)

2.2.4 SWITCHING DRUGS OF ABUSE OR DEPENDENCE

Switching drugs of abuse/dependence, usually to methadone, is a common strategy. *Table 2.2.6* may be of some use, although caution is obviously necessary regarding, e.g. the potency of individual samples of street drugs.

Advice:
1. Most of these equivalent doses are based on analgesic equivalents, which may differ by a factor of 10 to the dose needed to suppress opiate withdrawal symptoms.
2. The dose relationship may be non-linear, especially at higher doses and above BNF limits.

TABLE 2.2.5: BENZODIAZEPINE EQUIVALENT DOSES

See note in introduction regarding half lives

Diazepam	5 mg (oral, im, or iv)
Alprazolam	0.5 mg (0.25–0.5 mg)
Chlordiazepoxide	15 mg (10–25 mg)
Clobazam	10 mg
Clonazepam	0.5 mg (0.25–4)
Flunitrazepam	0.5 mg
Flurazepam	7.5–15 mg
Loprazolam	0.5–1 mg
Lorazepam	0.5–1 mg at 4 mg/d
	2 mg at 5 mg/d
Lormetazepam	0.5–1 mg
Nitrazepam	5 mg (2.5–20 mg)
Oxazepam	15 mg (10–40 mg)
Temazepam	10 mg

TABLE 2.2.6: METHADONE EQUIVALENT DOSES

Narcotics

Drug	Total daily dose	Equivalent daily dose of methadone in mg	Range quoted	
			Lower	Upper
Buprenorhine injection	0.3	8	8	8
Buprenorphine S/L	0.2	5	5	8
Codeine linctus 15mg/5ml in ml	1	0.2	0.2	0.2
Codeine phosphate	15	1	1	1
Dextropropoxyphene	32.5	2.145	2.145	2.145
Diamorphine BP injection	5	10	10	10
Diamorphine BP oral	10	10	10	20
Diconal tablets	1	5	4	5
Dihydrocodeine	30	2.5	2	3
Fentanyl patches in mcg/hr	25	2	1.65	2.5
Gee's Linctus	100	10	10	10
Hydromorphone oral	1	2.5	2.5	6.5
J Collis Brown's (in mls)	100	10	10	10
Morphine BP injection	10	10	10	10
Morphine BP oral	15	10	10	10
MST tablets	10	3.25	3.25	3.25
Oxycodone	1	0.8	0.4	1.32
Palfium	5	5	5	10
Papaveretum	10	4.4		
Pentazocine	25	2	2	2
Pethidone injection/tablets	50	4.25	4	5
Tramadol	50	1.6	1.6	8.25

3. Analgesic equivalents are mostly derived from single-dose studies, not long-term studies where a steady state has been achieved.
4. Total daily doses should be calculated.
5. These are definitely **not** starter doses, but may give an idea of a possible maximum. The person should be dose titrated and assessed, based on withdrawal symptoms and clinical response.
6. Analgesic equivalents for tramadol produce a much higher methadone equivalent. The tramadol dose here is based on a study showing tramadol 450mg/d is equivalent to 15mg/d methadone for suppressing opiate withdrawal symptoms (n = 70, RCT, d/b, Salehi et al, J Res Med Sci 2006;11:185–9). NB. SR, dispersable and liquid and tramadol may have different bioavailabilities.
7. Codeine is metabolised by 2D6 to active morphine, so any 2D6 slow or ultra-rapid

Switching methylphenidate preparations: *

IR-MPH, Equasym XL, Medikinet XL	Concerta XL equivalent dose
10mg/d	
15mg	18mg
20mg	
30mg	36mg
40mg	
45mg	54mg
50mg	72mg (unlicensed)

metabolisers will affect the equivalent dose.
8. Some texts recommend that when changing from weaker to stronger opioids, reduce the dose by up to 30–50%, as there is often incomplete cross tolerance due to different

binding profiles and also increased sedation.

9. Dihydrocodeine SR (DHC) is 95–100% absorbed so the total daily dose is the same for plain tablets (information from Napp).

2.2.5 SWITCHING ADHD TREATMENTS *

Methylphenidate to atomoxetine:
Although this switch can be done quickly, a slower switch is generally recommended to minimise adverse effects, as they can be given together. About 50% of methylphenidate non-responders will respond to atomoxetine and 75% methylphenidate responders will also respond to atomoxetine (Prasad and Steer, *Paediatr Drugs* 2008;**10**:39–47).

Week 1 = full-dose methylphenidate, plus atomoxetine 0.5 mg/kg/d

Week 2 = half-dose methylphenidate, plus atomoxetine 1.2 mg/kg/d

Week 3 = stop methylphenidate, atomoxetine 1.2 mg/kg/d

Ref: (n = 69 [c = 58], open, Quintana *et al, Clin Ther* 2007;**29**:1168–77).

2.2.6 SWITCHING ANTI-CHOLINESTERASES *

Switching anticholinesterases: *
Switching anticholinesterases may be necessary for tolerability, lack of efficacy or long-term loss of efficacy. There is no data on the last point. There are subtle differences in receptor modulation between the anticholinesterases and so lack of response to one does not necessarily exclude response to another. There is no published data on the outcome of switching to donepezil.

Donepezil to galantamine: *
One review suggested that the response rate to galantamine may be the same regardless of non-response to donepezil (Emre, *Int J Clin Pract Suppl* 2002;**127**:64–72) and is well tolerated (n = 4, Bartorelli *et al, Curr Med Res Opin* 2005;**21**:1809–18).

Donepezil to rivastigmine oral/patches: *
It has been reported that in donepezil non-response, around 50% will then respond to rivastigmine (n = 382, Auriacombe *et al, Curr Med Res Opin* 2002;**18**:129–38; n = 188, Bartorelli *et al, Curr Med Res Opin* 2005;**21**:1809–18). An

immediate switch from donepezil 5–10 mg/d to rivastigmine patches 4.6 mg/24 hours may be well tolerated and safe, but a slower switch might be appropriate with any pre-existing bradycardia or if concurrent beta-blockers are being taken, the incidence of nausea and vomiting being 4% and 1% respectively (open, Sadowsky *et al, Am J Alzheimer's Dis Other Demen* 2009;**24**:267–75). Abrupt switch from donepezil to oral rivastigmine (without washout) may be effective and well-tolerated (n = 146, open, 12/12, Figiel *et al, Prim Care Companion J Clin Psychiatry* 2008;**10**:363–7 and 291–8, MS; review of three switching studies; Sadowsky *et al, Int J Clin Pract* 2010;**64**:188–93).

Galantamine plain to galantamine XL: *
A manufacturer's computer simulation suggests that an abrupt switch should be acceptable (Hing *et al, Curr Med Res Opin* 2005;**21**:482–8).

Galantamine to rivastigmine patches: *
A review has concluded that galantamine can be switched abruptly to the patch, with nausea or vomiting in only 2–3% (Sadowsky *et al, CNS Neurosci Ther* 2010; **16**:51–60), and that response to rivastigmine can occur despite non-response to galantamine (n = 33, Bartorelli *et al, Curr Med Res Opin* 2005;**21**:1809–18).

Rivastigmine to galantamine: *
One review has suggested that the response rate to galantamine may be the same regardless of non-response to donepezil (Emre, *Int J Clin Pract Suppl* 2002;**127**:64–72).

Rivastigmine oral to rivastigmine patches: *
A review has concluded that rivastigmine oral high dose can be switched abruptly to the 9.5 mg/24-hour patch but low dose should be switched to 4.6 mg/24-hour for four weeks before increasing. The incidence of nausea and vomiting is 3% and 2% respectively (Sadowsky *et al, CNS Neurosci Ther* 2010;**16**:51–60). The first patch should be applied the day after the last oral dose:

Rivastigmine oral dose per day	Patch strength
3–6 mg	4.6 mg/24 hrs
9 mg (not stable/poorly tolerated)	4.6 mg/24 hrs
9 mg (stable and well-tolerated)	9.5 mg/24 hrs
12 mg	9.5 mg/24 hrs

Review: * expert consensus (Gauthier *et al, Curr Med Res Opin* 2003;**19**:707–14).

2.2.7 SWITCHING OR DISCONTINUING ANTIDEPRESSANTS

Switching from one antidepressant to another, either for reasons of side-effects, safety or lack of efficacy, can be problematical and present unexpected problems. Clinicians must be aware of these to eliminate avoidable adverse events.

1. Agomelatine to/from others

Agomelatine has no apparent significant problem with other antidepressants so should be able to be switched to and from with negligible risk (except fluvoxamine, which inhibits 1A2 and raises levels significantly). Until more data is available it is recommended to be careful.

2. SSRI to/from TCA

Fluoxetine, paroxetine and fluvoxamine (but probably not citalopram, escitalopram and sertraline at standard doses) can double or triple tricyclic levels (particularly of amitriptyline, imipramine, nortriptyline and clomipramine), by CYP2D6 inhibition and so great care is needed. Prescribing both drugs together over a change-over period is not advised unless the drugs and doses are chosen carefully and specific care is taken. Ideally, 'drop-and-stop' before starting the next drug is recommended.

Factors to be considered with an SSRI-tricyclic switch:

- Speed at which the switch is needed, e.g. faster switches can obviously be made, but additional monitoring, e.g. tricyclic levels and cardiac status is recommended.
- SSRI dose — CYP2D6 inhibition is dose-related for most drugs, e.g. paroxetine, fluoxetine.
- Tricyclic — stronger serotonin reuptake inhibitors are more likely to produce serotonin syndrome (e.g. clomipramine), and tertiary tricyclics (e.g. imipramine, amitriptyline, clomipramine) are also metabolised by CYP3A3/4 and CYP1A2, which are inhibited by fluvoxamine.
- P450 status of the patient ie slow or rapid metaboliser (see 4.2).
- Individual susceptibility to tricyclic and SSRI side-effects.

Factors to consider before choosing an antidepressant switching regimen

- Speed at which the switch is needed, e.g. with less urgency a more cautious regimen can be used, e.g. drugs that can be used in combination. Faster switches can obviously be made, but additional monitoring is recommended.
- Current dose of the first drug.
- Individual drugs and their effects, neurotransmitter effects, kinetics, etc.
- Individuals' susceptibility to (additive) ADRs.

Potential problems

- Cholinergic rebound, e.g. headache, restlessness, diarrhoea, nausea and vomiting (Lieberman, *Psychosomatics* 1981;**22**:253–4) from withdrawal of drugs blocking cholinergic receptors, e.g. tricyclics.
- Antidepressant withdrawal or discontinuation symptoms (see 13).
- Serotonin syndrome, for drugs affecting serotonin (see 6.9).
- Drug-drug interactions e.g. changed drug levels from altered metabolism (see 4.3).
- Discontinuation effects from the first drug being interpreted as side-effects of the second.

Switching drugs 'with care' means

- Drop and stop first drug.
- Leave a gap of a few days if possible.
- Warn the patient about potential complications and what to do about them, e.g. serotonin syndrome, cholinergic rebound, toxicity and discontinuation.

Main potential problems (see introduction for more details):

- Cholinergic rebound.
- Tricyclic/SSRI discontinuation symptoms (see reference 13).
- Serotonin syndrome (see 6.9).
- Increased tricyclic levels via CYP2D6 inhibition by SSRIs (see 4.3.1).

Suggested switch regimens:

Tricyclic to fluoxetine, paroxetine or fluvoxamine: Taper tricyclic dose to around 25–

50 mg/d, start SSRI at usual starting dose and discontinue tricyclic over next 5–7 days. Be wary of serotonin syndrome, raised tricyclic levels by P450 inhibition, cholinergic rebound and tricyclic withdrawal.

Tricyclic to citalopram, escitalopram or sertraline: Taper tricyclic as above, but there is a much lower potential for interactions so problems are less likely. A serotonin syndrome has been reported with sertraline and amitriptyline (Alderman et al, Ann Pharmacother 1996;**30**:1499–500).

Fluoxetine to tricyclic: Drop fluoxetine to 20 mg/d, then stop, wait several days for peak levels to fall, then add the tricyclic **cautiously at low dose** and build up slowly. Care is needed for up to four weeks as the interaction potential via 2D6 inhibition may be prolonged (see 4.3.2), e.g. an abrupt switch from fluoxetine 20 mg/d to amitriptyline 50–100 mg/d resulted in 14% dropping out due to adverse reactions, the rest tolerating the switch (Rutten et al, MI). Be wary of serotonin syndrome (especially with drugs such as clomipramine) and higher tricyclic levels via CYP2D6 inhibition.

Paroxetine to tricyclic: Leave a gap if possible or taper paroxetine to about 10 mg/d, and introduce the tricyclic at low dose. After several days, discontinue paroxetine and increase tricyclic dose to therapeutic levels. Be wary of paroxetine withdrawal (see 17), serotonin syndrome (especially with drugs such as clomipramine) and higher tricyclic levels via CYP2D6 inhibition.

Fluvoxamine to tricyclic: As paroxetine. Be wary of fluvoxamine withdrawal (rare, see 17), serotonin syndrome (especially with drugs such as clomipramine) and higher tricyclic levels via CYP1A2 and 3A3/4 inhibition (especially with tertiary tricyclics).

Citalopram, escitalopram or sertraline to tricyclic: If necessary, reduce to minimum doses of citalopram (20 mg/d), escitalopram (10 mg) or sertraline (50 mg/d). Stop the SSRI and introduce the tricyclic, titrating dose upwards as tolerated. With standard doses of these SSRIs, few problems should be seen. Be wary of SSRI withdrawal (rare, see reference 17), serotonin syndrome (especially with, e.g. clomipramine) and higher tricyclic levels via CYP2D6 inhibition (low risk).

3. Trazodone to/from others

Trazodone to SSRIs: Trazodone and fluoxetine have been used together but the risks include enhanced sedation (e.g. n = 8, Nirenberg et al, J Clin Psychiatry 1992;**53**:83), serotonin syndrome (n = 1, George and Godleski, Biol Psychiatry 1996;**39**:384–5) and slightly raised trazodone levels (see 4.3.2.2). A serotonin syndrome with low dose trazodone added to paroxetine (n = 1, Reeves and Bullen, Psychosomatics 1995;**36**:159–60) would indicate the need for similar care. For citalopram, there is a report of lack of a pharmacokinetic interaction, with no changes in plasma levels (n = 40 + 41 controls; Prapotnik et al, Int J Clin Pharmacol Ther 2004;**42**:120–4). There is no information on changing from trazodone to sertraline but a gradual switch, with close observation would seem sensible for all SSRIs. See 5.

Trazodone to tricyclics: Tricyclics: there are two isolated cases of hypomania after an abrupt change from trazodone to imipramine (n = 2, Haggerty and Jackson, J Clin Psychiatry 1985;**5**:342–3), so care is needed with the switch.

4. Tricyclic to/from tricyclic

No significant problems have been reported but a gradual switch is recommended as per normal practice.

5. SSRI to/from SSRI *

Any combination of SSRIs could precipitate a serotonin syndrome (see 6.9). Thus, careful observation initially and a gentle changeover is recommended. A washout period would further minimise the possibility of problems.

Fluoxetine to sertraline: be mindful of fluoxetine's long half-life, e.g. in outpatients abruptly swapped from fluoxetine to sertraline (20 mg:50 mg respectively dose substitution), 63% swapped successfully but 37% failed, including 18% with intolerable adverse effects (nervousness, jitters, diarrhoea, nausea and headache), suggestive of a serotonin-like syndrome (n = 54, Stock and Kofoed, Am J Hosp Pharm 1994;**51**:2279–81).

Fluoxetine to paroxetine: abrupt switching has produced an increased level of side-effects such as insomnia, nausea, dry mouth, nervousness and tremor in the immediate switch group when compared to a two-week washout, which was well tolerated (n = 240, d/b, Kreider et al, J Clin Psychiatry 1995;**56**:142–5; see also n = 9, Dominguez et al, J Clin Psychopharmacol 1996;**16**:320–3).

Fluvoxamine to paroxetine: * there is a case of rapidly increased fluvoxamine levels when paroxetine was started during a switch, probably via 2D6 inhibition (n = 1, Hori et al, World J Biol Psychiatry 2009;**10**:620–2).

6. Duloxetine *

Abruptly stopping an SSRI and starting **duloxetine** was as well tolerated and safe as tapered SSRI discontinuation and immediate duloxetine starting (n = 368, RCT, 10/52, Perahia et al, J Clin Psychiatry 2008;**69**:95–105). See also 8. Patients switching from SSRIs or venlafaxine to duloxetine have less nausea when starting than those starting de novo; immediate switching may be well-tolerated, although fluoxetine was surprisingly excluded from this Lilly study and would pose particular problems (n = 155, Wohlreich et al, Ann Clin Psychiatry 2005;**17**:259–68, MS).

7. MAOIs

MAOI to MAOI: A two-week gap is recommended, especially if switching to tranylcypromine. The literature for tranylcypromine recommends leaving at least a seven-day gap after stopping another antidepressant, then starting tranyl-cypromine at half the usual dosage for one week. Careful observation is essential. An open study of switching MAOIs with less than a 14-day gap showed that only one patient suffered adverse events, probably tranylcypromine withdrawal or a mild serotonin syndrome and so a shorter gap may be feasible with full dietary control, good compliance and close monitoring (n = 8, Szuba et al, J Clin Psychiatry 1997;**58**:307–10), although deaths have been reported (e.g. n = 1, Bazire, Drug Intell Clin Pharm 1986;**20**:954–56).

SSRIs to MAOIs: The time to wait between stopping an SSRI and starting an MAOI depends upon the SSRI. The literature for tranylcypromine recommends leaving at least a seven-day gap after stopping other antidepressants, then starting tranylcypromine at half the usual dosage

How to use *Table 2.2.7:*

i. Look down the vertical column headed 'from' and find the drug, or drug group, the patient is currently taking.

ii. Follow that line along until you come to the column of the drug, or drug group, to which you wish to change.

iii. The details there give the current known information. For further details look up the reference number quoted.

Example: Changing from tranylcypromine to a tricyclic requires a 14-day drug-free gap (reference 9), but changing from a tricyclic to tranylcypromine only requires a seven-day drug-free gap (reference 9).

for one week. The literature also recommends a two-week gap from an SSRI before an MAOI is started.

Fluvoxamine to MAOI: Fluvoxamine has a short half-life and so isocarboxazid/phenelzine may be started 4–5 days after stopping fluvoxamine (4–5 x half-life) or seven days for tranylcypromine.

Paroxetine to MAOI: A two-week gap is recommended (SPC).

Fluoxetine to MAOI: A serotonin syndrome has been reported when tranylcypromine was started six weeks after fluoxetine was stopped, due to the persistence of norfluoxetine (but not fluoxetine) in the blood (n = 1, Coplan and Gorman, Am J Psychiatry 1993;**150**:837). Since several reported interactions exist, it might be better to allow six weeks after stopping fluoxetine before starting an MAOI (Drug Ther Bull 1990;**28**:334). The isocarboxazid SPC recommends a gap longer than two weeks.

Sertraline to MAOI: A one-week gap should elapse before starting an MAOI. A serotonergic syndrome has been reported with sertraline and tranylcypromine (see SSRI interactions 4.3.2). The SPC states that at least a two-week gap between sertraline and MAOIs is needed.

Trazodone to MAOI: The literature recommends a one-week gap. A study of combined treatment did not show hypertensive reactions but an increase in side-effects e.g. sedation, and postural

TABLE 2.2.7: SWITCHING ANTIDEPRESSANTS *

NSPR = no significant problems reported, careful cross-taper; OP = occasional problems; SSP = serotonin syndrome possible

From \ To	Hydrazines (MAOI)	Tranylcypromine (MAOI)	Tricyclics	Citalopram/ escitalopram (SSRI)	Fluvoxamine (SSRI)	Fluoxetine (SSRI)	Sertraline (SSRI)	Paroxetine (SSRI)	Trazodone	Bupropion	Moclobemide	Venlafaxine	Duloxetine[5]	Mirtazapine	Agomelatine[13]	Reboxetine
Hydrazines		14/7[7]	7–14/7[7]	14/7[7]	14/7[7]	14/7[7]	14/7[7]	14/7[7]	14/7[7] or care	7/7[7]	Read text[7]	14/7[13]	14/7[6]	2/52[7]	NSPR[1]	2/52[7]
Tranylcypromine	14/7[7]		14/7[7]	14/7[7]	14/7[7]	14/7[7]	14/7[7]	14/7[7]	14/7[7]	7/7[7]	Read text[7]	14/7[13]	14/7[6]	2/52[7]	NSPR[1]	2/52[7]
Tricyclics	7/7[7]	7/7[7]		NSPR[4]	Great care[2]	Great care[2]	Care[2]	Great care[2]	NSPR[10]	NSPR[9]	Read text[7,8]	Care[13]	SSP[5]	NSPR[11]	NSPR[1]	NSPR[12]
Citalopram/ escitalopram	7/7[7]	7/7[7]	Care[2]	SSP	SSP[5]	SSP[5]	SSP[5]	SSP[5]	Care	NSPR[9]	7/7[8]	Care[13]	SSP[5]	NSPR[11]	NSPR[1]	NSPR[12]
Fluvoxamine	7/7[7]	7/7[7]	Great care[2]	SSP[5]		SSP[6]	SSP[5]	SSP[5]	Care	NSPR[9]	NSPR[8]	Care[13]	SSP[5]	NSPR[11]	Care[1]	NSPR[12]
Fluoxetine	4–5/7[7]	5/52[7]	Great care for 28/7[2]	SSP[5]	SSP[5]		SSP[5]	SSP[5]	Care	NSPR[10]	3/52[8]	Care[13]	SSP[6]	NSPR[11]	NSPR[1]	NSPR[12]
Sertraline	7–14/7[7]	7–14/7[7]	Great care[2]	SSP[5]	SSP[5]	SSP[5]		SSP[5]	Care	NSPR[9]	7–13/7[8]	Care[13]	SSP[6]	NSPR[11]	NSPR[1]	NSPR[12]
Paroxetine	14/7[7]	14/7[7]	Great care[2]	SSP[5]	SSP[5]	SSP[5]	SSP[5]		Care[6]	NSPR[9]	5/7[8]	Care[13]	SSP[6]	NSPR[11]	NSPR[1]	NSPR[12]
Trazodone	14/7[7]	14/7[7]	OP[3]	Care[3]	Care[3]	Care[3]	Care[3]	Care[3]		NSPR[9]	NSPR	Care[13]	SSP[6]	NSPR[11]	NSPR[1]	NSPR[12]
Bupropion[10]	7/7[8]	7/7[8]	Care	NSPR[9]	NSPR[9]	NSPR[9]	NSPR[9]	NSPR[9]	NSPR[9]		NSPR[9]	NSPR[13]	SSP[6]	NSPR[9,11]	NSPR[1]	NSPR[9]
Moclobemide	7/7[8]	NSPR[7]	OP[8]	NSPR[8]	NSPR[8]	NSPR[8]	NSPR[8]	NSPR[8]	NSPR[13]	NSPR		NSPR[13]	SSP[8]	NSPR[11]	NSPR[1]	NSPR[12]
Venlafaxine	7/7[13]	7/7[13]	NSPR[13]	Care[13]	Care[13]	Care[13]	Care[13]	Care[13]	Care[13]	NSPR[13]	NSPR[13]		Care SSP[5]	NSPR[11]	NSPR[1]	NSPR[12]
Duloxetine	5/7[6]	5/7[6]	SSP[5]	SSP[5] care	SSP[5]	SSP[5]	SSP[5]	SSP[5]	SSP[5]	SSP[5]	SSP[5]	SSP[5,13]		NSPR	NSPR[1]	NSPR[11]
Mirtazapine	7/7[7]	7/7[7]	NSPR[11]	NSPR[11]	NSPR[11]	NSPR[11]	NSPR[11]	NSPR[11]	NSPR[11]	NSPR[11]	NSPR[11]	NSPR[11]	NSPR		NSPR[1]	NSPR[11]
Agomelatine[1]	NSPR	NSPR	NSPR[1]	NSPR[1]	Care[1]	NSPR[1]	NSPR[1]	NSPR[1]	NSPR[1]	NSPR[1]	NSPR[1]	NSPR[1]	NSPR[1]	NSPR[1]		NSPR[1]
Reboxetine	1/52[12]	1/52[12]	NSPR[2]	NSPR[12]	NSPR[12]	NSPR[12]	NSPR[12]	NSPR[12]	NSPR[12]	NSPR[12]	NSPR[12]	NSPR[12]	NSPR[12]	NSPR[1]	NSPR[1]	
Just plain stopping[17]	Over 4/52[14]	Over 4/52[14]	Over 4/52[14]	Over 4/52	Over 4/52[14]	Drop to 20mg/d then stop[14]	Over 4/52[14]	Over 4/52[14] or longer	Over 4/52[14]	Over 4/52[14]	Over 4/52[14]	Over 4/52[14] or longer	Over 4/52[14] or longer	Over 4/52[14]	NSPR[14]	Over 4/52[14]

hypotension occurred (n = 13, Nierenberg and Keck, *J Clin Psychopharmacol* 1989;**9**:42).

Moclobemide to MAOI: Moclobemide has a half-life of 14 hours and so stopping it one day and starting an MAOI the next day is adequate.

Mirtazapine to MAOI: A one-week wash-out period is recommended by the manufacturers, although there are no reports of problems.

Trazodone to MAOI: The SPC recommends a two week gap after stopping trazodone before MAOIs.

Tricyclic to MAOI: A one-week gap is recommended and is advisable particularly if imipramine, clomipramine or tranylcypromine are involved. Low doses of the MAOI is essential.

MAOI to SSRIs: A two-week gap (*Drug Ther Bull* 1990;**28**:33–4) has been recommended (e.g. fluoxetine SPC) but longer may be safer as a severe serotonin syndrome has been reported with a two-week gap between stopping tranylcypromine and starting fluoxetine (n = 1, Ruiz, *Ann Emerg Med* 1994;**24**:983–5), even although tranylcypromine has a relatively short action (i.e. reversible MAO inhibition).

MAOI to moclobemide: A gap is not needed between stopping an MAOI and starting moclobemide, provided MAOI dietary restrictions are maintained for 10–14 days.

MAOI to mirtazapine: A two-week wash-out period is recommended.

MAOI to trazodone: The SPC recommends a two-week gap after stopping an MAOI before trazodone is started.

MAOIs to tricyclic: A 10–14-day gap is often recommended (isocarboxazid '1–2 weeks'), particularly if imipramine, clomipramine or tranylcypromine are involved. Using initial low doses of the tricyclic is essential.

8. Moclobemide to/from others *

Moclobemide to duloxetine: Immediate switching from moclobemide 400 mg/d to duloxetine 60 mg/d has induced serotonin syndrome within an hour (n = 1, Jimenez-Genchi, *J Clin Psychiatry* 2006;**67**:1821–2).

Moclobemide to fluoxetine: The fluoxetine SPC states that it can be started the day after moclobemide is stopped.

Moclobemide to tricyclic: Abrupt switching from moclobemide to tricyclics appears well tolerated

but switching to clomipramine has caused some problems.

SSRIs to moclobemide: The literature recommends a gap of 4–5 half-lives after stopping an SSRI before starting moclobemide, as serotonin syndromes have been reported (see *4.3.3.5*).

Citalopram/escitalopram to moclobemide: A seven-day gap is recommended.

Fluoxetine to moclobemide: With fluoxetine's long half-life, the gap should be as much as six weeks if five times the half-life of norfluoxetine is calculated. A gap of three weeks together with careful monitoring would seem a reasonably practical figure. However, in a study where up to 600 mg/d moclobemide was added to established fluoxetine therapy, there was no change in the number, intensity, or type of adverse events. Fluoxetine markedly inhibited the metabolism of moclobemide but did not lead to excessive accumulation, with no evidence of a 'serotonin syndrome' (n = 18, RCT, p/c, Dingemanse et al, *Clin Pharmacol Ther* 1998;**63**:403–13).

Fluvoxamine to moclobemide: A three-day gap is recommended (but see above).

Paroxetine to moclobemide: A five-day gap is recommended (but see above), although paroxetine's half-life can be longer in the elderly. A severe serotonin syndrome has been reported when moclobemide replaced paroxetine but with no washout (n = 1, Wu and Deng, *J Chin Med Assoc* 2009;**72**:446–9).

Sertraline to moclobemide: With the long half-life of desmethylsertraline, the gap should be up to 13 days, but only seven days is recommended by the sertraline SPC (but see above).

Tricyclic to moclobemide: A gap of 4–5 half-lives is recommended if the tricyclic concerned is a 5-HT reuptake inhibitor. However, healthy volunteers taking either clomipramine 100 mg/d or amitriptyline 75 mg/d for at least a week were swapped abruptly to moclobemide (150 mg first day, 300 mg/d thereafter) or placebo. There was no increase in the incidence or severity of side-effects or any significant pharmacokinetic interaction (n = 24, d/b, p/c, Dingemanse et al, *J Clin Psychopharmacol* 1995;**15**:41–8).

9. Bupropion *

Bupropion is contraindicated with **MAOIs**

as animal studies show that acute bupropion toxicity is enhanced by phenelzine. Co-administration of bupropion with drugs that are metabolised by CYP2D6 (e.g. **tricyclics, paroxetine** and **fluoxetine**) should be approached with caution and should be initiated at the lower end of the dose range of the concomitant medication. If bupropion is added to the treatment regimen of a patient already receiving a drug metabolised by CYP2D6, the need to decrease the dose of the original medication should be considered, particularly for those with a narrow therapeutic index.

Fluoxetine to bupropion: In fluoxetine non-responders, a switch to bupropion yielded 35% responders and 25% partial responders (n = 29, 12 + 8/52, open, Fava et al, Ann Clin Psychiatry 2003;**15**:17–22).

10. Tryptophan to/from others

Adding tryptophan to existing therapy is far more common than switching to tryptophan. Behavioural and neurological toxicity has been reported with concomitant high dose tryptophan and MAOIs, and so initial observation and care would seem advisable. With SSRIs, cases of central toxicity, agitation and nausea have occurred with the combination and are suggested as likely to occur with all SSRIs, and the possibility of a serotonergic syndrome developing should be considered.

11. Mirtazapine to/from others

Mirtazapine has multiple routes of metabolism (CYP2D6, 3A4 and 1A2) so switching problems will be unlikely in terms of P450 inhibition. The only recommendation is for MAOIs (see 7). Fluoxetine 20–40mg/d has been switched abruptly to mirtazapine 15mg/d, without problems (n = 40, Preskorn et al, Biol Psychiatry 1997;**41**:96S), although serotonin syndrome has been reported during a cross-over switch to venlafaxine (n = 1, Dimellis, World J Biol Psychiatry 2002;**3**:167).

12. SSRIs to/from reboxetine *

Fluoxetine to reboxetine: In fluoxetine non-responders, abrupt switch to reboxetine was well tolerated (n = 128, open, Fava et al, J Clin Psychopharmacol 2003;**23**:365–9).

13. Venlafaxine to/from others

MAOI to venlafaxine: The moclobemide SPC recommends a 14-day gap between stopping an MAOI and starting venlafaxine. This is appropriate as there are a number of reports of interactions, e.g. extreme agitation, diaphoresis, rapid respiration and raised CPK, e.g. after a 37.5 mg dose of venlafaxine seven days after phenelzine 45mg/d was stopped (Phillips and Ringo, Am J Psychiatry 1995;**15**:1400–1) and serotonin syndrome (e.g. n = 4, Diamond et al, Neurology 1998;**51**:274–6). In the first reported case, the reaction did not occur a further seven days later and strongly suggests that a 14-day gap is indeed required.

Venlafaxine to MAOI: The SPC recommends at least a seven-day gap (see above).

Venlafaxine to other drugs: No information, although agomelatine and mirtazapine have no reported or theoretical problems.

Tricyclic to venlafaxine: The venlafaxine SPC states that there is little problem between venlafaxine and tricyclics. There are no reports of any problems.

Other drugs to venlafaxine: No information, as above.

14. Withdrawal or discontinuation

Adverse discontinuation events have been reported for many antidepressants. Such symptoms are not, however, indicative of dependence, which usually requires three of the following:

• tolerance
• withdrawal symptoms
• use greater than needed
• inability to reduce doses
• excessive time taken procuring drug
• primacy of drug-taking over other activities
• continued use despite understanding of adverse consequences.

Discontinuation symptoms usually start within 1–2 days of stopping, resolve within 4–24 hours of restarting the drug, and are more common with longer courses or higher doses. They can occur with missed doses and about 30% of patients on SSRIs have dosing lapses of two or more days, long enough to produce discontinuation symptoms in patients on some short-acting SSRIs (n = 82, 3/12, Meijer *et al, Br J Psychiatry* 2001;**179**:519–22), but not fluoxetine (*Curr Prob* 2000;**26**:11–2). The *UK Drug and Therapeutics Bulletin* (1999;**37**:49–52) recommends:

- after less than eight weeks of treatment, withdraw over 1–2 weeks
- after 6–8 months of treatment, taper over a 6–8-week period
- after long-term maintenance treatment, reduce the dose by 25% every 4–6 weeks.

Options for the management of antidepressant withdrawal symptoms include:

1. Reduce the dose stepwise every week or so, stabilising between reductions, e.g. paroxetine 20mg/d, 10mg/d, then 10mg alternate days (but not less frequently). Use of the syrup, gradually diluted, may also be effective.
2. Transfer to a long half-life drug, e.g. fluoxetine (care with switching), then reduce (clomipramine case, Benazzi, *Am J Psychiatry* 1999 **156**:661–2; venlafaxine case, Giakas and David, *Psychiatr Ann* 1997;**27**:85–92).
3. Treat the emerging syndrome symptomatically, e.g. nausea, headache and diarrhoea have been managed with ondansetron (n = 1, Raby, *J Clin Psychiatry* 1998;**59**:621–2) and ginger root (Schechter, *J Clin Psychiatry* 1998;**59**:431–2).

Reviews: recognition, prevention and management of antidepressant withdrawal syndromes (Haddad, *Drug Safety* 2001;**24**:183–97), general (Haddad, *J Clin Psychiatry* 1998;**59**:541–8; Healy, *Prescriber* 2002;**13**:91–9).

Main withdrawal symptoms

Tricyclics: Cholinergic rebound, e.g. headache, restlessness, diarrhoea, nausea and vomiting (Lieberman, *Psychosomatics* 1981;**22**:253–4), flu-like symptoms, lethargy, abdominal cramps, sleep disturbance and movement disorders.

MAOIs: Psychosis, hallucinations, disorientation, catatonia, irritability, hypomania, nausea, sweating, palpitations, nightmares and delirium.

SSRIs: Dizziness, vertigo/lightheadedness, nausea, fatigue, headache, sensory disturbance, 'electric shocks' in the head, insomnia, abdominal cramps, chills, flu-like symptoms, increased or more vivid dreaming, anxiety/agitation and volatility, but not caused by anything else, e.g.

physical illness or other drugs.

Reviews: SSRI withdrawal (Healy, *Prescriber* 2002; **13**:91–9; Zajecka *et al, J Clin Psychiatry* 1997;**58**: 291–7).

Specific drugs

Comparative data: There have been a number of comparative studies between SSRIs. Interruption for 5–8 days of maintenance therapy produced few discontinuation symptoms with fluoxetine (long half-life), some with sertraline and most with paroxetine (n = 242, RCT, d/b, 4/52, Rosenbaum *et al, Biol Psychiatry* 1998;**44**:77–87; MS). In another study, suddenly discontinuing fluoxetine showed slightly more dizziness and somnolence at weeks 2–4, but no difference at week 6 compared to continuous treatment (n = 395, RCT, 12/52, Zajecka *et al, J Clin Psychopharmacol* 1998;**18**:193–7; review, Kendrick, *EBMH* 1999;**2**:31). A third study of a five-day interruption showed increased symptoms after a second missed dose with paroxetine, with impaired functional performance at five days, sertraline with less pronounced changes, and fluoxetine with no significant symptoms (n = 107, RCT, Michelson *et al, Br J Psychiatry* 2000;**174**: 363–8).

Citalopram: Even rapid discontinuation appears only to produce mild and transient effects (n = 225, RCT, d/b, 10/52, Markowitz *et al, Int Clin Psychopharmacol* 2000;**15**:329–33).

Escitalopram: * See citalopram. Electric shock-like sensations have been reported with escitalopram discontinuation (n = 1, Prakash and Dhar, *J Clin Psychopharmacol* 2008;**28**:359–60).

Fluoxetine: Fluoxetine has a long half-life and discontinuation problems are rare. There are reports of extreme dizziness 3–14 days after fluoxetine stopped (n = 1, Einbinder, *Am J Psychiatry* 1995;**152**:1235), of severe, dull, aching pain in the left arm after abrupt withdrawal, which remitted after reintroduction (n = 1, Lauterbach, *Neurology* 1994;**44**:983–4) and reversible delirium (Kasantikul, *J Med Assoc Thailand* 1995;**78**:53–4).

Fluvoxamine: A slow withdrawal may be preferred (Szabadi, *Br J Psychiatry* 1992;**160**:283–4).

Paroxetine: Paroxetine has been associated with more discontinuation reports than other SSRIs. A retrospective chart analysis showed that about 10% of people may get a significant discontinuation syndrome. This is more common with rapid withdrawal in people who got adverse reactions early in treatment (n = 385, Himei and Okamura, *CNS Drugs* 2006;**20**:665–72). Case reports include fever, severe fatigue, headache, nausea, vomiting and agitation and electrical, shock-like sensations (Frost and Lal, *Am J Psychiatry* 1995;**152**:180) and nocturnal enuresis (n = 1, Polimeni et al, *J Clin Psychopharmacol* 2008; **28**:589–91). It has presented as stroke (n = 2, Haddad et al, *J Psychopharmacol* 2001;**15**:139–41) and confused with dosulepin side-effects during a switch (n = 1, Haddad and Qureshi, *Acta Psychiatr Scand* 2000;**102**:466–8). This phenomenon may be more frequent because paroxetine has a short half-life and inhibits its own CYP2D6 metabolism. This dissipates much quicker than fluoxetine and sertraline (n = 45, RCT, open, Liston et al, *J Clin Psychopharmacol* 2002;**22**:169–73) and, as concentrations fall, metabolism is less inhibited and levels fall quicker, leading to a more rapid drop. Discontinuation symptoms tend to resolve in a few days or rapidly on reintroduction of paroxetine. The CSM recommends tapering if withdrawal symptoms occur, i.e. stop if problems occur then restart and taper over 12 weeks, with either half-tablet doses or alternate day (but not less frequently) therapy. However, even a four-week gradual dose reduction may not prevent significant symptoms of vertigo, light-headedness and gait instability, so care is needed (n = 5, Pacheco et al, *Br J Psychiatry* 1996;**169**:384).

Sertraline: Discontinuation reactions are relatively uncommon, e.g. fatigue, cramps, insomnia (which resolved on restarting and where tapering over 14 weeks was successful: Louie et al, *Am J Psychiatry* 1994;**151**:450–1), electrical shock-like sensations and postural hypotension (n = 1, Amsden and Georgian, *Pharmacotherapy* 1996;**16**:684–6). Abrupt sertraline 100 mg/d discontinuation has been enhanced by buspirone 15 mg/d (n = 1, Carrazana et al, *Am J Psychiatry* 2001;**158**:966–7).

Other antidepressants

Agomelatine: No discontinuation symptoms have been seen and so no tapering is required on discontinuation (MI).

Duloxetine: * The MHRA recommends that duloxetine should not be discontinued abruptly (*MHRA Drug Safety Update* 2007;1–9) and the UK SPC states that duloxetine should be tapered

over one to two weeks, reduced by a half on alternate days. Symptoms of abrupt withdrawal have been reported to occur in 44% people stopping duloxetine (cf. 23% for placebo), with dizziness (12%), nausea, headache, paraesthesia, vomiting, irritability, shock-like sensations (n = 1, Pitchot and Ansseau, *Ann Clin Psychiatry* 2008; **20**:175) and nightmares being the most common. Resolution occurs in a week in 65% (s = 6, Perahia et al, *J Affect Disord* 2005;**89**:207–12).

Mirtazapine: A withdrawal hypomania has been reported (n = 1, MacCall and Callender, *Br J Psychiatry* 1999;**175**:390; n = 1, Berigan, *Prim Care Companion J Clin Psychiatry* 2001; **3**:143).

Moclobemide: A discontinuation syndrome may present with influenza-like symptoms. Sertraline may not modify the symptoms, suggesting a different mechanism (n = 1, Curtin et al, *J Psychopharmacol* 2002;**16**:271–2).

Reboxetine: No withdrawal or discontinuation syndrome has been observed in studies with reboxetine, with few additional effects on abrupt withdrawal.

St John's wort: A withdrawal syndrome has been reported (Dean et al, *Ann Pharmacother* 2003; **37**:150).

Tryptophan: Many patients had their tryptophan stopped abruptly after it was withdrawn from the market in the UK without serious withdrawal problems, other than recurrence of depression.

Venlafaxine: * If used for more than six weeks, withdrawal over at least a week is recommended by the SPC, which describes withdrawal reactions from abrupt cessation, dose reduction or tapering of venlafaxine. These can include fatigue, nausea, vomiting, dizziness, dry mouth, diarrhoea, insomnia, nervousness, confusion, paraesthesia, sweating, vertigo, headache (e.g. n = 1, Mayr and Bonelli, *Ann Pharmacother* 2003;**37**:1145–6), electric shock-like symptoms (e.g. n = 2, Reeves et al, *Pharmacother* 2003;**23**:678–81), suicidal ideation (n = 2, Stone et al, *J Clin Psychopharmacol* 2007; **27**:94–5), delusions and psychosis (n = 1, Koga et al, *Acta Psychiatr Scand* 2009;**120**:329–31), and mania (n = 1, Fava and Mangelli, *Int J Neuropsychopharmacol* 2003;**6**:89–90). Other symptoms include abdominal distension and congested sinuses (n = 1, resolving within 12 hours of restarting, Farah and Lauer, *Am J Psychiatry* 1996;**153**:576), gastrointestinal upset (which responded to reintroduction and then slow reduction over 1–4 weeks, n = 3, Louie et al, Am J Psychiatry 1996;**153**:1652) and classic SSRI-type discontinuation symptoms (e.g. confusion, headache, agitation, abdominal distension and sweating) occurring 16 and 20 hours after stopping (n = 2, Agelink et al, Am J Psychiatry 1997;**154**:1473–4; review of similarity to SSRI symptoms, n = 13, Boyd, Med J Aus 1998;**169**:91–2). Discontinuation effects may also adversely effect driving abilities (Campagne, Med Gen Med 2005;**7**:22). An outpatient study showed that seven of the nine patients discontinuing sustained-release venlafaxine reported the emergence of adverse reactions, compared to two of the nine stopping placebo (n = 9, d/b, p/c, Fava et al, Am J Psychiatry 1997;**154**:1760–2). It may be resolved by sertraline (n = 1, Luckhaus and Jacob, Int J Neuropsychopharmacol 2001;**4**:43–4).

2.3 WEIGHT CHANGES WITH PSYCHOTROPIC DRUGS

Importance
Drug-induced weight gain is a potential threat to health, lowers self-esteem and the social embarrassment caused may lead to non-concordance (and hence risks relapse). Patients may become easily out-of-breath, have to spend money on new clothes, get embarrassed and often will not go out as a consequence.

The available data is difficult to compare due to the non-equivalence of collection and presentation. Some body weight gain is common with many psychotropic drugs and, although in most instances the gain is not 'clinically' significant (although it may be significant to the individual), the gain induced by some drugs, such as lithium and SGAs, can be clinically significant. Risk factors for weight increase have not yet been well

TABLE 2.3.1: RELATIVE WEIGHT GAIN WITH ANTIPSYCHOTICS

Drug	Long-term change †	Range (95% CI)	Change at 10/52 ‡
Perphenazine	5.8	0.4–11.1	–
Clozapine	5.7	4.3–7	4 (2.7–5.3)
Chlorpromazine	4.2	2.9–5.4	2.1 (0.9–3.4)
Olanzapine	4.2	3.7–4.6	3.5 (3.3–3.7)
Sertindole	2.9	2.7–3.2	3 (1.8–5.2)
Thioridazine	2.8	1.6–4	3.4 (1.8–5.2)
Quetiapine	2.5	<1.5–3.5	(0?)
Risperidone	1.7	1.4–2	2 (1.6–2.4)
Fluphenazine	1.1	0.1–2.2	0.4 (-0.7–1.5)
Non-drug controls	0.8	0.1–1.6	1.3 (0.8–1.8)
Polypharmacy	0.5	0.2–0.7	1.2 (0.4–2.1)
Haloperidol	0.5	0.2–0.8	0.5 (0.1–1)
Ziprasidone	0.3	-0.3–0.8	0 (-0.5–0.6)
Trifluoperazine	0.3	-0.9–1.5	–
Placebo	-1	-1.8–0.1	0.4 (-1.3–1.5)
Pimozide	-2.7	-9.3–3.9	–

(Allison et al, Am J Psychiatry 1999;**156**:1686–96, 96 refs, review by Fenton, EBMH 2000;**3**:58; n = 427, Brecher et al, In J Psychiatr Clin Pract 2000;**4**:287–91)
† longer-term weight change in kg (random effects mode)
‡ weight change at 10 weeks (fixed effects mode)
Please bear in mind that this is aggregated data, so is subject to error, weight was often measured at a different time and there may be a dose-relationship and a huge inter-individual variation.

characterised, although in general it is greatest in individuals with a past and/or family history of obesity (Ackerman and Nolan, *CNS Drugs* 1998;**9**:135–51), comorbid binge-eating, a greater number of depressive episodes, treatment with medications associated with weight gain and low exercise (Keck and McElroy, *J Clin Psychiatry* 2004;**64**:1426–35) and genetic disposition. The FDA definition of 'clinically significant' weight gain is 7% or greater increase over baseline weight.

A review of the relationship between mood disorders and obesity (McElroy et al, *J Clin Psychiatry* 2004;**65**:634–51) concludes:

- children and adolescents with MDD may be at increased risk of being overweight
- bipolars have elevated rates of overweight and obesity
- obese people seeking weight loss treatments have a greater incidence of depression
- atypical depression is more associated with weight gain than typical depression
- obesity is associated with depression in females
- most overweight people in the community do not have mood disorders.

There is, thus, an overlap between mood disorders and obesity, but it may be coincidental.

Reviews: general (Schwartz et al, *Obes Rev* 2004;**5**:115–21), treatment options (Schwartz et al, *Obes Rev* 2004;**5**:233–8), aetiology (Virks et al, *Obes Rev* 2004;**5**:167–70), mechanisms (Zimmermann et al, *J Psychiatr Res* 2003;**37**:193–220).

2.3.1 ANTIPSYCHOTICS

Table 2.3.1 provides an active comparison between drugs, but does not include all antipsychotics.

Most weight is gained during the first 12–16 weeks of therapy, although it can still continue for six months and can be maintained for at least two years, e.g. risperidone is associated with weight gain over five years, which increases over the first two years (mean 2 kg/m², range −8 to +18) then levels off to match the normal population's slight annual gain (n = 215, Neovius et al, *Acta Psychiatr Scand* 2007;**115**:277–85). A large US survey (schizophrenics n = 570, non-schizophrenic comparators n = 97 819) showed

male schizophrenics to be as obese as the general population, but female schizophrenics to be as, or more obese than the general population, suggesting that weight gain may be a problem, particularly for females taking antipsychotics (Allison et al, *J Clin Psychiatry* 1999;**60**:215–20). Initial antipsychotic response to clozapine and lower BMI has been associated with subsequent long-term weight gain as measured over eight years (n = 96 [c = 55], retrospective, Bai et al, *Am J Psychiatry* 2006;**163**:1276–9). **Asenapine** is associated with some weight gain. In short-term trials in schizophrenia 4.9% patients gained > 7% body weight (cf. 2% placebo), with a slightly lower gain in bipolar (US PI). In a 52-week study, 14.7% had > 7% increase in weight.

In a comparison of weight gain in drug-naïve first episode psychosis with haloperidol (3–9 mg/d), risperidone (3–6 mg/d) and olanzapine (5–20 mg/d), the gain was greatest at three months with olanzapine but after a year there were no significant differences (all around 10 kg), with 60% gaining excessive weight (n = 164 [c = 95], Perez-Iglesias et al, *Schizophr Res* 2007;**99**:13–22; comment by Saddichha, *EBMH* 2008;**11**:116). Risk factors for olanzapine, risperidone and clozapine weight gain include being female, younger, age increased parents' BMI, high patient's pre-morbid BMI, schizophrenia spectrum disorder diagnosis (trend) and being a non-smoker (n = 65, retrospective, Gebhardt et al, *J Psychiatry Res* 2009;**43**:620–6).

Reviews: general (Russell and Mackell, *CNS Drugs* 2001;**15**:537–51; Allison et al, *Am J Psychiatry* 1999;**156**:1686–96), comparative review (Wetterling, *Drug Safety* 2001;**24**:59–73, 93 refs), atypicals and weight gain (Nasrallah, *Psychoneuroendocrinology* 2003;**28**[Suppl 1]:S83–S96).

Management
See *Chapter 6*.

2.3.2 ANTIDEPRESSANTS

Weight change in depression is well known and weight loss or gain can be part of the presenting symptoms. Although weight gain with antidepressants may be the reversal of a pre-treatment weight loss in some people (although heavier people are more likely to gain weight if they become depressed), the main cause with tricyclics seems to be a decreased metabolic rate. There is also an association with tricyclics that have strong antihistaminic actions. Pooled data shows that more obese patients tend to lose more weight and that weight loss is directly proportional to baseline weight. Raised TNF-alpha (tumour necrosis factor) cytokinase levels are predictive of weight gain with psychotropics, but leptin is not with mirtazapine or venlafaxine (n = 20, open, Kraus et al, *Pharmacopsychiatry* 2002;**35**:220–5).

SSRIs

Overall, there is a tendency with SSRIs for weight loss over the first six weeks (increased metabolic rate, suppress appetite, and increased basal body temperature; n = 20, RCT, p/c, Bross and Hoffer, *Am J Clin Nutrition* 1995;**61**:1020–5), then gradually to regain this over six months, and then many may gain weight over the longer-term (reviewed by Sussman and Ginsberg, *Psychiatr Ann* 1998;**28**:89–97). **Fluoxetine** acute therapy is associated with modest (0.4 kg) initial weight loss over four weeks (n = 839, RCT, p/c, 12/12, Michelson et al, *Am J Psychiatry* 1999;**156**:1170–6) and in a trial of obese patients, fluoxetine 60 mg/d produced greater weight loss than placebo until 20 weeks, when this tended to wear off and the advantage of fluoxetine over placebo at 52 weeks was not clinically significant (n = 458, RCT, Goldstein et al, *Int J Obesity* 1994;**18**:129–35). A three-way clinical trial showed significant weight gain over six months with **paroxetine**, but not sertraline or fluoxetine (n = 284, RCT, 26–32/52, Fava et al, *J Clin Psychiatry* 2000;**61**:863–67). **Sertraline** may have a limited weight gain effect. No significant weight changes have been reported with **citalopram** (Milne and Goa, *Drugs* 1991;**41**:450–77), although carbohydrate craving and weight gain has been reported, particularly early on in treatment (n = 18, Bouwer and Harvey, *Int Clin Psychopharmacol* 1996;**11**:273–8). **Review:** general (Fava, *J Clin Psychiatry* 2000;**61** [Suppl 11]:37–41).

Tricyclics

Weight gain with tricyclics is well-documented

but is not as well known or appreciated as it should be. The two main causes are drug-induced carbohydrate craving (Paykel, *Br J Psychiatry* 1973; **123**:501–7) and a decreased metabolic rate (Fernstein et al, *Biol Psychiatry* 1985;**20**:688–92), rather than improved mood. Little comparative data is available, but weight gain has been reported with amitriptyline (89% of patients; see also n = 73, Christiansen et al, *Acta Psychiatr Scand* 1996;**93**:158–63) and nortriptyline (67%) in one of the few comparative studies (n = 73, RCT, 4/52, Fernstrom and Kupfer, *Psychiatr Res* 1988;**26**:256–71). It has also been reported with almost all tricyclics.

MAOIs and RIMAs

With the MAOIs, weight gain may be related to reduced blood glucose concentrations stimulating hunger or through central mechanisms. Weight gain is very rare with tranylcypromine and weight loss is more likely (n = 198, retrospective, Rabkin et al, *J Clin Psychopharmacol* 1985;**5**: 2–9). **Phenelzine** is the most widely implicated (45 reports, including 32 of over 15 lbs added). 15% of 62 patients on **moclobemide** gained weight, although overall there was a mean 0.1 kg weight loss in all patients (n = 129, RCT, 6/52 Guelfi et al, *Br J Psychiatry* 1992;**160**:519–24).

Other antidepressants

Agomelatine has no known weight gaining properties. **Venlafaxine** is usually associated with weight loss (e.g. Anon, *J Clin Psychiatry* 1993;**54**:119–26). Loss of appetite and weight has been reported in the available trials of **duloxetine**. There are only rare reports of weight changes with **trazodone** (Barnett et al, *J Clin Psychopharmacol* 1985;**5**:161–4), but not with **reboxetine**. Increased appetite and weight gain has been reported in patients treated with **mirtazapine**. One study showed increased appetite but without significant weight changes (n = 90, RCT, p/c, d/b, Claghorn and Lesem, *J Affect Disord* 1995;**34**:165–71) and another showed a slightly higher incidence than with amitriptyline (n = 150, RCT, d/b, p/c, Smith et al, *Psychopharmacol Bull* 1990;**26**:191–6). Overall, the incidence of weight gain with mirtazapine in all trials combined seems to be about 12%, with weight loss in 3% (review of mirtazapine weight-gain mechanisms; n = 14, Laimer et al, J Clin Psychiatry 2006;**67**:421–4).

Management
See *Chapter 6*.

2.3.3 MOOD STABILISERS

There is a high prevalence of obesity in bipolar patients, especially with drug treatment (44% gain > 5kg), so choose drugs unlikely to worsen this (n = 50, Fagiolini et al, J Clin Psychiatry 2002;**63**:528–33). Many risk factors are, however, involved, e.g. male gender, hypertension, arthritis (n = 644, McElroy et al, J Clin Psychiatry 2002;**63**:207–13) and drug-induced changes in food preference, especially high-energy fluids and carbohydrates, and so dietary advice is essential (n = 89, Elmslie et al, J Clin Psychiatry 2001; **62**:486–91).
Review: weight gain with mood stabilisers (Nemeroff, J Clin Psychiatry 2003;**64**:532–9).

Lithium
Weight gain, the second most common reason for non-compliance, is reported to occur in around 33% people (perhaps up to 65%, n = 70, open, Vendsborg et al, Acta Psychiatr Scand 1976;**53**:139–47), of which 25% are probably obese (review: Sachs and Guille, J Clin Psychiatry 1999;**60** [Suppl 21]:16–9). Weight increase occurs predominantly during the first two years of treatment, more often in people already overweight and may be more common in women than men. Increased thirst has been noted in 89% and strongly correlates with weight gain. Increased hunger/food intake has not been directly shown (J Psychopharmacol 1990;**4**:303) and so the predominant mechanism may be increased intake of high-calorie drinks. Thyroid status should also be assessed as a possible contributory cause. Lithium also increases insulin secretion, which may lead to more adipose tissue being produced, contributing to BMI gain. Weight gain may positively correlate with increased leptin levels (n = 15, 8/52, Atmaca et al, Neuropsychobiology 2002;**46**:67–9). Lithium-induced weight gain has been disputed by Armong (n = 42, open, Br J Psychiatry 1996;**169**:251–2) in a study that showed

no significant weight gain, even if taken with concomitant antipsychotics and antidepressants, a surprising finding. One study showed a non-significant BMI increase, with 27% actually showing a reduced BMI (n = 117, Mathew et al, Acta Psychiatr Scand 1989;**80**:538–40).

Management
See *Chapter 6*.

Carbamazepine
Studies have shown that 43% may gain some weight (n = 70, Corman et al, Can J Neurol Sci 1997;**24**:240–4) and 8% may gain over 5kg (n = 490, RCT, p/c, d/b, Mattson et al, NEJM 1992;**327**:765–71). This may be due to increased appetite, and is reversed by discontinuation but not by dieting (n = 4, Lampl et al, Clin Neuropharmacol 1991;**14**:251–5).

Valproate *
Weight gain with valproate is recognised as a common ADR and the literature says that weight gain can be marked and progressive. In a study against lamotrigine, significant weight gain (mean 12lb) occurred by week 10 and was maintained (n = 68, 32/52, Biton et al, Neurology 2001;**56**:172–7). Insulin resistance/hyperinsulinemia may be contributory, but leptin might not be involved independently (n = 81, survey, Pylvanen et al, Epilepsia 2002:**43**:514–7), although higher serum leptin and insulin levels were found in 15 patients becoming obese after one year of valproate, compared to the 25 who did not gain weight (n = 40, Verrotti et al, Neurology 1999;**53**:230–3; n = 20, RCT, 3/12, Demir and Aysun, Pediatr Neurol 2000;**22**:361–4). People who developed obesity with valproate (37%) have raised leptin, ghrelin and adiponectin, hormones involved in regulating balance between energy consumption and expenditure (n = 80, Greco et al, Neurology 2005;**65**:1808–9), and valproate has been shown to increase energy intake, particularly via fast food fat cravings (n=52, RCT, d/b, p/c, Martin et al, J Psychopharmacol 2008;**23**:814–25).

2.3.4 BENZODIAZEPINES

Weight gain has been reported with **alprazolam** (n = 17, Haney et al, Psychopharmacology 1997;

132:311–4) and **clobazam** (Ananth et al, Curr Ther Res 1979;**26**:119–26).

2.3.5 ANTICONVULSANTS

Reviews: mechanisms (Jallon and Picard, Drug Saf 2001;**24**:969–78; Biton, CNS Drugs 2003;**17**: 781–91).

Gabapentin
In a study of high-dose gabapentin, 23% patients gained more than 10% of their baseline weight, 15 gained 5–10%, 16 had no change and three lost 5–10%. Weight was gained in months 2–3 and tended to stabilise after 6–9 months, although the doses of gabapentin remained unchanged (n = 44, 12/12, DeToledo et al, Ther Drug Monit 1997;**19**:394–6). A mean weight gain of 6.9 kg (range 3.2–14.5 kg) has been noted (n = 11, open, Gidal et al, Ann Pharmacother 1995;**29**:1048).

Lamotrigine
In a study against valproate, weight gain with lamotrigine was low (1.3 +/- 11 lb) at week 10 (n = 68, 32/52, Biton et al, Neurology 2001; **56**:172–7), with no change from baseline in other studies (e.g. n = 122, open, < 5 years, Morrell et al, Epilepsy Res 2003;**54**:189–99; n = 38, RCT, d/b, 32/52, Biton et al, J Child Neurol 2003;**18**:133–9), and in another study, no effect on body weight when given as monotherapy or adjunctive in bipolar 1 (n = 1175 [c = 1139], open, 12/52, Zarzar et al, MedGenMed 2007;**9**:41).

Levetiracetam
Levetiracetam at normal doses is weight neutral (s = 4, n = 970, RCT, p/c, Gidal et al, Epilepsy Res 2003;**56**:121–6), but four cases of considerable weight loss (2.3–7 kg/month) have been reported (Hadjikoutis et al, Br Med J 2003;**327**:905) and weight gain is mentioned in the UK SPC.

Topiramate
Topiramate has been reported to produce weight loss, e.g. a dose-related weight loss occurred in 50% patients in a trial in bipolar disorder, with a mean 14.2 lb weight loss (n = 76, open, Ghaemi et al, Ann Clin Psychiatry 2001;**13**:185–9) and, compared to lithium and valproate, it produced an average of 1.2 kg weight loss (n = 214, open, chart, Chengappa et

al, Clin Ther 2002;**24**:1576–84). It has even been abused to try to promote weight loss (n = 1, Colom et al, J Clin Psychiatry 2001;**62**:475–6). The effect appears dose-related, with average amounts lost ranging from 1.1 kg/1.5% (up to 200 mg/d) to 5.9 kg/7% (800 mg/d or above). The effect peaks at 12–15 months, is greater in people with higher starting weights and is at least partially reversible (MI). Topiramate (mean 135 mg/d) may produce a modest loss in SSRI-induced weight gain (n = 15, open, 10/52, Van Ameringen et al, J Clin Psychiatry 2002;**63**:981–4), although it obviously has its own side-effects.

Other anticonvulsants *
Weight gain has been reported as a side-effect of **oxcarbazepine** and **pregabalin**, although reduced appetite and weight loss have been reported with (UK SPC). Adjunctive **tiagabine** may have no significant effect on body weight (n = 349, Hogan et al, Epilepsy Res 2000;**41**:23–8). About 35% people on zonisamide lose weight (> 5%) and about 14% gain weight (> 5%), which appears to be reversible on discontinuation (n = 157, Wellmer et al, Acta Neurol Scand 2009;**119**:233–8). Weight gain may occur in 5–40% patients prescribed **vigabatrin** long-term.

2.3.6 OTHER DRUGS *

No significant weight changes have been seen in clinical trials with **acamprosate**. A retrospective study showed weight loss with **methylphenidate** to occur more with heavier children and recommended that BMI percentile curves are used as the best measure of weight changes (study and review, Schertz et al, Pediatrics 1996; **98**:763–9). A mean body weight loss of 0.5 kg occurred with **atomoxetine** in 6–12-week studies with some normalisation over the longer-term (UK SPC). Weight loss may occur with **bupropion**, with 28% treated losing greater than 5 lb, but weight gain occurred in 9% patients (MI). Modest weight losses have been seen with long-term bupropion SR (n = 423, p/c, one year, Croft et al, Clin Ther 2002;**24**:662–72). Weight loss averaged 3.4 kg (maximum 31 kg) in people taking **oxybate** for narcolepsy (n = 54, two years, Husain et al, Sleep Med 2008;**10**:661–3).

3 PSYCHOTROPICS IN PROBLEM AREAS

3.1 BREAST-FEEDING

	LOWER RISK	MODERATE RISK	HIGHER RISK
Antipsychotics	Quetiapine[2] Sulpiride[5] Zuclopenthixol[4]	Amisulpride[5] Flupentixol[4] Haloperidol[6] Phenothiazines (LD)[7]	Aripiprazole[2] Asenapine[2] Clozapine[3] Olanzapine[2] Paliperidone[1] Pimozide[8] Phenothiazines HD[7] Risperidone[1] Ziprasidone[2] Zotepine[2]
Antidepressants	Flupentixol LD[4] Moclobemide[16] Tricyclics[12] (most) Tryptophan[16]	Agomelatine[11] Mianserin[16] Mirtazapine[11] SSRIs[9] St John's wort[16] Trazodone[13]	Doxepin?[12] Duloxetine[10] MAOIs[15] Reboxetine[14] Venlafaxine[10]
Anxiolytics and hypnotics	Benzodiazepines LD[17] Beta-blockers LD[20] Chloral[21] Temazepam LD[17] Zolpidem[19]	Benzodiazepines HD[17] Clomethiazole[21]	Buspirone[18] Hydroxyzine[18] Melatonin[21] Ramelteon[21] Zaleplon[19] Zopiclone[19]
Anticonvulsants	Carbamazepine[22] Phenytoin[24] Valproate[23]	Acetazolamide[28] Benzodiazepines[17] Gabapentin[26] Vigabatrin[27]	Ethosuximide[28] Lacosamide[27] Lamotrigine?[26] Levetiracetam[27] Oxcarbazepine[22] Phenobarbital[25] Pregabalin[27] Rufinamide[27] Tiagabine[27] Topiramate[27] Zonisamide[27]
Others	Methadone[35]	Anticholinergics[30] Atomoxetine[34] Buprenorphine[35] Disulfiram[31] Methylphenidate[34] Sodium oxybate[33]	Acamprosate[31] Anticholinesterases[29] Bupropion[36] Lithium?[32] Memantine[29] Modafinil[33]

GENERAL PRINCIPLES FOR MEDICATION IN BREAST FEEDING

1. All psychotropics pass into milk, so no decision is risk-free. Milk levels are usually around 1% of maternal plasma levels, but there have been few formal studies.

2. Breast milk is more acidic than plasma, so basic compounds may be retained and concentrations accumulate. Protein binding may also be a factor (in general, drug binding to milk proteins is less than to plasma proteins). The higher lipid content of the hind milk (second half of feed) makes it likely to have a higher drug concentration than the first half (fore milk).

3. Drugs should be avoided if the infant is pre-mature, or has renal, hepatic, cardiac or neurological impairment. Neonates (and particularly premature infants) are at greater risk from exposure to drugs via breast milk, because of an immature excretory function and the consequent risk of drug accumulation.

4. Avoid sedating drugs and those with long half-lives. Avoid drugs known to cause serious toxicity in adults or children. Drugs licensed for use in infants do not generally pose a hazard. It is best to avoid long-acting preparations, especially those of drugs likely to cause serious side-effects (eg. antipsychotic agents), as it is difficult to time feeds to avoid significant amounts of drug in breast milk. Avoid new drugs if a therapeutically equivalent alternative is available that has been more widely used.

5. Choose a regimen and route of administration which presents the minimum amount of drug to the infant. Since nearly all psychotropics can be given as a once-daily dose, this should be implemented as a single daily dose just before the infant's longest sleep period feed (eg. peak milk concentrations after oral administration: amitriptyline 1.5 hours, sertraline 8–9 hours), minimising actual concentration and maximising clearance before the next feed.

6. If a mother was taking a drug during pregnancy, it will not usually be necessary to switch drugs during breast-feeding, as the amount to which the infant is exposed will be less than that *in utero*.

7. Adverse effects will often be dose-related, so use the minimum effective maternal dose.

8. Polypharmacy may lead to enhanced adverse effects in the infant. Avoiding interacting drugs that raise plasma levels (even if asymptomatically) is essential. Multiple drug regimens may pose an increased risk, especially when adverse effects such as drowsiness are additive.

9. Drug effects on the development of the infant's brain are not clear and so monitor biochemical and behavioural parameters, especially if the infant shows signs of possible psychotropic side-effects (eg. sedation, tremulousness, colic) and take appropriate action, eg. dose reduction, drug change, etc.

10. Avoid unnecessary drug use and limit the use of over-the-counter (OTC) products.

A robust assessment of the balance of benefit to risk for a mother–child pair requires data both on the drug's passage into breast milk and its effects in infants: there is rarely enough information available about new drugs to allow such an assessment to be made.

Reviews: * mood stabilisers in breast-feeding (Gentile, *Bipolar Disord* 2006;**8**:207–20), bipolar disorder treatments in puerperium (Dodd and Berk, *Curr Drug Saf* 2006;**1**:25–33), practical recommendations for treating mood disorders during lactation (Eberhard-Gran et al, *CNS Drugs* 2006;**20**:187–98).

3.1.1 ANTIPSYCHOTICS

Review: * general (which concludes there is little difference between the available antipsychotics, and safety is not proven so chose the best one, except for avoiding clozapine and olanzapine; Gentile, *J Clin Psychiatry* 2008;**69**:666–73).

1. The UK SPCs for **risperidone** and **paliperidone** state that women should not breast-feed. In two cases the milk:plasma ratio for risperidone was <0.5 with a relative infant dose lower than the 10% level of concern (n = 2, Ilett et al, *Ann Pharmacother* 2004;**38**:273–6) and in another milk levels were 10 times higher than in the maternal serum but no adverse effects were seen in the infant and development was normal (n = 1, Aichhorn et al, *J Psychopharmacol* 2005;**19**:211–3; see also Hill et al, *J Clin Psychopharmacol* 2000;**20**:285–6).

2. * There is one reported human case, where **aripiprazole** milk levels were about 20% of maternal levels (15 mg/d producing 14 ng/ml in milk) giving a relatively low potential level to the infant (n=1, Schlotterbeck et al, *Int J Neuropsychopharmacol* 2007;**10**:433). It is excreted into rat milk. **Asenapine** is excreted in milk in animal

studies but until human data is available it should be used only with great caution in breastfeeding (US PI). **Olanzapine** is excreted in breast milk, with infants exposed to about 1% of a maternal dose of olanzapine (below the 10% nominal level of concern), with few adverse effects (n = 7, Gardiner et al, Am J Psychiatry 2003;**160**:1428–31; see also n = 3, Goldstein et al, J Clin Psychopharmacol 2000;**20**:399–403; n = 5, Croke et al, Int J Neuropsychopharmacol 2002;**5**:243–7; n = 1, Ambresin et al, J Clin Psychopharmacol 2004;**24**:93–5). However, in a breast-fed infant whose mum was taking olanzapine, plasma levels at four months were relatively high but declined to undetectable over the next four months, probably due to maturing of the hepatic systems (n = 1, Whitworth et al, J Psychopharmacol 2008;**22**:923–4) but even at 15 mg/d levels can be undetectable in the infant aged 5/12 (n = 1, Lutz et al, Ther Drug Monit 2008; **30**:399–401). Thus, the UK SPC recommends not breast-feeding while taking olanzapine. For **quetiapine**, there are several reports suggesting a low risk. A case series showed undetectable levels in milk, with low or undetectable levels in the infant's serum, the authors concluding that quetiapine posed only a low-level risk (n = 6, Misri et al, J Clin Psychopharmacol 2006;**26**:508–11). In another, milk levels at an oral dose of 200 mg/d were at a maximum of 0.43% of the weight-adjusted maternal dose and fell to pre-dose levels within two hours, appearing to be too small for significant pharmacological effects (n = 1, Lee et al, Am J Psychiatry 2004;**161**:1715–6) and an infant's plasma concentration was 6% of the mother's serum level and was exposed to less than 0.1% of the maternal dose, supporting the use of quetiapine following an appropriate risk:benefit analysis (n = 1, Rampono et al, Ann Pharmacother 2007;**41**:711–4). **Zotepine** and norzotepine may be secreted into breast milk (where milk levels can reach 50% of maternal plasma levels) and is incompatible with breast-feeding mothers. There is little data on **ziprasidone** apart from a case report (n = 1, Schlotterbeck et al, Int J Neuropharmacol 2009;**12**:437–8).

3. **Clozapine** is contraindicated as animal studies suggest it is excreted into milk and so it risks agranulocytosis in the infant. In the close study of one mother, there was some accumulation of clozapine in breast milk (possibly due to higher lipid concentrations), and so doses must be kept low (Barnas, Am J Psychiatry 1994;**151**:945) and the infant's plasma monitored if breast-feeding is essential. There are reports indicating that infants experience sedation if mothers take clozapine and breast-feed.

4.* A study showed that 0.6 mcg/kg or 1–2% of the maternal **flupentixol** dose might reach the infant and thus is probably safe at low dose, e.g. <2 mg/d (n = 6, Matheson and Skjaeraasen, Eur J Clin Pharmacol 1988;**35**:217–20). The **zuclopenthixol** UK SPC (updated 2008) states that breast-feeding can be continued during treatment as less than 1% of the weight-related maternal dose (in mg/kg) reaches the infant but observe the infant (especially during the first four weeks) for adverse effects.

5.* A mother taking **sulpiride** 100 mg/d is likely to give the child less than 1 mg/d. No adverse effects have been reported at higher doses (n = 28, p/c, d/b, 4/52, Ylikorkala et al, Br Med J 1982;**285**:249–51) but it is not recommended (UK SPC). There is no information for **amisulpride**.

6. **Haloperidol** is excreted into breast milk but levels are probably low, although infant levels may be the same as adults. Some element of delayed development has been detected (n = 5, Yoshida et al, Psychol Med 1998;**28**:81–91) and so the infant must be monitored carefully.

7. High doses of **phenothiazines** can produce drowsiness in the infant. **Chlorpromazine** has an inconsistent milk/plasma ratio, and drowsiness and lethargy are possible but not inevitable. With careful monitoring it should be safe, although some element of delayed development has been suggested (n = 3, Yoshida et al, Psychol Med 1998;**28**:81–91). In one case report the amount of **perphenazine** passed to an infant was about 0.1% of the adult dose in terms of mcg/kg body weight (Olesen et al, Am J Psychiatry 1990;**10**:1378–9), and this drug may become 'trapped' in milk due to its physiochemical properties.

8. **Pimozide** may be excreted into breast milk and use is not recommended (SPC).

3.1.2 ANTIDEPRESSANTS

Breast-feeding has many benefits, and the amount of antidepressant in milk varies according to the drug and what part of the milk is assayed, but maternal use at normal doses does not usually lead to substantial levels in the neonate, although they should be monitored for feeding difficulties, weight gain, and sleep or state changes (review by Yonkers, *Am J Psychiatry* 2007;**164**:1457–9), and infants have significantly lower weight if the mother has a depression lasting longer than two months (n = 78, naturalistic, 18/12, Hendrick *et al*, *J Clin Psychiatry* 2003;**64**:410–2), so there is a risk of **not** treating depression. In a review wittily entitled a 'pooled analysis of antidepressant levels in… breast milk' the conclusion was that fluoxetine produces the highest proportion (22%) of infant levels above 10% of the average maternal level, citalopram next at 17%, and that nortriptyline, paroxetine and sertraline may be the preferred choices, with citalopram relatively safe if doses are minimised (s = 67, Weissman *et al*, *Am J Psychiatry* 2004;**161**:1066–78).

Reviews: * extensive (s = 31, Lanza di Scalea and Wisner, *Clin Obstet Gynaecol* 2009;**52**:483–97).

9. Treatment with the **SSRIs** seems to be compatible with breast-feeding, although fluoxetine should probably best be avoided during lactation, unless also used during pregnancy.

Citalopram, escitalopram and **demethyl-citalopram** are excreted into milk. In one study, the mean combined dose (4.4–5.1% as citalopram equivalents) transmitted to infants was below the 10% notional level of concern, and infant levels appear low or undetectable (n = 11, Heikkinen *et al*, *Clin Pharmacol Ther* 2002:**72**:184–91). Another showed infant plasma concentrations to be very low or absent, with no adverse effects (n = 7, Rampono *et al*, *Br J Clin Pharmacol* 2000;**50**:263–8) and a prospective, observational, cohort study was unable to show any significant clinical events in mothers who took citalopram and breast-fed (n = 43, Lee *et al*, *Clin Pharmacol Ther* 2002;**71**:43). In eight women taking **escitalopram** 10 mg/d, the total dose reaching the infants was about 5% with no apparent adverse effects, and in the infants tested (n = 5), plasma levels were mostly below that detectable (Rampono *et al*, *Br J Clin Pharmacol* 2006;**62**:316–22). These data support the safety of the use of **citalopram** in breast-feeding women, provided doses are optimised.

Fluoxetine (s = 11, n = 190, Burt *et al*, *Am J Psychiatry* 2001;**158**:1001–9) plasma levels in the infant may range from undetectable to 340 ng/ml, but with no clear associations between maternal dose, age and plasma levels, so there is clearly some significant interpatient variability and adverse effects have been observed in breast-fed infants, e.g. colic. Plasma levels peak in breast milk at about eight hours post-dose and are dose-related, with 20 mg/d or less producing low infant serum levels (n = 19, Hendrick *et al*, *Biol Psychiatry* 2001;**15**:775–82), and probably less than 10% of the adult therapeutic dose of fluoxetine reaches the infant, below the notional level of concern (Nulman and Koren, *Teratology* 1996;**53**:304–8; careful study, n = 10 pairs, Suri *et al*, *Biol Psychiatry* 2002;**52**:446–51), with no developmental effects likely (n = 4, Yoshida *et al*, *Br J Psychiatry* 1998;**172**:175–9). Mean estimated infant exposures are 2.4–3.8% of the maternal plasma level (n = 11 + 10 controls, Heikkinen *et al*, *Clin Pharmacol Ther* 2003;**73**:330–7). Considering the potential for accumulation, careful monitoring of the infants is mandatory, especially in neonates exposed to these drugs *in utero* (n = 14, Kristensen *et al*, *Br J Clin Pharmacol* 1999;**48**:521–7).

Fluvoxamine levels in milk and infant plasma appear low in the few reported cases. The estimated daily intake by an infant is probably about 0.5% of the maternal dose (100 or 200 mg/d), it is thought to be of little risk, with no concerns about development up to 21 months (e.g. n = 2, Kristensen *et al*, *J Hum Lact* 2002;**18**:139–43; n = 1, Hägg *et al*, *Br J Clin Pharmacol* 2000;**49**:286–8).

Paroxetine has been well studied and maternal doses of 10–50 mg/d are found in milk, but at highly variable levels (sample n = 108, range 2–101 ng/ml). In 25 mother–infant sample sets, paroxetine was detected in all but one milk sample, but undetectable (i.e. < 0.1 ng/ml) in the infant's serum, with no adverse events reported (n = 24, Misri *et al*, *J Clin Psychiatry* 2000;**61**:828–32; n = 6, open, Ohman *et al*, *J Clin Psychiatry* 1999;**60**:519–23). Hindmilk concentrations may be 78% higher than foremilk (n = 16, Stowe *et al*, *Am J Psychiatry* 2000;**257**:185–9).

Sertraline and metabolite generally appear only at low levels in the infant (probably less than 2% of the maternal dose per day; n = 10, Dodd *et al*, *Hum Psychopharmacol* 2000;**15**:161–4), unlikely to cause any significant adverse effects (n = 8, Kristensen *et al*, *Br J Clin Pharmacol* 1998;**45**:453–7). Peak sertraline levels occur in milk at around 8–9 hours after the last dose, and discarding this peak reduces the infant's intake by 18% (n=26, 186 samples, Stowe et al, J Clin Psychiatry 2003;**64**:73–80). Higher levels have been reported rarely (Wisner et al, Am J Psychiatry 1998;**155**:690–2), as have rare withdrawal reactions in breast-fed children after the mother has abruptly stopped sertraline (Kent and Laidlaw, Br J Psychiatry 1995;**167**:412–3), implying that sertraline may appear in breast milk at levels sufficient to suppress withdrawal after birth, especially at higher doses, e.g. 200 mg/d (e.g. n = 12, Stowe et al, Am J Psychiatry 1997;**154**:1255–60).

10. * **Venlafaxine** levels peak at eight hours, with infant venlafaxine/desvenlafaxine plasma levels 37% of the maternal plasma levels, and highly variable but in excess of the notional 10% safety level (n = 13, Newport et al, J Clin Psychiatry 2009;**70**:1304–10). Previous studies suggested infant intake is lower (around 6.4%) than the 10% notional level of concern (n = 6 mothers, seven infants, Ilett et al, Br J Clin Pharmacol 2002;**53**:17–22), but there may be enough in milk to attenuate withdrawal symptoms (Koren et al, J Obstet Gynaecol Can 2006;**28**:299–302). Venlafaxine may be metabolised by infants, with no detectable adverse effects or apparent developmental issues (n = 2, Hendrick et al, Am J Psychiatry 2001;**158**:2089–90). **Duloxetine** is excreted into breast milk in animal studies but no human data is available so it is not recommended at the moment.

11.* In a careful study of breast-feeding mothers, a maximum of 1.5% of the adult **mirtazapine** dose (median 38 mg/d) reached the infants and of the four infants tested, only one had detectable plasma levels, well below the notional level of concern (n = 8, Kristensen et al, Br J Clin Pharmacol 2006;**6 3**:322–7). However, much higher levels have been reported, with one case where the infant had plasma levels approaching the adult range, with the authors suggesting close monitoring (n = 1, Toon et al, J Clin Psychopharmacol 2009;**29**:191–2). Hindmilk levels are slightly higher than foremilk (n = 1, Klier et al, Am J Psychiatry 2007;**164**:348–9). There is no data on **agomelatine** in breast milk, although it is excreted into rat milk, so should not be used in lactating mothers until more information is available (MI).

12. **Tricyclic antidepressants** should be used with care, but it does not seem warranted that breast-feeding should be discontinued completely (except for doxepin), as for tricyclics only about 1% of the maternal dose reaches the infant, with only minute amounts in the infant serum, no acute toxic effects and no evidence of developmental delay (n = 10, Yoshida et al, J Affect Disord 1997;**43**:225–37). For **imipramine**, a milk/plasma ratio of 0.05–0.08, based on high dose samples, would lead to 0.1% of the maternal daily dose appearing in milk. **Amitriptyline**/nortriptyline levels in the infant are probably very low (Breyer-Pfaff, Am J Psychiatry 1995;**152**:812–3). Two studies showed no detectable **nortriptyline** in the infant serum, despite some unusually high maternal plasma levels, although two infants had detectable levels of 10–hydroxy metabolites. None of the infants showed any adverse effects and so the risk could be considered very low (n = 12, Wisner and Perel, Am J Psychiatry 1996; **153**:295). Sertraline and nortriptyline were of equivalent efficacy in postpartum depression, with very low or undetectable levels in infant serum (n = 109 [c = 95], RCT, d/b, 8/52, Wisner et al, J Clin Psychopharmacol 2006;**26**:453–60). In two studies of a five-year follow-up of children who had received dothiepin/**dosulepin** via breast milk, no detectable adverse effects on cognitive development were detectable (compared to a variety of controls, n = 66 controls, Buist and Janson, Br J Psychiatry 1995;**167**:370–3), and the drug is unlikely to be a significant hazard for the infant (n = 5, Ilett et al, Br J Clin Pharmacol 1992;**33**:635–9). Case reports suggest that the infant may receive only up to 3.7% of the mother's **clomipramine** dose (n = 1, Pons et al, Clin Pharmacokinetics 1994;**27**:270–89), with no adverse effects (n = 4, Wisner et al, J Clin Psychiatry 1995;**56**:17–20). **Doxepin** has a longer-acting metabolite N-desmethyldoxepin, which may accumulate in breast-fed infants, causing severe drowsiness and near fatal respiratory depression (n = 1, Matheson et al, Lancet 1985;ii:1124;n = 1, Frey et al, Ann Pharmacother 1999;**33**:690–3). However, other reports failed to detect any effects in the infant with maternal doxepin doses of 150 mg/d (e.g. Kemp et al, Br J Clin Pharmacol 1995;**20**:497–9; Wisner et al, Am J Psychiatry 1996;**153**:1132) and so metabolic differences could explain these.

The general recommendation is to observe the child carefully for sedation and respiratory depression. A tricyclic with a short half-life for itself (and any active metabolites) would appear to be the best option. It has been recommended that amitriptyline and imipramine are the preferred tricyclics.

13. With **trazodone**, a 50mg single-dose study showed that 1% passed into the milk (n = 6, Verbeck et al, Br J Clin Pharmacol 1986;**22**:367–70). More information on, e.g. metabolites is needed, but it would appear to be of low risk. Drowsiness and poor feeding have been reported (n = 1, Yapp et al, Ann Pharmacother 2000;**34**:1269–72; n = 2, Dodd et al, Clin Psychopharmacol 2000;**20**:717–8). Caution is thus advised.

14. * Although **reboxetine** is excreted in breast milk, the amount excreted is low and so it is no longer contraindicated (SPC).

15. Minimal data is available for the **MAOIs**. **Tranylcypromine** is excreted in breast milk but levels are not thought to be significant. Some sources state that MAOI levels in milk are too small to affect the child, but this has not been supported by any studies other than with tranylcypromine.

16. In six lactating women, 0.06% of a single dose of **moclobemide** was excreted unchanged in the milk. It would seem unlikely this amount would produce adverse effects in the baby (Pons et al, Br J Clin Pharmacol 1990;**29**:27–31). **Mianserin** 40–60mg/d may produce only low milk and infant plasma levels with no untoward effects (Buist et al, Br J Clin Pharmacol 1993;**36**:133–4). In a prospective study, there were no significant problems in infants whose mothers took St John's wort while breast-feeding; there was no decrease in milk production or infant weight over the first year (n = 33 + 134 controls, Lee et al, J Clin Psychiatry 2003;**64**:966–8), and in a thorough study, hyperforin was only detected at low levels in milk, with infant exposure 0.9–2.5% of the maternal dose, comparable with other psychotropics and it thus appears relatively safe (n = 5, Klier et al, J Clin Psychiatry 2006;**67**:305–9). However, if possible, it should probably be avoided in breast-feeding (review by Dugoua et al, Can J Clin Pharmacol 2006;**13**:268–76). There are no known problems with **tryptophan**.

3.1.3 ANXIOLYTICS AND HYPNOTICS

17. Since **benzodiazepines** are excreted in breast milk, they should probably not be given to lactating mothers. Repeated doses of long-acting benzodiazepines can produce lethargy and weight loss but low and single doses are probably of low risk, provided the infant is monitored for drowsiness. Oxazepam seems to be preferable to diazepam in lactating women but, as with all anxiolytic benzodiazepines, infants should be observed for signs of sedation and poor suckling. **Diazepam, oxazepam, lorazepam, lormetazepam, nitrazepam** and **flunitrazepam** have all been shown in breast milk. Infant **temazepam** levels have been reported to be below detection levels at maternal doses of 10–20mg/d and no adverse effects have been seen (Lebedevs et al, Br J Clin Pharmacol 1992;**33**:204–6). Very little **midazolam** appears to reach breast milk (n = 5, Nitsun et al, Clin Pharmacol Ther 2006;**79**:549–57).

18. **Buspirone** should be avoided, based on excretion studies in rats, although there is no specific human data to show adverse effects. It is not known if **hydroxyzine** is excreted in human milk (UK SPC), so its use is not recommended.

19. **Zaleplon** is excreted in breast milk and should not be administered to breast-feeding mothers, although the actual amount likely to be transferred may be very low, e.g. 0.017% of the maternal dose (n = 5, Darwish et al, J Clin Pharmacol 1999;**39**:670–4). **Zopiclone** is contra-indicated in breast-feeding as it is excreted in appreciable amounts (up to 50% of maternal levels: n = 12, Matheson et al, Br J Clin Pharmacol 1990;**30**:267–71). Single occasional doses of 7.5mg are probably of low risk as accumulation is unlikely. The AAPCD considers **zolpidem** compatible with breast-feeding, as it is found only in minute amounts in milk due to its low lipophilic properties and rapid onset and excretion. In one study of women taking a (high) stat dose of 20mg, 3.8–19% of zolpidem was excreted into breast milk, nearly all within three hours of the dose, so 5–10mg should be relatively low risk (n = 5, Pons et al, Eur J Clin Pharmacol 1989;**37**:245–8). A low dose at bedtime and avoiding breast-feeding for the next 2–3 hours would minimise the potential effect on an infant.

20. For **beta-blockers**, the amounts excreted into breast milk are probably too small to affect the baby (<0.1% of maternal doses), but could produce bradycardia and hypoglycaemia in high doses.

21. **Clomethiazole** is excreted in insignificant amounts, based on IV and oral studies in pre-eclampsia (Acta Psychiatr Scand 1986;**73**[Suppl

329]:185–8). An infant might ingest active amounts and, although the sedative effects of this could be relevant, they are unlikely to be harmful. **Chloral hydrate** is excreted in breast milk and the sedation caused in the infant makes this a precaution, although only minimal sedation after large feeds has been reported (*Adv Drug React Bull* 1976;Dec:212). The American Academy of Pediatrics recommends that chloral can safely be used in lactating mothers, as do the authorities in many European countries. **Melatonin** is probably secreted into human breast milk and so use in lactating mothers is not recommended (SPC). **Ramelteon** is excreted into milk in animal studies but human data is not available yet.

3.1.4 ANTICONVULSANTS

Breast-feeding should be encouraged as bonding is especially important in epileptic mothers (Brodie, *Lancet* 1990;**336**:426–7). An extensive review (Hägg and Spigset, *Drug Safety* 2000; **22**:425–40, 88 refs) concluded:

- that carbamazepine, valproate and phenytoin are compatible with breast-feeding
- that ethosuximide, phenobarbital and primidone should be regarded as potentially unsafe and close clinical monitoring of the infant is recommended
- that data on the newer drugs is too sparse for reliable recommendations
- that occasional or short-term treatment with benzodiazepines could be considered compatible with breast-feeding, although maternal diazepam treatment has caused sedation in suckling infants after short-term use. During long-term use of benzodiazepines, infants should be observed for signs of sedation and poor suckling.

Reviews: * general (Sabers and Tomson, *Curr Opin Neurol* 2009;**22**:157–61, Pennell, *Neurology* 2003;**61** (Suppl 2):S35–42).

22. **Carbamazepine** has been classed by the AAPCD as compatible with breast-feeding, as levels have been found to be relatively low. This is, however, based only on case reports in epilepsy, with few reports when used as a mood stabiliser. The half-life is longer in infants, with levels in milk ranging from 7–95% of the mother's serum, but probably usually around 10%. There are cases of adverse effects in the infant (n = 1, Merlob et al,

Ann Pharmacother 1992;**26**:1563–5; n = 1, Frey et al, *Eur J Pediatr* 1990;**150**:136–8) and several of poor feeding. The mother should be informed of the potential signs of hepatic dysfunction and CNS effects (review, Chaudron and Jefferson, *J Clin Psychiatry* 2000;**161**:79–90). **Oxcarbazepine** is excreted into breast milk, the breast milk/plasma ratio for drug and metabolite being about 0.5, similar to carbamazepine (n = 1, Bulla et al, *Eur J Clin Pharmacol* 1988;**34**:311–3), and it is currently contraindicated.

23. **Valproate** has been classified by the AAPCD as compatible with breast-feeding, based on case reports in epilepsy. Infant serum levels usually range from 5–12% but can range from undetectable to 40% of the mother's serum level (n = 16, van Unruh et al, *Ther Drug Monit* 1984;**6**:272–6). In six mother–infant pairs, where infant exposure was exclusively during breast-feeding, mothers had valproate levels in the usual range for bipolar (39–79 mcg/mL) but the infants had low levels (0.7–1.5 mcg/mL), thus presenting a relatively low risk compared to the risk of relapse in the mother (n = 6, Piontek et al, *J Clin Psychiatry* 2000;**61**:170–2). Valproate thus appears relatively safe, although with the small but finite risk of haematological effects (Stahl et al, *J Pediatr* 1997;**130**:1001–3). Care and careful counselling is needed for higher doses (review, Chaudron and Jefferson, *J Clin Psychiatry* 2000;**161**:79–90).

24. Small quantities of **phenytoin** are excreted in breast milk, peaking at three hours, and have been considered clinically safe (*Adv Drug React Ac Pois Rev* 1982;**1**:255–87).

25. Larger doses of **phenobarbital** and **primidone** may accumulate in breast milk and cause unacceptable drowsiness.

26.* Extensive passage of **lamotrigine** into breast milk occurs, with slow elimination by the newborn. Lamotrigine is metabolised by glucuronidation, which is immature in neonates and may lead to accumulation, with concentrations in the infant. Infant plasma levels reported include 18% (peak four hours after the maternal dose; n = 30, Newport et al, *Pediatrics* 2008;**122**:223–31), 23–33% (milk to maternal serum ratio a consistent 0.6; n = 3, Ohman et al, *Epilepsia* 1998;**39** [Suppl 2]:21; review, Chaudron and Jefferson, *J Clin Psychiatry* 2000;**161**:79–90) and 30% (range 20–43%; n = 4, Liporace et al, *Epilepsy Behav* 2004;**5**:102–5), but with huge interindividual variations.

Gabapentin crosses into breast milk but appears of lower risk. In six mother–baby pairs, gabapentin levels were estimated to be 12% of the mother's plasma level, but with no adverse effects detected (n = 6, Ohman et al, *Epilepsia* 2005;**46**:1621–4) and in a single mother–infant pair, infant plasma level was 0.4mg/L (6% of maternal plasma level) and absolute dose 3% of children's dose (n = 1, Kristensen et al, *J Hum Lact* 2006;**22**:426–8).

27.* It is not known if **lacosamide** is excreted in breast milk (SPC). Animal studies indicate **levetiracetam** is excreted into breast milk and, since unusually high levels can occur (Pennell, *Neurology* 2003;**61**[6 Suppl 2]:S35–S42), breast-feeding is not recommended. **Pregabalin** is excreted into milk in animal studies but no human data exists, so is not recommended (SPC). No information is available for **rufinamide** (UK SPC). **Topiramate** and **tiagabine** are not recommended as no human information is currently available, although there is one healthy outcome with topiramate (n = 1, Gentile, *Clin Drug Investig* 2009;**29**:139–41). A small study suggested that the quantity of **vigabatrin** ingested through milk is small, at around 1–3% of the daily dose (n = 2, Tran et al, *Br J Clin Pharmacol* 1998;**45**:409–11). **Zonisamide** appears in breast milk, 41–57% being transferred, with a half-life in the two infants of 61–107 hours respectively (n = 2, Kawada et al, *Brain Dev* 2002;**24**:95–7), similar to the mother's plasma level. The UK SPC recommends avoiding breast-feeding during therapy and for a month afterwards.

28. **Ethosuximide** is excreted in breast milk, with detectable infant levels and should not be used.

3.1.5 OTHERS

29. There is no information available on **donepezil**, **galantamine** and **rivastigmine**, so should not be used in breast-feeding mothers. Human data is lacking but **memantine** is lipophilic and so is probably excreted into breast milk.

30.* There is no data for **anticholinergics** but the UK SPC for **orphenadrine** notes that as there is no information available, mothers should not breast feed.

31. No information is available to date on **disulfiram** in breast milk and so use must be with great caution. There is the possibility of interactions with alcohol in paediatric medicines (see *4.7.1*). **Acamprosate** is excreted in the milk of lactating animals and so the literature states that use in breast-feeding is a contraindication. No human data is available.

32. **Lithium** has been classified by the AAPCD as contraindicated in breast-feeding since 1989 but this is based on limited information. A recent systematic study, however, has shown relatively low milk and lower infant plasma levels with no serious or persistent adverse events noted, the authors suggesting that there is a need to reassess this widespread contraindication, provided careful monitoring is carried out (n = 10 mother-infant pairs, Viguera et al, *Am J Psychiatry* 2007;**164**:342–5). Breast milk levels may be approximately 40% (range 24–72%), with infant serum having levels 5–200% of the mother's serum concentrations and there have been case reports of adverse events (e.g. hypotonia and lethargy, possibly due to reduced renal clearance), although many of these may have been multifactorial. There is wide interindividual variability of the dose reaching an infant, and so informed choice, with careful monitoring (e.g. TDM of milk or infant plasma), considering poorer renal excretion and fluid balance/electrolytes and use of low doses, may help if the risk of bipolar relapse is high if stopping lithium (Moretti et al, *Ther Drug Monit* 2003;**25**:364–6).

Review: Chaudron Jefferson, *J Clin Psychiatry* 2000; **161**:79–90.

33. **Modafinil** is contraindicated in breast-feeding. **Sodium oxybate** is not recommended but there is no human data available (SPC).

34. In one report, no **methylphenidate** was detectable in breast milk 20–21 hours after the last dose of a plain tablet (probably because methylphenidate's short half-life of 2–3 hours), so breast-feeding before a morning dose should have a low risk (n = 1, Spigset et al, *Am J Psychiatry* 2007;**164**:348). The UK SPC recommends caution for **atomoxetine**.

35.* **Methadone** is now generally recommended, regardless of dose, as compatible with breast-feeding, based on three studies. Methadone concentrations in milk were unrelated to maternal dose, may peak about three hours post-dose but are small at 21–314ng/ml (n = 12, Jansson et al, *J Hum Lact* 2007;**23**:184–90). This is insufficient to prevent the development of a neonatal absence syndrome (n = 8 pairs, Begg et al, Br J Clin Pharmacol 2001;**52**:681–5) and even methadone doses as high as 50–105 mg/d (plus eight matched formula-fed infants) give low infant levels. Levels increase gradually over 30 days, there are no significant effects from breast-feeding on neurobehavioural outcomes (n = 8 + 8, 30/7, Jansson et al, Pediatrics 2008;**121**:106–14; see also n = 4, 6/52, Jansson et al, Breastfeed Med 2008;**3**:34–7), and a retrospective chart analysis showed that breast-feeding by drug-dependent mothers reduced neonatal abstinence syndrome (NAS), delayed onset of NAS, and decreased the need for pharmacological interventions, regardless of gestation and type of drug. Methadone maintenance also reduces the risk of poor quality street drugs being used, and stopping opiates is also dangerous as withdrawal reactions can damage the fetus more than methadone (for effect on the child in the first year, Abdel-Latif et al, Pediatrics 2006;**117**:1163–9). In breast-feeding mums, **buprenorphine** and norbuprenorphine levels are detectable in the infant's urine but the infant-exposed dose in mg/kg has been calculated at under 1%, supporting the use of buprenorphine during breast-feeding (n = 7, Lindemalm et al, J Hum Lact 2009;**25**:199–205; see also n = 1, 10 samples, Grimm et al, Ther Drug Monit 2005;**27**:526–30), although it is actually contraindicated in breast-feeding (UK SPC).

36. **Bupropion** and metabolites accumulate in breast milk at higher levels than the mother's plasma (SPC caution) and there is a report of an infant developing seizures from bupropion ingested via breast milk (n = 1, Prescrire Int 2005;**14**:144), although other reports indicate that bupropion is not detectable in the infant's plasma (n = 1, Briggs et al, Ann Pharmacother 1993;**27**:431–3; n = 2 pairs, Baab et al, J Clin Psychiatry 2002 **63**:910–1).

3.2 CARDIOVASCULAR DISEASE

	LOWER RISK	MODERATE RISK	HIGHER RISK
Antipsychotics	Quetiapine[2] Sulpiride[5]	Amisulpride[5] Aripiprazole[2] Flupentixol[4] Olanzapine[2] Paliperidone[1] Phenothiazines[7] Risperidone[1] Zuclopenthixol[4]	Clozapine[3] Haloperidol[6] Pimozide[8] Ziprasidone[2] Zotepine[2]
Antidepressants	Agomelatine[14] Duloxetine[10] Mianserin[16] Mirtazapine[11] St John's wort[16] SSRIs[9] Trazodone[13] Tryptophan[16]	Moclobemide[16] Reboxetine[14] Venlafaxine[10]	MAOIs[15] Tricyclics (especially dosulepin)[12]
Anxiolytics and hypnotics	Benzodiazepines[17] Buspirone[18] Melatonin[21] Ramelteon[21] Zaleplon[19] Zolpidem[19] Zopiclone[19]	Beta-blockers[20] Chloral hydrate[21] Clomethiazole[21] Pregabalin[27]	
Anticonvulsants	Benzodiazepines[17] Gabapentin[26] Lamotrigine[26] Tiagabine[27] Topiramate[27] Vigabatrin[27] Valproate[23]	Barbiturates[25] Carbamazepine[22] Lacosamide[27] Oxcarbazepine[22] Paraldehyde[28] Phenytoin[24] Pregabalin[27]	Fosphenytoin[24]
Others	Acamprosate[31] Memantine[29]	Anticholinergics[30] Anticholinesterases[29] Atomoxetine[34] Bupropion[36] Dextroamfetamine[35] Lithium[32] Methadone[37] Methylphenidate[34] Modafinil[33] Sodium oxybate[33]	Disulfiram[31]

GENERAL PRINCIPLES IN CARDIAC DISEASE
(adapted from *Maudsley Guidelines*)

1. Polypharmacy should be avoided where possible, particularly with drugs likely to effect cardiac rate and electrolyte balance.

2. Awareness of QT prolongation is increasing, and so care is essential with drugs likely to increase the QT interval.

3. Avoid drugs specifically contraindicated.
4. Start low and go slow is, as ever, good advice. Rapid dose escalation should be avoided.

Psychotropics in specific cardiac conditions

Angina

Avoid drugs causing orthostatic hypotension, which may exacerbate angina. Avoid drugs causing tachycardia, e.g. phenothiazines, clozapine and risperidone. Trazodone and tricyclics are best avoided, although most other antidepressants are thought to be of relatively low risk.

Arrhythmias

SSRIs are first choice antidepressants and are preferred to the tricyclics because of their lack of antiarrhythmic/proarrhythmic potential. Avoid phenothiazines, butyrophenones and pimozide. Sulpiride and olanzapine seem of low risk.

Congestive heart failure (CHF)

For chronic stable CHF, avoid beta-blockers and take care with drugs causing orthostatic hypotension, e.g. phenothiazines, clozapine, risperidone and tricyclics. For acute CHF, the cause will indicate which drugs are safer to use.

Hypertension

Drugs causing orthostatic hypotension should be monitored closely. Avoid MAOIs. Hypertension can occur with venlafaxine (high dose), clozapine and sometimes with tricyclics and antipsychotics.

Myocardial infarction (MI)

If essential, use SSRIs (except perhaps fluvoxamine) or agomelatine. Avoid high-dose antipsychotics and phenothiazines. Butyrophenones, thioxanthenes and benzamides are safer.

Reviews: cardiac effects of psychotropics (Chong et al, Ann Acad Med Singapore 2001;**30**:625–31), psychotropics and the heart (O'Brien and Oyebode, Adv Psychiatr Treat 2003;**9**:414–23).

QTc prolongation

Many antipsychotics are known to affect cardiac conduction, with a class IA antiarrhythmic-like effect. One way this manifests itself is by lengthening of the QT interval. This may then lead onto torsade de pointes, which may be asymptomatic or, in rare cases, may lead on to ventricular fibrillation and sudden death. The QT interval shortens with increased heart rate, and so a rate-correct value QTc is usually used. A QTc prolonged to about 450ms is considered of some concern, and above about 500ms to be of an unquantifiable risk of leading to torsade de pointes, which may be fatal, and should prompt review and possibly action. QTc varies markedly throughout the day, and so serial readings are necessary for accurate assessments.

Risk factors for antipsychotic-induced QTc prolongation:

- Recent introduction of an antipsychotic, dose increase or high doses (including overdose).
- Receiving other medicines associated with QT prolongation, including, e.g. some antiarrhythmic drugs, vasodilators, tricyclics, antipsychotics, macrolide and fluoroquinolone antibiotics, antimalarials, ketoconazole and antihistamines.
- Underlying cardiac disease, e.g. heart-failure, angina and cardiac myopathy.
- Bradycardia, or second or third degree heart block.
- Personal or family history of QTc prolongation, ventricular arrhythmias or torsade de pointes.
- Severe renal or hepatic impairment.
- Elderly or malnourished.
- History of heavy alcohol consumption or substance misuse.
- Electrolyte imbalance, especially hypokalaemia and hypomagnesaemia.
- Undergoing restraint and/or severe stress.
- Slow drug metabolisers.
- Female (QT prolongation may occur more frequently).

If a prolonged QT interval is predictable, monitoring of electrolytes and ECG may be indicated, but interpretation is dependent upon the timing (time since last dose, diurnal variation, postprandial state).

Reviews: * general (Harrigan et al, J Clin Psychopharmacol 2004;**24**:62–9), cardiac effects of psychotropics (Kovacs and Arora, Am J Ther 2008;**15**:474–83; Mackin, Hum Psychopharmacol 2008;**23**(Suppl 1):3–14).

3.2.1 ANTIPSYCHOTICS *

A massive retrospective cohort study showed the risk of sudden cardiac death was roughly double with antipsychotics (atypicals and typicals similar), although the effect wore off when stopped (n = 276907, Ray et al, N Engl J Med 2009;**360**:225–35). The ten-year incidence of CHD in CATIE showed:

- increased risk with olanzapine (0.5)
- increased risk with quetiapine (0.3)
- reduced risk with perphenazine (-0.5)
- reduced risk with risperidone (-0.6)
- reduced risk with ziprasidone (-0.6%)

(n = 1125, 18/12–10 years, part of CATIE, Daumit et al, Schizophr Res 2008;**105**:175–87).

Reviews: cardiovascular adverse effects of antipsychotics (Buckley and Sanders, Drug Safety 2000;**23**:215–28;80 refs), QTc, torsade de pointes and sudden death (Haddad and Anderson, Drugs 2002;**62**:1649–71) and antipsychotics and QTc prolongation (Taylor, Acta Psychiatr Scand 2003;**107**:85–95; 136 refs).

1. **Risperidone** should be used with caution due to orthostatic hypotension; low doses slightly drop bp and increase heart rate. It is best to introduce it slowly over several weeks. In the Medicaid cohort study (n = 95,632 + 29,086 controls, Hennessy et al, Br Med J 2002;**325**:1070–2), risperidone was the only drug that had higher rates than haloperidol for cardiac arrest and ventricular arrhythmia, especially at lower dose. The authors concluded that this was due to the frailest patients being given lowest doses. **Paliperidone** should be used with care in people with a familial history of CV disease or QT interval or co-prescribed with drugs thought to prolong the QTc interval (SPC).

2. * **Aripiprazole** may cause orthostatic hypotension and the UK SPC now lists QT prolongation, ventricular arrhythmias, sudden unexplained death, cardiac arrest, torsades de pointes and bradycardia as unwanted effects. Orthostatic hypotension and syncope have been reported with **asenapine** (US PI) especially early in treatment and so should be used carefully with any other drugs with cardiac effects, and those likely to prolong the QTc interval and in people with cardiac risk factors (n = 148, p/c, Chapel et al, J Clin Pharmacol 2009;**49**:1297–308). QTc prolongation of 2–5 msec has been shown but with none going over 500 msec.

Postural hypotension has been seen infrequently with **olanzapine**. Blood pressure monitoring is recommended periodically in patients over 65. One study showed that olanzapine (mean 14 mg/d) produced fasting triglyceride levels raised by a mean of 60 mg/dL (37%) (n = 25, 12/52, Osser et al, J Clin Psychiatry 1999;**60**:767–70), which, since triglycerides are a significant risk factor for exacerbation of CHD, needs care. An increase in the QTc interval has only been seen rarely, e.g. data from four RCTs showed the risk of QTc > 450 msec was approximately the same as at baseline, suggesting a minimal effect on QTc prolongation and hence fatal arrhythmias (n = 2700, Czekalla et al, J Clin Psychiatry 2001;**62**:191–8). UK SPC now cautions about the use of olanzapine with drugs known to increase the QTc interval. The literature for **quetiapine** recommends caution with drugs known to prolong the QTc interval and in patients with CV disease or conditions predisposing to hypotension. Trials have not shown sustained changes in the QTc interval but some sources list quetiapine as a moderate risk. Orthostatic hypotension is more common in the elderly, especially initially. **Ziprasidone** causes a well-publicised, dose-related prolongation of QTc interval (mean 10 msec), so should not be used in anyone with a known prolonged interval, recent MI or heart failure (review, Taylor, CNS Drugs 2003;**17**:423–30). **Zotepine** causes a dose-related QTc interval prolongation and caution is necessary with CHD and with other drugs known to cause QTc prolongation. Increased heart rate can occur so care in angina pectoris is necessary. Orthostatic hypotension can occur initially in treatment, so bp measuring is recommended. Caution is necessary in severe hypertension. Unlike other antipsychotics, it tends to cause a slight shortening of the QTc interval.

3. * **Clozapine** has well-established CV side-effects, e.g. tachycardia and postural hypotension (particularly early in treatment). The literature (Curr Probs Pharmacovig 2002;**28**:8; Layland et al, Med J Aust 2009;**190**:190–2) has warned that:

- patients who develop clozapine-induced cardiomyopathy should not be re-exposed to clozapine (data mining study, Coulter et al, Br Med J 2001;**322**:1207–9)
- it should only be started if severe heart disease has been excluded through a full history, examination and possibly an ECG

- myocarditis most commonly occurs in the first two months
- persistent tachycardia at rest, especially during first two months, should be followed up and the patient observed for other signs of cardiomyopathy/myocarditis
- ECG changes should be referred to a cardiologist for evaluation
- it should be discontinued in anyone where cardiomyopathy or myocarditis is suspected.

Studies of clozapine-associated myocarditis and cardiomyopathy have shown that:

- the median onset is 17 days (mean 6/12)
- 90% occur within dose range of 100–450mg/d (50% recovered but 10% died)
- symptoms are diverse and non-specific and a high degree of suspicion must be maintained (n = 116, Haas et al, Drug Saf 2007;**30**:47–57)
- it can occur in young healthy adults (from Australian database of 8000, Kilian et al, Lancet 1999;**354**:1841–5; n = 41 [10 fatal], La Grenade et al, NEJM 2001;**345**:224–5).

A 10-year naturalistic study showed patients on clozapine were also at risk of death from cardiovascular disease secondary to obesity, diabetes, hypertension and hyperlipidaemia (n = 96, 10 years, Henderson et al, J Clin Psychiatry 2005;**66**:1116–21). Regular ECG monitoring, especially at higher doses, may be very valuable (review of myocarditis and CV toxicity by Wooltorton, Can Med Assoc J 2002; **166**:1185–6). Prolonged QTc is also known with clozapine. Risk factors included increased age (but less so if there was a normal ECG with other antipsychotics). It is dose-dependent, often corrects itself with time, occurs mostly during the initial stages of treatment, is mostly benign, and pathological prolongation of QTc is rare (n = 61, Kang et al, J Clin Psychiatry 2000;**61**:441–6).

4.* There is a caution on the use of **flupentixol** in susceptible individuals (hypokalaemia, hypomagnesia, genetic disposition), or in people with a history of CV disorders (UK SPC). Cardiac disease is a precaution for **zuclopenthixol**.

5.* QTc prolongation can occur with **amisulpride** (e.g. in overdose; n = 4, Isbister et al, Med J Aust 2006;**184**:354–6), and it is now contraindicated with drugs that could cause torsade de pointes. There are no specific problems with **sulpiride**

but prolonged QT and torsade de pointes have been reported (n = 1, Huang et al, Int J Cardiol 2007;**118**:100–2; n = 1, Chang et al, Am J Emerg Med 2009;**27**:1016).

6.* **Haloperidol** is now contraindicated in patients with clinically significant cardiac disorders or used with other QT-interval prolonging drugs (SPC). Prolonged QT-interval has been reported (n = 596, Reilly et al, Lancet 2000;**35**:1048–52).

7. Some ECG abnormalities have been reported with **phenothiazines**, e.g. tachycardia, T-wave abnormalities, ST depression, QT prolongation and right bundle branch block. **Levomepromazine** (methotrimeprazine) causes orthostatic hypotension that can, on occasion, be prolonged and profound. Sudden death has also been reported.

8. **Pimozide** is contraindicated in QT prolongation, history of cardiac arrhythmias or torsades de pointes.

3.2.2 ANTIDEPRESSANTS *

Depression has been considered to be an independent risk factor for mortality in patients with CHD and for the development of heart disease. This is logical but not supported by the two most recent major studies (CBT +/- SSRIs, n = 2481, RCT, 6/12, ENRICHD, Berkman et al, JAMA 2003;**289**:3106–16; MIND-IT, n = 331, RCT, 18/12, van Melle et al, Br J Psychiatry 2007; **190**:460–6; for caveats see Carney and Freedland, Br J Psychiatry 2007;**190**:467–8), as treatment is associated with modest improvements (s = 11, Thombs et al, JAMA 2008;**300**:2161–71). However, only depression developing after a major cardiac event was associated with an increased risk of morbidity and mortality, but risk was substantial, i.e. seven times as high (n = 489, 12/12, Parker et al, Biol Psychiatry 2008;**64**:660–6). Studies suggest that depressed patients:

- are at 5-fold greater risk of cardiac mortality, but depression in the week preceding the MI is not (n = 588, mean 6.7 years, Dickens et al, Psychosom Med 2008;**70**:450–5; comment by Martens and de Jonge, EBMH 2009;**12**:8)
- are less likely to follow recommendations to reduce their cardiac risk during recovery from a myocardial infarction (n = 204, Ziegelstein et al, Arch Intern Med 2000;**160**:1818–23)
- are less likely to comply with

antihypertensives (n = 496, one year, Wang et al, J Gen Intern Med 2002;**17**:504–11)

- are at greater risk of new cardiac events within the first year after a heart attack (n = 528; 12/12, Kaptein et al, Psychosom Med 2006;**68**:662–8; comment by Huffman, EBMH 2007;**10**:42)
- may have may more than double the mortality over a seven-year follow-up if they have severe depression or fail to improve over 6/12 following ACS (acute coronary syndrome), so depression needs to be treated aggressively (n = 369, seven years, Glassman et al, Arch Gen Psychiatry 2009; **66**:1022–9)
- with more severe depression may have this as an independent risk factor for increased CHD mortality in older adults free of CHD at baseline (n = 660, mean 12 years, Ahto et al, Int J Ger Psychiatry 2007;**22**:757–63; comment by Gump, EBMH 2008;**11**:56)
- are 2.7 times more likely to die from ischaemic heart disease than those who do not, and although antidepressants did not seem to help cardiac outcomes (n = 19649, six years, Surtees et al, Am J Psychiatry 2008;**165**:515–23) they do help depressive outcomes (Thombs et al, JAMA 2008; **300**:2161–71)
- may be at greater risk of cardiac failure from untreated depression rather than from the antidepressants (n = 1005, O'Connor et al, Arch Intern Med 2008;**168**:2232–7).

Overall, sertraline, fluoxetine, citalopram, bupropion and mirtazapine appear safe after MI; use of sertraline and response to citalopram and mirtazapine may improve mortality; paroxetine and citalopram appear safe in coronary artery disease, and tricyclics should be avoided (Taylor, Acta Psychiatr Scand 2008;**118**:434–42).

Reviews: * depression after acute coronary syndrome (Carney and Freedland, Am J Psychiatry 2009;**166**:410–7), antidepressant cardiac side-effects (Sala et al, Curr Opin Investig Drugs 2006; **7**:256–63).

9.* Despite some reported cases of cardiac effects (e.g. a plasma-level related potential for conduction problems, e.g. AV block, QTc prolongation, etc; n = 114, Rodriguez de la Torre et al, Ther Drug Monit 2001;**23**:435–40), the **SSRIs** are generally considered safer to use in cardiac disease, with

robust data accumulating to support this. In a major study, **sertraline** was shown not to increase cardiac events in depressed patients with unstable angina or recent MI, and may even cut cardiac deaths post-MI by about 10% (n = 369, RCT, Glassman et al, JAMA 2002;**288**:701–9; review by Parissis et al, Expert Opin Pharmacother 2007;**8**:1529–37; see also n = 1080 + 4356, three years, Sauer et al, Circulation 2003;**108**:32–6), although augmentation with omega-3 fatty acids has no beneficial effect on depression (n = 122, RCT, d/b, 10/52, Carney et al, JAMA 2009;**302**:1651–7).

Several open trials have indicated **fluoxetine** up to 60 mg/day to have no significant adverse cardiac effects in patients with pre-existing CHF, conduction disease and/or ventricular arrhythmia (e.g. n = 27, average age 73, open, 7/52, Roose et al, Am J Psychiatry 1998;**155**:660–6) and fluoxetine 20 mg/d produced a modest reduction in bp, and patients with pre-existing, stable cardiovascular disease (including hypertension) showed no significant bp change (n = 796, 12/52, Amsterdam et al, J Clin Psychopharmacol 1999;**19**:9–14). Rare cases of, e.g. atrial fibrillation, bradycardia and syncope have been reported. **Paroxetine** may increase cholesterol (LDL-C) concentrations by around 11%, which might increase the risk of CHD in vulnerable individuals (n = 18, Lara et al, J Clin Psychiatry 2003;**64**:1455, IS). **Citalopram**, and presumably **escitalopram**, have no significant reported effect on blood pressure, cardiac conduction or heart rate (Milne and Goa, Drugs 1991;**41**:450–77), but exacerbation of pre-existing bradycardia has been reported (e.g. Myth et al, Acta Psychiatr Scand 1992;**86**:138–45), as has occasional postural dizziness (review of citalopram cardiac safety: Rasmussen et al, J Clin Psychopharmacol 1999;**19**:407–15).

10.* **Venlafaxine** has a dose-dependent effect on supine diastolic blood pressure, clinically significant at high doses (200–300 mg/d), probably as a result of noradrenergic potentiation (3% incidence at less than 100 mg/d [n = 17, Emul et al, J Psychopharmacol 2009;**23**:163–7], 7% for 150–200 mg/d and 13% above 300 mg/d). However, high dose venlafaxine (mean 346 mg/d, range 225–525) did not produce any significant effects on ECG parameters, although 12.5% developed hypertension and a dose-related association with heart rate (n = 37, Mbaya et al, Hum Psychopharmacol 2007;**22**:129–33). In the

UK, venlafaxine is no longer subject to excessive MHRA and SPC restrictions, as:

- it is only contraindicated in patients with an identified high risk of a serious cardiac ventricular arrhythmia or with uncontrolled hypertension (but is **not** contraindicated in controlled hypertension). There is a caution for use in established cardiac disease that may increase the risk of ventricular arrhythmias. No baseline ECG is needed but regular bp is recommended.

Duloxetine causes no QTc prolongation or major cardiac effects (n = 128, Wohlreich et al, Depress Anxiety 2007;**24**:41–52, MS), but is contraindicated in uncontrolled hypertension (SPC; MHRA Drug Safety Update 2007;1–9). In rare studies of supra-therapeutic doses, duloxetine up to 400 mg/d produced rises in bp and pulse (which might precipitate prehypertensive people to become hypertensive), but did not have severe clinically important ADRs (related studies: n = 117, RCT, d/b, p/c, c/o, 16/7, Derby et al, J Cardiovasc Pharmacol 2007;**49**:384–93; n = 117, RCT, d/b, p/c, Zhang et al, J Cardiovasc Pharmacol 2007;**49**:146–53, MS). Exacerbation of stable heart failure has been reported with duloxetine and venlafaxine (n = 2, Colucci and Berry, Ann Pharmacother 2008; **42**:882–7).

11. Although hypertension, hypotension and tachycardia have been reported with **mirtazapine**, the incidences of 6%, 4% and 2% respectively are the same as placebo (n = 150, RCT, d/b, p/c, 6/52, Smith et al, Psychopharmacol Bull 1990;**26**:191–6). No ECG changes have been observed in reported trials, or bp and heart rate changes in a depressed in-patient trial (n = 251, RCT, 6/12, Zivkov and Jongh, Hum Psychopharmacol 1995;**10**:173–80), and mirtazapine seemed safe and was superior to placebo on most measures in post-MI depression (n = 91, RCT, d/b, p/c, 24/52, Honig et al, Psychosom Med 2007;**69**:606–13). **Agomelatine** appears to have no cardiac effects, e.g. no QTc changes, ECG abnormalities, or other parameters (MI).

12.* **Tricyclics** produce orthostatic hypotension (and hence occasional myocardial infarction), have antiarrhythmic actions (quinidine-like) in high dose and antimuscarinic actions (raising heart rate). Thus, tricyclics should only be used with extreme caution in patients with ischaemic heart disease, ventricular arrhythmia, angina, recent MI and hypertension. Indeed, a study indicated that the odds ratio for developing IHD was significantly raised for patients who had ever received a TCA (even adjusting for other factors), with a further specific, significant and dose-related association with **dosulepin** (n = 922 with IHD, 5516 controls, Hippisley-Cox et al, Br Med J 2001;**323**:666–9). On average, starting tricyclics increases the QTc interval by 6.9 msec (including amitriptyline 8.5 ms and nortriptyline 35 msec) (n = 8222, van Noord et al, J Clin Psychopharmacol 2009;**29**:9–15). In patients with recurrent chest pain but normal coronary angiograms, **imipramine** therapy over 9–33 months produced no symptoms of a pro-arrhythmic effect, a slightly prolonged corrected QT interval and reduced chest pain (n = 58, Cannon et al, NEJM 1994;**330**:1411–7). Conversely, 150 mg/d of **amitriptyline** increased heart rate from 78 bpm to 93 bpm, and all other heart rate analysis parameters significantly worsened (n = 48, Rechlin et al, Psychopharmacology 1994;**116**:110–4). **Nortriptyline** has significant effects on cardiac vagal function and should only be used with care in IHD (n = 44, Yeragani et al, Neuropsychobiology 2002;**46**:125–35), especially in men who may be more susceptible to its cardiac side-effects (n = 78, 6/52, Pomara et al, Prog Neuropsychopharmacol Biol Psychiatry 2001;**25**:1035–48). **Doxepin**-induced torsade de pointes tachycardia has been reported (Alter et al, Ann Intern Med 2001;**135**:384–5).

13. Reversible ventricular tachycardia (n = 1, Vitullo et al, Chest 1990;**98**:247–8) and QT pro-longation has been reported with **trazodone** overdose (n = 1, Service and Waring, Clin Toxicol [Phila] 2008;**46**:71–3; n = 1, Dattilo and Nordin, J Clin Psychiatry 2007;**68**:1309–10), but is generally considered of low risk.

14. **Reboxetine** increased baseline heart rate in 20% of patients in short-term trials. Orthostatic hypotension occurs with increasing frequency at higher doses.

15. **Isocarboxazid, phenelzine** and **tranylcypro-mine** are contraindicated in severe cardiac disease.

16. Many cases of hypertension have been reported with **moclobemide** (e.g. Boyd, Lancet 1995;**346**:1498), so monitoring bp may be useful. Occasional hypertension with tyramine in patients with pre-existing labile hypertension has also occurred, and so caution in cardiac disease would be sensible. **St John's wort** does not affect heart rate variability, unlike amitriptyline 75 mg/d (n = 12,

RCT, d/b, c/o, 14/7 per arm, Siepmann et al, Br J Clin Pharmacol 2002;**54**:277–82). There are no apparent problems with **mianserin** and **tryptophan**.

3.2.3 ANXIOLYTICS AND HYPNOTICS

Anxiety and depression are inter-related predictors of ventricular arrhythmias in people with coronary artery disease and so treatment of these may be important (n = 940, Watkins et al, Psychosom Med 2006;**68**:651–6; comment by Rutledge and Linke, EBMH 2007;**10**:43).

17. **Benzodiazepines** are relatively safe but contra-indicated in acute pulmonary insufficiency. One study in elderly patients showed that temazepam (up to 30 mg/d) caused a fall in systolic blood pressure and an increase in heart rate (n = 12, Ford, Br J Clin Pharmacol 1990;**29**:61–7).

18. **Buspirone** may have some cardiac effects, e.g. rare cases of hypertension and tachycardia.

19. There are no apparent problems with **zaleplon**, **zolpidem** and **zopiclone**.

20.* The use of **beta-blockers** would depend upon the nature of the cardiac disease. In a prospective study of people with end-stage severe HF (61% with MDD), beta-blockers had a significant effect on reducing mortality but only if used with SSRIs, and had a negative effect if used with SNRIs or TCAs (n = 250 [c = 83], 18/12, Tousoulis et al, J Card Fail 2008;**14**:456–64).

21.* **Clomethiazole** is contraindicated in acute pulmonary insufficiency and should be used with care in chronic pulmonary insufficiency. **Chloral** is contraindicated in severe cardiac disease. No problems are anticipated for **melatonin** (SPC) although there is a study in patients with stable angina and arterial hypertension, but it's in Russian and the abstract doesn't make much sense to me, so you'd best take a stiff glass of vodka before trying to get your head round its finding (s = 2, n = 43, RCT, Zaslavskaia et al, Klin Med (Mosk) 2008;**86**:64–7).

3.2.4 ANTICONVULSANTS

22. Cardiovascular effects from **carbamazepine** are uncommon but there are reports of cardiac conduction changes, hypertension and atrio-ventricular block (n = 1, Labrecque et al, Am J Psychiatry 1992;**149**:572–3), enough to make a pacemaker ineffective (n = 1, Ambrosi et al, Lancet 1993;**342**:365). Patients on **oxcarbazepine** with cardiac insufficiency and secondary heart failure should have regular weight measurements to help detect any fluid retention and care is needed in patients with pre-existing conduction disturbances (UK SPC).

23.* **Valproate** appears to have no adverse effects on ECG, and it might even have some preventive or stabilising effects on ventricular conduction (n = 55, Kurt et al, J Psychopharmacol 2009;**23**:328–33).

24. **Phenytoin** has many cardiac effects and is a useful third-line treatment in cardiac arrhythmias. It is, however, contraindicated in sinus bradycardia, sino-atrial block, second and third degree A-V block and patients with Adams-Stokes syndrome. Severe cardiovascular ADRs have been reported with **fosphenytoin** IV, including asystole, VF and cardiac arrest, mostly within 30 minutes of an injection. The literature thus recommends (Curr Prob Pharmacovig 2000;**26**[May]:1):

- monitoring heart rate, bp and respiration during the infusion
- observing for at least 30 minutes after the infusion ends
- as hypotension may occur at recommended doses and rates, reduction of the dose or rate may be necessary
- reducing the loading dose and/or infusion rate by 10–25% in the elderly or those with hepatic or renal impairment.

25. IV **barbiturates** can cause hypotension. As there is no evidence that **primidone** causes QT-prolongation (and may actually shorten it), it may be the drug of choice in patients with QT-prolongation (Christidis et al, Seizure 2006; **15**:64–6).

26.* There is no evidence of any problems with **gabapentin** in cardiac disease. A self-styled thorough study showed that **lamotrigine** 100–400 mg/d had no QTc prolonging effect (n = 152, d/b, p/c, c/o, 11/52, Dixon et al, Br J Clin Pharmacol 2008;**66**:396–404), but ECG monitoring is recommended in cases of overdose (Buckley et al, Lancet 1993;**342**:1552–3).

27.* No significant changes in ECG, blood pressure or heart rate have been noted in initial clinical trials with **topiramate**, **vigabatrin** and **tiagabine**. There is now a caution for the use of **pregabalin** in severe CHF (SPC) and there are cases of heart failure exacerbation in people with clinically stable CHF taking pregabalin for neuropathic pain (n = 3 and review, Page et al, J Cardiovasc Med (Hagerstown) 2008;**9**:922–5). The UK SPC for **rufinamide** states it may shorten the QTc interval. Prolongations in PR interval have been observed with **lacosamide** and so caution is necessary in severe cardiac disease (SPC).

28. There have been reports of hypotension and tachycardia in young children given IV **paraldehyde** (Sinal and Crowe, Pediatrics 1976;**57**:158).

3.2.5 OTHERS

29.* The use of anticholinesterases has been associated with increased rates and risk of hospitalisation for bradycardia (n = 627, Park-Wyllie et al, PloS Med 2009;**6**:e1000157), syncope, bradycardia, pacemaker insertion, and hip fractures in older adults with dementia (n = 81,302, Gill et al, Arch Intern Med 2009;**169**:867–73). Heart block has been reported with **donepezil**, and so the UK SPC has recommended considering this before prescribing (Curr Prob Pharmacovig 1999;**25**:7). Analysis of four studies indicated that **rivastigmine** appears not to cause adverse ECG effects (n = 2149, d/b, p/c, 26/52, Morganroth et al, J Clin Pharmacol 2002;**42**:558–68), although rare cases of syncope and angina pectoris have been noted in trials. In a newer review of cardiac safety, rivastigmine produces a modest reduction in mean heart rate of 1.5–2 bpm, but no bradycardia or ECG abnormalities and appears to have a favourable cardiac safety profile (n = 661, Ballard et al, Int J Clin Pract 2006;**60**:639–45). **Galantamine** would appear relatively safe but caution is advised in people with cardiovascular conditions, e.g. sick sinus syndrome or other supraventricular cardiac conduction disturbances. There is little data on **memantine** in cardiac disease and use should be only with caution as it has been reported to cause bradycardia (n = 36, Gallini et al, Pharmacoepidemiol Drug Saf 2008;**17**:877–81).

30. **Anticholinergics** should be used with caution, particularly in those with a tendency to tachycardia. Sinus bradycardia has been reported with **benzatropine** (Voinov et al, Am J Psychiatry 1992;**149**:711) and **benzhexol/trihexyphenidyl** (n = 1, Blumensohn et al, Drug Intell Clin Pharm 1986;**20**:786–7).

31.* **Disulfiram** is contraindicated in cardiac failure, coronary artery disease, previous history of CVA and hypertension, and it can be cardiotoxic in overdose (n = 1, Jerónimo et al, Arq Bras Cardiol 2009;**92**:16–18). The Antabuse-alcohol reaction can cause cardiac arrest even in healthy adults. There are no known problems with **acamprosate**.

32.* **Lithium** rarely causes clinical problems although cardiac failure and sick sinus syndrome are contraindications. Usually benign cardiovascular side-effects may occur in 20–30% patients. The main problems with lithium can be T-wave flattening (or possibly inversion), ventricular ectopics, congestive myopathy, bradycardia (Farag et al, Lancet 1994;**343**:1371), ECG changes and conduction disturbances, e.g. sinus node dysfunction (Terao et al, Acta Psychiatr Scand 1996;**93**:407–8). On average, starting lithium increases the QTc interval by 18.6 msec (n = 8222, van Noord et al, J Clin Psychopharmacol 2009;**29**:9–15). An analysis, however, (n = 827, Ahrens et al, J Affect Disord 1995;**33**:67–75) showed that deaths from cardiac-related causes were no different in people taking lithium than in the general population, and so, despite the above reported problems, lithium can be considered not to have a significant risk in this situation (reviewed by Ananth, Lithium 1993; **4**:167–79). A pre-treatment ECG is very useful, especially in the elderly.

33. **Modafinil** is contraindicated in severe hypertension and arrhythmia and used with caution in patients with concurrent heart disease. Monitor heart rate and bp if used in moderate hypertension (MI; discussion by Heitmann et al, Clin Pharmacol Therapy 1999;**65**:328–35). **Sodium oxybate** contains a significant dose of sodium (0.75 g in 4.5 g dose) and so dietary restriction of sodium might be considered in hypertension and heart failure (SPC).

34.* The SPCs for **methylphenidate** preparations recommend caution in people with severe hypertension, and bp monitoring should be carried out in all patients. The EMEA (2009) also recommends screening for c/v problems before prescribing and periodically as stimulant and non-stimulant medication are associated with minor but statistically significant changes in heart rate and bp (n = 125, Wilens et al, J Clin Psychiatry 2005;**66**:253–9). Ongoing therapy at relatively high dose methylphenidate (1.5 mg/kg/d) can produce a small but significant increase in bp, especially during the first six weeks (n = 114 [c = 57], open, 6/12, Hammerness et al, J Pediatr 2009; **155**:84–9). **Atomoxetine** is associated with modest increases in bp (mean < 5 mmHg) and pulse (mean < 10 bpm), which stabilise over two years (UK SPC). Recent UK MHRA guidance is that atomoxetine should be used with caution in those with prolonged QT or a family history of QT prolongation, and care when used with other drugs that produce QT prolongation, drugs that can cause electrolyte disturbances and CYP2D6 inhibitors. QTc prolongation has been seen with atomoxetine overdose (n = 1, Sawant and Daviss, Am J Psychiatry 2004; **161**:757). Atomoxetine may produce a dramatic rise in blood pressure in people with central autonomic failure, even at very low doses (n = 3, RCT, p/c, c/o, Shibao et al, Hypertension 2007; **50**:47–53).

35. There is little evidence of developing hypertension with **dexamfetamine**, although regular bp testing has been recommended (ASDA, Sleep 1994; **17**:348–51). In adult ADHD, cardiovascular effects from amphetamine XR preps at < 60 mg/d were minimal (n = 223, < 24/12, Weisler et al, CNS Spectr 2005; **10**(suppl 20):35–43).

36.* **Bupropion** may cause small rises in supine blood pressure (n = 58, RCT, Kiev et al, Ann Clin Psychiatry 1994; **6**:107–15), but tends not to cause significant conduction complications, or to exacerbate ventricular arrhythmias and has a low rate of orthostatic hypotension (n = 36, open, Roose et al, Am J Psychiatry 1991; **148**:512–6). However, infrequent occurrences of orthostatic hypotension, tachycardia, stroke and vasodilation have been reported with bupropion. In mild untreated hypertension, bupropion up to 400 mg/d has no effect on blood pressure (n = 300, RCT, d/b, p/c, 4/52, Thase et al, J Clin Psychopharmacol 2008; **28**:302–7).

37.* **Methadone** can lengthen the QT interval and the CSAT (Center for Substance Abuse Treatment Cardiac Expert Panel) Consensus Guidelines has made five recommendations:

1. Inform patients of the risk of arrhythmia.
2. Enquire about any history of heart disease, arrhythmia or syncope.
3. Carry out pre-treatment ECG to measure QTc, repeated at 30 days and annually, with additional ECGs if the dose exceeds 100 mg/d or if unexplained syncope or seizures occur.
4. If the QTc is 451–499 ms, discuss with client and monitor more frequently. If QTc > 500 ms discontinue or reduce dose (although there appears to be no recommendation if the QTc is exactly 500 ms).
5. Clinicians be aware of interactions with other QT-prolonging or interacting drugs, e.g. 3A4 inhibitors.

(Krantz et al, Ann Intern Med 2009; **150**:387–95, 417–8; see also Ehret et al, Expert Opin Drug Saf 2007; **6**:289–303; George et al, Curr Drug Abuse Rev 2008; **1**:297–302; Stringer et al, Am J Health Syst Pharm 2009; **66**:825–33; n = 109, Fonseca et al, Drug Alcohol Depend 2009; **99**:327–32). However, to put it in perspective, a Finnish study showed that 4.6% of methadone-treated patients had a QTc > 500 msec, but that the maximum mortality attributable to QTc prolongation was low at 0.06 per 100 patient-years (n = 200, Anchersen et al, Addiction 2009; **104**:993–9). **Buprenorphine** is associated with less QTc prolongation than methadone (n = 165, RCT, d/b, 17/52, Wedam et al, Arch Intern Med 2007; **167**:2469–75), with some reports of no QTc prolongation with SuBoxone (n = 50, 2–4/52, Baker et al, Ann Pharmacotherapy 2006; **40**:392–6). It has been used safely in a patient with methadone-induced torsades de pointes (n = 1, Krantz et al, Pharmacotherapy 2005; **25**:611–4).

3.3 DIABETES

	LOWER RISK	MODERATE RISK	HIGHER RISK
Antipsychotics	Amisulpride[5] Aripiprazole[2] Asenapine[2] Butyrophenones[6] Paliperidone[1] Pimozide[8] Risperidone[1] Sulpiride[5] Ziprasidone[2]	Phenothiazines[7] Quetiapine[2] Thioxanthenes[4] Zotepine[2]	Clozapine[3] Olanzapine?[2]
Antidepressants	Agomelatine[14] Duloxetine[10] Moclobemide[16] Reboxetine[14] SSRIs[9] Trazodone[13] Tryptophan[16] Venlafaxine[10]	Fluoxetine[9] Mianserin[16] Mirtazapine[11] Tricyclics[12]	MAOIs[15]
Anxiolytics and hypnotics	Benzodiazepines[17] Buspirone[18] Chloral[21] Clomethiazole[21] Melatonin[21] Zaleplon[19] Zolpidem[19] Zopiclone[19]	Beta-blockers[20]	
Anticonvulsants	Barbiturates[25] Benzodiazepines[17] Carbamazepine[22] Ethosuximide[28] Gabapentin[26] Lamotrigine[26] Oxcarbazepine[22] Pregabalin[26] Rufinamide[27] Vigabatrin[27]	Acetazolamide[28] Phenytoin[24] Topiramate[27] Tiagabine[27] Zonisamide[27] Valproate[23]	Lacosamide[26]
Others	Acamprosate[31] Anticholinergics[30] Anticholinesterases[29] Atomoxetine[33] Buprenorphine[35] Lithium[32] Memantine[29] Methadone[35] Methylphenidate[33] Modafinil[33]	Bupropion[34] Disulfiram[31] Sodium oxybate[33]	

GENERAL PRINCIPLES IN DIABETES

1. Use drugs least likely to promote loss of diabetic control or alter glucose levels.
2. Warn that some side-effects may be interpreted as hypoglycaemia.
3. Check the family history
4. Monitor weight and glucose parameters

3.3.1 ANTIPSYCHOTICS *

People with schizophrenia are more liable to develop diabetes, with antipsychotics adding to that risk (n = 99, RCT, d/b, Saddichha et al, Acta Psychiatr Scand 2008;**117**:342–7) and especially with some of the newer agents, e.g. in a huge study of people taking antipsychotics (41% on typicals and 59% on atypicals [of which 48.4% were on olanzapine, 43.7% on risperidone, 5.3% on clozapine and 4.2% on quetiapine]), those on atypicals were 9% more likely to have diabetes than those on typicals. The prevalence was significantly increased for **clozapine, olanzapine** and **quetiapine** but not for **risperidone** (n = 38 632, Veterans, Sernyak et al, Am J Psychiatry 2002;**159**:561–6), although there may be no difference in new-onset diabetes between risperidone, quetiapine and olanzapine in veterans (n = 15767, Lambert et al, Am J Epidemiol 2006;**164**:672–81). In non-diabetic schizophrenics, glucose tolerance tests show elevated plasma glucose (compared to placebo or typicals) at all time points for olanzapine, partly raised for clozapine and only raised with risperidone compared to untreated non-schizophrenics, indicating an adverse effect by some atypicals on glucose regulation (n = 79, Newcomer et al, Arch Gen Psychiatry 2002;**59**:337–45). In diabetics, antipsychotics can worsen metabolic control and double the need for insulin, especially in the first two years (n = 2585, Spoelstra et al, J Clin Psychiatry 2004;**65**:674–8). In people aged over 65 with pre-existing diabetes, initiating any antipsychotic was associated with increased risk for hospitalisation for hyperglycaemia (n = 13817, Lipscombe et al, Arch Int Med 2009;**169**:1282–9).

1. There appears to be only a clinically insignificant effect from **risperidone** on blood biochemistry (n = 38 632, Veterans, Sernyak et al, Am J Psychiatry 2002;**159**:561–6) and is probably the least likely of the atypicals to exacerbate or cause diabetes (Gianfrancesco et al, J Clin Psychiatry 2002;**63**:920–30; n = 38 632, Veterans, Sernyak et al, Am J Psychiatry 2002;**159**:561–6; n = 79, Newcomer et al, Arch Gen Psychiatry 2002; **59**:337–45). **Paliperidone** has only a few rare reports of glucose-related adverse events (SPC).

2.* **Aripiprazole** is not thought to have any problems in diabetes although hyperglycaemia as an ADR has been added to the UK SPC and there is a report of diabetic ketoacidosis (n = 1, Makhzoumi et al, Pharmacotherapy 2008;**28**:1198–202). The incidence of hyperglycaemia in trials with **asenapine** (US PI) is less than 1% and so some care would be prudent, although it is only a precaution. **Olanzapine** seems to be the most likely of the newer agents to cause or exacerbate diabetes (see introduction), e.g. a cohort study indicated that the incidence of new-onset diabetes was about 1%, but 20% higher with olanzapine than risperidone, and 90% higher in the first three months of treatment (n = 33 946, three years, Caro et al, J Clin Psychiatry 2002;**63**:1135–9; see also odds ratio of 5.8 cf conventionals or non-antipsychotic treated; n = 19 637, Koro et al, Br Med J 2002;**325**:243–5). In 5000 patients with baseline non-fasting glucose levels of ≤7.8/L, the incidence of raised glucose (≥11 mmol/L, suggestive of diabetes) was 1% (cf 0.9% placebo). Raised levels (8.9–11 mmol/L; suggestive of hyperglycaemia) were 2% with olanzapine (cf 1.6% placebo) and so hyperglycaemia or exacerbation of pre-existing diabetes is in the 'very rare' spontaneous event (<0.01%) category in the UK SPC, although post-marketing surveillance in the UK has shown the incidence of diabetes mellitus to be about one in 1000 (eight cases in sample of 8858, Biswasl et al, J Psychopharmacol 2001;**15**:265–71). Olanzapine is also associated with the metabolic syndrome via e.g. weight gain, elevated levels of insulin, leptin and lipids (triglycerides and cholesterol), e.g. olanzapine (mean 14 mg/d) can produce fasting triglyceride levels raised by a mean of 60 mg/dL (37%) (n = 25, 12/52, Osser et al, J Clin Psychiatry 1999;**60**:767–70), which needs care since triglycerides are a risk factor for precipitation or exacerbation of diabetes. Insulin resistance is possibly the predominant mechanism, as the insulin secretory response to hyperglycaemic challenge is significantly decreased by olanzapine (n = 26, RCT, 14/7, Chiu et al, J Clin Psychopharmacol 2006;**26**:504–7; n = 10, Ebenbichler et al, J Clin Psychiatry 2003;**64**:1436–9; IS). Routine quarterly glucose monitoring is recommended with olanzapine, regardless of pre-existing diabetes (n = 590, Wirshing et al, J Clin Psychiatry 2002;63:856–65; reviews by eder-Ischia et al, Essent Psychopharmacol 2005;6:112–7; Koller and Doraiswamy, Pharmacotherapy 2002;22:841–52; Mir and Taylor, Int Clin Psychopharmacol 2001; 16:63–74).

There is evidence for a slightly increased risk of diabetes with quetiapine (n = 38 632, Veterans, Sernyak et al, Am J Psychiatry 2002;159:561–6). Occasional hypoglycaemia and hyperglycaemia have been reported with zotepine. Short-term treatment with ziprasidone appears to have little effect on glucose levels, and it may actually lower serum cholesterol and triglyceride levels (n = 37, 6/52, open, Kingsbury et al, J Clin Psychiatry 2001; 62:347–9).

3. Elevated glucose levels (in up to 23% in people with no PMH, n = 121, Sernyak et al, J Clin Psychiatry 2003;64:605–8) and diabetes have been shown with clozapine, and a dose-related effect noted, indicating a probable influence on insulin secretion and a causal relationship (n = 384, FDA MedWatch, Koller et al, Am J Med 2001;111:716–23). Clozapine may impair glucose control, independent of changes in insulin sensitivity and BMI (n = 20, open, 4/12, Howes et al, Am J Psychiatry 2004;161:361–3). Clozapine is also well-known to cause the metabolic syndrome, e.g. weight gain and lipid abnormalities (e.g. raised serum triglycerides) which are significant risk factors for developing diabetes (n = 82, naturalistic, five years, Henderson et al, Am J Psychiatry 2000; 157:975–81). Augmentation with quetiapine has been suggested as a possible management option (n = 65, open, 10/12, Reinstein et al, Clin Drug Invest 1999;18:99–104). Routine glucose monitoring is recommended with clozapine, regardless of pre-existing diabetes (n = 590, Wirshing et al, J Clin Psychiatry 2002;63:856–65; review by Mir and Taylor, Int Clin Psychopharmacol 2001;16:63–74).

4.* Lack of relationship between serum levels of zuclopenthixol (n = 9) and plasma insulin has been shown (Melkersson et al, J Clin Psychiatry 1999;60:783–91). The UK SPC for flupentixol notes that control of diabetes may be impaired and that an adjustment in antidiabetic therapy may be necessary.

5. There are no apparent problems with sulpiride and amisulpride.

6. There are no apparent problems with haloperidol.

7. A case-control study of cases of newly-treated diabetes indicated a modest and significant increased risk with chlorpromazine and perphenazine (n = 7227 + 6780, Wang et al, J Clin Psychiatry 2002;22:236–43) but lack of relationship between serum levels of perphenazine (n = 12) and plasma insulin has been shown (Melkersson et al, J Clin Psychiatry 1999;60:783–91; see also n = 850, Schwarz and Munoz, Am J Psychiatry 1968;125:253–5). Many phenothiazines cause weight gain and appetite stimulation which wouldn't help diabetic control.

8. There are no known problems with pimozide.

3.3.2 ANTIDEPRESSANTS *

Over one in four diabetics may develop depression and sertraline has been recommended as the drug of choice. Conversely, there is an increased incidence of diabetes with long-term (two years) antidepressant use (same for tricyclics and SSRIs) at moderate to high dose, but not with lower doses or shorter-use (n = 2243 + 8963 controls, Andersohn et al, Am J Psychiatry 2009;166:591–8). In the short-term, SSRIs may even decrease serum glucose levels by up to 30% and cause anorexia (reducing body weight), and in the short-term may enable people with diabetes to control hunger and eat better, via their serotonergic effects. By comparison, the tricyclics, often have an appetite-raising effect, e.g. in non-diabetic patients with MDD, imipramine caused an 11% increase in blood glucose (n = 60 [c = 43], RCT, d/b, 8/52, Ghaeli et al, J Clin Psychopharmacol 2004;24:386–8). In a two-year study of insulin-dependent diabetics, insulin use increased by 16%, but remained unchanged if treated with tricyclics and reduced by 13% if treated with an SSRI (n = 133, Knol et al, Pharmacoepidemiol Drug Saf 2008;17:577–86). So, it's not all bad then.

Reviews: * outcomes (n = 475, Ciechanowski et al, Gen Hosp Psychiatry 2003;25:246–52), meta-analysis (s = 24, Lustman et al, Diabetes Care 2000;23:934–42), general (Lustman, Curr Psychiatry Rep 2008;10:495–502).

9. No dose changes are recommended with citalopram/escitalopram. Citalopram has no significant effect on insulin sensitivity in women of reproductive age (n = 32, RCT, open, 8/52,

Kauffman et al, Gynecol Endocrinol 2005;**21**:129–37), and no changes in glycaemic control were seen in another trial (Sindrup et al, Clin Pharmacol Ther 1992;**52**:547–52). People with diabetes may become hypoglycaemic during **fluoxetine** treatment (Drug Ther Bull 1990;**28**:33) and its side-effects, eg. tremor, nausea, sweating and anxiety may be mistaken for hypoglycaemia. Most problems have been reported with the more common type 2 diabetes rather than the insulin dependent type 1 disease. If fluoxetine iş used, warn about this effect, noting a possible loss of hypoglycaemic awareness (n = 1, Sawka et al, J Pediatr 2000;**136**:394–6) and regularly check serum glucose levels. Fluoxetine has been shown to effectively reduce the severity of depression in people with diabetes with a trend towards better glycaemic control (n = 60, RCT, p/c, 8/52, Lustman et al, Diabetes Care 2000;**23**:618–23). There is a case of **fluvoxamine**-induced acute hyperglycaemia in a patient with diabetes (n = 1, Oswald et al, Int J Neuropsychopharmacol 2003;**6**:85–7). Little is reported with **paroxetine**. There have been no major reports of problems with **sertraline**, and maintenance dosing seems safe and effective in diabetes with a positive effect on the diabetes itself (n = 152, RCT, d/b, p/c, Lustman et al, Arch Gen Psychiatry 2006;**63**:521–9), especially in younger people (n = 152, d/b, p/c, Williams et al, Diabetes Care 2007;**30**:801–6). There are, however, cases of hypoglycaemia associated with sertraline (e.g. n = 1, Takhar and Williamson, Can J Clin Pharmacol 1999;**6**:12–4; n = 1, Pollak et al, Ann Pharmacother 2001;**35**:1371–4) and raised glucose levels in a person with diabetes (n = 1, Sansome and Sansome, Int J Psychiatr Med 2003;**33**:103–5).

10. There is no published evidence of problems with **venlafaxine** or **duloxetine**.

11.* **Mirtazapine** does not seem to influence glucose homeostasis (n = 14, Laimer et al, J Clin Psychiatry 2006;**67**:421–4) and glucose tolerance may improve but insulin sensitivity remains unchanged (n = 10, Hennings et al, Exp Clin Endocrinol Diabetes 2010;[in press]). Mirtazapine causes increased appetite which might be counterproductive. The mirtazapine UK SPC recommends care, a class labelling precaution.

12. * **Tricyclics** may adversely affect diabetic control as they increase serum glucose levels by up to 150%, increase carbohydrate craving and reduce the metabolic rate, but are generally considered safe unless the diabetes is very brittle. Hypoglycaemia has been associated with maprotiline (n = 1, Isotani and Kameoka, Diabetes Care 1999;**22**:862). Nortriptyline tends to worsen glycaemic control (n = 68, RCT, d/b, p/c, 8/52, Lustman et al, Psychosom Med 1997;**59**:241–50).

13. There are no apparent problems with **trazodone**.

14. There are no apparent problems with **reboxetine** nor **agomelatine**.

15. **MAOIs** may decrease serum glucose levels by up to 35% due to a direct influence on gluconeogenesis (Goodnick et al, J Clin Psychiatry 1995; **56**:128–36). Diabetes is a UK SPC precaution for **isocarboxazid**.

16. There is a case of **mianserin** dose-related hyperglycaemia in a non-diabetic woman (Marley and Rohan, Lancet 1993;**342**:1430–1). **Moclobemide** 600 mg/d did not modify the effect of glibenclamide on plasma glucose and insulin levels in healthy individuals (Amrein et al, Psychopharmacology 1992;**106**:S24–S31).

3.3.3 ANXIOLYTICS AND HYPNOTICS

17. There is a case of a person with diabetes presenting with a reduction in insulin requirements after discontinuing **clonazepam** (n = 1, Wagner et al, Diabetes Care 1999;**22**:2099).

18. There are no apparent problems with **buspirone**.

19. There are no apparent problems with **zaleplon**, **zolpidem** and **zopiclone**.

20. **Propranolol** may prolong the hypoglycaemic response to insulin and may effect hypoglycaemic episodes.

21. There are no apparent problems with **ramelteon**, **melatonin**, **clomethiazole** or **chloral hydrate**.

3.3.4 ANTICONVULSANTS

22. There is an isolated report of **carbamazepine**-induced urinary retention in two patients with diabetes, where withdrawal improved the condition (Steiner and Birman, Neurology 1993; **43**:1855–6). There are no apparent problems with **oxcarbazepine**.

23. **Valproate** may give false positives in urine tests for diabetes. Protein binding of valproate may be

lower in diabetes (Doucet et al, Eur J Clin Pharmacol 1993;**45**:577–9).

24. Hypoglycaemia has been reported with **phenytoin** and glucose metabolism can be affected. Protein binding of phenytoin may be lower in diabetes (Doucet et al, Eur J Clin Pharmacol 1993;**45**:577–9).

25. There are no apparent problems with **phenobarbital** or **primidone**.

26. There are no apparent problems with **lamotrigine** or **pregabalin**. Blood glucose fluc-tuations have been reported with **gabapentin** (e.g. n = 1, Penumalee et al, Am J Kid Dis 2003; **42**:E3–5).

27.* No information is available on **topiramate**, **zonisamide** and **tiagabine** and no problems noted for **rufinamide**. There is no information on **lacosamide** (UK SPC)

28. There are no apparent problems with **ethosuximide**. Hyperglycaemia has been reported with **acetazolamide** in diabetics and prediabetics, but probably not in non-diabetic patients, so some care may be necessary.

3.3.5 OTHERS

29. There are no apparent problems with **donepezil** or **galantamine**, but diabetes mellitus is a precaution for **rivastigmine**. No effect with **memantine** has been reported.

30. There are no known problems with the **anticholinergic agents**.

31. The literature for **disulfiram** recommends caution in diabetes mellitus. There are no apparent problems with **acamprosate**.

32. There is no problem with **lithium** in diabetes, but many patients on lithium develop polyuria and polydipsia, a diabetes insipidus-like syndrome via an effect on cAMP and vasopressin. This can be controlled by ensuring an adequate fluid and salt intake. There is a case of increased clearance of lithium in a patient with persistent hyperglycaemia, probably due to the subsequent osmotic diuresis increasing renal clearance (n = 1, Cyr et al, Ann Pharmacother 2002;**36**:427–9). Lithium may also increase insulin secretion.

33. There are no apparent problems with **methylphenidate** or **atomoxetine** but a transient loss of appetite may occur. There is no information on **sodium oxybate** and no apparent problems with **modafinil**.

34. Animal studies suggest some risks with **bupropion** and so caution is needed with use in type 2 diabetics (El-Dakhakhny et al, Arzneimittelforschung 1996;**46**:667–9).

35. There are no precautions for the use of **buprenorphine** in diabetes (UK SPC), or **methadone**, although the sugar-free liquid would be the presentation of choice for the latter.

3.4 EPILEPSY

	LOWER RISK	MODERATE RISK	HIGHER RISK
Antipsychotics	Amisulpride[5] Aripiprazole[2] Asenapine[2] Haloperidol[6] Pimozide[8] Risperidone?[1]	Olanzapine[2] Phenothiazines (most)[7] Quetiapine[2] Sulpiride[5] Ziprasidone[2] Zuclopenthixol[4]	Chlorpromazine[7] Clozapine[3] Zotepine[2]
Antidepressants	Agomelatine[14] MAOIs[15] Moclobemide?[16] Reboxetine[14] SSRIs[9] Tryptophan[16]	Duloxetine[10] Mianserin[16] Mirtazapine[11] Trazodone[13] Tricyclics (most)[12] Venlafaxine[10]	
Anxiolytics and hypnotics	Benzodiazepines[17] Beta-blockers[20] Chloral[21] Clomethiazole[21] Melatonin[21] Ramelteon[21] Zaleplon[19] Zolpidem[19] Zopiclone[19]	Buspirone[18]	
Others	Acamprosate[24] Anticholinergics[23] Methylphenidate[26] Modafinil[26]	Anticholinesterases[22] Atomoxetine[26] Disulfiram[24] Lithium[25] Memantine[22]	Bupropion[27] Sodium oxybate [26]

GENERAL PRINCIPLES FOR PRESCRIBING IN EPILEPSY (Pisani et al, Drug Safety 2002;**25**:91–110, 166 refs)

Risk factors for psychotropic-induced seizures:

- History of epilepsy (including febrile seizures) in the patient or their family.
- Neurological abnormalities (including brain injury, angioma cavernous, blood-brain barrier abnormality).
- Cerebral arteriosclerosis.
- Elderly.
- Reduced drug clearance.
- Pre-existing EEG alterations.
- Physical illness (eg malignant hypertension).
- Polypharmacy.

Practical recommendations in pre-existing epilepsy:

- Use anticonvulsants with psychotropic properties where possible (e.g. carbamazepine, lamotrigine or valproate).
- Avoid high-risk drugs.
- Start low and go slow, monitoring plasma levels and EEG where possible.
- Keep dosing simple and avoid polypharmacy.

3.4.1 ANTIPSYCHOTICS

General principles

1. Keep the daily dose as low as possible; the proconvulsive effect may be dose-related.
2. Take extra care where risk factors exist,

including head trauma, previous seizure history and concomitant drugs (especially other antipsychotics). The most susceptible patients are those with a history of epilepsy, any condition that predisposes to epilepsy and those withdrawing from central depressants, e.g. benzodiazepines and alcohol.

3. Use lowest risk drugs unless essential.

4. Use a slow rate of introduction and withdrawal. Anticonvulsant cover may be appropriate.

5. Dose changes should be small and gentle.

6. Avoid antipsychotics having more antihistaminic, antiserotonergic, sedative and antiadrenergic effects, which may have a greater seizure threshold lowering effect.

Review: * interventions for psychosis in epilepsy (Farooq and Sherin, *Cochrane Database Syst Rev* 2008;**4**:CD006118), general (Kanner, *Semin Neurol* 2008;**28**:279–88).

1. There is little adverse information about **risperidone**. Pre-marketing trials showed a seizure incidence of 0.3% (n = 2607) and it has been used successfully for psychosis in epilepsy (n = 1, Mahgoub, *J Neuropsychiatry Clin Neurosci* 2007;**19**:347–8). The SPC for **paliperidone** urges caution in people with risk factors or a history or seizures.

2. In pre-marketing trials, seizures occurred in only 0.1% patients taking **aripiprazole**, but should probably still be used with caution in epilepsy. Seizures have been reported in one patient on **asenapine** in trials (n = 851; 0.3%), compared with none with placebo (n = 706), and in long-term trials in five (n = 1953; 0.3%), so some care would be prudent but it is not an obvious problem (US PI). The literature for **olanzapine** states that it should be used cautiously in patients with a history of seizures. Unexplained seizures (i.e. patients without reported risk factors) occurred in 0.9% patients during pre-marketing trials (n = 2500). There may be a slightly higher risk of seizures in people over 65. The incidence of seizures during **quetiapine** trials has been equivalent to placebo but a short review suggested that it is associated with new-onset seizures in patients with seizurogenic conditions (Yalug et al, *J Neuropsychiatry Clin Neurosci* 2007; **19**:341–2). **Zotepine** has an established dose-related proconvulsive effect, with a higher risk at doses above 300 mg/d (open, n = 129, Hori

et al, *Jpn J Psychiatry Neurol* 1992;**46**:161–7). It should not be used in patients with a personal or family history of epilepsy. Seizures occurred in 0.4% patients during pre-marketing trials with **ziprasidone** (many with confounding factors), but it would be wise to use with caution in epilepsy.

3. **Clozapine** can cause dose-related seizures, the risk rising from 1% (< 300 mg/d), through 2.7% (300–600 mg/d) to 4.4% (> 600 mg/d). EEG changes occur in 75% people on clozapine, with up to 40% having paroxysmal discharges (reviewed by Pacia and Devinsky, *Neurology* 1994;**44**:2247–9). A more rapid dose-titration increases the risk. Valproate is the routine anticonvulsant cover of choice, at clozapine doses of 600mg/d or more. See also 4.2.2 and 6.3.

4.* **Zuclopenthixol** may have only mild-to-moderate effects, with few adverse reports, and may be one of the drugs of choice, although the UK SPC now note that they should only be used with caution in epilepsy. There is no mention in the **flupentixol** SPC.

5.* There are no known problems with **amisulpride**, but a spontaneously resolving generalised convulsion occurred after a 3 g overdose (n = 1, Tracqui et al, *Hum Exp Toxicol* 1995;**14**:294–8). **Sulpiride** may be a reasonable choice, with a few cases of convulsions reported and only minimal EEG effects. There is a new UK SPC warning on reducing seizure threshold so care is recommended in unstable epilepsy.

6. **Haloperidol** may have only mild-to-moderate effects, and may be a lower risk drug.

7. **Fluphenazine** may have a low proconvulsive effect, although status epilepticus has been reported (n = 1, Leksowski, *Psychiatr Pol* 1983; **17**:445–7). The incidence of seizures with **chlorpromazine** may be 9% at doses above 1 g/d and 0.5% at less than 1 g/d and is best avoided.

8. **Pimozide** may have a low effect as, although it may enhance spike activity at low dose, it may not do so at higher dose (Oliver et al, *Arch Gen Psychiatry* 1982;**39**:206–9). Epilepsy is not mentioned in the SPC.

3.4.2 ANTIDEPRESSANTS *

Unless a large scale trial is carried out (unlikely), the safest antidepressant in epilepsy will remain unknown. All patients require an individual assessment of their risk factors and recognition that there is a dose-dependent relationship between antidepressants and seizures. **A slow rate of introduction** reduces the risk. **Lamotrigine** has proved useful for interictal depression (n = 13, open, Kalogjera-Sackellares and Sackellares, *Epilepsy Behav* 2002;**3**:510–6), as well as in bipolar depression. In a post-hoc analysis of patients with MDD and TLE, antidepressants were effective, with no serious ADRs and no increase in seizures with citalopram, reboxetine and mirtazapine (n = 75, RCT, Kuhn *et al, Epilepsy Behav* 2003;**4**:674–9). There is a double risk of depression in seizure sufferers (13% vs 7%) (n = 130,880, Fuller-Thomson and Brennenstuhl, *Epilepsia* 2009;**50**:1051–8).

Reviews: * depression in epilepsy (Seethalakshmi and Krishnamoorthy, *Epileptic Disord* 2007;**9**:1–10; Mula *et al, Expert Opin Pharmacother* 2008;**9**: 3159–68).

9. * Serotonin function is unlikely to be of major importance in the genesis of seizures and so **SSRIs** are likely to have a low proconvulsive effect (review by Kondziella and Asztely, *Acta Neurol Scand* 2009;**119**:75–80). **Citalopram** and **escitalopram** have not been reported to interact with anticonvulsants or to have a proconvulsive effect, and citalopram has been used for interictal depression without an increase in seizure frequency or severity (n = 43, 8/52, Hovorka *et al, Epilepsy Behav* 2000;**1**:444–7; n = 75, RCT, Kuhn *et al, Epilepsy Behav* 2003;**4**:674–9). **Fluoxetine** has a probable seizure incidence of 0.2%, similar to other antidepressants, and may even have a positive effect (n = 17, open, add-on, Favale *et al, Neurology* 1995;**45**:1926–7). **Fluvoxamine** probably has a low proconvulsive effect, although this has been disputed (Vincenti, *Lancet* 1990;**336**:947) and there have been some literature reports of fits. **Paroxetine** appears to have a minimal potential for producing seizures at clinically useful doses (Sedgwick *et al, J Psychopharmacol* 1987;**1**:31–4; Milne and Goa, *Drugs* 1991;**41**:450–77). With **sertraline**, seizures occurred in early clinical trials at a similar frequency to placebo and only in people with a history of seizures, and it has been effective for depression in children and adolescents with epilepsy, with increased fits in only 6% (n = 36, Thomé-Souza *et al, Epilepsy Behav* 2007;**10**:417–25).

10. Seizures have been reported in 0.26% of patients treated with **venlafaxine** during clinical trials and so a slow introduction and withdrawal is recommended. For **duloxetine**, there is a UK SPC caution for epilepsy but no reported problems as such.

11. One grand mal seizure has been reported in a patient with a history of seizures receiving **mirtazapine** at a high dose of 80mg/d during a trial. More definite information would be needed before a cause-effect link could be made. Care and monitoring would thus be standard.

12. All **tricyclics** seem to lower the seizure threshold, with **amitriptyline** reputed to be the most proconvulsive and **doxepin** possibly of lowest risk. TDM of tricyclics minimises the risk of toxicity (review by Preskorn and Fast, *J Clin Psychiatry* 1992;**53**:160–2).

13.* The literature for **trazodone** now includes a caution in epilepsy, and a warning to avoid abrupt changes in dose.

14. **Reboxetine** may be particularly useful in epilepsy with a low interaction potential and a spontaneous incidence of seizures of <0.2% (n = 1500), with no seizures in overdose. There are no apparent problems with **agomelatine**.

15.* **MAOIs** are generally not considered epileptogenic at therapeutic doses and the UK SPC for **isocarboxazid** notes a varying effect, with some people having decreased seizures and others increased seizures. MAOI-induced myoclonic jerks and serotonin syndrome can occasionally be interpreted as seizures.

16. There have been no reports of problems with **moclobemide** or **tryptophan** in epilepsy to date. **Mianserin** is often quoted as being relatively safe in epilepsy (n = 40, Edwards and Glen-Bott, *Br J Clin Pharmacol* 1983;**15**:299S–311S). One study of 84 overdoses of 1 g or more showed no convulsions (*Curr Med Res Opin* 1980;**6**:44).

3.4.3 ANXIOLYTICS AND HYPNOTICS

17. For **benzodiazepines** in epilepsy, see *1.17*.

18. Animal studies show **buspirone** to have no anticonvulsant activity. The literature states buspirone to be contraindicated in epilepsy but there is no evidence that it is actually epileptogenic.

19. A weak anticonvulsant activity for **zopiclone** has been shown (Julou *et al, Pharmacol Biochem*

Behav 1985;**23**:653–9). **Zolpidem** is not reported to have any anticonvulsant activity. There is no data on **zaleplon**.

20. There are no apparent problems with the **beta-blockers**.

21. There are no apparent problems with **melatonin** or **ramelteon**. **Chloral hydrate** and **clomethiazole** have anticonvulsant properties (see *1.17.1*).

3.4.4 OTHERS

22. **Cholinomimetics** may have some potential for causing seizures so care is needed with **donepezil** in pre-existing seizure activity, although 10 mg/d had no adverse effects on seizures in one trial (n = 23, RCT, s/b, p/c, c/o, 3+3/12, Hamberger *et al, Epilepsia* 2007;**48**:1283–91). Care should be exercised with the use of **rivastigmine** in patients predisposed to seizures. There has been no increase in the incidence of seizures with **galantamine** in clinical trials. A single case report with **memantine** suggests it should only be used with caution.

23. There are no problems reported with the **anticholinergic** agents.

24. The literature for **disulfiram** recommends caution in epilepsy. The manufacturers report no known problems with **acamprosate** in epilepsy.

25. **Lithium** has a marked epileptogenic activity in overdose, but probably has no effect at standard dose. **Carbamazepine** and **valproate** may be suitable alternatives.

26.* **Methylphenidate** is not associated with a significant risk at therapeutic doses, e.g. there was no association between methylphenidate and seizure risk in children aged 6–17 years with ADHD and no prior seizures (n < 34727, McAfee *et al, Curr Drug Saf* 2008;**3**:123–31) and it is generally considered safe for seizure-free children with epilepsy although there are a few reports of exacerbation (Kaufmann *et al, J Child Neurol* 2009;**24**:727–33). The incidence of seizures during clinical trials is 0.1–0.2%, not significantly different to placebo and similar to population-based data (review by Wernicke *et al, Dev Med Child Neurol* 2007;**49**:498–502). **Sodium oxybate** has been reported to cause seizures and use is not recommended in epilepsy (SPC). The MHRA guidance is that **atomoxetine** should be introduced with caution in patients with a history of seizures and discontinuing considered if seizures start or increase in frequency. However, the incidence during clinical trials was 0.1–0.2%, not significantly different to placebo and similar to population-based data (Wernicke *et al, Dev Med Child Neurol* 2007;**49**:498–502) and there was no association between atomoxetine and the seizure risk in children aged 6–17 years with ADHD and no prior seizures (n < 34727, McAfee *et al, Curr Drug Saf* 2008;**3**:123–31). There are no apparent problems with **modafinil**.

27. **Bupropion** has some epileptogenic activity (literature warning: *Curr Prob Pharmacovig* 2001; **27**:5). The risk of seizures is about 0.4%, and it appears plasma level-related. Doses should not exceed 450 mg/d (although new-onset seizures can occur at therapeutic doses up to 450 mg/d, e.g. Pesola and Avasarala, *J Emerg Med* 2002;**22**:235–9), no single dose should be above 200 mg and doses should not be increased at more than 150 mg/d. It should be contraindicated in people with a history of seizures and concurrent eating disorder, known CNS tumor, and if abruptly withdrawing from benzodiazepines or alcohol. Other risk factors include concomitant use with any drug known to lower the seizure threshold, alcohol abuse, history of head trauma, diabetes treated with hypoglycaemics or insulin, and the use of stimulants or anorectics.

3.5 GLAUCOMA (narrow-angle)

	LOWER RISK	MODERATE RISK	HIGHER RISK
Antipsychotics	Asenapine[3] Butyrophenones[3] Paliperidone[3] Risperidone[3] Sulpiride[3] Thioxanthenes[2]	Aripiprazole[3] Clozapine[2] Phenothiazines[1] Ziprasidone[3] Zotepine[3]	Olanzapine[2]
Antidepressants	Agomelatine[5] Bupropion[5] Flupentixol[5] MAOIs[5] Moclobemide[5] Trazodone[5] Tryptophan[5]	Duloxetine[5] Mirtazapine[5] SSRIs[5] Venlafaxine[5]	Tricyclics[4]
Others	Acamprosate[8] Benzodiazepines[6] Clomethiazole[6] Disulfiram[8] Gabapentin[7] Lithium[8] Lofexidine[8] Memantine[8] Melatonin[8] Naltrexone[8] Phenobarbital[7] Phenytoin[7] Rufinamide[7] Tiagabine[7] Valproate[7] Z hypnotics[6]	Caffeine[8] Carbamazepine[7] Dexamfetamine[8] Lacosamide[7] Methylphenidate[8]	Atomoxetine[8] Anticholinergics[8] Topiramate[7]

Narrow-angle glaucoma (also called angle closure glaucoma) occurs in eyes with a narrow anterior chamber angle, where drainage of the aqueous fluid through the anterior chamber angle is reduced or blocked. Drugs with anticholinergic properties have the potential to either induce narrow-angle glaucoma or to worsen it. Although the degree of anticholinergic effects is of greater importance (review by Lam et al, Curr Opin Ophthalmol 2007;**18**:146–51).

GENERAL RECOMMENDATIONS
Patients with shallow anterior chamber and/or narrow angles, or with previously diagnosed glaucoma may be treated with drugs with anticholinergic properties, provided intraocular pressure is monitored, an ophthalmologist is involved and information is given on the symptoms of acute narrow-angle closure, with a recommendation to stop the drug and seek medical attention immediately should those symptoms occur. In a patient with a shallow anterior chamber and narrow angles, an ophthalmologist would normally perform an iridotomy or some type of drainage surgery to allow drug use. Treatment with miotic therapy, e.g. pilocarpine may not necessarily protect the patient with narrow angles against drug-induced angle closure, so monitoring is essential.

The main symptoms of acute narrow-angle glaucoma are blurred vision, 'coloured halos' around bright lights, intense pain, lacrimation, lid oedema, red eye, nausea and vomiting (review by Oshika, *Drug Saf* 1995;**12**:256–63). The incidence rises with age due to the ageing process, e.g. thickening of the lens, and most acute attacks occur in people who are unaware they have narrow iridocorneal angles. The peak effect from a drug on intraocular pressure can occur within 5–24 hours (or sooner).

Reviews: * general (Lee and Higginbotham *Am J Health Syst Pharm* 2005;**62**:691–9), drug-induced acute angle-closure glaucoma (Lachkar and Bouassida, *Curr Opin Ophthalmol* 2007;**18**:129–33), risk factors (Coleman and Kodjebacheva, *Open Ophthalmol J* 2009;**3**:38–42).

3.5.1 ANTIPSYCHOTICS

1. **Phenothiazines** have some anticholinergic effects so the potential for problems exists. Screening for glaucoma has been recommended before initiating therapy, although several studies have shown no detectable narrow-angle glaucoma in, e.g. 100 patients taking **thioridazine**, 98 on **fluphenazine** and 99 on **chlorpromazine** (Applebaum, *Arch Ophthalmol* 1963;**69**:578–80). Thus, there is need for routine care (see introduction). There are a few case reports of single high-dose injection of IV or IM chlorpromazine producing a transient decrease in intraocular pressure (mentioned in review by Bristow and Hirsch, *Drug Saf* 1993;**8**:136–48).

2. Other antipsychotics with similar anticholinergic effects would include **clozapine, flupentixol, zotepine** and **zuclopenthixol**. Olanzapine is contraindicated in narrow-angle glaucoma.

3.* Antipsychotics with little or no anticholinergic effect must still be considered to have a potential for problems, albeit probably at a low level, e.g. **sulpiride, haloperidol, risperidone** and **paliperidone**. Asenapine has no appreciable effect on muscarinic cholinergic receptors and so exacerbation of glaucoma is unlikely (US PI). No information is available on **ziprasidone** or **aripiprazole** but nothing would be expected.

3.5.2 ANTIDEPRESSANTS

4. **Tricyclics** generally have a greater anti-

cholinergic effect than phenothiazines, although most of the data is so old it should be pensioned off soon. If patients are at risk of narrow-angle glaucoma, pre-treatment examination by an ophthalmologist is recommended. Patients with a narrow anterior chamber angle who are receiving glaucoma treatment or who have had laser treatment should have few problems provided care (see introduction) is taken (Oshika, *Drug Saf* 1995;**12**:256–63). There is a report of patients with narrow angles developing acute-angle closure glaucoma with **imipramine** (n=4, Ritch et al, *Arch Ophthalmol* 1994;**112**:67–8), and with **clomipramine** (Schlingemann et al, *Lancet* 1996;**347**:465). A survey by Reid and Blouin (*Psychosomatics* 1976;**17**:83–5) showed no abnormal intraocular pressures in patients taking tricyclics, even in combination with **phenothiazines**. A postal survey of ophthalmologists and psychiatrists indicated that occasional, probably drug-induced, cases had been seen, most frequently associated with **amitriptyline** (review by Lieberman and Stoudemire, *Psychosomatics* 1987;**28**:145–8). See general recommendations.

5.* Antidepressants that can cause dilation of the pupil include the **SSRIs, mirtazapine, moclobemide, trazodone** (case of aggravated angle-closure glaucoma with low-dose trazodone: Pae et al, *Psych Clin Neurosci* 2003;**57**:127–8) and **MAOIs**. An extensive and arcane review has summarised six cases of angle-closure glaucoma with **paroxetine** (three in older people [aged 70–91] outside the normal life-period presentation; and three in younger people), one case with **fluvoxamine** (n=1, Jimenez-Jimenez et al, *Ann Pharmacother* 2001;**35**:1565–6), and two with **citalopram** (in younger women, n=1, Croos et al, *BMC Ophthalmol* 2005;**5**:23; n=1, Massaoutis et al, *Br J Ophthalmol* 2007;**91**:1086–7). There is a new UK SPC warning, uveal effusions and bilateral angle-closure glaucoma with **escitalopram** (n=1, Zelefsky et al, *Am J Ophthalmol* 2006;**141**:1144–7). There is one case with **fluoxetine** in a patient sensitive to anticholinergic effects and with a positive family history (Ahmad, *DICP Ann Pharmacother* 1991;**25**:436), and none with **sertraline** (review by Costagliola et al, *Curr Neuropharmacol* 2008;**6**:293–310). There is limited experience with **reboxetine** but the literature recommends close supervision. Raised intraocular pressure or narrow-angle glaucoma is a warning in the UK SPC for **venlafaxine,** and bilateral acute narrow-angle glaucoma has been reported as developing rapidly with venlafaxine (n = 1, Ng et al, Med J Aust 2002;**176**:241). Mydriasis has been reported with **duloxetine,** so caution is necessary in patients with raised intraocular pressure or at risk of acute narrow-angle glaucoma. No problems are expected with **agomelatine. Bupropion** has no effect on intraocular pressure or other parameters (Ghibellini et al, J Clin Pharmacol 2009; **49**:489–95).

3.5.3 HYPNOTICS

6. No problems are expected with the **benzodiazepines, zopiclone, zolpidem, melatonin** or **ramelteon.**

3.5.4 ANTICONVULSANTS

7.* There are no reported problems with any of the mood stabilisers, anxiolytics, hypnotics or anticonvulsants (no information on **lacosamide** yet), except **topiramate,** which has a particular problem. Although one study showed no evidence of topiramate-induced angle narrowing (n = 20, 4/52, Leung et al, Eye [Lond] 2009;**23**:2079–81), there are numerous reports of reversible acute secondary narrow-angle glaucoma (n = 86, Fraunfelder et al, Ophthalmology 2004;**111**:109–11; n = 1, Sachi and Vijaya, J Postgrad Med 2006;**52**:72–3) occurring within a month of starting treatment, bilateral angle-closure glaucoma (e.g. n = 1, Cruciani et al, Clin Ter 2009;**160**:215–6; n = 1, Singh et al, Kathmandu Univ Med J (KUMJ) 2007;**5**:234–6; n = 1, Levy et al, Can J Ophthalmol 2006;**1**:221–5; n = 1, Mansoor and Jain, Acta Ophthalmol Scand 2005;**83**:27–8; n = 1, Coats, J AAPOS 2003;**7**:303; discussion of possible mechanisms: Craig et al, Am J Ophthalmology 2004;**137**:193–5), possibly

enhanced by combination with citalopram (n = 1, Spaccapelo et al, Cases J 2009;**2**:87). The UK SPC notes that symptoms usually start within the first month and include decreased visual acuity and/or ocular pain. If this occurs, topiramate should be discontinued as soon as clinically feasible and appropriate measures to reduce intraocular pressure introduced (see also Curr Probs 2002;**28**:4).

3.5.5 OTHERS

8.* **Amfetamine** causes a transient rise in intraocular pressure, which is not associated with closure of the angle. **Caffeine** has been reported to cause a transient rise in intraocular pressure, which is not associated with closure of the angle. Average daily intakes of more than 180 mg/d caffeine (not a lot by the author's standards) may cause a clinically significant elevation of intraocular pressure (n = 28, Avisar et al, Ann Pharmacother 2002;**36**:992–5). **Methylphenidate** causes a transient rise in intraocular pressure but this is not associated with closure of the angle. There is a case of uneventful use of methylphenidate in a man with ADHD and primary open-angle glaucoma well-controlled by pilocarpine and betaxolol (Bartlik et al, Arch Gen Psychiatry 1997;**54**:188–9), but methylphenidate 60 mg/d has precipitated severe glaucoma requiring surgery (n = 1, Lu et al, J Chin Med Assoc 2006;**69**:589–90). The UK SPC lists glaucoma as a contraindication for **atomoxetine. Anticholinergics** are contraindicated in narrow-angle glaucoma. There is a case of angle-closure glaucoma after discontinuing **donepezil** (n = 1, Enzenauer and Bowers, J Geront A Biol Sci Med Sci 2005;**60**:1083). Glaucoma is not mentioned in the literature for **memantine.** There is no association with use of **ginkgo biloba** over last 12/12 and having glaucoma (Khoury et al, J Glaucoma 2009; **18**:543–5)

3.6 HEPATIC IMPAIRMENT

	LOWER RISK	MODERATE RISK	HIGHER RISK
Antipsychotics	Amisulpride[5] Aripiprazole[2] Flupentixol[4] Haloperidol[6] Paliperidone[1] Pimozide[8] Sulpiride[5] Ziprasidone[2] Zuclopenthixol[4]	Asenapine[2] Clozapine[3] Olanzapine[2] Risperidone[1] Phenothiazines[7] Quetiapine[2] Risperidone[1] Sertindole[2]	Zotepine[2]
Antidepressants	Agomelatine[14] Mianserin[16] Paroxetine[9] Tryptophan[16]	Duloxetine[10] Mirtazapine[11] Moclobemide[16] Reboxetine[14] SSRIs[9] St John's wort[16] Trazodone[13] Tricyclics[12] Venlafaxine[10]	Lofepramine[12] MAOIs[15]
Anxiolytics and hynpotics	Lorazepam LD[17] Melatonin[21] Oxazepam LD[17] Ramelteon[21] Temazepam LD[17]	Buspirone[18] Clomethiazole[21] Propranolol LD[20] Zaleplon[19] Zolpidem[19] Zopiclone[19]	Benzodiazepines (esp LA)[17] Chloral[21] Propranolol HD[20]
Anticonvulsants	Carbamazepine[22] Gabapentin[26] Pregabalin[27] Topiramate?[227] Vigabatrin[27]	Acetazolamide[28] Benzodiazepines[17] Lamotrigine[26] Levetiracetam[27] Oxcarbazepine[22] Paraldehyde[28] Rufinamide[27] Tiagabine[27]	Barbiturates[25] Ethosuximide[28] Fosphenytoin[24] Phenytoin[24] Valproate[23]
Others	Buprenorphine[36] Donepezil[29] Lithium[32] Memantine[29]	Acamprosate[31] Anticholinergics[30] Atomoxetine[34] Bupropion[35] Disulfiram[31] Galantamine[29] Methadone[36] Methylphenidate[34] Modafinil[33] Rivastigmine[29]	

LD = low dose   HD = high dose
SA = short-acting   LA = long-acting

GENERAL PRINCIPLES FOR PRESCRIBING IN HEPATIC IMPAIRMENT (adapted from *Maudsley Guidelines*)

1. The greater the degree of hepatic impairment, the greater the degree of impaired drug metabolism, and the greater the risk of drug toxicity, and so the starting and final dose should be lower. People may be more sensitive to common or predictable side-effects.
2. Start low, go slow, and monitor LFTs regularly (e.g. weekly).
3. LFTs do not necessarily correlate well with metabolic impairment, although they can give a reasonable indication.
4. Care is needed with drugs with a high first-pass clearance effect.
5. In severe liver disease, avoid drugs with the marked sedation and/or constipation.

Child-Pugh* is a measure of the severity and prognosis of cirrhosis, and is calculated from the severity of ascites and encephalopathy, bilirubin, albumin and clotting times:

Child-Pugh grade	A	B	C
Child-Pugh score	5–6	7–9	10–15
Description	Cirrhosis but functioning liver	significant functional compromise	decompensation of liver

3.6.1 ANTIPSYCHOTICS

1.* Unbound **risperidone** levels increase in hepatic impairment and so initial doses and dose increments should be halved, and 4 mg/d not exceeded. Risperidone-induced jaundice (n = 1, Oyewole et al, Int J Geriatr Psychiatry 1996;**11**:179) and rapid onset hepatotoxicity (n = 1, Phillips et al, Ann Pharmacother 1998;**32**:843) have been reported. **Paliperidone** is not extensively metabolised by the liver so no dose adjustments are needed in moderate hepatic impairment (n = 20, Boom et al, Int J Clin Pharmacol Ther 2009; **47**:606–16), but no data is available in severe impairment so caution is recommended (SPC).
2.* No changes in dose with **aripiprazole** seem necessary with mild, moderate or severe hepatic impairment. A single dose study showed that although the Cmax was lower in hepatic impairment there were no significant adverse effects (n = 25, Mallikaarjun et al, Clin Pharmacokinet 2008;**47**:533–42). **Asenapine** is not recommended in severe hepatic impairment (Child-Pugh C) as seven-fold increases in plasma levels have been shown. No dose changes are necessary in Child-Pugh A or B (US PI) as plasma levels are only increased by about 12%. A lower **olanzapine** starting dose of 5 mg/d may be appropriate. Transient, asymptomatic elevations in ALT and AST have been noted and monitoring of these in patients with risk factors (e.g. hepatic impairment, concomitant hepatotoxic drugs) may be appropriate. A lower starting dose of 150 mg/4 weeks should be considered for olanzapine pamoate in people with moderate (Child-Pugh A or B) hepatic impairment (SPC) and only increased with caution. The **quetiapine** SPC now says oral clearance is reduced by 25% in hepatic impairment, so start at 50 mg/d and increase at 50 mg/d according to response and tolerability. Discontinue if jaundice develops (Thyrum et al, Prog Neuropsychopharmacol Biol Psychiatry 2000;**24**:521–33). **Zotepine** levels may be 2–3 times higher with hepatic impairment, so start at 25 mg BD up to a maximum of 75 mg BD and measure LFTs weekly for the first three months. **Ziprasidone** is extensively metabolised and an extended half-life has been shown in Child-Pugh A or B, but dose adjustment is not necessary in mild-to-moderate impairment (n = 30, open, Everson et al, Br J Clin Pharmacol 2000;**49**(S3):21–6).
3. **Clozapine** is contraindicated in severe hepatic disease and so lower doses, regular plasma level monitoring and LFT monitoring would be necessary if used. There are reported cases of toxic hepatitis, with AST levels dramatically raised, eosinophilia developing early and full LFT normalisation within 4–5 weeks of stopping (e.g. Thatcher et al, Am J Psychiatry 1995;**152**:296–7).
4.* No dosage adjustments are necessary for **flupentixol** or **zuclopenthixol**, although both undergo hepatic metabolism and so some caution would be wise in significant hepatic impairment (UK SPC).
5. **Sulpiride** and **amisulpride** are virtually unmetabolised with little or no biliary excretion. There is a low incidence of liver toxicity reported,

with a transient rise in serum transaminase the only reported effect. Dosage adjustments are thus unnecessary (SPC).

6. There are no apparent problems with **haloperidol**, although the UK SPC states liver disease to be a caution.

7. **Phenothiazines** (particularly chlorpromazine) may cause hepatocanalicular cholestasis and there have been suggestions of immunological liver damage. They should be avoided where possible in hepatic dysfunction. Onset is usually during the first month of therapy. Coma may be precipitated due to increased cerebral neuron sensitivity.

8. **Pimozide** should be used with caution in hepatic impairment (UK SPC).

3.6.2 ANTIDEPRESSANTS

9. **Citalopram** and **escitalopram** are metabolised extensively by the liver, with three major metabolites. Doses at the lower end of the therapeutic range should be used (n = 1000, Milne and Goa, *Drugs* 1991;**41**:450–77), although no liver enzyme abnormalities were noted in this study. In hepatic impairment, alternate day dosing of **fluoxetine** is recommended. Patients with cirrhosis show higher plasma levels of fluoxetine and **norfluoxetine** and longer half-lives occur, and a 50% reduction in dose is recommended, especially if a low albumin is present. **Fluvoxamine** should be started at 50mg/d and monitored carefully, as raised hepatic enzymes have been reported. **Paroxetine** appears to be the safest option, using doses at the lower end of the therapeutic range, although cases of hepatitis (Benbow and Gill, *Br Med J* 1997;**314**:1387) and hepatotoxicity have been reported (n = 3, Azaz-Livshits et al, *Pharmacopsychiatry* 2002;**35**:112–5). **Sertraline** is extensively metabolised by the liver and is contraindicated in significant hepatic dysfunction. One study showed a 2.5–fold increase in half-life and a 1.6–fold increase in sertraline/desmethylsertraline peak levels in stable chronic cirrhosis (n = 20, Demolis et al, *Br J Clin Pharmacol* 1996;**42**:394–7; n = 1, Persky and Reinus, *Dig Dis Sci* 2003;**48**:939–44).

10. **Venlafaxine** clearance is reduced by about 35% in mild-to-moderate hepatic impairment, and so doses should be reduced by about 50% (UK SPC), although there is much interpatient variability (Anon, *J Clin Psychiatry* 1993;**54**:119–26) and it is not recommended in severe hepatic

impairment. **Duloxetine** is contraindicated in hepatic impairment (UK SPC). Moderate liver disease (Child-Pugh B) increases the half-life 2.3-fold and AUC 3.7-fold. The FDA in 2006 noted that duloxetine can cause hepatitis and jaundice, and people with pre-existing liver disease may be at risk of additional problems. There is no data in mild or severe hepatic insufficiency.

11. **Mirtazapine** clearance is reduced by 33% in moderate hepatic impairment (n = 16, single-dose study, Murdoch et al, *Br J Clin Pharmacol* 1993;**35**:76P), and so dosage reduction may be necessary. Transient asymptomatic raised liver enzymes (e.g. SGTP) have been noted in a few patients in early clinical trials.

12. Most **tricyclics** have a high first-pass clearance by the liver, and so lower starting doses are necessary. Increased sedation with tricyclics is likely to be due to decreased metabolism, e.g. **amitriptyline** plasma levels may be doubled or tripled in patients with cirrhosis and should be avoided. Increased blood levels may also occur with reduced plasma protein-binding if albumin levels are lower, as protein-binding is high with many tricyclics. Particular care is obviously needed if albumin levels are low. SSRIs such as paroxetine would appear to be easier to use than tricyclics in liver disease. Cholestatic jaundice has occasionally been noted with tricyclics. **Lofepramine** is contraindicated in severe liver disease.

13. **Trazodone** should be used with care in severe hepatic impairment, as hepatoxicity has been reported (n = 1, Rettman and McClintock, *Ann Pharmacother* 2001;**35**:1559–61).

14. **Reboxetine's** half-life and plasma levels appear to rise in severe hepatic insufficiency and dose adjustment may be necessary. A starting dose of 2mg BD is recommended (n = 12, Tran et al, *Clin Drug Invest* 2000;**19**:473–7). No problems are expected with **agomelatine**.

15. **MAOIs** are hepatotoxic and may precipitate coma. Patients may also be more sensitive to side-effects. If essential, start with a low dose, increase gradually and observe carefully. **Isocarboxazid** is contraindicated in any degree of impaired hepatic function.

16. **Moclobemide's** clearance can be reduced and half-life increased in cirrhosis and so doses should be reduced by 25–33% to avoid accumulation (Stoeckel et al, *Acta Psychiatr Scand* 1990;**360**[Suppl]:94–7). There are no apparent

problems with **mianserin** and **tryptophan**. St John's wort levels may rise in moderate cirrhosis, but absorption is decreased in mild cirrhosis (n = 16, Johne et al, Clin Pharmacol Ther 2002;**71**:P95). Hepatotoxicity has been reported (n = 1, Domínguez Jiménez et al, Gastroenterol Hepatol 2007;**30**:54–5).

3.6.3 ANXIOLYTICS AND HYPNOTICS

17. The metabolism of **diazepam** and **chlordiazepoxide** is impaired in liver disease. The half-lives of the metabolites desmethylchlordiazepoxide and demoxepam are reported to be prolonged to up to 346 hours and 150 hours respectively (n = 1, Barton et al, Med Tox Adv Drug Exp 1989;**4**:73–6) which may induce coma, and may be detectable two months after stopping treatment in patients with hepatic encephalopathy (Meier et al, Gastroenterology, 1991;**101**:274–5). Impaired metabolism has been reported with **alprazolam**, **clobazam** and **midazolam** (significantly impaired in cirrhosis, as it is metabolised by at least three different P450 enzymes, Wandel et al, Br J Anaesthesia 1994;**73**:658–61). The metabolism of **lorazepam**, **temazepam** and **oxazepam** is unchanged and in low dose these are probably the benzodiazepines of choice (reviewed by Peppers, Pharmacotherapy 1996;**16**:49–58).

18. **Buspirone** plasma levels are higher in patients with hepatic failure, with a good correlation between steady-state buspirone levels and serum albumin (open, Barbhaiya et al, Eur J Clin Pharmacol 1994;**46**:41–7). Caution is recommended with a history of hepatic impairment and it should not be used in severe hepatic disease.

19. Elimination of **zopiclone** can be reduced with hepatic dysfunction, producing enhanced adverse effects (n = 17, open, Parker and Roberts, Br J Clin Pharmacol 1983;**16**:259). A lower dose of 3.75 mg to 7.5 mg (but no higher) can be used with caution in hepatic disease. Plasma protein binding of **zolpidem** is reduced in hepatic impairment (n = 42, open, Pacifici, Int J Clin Pharmacol Ther Toxicol 1988;**26**:439–43) and it is contraindicated in severe hepatic insufficiency. Reduced doses are recommended in cirrhosis and other hepatic impairment (where half-life may rise to 10 hours). Hepatoxicity has been reported (n = 1, Karsenti et al, Br Med J 1999;**318**:1179). **Zaleplon** is contraindicated in severe hepatic insufficiency and

the dose reduced to 5 mg in mild-to-moderate hepatic impairment.

20. **Propranolol**'s metabolism is impaired in decompensated liver disease and by portal systemic shunting. High doses are potentially toxic and so reduced oral doses are needed. Propranolol may increase the risk of developing hepatic encephalopathy.

21. **Clomethiazole** clearance is reduced by 50% in moderate-to-severe heptic impairment, but with sedation not significantly enhanced in the majority (n = 24, Centerholt et al, Eur J Clin Pharmacol 2003;**59**:1117–22). In severe liver disease a ten-fold increase can occur, so reduce oral doses, e.g. a third of normal, and note that sedation can mask the onset of hepatic coma. **Chloral hydrate** is contraindicated in marked hepatic impairment. No problems are expected with **melatonin** or **ramelteon**.

3.6.4 ANTICONVULSANTS

Review: optimising anticonvulsants in hepatic dysfunction (Lalerda et al, Neurology 2006;**67**[12 Suppl 4]: S28–33).

22. Serious problems with **carbamazepine** are rare, but jaundice, hepatitis and liver function disorders have been reported, and so use should be with caution. Although **oxcarbazepine** is rapidly and extensively metabolised, no dose adjustments are generally needed in mild-to-moderate hepatic impairment. It has not been studied in severe hepatic impairment.

23. **Valproate** is contraindicated in active liver disease, as it can be hepatotoxic and liver failure can occur in about one in 10000 cases. The risk is higher early on in therapy and lessens after a couple of months (review by Eadie et al, Med Tox 1988;**3**:85–106). Electron-microscopy shows lipid droplets and a scarcity of cytoplasmic cells and normal mitochondria have been reported (n = 1, Caparros-Lefebvre et al, Lancet 1993;**341**:1604). Hepatotoxicity occurs mostly in children and presents as worsening epilepsy, drowsiness and with biochemical and/or clinical evidence of liver failure. Some fatal cases have been reported. Care needs to be taken if valproate is used in children, especially if used with other anticonvulsants. Valproate use may be possible in patients with hepatitis C, provided ALT is closely monitored (n = 564, Felker et al, Am J Psychiatry 2003;**160**:174–8).

24. **Phenytoin** is highly protein bound and extensively metabolised and so accumulation and toxicity may occur in severe liver disease. Use reduced doses and monitor for toxicity. In uraemia, protein-binding may be reduced but active/free levels remain unchanged so therapeutic control may be possible at plasma levels below the usual range. Severe cardiovascular ADRs have been reported with **fosphenytoin** IV (see 3.2.4), and a reduction in loading dose and/or infusion rate by 10–25% is recommended in hepatic impairment.

25. Increased cerebral sensitivity and impaired **barbiturate** metabolism may precipitate coma.

26. **Gabapentin** is virtually unmetabolised and so dose adjustments are unnecessary. No adjustment to initial and maintenance doses of **lamotrigine** is necessary for Child-Pugh grade A but should be reduced by 50% in moderate (Child-Pugh grade B) hepatic impairment, and by 75% in severe (Child-Pugh grade C) impairment (n = 36, Marcellin et al, Br J Clin Pharmacol 2001; **51**:410–4).

27.* No dose adjustment is needed with **lacosamide** in mild-to-moderate hepatic impairment, but there is no information on use in severe hepatic impairment (SPC). No dose adjustment of **levetiracetam** is necessary in Child-Pugh grade A and B, but in grade C start with half the normal dose as total clearance is reduced by about 57% (n = 16, Brockmoller et al, Clin Pharmacol Ther 2005; **77**:29–41). However, levetiracetam (dose 250 mg/d titrated to tolerance and response) was effective and produced no worsening of LFTs in epileptics with liver disease (n = 14 [c = 10], open, 3/12, Bilo et al, Clin Neuropharmacol 2008; **31**:221–5). No dose adjustments are necessary for **pregabalin** in hepatic impairment. No information is available for **rufinamide** but the UK SPC recommends slower dose titration in mild-to-moderate hepatic impairment and to avoid severe hepatic impairment. **Tiagabine** is metabolised by the liver. Initial doses in mild-to-moderate hepatic impairment should be lower, and so use in severe hepatic impairment is not recommended (n = 13, open, 8/7, Lau et al, Epilepsia 1997; **38**:445–51). **Topiramate** is not extensively metabolised and about 60% is excreted unchanged via the kidneys. In moderate-to-severe liver disease, clearance is reduced by about 26%, although the resultant changes in plasma levels have been considered clinically insignificant by the

manufacturers. **Vigabatrin** can cause decreased LFT levels but there is no evidence of hepatic toxicity. **Zonisamide** has not been studied in hepatic impairment so caution is needed.

28. The UK SPC for **ethosuximide** now requires extreme caution in impaired hepatic function. **Acetazolamide** should be used with caution. **Paraldehyde** elimination is slower in hepatic failure and so lower doses may be needed.

3.6.5 OTHERS

29. **Donepezil** 5 mg/d can be safely given in mild-to-moderate (Child-Pugh grade A or B) hepatic impairment (n = 35 [c = 32], Reyes et al, Br J Clin Pharmacol 2004; **58**[Suppl 1]:9–17, MS), and a 5 mg single-dose study indicated that compromised hepatic function did not significantly alter its kinetics (n = 20, Tiseo et al, Br J Clin Pharmacol 1998; **46**[Suppl 1]:51–5). **Rivastigmine** is contraindicated in severe liver impairment. **Galantamine** is not affected by mild hepatic impairment but clearance is reduced by 23% in moderate impairment and so care is necessary in moderate-to-severe impairment (n = 25, open, Zhao et al, J Clin Pharmacol 2002; **42**:428–36). Start with 4 mg/d, increasing slowly to a maximum of 8 mg BD. In severe impairment (Child-Pugh grade C), galantamine is contraindicated (due to current lack of safety data). There is no data on **memantine** in hepatic impairment but since it is metabolised only to a minor extent to inactive metabolites, mild-to-moderate hepatic impairment is unlikely to have a significant effect.

30. All the literature for the **anticholinergics** urges some caution in hepatic disease.

31. The literature for **disulfiram** recommends caution in liver disease. Although some evidence of further raised LFTs was noted, an open trial showed disulfiram was safe in patients with elevated LFTs and/or evidence of hepatitis C virus, provided LFTs were monitored regularly (n = 57, Saxon et al, J Clin Psych 1998; **59**:313–6). The literature for **acamprosate** states that use in severe hepatic failure (Child-Pugh grade C) is a contraindication, but the pharmacokinetics are not altered in mild-to-moderate hepatic dysfunction and this is only an SPC caution.

32. There are no problems with **lithium** in liver disease.

33. **Modafinil's** maximum dose of 400 mg/d should only be used in the absence of hepatic impairment. The starting dose of **sodium oxybate** should be halved in hepatic impairment as the elimination half-life is increased (UK SPC).

34. There is no data on **methylphenidate**. The UK SPC recommends possible **atomoxetine** dose modification in hepatic impairment and rare (one in 50 000) cases have been reported of severe acute hepatitis with markedly elevated hepatic enzymes and bilirubin (MHRA warning).

35. **Bupropion** is extensively metabolised and there are rare reports of abnormal LFTs, liver damage and hepatotoxicity, with some metabolite half-lives prolonged in cirrhosis.

Reduced initial doses and close monitoring is required, as a prolonged half-life has been reported in hepatic failure (n = 16, open, DeVane et al, J Clin Psychopharmacol 1990; **10**:328–32).

36. Cases of QT interval prolongation and torsades de pointes have been reported during treatment with **methadone** (particularly at doses > 100 mg/d) and liver disease (a risk factor for prolonged QTc) is a UK SPC caution. **Buprenorphine** is primarily metabolised by glucuronidation (Tegeder et al, Clin Pharmacokinet 1999; **37**:17–40) and so should have a low risk in mild-to-moderate hepatic impairment, although it is contraindicated in severe hepatic insufficiency as this may, in itself, possibly be associated with hepatic events (UK SPC).

3.7 OLD AGE

	LOWER RISK	MODERATE RISK	HIGHER RISK
Antipsychotics	Amisulpride[5] Aripiprazole[2] Paliperidone[1] Risperidone[1] Sulpiride[5] Ziprasidone[2]	Asenapine[2] Butyrophenones[6] Olanzapine[2] Quetiapine[2] Thioxanthenes[4]	Clozapine[3] Phenothiazines[7] Pimozide[8] Zotepine[2]
Antidepressants	Agomelatine[14] Duloxetine[10] Lofepramine[12] Mirtazapine[11] Moclobemide[16] SSRIs[9] Tryptophan[16] Venlafaxine[10]	Flupentixol[4] MAOIs[15] Mianserin[16] Nortriptyline[12] Reboxetine[14] Trazodone[13]	Tricyclics[12]
Anxiolytics and hynpotics	Alprazolam[17] Buspirone[18] Clobazam[17] Lorazepam[17] Melatonin[21] Oxazepam[17] Oxprenolol[20] Ramelteon[21] Zaleplon[19] Zopiclone[19]	Clomethiazole[21] Benzodiazepines, short-acting[17] Flunitrazepam[17] Flurazepam[17] Propranolol[20] Temazepam[17] Zolpidem[19]	Benzodiazepines, long-acting[17]
Anticonvulsants	Clobazam[17] Rufinamide[27] Tiagabine[27]	Barbiturates[25] Carbamazepine[22] Clonazepam[17] Gabapentin[26] Lamotrigine[26] Levetiracetam[27] Oxcarbazepine[22] Piracetam?[27] Pregabalin[27] Topiramate[27] Valproate[23]	Acetazolamide[28] Benzodiazepines (most)[17] Fosphenytoin[24] Paraldehyde[28] Phenytoin[24] Vigabatrin[27]
Others	Anticholinesterases[29] Bupropion[35] Memantine[29] Modafinil[33] Sodium oxybate [33]	Buprenorphine[36] Lithium[32] Methadone[36]	Acamprosate?[31] Anticholinergics[30] Methlyphenidate[34]

GENERAL PRINCIPLES FOR PRESCRIBING IN OLD AGE (adapted from *Maudsley Guidelines*)

1. Increased sensitivity to drugs occurs due to age-related changes in pharmacokinetics (ADME and protein binding) and pharmacodynamics (e.g. neuronal changes, and receptor binding). The over 70s have about twice as many ADRs as under 50s, e.g. postural hypotension, enhanced sedation with and increased sensitivity to anticholinergic side-effects (see 8).

2. Hepatic changes (e.g. reduced metabolism) and reduced renal clearance will affect many drugs.

3. The lowest effective dose should be used (so 'start low and go slow'), avoid polypharmacy and monitor effects (both positive and negative) regularly and frequently.

4. Avoid drugs with sedative and hypotensive effects, which can increase the under-rated risks of falls. A meta-analysis concluded that psychotropics are associated with a small increase in falls (s = 40, Leipzig et al, J Am Geriatr Soc 1999;**47**:30–9; reviewed by Shorr, EBMH 1999; **2**:95).

5. Use drugs only when necessary, decide a treatment aim, keep therapy simple, use the smallest effective doses and discontinue gradually if no apparent benefit can be seen, as accumulation of a drug can lead to the subtle and insidious development of side-effects.

6. Most drugs are highly lipophilic and an increased fat to lean body mass ratio, in addition to decreased metabolism and excretion, means that half-lives usually increase.

7. Consider other factors, e.g. potential poor compliance due to social or physical reasons, or use of OTC medicines.

8.* Avoid drugs with anticholinergic effects, as these increase the risk of cognitive decline and dementia (HR=1.65), although discontinuing decreases the risk (n = 6912, four years, Carrière et al, Arch Intern Med 2009;**169**:1317–24). Thus, avoid tricyclics, phenothiazines and anticholinergics.

9.* Monitor more carefully with pre-existing diabetes as in people aged > 66 initiating *any* antipsychotic was associated with increased risk of hospitalisation for hyperglycaemia (n = 13817, Lipscombe et al, Arch Int Med 2009;**169**:1282–9).

Review: geriatric psychopharmacology (Turnheim, Exp Gerontol 2003;**38**:843–53).

3.7.1 ANTIPSYCHOTICS *

The EMEA 2008 review of antipsychotics in elderly people with dementia concludes that:
- conventional antipsychotics are associated with excess mortality
- conventional antipsychotics are associated with excess mortality compared to atypicals
- no conclusion can be drawn on individual antipsychotics
- there is no known mechanism of cause.

The evidence for antipsychotics in old age includes:
- a Medicaid analysis was unable to show that "atypicals" (including risperidone) were more likely to cause CVEs than haloperidol or benzodiazepines (n = 8 million, Finkel et al, Int Psychogeriatr 2005;**17**;617–29)
- a prospective nursing home study failed to show that antipsychotics increased mortality in dementia (n = 273, 12/12, Suh et al, Int Psychogeriatr 2005;**17**:429–41)
- a large study showed the risk of death (all causes) in elderly people taking conventional antipsychotics is comparable to and possibly higher than that associated with atypicals (n = 37241, 180/7, Schneeweiss et al, CMAJ 2007;**176**:627–32).

The case against antipsychotics in the elderly:
- there is an increased risk of femur fracture in elderly institutionalised patients (n = 7393, Liperoti et al, J Clin Psychiatry 2007;**68**:929–34) and a 60% increased risk of pneumonia (n = 22944, Knol et al, J Am Geriatr Soc 2008; **56**:661–6)
- a one-year study showed that in patients with AD in residential care treated with antipsychotics, those that carried on had a survival probability of 70% compared to 77% in the switch-to-placebo group, clinically significant. In the follow-on study, the two-year survival was 46% vs 71%, and three-year was 30% vs 59%, even more marked (n = 128, RCT, p/c, 12/12, Ballard et al, Lancet Neurol 2009;**8**:151–7)
- the **haloperidol** SPC now states that in elderly people with dementia-related psychosis, the risk of death with atypicals is 1.6–1.7 times higher than with placebo (4.5% vs 2.6%) vs placebo, mostly cardiovascular or infections (s = 17, mean, 10/52, UK SPC).

Antipsychotics can relieve psychotic symptoms in older adults but pre-treatment assessment, repeated every 3–6 months, is recommended to detect common side-effects such as postural hypotension, anticholinergic effects and Parkinsonism. Single daily doses are usually appropriate once stable (as, indeed, they are in younger adults). Doses should be reviewed regularly, and a periodic reduction in dose (e.g. by 10–25% every four weeks) for some patients may be indicated.

Reviews: * atypicals in elderly (Bouman and Pinner, *Adv Psychiatr Treat* 2002;**8**:49–58), atypicals in the elderly (Burke and Tariot, *Expert Opin Pharmacother* 2009;**10**:2407–14), psychosis in the elderly with Parkinsonism (Hasnain et al, *Am J Med* 2009;**122**:614–22).

1. **Risperidone** is partially metabolised to an active metabolite and so lower doses may be needed only if hepatic impairment is present (see 3.6.1). Significant age-related differences have been noted, with higher plasma levels in patients over 40 years, and with a 30% increase per decade of life (n = 129, Aichhorn et al, *J Psychopharmacol* 2005;**19**:395–401). Risperidone is licensed for BPSD (see *Chapter 1* for dose and details). The same would apply to **paliperidone** but any renal impairment might require lower doses (see 3.9.1.1).

2.* In older adults with bipolar disorder, **aripiprazole** appears to be fairly well tolerated and have some efficacy (n = 20, open, 12/52, Sajatovic et al, *J Clin Psychiatry* 2008;**69**:41–6) and no dose adjustments are necessary in the elderly. There is a class warning for **asenapine** in dementia-related psychosis (US PI), and it is likely to cause postural hypotension in the elderly as plasma levels may be 30–40% higher than younger adults. The UK CSM recommends not using **olanzapine** in elderly demented people with behavioural problems, due to an increased risk of stroke (2% vs 1% on placebo), although the absolute risk is low, and the alternatives are not risk-free. The restriction does not apply to elderly demented people *without* behavioural problems, where a lower starting dose of 5 mg/d may be appropriate as the mean elimination half-life is 50% longer and clearance slightly reduced in otherwise healthy elderly patients. Periodic blood pressure monitoring is recommended and there may be a slightly higher risk of seizures in people

over 65. Transient sedation and somnolence were more marked in the elderly in pre-marketing trials. **Olanzapine pamoate** is not recommended for use in the elderly unless oral olanzapine has been used uneventfully before (SPC), and should not be used for people over 75. The UK SPC for **quetiapine** has been updated with a warning that quetiapine is not approved for the treatment of patients with dementia-related psychosis due to an approximately three-fold increased risk of cerebrovascular adverse events seen in RCTs with some antipsychotics in the dementia population. The mean clearance in elderly patients is 30–50% lower than healthy adults, so the starting dose should be 25 mg/d, with dose increments of 25–50 mg/d. Somnolence (32%), dizziness (13%) and postural hypotension (13%) are the most common side-effects in old age. Quetiapine (mean 200 mg/d, range 50–800 mg/d) can be effective and safe in elderly in-patients, but there is a wide and diagnosis-dependent (e.g. higher in functional psychosis) dosing range (n = 100 [c = 91], Yang et al, *J Psychopharmacol* 2005;**19**:661–6). **Zotepine** levels may be 2–3 times higher in elderly patients, so start at 25 mg BD up to a maximum of 75 mg BD. There are no dose changes needed for **ziprasidone**.

3.* **Clozapine** may be safe, reasonably well-tolerated (with slower dose titration) and effective in the elderly (n = 133, Barak et al, *Compr Psychiatry* 1999;**40**:320–5) at doses as low as 50–100 mg, with 6.25–50 mg/d suggested as the optimal dosage (review by Hoeh et al, *J Geriatr Psychiatry Neurol* 2003;**16**:213–8). There may be an increased incidence of agranulocytosis, so great care should be taken (review by Gareri et al, *Expert Opin Drug Saf* 2008;**7**:525–38).

4. **Zuclopenthixol** and **flupentixol** should be used with caution in renal disease. The UK SPC now recommends caution for flupentixol in people with risk factors for stroke, and lower dose increases and maximum (1.5 mg) may be needed due to altered kinetics (review: Jann et al, *Clin Pharmacokinet* 1985;**10**:315–33).

5.* Plasma levels for **amisulpride** in the elderly are similar to adults but the elderly may respond to lower plasma levels (n = 395, Müller et al, *J Psychopharmacol* 2009;**23**:278–86). Single doses of **sulpiride** are well tolerated and show a similar pharmacokinetic profile in healthy elderly and young subjects (n = 20, open, Hamon-Vilcot et *al, Eur J Clin Pharmacol* 1998;**54**:405–9), although renal function may have an effect.

6.* The **haloperidol** SPC now states that in elderly people with dementia-related psychosis, the risk of death with atypicals is 1.6-1.7 times higher than with placebo (4.5% vs 2.6%) vs placebo, mostly cardiovascular or infections (s = 17, mean, 10/52, UK SPC). Although the causes of death were varied, most of the deaths appeared to be either cardiovascular (e.g. heart failure, sudden death) or infections (e.g. pneumonia). An increased severity of side-effects including EPSE, sedation, hypotension and respiratory depression may occur and so lower starting doses are indicated.

7. It is generally recommended that 33–50% of the adult dose of **phenothiazines** should be used for elderly patients, who are more susceptible to Parkinsonian side-effects (n = 120, open, Caligiuri et al, J Clin Psychopharmacol 1999; **19**:322–8), and which are often then harder to manage. **Chlorpromazine** should be avoided. **Levomepromazine** is not recommended for use in people over 50 unless the risk of hypotension has been assessed.

8. Half the usual starting dose of **pimozide** should be used.

3.7.2 ANTIDEPRESSANTS *

Depression increases mortality in the elderly with cardiac disease, so it should not be ignored, especially if long-standing and severe (n = 652, Geerlings et al, Psychol Med 2002;**32**:609–18). Drugs with anticholinergic side-effects may further harm an already compromised cholinergic system. SSRIs and tricyclics (but not other antidepressants) may increase the risk of non-vertebral fractures in the elderly, although the number of cases was very small (n = 7983, > 55yo [mean 77yo], Ziere et al, J Clin Psychopharmacol 2008;**28**:411–7; comment by Diem, EBMH 2009; **12**:26). To put it into perspective, one review states that the magnitude of the risk of falling with an antidepressant is about the same as the excess risk found in people with untreated depression (Darowski et al, Drugs Aging 2009;**26**:381–94).

9.* **SSRIs** have obvious advantages over other antidepressants in the elderly but have some risks, including hyponatraemia, weight loss (review: Herrmann, Can J Clin Pharmacol 2000;**7**:91–5) and increased risk of falls and osteoporotic fractures in

the over 50s (n = 5008, 137 on SSRIs, Richards et al, Arch Int Med 2007;**167**:188–94). A prolonged **citalopram** half-life (up to 3.8 days) and raised steady-state plasma levels may be due to reduced metabolism, with side-effects more prevalent in the elderly, particularly bradycardia, nausea, sweating and headache (n = 1344, > 6/52, Barak et al, Prog Neuropsychopharmacol Biol Psychiatry 2003;**27**:545–8). Dose reduction (by up to 50%) has been suggested, but normal adult doses have been used in many studies with no apparent problem. However, in one study in people over 75, citalopram 10–40mg/d was no more effective than placebo, although there was huge inter-individual variation (n = 174, RCT, p/c, 8/52, Roose et al, Am J Psychiatry 2004;**161**:2050–9). For **escitalopram**, an initial dose of 5mg daily for the first two weeks of treatment is recommended, increasing to 10mg/d (UK SPC). It is well-tolerated in older adults (mean 68 years), albeit not superior to placebo (n = 268 [c = 205], RCT, d/b, p/c, 12/52, Bose and Gandhi, Am J Geriatr Psychiatry 2008; **16**:14–20), although in responders it reduces relapse (n = 225 [c = 171], open extension, one year, Kasper et al, Neuropsychobiology 2006; **54**:152–9). Escitalopram was also modestly effective for GAD in older people, but not significantly (n = 177 [c = 170], RCT, p/c, d/b, 12/52, Lenze et al, JAMA 2009;**301**:295–303). The half-life of **fluoxetine** appears not to be significantly different in the elderly. In an open study of depressed and physically ill hospitalised elderly patients with multiple pathology and polypharmacy, fluoxetine was claimed to be a safe and effective antidepressant in this difficult to treat cohort (n = 20, open, Evans and Lye, J Clin Exp Gerontol 1992;**14**:297–307). No pharmacokinetic differences have been seen with **fluvoxamine** in the elderly and so no dose alterations are necessary and 200mg/d seems as equally well-tolerated and effective in old age depression as sertraline 150mg/d (n = 93, RCT, d/b, 7/52, Rossini et al, J Clin Psychopharmacol 2005;**25**:471–5). Initially, lower doses of 10mg/d are recommended for **paroxetine**, as blood levels with 20mg/d in the elderly can be similar to those of 30mg/d in younger people (review in old age Holliday and Plosker, Drugs Aging 1993;**3**:278–99). **Sertraline's** clearance may be slightly reduced and half-life increased in elderly volunteers, but this does not seem to warrant dosage adjustment (n = 44, open,

30/7, Ronfeld et al, Clin Pharmacokin 1997;**32**[Suppl 1]:S22–S30), and it seems safe and effective in the elderly even with significant comorbid medical status (n = 752, RCT, d/b, p/c, 8/52, Sheikh et al, J Am Geriatr Soc 2004;**52**:86–92; review by Kurzthaler and Fleischhacker, EBMH 2004;**7**:82).

10.* **Venlafaxine** clearance is reduced by about 15% in the elderly, probably due to reduced renal function, but dosage adjustment is not generally considered necessary (Anon, J Clin Psychiatry 1993;**54**:119–26). However, venlafaxine (up to 150 mg/d) may be less well tolerated and possibly less safe than sertraline (up to 100 mg/d) in elderly frail populations (n = 32, RCT, d/b, Oslin et al, J Clin Psychiatry 2003;**64**:875–82; comment by Schneider, EBMH 2004;**7**:47). Postural hypotension may be more common. **Duloxetine's** half-life is about 25% longer in the elderly, but no dose adjustment is necessary and 60 mg/d was shown to have no adverse effects on cognition and depression in elderly (65–89) patients (n = 311, RCT, d/b, p/c, Wise et al, Int J Clin Pract 2007;**61**:1283–93). A pooled analysis of the sub-set of people over 65 taking part in larger trials for GAD showed duloxetine 60–120 mg/d to be effective but with a high discontinuation rate due to ADRs (s = 4, n = 73, RCT, d/b, p/c, < 10/52, Davidson et al, Hum Psychopharmacol 2008;**23**:519–26).

11. **Mirtazapine** dosage is the same in the elderly as younger adults, although the manufacturers recommend care with dosage increments, e.g. 15–45 mg/d has equivalent efficacy to sub-therapeutic amitriptyline 30–90 mg/d, but with relatively fewer cardiac effects (n = 115, d/b, Hoyberg et al, Acta Psychiatr Scand 1996;**93**:184–90). It appears to be slightly quicker acting and better tolerated than paroxetine in elderly depressed patients (n = 255, RCT, d/b, 8+16/52, Schatzberg et al, Am J Geriatr Psychiatry 2002;**10**:541–50).

12. Reduced initial doses of **tricyclics** are recommended, with perhaps slightly lower final doses, depending upon tolerance, as cognitive, anticholinergic and central effects are enhanced in the elderly. **Clomipramine** is as well-tolerated in patients 56–70 years old as in younger adults, although postural hypotension and anticholinergic side-effects are more common (n = 150, Stage et al, Acta Psychiatr Scand 2002;**105**:55–9). Single night-time doses of **dosulepin** have been used in the elderly with no increase in side-effects.

Higher serum levels occur with standard doses of **imipramine** (reviewed by Hicks et al, J Clin Psychiatry 1981;**42**:374–85) with reduced clearance and doubled half-life (open, Benetello et al, Int J Clin Pharmacol Res 1990;**10**:191–5). Elderly patients may respond to lower doses of **lofepramine** but in depressed elderly in-patients, low dose lofepramine (70 mg/d) appears no better than placebo, indicating that full, or at least higher, doses are necessary (n = 63. 4/52, Tan et al, Br J Clin Pharmacol 1994;**37**:321–4). **Nortriptyline** kinetics appear the same in the elderly as the young, although individual variation is high and the elderly may respond to lower doses (Kanba et al, Prog Neuropsychopharmacol Biol Psychiatry 1992;**16**:301–9). ECG changes may occur so care is needed in cardiovascular disease.

13. Single daily dosing of **trazodone** (except when used as a hypnotic) may not be appropriate in the elderly. 150 mg/d may be the optimum dose in the elderly, as higher plasma levels (n = 97, Prapotnik et al, Int J Clin Pharmacol Ther 2004;**42**:120–4) and a longer half-life occur in the elderly.

14. The incidence of side-effects with **reboxetine** is no greater in the elderly than in younger people, although the half-life may be doubled (Holm and Spencer, CNS Drugs 1999;**12**:65–83) and peak plasma levels are also over twice that in younger people (n = 12, Bergmann et al, Eur J Drug Metab Pharmacokinet 2000;**25**:195–8). The starting dose should probably be 2 mg BD. A delayed lowering of potassium levels and some treatment-emergent tachycardia has been reported. Frail elderly may need dose reductions. The UK SPC does not recommend use in the elderly, due to lack of safety data rather than the presence of negative data. No problems are expected with **agomelatine**.

15. **MAOIs** are often considered as more toxic in the elderly, mainly due to postural hypotension and dizziness, but they can be highly effective in resistant depression in the elderly (review by Volz and Gleiter, Drugs Aging 1998;**13**:341–55).

16. **Moclobemide** is considered to be safe, effective and having a seemingly beneficial effect on a range of cognitive functions (n = 694, d/b, p/c, Roth et al, Br J Psychiatry 1996;**168**:149–57). **Mianserin** elimination is highly variable and often prolonged in the elderly (n = 27, open, Begg et al, Br J Clin Pharmacol 1989;**27**:445–51). There are no apparent problems with **tryptophan**.

3.7.3 ANXIOLYTICS AND HYPNOTICS

A meta-analysis showed that improvements in sleep with the use of sedatives are significant in the elderly, albeit of small magnitude, but that ADRs and the risk of falls is clinically relevant (s = 24, n = 2417, RCT, Glass et al, Br Med J 2005; **331**:1169).

Review: management of insomnia in elderly (Bain, Am J Geriatr Pharmacother 2006;**4**:168–92).

17. All **benzodiazepines** should be used with care in the elderly, as side-effects are likely to be enhanced, e.g. sedation, disturbances in gait, daytime drowsiness, cognitive impairment, hypotension, memory impairment and reduced psychomotor performance. Half-lives are generally lengthened, sometimes only in men, although there is considerable interpatient variability. Prolonged half-lives in the elderly have been reported with **clonazepam, clobazam, flunitrazepam, nitraze-pam, flurazepam, chlordiazepoxide, clorazepate, bromazepam, diazepam** and **midazolam**. **Temazepam** is relatively safe over 8/52 and CBT may slightly improve the response (n = 60, RCT, 8/52, Morin et al, Hum Psychopharmacol 2003;**18**:75–82). Normal adult doses of **oxazepam** can be used as there are apparently no clinically significant pharmacokinetic changes in the elderly (n = 17, RCT, c/o, Dreyfuss et al, J Clin Psychiatry 1986;**47**:511–4). If used as a hypnotic, **lorazepam** doses should probably be slightly reduced. **Loprazolam** appears well-tolerated in the elderly, with a half-life similar to young adults, although peak levels are prolonged (n = 12, Dorling and Hindmarsh, Drugs Exp Clin Res 2001;**27**:151–9).

18. There do not appear to be any significant changes in the pharmacokinetics of **buspirone** in the elderly and so dose adjustments are not considered necessary (n = 48, open, Gammans et al, J Clin Pharmacol 1989;**29**:72–8).

19. Normal adult doses of **zopiclone** can be used (Goa and Heel, Drugs 1986;**32**:48–65). **Zolpidem** 5 mg is an effective hypnotic in the elderly, with no consistent memory or performance effects, or daytime drowsiness (n = 221, Roger and Attali, Clin Therap 1993;**15**:127–36), but doses of 10 mg or above slightly reduce REM sleep (n = 30, Scharf et al, J Clin Psychiatry 1991;**52**:77–83). Zolpidem causes less cognitive, memory and equilibrium adverse effects then zopiclone and lormetazepam and should be the preferred

hypnotic in the elderly (n = 48, RCT, d/b, p/c, c/o, Allain et al, Eur J Clin Pharmacol 2003;**59**:179–88). There appears to be no problem with **zaleplon** in the elderly.

20. Increased **propranolol** side-effects have been reported in the elderly and so reduced initial doses are generally recommended. No dose reduction is necessary for **oxprenolol**.

21. **Clomethiazole** doses should be reduced, as the half-life can be at least doubled and plasma levels up to five times normal can occur (Dehlin, Acta Psychiatr Scand 1986;**73**[Suppl 329]:112–5). No problems are expected with **melatonin** or **ramelteon**.

3.7.4 ANTICONVULSANTS

For anticonvulsants, it is best to avoid renally excreted drugs (e.g. **gabapentin**), as the renal excretion of some drugs may be significantly reduced in the elderly compared with younger people. Hepatically metabolised drugs, e.g. **carba-mazepine** and **lamotrigine** are not influenced by age and are to be preferred.

Reviews: management of epilepsy in old age (Brodie et al, Lancet Neurol 2009;**8**:1019–30; Marasco and Ramsay, Consult Pharm 2009;**24** (Suppl A):17–22).

22.* No significant changes have been shown with **carbamazepine** in the elderly, including ECG (n = 108 [c = 75], RCT, d/b, 40/52, Saetre et al, Epilepsia 2009;**50**:1841–9) and so dose requirements are likely to be the same, although a population-based pharmacokinetic model suggested doses may need to be lower (n = 171, Bondareva et al, J Clin Pharm Ther 2006;**31**:211–21). Although the AUC with **oxcarbazepine** may be 30–60% higher in the elderly, tolerability is comparable to that in adults (n = 52 cf 1574 adults, Kutluay et al, Epilepsy Behav 2003;**4**:175–80). No dose recommendations exist, other than gradual dose titration (n = 48, van Heiningen et al, Clin Pharmacol Ther 1991;**50**:410–9), a lower dose if the patient has compromised renal function and monitoring as it may cause hyponatraemia (review by Sommer et al, Expert Opin Drug Saf 2007;**6**:133–45).

23. **Valproate's** half-life may be doubled in the elderly and an extensive study of elderly nursing home residents on stable regimens, concluded that valproate doses may need to be lower

(by around 25%) in women, but higher with concurrent carbamazepine or phenytoin and if the syrup is used (n = 146, Birnbaum et al, Ther Drug Monit 2007;**29**:571–5). CNS side-effects and nausea are correlated with total and unbound levels, and hence likely to be increased in older people (n = 6, s/b, Felix et al, J Clin Psychopharmacol 2003;**23**:471–8).

24. Reduced doses of **phenytoin** may be needed with the elderly, e.g. by about 20%. (n = 92, open, Bauer and Blouin, Clin Pharmacol 1982;**31**:301–4). Careful monitoring is necessary, especially in those with hypoalbuminaemia or renal disease, as these individuals may have an increased level of side-effects and risk of toxicity, including cardiac arrhythmias. It may be that reduced doses are only needed with monotherapy, as opposed to anticonvulsant polypharmacy (review by Bachmann and Belloto, Drugs Aging 1999;**15**:235–50). Severe cardiovascular ADRs have been reported with **fosphenytoin** IV (see 3.2), and a reduction in the loading dose and/or infusion rate by 10–25% in the elderly is recommended.

25. The half-lives of **phenobarbital** and **primidone** are longer in the elderly due to reduced metabolism and so reduced doses should be used.

26.* **Lamotrigine** is hepatically metabolised and this is influenced by genetic factors rather than age. An increased volume of distribution in the elderly has been shown to increase the half-life of lamotrigine, thus increasing the chance of side-effects, and so reduced doses may be needed. When used in elderly patients with newly diagnosed epilepsy and no pre-existing AV conduction defects, lamotrigine had no significant effects on the ECG (n = 108 [c = 75], RCT, d/b, 40/52, Saetre et al, Epilepsia 2009;**50**:1841–9). In older epileptics suffering ADRs from existing AEDs, either adding lamotrigine or switching to lamotrigine was associated with improved tolerability and effectiveness, especially as monotherapy (n = 62, open, Evans et al, Am J Geriatr Pharmacother 2007;**5**:112–9). **Gabapentin** clearance is reduced in old age, probably via reduced renal clearance, although it seems to cause less cognitive impairment than carbamazepine in healthy adults (n = 34, RCT, c/o, Martin et al, Epilepsia 2001;**42**:764–71) but may cause ataxia (review by Sommer et al, Expert Opin Drug Saf 2007;**6**:133–45). It has been successful and well-tolerated as add-on therapy for neuroleptics or

valproate in geriatric mania (n = 7, open, Sethi et al, J Geriatr Psychiatry Neurol 2003;**16**:117–20).

27.* No dose reduction is needed with **lacosamide** in old age, although the AUC may be increased by 30–50%, but experience is limited (SPC). **Levetiracetam** seems well-tolerated in the elderly, e.g. it has been successful in 72% patients with new-onset seizures in advanced Alzheimer's (n = 25 [c = 24], open, Belcastro et al, Eur J Neurol 2007;**14**:1176–8), with only headache and tremor occurring more frequently (n = 3352, Cramer et al, Epilepsy Res 2003;**56**:135–45). Older adults (55–88 years) may, however, require 40% lower doses than younger adults to achieve the same serum levels (n = 308, retrospective, one year, Hirsch et al, Epilepsia 2007;**48**:1351–9), especially in renal impairment (see 3.9.4). No age-related changes in pharmacokinetics have been detected with **topiramate**, although it may cause significant cognitive impairment (review by Sommer et al, Expert Opin Drug Saf 2007;**6**:133–45). The half-life of **piracetam** is extended in the elderly (n = 10, open, Platt et al, Arzneimittel Forschung 1985;**35**:533–5). Reduced **pregabalin** doses may be necessary due to decreased renal function (see 3.9.4) but seems safe and effective for anxiety in older people (mean 72 years) within two weeks (n = 273, RCT, d/b, p/c, 8/52, Montgomery et al, Br J Psychiatry 2008;**193**:389–94). Although evidence is limited for **rufinamide**, dose adjustments are not required in people over 65 (UK SPC). There is no need to adjust the dose of **tiagabine** on the basis of age, although slightly higher plasma levels may occur in the elderly (n = 24, Snel et al, J Clin Pharmacol 1997;**37**:1015–20). **Vigabatrin** is renally excreted and reduced doses are recommended for Ccr <60 ml/min and so should be avoided in the elderly.

28. Lower **acetazolamide** doses are indicated (n = 12, open, Chapron et al, J Clin Pharmacol 1989;**29**:348–53). Deaths have been reported in debilitated patients given only 8 ml **paraldehyde**, and so use with the utmost caution (Baratham and Tinckler, Med J Aust, 1964;**51**:877).

3.7.5 OTHERS

29. There are no specific problems with **donepezil** and **rivastigmine**, provided the dose titration guidelines are followed. **Galantamine** levels are about 30–40% higher in elderly patients

than healthy young individuals. **Memantine** has a usual maximum dose of 20 mg/d.

30. Confusion can be induced in the elderly by further compromising brain cholinergic activity. An initial low dose is recommended for **trihexyphenidyl** (SPC now says use with extreme caution in elderly) and **orphenadrine**. Clearance of **procyclidine** should be reduced in the elderly (UK SPC) and so BD dosing may be more appropriate than TDS dosing (n = 6, RCT, p/c, Whiteman et al, *Eur J Clin Pharmacol* 1985; **28**:73–8).

31. **Acamprosate** should not be used in the elderly (UK SPC), due more to a lack of data rather than specific reported problems.

32. Reduced **lithium** clearance occurs in the elderly through reduced renal function and increased volume of distribution (review by Sproule et al, *Drugs Aging* 2000; **16**:165–77), so doses should be reduced by as much as 50%. The elderly may also develop symptoms of lithium toxicity at standard therapeutic blood levels (Nakra and Grossberg, *J Geriatr Drug Ther* 1987; **2**:47–63), but lithium can be safely used in the elderly if monitored closely and frequently. Just to prove it, a study in octogenarians showed lithium can be well-tolerated provided serum levels and renal and thyroid function are monitored regularly (n = 12, Fahy and Lawlor, *Int J Geriatr Psychiatry* 2001; **16**:1000–3). Hypothyroidism can also occur.

33. In the elderly, a **modafinil** starting dose of 100 mg/d is recommended. **Sodium oxybate** may cause cognitive impairment so care might be needed (SPC).

34. There is no data for **methylphenidate**, but it has been used for depression in the elderly.

35. **Bupropion** can be effective and well-tolerated in the elderly (n = 100, RCT, Weihs et al, *J Clin Psychiatry* 2000; **61**:196–202), although accumulation and greater side-effects can occur.

36. Caution is recommended with repeated doses of **methadone,** but there are no recommendations for **buprenorphine**.

3.8 PREGNANCY

	LOWER RISK (FDA=A)	MODERATE RISK (FDA=B OR C)	HIGHER RISK (FDA=D OR X)
Antipsychotics		Aripiprazole[2] Butyrophenones[6] Clozapine[3] Olanzapine[2] Paliperidone[1] Phenothiazines[7] Quetiapine[2] Risperidone[1] Sulpiride[5] Thioxanthenes[4] Ziprasidone[2]	Zotepine[2]
Antidepressants	Flupentixol?[24] Tryptophan?[16]	Agomelatine[14] Duloxetine[10] MAOIs[15] Mianserin[16] Mirtazapine[11] Moclobemide[16] SSRIs (except paroxetine)[9] St John's wort[16] Trazodone[13] Tricyclics[12] Venlafaxine[10]	Paroxetine[9] Reboxetine[14]
Anxiolytics and hynpotics	Chloral[21] Clomethiazole[21] Melatonin[21] Zolpidem[19]	Beta-blockers[20] Buspirone[18] Chlordiazepoxide[17] Clonazepam[17] Oxazepam[17] Promethazine[21] Zaleplon[19] Zopiclone[19]	Alprazolam[17] Hydroxyzine[17] Lorazepam[17] Ramelteon[21] Temazepam[17]
Anticonvulsants		Acetazolamide[28] Clonazepam?[17] Gabapentin[26] Lamotrigine[26] Levetiracetam[27] Oxcarbazepine[22] Paraldehyde[28] Pregabalin?[27] Tiagabine[27]	Benzodiazepines[17] Carbamazepine[22] Ethosuximide[28] Fosphenytoin[24] Lacosamide[27] Phenobarbital[25] Phenytoin[24] Rufinamide[27] Topiramate[27] Valproate[23] Vigabatrin[27] Zonisamide[27]

Others		Acamprosate[31]	Lithium[32]
		Anticholinergics[30]	Methadone HD[34]
		Anticholinesterases[29]	
		Atomoxetine[35]	
		Buprenorphine[34]	
		Bupropion[36]	
		Dextroamfetamine[35]	
		Disulfiram[31]	
		Memantine[29]	
		Methylphenidate[35]	
		Modafinil[33]	
		Methadone LD[34]	
		Sodium oxybate[33]	

The **FDA** has established five categories to indicate a drug's potential for teratogenicity, and, where known, these classifications are noted in the text:

A Controlled studies in women fail to show a risk in the first trimester and the risk of fetal harm seems remote.

B Either animal tests do not show a risk but there are no human studies **or** animal studies show a risk but human studies have failed to show a risk to the fetus.

C Either animal studies show teratogenic or embryocidal effects but there are no controlled studies in humans **or** there are no studies in either animals or humans.

D Definite evidence of a risk to the fetus exists, but the benefits in certain circumstances (e.g. life-threatening situations) may make use acceptable.

X Fetal abnormalities have been shown in animals or humans or both and the risk outweighs any possible benefits.

The **Australian (ADEC) pregnancy category definitions** (in brief) are:

A Drug has been taken by a large number of pregnant women with no proven increase in malformations or other direct or indirect harmful effects on the fetus.

B1 Drug has been taken by a limited number of pregnant women with no proven increase in malformations or other direct or indirect harmful effects on the fetus. Animal studies have not shown evidence of fetal damage.

B2 As B1, but animal studies are inadequate or lacking, but other evidence shows no evidence of fetal damage.

B3 As B1, but animal studies have shown evidence of an increased occurrence of fetal damage of uncertain significance.

C Drugs that have caused or are suspected of causing an increase in fetal malformations or irreversible damage.

D As 'C' but also may be expected to cause an increase in fetal malformations or irreversible damage, and have adverse pharmacological effects.

X High risk of causing permanent damage so should not be used in pregnancy or where there is a possibility of pregnancy.

Where known, both the FDA and ADEC categories are quoted.

Further information should be sought on individual drugs to balance the risk-benefit ratio in a particular individual patient. The FDA and ADEC risk classification systems may not always be a reliable source of information (Addis *et al*, *Drug Saf* 2000;**23**:245–53).

Reproductive toxicity falls into five domains (Wisner *et al*, *Am J Psychiatry* 2000;**157**:1933–40):

1. Intrauterine fetal death/miscarriage.
2. Physical malformations.
3. Growth impairment.
4. Behavioural toxicity (post-birth).
5. Neonatal toxicity, e.g. withdrawal or direct adverse effects.

For the record, spontaneous major or gross malformations (usually defined as incompatible with life or requiring surgical correction) occur in

2–3% of pregnancies and spontaneous abortions in about 10–20% of clinically recognised pregnancies. In the first trimester, teratogenicity is the main drug risk, and growth retardation and neurological damage may occur in the second and third trimesters. After birth, drug withdrawal effects may occur. Although there are a few reports that pregnancy may protect against the risk of, e.g. bipolar disorder, other papers show an increased risk (reviewed by Viguera and Cohen, *Psychopharmacol Bull* 1998;**34**:339–46).

Assessing risk: Recent retrospective studies are more useful pointers to risk than the length of time a drug has been on the market or anecdotal case reports.

GENERAL PRINCIPLES FOR PRESCRIBING IN PREGNANCY (adapted from *Maudsley Guidelines*)

Planning for possible pregnancy provides time for informed decisions. In bipolar disorder, pregnancy and the postpartum periods can be considered as separate risk periods, and treatment plans may need to be different for each. See also an additional section under anticonvulsants (*3.8.4*).

Pre-conception

1. For planned conception, discuss the risks and benefits of discontinuing or continuing medication, e.g. relapse, teratogenicity, etc, the unpredictability of the pre-conceptual duration, and that no decision is risk-free. Avoiding all drugs during the first trimester is the ideal but may risk relapse. Other options include continuing at the lowest possible dose (or switching to a drug with the shortest possible half-life) until a positive pregnancy test, or continuing throughout pregnancy at the lowest viable dose.
2. Consider the risk of pregnancy even if not currently planned, e.g. carry out a pregnancy test before starting teratogenic drugs in a woman of child-bearing potential. As up to 50% of pregnancies are unplanned:
   - document the woman's birth control method
   - document the potential risks for exposure to drug(s) during pregnancy
   - encourage proper nutrition, exercise and vitamin supplementation

- note any other substances taken (e.g. excess caffeine, alcohol and natural products)
- educate the patient about the potential risks
- inquire about any pregnancy plans and emphasise the need for a pre-pregnancy consultation.

3. For drugs of known significant risk or where there is little data, consider switching to a lower-risk drug before conception.
4. Avoid polypharmacy, as synergistic teratogenicity can occur (up to 16% with multiple AEDs, n = 172, Kaneko *et al*, *Epilepsia* 1988;**29**:459–67).

Pregnancy

1. Avoid all drugs during the first trimester if possible. The maximum teratogenic potential is from days 17–60 (2–9 weeks) after conception, and decisions must balance the relative versus absolute risk.
2. Behavioural teratogenesis and subtle functional disturbances (e.g. learning difficulties, neurological deficits and developmental delay), and an effect on labour and delivery may occur in the second and third trimesters.
3. Use the lowest possible (maintenance) dose and monitor effects (adverse and desired) carefully. Maintain a low threshold for reintroduction or dose increase.
4. In many cases, the risk of relapse (and subsequent higher dose drug use) will be higher than the risk of fetal damage.
5. The pharmacokinetics of drugs may change during pregnancy and so doses may need to be adjusted (see e.g. lithium, tricyclics).
6. Discontinuation effects have been reported in the newborn (e.g. benzodiazepines, antidepressants and opiates) and these psychotropics should, if possible, be gradually reduced or withdrawn over the weeks before delivery is due.

Unexpected pregnancy

If a woman discovers or reports that she is pregnant while taking a drug:
1. Don't panic.
2. If before day 17, consider immediate stopping or temporary discontinuation.

3. If after day 60, the major risk has passed and so decisions are less urgent.
4. Institute immediate nutritional supplements (e.g. folic acid).
5. Reduce the dose if possible, at least during the high risk period.
6. Discontinue any non-essential treatments, particularly any that might be at sub-therapeutic doses.
7. Do not stop lithium abruptly (see point 32), and beware of stopping some SSRIs and anticonvulsants.
8. Seek specific specialist advice, and discuss the risk of the possible consequences of relapse versus the published risk to the fetus.

Reviews: * *Drugs in Pregnancy and Lactation: A Reference Guide to Fetal and Neonatal Risk*, by Briggs et al, Williams and Wilkins, Baltimore, MD; general (Kohen, *Adv Psychiatr Treat* 2004;**10**:59–66, 55 refs), psychotropics in pregnancy in bipolar disorder (Nguyen et al, *Adv Ther* 2009;**26**:281–94; Dodd and Berk, *Curr Drug Saf* 2006;**1**:25–33; Yonkers et al, *Am J Psychiatry* 2004;**161**:608–20).

3.8.1 ANTIPSYCHOTICS *

With more prolactin-sparing antipsychotics available, more women have been planning to (or have) become pregnant (McKenna et al, *Vet Hum Toxicol* 2004;**46**:44–6). However, low folate intake and low serum folate levels have been shown in women taking atypicals, increasing the risk of neural tube defects (Koren et al, *Am J Psychiatry* 2002;**159**:136–7) and so dietary advice and folate supplements pre-conception are **essential**. One systematic review suggested that women with schizophrenia have a greater risk of poor pregnancy outcomes than other women, with an increased risk with phenothiazines, although the review omitted two major studies that show no increased risk with phenothiazines (Patton et al, *Can J Psychiatry* 2002;**47**:959–65; comment by Levinson, *EBMH* 2003;**6**:89). Similarly, an extensive Swedish study (1995–2005) showed no difference in the MCM rate between women taking antipsychotics or not, a consistent finding with other large studies, although the rate was higher in women also taking anticonvulsants (infants n = 973,767, Reis and Kallen, *J Clin Psychopharmacol* 2008;**28**:279–88; comment by Einarson and Einarson, *EMBH*

2009;**12**:29). However, a prospective study suggested atypical antipsychotic exposure in pregnancy may increase infant birth weight and risk of larger gestational age (n = 108, Newham et al, *Br J Psychiatry* 2008;**192**:333–7).

The placental passage ratio for transfer (based on umbilical cord cf. maternal plasma) for the major atypicals is:

- olanzapine 72% (highest)
- haloperidol 66%
- risperidone 49%
- quetiapine 24% (lowest).

There is a tendency for lower birth rates and SCBU admissions with olanzapine (n = 54, Newport et al, *Am J Psychiatry* 2007;**164**:1214–20).

Reviews: * general (Einarson and Boskovic, *J Psychiatr Pract* 2009;**15**:183–92: Gentile, *Ann Pharmacother* 2004;**38**:126–71).

1.* **Risperidone** (FDA = C; ADEC = B3) has no reported teratogenicity in animal tests. A prospective cohort study of showed no increase in malformations in women who took risperidone (n = 49, McKenna et al, *J Clin Psychiatry* 2005;**66**:444–9; comment by Howard, *EBMH* 2005;**8**:115). There are several published reports of normal pregnancies and postnatal development with oral or Consta given throughout pregnancy (n = 1, Dabbert and Heinze, *Pharmacopsychiatry* 2006;**39**:235; n = 1, Kim et al, *Prog Neuropsychopharmacol Biol Psychiatry* 2007;**30**:543–5; two successive pregnancies; n = 1, Mendhekar and Lohia, *J Neuropsychiatry Clin Neurosci* 2008;**20**:485–6; n = 1, Rodríguez-Salgado, *Actas Esp Psiquiatr* 2008;**36**:366–8). **Paliperidone** (FDA=C) is not teratogenic in animal studies but some reversible developmental effects have been seen, so is not recommended, but should not be stopped abruptly during pregnancy (SPC).

2.* There is limited adequate data on **aripiprazole** (FDA = C), although data is currently unremarkable. Healthy children have been born with aripiprazole throughout pregnancy (n = 1, Doulgeraki et al, *Eur Psychiatry* 2007;**22**(suppl 1):S206), from week 29 to term (n = 1, Mendhekar et al, *Ann Pharmacother* 2006;**40**:575), from week 8 to term (n = 1, Mervak et al, *Arch Women's Ment Health* 2008;**11**:249–50), and with aripiprazole 10–15mg/d from 0–8 weeks and then 20 weeks to term (n = 1, Mendhekar et al, *Bipolar Disord* 2006;**8**:299–300), although there was a lactation failure in this last case, possibly due to aripiprazole-induced regulation of prolactin.

Asenapine (FDA = C) is not teratogenic in animal studies but human data is not yet available (US PI).

Olanzapine (FDA = C; ADEC=B3): From 516 documented pregnancies to May 2008 (MI) 65.1% were normal, 10.3% premature, 8.7% spontaneous abortions, 8.3% had perinatal complications, 4.7% MCMs and 2.9% others. All these are reported as being within normal ranges (n = 23, Goldstein et al, J Clin Psychopharmacol 2000;**20**:399–403). A prospective cohort study showed no increase in malformations in women who took olanzapine (n = 60, McKenna et al, J Clin Psychiatry 2005;**66**:444–9; comment by Howard, EBMH 2005;**8**:115). Use should only be when the potential benefit outweighs the potential risk. Atrioventricular canal defect and unilateral clubfoot has been reported with a mother who took olanzapine 10 mg/d (Yeshayahu, Am J Psychiatry 2007;**164**:1759–60). In a woman who took olanzapine throughout pregnancy, the newborn's plasma levels were about a third of the mother's (11 ng/ml vs 25–34 ng/ml), with normal development over the first six months (n = 1, Aichhorn et al, J Psychopharmacol 2008; **22**:923–4).

Quetiapine (FDA = C); the literature recommends using only if the benefits justify the risk but the available data shows no major cause for concern. A prospective cohort study showed no increase in malformations in women who took quetiapine (n = 36, McKenna et al, J Clin Psychiatry 2005;**66**:444–9; comment by Howard, EBMH 2005;**8**:115). There are cases of 400 mg/d (n = 1, Tényi et al, Am J Psychiatry 2002;**159**:674), 200–300 mg/d (n = 1, Taylor et al, Am J Psychiatry 2003;**160**:587–8) and 1200 mg/d (starting from week 21, n = 1, Cabuk et al, Arch Women's Ment Health 2007;**10**:235–6) taken throughout pregnancy without complications and with normal development at six months. Other reports note a low placental transfer (n = 21, Newport et al, Am J Psychiatry 2007;**164**:1214–20) and uneventful use with risperidone (n = 4, Gentile et al, Ann Pharmacother 2004;**38**:1265–71).

Others: There are no adequate human studies during pregnancy with **ziprasidone** (FDA = C). **Zotepine** crosses the placenta and although there are no indications of teratogenicity, there is insufficient data in humans and the drug is contraindicated in pregnancy.

3. Women are more likely to conceive on **clozapine** (FDA = B; ADEC = C) than most other antipsychotics due to an absence of raised prolactin. In the close study of one patient, there was clear accumulation of clozapine in the infant, possibly due to higher albumin concentrations (n = 1, Barnas, Am J Psychiatry 1994;**151**:945). Of 84 reports of pregnancy with clozapine with known outcomes, there were 51 births, seven miscarriages and 14 elective terminations, of which one was due to known abnormalities (patient taking clozapine 25 mg/d plus lithium). Of the 51 births, 43 were born healthy and normal and eight had abnormalities, ranging from low glucose levels through to malformations. Clozapine is known to pass the placental barrier in animals and is assumed to do so in humans. No clear conclusion can be drawn, although combined with animal studies it would appear clozapine is not a major teratogen, but not recommended in pregnancy as such.

4.* **Thioxanthenes: Flupentixol** (ADEC = C) passes across the placenta and fetal levels are about a quarter of the mother's levels (n = 5, open, Kirk and Jorgensen, Psychopharmacology 1980;**72**:107–8). There is no positive evidence of teratogenicity, although Lundbeck do not recommend its use. Studies in three species have not shown malformations. The UK SPC now states that **zuclopenthixol** should not be administered during pregnancy unless the benefit outweighs the theoretical risk to the fetus. Animal studies have not shown any increase in fetal effects but lethargy, tremor, hyperexcitability and low Apgar scores have been reported (SPC).

5.* **Sulpiride** has been used as an antinauseant in pregnancy. Limited human data has shown some possible adverse effects but these are probably not drug-related and animal studies have not shown direct or indirect adverse effects (the UK SPC now recommends appropriate monitoring of the neonate). **Amisulpride** shows no animal reproductive toxicity but is contraindicated in pregnancy in humans.

6. **Butyrophenones:** The safety of **haloperidol** (FDA = C; ADEC = C) in pregnancy has not been fully established, but a prospective study showed that of 188 haloperidol pregnancies, there was no significant increase in MCMs (cf control group) even if taken in the first trimester (although there were two limb defects), but there was a higher incidence of therapeutic termination, preterm

birth and low birth weight (n = 188, Diav-Citrin et al, J Clin Psychiatry 2005;**66**:317–22). There is a case of dyskinesia in a newborn after haloperidol monotherapy (n = 1, Collins and Comer, Am J Health Syst Pharm 2003;**60**:2253–5).

7. **Phenothiazines:** (ADEC: chlorpromazine = C, promazine = C, trifluoperazine = C, fluphenazine = C, thioridazine = C)

The teratogenicity of phenothiazines has been investigated in some studies, although most of the data is based on low doses and thus not necessarily applicable to higher dose use. The phenothiazines are considered by some to be of low risk, although the potential for hypotension, sedation and anticholinergic effects means that any use must be with extreme care. Severe MCMs were not significantly different in the studies of 543 women taking low-dose phenothiazines, other than **prochlorperazine** (FDA = C) for nausea (Miklovich and van den Berg, Am J Obstet Gynecol 1976;**125**:244–8), and in 1309 mothers mostly taking prochlorperazine (prospective, Slone et al, Am J Obstet Gynecol 1977;**128**:486–8). The largest study of 315 pregnancies where phenothiazines were taken in the first trimester, showed a statistically significant difference in the malformation rate of 3.5% in the aliphatic (**chlorpromazine** and **promazine**) phenothiazine-treated group (11 malformed infants), compared with 1.6% in the control group. There was no apparent trend in the type of abnormality and the risk is still considered low. There was no difference with the other phenothiazines, which appear to have an incidence of malformations similar to the background incidence (Teratology 1977;**15**:57–64). Although **levomepromazine** (methotrimeprazine) is an aliphatic phenothiazine, it has generally been considered safe for both mother and fetus if used occasionally in low dose later in pregnancy. A follow-up of trifluoperazine pregnancies showed no teratogenic effects (Moriarity, Can Med Assoc J 1963;**88**:97). In the neonate, lethargy and extrapyramidal symptoms have been reported, as has respiratory depression when given in high dose (above 500 mg chlorpromazine equivalents) close to term.

Postnatal development: In the longer term, a lack of impaired mental or physical development has been shown at two and seven years in a follow-up study (n = 16, Ayd, Int Drug Ther Newsletter 1976;**11**:5).

8. Animal studies of **pimozide** have shown no teratogenicity but use is not advisable (SPC).

3.8.2 ANTIDEPRESSANTS *

It is still unclear which is worse; untreated antenatal depression (e.g. higher incidence of SIDS, poor engagement and self-care) or antidepressant exposure during pregnancy (e.g. neonatal syndrome from antidepressant exposure), so no decision is risk-free (summary by Freeman, J Clin Psychiatry 2007;**68**:1277–8). Overall, the adverse effects of antidepressants in general in pregnancy have been reported as:

- There was no consistent link with MCMs if used in the first trimester, but if used in the third trimester there is an increased risk of perinatal complications (n = 2201, Davis et al, Pharmacoepidemiol Drug Saf 2007;**16**:1086–94).

- In women aged 15–45 who had used an antidepressant for at least a month in the year before pregnancy, there was no association with an increased risk of MCMs compared to no antidepressants (n = 2329, 21/12, Ramos et al, Br J Psychiatry 2008;**199**:344–50; comment by Howard, EBMH 2009;**12**:28).

- In mothers who took a tricyclic [n = 80], fluoxetine [n = 55] or nothing [n = 84], Nulman et al, NEJM 1997;**336**:258–62) there seems to be no effect on the neurological development or intelligence of their children (see 20 below).

- In first trimester exposure to antidepressants, MCMs were 3.2% in antidepressant group and 3.3% in matched controls, so there was no association with increased MCM (n = 2486, Einarson et al, Can J Psychiatry 2009;**54**:242–6).

- Third trimester exposure to antidepressants was not associated with a significant increase in postpartum hemorrhage (n = 28863 [PPH n = 2460 vs 26403 controls], Salkeld et al, J Clin Psychopharmacol 2008;**28**:230-4; comment by Heerdink, EBMH 2008;**11**:125).

A 2009 US report on the management of depression during pregnancy recommends:

Women thinking of getting pregnant: *
- If mild or no symptoms for 6/12 or longer consider tapering and discontinuation before becoming pregnant.
- This may not be appropriate if the depression is severe or recurrent (including psychosis, bipolar, history of suicide).
- Women with suicidal or acute psychosis should be referred to secondary care for 'aggressive' treatment.

Pregnant women currently taking antidepressants: *
- Psychiatrically stable women who want to stay on medication may be able to after discussion with a psychiatrist and obstetrician.
- Women who want to discontinue may attempt tapering, and stopping if no symptoms occur.
- Women with recurrent depression, or who have symptoms despite antidepressants, may be helped by psychological therapies as a replacement or augmentation
- Women with severe depression (with e.g. suicidal attempts, weight loss) should remain on antidepressants.

Pregnant women depressed and not currently on antidepressants: *
- Psychotherapy may be helpful if woman prefers to avoid antidepressants.
- If preferring antidepressants, choose carefully based on e.g. trimester, history of depression, comorbidity.

All pregnant women: *
- Seek psychiatric help urgently if suicidal or psychotic symptoms develop.

(Yonkers et al, Gen Hosp Psychiatry 2009;**31**:403–13; Yonkers et al, Obstet Gynecol 2009;**114**:703–13).

Reviews: * general (Osborne and O'Keane, Prog Neurol Psychiatry 2009;**13**:6–12; Källén, Expert Opin Drug Saf 2007;**6**:357–70), risks of untreated depression (Bonari et al, Can J Psychiatry 2004;**49**:726–35), depression during pregnancy and postpartum (Cohen et al, CNS Spectr 2004;**9**:209–16).

9.* **SSRIs**: (FDA: citalopram = C, escitalopram = C, fluoxetine = C, fluvoxamine = C, paroxetine = D, sertraline = C, ADEC: citalopam = C, fluoxetine = C, paroxetine = B3, sertraline = B3)

There is a significant body of data on SSRIs in pregnancy:

First trimester use: *
- A prospective, multicentre cohort study of 267 women exposed to an SSRI (fluvoxamine, sertraline or paroxetine) during pregnancy and 267 controls, exposure to SSRIs at recommended doses did not appear to be associated with increased teratogenicity (relative risk 1.06, 95% CI, 0.43–2.62) or higher rates of miscarriage, stillbirth or prematurity. (prospective, Kulin et al, JAMA 1998;**279**:609–10).
- A prospective controlled study of SSRIs in the first trimester showed a higher rate of abnormalities with paroxetine (5.2%, n = 410) and fluoxetine (4.7%, n = 314) compared to placebo (2.5%, n = 1467), particularly cardiovascular abnormalities; 2%, 2.8%, 0.6% respectively (n = 2191, Diav-Citrin et al, Br J Clin Pharmacol 2008;**66**:695–705).
- First trimester use of SSRIs has been associated with two-fold higher risk of mild nonsyndromic heart defects (n = 235 + 67636, Merlob et al, Birth Defects Res A Clin Mol Teratology 2009;**85**:837–41).
- In a population-based cohort study, the incidence of septal heart defects was 0.5% (n = 2315) in unexposed children, 0.9% (n = 12) with SSRIs and 2.1% (n = 4) in children exposed to more than one SSRI, with the risk being greater with sertraline and citalopram in the first trimester (n = 493113, Pedersen et al, BMJ 2009;**339**:b3569).
- A review of 138 pregnancies concluded that the rates of MCMs, low birth weight and preterm births were the same as in the general population, although high-dose fluoxetine (40–80 mg/d) may be associated with a risk of lower birth weight (n = 138, Hendrick et al, Am J Obstet Gynaecol 2003; **188**:812–15).
- The overall rate of MCMs is 1.4%, similar to that seen in the general population, e.g. there were no general increases in heart defects and other birth defects with first-trimester exposure to SSRIs. There was a slight association of sertraline with omphalocele and septal defects, and between paroxetine and right ventricular obstruction defects,

but these specific defects are rare and the absolute risk small (n = 15,709, Louik et al, N Engl J Med 2007;**356**:2675–83).

Second and third trimesters: *

- One study showed an increased incidence of gestational hypertension in pregnant women taking SSRIs (19% vs 9%), especially if used in the third trimester, although a causal link was not established (n = 5731, Toh et al, Am J Psychiatry 2009;**166**:320-8).

- In a prospective study, exposure to SSRIs was associated with an increased risk of pre-term delivery, a lower 5-min Apgar score and SCBU admission (n = 329, + 4902 controls, Lund et al, Arch Pediatr Adolesc Med 2009;**163**:949–54).

- There is an association between SSRI use after 20 weeks' gestation and PPHN (persistent pulmonary hypertension in the newborn), with the absolute risk being around 1%, but not with other antidepressants or use up to 20 weeks (n = 1213, Chambers et al, N Engl J Med 2006;**354**:579–87).

- In a retrospective study, apparent prenatal SSRI exposure, slightly earlier delivery (0.9 week) and decreased birth weight (175 g) were noted and third trimester exposure to SSRIs was associated with a 0.29 decrease in mean Apgar scores at five minutes (n = 185, controls n = 185, Simon et al, Am J Psychiatry 2002;**159**:2055–61). Caution is advised and use should only be if clearly needed.

Birth: *

- A Canadian study has concluded that the risk adverse neonatal outcomes (e.g. gestation duration and low birth rate, but not length of hospital stay, convulsions or feeding difficulties) is more related to the duration of SSRI exposure during pregnancy, rather than the timing of the exposure, a confusing finding (n = 3500, one year, Oberlander et al, Br J Psychiatry 2008;**192**:338–43; comment by Gentile, EBMH 2009;**12**:27).

- Serotonergic drugs may increase the risk of CNS serotonergic adverse effects (tremor, restlessness, rigidity), but these subside quickly without treatment and may be due to serotonergic hyperstimulation rather than withdrawal (prospective, n = 40, p/c, Laine et al, Arch Gen Psychiatry 2003;**60**:720–6).

- Neonatal withdrawal symptoms (irritability, constant crying, shivering, increased tonus, eating and sleeping difficulties and con-vulsions) have been reported after in utero exposure to paroxetine (n = 3), citalopram (n = 1) and fluoxetine (n = 1), four requiring calming with chlorpromazine (Nordeng et al, Acta Paediatrica 2001;**90**:288–91).

Postnatal development: *

- In a retrospective study, apparent prenatal SSRI exposure was not associated with malformation or any developmental delay (n = 185, controls n = 185, Simon et al, Am J Psychiatry 2002;**159**:2055–61).

Citalopram and **escitalopram** (review by Gentile, Clin Drug Investig 2008;**28**:735–9): * of 125 women who took citalopram in the first trimester (including 71 who also took it throughout pregnancy), there were 86% normal live births, 11% spontaneous abortions, 1.5% elective terminations and 1.5% stillbirths, plus one male infant born with MCMs and there was an overall increased risk of admission to a SCBU (n = 125, Sivojelezova et al, Am J Obstet Gynecol 2005;**193**:2004–9). Occasionally, slightly increased doses of citalopram may be needed in pregnancy (n = 11, Heikkinen et al, Clin Pharmacol Ther 2002;**72**:184–91).

Fluoxetine: * There is a mass of safety data on fluoxetine-exposed pregnancies reported in three prospective cohort-controlled studies and four prospective surveys. Based on published studies, use in the first trimester is not associated with increased risk of major malformations (meta-analysis by Addis and Koren, Psychol Med 2000;**30**:89–94; critical review by Gijsman, EBMH 2000;**3**:122). There is an absence of perinatal sequelae and no evidence of an increase in major malformations, spontaneous abortion, poor perinatal state or neurodevelopmental delay. Studies have shown first-trimester exposure produces no statistical differences in pregnancy outcome, age or weight, but a slight tendency to miscarriage with both drug groups (SSRI 14.8%, TCA 12.2%, no drug 7.8%; n = 312, Pastuszak et al, JAMA 1993;**269**:2246–8), and with perinatal major malformation and post-perinatal mal-formation rates similar to the unexposed population (Goldstein and Marvel, JAMA, 1993; **270**:2177–8), but miscarriage rates double that in the control group (n = 228, Chambers et al, NEJM 1996;**335**:1010–5). A prospective study showed a possible association between cardiovascular abnormalities and first-trimester exposure to fluoxetine (n = 314, risk 2.8%), but not quite with paroxetine (n = 410, risk 2%), compared to controls (n = 1467, risk 0.6%) (Diav-Citrin et al, Br J Clin Pharmacol 2008;**66**:695–705).

Postnatal development: A careful prospective study of children (assessed between 18 and 86 months) whose mothers had taken either fluoxetine (n = 55) or no drug (n = 84) showed fluoxetine to have no effect on global IQ, language development or behavioural development (n = 139, Nulman et al, NEJM 1997;**336**:258–62). Further data on exposure to fluoxetine throughout pregnancy shows no detectable adverse affect on cognition, language development or temperament, whereas untreated depression was associated with poorer cognitive and language achievement in their children (TCA n = 46, fluoxetine n = 40, control n = 36; open, Nulman et al, Am J Psychiatry 2002;**159**:1889–95). Relatively low plasma fluoxetine levels have been reported in pregnancy, which might lead to therapeutic failure at standard doses, with infant fluoxetine and norfluoxetine plasma levels 65% and 72% respectively at birth (n = 11 + 10 controls, Heikkinen et al, Clin Pharmacol Ther 2003;**73**:330–7).

Paroxetine: * A review from respected authors of the use of paroxetine in early pregnancy concludes that the data is inconsistent and inconclusive (s = 25, Gentile and Bellantuono, J Clin Psychiatry 2009;**70**:414–22; see also meta-analysis showing no increased risk of cardiac malformations from first trimester exposure; s = 9, n = 97,656, O'Brien et al, J Obstet Gynaecol Can 2008;**30**:696–70), whereas a meta-analysis has suggested that first-trimester exposure to paroxetine may be associated with an increased risk of cardiac malformations (Bar-Oz et al, Clin Ther 2007;**29**:918–26), although it is clearly not a major risk, although a mild-to-moderate association could not be excluded (n = 182 exposed infants, Davis et al, Pharmacoepidemiol Drug Saf 2007;**16**:1086–94). Another study suggested that first trimester exposure to paroxetine does not appear to be associated with increased cardiac effects (paroxetine 0.7%, unexposed group 0.7%) unlike antidepressants

in general (n = 2061, 1.5%), when the usual population incidence is around 1% (n = 1174, Einarson et al, Am J Psychiatry 2008;**165**:749–52). However, the UK SPC now states that paroxetine use in the first trimester is associated with increased risk of cardiovascular defects (increase from about 1% to less that 2%), but the MHRA do not recommend stopping paroxetine abruptly if a woman is pregnant as this could precipitate discontinuation symptoms, but to discuss the risks and benefits at the next appointment. When used in the third trimester, paroxetine may cause a high rate of neonatal complications, probably due to a withdrawal syndrome, e.g. a careful prospective study showed 22% neonates had complications (9 = respiratory distress, 2 = hypoglycaemia) requiring intensive treatment and hospitalisation, although all symptoms had disappearing within 1–2 weeks (n = 55 + controls; Costei et al, Arch Pediatr Adolesc Med 2002;**156**:1129–32; more severe case, Morag et al, J Toxicol Clin Toxicol 2004; **42**:97–100). Finally, in women who are extensive or ultra-rapid 2D6 metabolisers, paroxetine levels steadily decrease throughout pregnancy at 0.3 mcg/L per week, whereas in intermediate and poor metabolisers plasma paroxetine levels increase by 0.82 mcg/L per week. Accumulation can thus occur in some women, which might have adverse consequences (n = 74, Ververs et al, Clin Pharmacokinet 2009;**48**:677–83).

Review: (n = 22, Wurst et al, Birth Defects Res A Clin Mol Teratol 2009;[in press]).

Sertraline * has been included in a number of studies, e.g. in a prospective, multicentre cohort study of 267 women exposed to an SSRI (fluvoxamine, sertraline or paroxetine) during pregnancy and 267 controls, exposure to SSRIs at recommended doses did not appear to be associated with increased teratogenicity (relative risk 1.06, 95% CI, 0.43–2.62) or higher rates of miscarriage, stillbirth or prematurity. Gestational ages and birth weights were similar among offspring of both groups of women (n = 534, Kulin et al, JAMA 1998;**279**: 609–10). Sertraline levels and AUC remain fairly constant throughout pregnancy and postpartum, although they fall slightly in the third trimester (n = 11, Freeman et al, J Clin Psychopharmacol 2008;**28**:646–53).

10. * Prospective data on 150 **venlafaxine** (FDA = C; ADEC = B2) pregnancies showed 125 live births, 18 spontaneous abortions,

seven therapeutic abortions and two major malformations, suggesting that the base-rate of malformations does not rise above the spontaneous rate but, as with the SSRIs, the spontaneous abortion rate is slightly higher (venlafaxine n = 150; SSRIs n=150; controls n=150; Einarson et al, Am J Psychiatry 2001;**158**:1728–30). Neonatal discontinuation signs start as soon as infant plasma levels decline; respiratory symptoms tend to start early and may contribute to PPHN (n = 5, Boucher et al, Ther Drug Monit 2009;**31**:404–9). It is no longer contraindicated in pregnancy in the UK SPC, although there is a warning of the potential for withdrawal symptoms in the neonate (e.g. case that resolved with use of 1 mg/d for 8/7; n = 1, de Moor et al, Ned Tijdschr Geneeskd 2003;**147**:1370–2). Animal studies with **duloxetine** (FDA = C) suggest some adverse behavioural effects in one animal species. In a published human case, duloxetine used from the middle of the second trimester showed no adverse effects on the infant at birth or for a month afterwards (n = 1, Briggs et al, Ann Pharmacother 2009;**43**:1898–902). However, a case has been reported of neonatal withdrawal syndrome similar to SSRIs (e.g. jitteriness, poor muscle tone, weak cry, respiratory distress, hypoglycaemia, low Apgar score and seizure) lasting several weeks but with normal development at two years (n = 1, Eyal and Yaeger, Am J Psychiatry 2008;**165**:651).

11. * For **mirtazapine** (FDA = C; ADEC = B3) a recent comprehensive and prospective study has shown no increase in the baseline rate of major malformations but a slight increase in spontaneous abortions (19% vs 17% vs 11%) and preterm births (10% vs 7% vs 2%) (n = 104 mirtazapine, vs n=104 other antidepressants vs. control group, Djulus et al, J Clin Psychiatry 2006;**67**:1280–4). Animal tests do not show any teratogenicity or fetal harm. There are two cases of recurrent hypothermia lasting for 10 days in identical twins born to mother who took mirtazapine throughout pregnancy (n = 2, Sokolover et al, Can J Clin Pharmacol 2008;**15**:188–90). When used for depression, anxiety and hyperemesis gravidarum in seven pregnancies, all women improved and all babies were born healthy at term (n = 7, Saks, Arch Women's Ment Health 2001;**3**:165–170; see also n = 2, Kesim et al, Teratology 2002;**66**:204).

12. **Tricyclic antidepressants:** (FDA: clomipramine = C, desipramine =C, doxepin = B,

maprotiline = B, trimipramine = C; ADEC: amitriptyline = C, clomipramine = C, dosulepin = C, doxepin = C, imipramine = C, nortriptyline = C, trimipramine = C)

In the most recent retrospective study, prenatal tricyclic exposure was not associated with MCMs, developmental delay or any adverse perinatal outcomes (n = 209, controls n = 209, Simon et al, Am J Psychiatry 2002;**159**:2055–61), confirming an earlier meta-analysis (n = 414 from 414 000 live births), although withdrawal symptoms were noted.

In pregnancy, mild toxicity in the infant has been seen with **imipramine**, e.g. respiratory distress, hypotonia, irritability, tremors, convulsions and jerky movements (e.g. n = 2, Ware and DeVane, J Clin Psychiatry 1990;**51**:482–4). Phenobarbital can improve these symptoms, which can persist for a total duration of up to two weeks. **Amitriptyline** and **imipramine** are considered the tricyclics of choice, based on cumulative data on their relative safety.

Discontinuation effects have been noted in the neonate, sometimes requiring active treatment, e.g. clomipramine discontinuation has caused jittery/twitchy infants which resolves upon introduction of the drug, i.e. either via a drip or via breast milk (n = 1, Schimmel et al, Clin Toxicol 1991;**29**:479–84). Abrupt discontinuation of clomipramine 150 mg/d by a mother resulted in a lethargic and cyanotic baby, who had abnormal movements, feeding difficulties and fetal seizures unresponsive to phenobarbital and phenytoin, but which settled when clomipramine was started (Bromiker and Kaplan, JAMA 1994;**272**:1722–3). **Postnatal development:** A careful study of children (assessed between 18 and 86 months) whose mothers had taken either a tricyclic (n = 84) or no drug (n = 80) showed tricyclics to have no adverse effect on global IQ, language development or behavioural development compared to no drug (n = 164, Nulman et al, NEJM 1997;**336**:258–62). Further data shows no adverse affect on cognition, language development or temperament, whereas untreated depression is associated with poorer cognitive and language achievement in their children (tricyclic n=46, fluoxetine n=40, control n = 36, open, Nulman et al, Am J Psychiatry 2002; **159**:1889–95).

13. For **trazodone** (FDA = C) at very high doses

(15+ times the maximum human dose), there appears to be some fetal resorption and MCMs in animals but little human data exists to support this.

14.* No teratogenic effects have been noted with **reboxetine** (and so it is no longer contraindicated). For **agomelatine**, little human data exists so the drug should be avoided in pregnancy.

15. **MAOIs**: (FDA: isocarboxazid = C; ADEC: isocarboxazid = B3, phenelzine = B3, tranylcypromine = B2)

There are no reports of human teratogenicity with **phenelzine** or **tranylcypromine**, although it has been suggested that the risk may be roughly doubled if tranylcypromine is taken in the first trimester (AAPCD, *Pediatrics* 1982;**69**:241–3). Growth retardation and fetal toxicity have been reported. If at all possible, MAOIs should be avoided due to maternal toxicity and lack of published safety data. MAOIs may also interact with drugs used in labour (see also *4.3.4*).

16.* There is no evidence of teratogenicity with **mianserin** (ADEC = B2) in animals except at toxic doses but little human data is available. No firm data is available on the use of **moclobemide** in pregnancy, but there is a case of 300 mg/d taken throughout pregnancy with no problems and normal development within the first 14 months (n = 1, Rybakowski, *Pharmacopsychiatry* 2001;**34**:82–3). No human data is available for **tryptophan**, but it is a naturally occurring substance in food. In **St John's wort**-exposed pregnancies (n = 54), the MCM rate was 5%, comparable to other antidepressants (4%, n = 54) and controls (0%, n = 54), not considered statistically different from each other (n = 162, Moretti *et al, Reprod Toxicol* 2009;**28**:96–9).

3.8.3 ANXIOLYTICS AND HYPNOTICS

Review: general (Vythilingum, *Curr Psychiatry Rep* 2008;**10**:331–5)

17. **Benzodiazepines**: (FDA: alprazolam = D, clonazepam = D, lorazepam = D, temazepam = X; ADEC: clonazepam = C, diazepam = C, flunitrazepam = C, lorazepam = C, oxazepam = C, temazepam = C)

Assessment of 104 000 births in the USA has shown a higher incidence of teratogenicity in women taking a variety of benzodiazepines, but multiple alcohol and illicit substance exposure could account for this (Bergman *et al, Lancet* 1992;**340**:694–6). For individual BDZs, a population-based case-control study indicated that **nitrazepam**, **medazepam**, **alprazolam** and **clonazepam** taken during pregnancy did not present a detectable teratogenic risk (n = 38,151, Eros *et al, Eur J Obstet Gynecol Reprod Biol* 2002; **101**:147–54). With **chlordiazepoxide**, there was slight increase in MCMs with use in the second to third months, but no specific type or pattern was seen, and so the risk is unlikely to be substantial (n = 469, Czeizel *et al, Neurotoxicol Teratol* 2004;**26**:593–8). **Clobazam** is known to cross the placenta and benzodiazepine withdrawal symptoms in the neonate have been suggested but no teratogenicity has been reported. For **diazepam**, studies show a varying risk of oral clefts, with the worst case scenario bringing the risk to seven in 1000. In late pregnancy, doses of 30 mg or more of diazepam IM or IV during the last 15 hours of labour can induce neonatal respiratory depression and feeding problems, although 10 mg given IV within 10 minutes of birth has been shown not to affect Apgar scores (n = 23, open, McAllister, *Br J Anaesth* 1980;**52**:423–7). As with other benzodiazepines, withdrawal symptoms in the neonate have been seen (n = 3, Rementeria and Bhatt, *J Pediatr* 1977;**90**:123–6). As **lorazepam** crosses the placenta, the floppy baby syndrome and respiratory depression can occur, especially if IV doses are used close to birth. Oral use during later pregnancy may show delayed feeding in full-term infants, but premature infants may have lower Apgar scores and respiratory depression (n = 53, open, Whitelaw *et al, Br Med J* 1981;**282**:1106–8).

The UK CSM has noted the danger of benzodiazepine use during pregnancy or labour due to the effects on the neonate, such as hypothermia, hypotonia, respiratory depression and withdrawal symptoms (*Curr Prob* 1997; **23**:10). Shorter-acting benzodiazepines on a 'when required' basis may be acceptable later in pregnancy, but the first trimester should be avoided if possible. After birth, benzodiazepine withdrawal symptoms have been noticed in the neonate with many benzodiazepines. The 'floppy baby' syndrome, as it is often termed, includes facial features and CNS dysfunction and can occur particularly with higher doses (eg. > 30 mg diazepam equivalent per day) of longer-acting benzodiazepines (n = 8, Laegreid et al, J Pediatrics 1989;**114**:126–31).

Overdoses: *

- **Alprazolam:** In cases of attempted suicide by alprazolam overdose (7.5–100mg, mean 30mg) there was no significantly higher rate of MCMs, although there were only 10 live births assessed and association cannot be excluded for one multiple abnormality (n = 10, Gidai et al, Toxicol Ind Health 2008; **24**:53–60).

- **Chlordiazepoxide:** In women who took large overdoses of CDZ during pregnancy, there was no evidence of a higher rate of MCMs but a dose-dependent intrauterine growth retardation was seen, with lower birth weight newborns (n = 88, live births = 35, Gidal et al, Toxicol Ind Health 2008;**24**:41–51).

- **Diazepam:** In a study of women who overdosed on diazepam as suicide attempts, doses of 25–800mg produced 13.4% MCMs (cf 7.1% matched controls) but the overdoses taken during the first trimester critical periods did not show excess abnormalities, suggesting the observations were unrelated to diazepam (n = 229; 112 live births, Gidai et al, Toxicol Ind Health 2008; **24**:29–39).

18. There is no evidence of a teratogenic effect from **buspirone** (FDA = B; ADEC = B1) but some effects on survival and weights have been noted in some, but not all, animal tests. **Hydroxyzine** is contraindicated in early pregnancy as very high-dose animal tests induced fetal abnormalities (UK SPC).

19. **Zopiclone** has not been contraindicated in pregnancy. Animal tests have shown no abnormalities and the limited human data is unremarkable. Little information is currently available on **zaleplon** (FDA = C). **Zolpidem** (FDA = C; ADEC = B3) crosses the placenta but clears rapidly from the fetal circulation, and there is a (statistically) non-significant increase in pre-term delivery (27% vs 13%) and low birth weight (16% vs 5%) from regular zolpidem compared to matched controls (n = 45, Juric et al, Arch Women's Ment Health 2009; **12**:441–6). In an unusual case, maternal use of high-dose zolpidem (at least 1000mg over at least one month) was studied; cord levels were less than the mean maternal plasma levels likely from a single 5mg dose, and the neonate was alert and with no apparent withdrawal symptoms over the first 48 hours (n = 1, Askew, Pharmacotherapy 2007;**27**:306–8).

None of these three hypnotics are contraindicated in pregnancy and short-term 'when required' use of zolpidem would appear to present only minimal risk.

20. **Beta-blockers:** (FDA: propranolol = C; ADEC = C)

Beta-blockers are not generally considered teratogens but a connection between **propranolol** use in pregnancy and tracheosophageal fistulas and intrauterine growth retardation has been proposed but not substantiated. Direct effects of beta-blockade on the fetus would also occur, e.g. bradycardia. Use in the second and third trimesters may aggravate or produce neonatal hypoglycaemia. Fetal and neonatal bradycardia may occur, especially in pregnancies already complicated by placental insufficiency (e.g. severe maternal hypertension). Due to direct cardiac effects, hypoglycaemia and apnoea from beta-blockers, it may be prudent to discontinue treatment 1–2 weeks before delivery.

21. * Maternally administered **chloral** (ADEC = A) appears relatively safe as no increase in MCMs was seen in a study of 71 women who took chloral in the first four months of pregnancy, or to 358 women who took chloral at some time in pregnancy (Heinonen et al, Birth Defects and Drugs in Pregnancy, Publishing Sciences Group 1977:336–7). The UK manufacturers state that **clomethiazole** (ADEC = A) should not be used, particularly in the first and third trimesters, although it has been used widely for pre-eclampsia. Platelet aggregation in the neonate has been reported with **promethazine** (FDA = C; ADEC = C). In pregnant women attempting suicide by taking up to 1780mg promethazine, there was no evidence of teratogenicity, lower IQ or development, although the total MCM rate was very high in the cohort (n = 32 from 1044 overdoses, Petik et al, Toxicol Ind Health 2008;**24**:87–96). **Melatonin** has no apparent teratogenic effects but use is not recommended at the moment (SPC).

3.8.4 ANTICONVULSANTS

Pregnant women with epilepsy are at increased

risk of complications and 25–33% have an increased risk of seizures. One of the main reasons for this increase is the marked alterations in plasma protein-binding of drugs as pregnancy progresses, resulting in declining plasma levels. A number of prospective and retrospective studies have shown that there are a wide range of risks associated with anticonvulsants (some used as mood stabilisers) used throughout pregnancy. Most have an uncomplicated pregnancy and normal healthy offspring (n = 151 pregnancies, 124 women, retrospective, Sabers et al, Acta Neurol Scand 1998;**97**:164–70), but there is an association with an increased risk of major MCMs with most AEDs, in particular, valproate, carbamazepine and benzodiazepines (n = 1411, Samren et al, Ann Neurol 1999;**46**:739–44). Polytherapy carries additional risks, e.g. it is associated with a (partly reversible) decline in body dimension (n = 963, Swedish survey, Wide et al, Epilepsia 2000;**41**:854–61), including the risk of pre-term delivery, lower birthweight, length and head circumference (n = 193, controls n = 24094, Hvas et al, Br J Obstet Gynaecol 2000; **107**:896–902).

Postnatal development: Three recent studies have shown some specific effects on post-natal development of children exposed to anticonvulsants during pregnancy. One survey suggested a higher frequency of educational needs statements (10.3% drug exposed cf. 5.7% non-drug-exposed). The figures for **valproate** (30%), and possibly also polypharmacy, were much higher, supporting the possibility of a drug-related effect (n = 400 school-age children: 150 exposed to monotherapy, 74 to polytherapy and 176 to none; Adab et al, J Neurol Neurosurg Psychiatry 2001;**70**:15–21). Another study concluded that while there were no global score differences, phenytoin (n = 16, but not CBZ n = 35) caused a significant albeit subtle reduction in psychomotor development, which may be more obvious at school age (n = 76 exposed, c/w 71 unexposed, Wide et al, Acta Paediatrica 2002;**91**:409–14). Finally, in a review of the long-term health and neurodevelopment in children exposed to antiepileptic drugs before birth, developmental delay was seen in 24% of exposed children (cf. 11% non-exposed siblings), childhood medical problems in 31% (cf. 13% of non-exposed siblings) and behaviour disorders

in 20% (cf. 5% of non-exposed), concluding that prenatal antiepileptic drug exposure is associated with developmental delay and later childhood morbidity, in addition to MCMs (n = 129 mothers, 293 children, Dean et al, J Med Genet 2002;**39**:251–9).

Facial dysmorphism has been described in patients with uncontrolled seizures, as well as with phenytoin, phenobarbital, primidone, valproate, benzodiazepines and carbamazepine. All appear quite similar, not really drug-specific and some effects, especially digital, appear to resolve with age, although a review and huge multicentered study concluded that the distinctive pattern of physical abnormalities are associated with anticonvulsants rather than epilepsy itself (n = 128049, Holmes et al, NEJM 2001;**344**:1132–8).

Summary of the risks of pregnancy in women with epilepsy:

- 25–33% increase in maternal seizure frequency
- 10% risk of vaginal bleeding
- 7% risk of neonatal haemorrhage if no vitamin K is given
- 10% risk of infant facial dysmorphism.
- 4–6% risk of major malformations (30% of which are oral facial defects)
- 1–2% risk of spina bifida with valproate
- 0.5–1% risk of spina bifida with carbamazepine.

(Yerby, Epilepsia 1992;**33**[Suppl 1]:S23–S27.)

UK epilepsy and pregnancy register

A prospective study (n = 3607, Morrow et al, J Neurol Neurosurg Psychiatry 2006;**77**:193–8) has shown that only 4.2% of children born to mothers with epilepsy and taking AEDs had MCMs, subdivided as follows:

- 6% polytherapy exposures had MCMs
- 3.7% monotherapy exposures had MCMs
- more polytherapies with MCM had valproate than those that did not include valproate.

Relative risks of MCMs with monotherapy:

- 2.2% carbamazepine (least risk)
- 3.2% lamotrigine (> 200 mg/d had higher risk)
- 6% valproate (higher with > 1000 mg/d at 9%).

Summary of risk minimisation strategies:

1. Pre-conception:

- Education of the patient as to the risks and benefits of continued treatment. This should be documented and supported with written information (n = 300, survey, Fairgrieve et al, Br Med J 2000;**321**:674–5).

- Adequate oral contraceptive dosage (see individual drugs' interactions, 4.5) until conception is planned, e.g. 50 mcg of ethinylestradiol.

- Start regular multivitamins with folate (4–5 mg/d from before oral contraceptives are stopped, until at least 12 weeks of gestation) to reduce the chance of spina bifida. Folic acid antagonists (e.g. carbamazepine, phenytoin, phenobarbital) taken during pregnancy increase the risk of cardiovascular birth defects and oral clefts, and oral folic acid (e.g. in multivitamins) may reduce the risks of these defects (n = 6932, Hernandez-Diaz et al, NEJM 2000;**343**:1608–14), although folic acid is not always successful with valproate (n = 2, Duncan et al, Epilepsia 2001;**42**:750–3).

- Minimise the exposure to drugs with known associated risks, e.g. phenobarbital, valproate, carbamazepine and benzodiazepines.

- Seizure control with the lowest dose monotherapy should be targeted.

- Diagnosis should be verified and the need for anticonvulsants confirmed.

2. After conception:

- Education of the patient about risk minimisation, e.g. vitamin supplementation.

3. Seizure control without toxicity during pregnancy:

- Do not change drugs if the patient is stabilised.

- Continue multivitamins with folate.

- Frequent monitoring of free anticonvulsant concentrations and dose adjustment if necessary.

- Monotherapy should be continued if possible.

- Vitamin K should be given during last week of pregnancy if possible.

- Ultrasound and AFPs should be carried out.

It is worth noting that one study showed that only 38% of female epileptics were able to recall any pre-pregnancy counselling, only 44% had planned the pregnancy (24% reported contraceptive failure) and only 11% took folate appropriately. Most published advice is directed at neurologists, rather than the GPs caring for many patients. The net result was malformation rates double the background rate and there was an excess of premature deliveries cf. controls (n = 300, survey, Fairgrieve et al, Br Med J 2000; **321**:674–5).

Reviews: * general (Crawford, Drug Saf 2009; **32**:293–307; Pennell, Epilepsia 2008; **49**(Suppl 9):43–55; Hovinga and Pennell, Int Rev Neurobiol 2008;**83**:241–58; Harden, Int Rev Neurobiol 2008; **83**:205–13; Sabers and Tomson, Curr Opin Neurol 2009;**22**:157–61), optimising therapy (Kalviainen and Tomson, Neurology 2006 **67**(12 Suppl 4): S59–63), postnatal development (Meador et al, N Engl J Med 2009;**360**:1597–605).

22. **Carbamazepine** (FDA = D; ADEC = D) is now considered to have a higher risk. In a pooled data study of 1255 exposures (Matalon et al, Reprod Toxicol 2002;**16**:9–17), carbamazepine was associated with:

- an increased rate of MCMs, mainly neural tube defects (e.g. spina bifida, 1% incidence; Rosa, NEJM 1991;**324**:674–7), cardiovascular and urinary tract anomalies, and cleft palate (a 'carbamazepine syndrome': Ornoy and Cohen, Arch Dis Child 1996;**75**:517)

- some minor abnormalities

- some reduced gestational age at delivery

- an increased risk with polytherapy

- a negative influence on body dimensions (n = 963, Wide et al, Epilepsia 2000;**41**: 854–61).

Children exposed to carbamazepine may also have subtle but distinctive facial features (n = 274, Kini et al, Arch Dis Child Neonatal Ed 2006;**91**:90–5), although 45% unexposed children also had some facial features. Other problems include craniofacial defects (11%), fingernail hypoplasia (27%) and developmental delay (20%) (n = 72, retrospective, Jones et al, NEJM 1989;**320**:1661–6, + correspondence in NEJM, 1989;**321**:1480–1). Population studies indicate a two-fold increase in major MCMs and a slight reduction in birth weight (n = 210, 629 controls, Diav-Citrin et al, Neurology 2001;**57**:321–4). However, the UK epilepsy and pregnancy register showed that carbamazepine monotherapy may still have a low risk of major malformations (n = 3607, Morrow et al, J Neurol Neurosurg Psychiatry 2006; **7**:193–8). The literature recommends the need for counselling and screening for neural tube defects, which can detect 90–95% of neural tube defects if carried out with AFP levels at 16–18 weeks. In late pregnancy, routine vitamin K to mothers and the neonates is usually recommended.

Postnatal development: In a controlled study of *in utero* exposure, 36 children born to mothers taking carbamazepine were compared to matched controls. Allowing for variables, the carbamazepine children had similar IQs and language abilities to those of the controls (n = 36, Scolnik et al, *JAMA* 1994;**271**:767), and a long-term follow-up over up to 10 years showed normal intelligence in children exposed to carbamazepine monotherapy within normal plasma ranges during pregnancy compared to matched controls (n = 323; CBZ n = 86, Gaily et al, *Neurology* 2004;**13**:28–32), suggesting the lack of a clinically important adverse effect on cognitive development.

Oxcarbazepine (FDA = C) is closely related to carbamazepine. The placenta may contribute to the metabolism of oxcarbazepine (Pienimaki et al, *Epilepsia* 1997;**38**:309–16) and data indicate that oxcarbazepine may cause serious birth defects, and there is significant transfer through the placenta in humans (n = 12, Myllynen et al, *Epilepsia* 2001;**42**:1482–5). However, a large study from Argentina suggested that oxcarbazepine had a lower risk of teratogenicity than older AEDs (n = 114, Meischenguiser et al, *Epilepsy Behav* 2004;**5**:163–7). There is a report of an uneventful pregnancy and healthy child with oxcarbazepine taken throughout pregnancy (n = 1, Eisenschenk, *Neurologist* 2006; **12**:249–54). There is a significant decrease in ratio of plasma levels of oxcarbazepine MHD and dose in the first (26%), second (37%) and third (38%) trimesters, leading to seizures in eight patients (n = 10[13 pregnancies], Petrenaite et al, *Epilepsy Res* 2009;**84**:245–9).

In the third trimester there is a higher risk of seizures and higher doses are needed in mothers taking oxcarbazepine (n = 1956, EURAP Study Group, *Neurology* 2006;**66**:354–60), because plasma oxcarbazepine and metabolite (MHD) levels drop to 72% in the first trimester, 74% in the second trimester and down to 64% in the third trimester, rising to 108% after pregnancy (n = 7, Christensen et al, *Neurology* 2006;**67**:1497–9).

Careful monitoring throughout pregnancy and immediately afterwards is essential (n = 5, Mazzucchelli et al, *Epilepsia* 2006;**47**:504–9).

23. * **Valproate** (FDA = D; ADEC = D) crosses the placenta easily and is now well-established as both teratogenic and causing developmental problems and should not be used in women of child-bearing potential. There is undoubtedly a pharmacogenetic component to teratogenic and neurodevelopmental effects (Duncan, *Curr Opin Neurol* 2007;**20**:175–80):

- **First trimester:** The North American Antiepileptic Drug Pregnancy Registry has shown an increased relative risk of 7.3 of major malformations after first trimester exposure to valproate (10.7% had major malformations cf. 2.9% controls; n = 149, n = 1048 controls, Wyszynski et al, *Neurology* 2005;**64**:961–5). These include facial dysmorphia, hypospadias, limb malformations and spina bifida. However, dysmorphic features, developmental delay and structural anomalies may only be found in children exposed to maternal valproate doses above 1000 mg/d (n = 69, Mawer et al, *Seizure* 2002;**11**:512–8), an important observation.

- **Second/third trimester:** * reduced mean birth-weight-adjusted mean head circumference has been shown, although the significance of this is unknown, but has not been shown for phenytoin, clonazepam, lamotrigine and gabapentin (n = 900 000, Almgren et al, *Seizure* 2009;**18**:672–5).

- **Birth:** The literature now states that there have been rare reports of haemorrhagic syndrome in neonates whose mothers took valproate in pregnancy.

- **Postnatal development:** * The Liverpool and Manchester study of children aged 6–16 showed that those exposed to valproate *in utero* were more likely to have an IQ below 69 and a poorer memory compared to exposure to other AEDs or none. The mother's IQ and number of GTC seizures during pregnancy were significant predictors of verbal IQ in the children (n = 249, Vinten et al, *Neurology* 2005;**64**:949–54). Additional findings from this group also conclude that there is a seven times higher incidence cf. the control group of autism (6.3% vs 0.9%)

if valproate is used as monotherapy (n = 620 mothers, n = 632 live births, Bromley et al, Neurology 2008;**71**:1923–24). Exposure to valproate in utero may lead to a higher than expected incidence of education needs statements (n = 400 school-age children: 150 exposed to monotherapy, 74 to polytherapy and 176 to none, Adab et al, J Neurol Neurosurg Psychiatry 2001;**70**:15–21). A long-term follow-up over up to 10 years showed some evidence of reduced verbal intelligence in children exposed to valproate and AED polytherapy during pregnancy compared to matched controls (n = 323; valproate n = 13, polytherapy n = 30, Gaily et al, Neurology 2004;**13**:28–32). These support other studies showing an association with a risk of developmental delay (n = 400, Adab et al, J Neurol Neurosurg Psychiatry 2001;**70**:15–21; Dean et al, J Med Genet 2002;**39**:251–9; Finish registry study; n = 13, Viinikainen et al, Epilepsy Behav 2006;**9**:636–40). A prospective five-year study showed that at three years old, children exposed to valproate in utero had lower mean IQ scores (lamotrigine 101, phenytoin 99, carbamazepine 98, valproate 92) than with other AEDs (n = 309, Meador et al, N Engl J Med 2009;**360**:1597–605).

- Polycystic ovary syndrome (PCOS): There is an association between valproate and PCOS which may have some effect on reproductive capacity (n = 32, O'Donovan et al, J Clin Psychiatry 2002;**63**:322–30; review by Genton et al, Epilepsia 2001;**42**:295–304), but this may just be because valproate causes weight gain, a risk factor for PCOS.

The UK MHRA noted in September 2003 (Curr Prob Pharmacovig 2003;**29** [Sept]:6) that:

- specialist consultation should be sought for women likely to become pregnant on valproate
- if used in pregnancy, use the lowest effective dose (below 1000 mg/d)
- monotherapy
- use divided daily doses (2–3 times a day)
- give as an MR prep to reduce peak levels
- 5 mg folic acid should be started as soon as contraception is discontinued.

(Ornoy, Reprod Toxicol 2009;**28**:1–10).

NICE has recommended (Bipolar Guidelines, 2006) that valproate should not be used in women of child-bearing potential.

Reviews: general (Duncan, Curr Opin Neurol 2007;**20**:175–80; Genton et al, Drug Saf 2006; **29**:1–21).

24. **Phenytoin** (FDA = D; fosphenytoin = D; ADEC: phenytoin = D) crosses the placenta freely and teratogenicity is well-established, particularly the 'fetal hydantoin syndrome'. This syndrome includes growth retardation, microcephaly, mental retardation, facial defects, including cleft lip and/ or palate, digit and nail hypoplasia, rib anomalies, hirsuitism, low hairlines and inguinal hernia, plus cardiovascular, gastrointestinal or genitourinary anomalies (n = 2 and review: Ozkinay et al, Turk J Pediatr 1998;**40**:273–8). The full syndrome occurs in about 8–10% of children born to mothers who took phenytoin in the first trimester (n = 88, Rodriguez-Palomares et al, Arch Med Res 1995; **26**:371–7), and a part syndrome in a further 30% of children (controlled prospective study, n = 34, Nulman et al, Am J Med Genet 1997; **68**:18–24). It appears not to be dose-related (n = 88, Rodriguez-Palomares et al, Arch Med Res 1995;**26**:371–7). Prediction of the teratogenic risk may be possible by measuring microsomal epoxide hydrolase activity (n = 19, Buehler et al, NEJM 1990;**332**:1567–72).

The syndrome may be related to phenytoin-induced reduction in GSH levels, enhancing peroxidative damage to the fetus via the placental circulation (n = 52, controlled, Lui et al, Human Toxicol 1997;**16**:177–81). It has also been noted that epileptic fathers taking phenytoin have increased rates of malformed children (Friis, Acta Neurol Scand 1983;**94**[Suppl]:39–43).

The kinetics of phenytoin change in pregnancy. Elimination increases (single dose study, n = 5, Dickinson et al, Br J Clin Pharmacol 1989;**28**:17–27) and plasma levels fall steadily as the pregnancy progresses, with a possible change in the seizure frequency. Bound levels may be reduced with free (i.e. active) levels unchanged in pregnancy and so care with plasma level interpretation is needed (review of phenytoin disposition and metabolism in pregnancy, Eadie et al, Eur J Clin Pharmacol 1992;**43**:389–92).

Risk reduction with phenytoin: The general consensus seems to be that where documented seizures are proven to be controlled by phenytoin, the risks of withdrawal are probably greater than with the continued use of phenytoin, with the following precautions:

1. **Use of minimal effective doses.** At least monthly blood level monitoring (including free levels) during pregnancy (and for up to six months after) is essential to avoid toxicity and an increased teratogenic risk.

2.* **Use of folic acid 5 mg/d** from before conception. One study resulted in no birth defects in the 33 mothers who took folic acid from before conception, or immediately upon becoming pregnant, but there were 10 children with malformations from the 66 born to mothers who did not take folic acid, a **significant** and highly important difference (n = 66 retrospective, n = 22 prospective, Biale and Lewenthal, *Eur J Obstet Gynecol Reprod Biol* 1984;**18**:211). The neural tube closes around the time of the first missed period and so folic acid supplements need to be started **before** pregnancy is detected. However, not everyone agrees that folic acid supplementation reduces the risk, as other mechanisms may be responsible other than folic acid metabolism (n = 1935, Morrow et al, *J Neurol Neurosurg Psychiatry* 2009;**80**:506–11), but it is a low risk strategy either way.

3. **Vitamin K supplementation.** Phenytoin inhibits the synthesis of vitamin K-dependent clotting factors and neonatal haemorrhage may occur. Vitamin K deficiency may also be the cause of abnormal facial development, via abnormal development of the cartilaginous nasal septum. Early vitamin K supplementation in at-risk pregnancies is thus recommended and to the neonate after birth.

After birth, a withdrawal syndrome, including irritability and haemorrhage has been reported (prospective, Hill et al, *Am J Dis Child* 1974;**127**: 645–53).

Postnatal development: One study has indicated a negative neurodevelopmental effect from phenytoin. In a controlled study of *in utero* exposure, 34 children born to mothers taking phenytoin and 36 children born to mothers taking carbamazepine were compared to matched controls. Allowing for other variables, the phenytoin children had a significantly lower mean IQ and language ability, the carbamazepine children being similar to controls (Scolnik et al, *JAMA* 1994;**271**:767). Reports of malignancies in the infant have probably been disproven (Koren et al, *Teratology* 1989;**40**:157–62).

25.* **Phenobarbital** (FDA = D) has been implicated as a teratogen (see introduction to *3.8.4*), although in many reported cases it has been as part of a combination therapy. Minor digital deformities (finger-like thumbs, rudimentary or missing nails), as well as hip and facial abnormalities have been reported. In a study of pregnant women who attempted suicide by a barbiturate overdose, single very large doses did not appear to have any teratogenic, growth retardation or development adverse effects (n = 367, Timmermann et al, *Toxicol Ind Health* 2008;**24**:109–19; n = 88, Timmermann et al, *Pharmacoepidemiol Drug Saf* 2009;**18**:815–25). Withdrawal symptoms, such as seizures and irritability have occurred in the neonate, some delayed by up to two weeks after birth. Neonatal bleeding in the first 24 hours has been reported, as has respiratory depression. However, antenatal phenobarbital exposure does not appear to affect the neurodevelopmental outcome of premature infants at 18–22 months of age (n = 578, Shankaran et al, *Am J Obstet Gynecol* 2002;**187**:171–7).

Postnatal development: There is some evidence of a direct neurotoxic effect by phenobarbital on developing fetal neurons, which may be responsible for some cognitive or CNS abnormalities. Prenatal exposure to combined phenobarbital and phenytoin (n = 172) compared to controls (n = 168) produced smaller head size at birth and persistent learning problems (12%) compared to controls (1%) in one study (Dessens et al, *Acta Paediatrica* 2000;**89**:533–41). In the longer-term, a smaller head circumference and an impaired cognitive development has been suggested in two studies (n = 122, van der Pol et al, *Am J Obstet Gynecol* 1991;**164**:121–8).

26. * For **lamotrigine** (FDA = C; ADEC = B3), teratogenicity data from the North American Antiepileptic Drug Pregnancy Registry led the UK MHRA to issue a warning in June 2006 about an increased risk of oral clefts, although they note that this now needs confirming by other database analyses. Two of these confuse matters, e.g. the MCM level for lamotrigine was 2.3%, with an increased risk of isolated cleft palate or cleft lip deformity (n = 684, Holmes et

al, Neurology 2008;**70**:2152–8), but there was no evidence of a specific increased risk of isolated orofacial clefts compared to other lamotrigine associated malformation (n = 72 live births, Dolk *et al, Neurology* 2008;**71**:714–22). Previously, the incidence of major malformations with first-trimester exposure had been reported to be 1.8% (eg. n = 51, Sabers *et al, Acta Neurol Scand* 2004;**109**:9–13). When used as an anticonvulsant, extreme care is needed as plasma levels change throughout pregnancy:

- **First trimester:** LTG clearance increases by 197%, reducing levels by about 20% (n = 11, Franco *et al, Ther Drug Monit* 2008;**30**:544-7)
- **Second trimester:** clearance is increased 236%
- **Third trimester:** clearance is increased 248%
- **Delivery:** clearance is increased 264%.

The average lamotrigine dose increase necessary was 250% to maintain therapeutic plasma levels (n = 9, Fotopoulou *et al, Epilepsy Res* 2009; **85**:60–4; see also n = 6, Tomson *et al, Neurology* 2006;**67**:1297–9; n = 11, Petrenaite *et al, Epilepsy Res* 2005;**65**:185–8; n = 1956, EURAP Study Group, *Neurology* 2006;**66**:354–60). Levels revert rapidly to normal after delivery so reduce doses again, e.g. there is a case of severe apnoea and need for resuscitation in an infant having been breast-fed, with the mother using increasing doses of lamotrigine 850 mg/d before pregnancy (n = 1, Nordmo *et al, Ann Pharmacother* 2009; **43**:1893–7). In six mother–baby pairs, fetal **gabapentin** (FDA = C, ADEC = B1) levels were estimated to be 0.2–1.3 mg/kg/d (1.3–3.8% of mother's dose), with no adverse effects detected (n = 6, Ohman *et al, Epilepsia* 2005;**46**:1621–4), and there were no MCMs in the 11 babies born to mothers taking gabapentin in the first trimester in the Southampton PMSS (n = 3100, Wilton and Shakir, *Epilepsia* 2002;**43**:983–92).

27.* **Lacosamide** should not be used in pregnancy unless clearly indicated (SPC). Although some animal studies show reproductive toxicity, early results from the UK Epilepsy and Pregnancy Register show that in 117 infants exposed to **levetiracetam** (FDA = C), three (2.7%) had MCMs. Although all three had also been exposed to other AEDs (n = 117, Hunt *et al, Neurology* 2006;**67**:1876–9), it should not be used unless clearly necessary. In another study, the infant dose was equivalent to 2.4 mg/kg/d, equivalent to 7.9%

of weight-normalised maternal dose. Plasma concentrations in the infant were around 13% of mother's plasma levels, the author concluding that significant transfer and slow elimination can occur so TDM might be appropriate (n = 15, Abou-Khalil, *Epilepsy Curr* 2008;**8**:62–3). Limited data suggests that a significant fall in levetiracetam levels may occur during pregnancy (Tomson and Battino, *Clin Pharmacokinet* 2007;**46**:209–19). Animal studies have shown some animal reproductive toxicity with **pregabalin** (FDA = C) at high dose but the human risk is not known (SPC). The UK SPC recommends avoiding **rufinamide** in pregnancy and ensuring adequate contraception measures during treatment as the incidence of malformations is 2–3 times greater than the general spontaneous rate (UK SPC). No human data is available on **tiagabine** (FDA = C; ADEC = B3) in pregnancy and so use should only be where clearly indicated. **Topiramate** (FDA = C; ADEC = B3) passes across the placenta. Topiramate levels may rise in the first trimester by around 32%, by 81% in the second and by 75% in the third trimester, with significant interindividual variation (n = 10, Ohman *et al, Epilepsy Res* 2009;**87**:124–9), so TDM and assessing doses is advised to avoid the risk of increased seizures (n = 12, Westin *et al, Epilepsia* 2009;**50**:480–5). Preliminary experience from the UK Epilepsy and Pregnancy Register showed 31 (17%) abnormalities from 178 live births, including 16 with MCMs (n = 203, Hunt *et al, Neurology* 2008;**71**:272–6). The incidence of oral clefts was 2.2%, about 11 times the background rate. Another study of 52 pregnancies had 41 live births with reduced birth weight but no increase in structural defects (n = 52, Ornoy *et al, Reprod Toxicol* 2008;**25**:388–9). **Vigabatrin** is contraindicated due to a slight increase in the incidence of cleft palate at high doses in one animal test. **Zonisamide** is transferred to the infant via the placenta, the transfer rate being 92% (n = 2, Kawada *et al, Brain Dev* 2002;**24**:95–7) and adequate contraception in women is necessary during treatment and for one month afterwards. One case and a case series suggest a significant increase in clearance at the end of the second trimester to TDM and increased doses may be appropriate (n = 1, Oles and Bell, *Ann Pharmacother* 2008;**42**:1139–41).

28. For **acetazolamide** (FDA = C; ADEC = B3),

animal tests indicate that it is teratogenic and can increase miscarriages when taken at toxic doses. If use is essential, maternal electrolyte balance should be monitored. There are reported cases of malformations with **ethosuximide** (ADEC = D) alone, and some when combined with other drugs but no cause-effect relationship has been proven. Although animal studies in rats have raised some concerns, no systematic human data is available. Little data is available for **paraldehyde** (FDA = C).

3.8.5 OTHERS

29. Very high doses of **donepezil** (FDA = C; ADEC = B3) may have some minor effects in pregnancy but no teratogenicity has been detected. The safety of **rivastigmine** (FDA = B) in pregnancy has not been established. There is no data on **galantamine** (FDA = B) in pregnancy, although animal studies show a slight delay in fetal and neonatal development. Human data is lacking with **memantine** (FDA = B) but animal data suggests potentially reduced interuterine growth.

30.* **Anticholinergics**: (ADEC: benzatropine = B2, procyclidine = A)

There is little data available on these drugs. A 'small left colon syndrome' has been reported in two children born to mothers who took benzatropine and other psychotropic drugs late in pregnancy (Falterman and Richardson, *J Paediatr* 1980;**92**:308–10), although a cause-effect relationship was not established. The UK SPC notes that there no studies with **orphenadrine** and so should only be used if there is no safer alternative.

31. For **disulfiram** (ADEC = B2) there have been isolated reports of MCMs (e.g. Gardner and Clarkson, *N Z Med J* 1981;**93**:184–6), although other drugs were often taken and the symptoms were similar to the fetal alcohol syndrome. In animals, disulfiram has been shown to be embryotoxic. The risk-benefit ratio for the risks of alcoholism against disulfiram for the fetus must be assessed carefully. The UK SPC for **acamprosate** (FDA = C) states that use in pregnancy is a contraindication, but animal studies have not shown any evidence of teratogenicity.

32. * **Lithium** (FDA = D; ADEC = D) completely equilibrates across the placenta. Some studies show that the overall MCM rates with lithium (2.8%) are similar to control rates (2.4%), and suggest that lithium is not an important human teratogen if used with adequate screening (including level II ultrasound and fetal echocardiography) to detect Ebstein's anomaly (n = 148, prospective Jacobson et al, *Lancet* 1992;**339**:530–3; see also n=225, Yacobi and Ornoy, *Isr J Psychiatry Relat Sci* 2008;**45**:95–106). The malformation risk in the first trimester is in the order of 4–12% and, hence, still greater than the general population. The risk of Ebstein's anomaly (a rare congenital downward displacement of the tricuspid valve into the right ventricle) exists if lithium is taken during weeks two to six post-conception. Ebstein's anomaly is often quoted as 20 times more common with lithium, but remains rare as the risk rises from one in 20 000 to one in 1000. However, this risk must be weighed against the 50% chance of relapsing if lithium is stopped abruptly. An important study (n = 101, retrospective, Viguera et al, *Am J Psychiatry* 2000;**157**:179–84) noted that:

- the heart is formed very early, so stopping lithium when pregnancy is confirmed is too late anyway
- the relapse rates in the 40 weeks after lithium discontinuation are similar for pregnant (52%) and non-pregnant (58%) women, but much higher than the year before discontinuation (21%), so stopping lithium raises the risk of release 2–3-fold but pregnancy itself is relatively 'risk neutral'
- women who remained stable over the first 40 weeks after lithium discontinuation were 2.9 times more likely to relapse than non-pregnant women during weeks 41–62 (70% vs 24%)
- the relapse rates are much higher in rapid rather than gradual lithium discontinuation
- the > 50% relapse rate in the first 40 weeks is high, and the risk from consequentially needed drugs is high
- there were no major malformations in the children born to the women (n = 9) who continued lithium throughout pregnancy
- an unstudied option might be to stop lithium gradually as soon as pregnancy is known, then reintroduce it in the third trimester.

NICE (Antenatal and Postnatal Mental Health Guideline, 2007) recommends advising a woman to stop lithium if she is planning a pregnancy, is well and not at high risk of relapse. NICE also recommends that if a woman taking lithium becomes pregnant, is well and not at high risk of relapse, lithium should be stopped gradually over four weeks, and then informed that this may not remove the risk of cardiac defects in the fetus (although the author of this book fails to fully comprehend the logic of this bearing in mind the Viguera study mentioned above). If the woman is not well or at high risk of relapse, NICE recommends switching to an antipsychotic, stopping lithium and restarting in the second trimester, or continuing lithium if at high risk of relapse (for which rapid withdrawal would be a risk factor). Renal clearance is increased during pregnancy and so higher doses are needed, but then lithium clearance reduces markedly near the end of term, doses may need to be reduced by up to 30–50% in the last few weeks (or a few doses omitted close to delivery) and plasma levels monitored carefully and frequently (n = 10 + 32, Newport et al, Am J Psychiatry 2005;**162**:2162–70). NICE recommends monitoring levels every four weeks until the 36th week, then weekly, then within the first 24 hours after childbirth, with doses adjusted according to those serum levels, and adequate fluid intake maintained.

Postnatal development: A study of healthy children born to mothers who took lithium during the first trimester did not reveal any increased frequency of physical or mental anomalies among the lithium children compared to their non-lithium exposed siblings over 5–10 years (n = 60, Schou, Acta Psychiatr Scand 1976;**54**:193–7; see also Pinelli et al, Am J Obstet Gynecol 2002;**187**:245–9).

Reviews: Llewellyn et al, J Clin Psychiatry 1998; **59**[Suppl 6]:S57–S64; Yonkers et al, CNS Drugs 1998;**9**:261–9.

33. **Modafinil** (FDA = C) is contraindicated in pregnancy. Pre-clinical studies have shown no teratogenicity but more information is required. There is limited data on **sodium oxybate** (FDA = B), with no evidence of malformations or toxicity after second and third trimester exposure, but there is no data in the first trimester and so it is not recommended (SPC).

34.* **Methadone** (ADEC = C) maintenance throughout pregnancy is associated with reduced risk of poor quality street drug use, earlier and better antenatal care and improved treatment

retention (n = 2993, Burns et al, Addiction 2007; **102**:264–70) than tapered withdrawal (n = 175, Jones et al, Am J Addict 2008;**17**:372–86).

- **First trimester:** With potential illicit drug-using mothers, teratogenicity with methadone will obviously be very difficult to ascertain, but there does not appear to be a clear association with malformations (e.g. study by Newman et al, Am J Obstet Gynecol 1975;**121**:233–7). Stopping opiates abruptly is dangerous, as withdrawal reactions can damage the fetus more than methadone.

- **Second/third trimester:** Methadone clearance can be increased, with trough plasma levels dropping to 58%, which may require higher doses (n = 9, Wolff et al, Eur J Clin Pharmacol 2005;**61**:763–8). In a study of methadone maintenance in pregnancy, head circumference and birth weight were slightly lower with methadone compared to controls (n = 32, Brown et al, Am J Obstet Gynecol 1998;**179**:459–63).

- **NAS (neonatal abstinence syndrome):*** Symptoms include tremor, irritability, hyperactivity, jitteriness, shrill cry, vomiting, diarrhoea and convulsions. About 45% of infants develop NAS with maternal methadone requiring treatment (median stay 10/7), and the incidence can be reduced by breast-feeding (n = 450, Dryden et al, BJOG 2009;**116**:665–71). Although logically dose-related, high-dose methadone appears not to be associated with an increased risk of NAS compared to lower doses (e.g. n = 159, Simmat-Durand et al, Eur J Obstet Gynecol Reprod Biol 2009;**142**:119–23), but rather to overall maternal drug use (n = 81, McCarthy et al, Am J Obstet Gynecol 2005;**193**:606–10; see also breast-feeding, 3.1).The incidence of NAS may be higher with buprenorphine than methadone (67% vs 58%, n = 41 [c = 38], Bakstad et al, Eur Addict Res 2009;**15**:128–34) or vice versa (methadone 78% vs 40%, n = 47, Kakko et al, Drug Alcohol Depend 2008;**96**:69–78), although may be lower if buprenorphine is started pre-conception. Slow-release morphine is no better at reducing neonatal withdrawal symptoms than methadone (n = 48, Fischer et al, Addiction 1999;**94**:231–9). Cochrane concluded that there was no proven significant difference between the available opiate agonists with regard to NAS and birth weight, but the data sample was small (s = 3, n = 96, Minozzi et al, Cochrane Database Syst Rev 2008;**2**:CD006318). Each 1 mg increase in methadone dose taken before delivery adds an extra 0.18 days to neonatal abstinence syndrome duration or, to put it another way, each 5.5 mg adds a day to the NAS (n = 68, retrospective, Lim et al, Am J Obstet Gynecol 2009;**200**:e1–5). Clonidine and chloral hydrate (n = 29) have been used successfully as a short-term alternative to morphine and phenobarbital (n = 64) for NAS (n = 133, Esmaeili et al, Acta Paediatr 2010:[in press]).

- Postnatal development: Long-term developmental outcome seems unaffected by methadone (Kaltenbach and Finnegan, Neurotoxicol Teratol 1987;**9**:311–3; effect in the first year see Arch Dis Childhood 1989;**64**:235–45).

Buprenorphine * (FDA = C; ADEC = C) may have some advantages in pregnancy (Nocon, Addiction 2006;**101**:608). In weeks 24–29, buprenorpine had a higher retention rate than methadone, but higher additional opioid use with an earlier onset of NAS occurring with methadone (mean 60 hours) than buprenorphine (72 hours) (n = 18[c = 14], RCT, d/b, Fischer et al, Addiction 2006;**101**:275–81). There is evidence for increased buprenorphine renal elimination in the third trimester, but with significant intrasubject differences (n=9, Kacinko et al, Clin Chem 2009;**55**:1177–87). Women on high-dose buprenorphine (n = 159) throughout pregnancy (compared to methadone), surprisingly showed that there was no relationship between dose and the duration or severity of NAS (n = 251, Simmat-Durand et al, Eur J Obstet Gynecol Reprod Biol 2008;**142**:119–23).

Review: * extensive review of methadone, naltrexone and buprenorphine (Farid et al, Curr Neuropharmacol 2008;**6**:125–50).

35. No teratogenic effects have been reported in women who took **dexamfetamine** (FDA = C) before knowing they were pregnant (Guilleminault, Sleep 1993;**16**:199–201). There is little information available for **methylphenidate** (FDA = C; ADEC = B2) and the few reported cases are unremarkable, but the literature advises caution. The UK SPC recommends use of **atomoxetine** (FDA = C) only where the benefit justifies the potential risk (short review of evidence for all ADHD treatments: Humphreys et al, Can Fam Physician 2007;**53**:1153–5).

36. There have been reports of a higher than expected incidence of neonatal malformations with **bupropion** (FDA = C), especially cardiac (n = 10, Anon, Prescrire Int 2005;**14**:225), but a large US study (1995–2004) showed that exposure to bupropion in the first trimester (n = 1213) and second and third trimesters (n = 1049) was not associated with an increased risk of cardiovascular or other malformations, compared to other antidepressant (n = 4743) first trimester exposures (Cole et al, Pharmacepidemiol Drug Saf 2007;**16**:474–84).

3.9 RENAL IMPAIRMENT (SEE ALSO BNF)

	LOWER RISK (FDA=A)	MODERATE RISK (FDA=B OR C)	HIGHER RISK (FDA=D OR X)
Antipsychotics	Asenapine[2]	Aripiprazole[2] Butyrophenones[6] Clozapine[3] Olanzapine[2] Phenothiazines[7] Pimozide[8] Quetiapine[2] Thioxanthenes[4] Ziprasidone[2]	Amisulpride[5] Paliperidone[1] Risperidone[1] Sulpiride[5] Zotepine[2]
Antidepressants	Agomelatine[14] Mianserin[16] Moclobemide[16] Tricyclics[12] Trazodone[13] Tryptophan[16]	Duloxetine[10] MAOIs[15] Mirtazapine[11] Reboxetine[14] SSRIs[9]	Fluoxetine[9] Venlafaxine[10]
Anxiolytics and hypnotics	Benzodiazepines (some)[17] Zaleplon[19] Zopiclone[19]	Benzodiazepines[17] Beta-blockers[20] Clomethiazole[21] Hydroxyzine[18] Melatonin[21] Zolpidem[19]	Buspirone[18] Chloral[21]
Anticonvulsants	Phenytoin[24] Rufinamide[27] Tiagabine[27]	Barbiturates[25] Benzodiazepines[17] Carbamazepine[22] Fosphenytoin[24] Lacosamide[27] Lamotrigine[26] Piracetam[27] Topiramate[27] Zonisamide[27]	Acetazolamide[28] Ethosuximide[28] Gabapentin[26] Levetiracetam[27] Midazolam[17] Oxcarbazepine[22] Pregabalin[27] Valproate[23]
Others	Anticholinesterases[29] Sodium oxybate[33]	Anticholinergics[30] Atomoxetine[35] Bupropion[34] Disulfiram[31] Memantine[29] Modafinil[33]	Acamprosate[31] Lithium[32] Methylphenidate[35]

Grade	GFR ml/min	Serum creatinine micromo/L
Mild	20–50	150–300
Moderate	10–20	300–700
Severe	<10	>700

GENERAL PRINCIPLES FOR PRESCRIBING IN RENAL IMPAIRMENT (adapted from *Maudsley Guidelines*)

1. The greater the renal impairment, the greater the potential for accumulation of drugs. Adverse effects such as postural hypotension, sedation and confusion may be more common.

2. Serum creatinine may not be raised in the elderly, although renal impairment may be present.

3. Care is needed with drugs or active metabolites predominantly cleared by the kidney, e.g. antidepressants and antipsychotics (except substituted benzamides).

4. Start low and go slow, adjusting doses to tolerance.

5. Care is needed with drugs with marked anticholinergic activity, which may cause urinary retention and interfere with U&E measurements.

3.9.1 ANTIPSYCHOTICS

Lower doses of all antipsychotics should be used, due to increased cerebral sensitivity and EPS.

1. **Risperidone** elimination is reduced in renal disease and so initial doses and dose increments should be halved, up to a maximum of about 4 mg/d. Haemodialysis has resulted in reduced risperidone levels, leading to relapse (n = 1, Railton et al, *Ther Drug Monit* 2005;**27**:558–61). In mild renal impairment (Ccr 50–79 ml/min), start with **paliperidone** 3 mg/d and increase carefully. If 30–49 ml/min stay at 3 mg/d, if 10–29 ml/min, use 3 mg on alternate days and it is not recommended for < 10 ml/min.

2. * Dose adjustment with **aripiprazole** is not necessary even in severe renal impairment, e.g. although the Cmax for a single dose of aripiprazole 15 mg was 40% higher in severe renal impairment, there were no significant adverse effects (n = 13, Mallikaarjun et al, *Clin Pharmacokinet* 2008; **47**:533–42). For **asenapine**, 50% is renally excreted but no dose alterations are necessary in renal impairment (US PI). **Olanzapine** is excreted primarily (57%) via the renal pathway and 30% in faeces. A lower olanzapine starting dose of 5 mg/d may be appropriate in renal impairment (review: Callaghan et al, *Clin Pharmacokinetics* 1999;**37**:177–93). If creatinine clearance is < 10 ml/

min, there is only a slight (11%) increase in half-life and 17% reduction in clearance. For olanzapine pamoate, a lower starting dose of 150 mg/4 weeks should be considered in people with renal impairment (SPC). The UK SPC for **quetiapine** now states that oral clearance is reduced by 25% in renal impairment (UK SPC), so start at 50 mg/d (25 mg/d in severe) and increase at 50 mg/d according to response and tolerability (e.g. n = 8, Thyrum et al, *Prog Neuropsychopharmacol Biol Psychiatry* 2000;**24**:521–33). 17% of a dose of **zotepine** is excreted through the kidneys and levels may be 2–3 times higher in patients with renal impairment. Start at 25 mg BD up to a maximum of 75 mg BD. Only 1% of a **ziprasidone** dose is excreted unchanged via urine (20% excreted as metabolites), so dosage adjustment is not required in renal impairment.

3. **Clozapine** is contraindicated in severe renal disease. Start at 12.5 mg/d and increase slowly in mild-to-moderate renal failure.

4. * **Zuclopenthixol** and **flupentixol** should be used with caution in renal impairment, as some accumulation of metabolites has been reported. Flupentixol has not been studied in renal impairment.

5. **Sulpiride** is mainly cleared by the kidneys and its half-life can range from 6–25 hours, depending upon renal function. Reduce the dose by 35–70% or extend the dosage interval by a factor of 1.5 to 3 if necessary (n = 24, open, Bressolle et al, *Clin Pharmacokinet* 1989; **17**:367–73). **Amisulpride** is principally cleared unchanged through the kidneys, so care is needed in moderate-to-severe renal insufficiency (GFR 10–30 ml/min). It is not appreciably removed during haemodialysis.

6. There are no apparent problems with **haloperidol** although the literature recommends caution as some accumulation might occur.

7. There is little information on **phenothiazines**, but excretion may be slower and accumulation may occur, causing sedation or postural hypotension. **Levomepromazine** (methotrimeprazine) should be used with care in renal disease, and chlorpromazine avoided.

8. The UK SPC for **pimozide** recommends caution in renal impairment.

3.9.2 ANTIDEPRESSANTS

Review: * antidepressants in chronic kidney

disease (Raymond et al, Nephrol Nurs J 2008;**35**: 257–63).

9. Renal clearance accounts for about 20% of total **citalopram** elimination, and although half-life increases slightly, no reduction of citalopram dosage is warranted in patients with moderately impaired renal function, but slight reduction in severe renal failure may be prudent (RCT, Joffe et al, Eur J Clin Pharmacol 1998;**54**:237–42). Haemodialysis had an insignificant effect on plasma levels (n = 12, open, Spigset et al, Eur J Clin Pharmacol 2000;**56**:699–703). Dosage adjustment with **escitalopram** is not necessary in patients with mild or moderate renal impairment. Caution is advised in patients with severely reduced renal function (Ccr < 30 ml/min). The UK SPC for **fluoxetine** notes that when given 20 mg/day for two months, patients with severe renal failure (GFR < 10 ml/min) requiring dialysis showed no difference in plasma levels of fluoxetine or norfluoxetine compared to controls with normal renal function. **Fluvoxamine** should be used with care, starting at 50 mg/d and increasing only slowly. Plasma levels of fluvoxamine are reduced by about 22% by haemodialysis, so higher doses might be needed (n = 7, Kamo et al, Psychiatr Clin Neurosci 2004;**58**:133–7). In moderate renal impairment, reduce the initial dose of **paroxetine** to 10 mg/d and increase only if necessary. Use of **sertraline** is not recommended by the SPC, although Pfizer had 'data on file' of a single dose study which showed no significant changes in kinetics in mild, moderate or severe renal failure.

10. About 1–10% of a **venlafaxine** dose is cleared unchanged by the kidney and 30% renally excreted as the major metabolite. Total clearance is reduced by about 35% in mild-to-moderate renal impairment (GFR 10–30 ml/min) and so doses should be reduced by about 25–50%, although there is much inter-patient variability in renal impairment (Anon, J Clin Psychiatry 1993;**54**:119–26). A study (12 with renal impairment, eight on dialysis and 18 matched controls) showed that clearance was reduced by about 55% in moderate-to-severe renal disease, and the authors suggested a 50% reduction in venlafaxine dose, given once a day, where GFR was less than 30 ml/min (n = 38, open, Troy et al, Clin Pharmacol Therapeut 1994;**56**:14–21). Daily doses should also be reduced by 50% in dialysis and doses withheld until after dialysis is complete. Venlafaxine is not

recommended in severe renal failure. No dose adjustment is needed for **duloxetine** in mild-to-moderate renal disease (Ccr 30–80 ml/min), but is contraindicated in severe (Ccr < 30 ml/min) renal disease where plasma levels are doubled.

11.* **Mirtazapine** clearance was reduced by 33% in moderate and by 50% in severe renal failure, but not in mild renal impairment in a single dose study (n = 40, Bengtsson et al, Hum Psychopharmacol 1998;**13**:357–65). Care with higher doses is recommended. Mirtazapine is largely unaffected by haemodialysis as, since 85% is protein-bound, only 15% is likely to be dialysed, and there is a report of dialysis having no effect on mirtazapine levels (n = 1, Schlotterbeck et al, Pharmacopsychiatry 2008;**41**:259–60).

12. **Tricyclics** should be started at low dose and increased slowly, with divided doses. Avoid **lofepramine** in severe renal impairment, as 50% is renally excreted.

13. No dosage adjustment is necessary for **trazodone**.

14. **Reboxetine's** half-life and plasma levels appear to rise (up to two-fold) in severe renal impairment, where dose adjustment may be necessary. In a single-dose study, a reduction in starting dose to 2 mg BD in patients with moderate-to-severe renal dysfunction has been suggested (n = 18, open, Coulomb et al, J Clin Pharmacol 2000; **40**: 482–7). No dose adjustments are needed with **agomelatine**.

15. No dosage adjustments are usually necessary for the **MAOIs**, although **isocarboxazid** should be used with caution with impaired renal function to prevent accumulation.

16. Dosage adjustments in renal disease are not necessary for **moclobemide** (n = 12, open, Stoeckel et al, Acta Psychiatr Scand 1990;**360**[Suppl]:S94–S97), **mianserin** or **tryptophan**.

3.9.3 ANXIOLYTICS AND HYPNOTICS

17. Low dose anticonvulsant use of **benzo-diazepines** may be acceptable, as higher doses produce an increase in CNS sedative side-effects. **Chlordiazepoxide** can be given in normal doses and is not affected by haemodialysis (review, Bennett et al, Am J Kidney Dis 1983;**3**:155). In severe renal failure, doses of **oxazepam** should be reduced to 75%. In end-stage renal failure and haemodialysis, **clobazam** and metabolite

concentrations appear no different to those with normal renal function so there may be no need to change doses in any degree of renal failure or in haemodialysis (n = 1, Roberts and Zoanetti, *Ann Pharmacother* 1994;**28**:966–7). Accumulation of metabolites of **midazolam** may be responsible for prolonged sedation, not reversible by flumazenil (n = 5, Bauer et al, *Lancet* 1995;**346**:145–7).

18. **Buspirone** plasma levels have been shown to be higher in patients with renal failure, with a good correlation between steady-state levels and serum albumin (n = 54, open, Barbhaiya et al, *Eur J Clin Pharmacol* 1994;**46**:41–7). It is contraindicated in moderate or severe renal impairment. **Hydroxyzine** should be used with caution in patients with impaired renal function (UK SPC).

19. Plasma protein-binding of **zolpidem** is reduced in renal failure (n = 54, open, Pacifici, *Int J Clin Pharmacol Ther Toxicol* 1988;**26**:439–43). The half-life may be doubled but no dosage adjustments are recommended in mild renal dysfunction. The pharmacokinetics of **zaleplon** and **zopiclone** are not significantly different in renal impairment, and dose alteration is not required.

20. In severe renal disease, plasma levels of **beta-blockers** may be higher and so starting doses should be lower. Beta-blockers may also reduce renal blood flow and adversely affect renal function.

21. * Caution is needed with **clomethiazole** in chronic renal disease. **Chloral** is contraindicated in moderate to marked renal impairment. **Melatonin** has not been studied in renal impairment (SPC) but 3 mg/d improves sleep-wake rhythm in people undergoing haemodialysis (c = 20, RCT, d/b, p/c, c/o, 3 × 6/52, Koch et al, *Br J Clin Pharmacol* 2009; **67**:68–75).

3.9.4 ANTICONVULSANTS

Review: optimising AEDs in renal dysfunction (Lalerda et al, *Neurology* 2006;**67**(12 Suppl 4): S28–33).

22. **Carbamazepine** rarely causes renal disturbances, although it has been suggested that doses should be reduced by 25% in severe renal failure. The UK SPC has renal impairment as a precaution. For **oxcarbazepine** in renal impairment (Ccr <30 ml/min), start at half the usual dose

(300 mg/day), increasing no more frequently than at weekly intervals. In patients with pre-existing renal conditions associated with low sodium or in patients treated concomitantly with sodium-lowering drugs (e.g. diuretics, desmopressin) as well as NSAIDs, serum sodium levels should be monitored carefully.

23. * **Valproate** is eliminated mainly through the kidneys and the literature states that it may be necessary to decrease dosage in renal insufficiency. There are two cases of valproate used successfully in renal failure of haemodialysis (n = 2, Gupta and Annadatha, *Clin Pract Epidemol Ment Health* 2008;**4**:21).

24. No specific dose adjustments are required for **phenytoin**, but protein-binding is altered in uraemia, which can be problematic in accurately assessing serum levels. Severe cardiovascular ADRs have been reported with **fosphenytoin** IV in renal impairment (see 3.2) and so a reducing loading dose and/or infusion rate by 10–25% is recommended.

25. **Phenobarbital** causes increased sedation and the dosage interval should be no more frequently than 12–16 hours in severe renal failure. Large doses of **primidone** should be avoided. Active metabolites of **amylobarbital** accumulate in severe renal disease.

26. * **Gabapentin** is mainly excreted unchanged in the urine (n = 12, open, Hooper et al, *Br J Clin Pharmacol* 1991;**31**:171–4). The manufacturer recommends dose reductions as follows:

Creatine clearance	Gabapentin dosage and frequency
60–90 ml/min	400 mg TDS
30–59 ml/min	300 mg BD
15–29 ml/min	300 mg/d
<15 ml/min	300 mg alternate days

Patients undergoing haemodialysis should receive a gabapentin loading dose of 400 mg, plus 200–300 mg for every four hours of dialysis. Alternatively, a single-dose study of gabapentin 400 mg in adults with varying degrees of renal function (but none on dialysis) showed that clearance correlated well with creatinine clearance, with increased half-life with poorer renal function. The authors of this study suggested normal gabapentin doses for creatinine clearance of 60 ml/min, 600 mg/d for 30–59 ml/min, 300 mg/d for 15–29 ml/min and 150 mg/d for CLcr less than 15 ml/min (n = 60, open, Blum et al, Clin Pharmacol Therapeut 1994;**56**:154–9). There are reported cases of significantly impaired consciousness (n = 1, Miller and Price, Pain Med 2009;**10**:190–2) and reversible hearing loss (n = 1, Pierce et al, Clin Ther 2008;**30**:1681–4), so reducing doses is important. A reduced maintenance dose of **lamotrigine** is usually recommended in severe renal impairment, but the dose probably needs little adjustment in mild-to-moderate impairment (n = 21, Wootton et al, Br J Clin Pharmacol 1997;**43**:23–7), and even in end-stage renal failure, although the major glucuronide metabolite levels may increase eight-fold due to reduced renal clearance.

27. * No dose adjustment is needed with **laco-samide** in mild-to-moderate renal impairment, but 250 mg/d is the maximum in severe renal impairment (SPC) as the AUC is increased by about 30%. Supplements are needed in haemodialysis. Since 66% of a dose of **levetiracetam** is excreted unchanged in the urine, dose reductions are necessary in impaired renal function as follows (UK SPC):

Renal function	Creatinine clearance	Levetiracetam maximum dose
Normal	80 ml/min	500–1500 mg BD
Mild	50–79 ml/min	500–1000 mg BD
Moderate	30–49 ml/min	250–750 mg BD
Severe	< 30 ml/min	250–500 mg BD
End-stage renal disease, undergoing dialysis *	–	500–1000 mg OD

* Following dialysis, a 250–500 mg supplemental dose is recommended.

Piracetam is excreted unchanged via the kidneys and dose adjustments may be needed in renal impairment (review: Tacconi and Wurtman, Adv Neurol 1986;**43**:675–85). **Pregabalin** is mainly

excreted unchanged by the kidney, clearance being directly proportional to creatinine clearance (n = 50, Randinitis et al, J Clin Pharmacol 2003;**43**:277–83), so doses in renal impairment must be individually calculated (see SPC) as a few cases of reversible renal failure have been reported. Supplementary doses are necessary after every four-hour haemodialysis (SPC). No dose adjustment is needed for **rufinamide** in people with severe renal impairment (UK SPC) as it is almost entirely metabolised, but levels are reduced by about 30% by haemodialysis. There are no apparent problems with **tiagabine** (n = 25, Cato et al, Epilepsia 1998;**39**:43–7). About 60–70% of a **topiramate** dose is excreted unchanged via the kidneys. Time to steady state may be 10–15 days in severe renal impairment instead of 4–8 days with normal renal function. Dose titration may thus need to be more careful. Supplemental doses of 50% of the daily dose should be given on haemodialysis days. There is an increased risk of renal stone formation, via its carbonic anhydrase inhibition; carbonic anhydrase being a known inhibitor of renal crystallisation. Care is needed to ensure adequate fluid throughput, especially in patients with known disposition to this problem (Wasserstein et al, Epilepsia 1995;**36**[Suppl 3]: S153). **Vigabatrin** is renally excreted and so reduced doses are recommended with a Ccr < 60 mL/min. **Zonisamide** and metabolite are excreted renally and should not be used in acute renal failure or where serum creatinine is significantly raised. Zonisamide AUC is increased by 35% in people where Ccr < 20 ml/min. It may cause symptomatic renal calculus.

28. The UK SPC for **ethosuximide** now requires use only with extreme caution in impaired renal function, and doses should be reduced by at least 25% in severe renal failure.

3.9.5 OTHERS

29. No change in dose is necessary with **donepezil** in mild-to-moderate renal impairment and a 5 mg single-dose study indicated that even moderate-to-severe renal impairment did not significantly alter donepezil kinetics (open, n = 22, Tiseo et al, Br J Clin Pharmacol 1998;**46**[Suppl 1]:S56–S60). There are no reported problems with **rivastigmine**. No dosage reduction of **galantamine** is necessary for creatinine clearance

greater than 9 ml/min. In severe impairment (<9 ml/min) galantamine is contraindicated (due to a lack of safety data). **Memantine** can be used in renal failure with no dosage adjustments, although 5 mg BD is recommended in severe renal failure (n = 32 [c = 31], Periclou et al, *Clin Pharmacol Ther* 2006;**79**:134–43).

30. * The literature recommends some caution in renal disease with the **anticholinergics**. **Orphenadrine** is mainly excreted in the urine.

31. The SPC for **disulfiram** recommends caution in renal disease. The UK SPC contraindicates **acamprosate** in renal insufficiency (serum creatinine >120 micromol/L).

32. * **Lithium** is contraindicated in severe renal impairment but if use is unavoidable, use alternate-day dosing, very low doses (25–75% normal) and frequently estimate levels (e.g. 125 mg on alternate days in a 78-year-old woman, n = 1, Gash et al, *J Affect Disord* 1995;**34**:51–3).

A review of lithium and chronic kidney disease (Kripalani et al, *BMJ* 2009;**339**:b2452) notes that the renal markers that should prompt nephrology advice and stopping lithium include:

- fall in GFR to below 45 ml/min/1.732 body surface or a rapidly falling rate or heavy proteinuria
- steady or persistent fall in GFR (rather than a single measurement)
- stages 4 and 5 of chronic kidney disease.

Review: * lithium nephrotoxicity (Grünfeld and Rossier, *Nat Rev Nephrology* 2009;**5**:270–6).

33. The maximum **modafinil** dose of 400 mg/d should only be used in the absence of renal impairment. **Sodium oxybate** contains a significant dose of sodium (0.75 g in 4.5 g dose) and so dietary restriction of sodium might be considered, but since the kidney is not involved in excretion no dose reduction is thought to be necessary (SPC).

34. **Bupropion** and metabolites are almost exclusively (85%) excreted through the kidneys and so, in renal failure, the initial dose should be reduced and close monitoring for toxicity carried out.

35. For **atomoxetine**, 80% of a dose is excreted in urine and the UK SPC recommends possible dose reduction in renal impairment. The SPCs for **methylphenidate** note that there is no experience of use in renal failure.

DRUG INTERACTIONS

Full reviews, assessments and references for most of these interactions can be found in standard reference books. Resources include *Drug Interactions Facts, Drug Interactions* by Ivan Stockley (Blackwell Scientific, Oxford), or *Drug Interactions in Psychiatry*, edited by Ciraulo, Shader, Greenblatt and Creelman (Williams & Wilkins, Maryland).

Absolute classification of interactions is impossible. Many factors, e.g. age, concurrent illness, P450 status, etc are important. Single case reports merely suggest a possible interaction, and more structured formal studies may show the probable likelihood of an interaction. For completeness, some drugs available worldwide are included and may not be marketed in all countries. To give some guidance, interactions with the drugs in **CAPITAL LETTERS** are those that could be:

- potentially hazardous
- where a dosage adjustment is likely to have to be made
- well-established and documented
- of clinical significance
- rare but important.

How to use this section:

1. Look up the psychiatric drug or group.
2. Look up the drug group of the interacting drug.
3. If no entry there, look up the actual drug.
4. If still no entry, little or nothing has been reported to date.

Review: general psychotropics (Chadwick *et al*, *Adv Psychiatr Treat* 2005;**11**:440–9).

4.1 ANXIOLYTICS AND HYPNOTICS

Reviews: clinically important drug interactions with zopiclone, zaleplon and zolpidem (Hesse *et al*, *CNS Drugs* 2003;**17**:513–32), pharmacokinetics and pharmacodynamics (Drover, *Clin Pharmaco-kinet* 2004;**43**:227–38).

4.1.1 BENZODIAZEPINES

Benzodiazepines are mainly metabolised by CYP2C and CYP3A3/4.

Review: * Herbal medication interactions with midazolam (Tweddell and Boyle, *Dent Update* 2009;**36**:175–8)

Acamprosate + benzodiazepines
See acamprosate (*4.6.1*).

Agomelatine + benzodiazepines
See agomelatine (*4.3.3.1*).

ALCOHOL + BENZODIAZEPINES
See alcohol (*4.7.1*).

Alosetron + alprazolam
Alosetron, a 5–HT3 receptor antagonist, has no effect on the kinetics of alprazolam (n = 12, RCT, open, D'Souza *et al*, *J Clin Pharmacol* 2001; **41**:452–4).

Amfetamines + benzodiazepines
Amfetamine significantly reverses the sedative and memory-impairing effects of triazolam (n = 20, p/c, d/b, c/o, Mintzer and Griffiths, *J Psychopharmacol* 2003;**17**:17–29, 146).

Amiodarone + clonazepam
Amidarone has been reported to cause clonazepam toxicity at low dose (n = 1, Witt *et al*, *Ann Pharmacother* 1993;**27**:1463–4).

Antacids + benzodiazepines
Benzodiazepine absorption is slightly delayed by antacids, but total absorption remains the same.

Anticholinergics + benzodiazepines
Benzodiazepine absorption may be delayed by anticholinergics, but the AUC remains unchanged.

Anticoagulants + benzodiazepines
Lack of an interaction has been demonstrated and benzodiazepines. Isolated cases of adverse reactions have been reported, e.g. no interaction has been reported with warfarin but is theoretically possible (mentioned in Sayal *et al*, *Acta Psychiatr Scand* 2000;**102**:250–5).

Antihistamines + benzodiazepines
Enhanced sedation is possible.

Antihypertensives + benzodiazepines
Enhanced hypotension is possible.

Antipsychotics + benzodiazepines
See individual drugs and antipsychotics (*4.2.1*).

Antiretrovirals + benzodiazepines
Maraviroc levels have not been measured, but although midazolam levels change slightly no significant interaction is expected.

Atomoxetine + benzodiazepines
See atomoxetine (4.6.4).

Atropine + benzodiazepines
No interaction is thought to occur.

Baclofen + benzodiazepines
Enhanced sedation can occur.

Barbiturates + benzodiazepines
Enhanced sedation and increased benzodiazepine clearance may occur via CYP3A4 induction. Dose adjustment may be necessary.

Beta-blockers + benzodiazepines
Propranolol and metoprolol produce a small but significant reduction in diazepam clearance. Propranolol and labetolol have no effect on oxazepam (n = 6, Sonne et al, Br J Clin Pharmacol 1990;**29**:33–7) and metoprolol has no effect on lorazepam (n = 12, open, Scott et al, Eur J Clin Pharmacol 1991;**40**:405–9).

Buprenorphine + benzodiazepines
Buprenorphine does not inhibit the metabolism of flunitrazepam and so any interaction is likely to be pharmacodynamic rather than metabolic, although deaths have been reported with concomitant buprenorphine and benzodiazepines (n = 6, Reynaud et al, Addiction 1998;**93**:1385–92).

Buspirone + benzodiazepines
See buspirone (4.1.2).

CALCIUM-CHANNEL BLOCKERS + BENZODIAZEPINES
Diltiazem significantly increases diazepam levels, probably via CYP3A4 inhibition (n = 13, RCT, d/b, c/o, Kosuge et al, Drug Metab Dispos 2001;**29**:1284–9). Both diltiazem and verapamil significantly raise midazolam levels and half-life, via 3A4 inhibition, increasing sedative side-effects, and so a 50% midazolam dose reduction has been recommended (n = 9, RCT, d/b, c/o, 2/7, Backman et al, Br J Clin Pharmacol 1994;**37**:221–5).

Cannabis + benzodiazepines
See cannabis (4.7.2).

Carbamazepine + benzodiazepines
See carbamazepine (4.5.1).

Charcoal, activated + benzodiazepines
25 g of activated charcoal given 30 minutes after diazepam 5 mg reduces diazepam AUC by 27%, but not the peak levels. Concurrent gastric lavage does not provide any additional reductions (n = 9, RCT, Lapatto-Reiniluoto et al, Br J Clin Pharmacol 1999;**48**:148–53).

Citalopram + benzodiazepines
See citalopram/escitalopram (4.3.2.1).

Clarithromycin + benzodiazepines
Higher dose clarithromycin (2.5 g/d) may increase the availability of midazolam, probably via CYP3A4 inhibition (n = 16, open, 8/7, Gorski et al, Clin Pharmacol Ther 1998;**64**:133–43).

CLOZAPINE + BENZODIAZEPINES
See clozapine (4.2.3).

Cyclophosphamide + benzodiazepines
Cyclophosphamide toxicity has been proposed in animals but not reported in humans.

Dehydroepiandrosterone + benzodiazepines
Alprazolam rapidly and significantly increases dehydroepiandrosterone levels (n = 38, Kroboth et al, J Clin Psychopharmacol 1999;**19**:114–24).

Dextropropoxyphene + alprazolam
Increased sedation can occur with alprazolam.

Digoxin + benzodiazepines
Lack of interaction has been shown.

Disulfiram + benzodiazepines
See disulfiram (4.6.8).

Escitalopram + benzodiazepines
See citalopram/escitalopram (4.3.2.1).

Ethambutol + diazepam
Lack of interaction has been shown.

Fluoxetine + benzodiazepines
See fluoxetine (4.3.2.2).

Fluvoxamine + benzodiazepines
See fluvoxamine (4.3.2.3).

Food + benzodiazepines
Food delays the absorption of benzodiazepines; only significant if rapid onset of action is needed.

Gabapentin + benzodiazepines
See gabapentin (4.5.3).

Gingko biloba + benzodiazepines
GB may inhibit CYP3A4 and increase midazolam's AUC by 25–30%, possibly significantly (n = 10, 4/52, c/o, Uchida et al, J Clin Pharmacol 2006; **46**:1290–8; n = 14, 2/52, Robertson et al, Curr Med Res Opin 2008;**24**:591–9).

Grapefruit juice + benzodiazepines
200 ml normal-strength grapefruit juice increases plasma triazolam levels, and repeated consumption produces a greater increase (n = 12, RCT, Lilja et al, Eur J Clin Pharmacol 2000;**56**:411–5).

H2-blockers + benzodiazepines
Cimetidine inhibits the CYP3A4 metabolism of long-acting benzodiazepines, but not lorazepam, oxazepam and temazepam. The clinical effect is probably negligible. The other H2-blockers do not interact this way (e.g. ranitidine, n = 9, RCT, d/b, c/o, 4/7, Klotz et al, J Clin Pharmacol

1987;**27**:210–2), although ranitidine may slightly reduce the absorption of diazepam (n = 30, RCT, open, 3/7, O'Connor-Semmes et al, Clin Pharmacol Ther 2001;**70**:126–31).

Heparin + benzodiazepines

A transient rise in benzodiazepine levels could occur (n = 14, open, Desmond et al, Br J Clin Pharmacol 1980;**9**:171–5).

Indometacin + diazepam

Increased dizziness may occur (d/b, Nuotto and Saariolho, Pharmacol Toxicol 1988;**62**:293–7).

Isoniazid + benzodiazepines

Isoniazid reduces the clearance of diazepam but not of oxazepam (n = 9, Ochs et al, Clin Pharmacol Ther 1981;**29**:671–8).

Itraconazole/ketoconazole/posaconazole + benzodiazepines *

Increased chlordiazepoxide oral bioavailability and midazolam AUC can occur, up to eight-fold higher (e.g. n = 10, RCT, 12/7, Lam et al, J Clin Pharmacol 2003;**43**:1274–82). Midazolam levels were significantly higher with itraconazole 200 mg/d for four days, the effect being detectable up to four days after cessation of treatment (n = 9, open, Backman et al, Eur J Clin Pharmacol 1998;**54**:53–8). Posaconazole is a less potent inhibitor of 3A4 than ketoconazole but can cause an up to 2.4-fold increase in midazolam levels (n = 12, open, Krishna et al, Clin Ther 2009;**31**:286–98).

Lamotrigine + benzodiazepines

See lamotrigine (4.5.5).

LEVODOPA + BENZODIAZEPINES

Levodopa can be antagonised by diazepam, nitrazepam and chlordiazepoxide (Yousselson et al, Ann Intern Med 1982;**96**:259–60): observe for worsening of symptoms.

Lithium + benzodiazepines

See lithium (4.4).

MAOIs + benzodiazepines

See MAOIs (4.3.4).

Melatonin + benzodiazepines

See melatonin (4.1.4).

Methadone + benzodiazepines

See methadone (4.6.10).

Metronidazole + benzodiazepines

Lack of interaction has been reported.

Mianserin + benzodiazepines

See mianserin (4.3.3.3).

Mirtazapine + benzodiazepines

See mirtazapine (4.3.3.4).

Moclobemide + benzodiazepines

See moclobemide (4.3.3.5).

Modafinil + benzodiazepines

See modafinil (4.6.12).

Muscle relaxants + benzodiazepines

Variable relatively minor effects have been reported (n = 113, Driessen et al, Acta Anaesthesiol Scand 1986;**30**:642–6). Diazepam may hasten the onset and prolong the duration of action of vecuronium (n = 20, RCT, Yuan et al, Chung Hua I Hsueh Tsa Chih (Taipei) 1994;**54**:259–64), but midazolam appears not to do this (n = 10, Husby et al, Acta Anaesthesiol Scand 1989;**33**:280–2).

Nimodipine + benzodiazepines

Lack of a clinically significant interaction during chronic oral administration has been reported (n = 24, RCT, c/o, 3×5/7, Heine et al, Br J Clin Pharmacol 1994;**38**:39–43).

Olanzapine + benzodiazepines

See olanzapine (4.2.4).

Ondansetron + benzodiazepines

Lack of interaction has been shown with temazepam (n = 24, RCT, d/b, c/o, 2/7, Preston et al, Anesthesia 1996;**51**:827–30).

Opioids + benzodiazepines

Synergism (e.g. n = 95, RCT, d/b, Kissin et al, Anesth Analg 1990;**71**:65–9) and changes in haemodynamic status have been reported. A fatal interaction has been reported with clonazepam and oxycodone, although the mechanism is unclear (n = 1, Burrows et al, J Forensic Sci 2003; **48**:683–6).

Oral contraceptives + benzodiazepines

OCs may increase the effects of longer-acting benzodiazepines, probably of minimal significance.

Paraldehyde + benzodiazepines

Enhanced sedation would be expected.

Paroxetine + benzodiazepines

See paroxetine (4.3.2.4).

Passiflora incarnata + benzodiazepines *

See valerian + benzodiazepines.

Phenytoin + benzodiazepines

See phenytoin (4.5.9).

Physostigmine + benzodiazepines

Physostigmine may reverse diazepam-induced sleep (Speeg et al, J Neurochem 1980;**34**:856–5) and midazolam-induced somnolence (Ho et al, Ma Tsui Hsueh Tsa Chi 1991;**29**:643–7).

Pregabalin + benzodiazepines

See pregabalin (4.5.11).

Probenecid + lorazepam *

Administration of probenecid with lorazepam can lead to a more rapid onset and prolonged effect and so lorazepam doses should be reduced by 50% (SPC 2009).

Progabide + clonazepam

Lack of interaction has been reported.

Propofol + benzodiazepines

Propofol increases the half-life of midazolam by 61%, probably by inhibiting CYP3A4 (n = 24, RCT, Hamaoka et al, Clin Pharmacol Ther 1999;**66**:110–7).

Proton–pump inhibitors + benzodiazepines

Omeprazole, but not pantoprazole (review: Steinijans et al, Int J Clin Pharmacol Ther 1996; **34**:S31–S50), can reduce diazepam clearance by up to 50% (n = 12, 1/52, Andersson et al, Eur J Clin Pharmacol 1990;**39**:51–4), probably by 3A4 inhibition (Zomorodi and Houston, Br J Clin Pharmacol 1996;**42**:157–62).

Quetiapine + benzodiazepines

See quetiapine (4.2.5).

Ramelteon + benzodiazepines

See ramelteon (4.1.5).

Reboxetine + benzodiazepines

See reboxetine (4.3.3.6).

Rifampicin + benzodiazepines

CYP3A4 induction by rifampicin can lead to increased diazepam clearance (n = 21, 7/7, Ohnhaus, Clin Pharmacol Ther 1987;**42**:148) and reduced midazolam levels (n = 9, 9/7, Backman et al, Eur J Clin Pharmacol 1998;**54**:53–8).

Ritonavir + benzodiazepines

The UK SPC now contraindicates ritonavir with clorazepate, diazepam, estazolam, flurazepam, oral (parenteral is just a warning) midazolam and triazolam due to the risk of extreme sedation and respiratory depression.

Rivastigmine + benzodiazepines

See rivastigmine (4.6.3.3).

Rufinamide + benzodiazepines

See rufinamide (4.5.12).

Selegiline + benzodiazepines

Selegiline transdermal system (STS) had no effects on the pharmacokinetics of alprazolam (open, RCT, c/o, Azzaro et al, J Clin Pharmacol 2007;**47**:146–58).

Sertraline + benzodiazepines

See sertraline (4.3.2.5).

Smoking + benzodiazepines

See smoking (4.7.4).

Sodium oxybate + benzodiazepines

See sodium oxybate (4.6.13).

St John's wort + benzodiazepines

See St John's wort (4.3.3.10).

Tiagabine + benzodiazepines

See tiagabine (4.5.13).

Tricyclics + benzodiazepines

Enhanced sedation has been reported and would be expected. Reduced hydroxylation of clomipramine has been reported and dose reduction may be necessary (Pharmaceutisch Weekblad 1992;**14**[4] Suppl D:D3).

Valerian + benzodiazepines *

Tremor, dizziness and fatigue have been reported in someone on lorazepam after taking valerian officinalis and Passiflora incarnate (n = 1, Carrasco et al, Phytother Res 2009;**23**:1795–6).

Valproate + benzodiazepines *

Valproate displaces diazepam from plasma protein-binding sites and so doses may need to be reduced. Valproate increases lorazepam levels by up to 20–40% (n = 16, RCT, Samara et al, J Clin Pharmacol 1997;**37**:442–50; SPC change 2009) and coma has been reported with the combination, possibly via reduced lorazepam clearance (n = 1, Lee et al, Seizure 2002;**11**:124–5). Valproate increases clonazepam clearance by 14% and reduces valproate clearance by 18% (n = 317, Yukawa et al, J Clin Pharm Ther 2003;**28**:497–504), probably of minimal significance (n = 4, Wang and Wang, Ther Drug Monit 2002;**24**:532–6).

Venlafaxine + benzodiazepines

See venlafaxine (4.3.3.9).

Xanthines + benzodiazepines

Xanthines, e.g. theophylline, aminophylline and caffeine antagonise the sedative (and possibly anxiolytic) effects of benzodiazepines (e.g. midazolam 12mg is moderately antagonised by 250mg caffeine, n = 114, Mattila et al, Int J Clin Pharmacol Ther 2000;**38**:581–7). This can be useful in the treatment of benzodiazepine overdose, but care must be taken if a patient on a benzodiazepine has theophylline stopped, as respiratory depression could then occur.

Ziprasidone + benzodiazepines

See ziprasidone (4.2.8).

Zotepine + benzodiazepines

See zotepine (4.2.9).

4.1.2 BUSPIRONE

Buspirone is metabolised by CYP3A4 and has an active metabolite 6-hydroxybuspirone (n = 13, Dockens et al, J Clin Pharmacol 2006;**46**:1308–12).

Alcohol + buspirone
See alcohol (4.7.1).

Benzodiazepines + buspirone
Two studies with diazepam have shown only a minimal enhanced sedation. Alprazolam appears not to interact with buspirone (n = 24, 7/7, Buch et al, J Clin Pharmacol 1993;**33**:1104–9).

Beta-blockers + buspirone
Buspirone appears not to displace propranolol from plasma-binding sites (review: Gammans et al, Am J Med 1986;**80**[Suppl 3B]:41–51).

Calcium–channel blockers + buspirone
Verapamil and diltiazem increase buspirone plasma concentrations three-fold and five-fold respectively. Peak plasma levels are also raised, probably by CYP3A4 inhibition, potentially enhancing the side-effects of buspirone (n = 9, RCT, p/c, c/o, Lamberg et al, Clin Pharmacol Ther 1998;**63**:640–5).

Cimetidine + buspirone
Lack of interaction has been reported (n = 10, open, Gammans et al, Pharmacotherapy 1987; **7**:72–9).

Citalopram + buspirone
See citalopram/escitalopram (4.3.2.1).

Clozapine + buspirone
Near fatal gastrointestinal bleeding and hyperglycaemia occurring one month after buspirone was added to a stable clozapine regimen has been reported, but no firm explanation found (n = 1, Good, Am J Psychiatry 1997;**154**:1473).

Erythromycin + buspirone
Erythromycin and itraconazole may increase plasma buspirone levels dramatically, probably via CYP3A4 inhibition, with increased side-effects noted (n = 8, Kivisto et al, Clin Pharmacol Ther 1997;**62**:348–54).

Escitalopram + buspirone
See citalopram/escitalopram (4.3.2.1).

Fluoxetine + buspirone
Reduced anxiolytic effect, dystonia, akathisia (n = 1, Metz, Can J Psychiatry 1990;**35**:722–3) and anorgasmia (n = 20, open, 8/52, Jenike et al, J Clin Psychiatry 1991;**52**:13–4) have been reported.

Fluvoxamine + buspirone
Fluvoxamine 100mg/d raises buspirone levels, probably via CYP3A4 inhibition, but this is of limited significance (n = 10, RCT, Lamberg et al, Eur J Clin Pharmacol 1998;**54**:761–6).

Grapefruit juice + buspirone
200ml double-strength grapefruit juice raised peak buspirone plasma levels four-fold, probably via CYP3A4 inhibition or delayed gastric emptying, so avoid buspirone and, at least, large amounts of grapefruit juice, or adjust doses (n = 10, RCT, Lilja et al, Clin Pharmacol Ther 1998;**64**:655–60).

Itraconazole + buspirone
See erythromycin + buspirone (above).

MAOIs + BUSPIRONE
See MAOIs (4.3.4).

NSAIDs + buspirone
GI side-effects and headache may be slightly more common with the combination (n = 150, Kiev and Domantay, Curr Ther Res 1989;**46**:1086–90).

Phenytoin + buspirone
Buspirone does not appear to displace phenytoin from plasma-binding sites (review: Gammans et al, Am J Med 1986;**80**[Suppl 3B]:41–51).

Rifampicin + buspirone
The buspirone UK SPC now states that rifampicin decreases buspirone plasma levels, probably via CYP3A4 induction. Significant changes in psychomotor tests have been noted and so dose adjustment may be necessary (n = 10, Lamberg et al, Br J Clin Pharmacol 1998;**45**:381–5).

Ritonavir + buspirone
Severe EPSE have appeared after ritonavir was added to buspirone (n = 1, Clay and Adams, Ann Pharmacother 2003;**37**:202–5).

St John's wort + buspirone
There is a possible case of serotonin syndrome (n = 1, Dannawi, J Psychopharmacol 2002;**16**:401).

Terfenadine + buspirone
No interaction occurs (n=10, RCT, p/c, c/o, 3/7, Lamberg et al, Pharmacol Toxicol 1999;**84**:165–9).

Trazodone + buspirone
There are some isolated reports of raised SGPT/ALT levels and a case of serotonin syndrome (n = 1, Goldberg and Huk, Psychosomatics 1992;**3**:235).

Warfarin + buspirone
Buspirone does not appear to displace warfarin from plasma-binding sites (review: Gammans et al, Am J Med 1986;**80**[Suppl 3B]:41–51).

Zidovidine + buspirone
The combination has been used safely (n = 2, Batki, J Clin Psychopharmacol 1990;**10**[Suppl 3]: 111S–5S).

4.1.3 CHLORAL HYDRATE

Chloral is probably metabolised by CYP2E1.

ALCOHOL + CHLORAL HYDRATE
See alcohol (4.7.1)

Fluvoxamine + chloral hydrate
See fluvoxamine (4.3.2.3).

Furosemide + chloral hydrate
Diaphoresis, facial flushing and agitation occurred with chloral hydrate and IV furosemide, which stopped when the chloral was discontinued (n = 1, Dean et al, Clin Pharm 1991;**10**:385–7).

MAOIs + chloral hydrate
See MAOIs (4.3.4).

Methadone + chloral hydrate
See methadone (4.6.10).

Phenytoin + chloral hydrate
See phenytoin (4.5.9).

Nicoumalone + chloral hydrate
An enhanced anticoagulant effect can occur. See also warfarin + chloral hydrate.

Warfarin + chloral hydrate
The anticoagulant effects of warfarin are increased slightly by chloral hydrate, probably by plasma protein displacement (BCDSP, N Engl J Med 1972;**286**:53–5). This can be important if chloral hydrate is given as a PRN hypnotic.

4.1.4 MELATONIN

Melatonin is metabolised by 1A2 and possibly 2C9/19 to a minor extent (Facciola et al, Eur J Clin Pharmacol 2001;**56**:881–8) and induces 3A4, possibly 2C19, but has no effect on 1A2.

Alcohol + melatonin
Alcohol reduces the effect of melatonin (SPC).

Antipsychotics + melatonin
Muzzy-headedness has been reported with thioridazine and melatonin (SPC).

Benzodiazepines + melatonin
Melatonin can enhance the sedative effects (SPC).

Carbamazepine + melatonin
Carbamazepine may decrease melatonin levels (SPC) via 1A2 induction.

Cimetidine + melatonin
Cimetidine may raise melatonin levels (SPC).

Citalopram/escitalopram + melatonin
See citalopram/escitalopram (4.3.2.1).

Estrogens + melatonin
Estrogens (e.g. oral contraceptives or HRT) may increase melatonin levels (SPC).

FLUVOXAMINE + MELATONIN
Fluvoxamine 50 mg inhibits the metabolism of oral melatonin 5 mg, increasing plasma levels (n = 5, open, Hartter et al, Clin Pharmacol Ther 2000;**67**:1–6), supported by a further case, where combining the treatments improved sleep (n = 1, Grozinger et al, Arch Gen Psychiatry 2000; **57**:812–3). The UK SPC states that fluvoxamine may raise melatonin levels, with AUC 17-fold higher and Cmax 12-fold higher (SPC).

Methoxypsoralen + melatonin
Melatonin levels can be raised (SPC).

Quinolones + melatonin
Quinolones may increase melatonin levels via 1A2 inhibition (SPC).

Rifampicin + melatonin
Rifampicin may decrease melatonin levels (SPC) via 1A2 induction.

Smoking + melatonin
Smoking may decrease melatonin levels (SPC) via 1A2 induction.

Tricyclics + melatonin
Increased feelings of tranquillity have been reported with imipramine and melatonin (SPC).

Zaleplon + melatonin
Melatonin can enhance the sedative effects of zaleplon (SPC).

Zolpidem + melatonin
Melatonin can enhance the sedative effects of zolpidem (SPC).

Zopiclone + melatonin
Melatonin can enhance the sedative effects of zopiclone (SPC).

4.1.5 RAMELTEON

Ramelteon is primarily oxidised to a number of metabolites. CYP1A2 is the major isoenzyme, with 2C9/19 and 3A4 having a minor effect. Lack of meaningful interaction has been shown with theophylline, dextromethorphan, omeprazole, digoxin and warfarin.

Alcohol + ramelteon
Although ramelteon and alcohol produce no significant pharmacokinetic interaction, there may be some additive psychomotor impairment.

Benzodiazepines + ramelteon
There is no significant interaction with midazolam.

Fluconazole + ramelteon
Fluconazole increases the AUC and Cmax of

ramelteon by about 150% so care is needed with the combination.

Fluoxetine + ramelteon

No significant interaction occurs.

FLUVOXAMINE + RAMELTEON

Fluvoxamine 200 mg/d increases the AUC for ramelteon by 190-fold and Cmax 70-fold so this combination should be avoided.

Ketoconazole + ramelteon

Ketoconazole increases the AUC and Cmax of ramelteon by about 84% and 36% respectively, so care is needed with the combination.

Rifampicin + ramelteon

Rifampicin 600 mg/d reduces ramelteon levels by about 80%, some care is needed.

4.1.6 ZALEPLON

Zaleplon is primarily metabolised by aldehyde oxidase, and a small amount by CYP3A4 to inactive metabolites. As with other such drugs, use with other CNS-depressants needs care.

Alcohol + zaleplon

See alcohol (4.7.1).

Antipsychotics + zaleplon

Additive psychomotor effects may occur with thioridazine (n = 12, RCT, Hetta *et al, Eur J Clin Pharmacol* 2000;**56**:211–7).

Carbamazepine + zaleplon

Co-administration may reduce zaleplon's efficacy through CYP3A4 induction.

Cimetidine + zaleplon

Raised zaleplon levels can occur with cimetidine, via aldehyde oxidase and CYP3A4 inhibition.

Digoxin + zaleplon

Lack of interaction has been shown (n = 20, Sanchez-Garcia *et al, Am J Health Syst Pharm* 2000;**57**:2267–70).

Erythromycin + zaleplon

Raised zaleplon levels can occur, via 3A4 inhibition.

Ibuprofen + zaleplon

Lack of significant interaction has been shown (n = 17, open, Sanchez–Garcia *et al, Am J Health Syst Pharm* 2000;**57**:1137–41).

Ketoconazole + zaleplon

Raised zaleplon levels can occur, via 3A4 inhibition.

Melatonin + zaleplon

See melatonin (4.1.4).

Opioids + zaleplon

Enhanced euphoria is possible.

Phenobarbital + zaleplon

Reduced zaleplon levels can occur, via CYP3A4 induction.

Rifampicin + zaleplon

A four-fold reduction in zaleplon levels can occur, via CYP3A4 induction.

Warfarin + zaleplon

No interaction occurs.

4.1.7 ZOLPIDEM

Zolpidem is mainly metabolised by CYP3A4 but has no effect on 1A2, 2B6, 2C9, 2D6 and 3A4. Enhanced sedation would be expected with concurrent use with any CNS depressant.

Alcohol + zolpidem

See alcohol (4.7.1).

Antipsychotics + zolpidem

Excessive sedation has been reported with chlorpromazine (n = 6, d/b, single-dose, Desager *et al, Psychopharmacol* 1988;**96**:63–6).

Bupropion + zolpidem

See bupropion (4.6.6).

Caffeine + zolpidem

In a parallel group study, 300 mg caffeine did not antagonise the sedative effects of zolpidem given during the day (n = 45+, d/b, p/c, Mattila *et al, Eur J Clin Pharmacol* 1998;**54**:421–5).

Clarithromycin + zolpidem *

Clarithromycin has no effect on the kinetics or dynamics of zolpidem (n = 10, c/o, Farkas *et al, Clin Pharmacol Ther* 2009;**85**:644–50).

Fluconazole + zolpidem

See itraconazole + zolpidem.

Food + zolpidem

The rate of absorption of zolpidem is slowed significantly by food.

H2-blockers + zolpidem

Lack of a significant interaction has been shown with cimetidine and ranitidine (n = 6, c/o, 18/7, Hulhoven *et al, Int J Clin Pharmacol Res* 1988;**8**:471–6).

Itraconazole + zolpidem

Single doses of itraconazole or fluconazole slightly lengthen the half–life of zolpidem (n = 12, RCT, Greenblatt *et al, Clin Pharmacol Ther* 1998;**64**:661–71). However, itraconazole 200 mg/d for four days had no marked effect on the pharmacokinetics of zolpidem, although central effects were slightly increased (n = 10, Luurila *et al, Eur J Clin Pharmacol* 1998;**54**:163–6).

Ketoconazole + zolpidem

See itraconazole + zolpidem.

Melatonin + zolpidem

See melatonin (4.1.4).

Oral Contraceptives + zolpidem

Zolpidem clearance is slightly higher and half–life slightly shorter in women using OCs (n = 16, Olubodun et al, J Clin Pharmacol 2002;**42**:1142–6).

Rifampicin + zolpidem

Rifampicin significantly reduces zolpidem's plasma levels and therapeutic effect, via CYP3A4 induction (n = 8, RCT, Villikka et al, Br J Clin Pharmacol 1997;**43**:629–34).

Smoking + zolpidem

Zolpidem's half–life may be 30% shorter in smokers than non–smokers, of low clinical significance (due to CYP1A2 induction; n = 16, Olubodun et al, J Clin Pharmacol 2002; **42**:1142–6).

Sodium oxybate + zolpidem

See sodium oxybate (4.6.13).

SSRIs + zolpidem

SSRIs may enhance zolpidem-associated hallucinations (n = 5, Elko et al, J Toxicol Clin Toxicol 1998;**36**:195–203; n = 1 Coleman and Ota, J Forensic Sci 2004;**49**:392–3). One study showed a minimal pharmacokinetic interaction between **fluoxetine** and regular zolpidem in healthy women, with no significant psychomotor function changes, although zolpidem's half–life increased slightly (n = 29, 5/52, Allard et al, Drug Metab Dispos 1998;**26**:617–22). Visual hallucinations and amnesia triggered by **fluvoxamine** have been reported (n = 1, Kito and Koga, Int Psychogeriatr 2006;**18**:749–51). The combination with **sertraline** may lead to a shorter onset of action and an increased effect from zolpidem (n = 28, RCT, Allard et al, J Clin Pharmacol 1999;**39**;184–91).

Valproate + zolpidem

Somnambulism has been reported with the combination in a 47-year-old male (n = 1, Sattar et al, Ann Pharmacother 2003;**37**:1429–33).

4.1.8 ZOPICLONE

Zopiclone is mainly metabolised by CYP3A4 to active metabolites, with 2C8 a minor metaboliser. It is excreted via the urine (80%) and faeces (16%).

Alcohol + zopiclone

See alcohol (4.7.1).

Aspirin + zopiclone

Lack of interaction has been shown.

Caffeine + zopiclone

Caffeine may moderately antagonise the psychomotor impairment caused by zopiclone (d/b, Mattila et al, Pharmacol Toxicol 1992; **70**:286–9).

Erythromycin + zopiclone

Erythromycin accelerates zopiclone absorption, leading to a more rapid onset, which could be clinically significant in the elderly (n = 10, Aranko et al, Br J Clin Pharmacol 1994;**38**:363–7).

Itraconazole + zopiclone

Itraconazole significantly increased zopiclone plasma levels by 28% and half-life by 40%, but had no clinically significant effect (n = 10, d/b, p/c, c/o, Jalava et al, Eur J Clin Pharmacol 1996;**51**:331–4).

Melatonin + zopiclone

See melatonin (4.1.4).

Ranitidine + zopiclone

Lack of interaction has been shown.

Rifampicin + zopiclone

Rifampicin significantly reduces zopiclone plasma levels and therapeutic effect, via CYP3A4 induction (n = 8, RCT, Villikka et al, Br J Clin Pharmacol 1997;**43**:471–4).

Tricyclics + zopiclone

One study showed decreased levels of trimipramine and zopiclone, of minimal significance (n = 10, RCT, Caille et al, Biopharm Drug Dispos 1984;**5**:117–25).

4.2 ANTIPSYCHOTICS

Aripiprazole (4.2.2), asenapine (4.2.3) clozapine (4.2.4), olanzapine (4.2.5), quetiapine (4.2.6), risperidone (4.2.7), ziprasidone (4.2.8) and zotepine (4.2.9) also have their own sections

4.2.1 ANTIPSYCHOTICS — GENERAL *

There are few specific interactions reported for some antipsychotics, other than additive sedation. Sulpiride has no significant effect on 1A2, 2C9, 2C19, 2D6 2E1 or 3A4 enzymes (Niwa et al, Biol Pharm Bull 2005;**28**:188–91). **Haloperidol** is metabolised by 3A4, 2D6 and by glucuronidation, and is susceptible to interaction with drugs affecting these enzymes. Use of haloperidol with other drugs known to prolong the QTc interval is not recommended (UK SPC, 2009), e.g:

- Class IA (quinidine, disopyramide, procainamide)
- Class III (e.g. amiodarone, sotalol, dofetilide)
- Some antimicrobials (moxifloxacin, IV erythromycin)
- Tricyclics, other neuroleptics (e.g. pimozide, phenothiazines), bretylium, quinine, mefloquine.

ACE inhibitors + antipsychotics
An enhanced hypotensive effect with severe postural hypotension has been reported, e.g. captopril plus chlorpromazine (White, *Arch Int Med* 1986; **146**:1833–4).

Activated charcoal + phenothiazines
Decreased antipsychotic absorption is likely.

ALCOHOL + ANTIPSYCHOTICS
See alcohol (4.7.1).

Amfetamines + antipsychotics
The antipsychotic effects of phenothiazines can be antagonised by amfetamines, although haloperidol and other antipsychotics can be used to treat amfetamine-induced psychosis.

Amiodarone + phenothiazines *
The literature notes an increased risk of ventricular arrhythmias with phenothiazines. A small but potentially significant QTc prolongation (but not ventricular arrhythmia) has been seen with amiodarone and haloperidol (n=49, Bush et al, *Am J Health Syst Pharm* 2008; **65**:2232–6).

Antacids + antipsychotics
Antacids may reduce chlorpromazine and possibly haloperidol serum levels. Sulpiride absorption may be reduced by sucralfate or aluminium-containing antacids. Separate doses by a couple of hours minimises the effect.

Anticholinergics + antipsychotics *
Anticholinergics may reduce the efficacy of antipsychotics, probably by lowering the serum levels of oral and depot antipsychotics (n=25, Bamrah et al, *Br J Psychiatry* 1986; **149**:726–33). Additive anticholinergic effects, e.g. acute intestinal pseudo-obstruction have been reported with benzatropine and haloperidol (n=1, Sheikh et al, *Am J Gastroenterol* 2001; **96**:934–5). The UK SPC now recommends anticholinergics are not used with olanzapine.

ANTICONVULSANTS + ANTIPSYCHOTICS
Antipsychotics lower the seizure threshold and may thus antagonise anticonvulsant actions. See also individual anticonvulsants (4.5).

ANTIHISTAMINES + ANTIPSYCHOTICS
Loratadine and fexofenadine are currently considered suitable, although there are three unproven reports of arrhythmia with loratadine.

Antihypertensives + phenothiazines
Combined hypotensive effect may occur.

Antimalarials + chlorpromazine
One study showed markedly increased chlorpromazine levels with anti-malarials, e.g. chloroquine and 'Fansidar' (open, Makanjuola et al, *Trop Geogr Med* 1988; **40**:31–3).

Aripiprazole + antipsychotics (other)
See aripiprazole (4.2.2).

Ascorbic acid + fluphenazine
An isolated case exists of reduced fluphenazine levels (Dysken et al, *JAMA* 1979; **241**:2008) with 1 g/d of ascorbic acid.

BARBITURATES + ANTIPSYCHOTICS
Additive sedative effects can occur acutely with this combination, and death has been reported (n=1, Hino et al, *Leg Med* (Tokyo) 1999; **1**:48–51). Barbiturates may induce the metabolism of many antipsychotics, e.g. haloperidol levels are reduced by 40–75%. Antagonism of the anticonvulsant effects may also occur.

Benzodiazepines + antipsychotics *
Enhanced sedation and impaired psychomotor function can occur (see 1.1) and death has been reported after an overdose of triazolam and promazine in an older woman (n=1, Rossi et al, *Med Sci Law* 2009; **49**:65–8).

Beta-blockers + antipsychotics
Generally, raised antipsychotic plasma levels occur, of possible clinical significance, e.g. chlorpromazine levels may rise by up to 100–500% with propranolol (Peet et al, *Lancet* 1980; **ii**:978), although pindolol has no significant effect on haloperidol levels (n=26, open, Greendyke and Gulya, *J Clin Psychiatry* 1988; **49**:105–7).

Betel nut + antipsychotics
Betel nut (*Areca catechu*), which contains the cholinergic alkaloid arecoline, has been reported to cause EPSE, bradykinesia, stiffness and akathisia with flupentixol and fluphenazine (n=1, Deahl, *Mov Disord* 1998; **4**:330–3).

Bromocriptine + antipsychotics
A predictable reversal of the antipsychotic effect may occur. Antipsychotics may also antagonise the hypoprolactinaemic and antiparkinsonian effects of bromocriptine.

Calcium-channel blockers + antipsychotics
Increased antipsychotic plasma levels or enhanced hypotension have been predicted (review by Markowitz et al, Ann Pharmacother 1995;**29**:603–9).

Cannabis + antipsychotics
See cannabis (4.7.2).

CARBAMAZEPINE + ANTIPSYCHOTICS
See carbamazepine (4.5.1).

Citalopram + antipsychotics
See antipsychotics + citalopram/escitalopram (4.3.2.1).

CLARITHROMYCIN + ANTIPSYCHOTICS
References report an increased risk of arrhythmias with phenothiazines and recommend avoiding the combination. Death has been reported when clarithromycin was added to pimozide in a man with a documented prolonged QT interval (n = 1, Flockhart et al, J Clin Psychopharmacol 2000;**20**:317–24).

Clonidine + antipsychotics
Animal studies have shown phenothiazines and haloperidol (but not pimozide) to antagonise the hypotensive effect of clonidine. Severe hypotension (Fruncillo et al, Am J Psychiatry 1985;**142**:274) and delirium have been reported (review by Markowitz et al, Ann Pharmacother 1995;**29**:603–9).

CLOZAPINE + ANTIPSYCHOTICS
See clozapine (4.2.4).

Cocaine + antipsychotics
See cocaine (4.7.3).

Desferrioxamine + prochlorperazine
Prolonged unconsciousness may occur.

Diazoxide + chlorpromazine
Enhanced hypoglycaemia has been reported (n = 1, Aynsley-Green and Illig, Lancet 1975;**2**:658).

Disopyramine + antipsychotics
Increased anticholinergic effects may occur.

Disulfiram + antipsychotics
See disulfiram (4.6.8).

Domperidone + antipsychotics
There is an enhanced risk of EPSE.

Donepezil + antipsychotics
See donepezil (4.6.3.1).

Erythromycin + antipsychotics
See clarithromycin + antipsychotics.

Escitalopram + antipsychotics
See citalopram/escitalopram (4.3.2.1).

FLUOXETINE + ANTIPSYCHOTICS
Severe EPSE have been reported with fluoxetine and **haloperidol** (n = 1, Tate, Am J Psychiatry 1989; **146**:399–400), dystonia with **fluphenazine**, and stupor, confusion (n = 1, Hansen–Grant et al, Am J Psychiatry 1993;**150**:1750–1), and severe bradycardia and drowsiness (n = 1, Friedman, Can J Psychiatry 1994;**39**:634) with **pimozide**. The probable mechanism is CYP2D6 inhibition so the combination should be avoided if possible (Ahmed et al, Can J Psychiatry 1993;**38**:62–3). Citalopram, escitalopram and sertraline would be suitable alternatives.

Fluvoxamine + antipsychotics
See fluvoxamine (4.3.2.3).

Ginseng + haloperidol
Ginseng may potentiate the general effects of haloperidol (Mitra et al, Indian J Exp Biol 1996; **34**:41–7).

H2-blockers + antipsychotics
Chlorpromazine levels may be reduced by 30% by cimetidine (Howes et al, Eur J Clin Pharmacol 1983;**24**:99–102), but not ranitidine.

Haloperidol + chlorpromazine
Chlorpromazine may significantly increase haloperidol levels, probably via CYP2D6 inhibition (n = 43, Suzuki et al, Ther Drug Monit 2001;**23**:363–8).

Hydroxyzine + phenothiazines
The effect of phenothiazines may be decreased (Ross and Priest, Dis Nerv Syst 1970;**31**:412).

Hypoglycaemics + chlorpromazine
Chlorpromazine can induce hyperglycaemia and disrupt the control of diabetes (Schwarz and Munoz, Am J Psychiatry 1968;**125**:253).

Indometacin + haloperidol
One study showed profound drowsiness and confusion on the combination (Bird et al, Lancet 1983;**i**:830–1).

Itraconazole + haloperidol
Itraconazole 200 mg/d for seven days significantly increases haloperidol and metabolite levels, leading to increased side-effects, presumably due to CYP3A4 inhibition (n = 13, Yasui et al, J Clin Psychopharmacol 1999;**19**:149–54).

LEVODOPA + ANTIPSYCHOTICS
The therapeutic effect of levodopa is antagonised by antipsychotics and vice versa. Levodopa may worsen antipsychotic-induced EPSE.

Lithium + antipsychotics
See antipsychotics + lithium (4.4).

MAOIs + antipsychotics
See antipsychotics + MAOIs (4.3.4).

Melatonin + antipsychotics
See melatonin (4.1.4).

Memantine + antipsychotics
See memantine (4.6.9).

Methadone + sulpiride *
The sulpiride SPC now states that it should be used with caution with drugs that can prolong QTc, e.g. methadone and halofantrine.

Metirosine + antipsychotics
An enhanced risk of EPSE exists.

Metoclopramide + antipsychotics
An enhanced risk of EPSE exists.

Minocycline + phenothiazines
There is a case of pigmented galactorrhoea with the combination (n = 1, Basler and Lynch, *Arch Dermatol* 1985;**121**:417).

Naltrexone + phenothiazines
Severe drowsiness may occur with chlorpromazine.

Olanzapine + antipsychotics (other)
See olanzapine (4.2.5).

Oral contraceptives + chlorpromazine
There is a report of a combined OC raising chlorpromazine levels six-fold (n = 1, Chetty and Miller, *Ther Drug Monit* 2001; **23**:556–8).

Orlistat + haloperidol
A small trial suggested a lack of interaction (n = 8, open, 8/52, Hilger et al, *J Clin Psychopharmacol* 2002;**22**:68–70).

Oxcarbazepine + antipsychotics
See oxcarbazepine (4.5.7).

Paroxetine + antipsychotics
See antipsychotics + paroxetine (4.3.2.4).

Pethidine + phenothiazines
Increased CNS toxicity and hypotension can occur (n = 10, open, c/o, Stambaugh and Wainer, *J Clin Pharmacol* 1981;**21**:140–6).

PHENYTOIN + ANTIPSYCHOTICS
Phenytoin may reduce haloperidol levels by 40–75%, probably via enzyme induction (n = 30, open, Linnoila et al, *Am J Psychiatry* 1980;**137**:819). Chlorpromazine may increase phenytoin levels by up to 50% (n = 27, open, Sands et al, *Drug Intell Clin Pharm* 1987;**21**:267–72), although other studies show a nil or opposite effect. Antipsychotics lower the seizure threshold and may antagonise the anticonvulsant effect of phenytoin.

Piperazine + chlorpromazine
The validity of a single case of convulsions with the combination has been queried by a small study (Sturman, *Br J Pharmacol* 1974;**50**:153–5).

Polymyxin + phenothiazines
The neuromuscular blocking effects of polymyxin antibiotics may be increased by phenothiazines with prolonged respiratory depression possible (Pohlmann, *JAMA* 1966;**196**:181).

Procarbazine + antipsychotics
Enhanced sedation is possible.

Quetiapine + antipsychotics (other)
See quetiapine (4.2.6).

Reboxetine + antipsychotics
See reboxetine (4.3.3.6)

RIFAMPICIN + HALOPERIDOL
Rifampicin may reduce haloperidol serum levels by a third (n = 17, Kim et al, *J Clin Psychopharmacol* 1996;**16**:247–52), a clinically significant effect. Care would also be needed if rifampicin were stopped.

Sertraline + antipsychotics
See sertraline (4.3.2.5).

Smoking + antipsychotics
See smoking (4.7.4).

Suxamethonium + promazine
Prolonged apnoea has been reported (n = 1, Regan and Aldrete, *Anesth Analg* 1967;**46**:315–8).

Sucralfate + antipsychotics
See antacids + antipsychotics (4.2.1).

Tea or coffee + antipsychotics
Typical antipsychotics precipitate out of solution to form a tannin complex with tea and coffee, almost certainly of minimal clinical significance (Bowen et al, *Lancet* 1981;**i**:1217–8).

Tetrabenazine + antipsychotics
A single predictable case exists of enhanced EPSE in a Huntington's patient (Moss and Stewart, *Can J Psychiatry* 1986;**31**:865–6).

Trazodone + antipsychotics
See trazodone (4.3.3.7).

Tricyclics + antipsychotics
See tricyclics (4.3.1).

Valproate + antipsychotics
No interaction occurs with **aripiprazole** (Citrome et al, *Int J Neuropsychopharmacol* 2002;**5**[Suppl 1]:S187). **Chlorpromazine** may inhibit the metabolism of valproate and so monitoring of valproate levels may be appropriate (open, Ishizaki et al, *J Clin Psychopharmacol* 1984;**4**:254–61). Valproate has no significant effect on the plasma levels of **haloperidol** (n = 27, 4/52, Hesslinger et al, *J Clin Psychopharmacol* 1999;**19**:310–5) or **risperidone** and 9–hydroxyrisperidone (n = 22, s/b, p/c, 28/7, Ravindran et al, *Clin Pharmacokinet*

2004;**43**:733–40; n=12, Yoshimura *et al, Pharmacopsychiatry* 2007;**40**:9–13), but there are cases of dose-related generalised oedema with risperidone and valproate (n=2, Sanders and Lehrer, *J Clin Psychiatry* 1998;**59**:689–90). Two studies have shown that valproate produces a clinically insignificant rise in **clozapine**, but lower norclozapine levels (n=37+6, Facciola *et al, Ther Drug Monit* 1999;**21**:341–5). Although valproate is often used as anticonvulsant cover for higher doses of clozapine, a careful study showed valproate to produce a 15% drop in clozapine levels and a 65% drop in norclozapine levels (n=7, Longo and Salzman, *Am J Psychiatry* 1995;**152**:650), although raised clozapine levels have been reported (n=1, Costello and Suppes, *J Clin Psychopharmacol* 1995;**15**:139–41). Since norclozapine is more toxic than clozapine, this may be a useful effect with careful manipulation of the dose. Clozapine may, of course, also lower the seizure threshold and antagonise the anticonvulsant effect of valproate.

Venlafaxine + antipsychotics
See venlafaxine (*4.3.3.9*).

Warfarin + antipsychotics
An interaction is theoretically possible (see Sayal *et al, Acta Psychiatr Scand* 2000;**102**:250–5).

Zaleplon + antipsychotics
See zaleplon (*4.1.6*).

Zolpidem + antipsychotics
See zolpidem (*4.1.7*).

Zotepine + antipsychotics (other)
See zotepine (*4.2.9*).

4.2.2 ANTIPSYCHOTICS — ARIPIPRAZOLE *

Aripiprazole is metabolised mainly by CYP2D6 (n=80, Kim *et al, Br J Clin Pharmacol* 2008;**66**:802–10) and 3A4, but not CYP1A1, 1A2 or 2C9/19. It has no effect on CYP2C9, 2C19, 2D6 and 3A4. 3A4 inducers lower aripiprazole lowers levels by about 60%, 3A4 inhibitors increase levels by about 45% (samples=361, Waade *et al, Ther Drug Monit* 2009;**31**:233–8). The UK SPC now says caution is necessary with drugs known to cause QTc prolongation or electrolyte imbalance.

Alcohol + aripiprazole
See alcohol (*4.7.1*).

Antipsychotics (other) + aripiprazole *
There is a theoretical interaction with potent D2 antagonists such as older neuroleptics and risperidone with aripiprazole. Aripiprazole has a very high affinity for D2 receptors and would displace almost any other antipsychotic from these receptors. There is a case of asymptomatic QTc prolongation with aripiprazole and haloperidol (n=1, Leo *et al, J Clin Psychiatry* 2008;**69**:327–8). See also combinations in C1.23.

CARBAMAZEPINE + ARIPIPRAZOLE
See antipsychotics + carbamazepine (*4.5.1*).

Citalopram + aripiprazole
See antipsychotics + citalopram (*4.3.2.1*).

Dextromethorphan + aripiprazole
Lack of interaction has been shown.

H2-blockers + aripiprazole
Lack of significant interaction has been shown with famotidine.

Itraconazole + aripiprazole
Although itraconazole is a potent CYP3A4 inhibitor, it made no clinically significant difference to aripiprazole levels in one study (n=24, Kubo *et al, Drug Metab Pharmacokinet* 2005;**20**:55–64).

Ketoconazole + aripiprazole
Ketoconazole decreases aripiprazole metabolism and so aripiprazole doses should be decreased by a half during co-administration.

Lamotrigine + aripiprazole *
See aripiprazole + lamotrigine (see *4.5.5*).

Lithium + aripiprazole
See antipsychotics + lithium (*4.4*).

Omeprazole + aripiprazole
Lack of interaction has been shown.

Quinidine + aripiprazole
Quinidine decreases aripiprazole metabolism and so aripiprazole doses should be halved.

Smoking + aripiprazole
See smoking (*4.7.4*)

Tamoxifen + aripiprazole
There is a case of tardive dyskinesia occurring with the combination (n=1, Evcimen *et al, Am J Psychiatry* 2007;**164**:1436–7).

Valproate + aripiprazole
See valproate + antipsychotics (*4.2.1*).

Warfarin + aripiprazole
Lack of interaction has been shown.

4.2.3 ANTIPSYCHOTICS — ASENAPINE *
Asenapine is primarily metabolised by UGT1A4 and 1A2.

Cimetidine + asenapine *
Lack of interaction has been shown (US PI).

Carbamazepine + asenapine *
See antipsychotics + carbamazepine (4.5.1).
Fluvoxamine + asenapine *
See antipsychotics + fluvoxamine (4.3.2.3).
Imipramine + asenapine *
Lack of interaction has been shown (US PI).
Paroxetine + asenapine
Lack of interaction has been shown (US PI).
Valproate + asenapine *
Lack of interaction has been shown (US PI).
Smoking + asenapine *
Lack of interaction has been shown (US PI).

4.2.4 ANTIPSYCHOTICS — CLOZAPINE *
See 4.2.1 for other, more general interactions

The major metabolic route of clozapine is to norclozapine, which is more stable but more toxic to stem cells (Gerson et al, Br J Haematology 1994;**86**:555–61). CYP1A2 is the major metabolising enzyme, with 2D6, 3A4, 2C9/19 and FMO enzymes also involved (Urichuk et al, Curr Drug Metab 2008;**9**:410–8).
Review: general (Chetty and Murray, Curr Drug Metab 2007;**8**:307–13).
ACE inhibitors + clozapine
Clozapine plus diltiazem or enalapril (Aronowitz et al, J Clin Psychopharmacol 1994;**14**:429–30) have been reported to produce additional hypotension. There is also a well-documented case of a clinically important rise in clozapine and norclozapine levels with lisinopril, via an unknown mechanism (n=1, Abraham et al, Am J Psychiatry 2001;**158**:969).
Alcohol + clozapine
See antipsychotics + alcohol (4.7.1).
Amiodarone + clozapine
Raised clozapine levels have been reported with concurrent amiodarone (n=1, Stevens et al, Psychosomatics 2008;**49**:255–7).
ANTIBIOTICS + CLOZAPINE
(see also erythromycin) *
Antibiotics reported to cause leucopenia/neutropenia may enhance the likelihood of clozapine-induced neutropenia and should, if possible, be avoided. It should be noted however, that respiratory infections can themselves inhibit CYP1A2, raising clozapine levels, and so antibiotics may not always be the cause of apparent interactions (Leon, J Clin Psychiatry 2004;**65**:1144–5).

1. Antibiotics LESS likely to cause neutropenia (safer to use): penicillins (all except benzylpenicillin G), all tetracyclines, aminoglycosides, macrolides, clarithromycin, some anti-TBs (ethambutol, pyrazinamide, streptomycin), clofazimide, hexamine, sodium fusidate, spectinomycin, colistin, polymixin B and cycloserine.
2. Antibiotics MORE likely/CAN cause leucopenia and/or neutropenia (less safe to use): cephalosporins and cephamycins, clindamycin, lincomycin, sulphonamides and trimethoprim, some anti-TBs (capreomycin, isoniazid, rifampicin), dapsone, metronidazole, tinidazole, nitrofurantoin, chloramphenicol, vancomycin, teicoplanin and the 4-quinolones (ciprofloxacin, nalidixic acid, etc), e.g. there is a case of clozapine levels falling by nearly 50% when ciprofloxacin was stopped, probably due to CYP1A2 inhibition (Markowitz et al, Am J Psychiatry 1997;**153**:881) and cases of doubling of clozapine levels a few days after ciprofloxacin added, presumably by 1A2 and 3A4 inhibition (n=2, Brouwers et al, Clin Drug Invest 2009;**29**:59–63). Where possible, choose antibiotics from the first list and be aware of the potential for problems if drugs from the second list must be used. See also individual drugs for other interactions.
Anticholinergics + clozapine
See antipsychotics (4.2.1).
Antihypertensives + clozapine
Potentiation of the antihypertensive effects may occur. This can be particularly important during the upward dose titration period.
ANTIPSYCHOTICS (other) + CLOZAPINE *
A 15% reduction in clozapine levels has been reported with **aripiprazole** (n=94, Englisch and Zink, Prog Neuropsychopharmacol Biol Psychiatry 2008;**32**:1386–92). **Amisulpride** has no apparent effect on plasma clozapine concentrations (Bergemann et al, J Clin Psychopharmacol 2005;**25**:494–7). There is an enhanced risk of agranulocytosis with some antipsychotics, e.g. **phenothiazines**, which would additionally be complicated by the long-term nature of any given as a depot. Examples include thrombocytopenia with **fluphenazine** and clozapine (n=1, Mihaljevic-Peles et al, Nord J Psychiatry 2001;**55**:449–50) and significantly lower clozapine plasma levels with **levomepromazine** (n=2, Bugamelli et al, Prog Neuropsychopharmacol Biol Psychiatry 2007;**31**:567–70). Elevated **haloperidol** levels have been reported in

combination with clozapine (n = 1, Allen, *J Clin Pharmacol* 2000;**40**:1296–7), as have myoclonic and GTC seizures (n = 1, Haberfellner, *Eur Psychiatry* 2002;**17**:55–6). Although there have been case reports, eg. (n = 18, Raaska *et al, Eur J Clin Pharmacol* 2002;**58**:587–91; n = 1, Kontaxakis *et al, Prog Neuropsychopharmacol Biol Psychiatry* 2002;**26**:407–9), a study was unable to show any kinetic interactions between **risperidone** and clozapine (n = 20, Chetty *et al, Br J Clin Pharmacol* 2009;**68**:574–9). The mechanism cannot be explained by inhibition of CYP1A2, 2D6 or 2C19 (n = 8, Eap *et al, Ther Drug Monit* 2001;**23**:228–31). See also antipsychotics + quetiapine (*4.2.5*) and combinations (*1.23*).

BENZODIAZEPINES + CLOZAPINE

There are rare cases of severe hypotension and respiratory depression (e.g. n = 3, Friedman *et al, N Engl J Med* 1991;**325**:518–9), sudden death after IV lorazepam (n = 1, Klimke and Klieser, *Am J Psychiatry* 1994;**151**:780), sedation (n = 2, Cobb *et al, Am J Psychiatry* 1991;**148**:1606–7) and delirium with lorazepam (n = 3, Jackson *et al, Ann Clin Psychiatry*1995;**7**:139–41). Monitor for enhanced sedation and take particular care when a clozapine dose is being increased.

Buspirone + clozapine

See buspirone (*4.1.2*).

Caffeine + clozapine

Caffeine and clozapine are both metabolised by CYP1A2 and so some competitive inhibition of metabolism may occur. Caffeine, in doses of 400–1000 mg, inhibits the metabolism of clozapine to an extent that might be significant in some people (n = 12, RCT, open, Hagg *et al, Br J Clin Pharmacol* 2000;**49**:59–63), e.g. mean serum trough levels of clozapine increased by about 26% have been reported, probably of minor clinical significance in most patients (n = 12[c = 6], RCT, d/b, Raaska *et al, Basic Clin Pharmacol Toxicol* 2004;**94**:13–8), causing drowsiness and siallorrhoea, with clozapine levels halving when caffeine was stopped (n = 1, Odom–White and de Leon, *J Clin Psychiatry* 1996;**57**:175–6).

Cannabis + clozapine

See antipsychotics + cannabis (*4.7.2*).

CARBAMAZEPINE + CLOZAPINE

See antipsychotics + carbamazepine (*4.5.1*).

Chloramphenicol + clozapine

There is an enhanced risk of agranulocytosis.

CIPROFLOXACIN + CLOZAPINE

See antibiotics + clozapine (above).

Citalopram + clozapine

See antipsychotics + citalopram/escitalopram (*4.3.2.1*).

Clonidine + clozapine

See clonidine + antipsychotics (*4.2.1*).

Cocaine + clozapine

See antipsychotics + cocaine (*4.7.3*).

Co-trimoxazole + clozapine

There is an enhanced risk of agranulocytosis.

Cytotoxic agents + clozapine

Although there is an increased risk of neutropenia, there may be no need to discontinue clozapine. Patients receiving chemotherapy should be assessed on an individual basis and special monitoring should be carried out, e.g. monitor for symptoms of infection, increase frequency of testing schedule and establish thresholds for stopping those treatments, in collaboration with medical and haematological specialists.

Digoxin + clozapine

The SPC for clozapine advises caution with highly bound drugs, which would include digoxin. Monitor for adverse effects and adjust doses as necessary.

ERYTHROMYCIN + CLOZAPINE

Raised clozapine levels have been reported, with seizures seven days after erythromycin 250 mg/d was added to clozapine 800 mg/d, with levels falling by 50% when erythromycin was stopped (Funderburg *et al, Am J Psychiatry* 1994;**151**:1840) and increased toxicity, e.g. somnolence and leukocytosis (n = 1, Cohen *et al, Arch Intern Med* 1996;**156**:675–7). Reduced clozapine metabolism via CYP1A2 is the probable mechanism

Escitalopram + clozapine

See antipsychotics + citalopram/escitalopram (*4.3.2.1*).

FLUOXETINE + CLOZAPINE

Fluoxetine produces significant increases in plasma clozapine and norclozapine levels, with some inter-individual variation (n = 80, open, Centorrino *et al, Am J Psychiatry* 1996;**153**:820–2). There are many case reports (e.g. n = 6, Centorrino *et al, Am J Psychiatry* 1994;**151**:123–5), including death (n = 1, Ferslew *et al, J Forensic Sci* 1998;**43**:1082–5) and uncontrollable myoclonic jerks (n = 1, Kingsbury and Puckett, *Am J Psychiatry* 1995;**152**:473–2). The mechanism is possibly CYP2D6 inhibition. The risk of clozapine toxicity must be considered and measuring clozapine levels may be useful.

FLUVOXAMINE + CLOZAPINE

This is an important and significant interaction. Fluvoxamine inhibition of CYP1A2 leads to clozapine levels increased by up to 900% and AUC by 40% (e.g. n = 2, Dequardo and Roberts, *Am J Psychiatry* 1996;**153**:840–1; n = 1, Armstrong and Stephans, *J Clin Psychiatry* 1997;**58**:499) although peak levels may remain unchanged (n = 9, Wang et al, *J Clin Pharmacol* 2004;**44**:785–92). So predictable is the effect that fluvoxamine has been used to counteract 1A2 induction by smoking, which can lead to clozapine non–response (n = 3, Bender and Eap, *Arch Gen Psychiatry* 1998;**55**:1048–50) in 1A2 ultra–rapid metabolisers. Close pharmacokinetic monitoring is thus necessary, as the effect can be dramatic over a few days in some patients even with very low doses, e.g. 10–20 mg/d fluvoxamine.

Grapefruit juice + clozapine

Grapefruit juice has no effect on clozapine levels (n = 15, open, 12/52, Lane et al, *Drug Metabol Drug Interact* 2001;**18**:263–78).

H2-blockers + clozapine

Clozapine levels may rise by over 50% with cimetidine (n = 1, Czymanski et al, *J Clin Psychiatry* 1991;**52**:21). Ranitidine is a safer alternative.

Influenza vaccine + clozapine

Influenza vaccine has no effect on clozapine levels (n = 14, Raaska et al, *Eur J Clin Pharmacol* 2001;**57**:705–8).

Isoniazid + clozapine *

There is a case of increased plasma levels of clozapine after the addition of isoniazid (n = 1, Angelini et al, *J Clin Psychopharmacol* 2009; **29**:190–1).

Itraconazole/ketoconazole + clozapine

Itraconazole 200 mg/d had no effect on plasma clozapine and norclozapine levels (RCT, n = 7, 7/7, Raaska and Neuvonen, *Eur J Clin Pharmacol* 1998; **54**:167–70), and ketoconazole also has no effect on clozapine (Lane et al, *Drug Metabol Drug Interact* 2001;**18**:263–78).

Lamotrigine + clozapine

Lamotrigine 200 mg/d for 8/52 had no effect on stable clozapine levels (n = 11, Spina et al, *Ther Drug Monit* 2006;**28**:599–602), but an unexplained three-fold increase in clozapine levels was seen two weeks after lamotrigine 100 mg/d was added to a stable clozapine 400 mg/d regimen (n = 1, Kossen et al, *Am J Psychiatry* 2001;**158**:1930).

Lithium + clozapine

See antipsychotics + lithium (*4.4*).

MAOIs + clozapine

See antipsychotics + MAOIs (*4.3.4*).

Mirtazapine + clozapine

See mirtazapine (*4.3.3.4*).

Oral contraceptives + clozapine

Elevated plasma clozapine levels have been reported with norethindrone, resolving on OC discontinuation (n = 1, Gabbay et al, *J Clin Psycho–pharmacol* 2002;**22**:621–2).

Orlistat + clozapine

A small trial suggested lack of interaction (8/52, Hilger et al, *J Clin Psychopharmacol* 2002;**22**:68–70).

Oxcarbazepine + clozapine

See antipsychotics + oxcarbazepine (*4.5.7*).

PAROXETINE + CLOZAPINE

Paroxetine produces significant increases in plasma clozapine and norclozapine levels (n = 60, open, Centorrino et al, *Am J Psychiatry* 1996;**153**:820–2), and so the risk of clozapine toxicity must be considered carefully. NMS with no leukocytosis and normal CPK has also been reported with the combination (n = 1, Gambassi et al, *Aging Clin Exp Res* 2006;**18**:266–70).

Penicillamine + clozapine

There is an enhanced risk of agranulocytosis (mandatory precaution in SPC).

Phenobarbital + clozapine

Elevated plasma clozapine levels (requiring dose reduction) have been reported after discontinuation of phenobarbital, presumably from removal of CYP1A2 induction (n = 1, Lane et al, *J Clin Psychiatry* 1998;**59**:131–3).

Phenylbutazone + clozapine

There is an enhanced risk of agranulocytosis (mandatory precaution in SPC).

PHENYTOIN + CLOZAPINE

Serum concentrations of clozapine may be markedly reduced by phenytoin (n = 2, Miller et al, *J Clin Psychiatry* 1991;**52**:23) via CYP1A2 induction, so monitor for reduced effect.

Proton pump inhibitors + clozapine

A switch from omeprazole to pantoprazole does not alter average clozapine plasma levels, although some individual increases may be seen (n = 13, Mookhoek and Loonen, *Br J Clin Pharmacol* 2002;**53**:545P).

Pyrazolone analgesics + clozapine

There is an enhanced risk of agranulocytosis (mandatory precaution in SPC).

Quetiapine + clozapine
See quetiapine (*4.2.5*).

Reboxetine + clozapine
See reboxetine (*4.3.3.6*).

Rifampicin + clozapine
There is a case of a 600% reduction in clozapine levels 2–3 weeks after rifampicin was started, probably via 1A2 and 3A4 induction (n = 1, Joos et al, *J Clin Psychopharmacol* 1998;**18**:83–5).

SERTRALINE + CLOZAPINE
Sertraline may produce significant increases in plasma clozapine and norclozapine levels, with some inter–individual variation (n = 80, Centorrino et al, *Am J Psychiatry* 1996;**153**:820–2). There is a case of sudden death with the combination, probably as a result of cardiac arrhythmia (n = 1, Hoehns et al, *Ann Pharmacother* 2001;**35**:826–6). The risk of clozapine toxicity must be considered.

Smoking + clozapine
See antipsychotics + smoking (*4.7.4*).

Sulphonamides + clozapine
There is an enhanced risk of agranulocytosis (mandatory precaution in SPC).

Topiramate + clozapine
See antipsychotics + topiramate (*4.5.13*).

Tricyclics + clozapine
See antipsychotics + tricyclics (*4.3.1*).

Valproate + clozapine
See valproate + antipsychotics (*4.2.1*).

Venlafaxine + clozapine
See venlafaxine (*4.3.3.9*).

Warfarin + clozapine
The SPC for clozapine advises caution with highly bound drugs, which would include warfarin (mentioned in Sayal et al, *Acta Psychiatr Scand* 2000;**102**:250–5), so monitor and adjust doses as necessary.

4.2.5 ANTIPSYCHOTICS — OLANZAPINE *
See *4.2.1* for other, more general, interactions

Olanzapine is metabolised by CYP1A2 and 2D6, 2D6 and 3A4 (Urichuk et al, *Curr Drug Metab* 2008;**9**:410–8), with little or no effect on 1A2, 2D6, 2C19, 2C9 and 3A4 at normal doses. It is highly bound to albumin (90%) and alpha 1-acid glycoprotein (77%), and interactions may be possible through this mechanism. Olanzapine also undergoes N-glucuronidation by UGT1A4. Olanzapine is approximately 60% excreted in urine and 30% in faeces. Fixed doses appear to give higher levels in women. The UK SPC now cautions about the use of olanzapine with drugs known to increase the QTc interval.

Review: extensive, of pharmacokinetics and pharmacodynamics (Callaghan et al, *Clin Pharmacokinetics* 1999;**37**:177–93, 56 refs).

Alcohol + olanzapine
See antipsychotics + alcohol (*4.7.1*).

Antacids + olanzapine
Antacids have no effect on olanzapine bio–availability.

Anticholinergics + olanzapine *
The UK SPC now recommends that anti-cholinergics are not used with olanzapine.

Antipsychotics (other) + olanzapine
An interaction has been suggested with **halo–peridol** and olanzapine (Gomberg, *J Clin Psychopharmacol* 1999;**19**:272–3) and NMS has been reported (n = 1, Mujica and Weiden, *Am J Psychiatry* 2001;**158**:650–1). Seizures have been reported with **quetiapine** and olanzapine (n = 1, Hedges and Jeppson, *Ann Pharmacother* 2002;**36**:437–9). Unchanged olanzapine levels with **flupentixol** were mentioned in one study (Bergemann et al, *Pharmacopsychiatry* 2004; **37**:63–8).

Benzodiazepines + olanzapine
Single dose studies show no effect of olanzapine on the metabolism of **diazepam**. Mild increases in heart rate, sedation and dry mouth were noted, but no dose adjustment considered necessary. Unchanged olanzapine levels with **lorazepam** were mentioned in one study (Bergemann et al, *Pharmacopsychiatry* 2004; **37**:63–8). Concomitant IM olanzapine and IM BDZs are contraindicated (UK SPC) and must be separated by at least one hour. There is one case report of significant hypotension (down to 66/30 within four hours) lasting 12 hours in a patient given olanzapine IM with lorazepam 2mg IM 30 minutes later (n = 1, Zacher and Roche–Desilets, *J Clin Psychiatry* 2005;**66**:1614–5).

Carbamazepine + olanzapine
See antipsychotics + carbamazepine (*4.5.1*).

Charcoal (activated) + olanzapine
Activated charcoal reduces olanzapine bio–availability by 50–60%.

Cimetidine + olanzapine
There is no effect on olanzapine bioavailability.

Ciprofloxacin + olanzapine
Raised olanzapine levels have been reported,

possibly caused by ciprofloxacin (n = 1, Marko-witz and DeVane, *J Clin Psychophamacol* 1999; **19**:289–91).

Duloxetine + olanzapine *

There is a case of urinary retention with the combination, resolving when duloxetine was switched to venlafaxine (n = 1, Englisch *et al*, *Clin Neuropharmacol* 2008;**31**:308–9).

Lamotrigine + olanzapine

Lamotrigine 200mg/d for 8/52 produced a statistically significant but probably clinically insignificant rise in stable olanzapine levels (n = 11, Spina *et al*, *Ther Drug Monit* 2006;**28**:599–602).

Lithium + olanzapine

See antipsychotics + lithium (4.4).

MAOIs + olanzapine

See antipsychotics + MAOIs (4.3.4).

Mirtazapine + olanzapine

See olanzapine + mirtazapine (4.3.3.4).

Opioids + olanzapine

Opioid-induced delirium has been reported with the combination (n = 2, Estfan *et al*, *J Pain Symptom Manage* 2005;**29**:330–2).

Oxcarbazepine + olanzapine

See antipsychotics + oxcarbazepine (4.5.6).

Probenecid + olanzapine

Probenecid appears to decrease olanzapine glucuronidation (n = 12, RCT, d/b, c/o, Markowitz *et al*, *Clin Pharmacol Ther* 2002;**71**:30–8).

Reboxetine + olanzapine

See antipsychotics + reboxetine (4.3.3.6).

Rufinamide + olanzapine

See olanzapine + rufinamide (4.5.12).

Selegiline + olanzapine

Selegiline transdermal system (STS) had no effects on the pharmacokinetics of olanzapine (open, RCT, c/o, Azzaro *et al*, *J Clin Pharmacol* 2007;**47**:146–58).

Smoking + olanzapine

See antipsychotics + smoking (4.7.4).

SSRIs + olanzapine

Fluvoxamine (but not **sertraline**) inhibits the metabolism of olanzapine, probably via CYP1A2 (n = 165, Weigmann *et al*, *Ther Drug Monit* 2001;**23**:410–13; Bergemann *et al*, *Pharmacopsychiatry* 2004;**37**:63–8), with 100mg/d raising peak levels by 49%, AUC by 70%, half–life by 40% and steady-state olanzapine levels by 12–112% and so care is needed (n = 10, Chiu *et al*, *J Clin Pharmacol* 2004;**44**:1385–90, n = 12, Wang *et al*, *J Clin Pharmacol* 2004;**44**:785–92).

Use of fluvoxamine 25 mg/d has allowed a 26% reduction in olanzapine dose for the same plasma level, or could have increased OLZ levels by 25% without increasing the dose (n = 10, 6/52, open, Albers *et al*, *J Clin Psychopharmacol* 2005;**25**:170–4). This could be a useful trick for keeping olanzapine doses within BNF limits with the MHA commissioners around. Higher doses of **fluoxetine** may slightly increase olanzapine levels, probably via CYP2D6 inhibition (n = 15, Gossen *et al*, *AAPS PharmSci* 2002;**4**:E11). Melancholic depression has been reported with fluoxetine and olanzapine (n = 1, Nelson and Swartz, *Ann Clin Psychiatry* 2000;**12**:167–70), although the combination has been licensed in the USA for psychotic depression.

Topiramate + olanzapine

See antipsychotics + topiramate (4.5.14).

Tricyclics + olanzapine

See antipsychotics + tricyclics (4.3.1).

Valproate + olanzapine

Valproate lowers the plasma levels of olanzapine (Bergemann *et al*, *J Clin Psychopharmacol* 2006; **26**:432–4).

Warfarin + olanzapine

Single dose studies show no effect of olanzapine on the metabolism of warfarin, although it could be possible (mentioned in Sayal *et al*, *Acta Psychiatr Scand* 2000;**102**:250–5).

Xanthines + olanzapine

Lack of interaction has been shown with aminophylline and theophylline (n = 19, RCT, Macias *et al*, *Pharmacotherapy* 1998;**18**:1237–48).

4.2.6 ANTIPSYCHOTICS — QUETIAPINE *

See 4.2.1 for other, more general, interactions

Quetiapine is metabolised primarily by CYP3A4. The quetiapine UK SPC now advises caution when used with drugs known to increase the QTc interval or cause electrolyte imbalances.

Alcohol + quetiapine

See alcohol (4.7.1).

Antipsychotics (other) + quetiapine

Haloperidol 15mg/d and **risperidone** 6mg/d have no effect on quetiapine levels (n = 36, RCT, 9/7, Potkin *et al*, *J Clin Psychopharmacol* 2002;**22**:121–30). Lower quetiapine doses when used with **clozapine** have been recommended in a TDM service analysis (n = 1179, Castberg *et al*, *J Clin Psychiatry* 2007;**68**:1540–5). See also 4.2.4.

Antiretrovirals + quetiapine *

The UK SPC states that caution is necessary with this combination, as quetiapine levels can rise via CYP3A4 induction by, eg, fosamprenavir, indinavir, nelfinavir and ritonavir. Rapid but reversible weight gain and sedation have been reported when atazanavir/ritonavir have been used with quetiapine, presumably via 3A4 inhibition (n = 2, Pollack et al, Pharmacother 2009; **29**:1386–91).

Baclofen + quetiapine *

There is a case of cranial diabetes insipidus after an overdose of baclofen and quetiapine (n = 1, Silverstone and Scott, Anaesth Intensive Care 2009; **37**:319–20).

Barbiturates + quetiapine

Lower levels of quetiapine would be expected, due to CYP3A4 induction by barbiturates.

Benzodiazepines + quetiapine

Single doses of lorazepam and diazepam are unaffected by quetiapine.

Carbamazepine + quetiapine

See antipsychotics + carbamazepine (4.5.1).

Cimetidine + quetiapine

No interaction occurs (n = 13, open, Strakowski et al, J Clin Psychopharmacol 2002; **22**:201–5).

Clarithromycin + quetiapine *

There is a case of major increase in quetiapine plasma levels when clarithromycin was started (n = 1, Schulz–Du Bois et al, Pharmacopsychiatry 2008; **41**:258–9).

Erythromycin + quetiapine

Raised quetiapine levels are likely via CYP3A4 inhibition.

KETOCONAZOLE + QUETIAPINE

Ketoconazole 200 mg/d increases quetiapine plasma levels 3.5-fold, by CYP3A4 inhibition, potentially clinically significant (n = 12, Grimm et al, Br J Clin Pharmacol 2006; **61**:58–69).

Lithium + quetiapine

See antipsychotics + lithium (4.4).

Lovastatin + quetiapine

A prolonged QTc interval has been reported with the combination (n = 1, Furst et al, Biol Psychiatry 2002; **51**:264–5).

MAOIs + quetiapine

See antipsychotics + MAOIs (4.3.4).

Methadone + quetiapine

See quetiapine + methadone (4.6.10).

Phenytoin + quetiapine

Lower levels of quetiapine would be expected, due to CYP3A4 induction by phenytoin.

Reboxetine + quetiapine

See antipsychotics + reboxetine (4.3.3.6).

Rifampicin + quetiapine

Lower levels of quetiapine would be expected, due to CYP3A4 induction by rifampicin.

Smoking + quetiapine

See quetiapine + smoking (4.7.4).

SSRIs + quetiapine

Fluoxetine 60 mg/d has no significant effect on quetiapine kinetics (n = 26, RCT, Potkin et al, J Clin Psychopharmacol 2002; **22**:174–82) but a case of rhabdomyolysis has been reported with the combination (n = 1, Himmerrich et al, J Clin Psychopharmacol 2006; **26**:676–7). Lower quetiapine doses when used with fluvoxamine have been recommended in a TDM service analysis (n = 1179, Castberg et al, J Clin Psychiatry 2007; **68**:1540–5).

Topiramate + quetiapine

See antipsychotics + topiramate (4.5.13).

Tricyclics + quetiapine

Imipramine 150 mg/d has no significant effect on quetiapine (n = 26, RCT, Potkin et al, J Clin Psychopharmacol 2002; **22**:174–82) but quetiapine has caused a falsely elevated estimation of nortriptyline levels (n = 1, Schussler et al, Am J Psychiatry 2003; **160**:589).

Valproate + quetiapine

There is a case of cervical dystonia with the combination (n = 1, Habermeyer et al, J Clin Psychopharmacol 2007; **27**:396–7).

Warfarin + quetiapine

No interaction is likely to occur routinely (mentioned in Sayal et al, Acta Psychiatr Scand 2000; **102**:250–5), but an isolated case has been reported (n = 1, Rogers et al, J Clin Psycho-pharmacol 1999; **19**:382–3).

4.2.7 ANTIPSYCHOTICS — RISPERIDONE AND PALIPERIDONE *

See 4.2.1 for other, more general, interactions

Risperidone is metabolised by CYP2D6 to 9-hydroxy-risperidone n = 218, Mannheimer et al, Ther Drug Monit 2010; [in press]).

Reviews: general (DeVane and Nemeroff, J Clin Psychopharmacol 2001; **21**:408–16), P450 metabolism (Berecz et al, Curr Drug Targets 2004; **5**:573–9).

Aripiprazole + risperidone/paliperidone

See antipsychotics (other) + aripiprazole (4.2.2).

Caffeine + risperidone/paliperidone

Caffeine appears to have no effect on plasma risperidone levels (n = 136, Kakihara et al, Int Clin Psychopharmacol 2005;**20**:71–8).

CARBAMAZEPINE + RISPERIDONE/ PALIPERIDONE

See antipsychotics + carbamazepine (4.5.1).

Citalopram/escitalopram + risperidone/ paliperidone

See citalopram/escitalopram (4.3.2.1).

Clindamycin + risperidone/paliperidone *

Abnormal movements have been seen when clindamycin was added to risperidone in a girl with autism (n=1, Malone and Harvery, J Child Adolesc Psychopharmacol 2008;**18**:221–2).

CLOZAPINE + RISPERIDONE/PALIPERIDONE

See antipsychotics + clozapine (4.2.4).

Dexamfetamine + risperidone *

There is a report of an acute dystonic reaction when dexamfetamine was stopped from the combination (n=1, Keshen and Carandang, J Child Adolesc Psychopharmacol 2007;**17**:867–70; see also Benjamin and Salek, J Am Acad Child Adolesc Psychiatry 2005;**44**:510–2).

Donepezil + risperidone/paliperidone

See antipsychotics + donepezil (4.6.3.1).

FLUOXETINE + RISPERIDONE/PALIPERIDONE*

Fluoxetine 20mg/d has caused a 75% increase in risperidone levels over four weeks, resulting in side-effects in 30% (n = 10, Spina et al, J Clin Psychopharmacol 2002;**22**:419–23). Severe EPSE, urinary retention (n = 1, Bozikas et al, J Psychopharmacol 2001;**15**:142–3) and nasal bleeding (n = 1, Mowla et al, Pharmacopsychiatry 2009;**42**:204–5) have also been reported.

Fluvoxamine + risperidone/paliperidone

See antipsychotics + fluvoxamine (4.3.2.3).

Galantamine + risperidone/paliperidone

See antipsychotics + galantamine (4.6.3.2).

Gingko biloba + risperidone/paliperidone

Priapism has been associated with the combination (n = 1, Lin et al, Mayo Clin Proc 2007; **82**: 1289–90).

Itraconazole + risperidone/paliperidone

One week of itraconazole 200mg/d raised risperidone and metabolite levels by around 70–75%, presumably via 3A4 inhibition, returning to normal over the next week (n = 19, 2/52, Jung et al, Clin Pharmacol Ther 2005;**78**:520–8).

Lamotrigine + risperidone/paliperidone

Increasing lamotrigine from 175mg/d to 225mg/d produced a rise in risperidone levels from 70ng/ml to 412ng/ml in one patient also on clozapine, although the mechanism was unknown (n = 1, Bienentreu and Kronmüller, Am J Psychiatry 2005;**162**:811–2). Others have disputed this (n = 15 + 211 controls, Castberg and Spigset, J Clin Psychiatry 2006;**67**:1159) as lamotrigine 200mg/d for 8/52 had no effect on stable risperidone levels in another study (n = 10, Spina et al, Ther Drug Monit 2006;**28**:599–602).

Lithium + risperidone/paliperidone

See antipsychotics + lithium (4.4).

Methadone + risperidone/paliperidone

See methadone (4.6.10).

MAOIs + risperidone/paliperidone

See antipsychotics + MAOIs (4.3.4).

Mirtazapine + risperidone/paliperidone

See mirtazapine (4.3.3.4).

Oxcarbazepine + risperidone/paliperidone

See antipsychotics + oxcarbazepine (4.5.7).

Paroxetine + risperidone/paliperidone *

Paroxetine causes a dose-dependent rise in risperidone and metabolite levels (up to double with paroxetine 40mg/d), and so risperidone dose reduction might be needed should side–effects occur (n = 12, open, 12/52, Saito et al, J Clin Psychopharmacol 2005;**25**:527–32; n = 10, open, 4/52, Spina et al, Ther Drug Monit 2001;**23**:223–7; n = 1, Barnhill et al, Pharmacopsychiatry 2005;**38**: 223–5). There seems to be no clinically relevant interaction with single doses of paliperidone (RCT, c/o, Berwaerts et al, Pharmacopsychiatry 2009;**42**:158–63).

Phenothiazines + risperidone/paliperidone

Levomepromazine has no effect on risperidone plasma levels (n = 20, 2/52, Yoshimura et al, Pharmacopsychiatry 2005;**38**:98–100).

Phenytoin + risperidone/paliperidone

Severe EPSE have been reported (n = 1, Sanderson, J Clin Psychiatry 1996;**57**:177).

Probenecid + risperidone/paliperidone

Probenecid has no effect on risperidone kinetics (n = 12, RCT, d/b, c/o, Markowitz et al, Clin Pharmacol Ther 2002;**71**:30–8).

Quetiapine + risperidone/paliperidone

See antipsychotics + quetiapine (4.2.6).

Reboxetine + risperidone/paliperidone

See antipsychotics + reboxetine (4.3.3.6).

RIFAMPICIN + RISPERIDONE/PALIPERIDONE

Rifampin reduces risperidone AUC by 72% and reduces Cmax by 50%, probably by 3A4 and

2D6 induction (n = 10, RCT, open, c/o, 2×5/7, Mahatthanatrakul *et al, J Clin Pharm Ther* 2007; **32**:161–7).

Ritonavir/indinavir + risperidone/paliperidone

Addition of ritonavir/indinavir to risperidone has led to severe EPSE, dystonia (n = 1, Kelly *et al, Ann Pharmacother* 2002;**36**:827–30) and reversible coma (n = 1, Jover *et al, Clin Neuropharmacol* 2002; **25**:251–3), probably via risperidone toxicity.

Selegiline + risperidone/paliperidone

Selegiline transdermal system (STS) had no effects on the pharmacokinetics of risperidone (open, RCT, c/o, Azzaro *et al, J Clin Pharmacol* 2007;**47**:146–58).

Sertraline + risperidone/paliperidone *

High doses of sertraline (150 mg/d) can elevate risperidone levels by about 40%, presumably via 2D6 inhibition (n = 11, open, Spina *et al, Ther Drug Monit* 2004;**26**:386–90). Risperidone has no effect on sertraline kinetics (n = 10, 4/52, Yoshimura *et al, Hum Psychopharmacol* 2008;**23**:707–13).

Smoking + risperidone/paliperidone

See antipsychotics + risperidone (4.7.4).

Topiramate + risperidone/paliperid one

See antipsychotics + topiramate (4.5.14).

Tricyclics + risperidone/paliperidone

See antipsychotics + tricyclics (4.3.1).

Valproate + risperidone/paliperidone

See antipsychotics (4.2.1).

Venlafaxine + risperidone/paliperidone

See antipsychotics + venlafaxine (4.3.3.9).

4.2.8 ANTIPSYCHOTICS — ZIPRASIDONE

Ziprasidone is partly metabolised by CYP3A4 (with a minor amount from 1A2), plus around 65% via aldehyde reductase. It has no effect on CYP1A2, 2C9/19, 2D6 or 3A4. It is 99% plasma bound. Due to the QTc-prolonging effect, ziprasidone should not be used with drugs also likely to prolong the QTc interval, e.g. sotalol, quinidine, other class Ia and III anti-arrhythmics, phenothiazines, tricyclics, pimozide, mefloquine and dolasetron (see SPC).

Antacids + ziprasidone

Lack of interaction has been shown with 30 ml Maalox (n = 11, RCT, Wilner *et al, Br J Clin Pharmacol* 2000;**49**[S3]:57–60).

Anticholinergics + ziprasidone

Lack of interaction has been shown with benzatropine.

Benzodiazepines + ziprasidone

Lack of interaction with lorazepam has been shown.

Beta-blockers + ziprasidone

Lack of interaction has been shown with propranolol.

Carbamazepine + ziprasidone

See antipsychotics + carbamazepine (4.5.1).

Cimetidine + ziprasidone

Lack of interaction has been shown (n = 11, RCT, Wilner *et al, Br J Clin Pharmacol* 2000;**49**[S3]: 57–60).

Dextromethorphan + ziprasidone

Lack of interaction has been shown (Wilner *et al, Br J Clin Pharmacol* 2000;**49**(S3):43–8).

Ketoconazole + ziprasidone

Ketoconazole decreases ziprasidone AUC by about 35%, which may require slightly raised doses.

Levodopa + ziprasidone

Ziprasidone may antagonise the effects of levodopa and other dopaminergic agents.

Lithium + ziprasidone

See antipsychotics + lithium (4.4).

Oral contraceptive + ziprasidone

Lack of interaction has been shown with a combined OCs (n = 19, d/b, p/c, c/o, Muirhead *et al, Br J Clin Pharmacol* 2000;**49**[S3]:49–56).

Smoking + ziprasidone

See antipsychotics + smoking (4.7.4).

Warfarin + ziprasidone

Lack of interaction has been shown.

4.2.9 ANTIPSYCHOTICS — ZOTEPINE

See 4.2.1 for other, more general, interactions

Zotepine is metabolised by CYP1A2 and 3A4 to norzotepine and both have a plasma protein binding of 97%, making protein-displacement interactions unlikely. Zotepine has no significant effect on CYP2D6.

Alcohol + zotepine

Zotepine should not be used in people with alcohol intoxication.

Anticholinergics + zotepine

Biperiden had no effect on zotepine kinetics, side-effects or efficacy in one study (n = 21, Otani *et al, Br J Psychiatry* 1990;**157**:128–30).

Anticonvulsants + zotepine

Zotepine lowers the seizure threshold, particularly at doses above 300 mg/d.

Anticoagulants + zotepine
Zotepine has been reported to enhance the risk of bleeding when given with anticoagulants, e.g. with nicoumalone, dicoumarol and warfarin, possibly via a change in protein binding.

Antipsychotics (other) + zotepine
Co-prescribing other antipsychotics with zotepine can raise the incidence of seizures.

Benzodiazepines + zotepine
Diazepam increases zotepine levels by 10% (higher in Japanese patients) and doubles norzotepine levels (n=17, open, Kondo et al, Psychopharmacol [Berl] 1996;**127**:311–4), possibly via CYP3A4 inhibition.

Carbamazepine + zotepine
See antipsychotics + carbamazepine (4.5.1).

Clonidine + zotepine
The Japanese SPC notes that zotepine has alpha-1-adrenergic antagonist properties, which may decrease the hypotensive actions of clonidine and other hypotensive agents.

Hypotensive drugs + zotepine
See clonidine.

Phenytoin + zotepine
The Japanese SPC notes that zotepine may increase phenytoin plasma levels, so more frequent monitoring is required.

Smoking + zotepine
See antipsychotics + smoking (4.7.4).

SSRIs + zotepine
Fluoxetine increases zotepine levels by 10% and doubles norzotepine levels. Deep vein thrombosis, possibly linked to concurrent paroxetine and zotepine, has been reported (n=2, Pantel et al, Pharmacopsychiatry 1997;**30**:109–11).

4.3 ANTIDEPRESSANTS

Review: significant drug interactions with antidepressants in the elderly (Spina and Scordo, Drugs Aging 2002;**19**:299–320, 95 refs).

4.3.1 TRICYCLIC ANTIDEPRESSANTS

Tricyclics are metabolised by a range of P450 enzymes, e.g. CYP1A2, 2D6 and 3A3/4. Some tricyclics have several metabolic routes, which may vary with concentration and where another might take over should one be inhibited.

Acamprosate + tricyclics
See acamprosate (4.6.1).

Acetazolamide + tricyclics

An interaction is unlikely to occur.

Adrenaline + tricyclics *
Tricyclics may potentiate the effects of adrenaline injection increasing the risk of hypertension and cardiac arrhythmias (SPC).

ALCOHOL + TRICYCLICS
See alcohol (4.7.1).

Amiodarone + tricyclics
The literature notes an increased risk of ventricular arrhythmias with tricyclics.

Anaesthetics + tricyclics
Halothane, pancuronium or gallamine should be used with care with tricyclics with strong anticholinergic actions. Enflurane may be a safer alternative.

Anticholinergics + tricyclics
Enhanced anticholinergic effects may occur, especially in the elderly.

Antihistamines + tricyclics
Enhanced sedation and anticholinergic effects are possible.

Antipsychotics + tricyclics
Tricyclic levels may be up to twice as high if haloperidol is taken concurrently, e.g. with desipramine, nortriptyline and imipramine. Tricyclic levels may also rise with phenothiazines (eg. Siris et al, Am J Psychiatry 1982;**143**:104–6) giving enhanced side-effects, e.g. perphenazine increased nortriptyline levels by about 25%, probably by CYP2D6 inhibition (n=25, Mulsant et al, J Clin Psychopharmacol 1997;**17**:318–21). No significant interaction has been reported with the thioxanthenes, although raised imipramine levels with flupentixol have occurred (n=1, Cook et al, Can J Psychiatry 1986;**31**:235–7). Single dose studies show no effect of olanzapine on the metabolism of imipramine (n=9, open, Callaghan et al, J Clin Pharmacol 1997;**37**:971–8). Seizures have been reported with olanzapine and clomipramine (Deshauer et al, J Clin Psychopharmacol 2000;**20**:283–4). Lower olanzapine levels with trimipramine, but unchanged levels with amitriptyline were mentioned in one study (Bergemann et al, Pharmacopsychiatry 2004;**37**:63–8). Up to 100mg/d amitriptyline may have no effect on risperidone (n=12, open, Sommers et al, Int Clin Psychopharmacol 1997;**12**:141–5) but risperidone may raise maprotiline levels, not a thing you would want to do accidentally (Normann et al, J Clin Psychopharmacol 2002;**22**:92–4).

Asenapine + imipramine *

See imipramine + asenapine (4.2.3).

Aspirin + imipramine

Imipramine plasma levels may rise and ADRs increase when aspirin is added to imipramine (n = 20, Juarez–Olguin et al, Clin Neuropharmacol 2002;**25**:32–6).

Atomoxetine + tricyclics

See atomoxetine (4.6.4).

Baclofen + tricyclics

A patient with MS lost muscle tone when nortriptyline and imipramine were added to baclofen (n = 1, Silverglat, JAMA 1981;**246**:1659).

BARBITURATES + TRICYCLICS

Barbiturates can reduce the serum levels of amitriptyline, protriptyline and nortriptyline by 14–60%, via CYP3A4 induction. Pentobarbital may affect nortriptyline metabolism within two days, both when starting (induction) and on discontinuation (n = 6, von Bahr et al, Clin Pharmacol Ther 1998;**64**:18–26). Use an alternative to barbiturates or monitor tricyclic levels.

Benzodiazepines + tricyclics

See benzodiazepines (4.1.1).

Beta–blockers + tricyclics

Enhanced maprotiline toxicity has been reported, labetolol increases imipramine plasma levels by 28% (n = 12, RCT, p/c, c/o, Hermann et al, J Clin Pharmacol 1992;**32**:176–83) and there are cases of propranolol possibly raising imipramine levels in children (n = 2, Gillette and Tannery, J Am Acad Child Adolesc Psychiatry 1994;**33**:223–4), possibly via 2D6 inhibition. This would appear to be a rare but possible interaction.

Buprenorphine + amitriptyline

No enhanced CNS depression or respiratory effects have been seen (n = 12, d/b, p/c, c/o, Saarialho–Kere et al, Eur J Clin Pharmacol 1987; **33**:139–46).

Bupropion + tricyclics

See bupropion (4.6.6).

Calcium-channel blockers + tricyclics

Amitriptyline clearance was reduced by diltiazem and verapamil in one study, with adverse effects increased (n = 32, Hermann et al, J Clin Pharmacol 1992;**32**:176–83). Diltiazem may increase nor–triptyline concentrations (n = 1, Krahenbuhl et al, Eur J Clin Pharmacol 1996;**49**:417–9). Enhanced cardiac side-effects are also possible.

Cannabis + tricyclics

See antidepressants + cannabis (4.7.2).

CARBAMAZEPINE + TRICYCLICS

See carbamazepine (4.5.1).

Charcoal, activated + tricyclics

5–10g may reduce the absorption of tricyclics by up to 75% if given within 30 minutes and may be an effective treatment for overdose, even up to two hours after the overdose is taken (open, Dawling et al, Eur J Clin Pharmacol 1978;**14**:445–7).

Cholestyramine + doxepin

Plasma levels of doxepin may be reduced to a third by cholestyramine (n = 1, Geeze et al, Psychosomatics 1988; **29**:233–5).

CLONIDINE + TRICYCLICS

Tricyclics can be expected to antagonise the hypotensive effects of clonidine (e.g. Hui, J Am Geriatr Soc 1983;**31**:164–5).

Cocaine + tricyclics

See antidepressants + cocaine (4.7.3).

Codfish + clomipramine

In the never-ending quest for completeness, it is (probably) worth reporting that a generalised urticaria (Naranjo 'probable') has occurred after someone ate codfish while taking clomipramine 75–100 mg/d (n = 1, Gallelli et al, Pharmacopsychiatry 2006;**39**:154–6).

Co-trimoxazole + tricyclics

Five cases of relapse have been reported when co-trimoxazole was added to antidepressant therapy (L'Encephale 1987;**8**:123–6).

Dextropropoxyphene + doxepin

There are reports of doxepin plasma levels raised by up to 150% with dextropropoxyphene, via 2D6 inhibition.

Disopyramide + tricyclics

Increased anticholinergic effects may be seen (Hartel et al, Clin Pharmacol Ther 1974;**15**:551–5) and the BNF notes an increased risk of ventricular arrhythmias.

Disulfiram + tricyclics

Amitriptyline may enhance the effects of disulfiram (MacCallum, Lancet 1969;i:313) and tricyclic levels may be increased by about 30% by CYP1A2 inhibition (n = 2, Ciraulo et al, Am J Psychiatry 1985;**142**:1373–4).

Duloxetine + tricyclics

See duloxetine (4.3.3.2).

Fibre + tricyclics

There are several cases of a high fibre diet reducing tricyclic levels by up to a third (and hence to inactive levels), e.g. with doxepin. This might explain non-response in some patients.

Fluconazole + tricyclics

Inhibition of CYP3A4 by fluconazole has resulted in cases of elevated, toxic nortriptyline levels (n = 1, Gannon, *Ann Pharmacother* 1992; **26**:1456–7) and syncope (Robinson *et al*, *Ann Pharmacother* 2000;**34**:1406–9). Delirium (Duggal, *Gen Hosp Psychiatry* 2003;**25**:297–8) has been associated with concurrent amitriptyline and fluconazole therapy.

Glyceryl trinitrate + tricyclics

See nitrates + tricyclics (below).

H2-blockers + tricyclics

CYP1A2 inhibition by **cimetidine** may decrease the metabolism and increase the half-life and plasma levels of tricyclics, e.g. amitriptyline (by 37–80%, Curry *et al*, *Eur J Clin Pharmacol* 1985;**29**:429–33), doxepin (by 30%, n = 10, RCT, Abernethy and Todd, *J Clin Psychopharmacol* 1986;**6**:8–12), imipramine (by over 100%, n = 12, RCT, d/b, p/c, c/o, Wells *et al*, *Eur J Clin Pharmacol* 1986;**31**:285–90) and nortriptyline (by 20%, Henauer and Hollister, *Clin Pharmacol Ther* 1984;**35**:183–7). Other H2-blockers, e.g. **ranitidine**, do not appear to interact this way (n = 6, open, Sutherland *et al*, *Eur J Clin Pharmacol* 1987;**32**:159–64).

Hypoglycaemics + tricyclics

There are two isolated cases of enhanced hypoglycaemia with doxepin and nortriptyline (n = 2, True *et al*, *Am J Psychiatry* 1987;**144**:1220–1), so monitor blood glucose regularly.

Levodopa + tricyclics

A small reduction in the effect of levodopa may be seen (open, Morgan *et al*, *Neurology* 1975; **25**:1029), of minimal clinical significance.

Levothyroxine + tricyclics

This is usually a synergistic interaction (see *1.14*) but a few isolated cases of tachycardia and hypothyroidism have been reported.

Lithium + tricyclics

The combination is well used (see depression, *1.14*) but some adverse reactions have been reported, e.g. myoclonus (Devanand *et al*, *J Clin Psychopharmacol* 1988;**8**:446), neurotoxicity with motor symptoms and seizures (e.g. Austin *et al*, *J Clin Psychiatry* 1990;**51**:344) and NMS with amoxapine (n = 1, Gupta and Racaniello, *Ann Clin Psychiatry* 2000;**12**:107–9).

MAOIs + TRICYCLICS

See MAOIs (*4.3.4*).

Melatonin + tricyclics

See melatonin (*4.1.4*).

Methadone + tricyclics

See methadone (*4.6.10*).

Methyldopa + desipramine

The hypotensive effect of methyldopa may be decreased, with possible tachycardia and CNS stimulation (Van Spanning *et al*, *Int J Clin Pharmacol Biopharm* 1975;**11**:65–7).

Methylphenidate + tricyclics

See methylphenidate (*4.6.11*).

Mirtazapine + tricyclics

See mirtazapine (*4.3.3.4*) .

Moclobemide + tricyclics

See moclobemide (*4.3.3.5*).

Modafinil + tricyclics

See modafinil (*4.6.12*).

Morphine + tricyclics

Tricyclics such as amitriptyline increase the bioavailability of morphine and potentiate the analgesic effect, usually a beneficial combination (Ventafridda *et al*, *Lancet* 1987;**i**:1204).

Nitrates (sublingual) + tricyclics

Dry mouth may reduce the dissolution of sublingual nitrates.

Olanzapine + tricyclics

See olanzapine (*4.2.5*).

Oral contraceptives/estrogens + tricyclics

Akathisia (n = 3, Krishnan *et al*, *Am J Psychiatry* 1984;**141**:696–7), reduced tricyclic effectiveness and enhanced tricyclic toxicity have been reported. Best to monitor the tricyclic closely.

Orlistat + tricyclics

A small trial suggested lack of interaction with clomipramine (n = 8, 8/52, Hilger *et al*, *J Clin Psychopharmacol* 2002;**22**:68–70).

Phenindione + tricyclics

An enhanced risk of bleeding may occur.

Phenylbutazone + tricyclics

Tricyclic absorption may get delayed or reduced by phenylbutazone (Consolo *et al*, *Eur J Pharmacol* 1970;**10**:239–42).

PHENYTOIN + TRICYCLICS

See phenytoin (*4.5.9*).

Quetiapine + tricyclics

See quetiapine (*4.2.6*).

Quinine/quinidine + tricyclics

Studies have shown raised nortriptyline levels with quinidine and quinine (n = 10, Steiner *et al*, *Clin Pharmacol Ther* 1988; **43**:577–81), via 2D6 inhibition. Best to monitor tricyclic levels.

Reboxetine + tricyclics

See reboxetine (*4.3.3.6*).

Smoking + tricyclics

See smoking (4.7.4).

Sodium oxybate + tricyclics

See sodium oxybate (4.6.13).

SSRIs + TRICYCLICS *

Tricyclics are predominantly metabolised by CYP2D6 and SSRIs produce a dose-related inhibition of this enzyme. **Fluoxetine, paroxetine** and **fluvoxamine** all cause significant inhibition at therapeutic doses, whereas citalopram/escitalopram and sertraline cause little clinically significant 2D6 inhibition at standard doses. **Citalopram** (and presumably **escitalopram**) has no effect on some tricyclic levels (n = 5, Baettig et al, Eur J Clin Pharmacol 1993;**44**:403–5), although desipramine (but not imipramine) levels may rise slightly (e.g. n = 1, Ashton, J Clin Psychiatry 2000;**61**:144). **Fluoxetine** may double or triple tricyclic levels, e.g. with amitriptyline (e.g. fatality reported by Preskorn and Baker, JAMA 1997; **277**:1682; n = 29, open, Vandel et al, Pharmacol Res 1995; **31**:347–53), clomipramine (n = 4, Vandel et al, Neuropsychobiology 1992;**25**:202–7), imipramine (Leroj and Walentynowicz, Can J Psychiatry 1996;**41**:318–9), even if the tricyclic is used after an extended interval (Extein, Am J Psychiatry 1991;**148**:1601–2). Tricyclic doses should be reduced by up to 75% if used with fluoxetine (n = 3, Wester-Meyer, J Clin Pharmacol 1991;**31**:388–92). **Fluvoxamine** increases amitriptyline (n=22, Vezmar et al, J Pharmacol Sci 2009;**110**:98–104), clomipramine (n = 1, Bertschy et al, Eur J Clin Pharmacol 1991;**40**:119–20) and imipramine levels (Maskall and Lam, Am J Psychiatry 1993; **50**:1566), also by inhibiting both hydroxylation and N-demethylation (Hartter et al, Psychopharmacology 1993;**110**:302–8). **Paroxetine** significantly reduces the metabolism of amitriptyline and imipramine (e.g. Skjelbo and Brosen, Br J Clin Pharmacol 1992;**34**:256–61), resulting in enhanced tricyclic toxicity. **Sertraline** 50 mg/d may produce a 31–60% increase in desipramine levels (n = 18, RCT, 7/52, Preskorn et al, J Clin Psychopharmacol 1994;**14**:90–8) but a 200–300% increase has been seen (n=4, Zussman et al, Br J Clin Pharmacol 1995;**39**:S530–S551; See also n = 12, RCT, open, Kurtz et al, Clin Pharmacol Ther 1997;**62**:145–56) so the potential for interaction is present. A serotonin syndrome has been reported with many SSRI-tricyclic combinations (see 5.14).

St John's wort + tricyclics

See St John's wort (4.3.3.10).

Sucralfate + amitriptyline

One small study showed a marked reduction in amitriptyline absorption (Fed Proc 1986;**45**:205).

Tea or coffee + tricyclics

Studies have shown that some tricyclics (e.g. amitriptyline and imipramine) precipitate out of solution to form a tannin complex with tea and coffee (J Pharm Sci 1984;**73**:1056–8). The clinical significance is thought to be minimal (Bowen et al, Lancet 1981;**i**:1217–8).

Terbinafine + tricyclics

Terbinafine, a potent 2D6 inhibitor, may triple desipramine plasma levels (n = 1, O'Reardon et al, Am J Psychiatry 2002;**159**:492) and induce imipramine (e.g. n = 1, Teitelbaum and Pearson, Am J Psychiatry 2001;**158**:2086) and nortriptyline toxicity (n = 1, van der Kuy et al, Ann Pharmacother 2002;**36**:1712–4). A significant rise may occur in amitriptyline levels, an effect that may, extraordinarily, last for up to three to six months after stopping terbinafine (n = 1, Castberg et al, Ther Drug Monit 2005;**27**:680–2).

Valproate + tricyclics

See antidepressants + valproate (4.5.15).

VASOCONSTRICTOR SYMPATHOMIMETICS + TRICYCLICS

A greatly enhanced response, e.g. hypertension and arrhythmias, to norepinephrine and phenylephrine in patients taking tricyclics has been shown in many reports. Doxepin may have a lesser effect. Local anaesthetics with epinephrine appear safe. Moderate doses of cold cures containing sympathomimetics should present little risk in healthy patients.

Venlafaxine + tricyclics

Venlafaxine increases imipramine levels, showing a consistent but probably clinically modest effect (n=8, Albers et al, Psychiatr Res 2000;**6**:35–43). Serotonin syndrome has been reported with venlafaxine and amitriptyline (n = 1, Postgrad Med J 2000;**76**:254–6) and a GTC fit with venlafaxine and trimipramine (n=1, Schlienger et al, Ann Pharmacother 2000;**34**: 1402–5).

Warfarin + tricyclics

Normally there is no problem, but occasional control problems have been reported with lofepramine (mentioned in Sayal et al, Acta Psychiatr Scand 2000;**102**:250–55 and Duncan et al, Int Clin Psychopharmacol 1998;**13**:87–94).

Yohimbine + tricyclics
Tricyclics can potentiate the blood pressure changes caused by yohimbine, especially if blood pressure is already raised (mentioned in Fugh-Berman, *Lancet* 2000;**355**:134–8).
Zopiclone + tricyclics
See zopiclone (4.1.8).
Zotepine + tricyclics
See zotepine (4.2.9).

4.3.2 SSRIs (SELECTIVE SEROTONIN REUPTAKE INHIBITORS)

Drug interactions involving the P450 system have been described for all SSRIs, but there are significant differences in the isoenzymes inhibited and the degree of inhibition.

The *in vitro* inhibition of 2D6 on a molar basis is: paroxetine (most potent), norfluoxetine, fluoxetine, sertraline, fluvoxamine and citalopram (least potent). *In vivo* is probably broadly similar. Fluoxetine and paroxetine are probably broadly similar in 2D6 inhibition, but with some variation (n=31, RCT, using multiple-dose fluoxetine 60mg/d, fluvoxamine 100mg/d, paroxetine 20mg/d, or sertraline 100mg/d; Alfaro et al, *J Clin Psychopharmacol* 1999;**19**:155–63).
Review: overview and review of SSRI interactions and P450 effects (Hemeryck and Belpaire, *Curr Drug Metab* 2002;**3**:13–37).

4.3.2.1 CITALOPRAM AND ESCITALOPRAM
Citalopram is a weak inhibitor of CYP2D6 and is metabolised mainly by 3A4 (also 2D6 and 2C19). A review (Brosen and Naranjo, *Eur Neuropsychopharmacol* 2001;**11**:275–83) concludes that citalopram is neither a source nor a cause of clinically important drug–drug interactions. Escitalopram would be expected to have similar characteristics.
Acenocoumarol + citalopram/escitalopram
There is a reported case of interaction (n=1, Borras-Blasco et al, *Ann Pharmacother* 2002; **36**:345).
Alcohol + citalopram/escitalopram
See alcohol (4.7.1).
Alimemazine (trimeprazine) + citalopram/escitalopram
See antipsychotics + citalopram/escitalopram in this section.
Antipsychotics + citalopram/escitalopram

Urinary obstruction has been reported in an elderly patient taking citalopram and **aripiprazole** (n=1, Padala et al, *J Clin Psychopharmacol* 2006; **26**:667–8). **Levomepromazine** may increase plasma levels of citalopram by about a third (Milne and Goa, *Drugs* 1991;**41**:450–77), possibly via enzyme inhibition and of minimal clinical significance. There has been no detectable effect from citalopram on the plasma levels of other antipsychotics (n=90, d/b, Syvalahti et al, *J Intern Med Res* 1997;**25**:24–32), e.g. citalopram 40mg/d had no effect on the plasma levels of **clozapine** (n=8, 200–400mg/d), **risperidone** (n=7, 4–6mg/d) in patients with chronic schizophrenia (8/52, Avenoso et al, *Clin Drug Investigation* 1998;**16**:393–8), although torsades de pointes with risperidone and citalopram has been reported (n=1, Blaschke et al, *Pharmacopsychiatry* 2007;**40**:294–5). Despite this, the FDA has issued a warning about citalopram raising **clozapine** levels by clinically significant levels.
Atomoxetine + citalopram/escitalopram
See SSRIs + atomoxetine (4.6.4).
Benzodiazepines + citalopram/escitalopram
No pharmacokinetic interaction could be demonstrated between citalopram and the CYP3A4 substrate triazolam (n=18, open, Nolting and Abramowitz, *Pharmacother* 2000; **20**:750–5) and citalopram does not prolong the half-life of alprazolam (Hall et al, *J Clin Psychopharmacol* 2003;**23**:349–57).
Beta-blockers + citalopram/escitalopram
Escitalopram is a weak 2D6 inhibitor, but can increase metoprolol's AUC by 89% (Preskorn et al, *J Clin Psychopharmacol* 2007;**27**:28–34).
Buspirone + citalopram/escitalopram
Hyponatraemia and serotonin syndrome has been reported with this combination (Spigset and Adielsson, *Int Clin Psychopharmacol* 1997; **12**:61–3).
Carbamazepine + citalopram/escitalopram
Carbamazepine may reduce the proportion and concentration of the escitalopram isomer (n=6, Steinacher et al, *Eur Neuropsychopharmacol* 2002;**12**:255–60). Citalopram has no effect on carbamazepine kinetics (n=12, open, Moller et al, *J Clin Psychophamacol* 2001;**21**:493–9).
Charcoal, activated + citalopram/escitalopram
25 g activated charcoal given 30 minutes after citalopram reduced citalopram AUC by 51%,

and peak levels by over 50%. Concurrent gastric lavage did not provide any additional reductions (n = 9, RCT, Lapatto-Reiniluoto *et al*, *Br J Clin Pharmacol* 1999;**48**:148–53).

Ciclosporin + citalopram/escitalopram
Citalopram has no effect on ciclosporin kinetics (Liston *et al*, *Psychosomatics* 2001;**42**:370–2).

Cimetidine + citalopram/escitalopram
Cimetidine increases escitalopram levels but this is unlikely to be clinically significant (n = 16, RCT, p/c, Malling *et al*, *Br J Clin Pharmacol* 2005;**60**:287–90).

Digoxin + citalopram/escitalopram
Steady state citalopram 40mg/d had no effect on the kinetics of single doses of digoxin 1mg (n = 11, open, c/o, 50/7, Larsen *et al*, *J Clin Pharmacol* 2001;**41**:340).

Donepezil + citalopram/escitalopram
See SSRIs + donepezil (4.6.3.1).

Duloxetine + citalopram/escitalopram
See SSRIs + duloxetine (4.3.3.2).

Fluconazole + citalopram/escitalopram *
Serotonin syndrome has been reported with this combination, probably via 2C19 inhibition (n = 2, Levin *et al*, *Gen Hosp Psychiatry* 2008;**30**:372–7).

Fluvoxamine + citalopram/escitalopram
Fluvoxamine may increase the ratio of escitalopram to R-citalopram, enhancing its action (n = 7, open, Bondolfi *et al*, *Psychopharmacol* [Berl] 1996;**128**:421–5).

Itopride + escitalopram *
Tardive dyskinesia has been reported after long–term co-administration of escitalopram and the D2 antagonist antinauseant itopride (n = 1, *Prog Neuropsychopharmacol Biol Psychiatry* 2009;**33**: 380–1).

Ketoconazole + citalopram/escitalopram
Single doses of ketoconazole have no effect on the kinetics of citalopram (n = 18, RCT, d/b, c/o, Gutierrez and Abramowitz, *Pharmacotherapy* 2001;**21**:163–8).

Lamotrigine + citalopram/escitalopram
Myoclonus has been reported with the combination (n = 1, Rosenhagen *et al*, *J Clin Psychopharmacol* 2006;**26**:346–7).

Linezolid + citalopram/escitalopram
In people taking SSRIs, serotonin syndrome may occur about nine days after the introduction of linezolid (longer the older you are); symptoms may resolve in three days or longer (n = 12, Morales–Molina *et al*, *J Antimicrob Chemother* 2005;**56**:1176–8; n = 1, Tahir, *J Am Med Dir*

Assoc 2004;**5**:111–3; n = 1, Bergeron *et al*, *Ann Pharmacother* 2005;**39**:956–61).

Lithium + citalopram/escitalopram
No pharmacokinetic interaction was noted in one study (n = 24, open, Gram *et al*, *Ther Drug Monit* 1993;**15**:18–24).

MAOIs + citalopram/escitalopram
See MAOIs (4.3.4).

Melatonin + citalopram/escitalopram
Citalopram may slow the metabolism of exogenous melatonin (n = 15, RCT, d/b, p/c, 21/7, Huuhka *et al*, *Methods Find Exp Clin Pharmacol* 2006;**28**:447–50).

Metoclopramide + citalopram/escitalopram
See metoclopramide + fluvoxamine (4.3.2.3).

Moclobemide + citalopram/escitalopram
See SSRIs + moclobemide (4.3.3.5).

NSAIDs + citalopram/escitalopram
See NSAIDs + fluoxetine (4.3.2.2).

Omeprazole + citalopram/escitalopram
Omeprazole increases escitalopram levels but this is unlikely to be clinically significant (n = 16, RCT, p/c, Malling *et al*, *Br J Clin Pharmacol* 2005;**60**:287–90).

Oxcarbazepine + citalopram/escitalopram
See oxcarbazepine (4.5.7).

Perhexiline + citalopram/escitalopram
Perhexiline toxicity with citalopram has been reported (n = 1, Nyfort–Hansen, *Med J Aust* 2002;**176**:560–1).

Propafenone + citalopram/escitalopram *
There is a case of citalopram enhancing propafenone's side-effects such as dizziness, and mimicking coronary artery disease (n = 1, Garcia, *Am J Geriatr Pharmacother* 2008;**6**:96–9).

Rasagiline + escitalopram *
Lack of significant interaction has been shown, although the AUC for rasagiline was increased by 42% (n = 12, 17/7, Hilli *et al*, *Prog Neuropsychopharmacol Biol Psychiatry* 2009; **33**:1526–32). Confusion and hallucinations have been reported with the combination (n = 1, Bandrés *et al*, *Farm Hosp* 2009;**33**:173–5).

Ritonavir + citalopram/escitalopram
No pharmacokinetic interaction occurs (n = 21 [c = 18], RCT, open, c/o, Gutierrez *et al*, *Clin Ther* 2003;**25**:1200–10).

Selegiline + citalopram/escitalopram
One study showed the lack of a clinically significant interaction (n = 18, RCT, Laine *et al*, *Clin Neuropharmacol* 1997;**20**:419–33).

Sibutramine + citalopram/escitalopram
A case of hypomania has been reported with this combination (n = 1, Benazzi, *J Clin Psychiatry* 2002;**63**:165).

St John's wort + citalopram/escitalopram
See SSRIs + St John's wort (*4.3.3.10*).

Sympathomimetics + citalopram/escitalopram
Augmentation of amfetamines is theoretically possible (see sympathomimetics + fluoxetine).

Tamoxifen + citalopram/escitalopram *
A nested case-control study showed that long-term citalopram does not reduce tamoxifen's breast cancer protective effect (n = 368, Lash *et al*, *Br J Cancer* 2008;**99**:616–21).

Topiramate + citalopram/escitalopram *
See citalopram + topiramate (*4.5.14*).

Tramadol + citalopram/escitalopram
Serotonin syndrome has been reported with tramadol 50 mg/d and citalopram 10 mg/d in a patient with slow metabolising 2D6 and 2C19 enzymes (n = 1, Mahlberg *et al*, *Am J Psychiatry* 2004;**161**:1129).

Trazodone + citalopram/escitalopram
No pharmacokinetic interaction occurs (n = 41, Prapotnik *et al*, *Int J Clin Pharmacol Ther* 2004; **42**:120–4).

Tricyclics + citalopram/escitalopram
See SSRIs + tricyclics (*4.3.1*).

Triptans + citalopram/escitalopram
The literature notes an increased risk of CNS toxicity with sumatriptan and recommends avoiding the combination. See also triptans + fluoxetine (*4.3.2.2*).

Warfarin + citalopram/escitalopram
Citalopram 40 mg/d may produce a small increase in prothrombin time (n = 12, Preskorn *et al*, *Br J Clin Pharmacol* 1997;**44**:199–202), but this is probably clinically insignificant (Sayal *et al*, *Acta Psychiatr Scand* 2000;**102**:250–5).

Zolpidem + citalopram/escitalopram
See SSRIs + zolpidem (*4.1.7*).

4.3.2.2 FLUOXETINE
Fluoxetine is 95% protein bound and substantially inhibits CYP2D6 and probably 2C9/10, moderately inhibits 2C19 and weakly inhibits 3A3/4 and has a higher incidence of interactions with drugs metabolised by these enzymes. Norfluoxetine is a potent CYP3A4 inhibitor and a moderate inhibitor of 2D6.

Alcohol + fluoxetine
See alcohol (*4.7.1*).

Alosetron + fluoxetine
There is no significant effect from the 5-HT3 antagonist alosetron on fluoxetine kinetics (n = 12, D'Souza *et al*, *J Clin Pharmacol* 2001;**41**:455–8).

Amfetamines + fluoxetine
See sympathomimetics + fluoxetine.

ANTIPSYCHOTICS + FLUOXETINE
See antipsychotics (*4.2.1*), asenapine (*4.2.3*), clozapine (*4.2.4*), olanzapine (*4.2.5*), quetiapine (*4.2.6*) and risperidone (*4.2.7*).

Atomoxetine + fluoxetine
See SSRIs + atomoxetine (*4.6.4*).

Beta-blockers + fluoxetine
Bradycardia may occur in people taking fluoxetine and metoprolol, possibly due to CYP2D6 inhibition. Atenolol or sotalol may be suitable alternatives (n = 2, Proudlove, *Lancet* 1993;**341**:967). Fluoxetine may inhibit the metabolism of R-carvedilol (rather than S-carvedilol), but this appears to have little clinical significance (n = 10, RCT, d/b, c/o, 28/7, Graff *et al*, *J Clin Pharmacol* 2001;**41**:97–106).

Benzodiazepines + fluoxetine
Fluoxetine may slightly increase the plasma levels of some benzodiazepines (e.g. **diazepam**: n = 10, Lemberger *et al*, *Clin Pharmacol Ther* 1988;**43**:412–9), although probably not **midazolam** (n = 10, RCT, 12/7, Lam *et al*, *J Clin Pharmacol* 2003;**43**:1274–82). Desmethyldiazepam levels may be lower, which may explain the lack of additive psychomotor impairment (review: Ciraulo and Shader, *J Clin Psychopharmacol* 1990;**10**:213–7). Fluoxetine increases **alprazolam's** half-life by 16% (Hall *et al*, *J Clin Psychopharmacol* 2003;**23**:349–57) due to decreased clearance (RCT, p/c, Greenblatt *et al*, *Clin Pharmacol Ther* 1992;**52**:479–86). The clinical significance is minor.

Bupropion + fluoxetine
See bupropion (*4.6.6*).

Buspirone + fluoxetine
See buspirone (*4.1.2*).

Calcium-channel blockers + fluoxetine
Oedema, weight gain and headache have occurred with verapamil and fluoxetine (n = 2, Sternbach, *J Clin Psychopharmacol* 1991;**11**:390). Lowering doses is recommended if an interaction is suspected.

Cannabis + fluoxetine
See antidepressants + cannabis (*4.7.2*).

Carbamazepine + fluoxetine
Two studies have shown that fluoxetine and norfluoxetine inhibit carbamazepine metabolism, increasing levels by up to 25% (n = 14, Gidal et al, Ther Drug Monit 1993;**15**:405–9), but a small study showed fluoxetine 20mg/d to have no effect on carbamazepine levels (n = 8, open, Spina et al, Ther Drug Monit 1993;**15**:247–50). A toxic serotonin syndrome has been reported (n = 1, Dursun et al, Lancet 1993;**342**:442–3).

Ciclosporin + fluoxetine
Ciclosporin plasma concentrations were nearly doubled by fluoxetine 20mg/d in one report, probably by CYP3A4 inhibition (n = 1, Holton and Bonser, Br Med J 1995;**311**:422).

Clarithromycin + fluoxetine
Acute delirium has been reported when clarithromycin was added to fluoxetine (e.g. n = 1, Tracy and Johns Cupp, Ann Pharmacother 1996;**30**:1199–200), probably via CYP3A4 inhibition.

Cocaine + fluoxetine
See antidepressants + cocaine (4.7.3).

Cyproheptadine + fluoxetine
Patients treated with cyproheptadine for fluoxetine-induced anorgasmia may relapse (n = 3, Feder, J Clin Psychiatry 1991;**52**:163–4), and interaction has been reported in a bulimic patient (n = 2, Goldbloom and Kennedy, J Clin Psychiatry 1991;**52**:261–2).

Dextromethorphan + fluoxetine
Visual hallucinations lasting 6–8 hours occurred in a patient taking fluoxetine 20mg/d who also took a cough mixture containing dextromethorphan (n=1, Achamallah, Am J Psychiatry 1992;**149**:1406), and a serotonin syndrome has been reported in a patient also taking lithium (n = 1, Navarro et al, Gen Hosp Psychiatry 2006;**28**:78–80).

Digoxin + fluoxetine
In a nested case-control study, there was no apparent increased risk of digoxin toxicity after initiation of paroxetine, fluoxetine, sertraline and fluvoxamine compared to tricyclics and benzodiazepines (n = 3144, Juurlink et al, Br J Clin Pharmacol 2005;**59**:102–7).

Donepezil + fluoxetine
See SSRIs + donepezil (4.6.3.1).

Duloxetine + fluoxetine
See SSRIs + duloxetine (4.3.3.2).

Lamotrigine + fluoxetine *

There is a case of delirium occurring within two weeks of a lamotrigine dose being increased from 200mg/d to 400mg/d in a lady taking fluoxetine 40mg/d (n = 1, Chistyyakova and Amos, Am J Psychiatry 2008;**165**:918–9).

Lithium + fluoxetine
See lithium (4.4).

LSD + fluoxetine
GTC convulsions occurred in one patient who took a double dose of LSD while on fluoxetine 20mg/d, having previously taken single doses of LSD uneventfully (n = 1, Achamallah, Am J Psychiatry 1992;**149**:843–4).

MAOIs + FLUOXETINE
See MAOIs (4.3.4)

Methadone + fluoxetine
See methadone (4.6.10).

Methylphenidate + fluoxetine *
See fluoxetine + methylphenidate (4.6.11).

Metoclopramide + fluoxetine
Fluoxetine increases metoclopramide plasma levels, increasing Cmax by 42% and half-life by 53% (n = 24, c/o, Viase et al, Biopharm Drug Dispos 2006;**27**:285–9). See also fluvoxamine.

Mirtazapine + fluoxetine
See mirtazapine (4.3.3.4).

Moclobemide + fluoxetine
See SSRIs + moclobemide (4.3.3.5).

Morphine + fluoxetine
Fluoxetine may mildly enhance the analgesic effects of morphine and reduce its side-effects (n = 15, d/b, Erjavec et al, J Clin Pharmacol 2000; **40**:1286–95).

NSAIDs + SSRIs *
There is a three-fold increase in upper GI bleeding, although the absolute risk remains low, e.g. NNH = 411 for SSRIs alone, NNH = 106 for an SSRI plus NSAID (s = 4, n = 153,000, Loke et al, Aliment Pharmacol Ther 2008;**27**:31–40). So, use NSAIDs and SSRIs together with caution in the over 80s, in those with a history of GI bleeding and in those taking aspirin or other NSAIDs (Drug Ther Bull 2004;**42**:17–8).

Olanzapine + fluoxetine
See SSRIs + olanzapine (4.2.5).

Oral contraceptives + fluoxetine
Lack of interaction has been shown (n = 1698, Koke et al, Am J Obstet Gynecol 2002;**187**:551–5).

Pentazocine + fluoxetine
Rapid toxicity has been reported, although an interaction was not proven (n = 1, Hansen et al,

Am J Psychiatry 1990;**147**:949–50).

PHENYTOIN + FLUOXETINE

See phenytoin (4.5.9).

Quetiapine + fluoxetine

See SSRIs + quetiapine (4.2.6).

Ramelteon + fluoxetine

See ramelteon (4.1.5).

Reboxetine + fluoxetine

See reboxetine (4.3.3.6).

RISPERIDONE + FLUOXETINE

See risperidone (4.2.7).

Rivastigmine + fluoxetine

See rivastigmine (4.6.3.3).

Selegiline + fluoxetine

There are isolated cases of toxic reactions, e.g. hypomania, hypertension and shivering (n=1, Suchowersky and de Vries, *Can J Psychiatry* 1991;**35**:571–2), ataxia (n=1, Jermain et al, *Ann Pharmacother* 1992;**26**:1300) and hypertension (Montastruc et al, *Lancet* 1993; **341**:555).

Sertraline + fluoxetine

See sertraline (4.3.2.5).

St John's wort + fluoxetine

See SSRIs + St John's wort (4.3.3.10).

Sympathomimetics + fluoxetine

An interaction has been suggested by reports of extreme restlessness, agitation and psychotic symptoms apparently caused by fluoxetine augmentation of amfetamines (n=2, Barrett et al, *Br J Psychiatry* 1996;**168**:253).

Tolterodine + fluoxetine

Fluoxetine has been shown to inhibit the metabolism of tolterodine (n=13, open, Brynne et al, *Br J Clin Pharmacology* 1999;**48**:553–63), probably via 2D6.

Tramadol + fluoxetine

Serotonin syndrome and mania have been reported with this combination (n=1, Kesavan and Sobala, *J Roy Soc Med* 1999;**92**:474–5; n=1, Gonzalez–Pinto et al, *Am J Psychiatry* 2001; **158**:964–5).

Trazodone + fluoxetine

No pharmacokinetic interaction occurs (n=16, Prapotnik et al, *Int J Clin Pharmacol Ther* 2004; **42**:120–4), although trazodone toxicity (e.g. Neirenberg et al, *J Clin Psychiatry* 1992;**53**:83) and myoclonus have been reported (n=1, Darko et al, *Vet Hum Toxicol* 2001;**43**:214–5).

TRICYCLICS + FLUOXETINE

See SSRIs + tricyclics (4.3.1).

Triptans + fluoxetine *

The literature notes an increased risk of CNS toxicity with all SSRIs and recommends avoiding the combination, e.g. post-marketing surveillance in Canada indicated that a serotonin-like syndrome may occur rarely with the combination (n=22, Joffe and Sokolov, *Acta Psychiatr Scand* 1997;**95**:551–2). While there is a possible problem, to ban triptans in people taking SSRIs denies them highly effective drugs for a disabling (for a day or so) and painful condition (and the author is speaking here from personal experience). Triptans with low lipid solubility and a short half-life (e.g. sumatriptan, rizatriptan or zolmitriptan) may in theory be a safer choice than others (e.g. frovatriptan, which has a long half-life). However, lack of significant interaction has been reported with sumatriptan (n=14, open, Blier and Bergeron, *J Clin Psychopharmacol* 1995;**15**:106–9), and fluoxetine 60 mg/d had only a modest effect on almotriptan peak levels, with no clinically significant side-effects or changes in vital signs or ECGs (n=14, RCT, c/o, 8/7, Fleishaker et al, *J Clin Pharmacol* 2001;**41**:217–23).

Tryptophan + fluoxetine

Central toxicity has been reported (n=5, Steiner and Fontaine, *Biol Psychiatry* 1986;**21**:1067–71).

Valproate + fluoxetine

Valproate levels may rise by up to 50% if fluoxetine is added, although the mechanism is not established (e.g. Lucena et al, *Am J Psychiatry* 1998;**155**:575) and reduced valproate levels have been reported (Droulers et al, *J Clin Psychopharmacol* 1997;**17**:139–40).

Venlafaxine + fluoxetine

Serotonin syndrome has been reported when venlafaxine was started immediately after fluoxetine was discontinued (n=1, Bhatara et al, *Ann Pharmacother* 1998;**32**:432–6), as have severe anticholinergic side–effects (n=4, Benazzi, *J Clin Psychopharmacol* 1999;**19**:96–8, letter).

WARFARIN + FLUOXETINE

An *in vitro* study indicated fluoxetine has a potentially significant effect on warfarin (Schmider et al, *Br J Clin Pharmacol* 1997;**44**:495–8). Raised INR has been reported within ten days of starting fluoxetine (n=2, Woolfrey et al, *Br Med J* 1993; **307**:241) and two patients on warfarin with stable INRs experienced dramatic increases in INR when fluoxetine 20 mg/d was added (n=2, Hanger and Thomas, *N Z Med J* 1995;**108**:157). There is also a case report of an elderly man prescribed warfarin, diazepam and fluoxetine who developed an elevated INR and died from a cerebral haemorrhage (n = 1, Dent and Orrock, *Pharmacotherapy* 1997;**17**:170–2).

Zolpidem + fluoxetine
See SSRIs + zolpidem (*4.1.7*).

Zotepine + fluoxetine
See SSRIs + zotepine (*4.2.9*).

4.3.2.3 FLUVOXAMINE
Fluvoxamine is 80% protein bound and strongly inhibits CYP1A2, 2D6, 3A4 and 2C19 (and possibly 2C8 weakly) and may have a high incidence of interactions with drugs metabolised by these enzymes (n = 20, *Clin Pharmacol Ther* 1998;**64**:257–68). It is probably only metabolised by CYP2D6 to fluvoxamino alcohol, then by alcohol dehydrogenase (Miura and Ohkubo, *Xenobiotica* 2007;**37**:169–79).

AGOMELATINE + FLUVOXAMINE
See agomelatine (*4.3.3.1*).

Alcohol + fluvoxamine
See alcohol (*4.7.1*).

AMINOPHYLLINE + FLUVOXAMINE
See theophylline + fluvoxamine.

Antipsychotics + fluvoxamine *
Fluvoxamine is a 1A2 inhibitor and asenapine plasma levels may rise by up to 29% (US PI). Seizures have been reported with levomepromazine and fluvoxamine (n = 1, Grinshpoon et al, *Int Clin Psychopharmacol* 1993;**8**:61–2), although levomepromazine does not appear to increase fluvoxamine levels (n = 15, Yoshimura et al, *Int Clin Psychopharmacol* 2000;**15**:233–5). Fluvoxamine 100 mg/d had no effect on plasma levels of risperidone 3–6 mg/d but 200 mg/d increased concentrations by 26% (n = 11, open, 8/52, D'Arrigo et al, *Pharmacol Res* 2005;**52**:497–501) and neurotoxicity (e.g. confusion, diaphoresis and myoclonus) has been reported within two days when fluvoxamine was added to risperidone (n = 1, Reeves et al, *Ann Pharmacother* 2002; **36**:440–3). Fluvoxamine produces a dose-dependent increase in haloperidol levels, 150 mg/d raising levels by 60%, although this was without additional side-effects at 6 mg/d (n = 12, Yasui–Furukori et al, *Psychopharmacol* [Berl] 2003;**171**:223–7). See also clozapine (*4.2.4*).

Benzodiazepines + fluvoxamine *
Plasma concentrations of bromazepam are doubled by fluvoxamine, but lorazepam is unaffected (van Harten et al, mentioned in *Clin Pharmacokinet* 1993;**24**:203–20). A study showed that fluvoxamine 100 mg/d increased alprazolam plasma levels by 100%, and so reduced doses of alprazolam should be used (n = 60, Fleishaker and Hulst, *Eur J Clin Pharmacol* 1994;**46**:35–9), and the effect may be 30% greater in non-smokers compared to smokers (n = 49, Sugahara et al, *Eur J Clin Pharmacol* 2009;**65**:699–704). A slight increase (66%) in midazolam (n = 10, RCT, 12/7, Lam et al, *J Clin Pharmacol* 2003;**43**:1274–82) and quazepam levels (n = 12, RCT, d/b, c/o, p/c, 14/7, Kanda et al, *J Clin Pharmacol* 2003;**43**:1392–7) has been reported.

Beta-blockers + fluvoxamine
Lack of significant interaction has been shown with atenolol. Propranolol plasma levels can be raised by fluvoxamine by up to 500%, but apparently without major clinical effect (reviewed by Benfield and Ward, *Drugs* 1988;**32**:313–34).

Buspirone + fluvoxamine
See buspirone (*4.1.2*).

Caffeine + fluvoxamine
Even low-dose fluvoxamine (10–20 mg/d) inhibits the metabolism of caffeine, presumably via 1A2 inhibition (n = 10, Christensen et al, *Clin Pharmacol Ther* 2002;**71**:141–52), and half-life may rise from five hours to 22 hours (Slaughter and Edwards, *Ann Pharmacother* 1995;**29**:619–24), unlikely to be significant (n = 10, Spigset, *Eur J Clin Pharmacol* 1998;**54**:665–6). Caffeine decreases plasma levels of fluvoxamine but not its pharmacodynamic effects (n = 12, RCT, 11/7, d/b, p/c, c/o, Fukasawa et al, *Ther Drug Monit* 2006; **28**:308–11).

Carbamazepine + fluvoxamine
One small study showed fluvoxamine 100 mg/d to have no effect on carbamazepine levels (n = 15, RCT, Spina et al, *Ther Drug Monit* 1993;**15**:247–50), although increased carbamazepine levels and toxicity have been reported (e.g. Martinelli et al, *Br J Clin Pharmacol* 1993;**36**:615–6).

Chloral + fluvoxamine
Lack of interaction has been reported (Wagner et al, *Adv Pharmacother* 1986;**2**:34–56).

Ciclosporin + fluvoxamine
There is a case report of ciclosporin levels elevated by the introduction of fluvoxamine to a ciclosporin-treated allograft recipient, probably via CYP3A4 inhibition. Intensive monitoring of the serum creatinine and ciclosporin level was

recommended, along with appropriate dose reductions (Vella and Sayegh, *Am J Kidney Dis* 1998;**31**:320–3).

Citalopram/escitalopram + fluvoxamine
See citalopram/escitalopram (*4.3.2.1*).

CLOZAPINE + FLUVOXAMINE
See clozapine (*4.2.4*).

Digoxin + fluvoxamine
See digoxin + fluoxetine (*4.3.2.2*).

Donepezil + fluvoxamine
See SSRIs + donepezil (*4.6.3.1*).

DULOXETINE + FLUVOXAMINE
See SSRIs + duloxetine (*4.3.3.2*).

Enoxacin + fluvoxamine
Enoxacin appears to increase the sleepiness caused by fluvoxamine (n = 10, RCT, d/b, c/o, 11/7, Kunii et al, *Ther Drug Monit* 2005;**27**:349–53).

Glimepiride + fluvoxamine
Fluvoxamine may produce a modest increase in glimepiride plasma concentrations (n = 12, RCT, d/b, c/o, 4/7, Niemi et al, *Clin Pharmacol Ther* 2001;**69**:194–200).

Lansoprazole + fluvoxamine
Fluvoxamine increases lansoprazole levels 2–3-fold in extensive (but not poor) metabolisers, probably by 2C19 inhibition (n = 18, RCT, p/c, Yasui–Furukori et al, *J Clin Pharmacol* 2004; **44**:1223–9; n = 18, Muira et al, *Br J Clin Pharmacol* 2005;**60**:61–8).

Lidocaine + fluvoxamine
Lidocaine metabolism is reduced by fluvoxamine, leading to potential toxicity (n = 8, RCT, d/b, p/c, c/o, Isohanni et al, *Basic Clin Pharmacol Toxicol* 2006;**99**:168–72), although the effect of the interaction lessens as liver function worsens (n = 30, RCT, d/b, c/o, Orlando et al, *Clin Pharmacol Ther* 2004;**75**:80–8).

Lithium + fluvoxamine
Although lack of interaction has been reported (Hendrickx and Floris, *Curr Ther Res* 1991;**49**:106–10), case reports exist of serotonin syndrome (n = 1, Ohman and Spigset, *Pharmacopsychiatry* 1993;**26**:263–4), irresistible somnolence (n = 1, Evans and Marwick, *Br J Psychiatry* 1990;**156**:286) and diurnal somnolence (n = 1, Marchesi et al, *Pharmacopsychiatry* 2005;**38**:145–6).

MAOIs + FLUVOXAMINE
See MAOIs (*4.3.4*).

MELATONIN + FLUVOXAMINE
See melatonin (*4.1.4*).

Methadone + fluvoxamine
See methadone (*4.6.10*).

Metoclopramide + fluvoxamine
The combination metoclopramide with **fluoxetine**, **sertraline** (n = 1, Fisher and Davies, *Ann Pharmacother* 2002;**36**:67–71) or **fluvoxamine** may increase the incidence of serotonin syndrome (SPC). Acute dystonia has been associated with the combination (n = 1, Palop et al, *Ann Pharmacother* 1999;**33**:382).

MIRTAZAPINE + FLUVOXAMINE
See mirtazapine (*4.3.3.4*).

Moclobemide + fluvoxamine
See SSRIs + moclobemide (*4.3.3.5*).

NICOUMALONE + FLUVOXAMINE
The anticoagulant effects may be enhanced by fluvoxamine.

NSAIDs + FLUVOXAMINE
See NSAIDs + fluoxetine (*4.3.2.2*).

Olanzapine + fluvoxamine
See olanzapine (*4.2.5*).

Oxycodone + fluvoxamine
Serotonin syndrome has been reported with the combination (n = 1, Karunatilake and Buckley, *Ann Pharmacother* 2006;**40**:155–7).

PHENYTOIN + FLUVOXAMINE
See phenytoin (*4.5.9*).

Pipamperone + fluvoxamine
ECG changes have occurred as a result of acute overdose with this combination (Gallerani et al, *Clin Drug Invest* 1998;**15**:64–8).

Quetiapine + fluvoxamine
See quetiapine (*4.2.6*).

Quinidine + fluvoxamine
Fluvoxamine significantly inhibits the clearance of quinidine, probably by 3A4 inhibition (n = 6, open, Damkier et al, *Eur J Clin Pharmacol* 1999; **55**:451–6).

RAMELTEON + FLUVOXAMINE
See ramelteon (*4.1.5*).

Ramosetron + fluvoxamine *
Fluvoxamine increases ramosetron Cmax and AUC 1.42-fold and 2.78-fold respectively (open, 11/7, Kadokura et al, *Eur J Clin Pharmacol* 2008; **64**:691–5).

Reboxetine + fluvoxamine
See reboxetine (*4.3.3.6*).

Risperidone + fluvoxamine
See antipsychotics + risperidone (*4.2.7*).

Rosiglitazone + fluvoxamine
There appears no significant interaction, although rosiglitazone levels may rise in some

people (n = 23, open, c/o, Pedersen *et al*, *Br J Clin Pharmacol* 2006;**62**:682–9).

Sildenafil + fluvoxamine
Fluvoxamine increases sildenafil AUC by 40% and half–life by 19%, probably via CYP3A4 inhibition (n = 12, Hesse *et al*, *J Clin Psychopharmacol* 2005; **25**:589–92).

Smoking + fluvoxamine
See smoking (*4.7.4*).

St John's wort + fluvoxamine
See SSRIs + St John's wort (*4.3.3.10*).

Sympathomimetics + fluvoxamine
Augmentation of amfetamines is theoretically possible (see also fluoxetine, *4.3.2.2*).

THEOPHYLLINE + FLUVOXAMINE
Several cases of theophylline toxicity have been reported (eg. Devane *et al*, *Am J Psychiatry* 1997;**154**:1317–18), probably via CYP1A2 inhibition. The literature recommends avoiding the combination (*Curr Prob* 1994;**20**:12).

TIZANIDINE + FLUVOXAMINE
Fluvoxamine increases tizanidine's AUC 33-fold and peak levels 12-fold, a dramatic and important interaction (n = 10, RCT, d/b, c/o, 4/7, Granfors *et al*, *Clin Pharmacol Ther* 2004;**75**:331–41).

Tolbutamide + fluvoxamine
Fluvoxamine 150 mg/d may increase tolbutamide levels by about 20% (n = 14, RCT, Madsen *et al*, *Clin Pharmacol Ther* 2001;**69**:41–7).

Topiramate + fluvoxamine *
There is a case of rapidly reversible tremor and myoclonus with the combination (n = 1, Oulis *et al*, *Clin Neuropharmacol* 2008;**31**:366–7).

TRICYCLICS + FLUVOXAMINE
See SSRIs + tricyclics (*4.3.1*).

Triptans + fluvoxamine
See triptans + fluoxetine (*4.3.2.2*).

Tryptophan + fluvoxamine
Central toxicity has been suggested with fluvoxamine (n = 5, Steiner and Fontaine, *Biol Psychiatry* 1986;**21**:1067–71).

Valproate + fluvoxamine
Augmentation of fluvoxamine has been claimed with valproate (Corrigan, *Biol Psychiatry* 1992; **31**:1178–9).

WARFARIN + FLUVOXAMINE
An *in vitro* study indicated fluvoxamine has the most potent effect on warfarin of the SSRIs (Schmider *et al*, *Br J Clin Pharmacol* 1997;**44**:495–8), e.g. it can increase warfarin levels by up to 65%, increasing prothrombin time (Benfield and Ward,

Drugs 1986;**32**:313–34; n = 1, Limke *et al*, *Ann Pharmacother* 2002;**36**:1890–2). Elevated INR has occurred up to two weeks after fluvoxamine was stopped, a prolonged effect (n = 1, Yap and Low, *Singapore Med J* 1999; **40**:480–2).

Zolpidem + fluvoxamine
See SSRIs + zolpidem (*4.1.7*).

Zotepine + fluvoxamine
See SSRIs + zotepine (*4.2.9*).

4.3.2.4 PAROXETINE
Paroxetine is 95% protein bound and probably the most potent SSRI inhibitor of CYP2D6, although this is rapidly reversible. It does not appear to inhibit any other P450 enzyme. The main metabolite has approximately one third the CYP2D6 inhibition potency of paroxetine.

Agomelatine + paroxetine
See agomelatine (*4.3.3.1*).

Alcohol + paroxetine
See alcohol (*4.7.1*).

Anticholinergics + paroxetine
See SSRIs + anticholinergics (*4.6.2*).

Antipsychotics + paroxetine *
Lack of interaction has been shown between paroxetine and haloperidol (Cooper *et al*, *Acta Psychiatr Scand* 1989;**80**[Suppl 350]:53–5), thiothixene (a thioxanthene; n = 10, Guthrie *et al*, *J Clin Pharm Ther* 1997;**22**:221–6) and with asenapine (US PI). See also clozapine (*4.2.3*).

Atomoxetine + paroxetine
See SSRIs + atomoxetine (*4.6.4*).

Benzodiazepines + paroxetine
Lack of interaction has been shown (Boyer and Blumhardt, *J Clin Psychiatry* 1992;**53**[Suppl 2]:132–24), e.g. with oxazepam (Cooper *et al*, *Acta Psychiatr Scand* 1989;**80**[Suppl 350]: 53–5) and alprazolam (n = 25, d/b, p/c, c/o, 4 x 15/7, Calvo *et al*, *J Clin Psychopharmacol* 2004;**24**:268–76), but NMS has been reported with paroxetine 20 mg/d and alprazolam 1.2 mg/d (n = 1, Naranjo = 6, Tanii *et al*, *Prog Neuropsychopharmacol Biol Psychiatry* 2006;**30**:1176–8). Serotonin syndrome has been reported in a person taking maintenance paroxetine after a single dose clonazepam (Rella and Hoffman, *J Toxicol Clin Toxicol* 1998;**36**:257–8).

Beta-blockers + paroxetine *
CYP2D6 inhibition by paroxetine 20 mg/d leads to an accumulation of S metoprolol, and so a reduced metoprolol dose might be needed (n = 8, open, Hemeryck *et al*, *Clin Pharmacol Ther*

2000;**67**:283–91) and complete atrioventricular block has been reported with the combination (n = 1, Onalan et al, Mayo Clin Proc 2008;**83**:595–9). Raised paroxetine levels after the addition of pindolol have been reported, probably via 2D6 inhibition (n = 1, Olver and Burrows, Int J Psych Clin Pract 1998;**2**:225–7).

Bupropion + paroxetine
See bupropion (4.6.6).

Carbamazepine + paroxetine
Lack of significant interaction has been shown (n = 20, s/b, p/c, c/o, 23/7, Andersen et al, Epilepsy Res 1991;**10**:201–4), although hyponatraemia has been reported (n = 1, Sempere I Verdu et al, Aten Primaria 2004;**33**:473–4).

Cimetidine + paroxetine
Cimetidine may inhibit the first-pass metabolism of paroxetine, increasing bioavailability by up to 50% (Bannister et al, Acta Psychiatr Scand 1989; **80**[Suppl 350]:102–6), so use ranitidine instead.

CLOZAPINE + PAROXETINE
See clozapine (4.2.4).

Dextromethorphan + paroxetine
Paroxetine would be expected to increase dextromethorphan levels by CYP2D6 inhibition (see reported case with fluoxetine, 4.3.2.2).

Digitalis + paroxetine
Digitalis toxicity five days after starting paroxetine has been reported (n = 1, Yasui-Fukukori and Kaneko, Lancet 2006;**367**:788), although this may just have been hospital-induced compliance (Bateman et al, Lancet 2006;**368**:1962–3).

Digoxin + paroxetine
See digoxin + fluoxetine (4.3.2.2).

Donepezil + paroxetine
See SSRIs + donepezil (4.6.3.1).

Duloxetine + paroxetine
See SSRIs + duloxetine (4.3.3.2).

Ecstasy (MDMA) + paroxetine
In people treated with paroxetine 20 mg/d, the physiological and psychological effects of ecstasy were significantly attenuated, which could lead users to take higher (and hence toxic) doses to achieve the same effects (n = 12, RCT, d/b, p/c, c/o, 2×3/7, Farré et al, J Pharmacol Exp Ther 2007;**323**:954–62).

Flecainide + paroxetine *
Paroxetine inhibits flecainide's metabolism and flecainide toxicity has led to delirium (n = 1, Tsao and Gugger, Ann Pharmacother 2009;**43**:1366–9).

Galantamine + paroxetine

See galantamine (4.6.3.2).

Interferon alfa + paroxetine
A previous good response to paroxetine and trazodone was reversed by interferon alfa, which has anti–serotonergic actions (n = 1, McAllister-Williams et al, Br J Psychiatry 2000;**176**:93).

Lithium + paroxetine
There are some cases of a possible serotonin syndrome (n = 17, Fagiolini et al, J Clin Psychopharmacol 2001;**21**:474–8).

Methadone + paroxetine
Steady-state plasma methadone levels may rise with paroxetine, but only in poor 2D6 metabolisers (n = 10, 12/7, Begre et al, J Clin Psychopharmacol 2002;**22**:211–5).

Methylene blue + paroxetine
Postoperative serotonin syndrome has been reported after methylene blue was used in someone taking paroxetine (n = 1, Ng et al, Can J Anaesth 2008;**55**:36–41;see also Ramsay et al, Br J Pharmacol 2007;**152**:946–51).

Metoclopramine + paroxetine
See metoclopramide + fluvoxamine (4.3.2.3).

Mirtazapine + paroxetine
See mirtazapine (4.3.3.4).

Moclobemide + paroxetine
See SSRIs + moclobemide (4.3.3.5).

MAOIs + PAROXETINE
See MAOIs (4.3.4).

NSAIDs + SSRIs
See NSAIDs + fluoxetine (4.3.2.2).

Oral contraceptives + paroxetine
Lack of interaction has been shown (Boyer and Blumhardt, J Clin Psychiatry 1992;**53**[Suppl 2]: 132–4).

Phenytoin + paroxetine
Paroxetine bioavailability may be decreased slightly (Andersen et al, Epilepsy Res 1991;**10**: 201–4).

Phenobarbital + paroxetine
Paroxetine bioavailability may be decreased slightly, resulting in a 25% decrease in plasma concentrations (Bannister et al, Acta Psychiatr Scand 1989;**80**[Suppl 350]:102–6). No interaction occurs with amylobarbital (Cooper et al, Acta Psychiatr Scand 1989;**80**[Suppl 350]:53–5).

Risperidone + paroxetine
See risperidone (4.2.7).

St John's wort + paroxetine
See SSRIs + St John's wort (4.3.3.10).

Sympathomimetics + paroxetine
Augmentation of amfetamines is theoretically

possible (see sympathomimetics + fluoxetine 4.3.2.2).

Tamoxifen + paroxetine *

Paroxetine may inhibit the CYP2D6 metabolism of tamoxifen to its active metabolite and so may reduce efficacy (UK SPC).

Terbinafine + paroxetine

Terbinafine 150 mg/d increases the Cmax of paroxetine 2-fold and increases half-life 48% from 15–23 hours (n = 12, 2 × 6/7, Yasui-Furukori et al, Eur J Clin Pharmacol 2007;**63**:51–6).

TRICYCLICS + PAROXETINE

See SSRIs + tricyclics (4.3.1).

Triptans + paroxetine

The literature notes an increased risk of CNS toxicity and recommends avoiding sumatriptan and paroxetine, although almost complete lack of interaction has been shown with rizatriptan and paroxetine (n = 12, RCT, 14/7, Goldberg et al, J Clin Pharmacol 1999;**39**:192–9). See also fluoxetine (4.3.2.2).

Valproate + paroxetine

No significant interaction occurs (n = 20, s/b, p/c, c/o, 23/7, Andersen et al, Epilepsy Res 1991; **10**:201–4).

Warfarin + paroxetine

An in vitro study indicated that all SSRIs have an effect on warfarin (Schmider et al, Br J Clin Pharmacol 1997;**44**:495–8), eg. up to a three-point rise in INR has been reported in several patients (mentioned by Askinazi, Am J Psychiatry 1996;**153**:135–6).

Zolpidem + paroxetine

See SSRIs + zolpidem (4.1.7).

Zotepine + paroxetine

See SSRIs + zotepine (4.2.9).

4.3.2.5 SERTRALINE

Sertraline is 98% protein bound and has a dose-related inhibition of CYP2D6 but has little, if any, effect on CYP1A2, 2C9/10, 2C19 or 3A3/4. It appears a less potent inhibitor of CYP2D6 than most other SSRIs (Baettig et al, Eur J Clin Pharmacol 1993;**44**:403–5) and has, at 50–100 mg/d, a low incidence of interactions with drugs metabolised by 2D6. It is metabolised mainly by 3A4 but also other P450 enzymes, plus monoamine oxidase and UGT2B7 (Obach et al, Drug Metab Disp 2005;**33**:262–70).

Alcohol + sertraline

See alcohol (4.7.1).

Anticholinergics + sertraline

See SSRIs + anticholinergics (4.6.2).

Antipsychotics + sertraline

There were no changes in a range of antipsychotic levels when sertraline 50–100 mg/d was added (n = 48, RCT, d/b, p/c, 6/52, Pierson et al, Can J Psychiatry 2006;**51**:715–8). Sertraline (up to 200 mg/d) may cause **pimozide** levels to rise by 35%, but with no prolonged QTc (n = 15, Alderman, Clin Ther 2005;**27**:1050–63). See also individual drugs.

Atomoxetine + sertraline

See SSRIs + atomoxetine (4.6.4).

Ayurvedic medicines + sertraline *

There is a case of a patient twice suffering relapses after starting Ayurvedic herbal mixtures, probably due to either Terminalia chebula or Commiphora wighteii (n = 1, Prasad et al, J Psychopharmacol 2009;**23**:216–9).

Benzodiazepines + sertraline

A study in male volunteers showed no effect of sertraline on diazepam and suggested no effect on the CYP2C and CYP3A4 enzymes (n = 20, RCT, d/b, p/c, c/o, Gardner et al, Clin Pharmacokinetics 1997; **31**[Suppl 1]:43–9), but a slight decrease in plasma levels by 13% may occur (review: Warrington, Int Clin Psychopharmacol 1991;**6**[Suppl 2]:11–21).

Beta-blockers + sertraline

No pharmacodynamic interaction has been found with atenolol (e.g. n = 10, RCT, Ziegler and Wilner, J Clin Psychiatry 1996;**57**[Suppl 1]:12–15), but sertraline can increase metoprolol AUC by 48–67% (17/7, Preskorn et al, J Clin Psychopharmacol 2007;**27**:28–34).

Bupropion + sertraline

See bupropion (4.6.6).

Carbamazepine + sertraline

Lack of significant interaction has been reported, but there are cases where sertraline 100 mg/d increased carbamazepine (600 mg/d) plasma levels, probably via 3A4 inhibition (d/b, p/c, Joblin, N Z Med J 1994;**107**:43; Lane, N Z Med J 1994; **107**:209). Non-response to sertraline has been due to low plasma levels associated with carbamazepine use, possibly via CYP3A4 induction (n = 2, Khan et al, J Clin Psychiatry 2000; **61**:526–7).

Clozapine + sertraline

See clozapine (4.2.3).

Digoxin + sertraline

See digoxin + fluoxetine (4.3.2.2).

Dolasetron + sertraline

A serotonin syndrome has been reported with the combination (n = 1, Sorscher, *J Psycho-pharmacol* 2002;**16**:191).

Donepezil + sertraline

See SSRIs + donepezil (4.6.3.1).

Duloxetine + sertraline

See SSRIs + duloxetine (4.3.3.2).

Erythromycin + sertraline

Serotonin syndrome has been reported with the combination, possibly via CYP3A4 inhibition (n = 1, Lee and Lee, *Pharmacother* 1999;**19**:894–6).

Fluoxetine + sertraline

A possible serotonin syndrome has been reported (see switching antidepressants, 2.2.5).

Lamotrigine + sertraline

See lamotrigine (4.5.5).

Linezolid + sertraline

A case of serotonin syndrome has been reported (n = 1, Clark *et al*, *Pharmacotherapy* 2006;**26**:269–76).

Lithium + sertraline

See SSRIs + lithium (4.4).

MAOIs + SERTRALINE

See MAOIs (4.3.4).

Methylphenidate + sertraline *

See sertraline + methylphenidate (4.6.11).

Metoclopramide + sertraline

See metoclopramide + fluvoxamine (4.3.2.3).

Mirtazapine + sertraline

See SSRIs + mirtazapine (4.3.3.4).

Moclobemide + sertraline

See SSRIs + moclobemide (4.3.3.5).

NSAIDs + sertraline

See NSAIDs + fluoxetine (4.3.2.2).

Olanzapine + sertraline

See SSRIs + olanzapine (4.2.5).

Oxycodone + sertraline

Visual hallucinations and tremor have been reported with the combination in a bone marrow transplant patient (n = 1, Rosebraugh *et al*, *J Clin Pharmacol* 2001;**41**:224).

Phenytoin + sertraline

Lack of significant interaction has been shown (n = 30, RCT, Rapeport *et al*, *J Clin Psychiatry* 1996;**57**[Suppl 1]:24–8), but dramatically raised phenytoin levels have been reported after the addition of sertraline (n = 2, Haselberger *et al*, *J Clin Psychopharmacol* 1997;**17**:107–9), as

has a significant reduction in sertraline levels by phenytoin (Pihlsgard and Eliasson, *Eur J Clin Pharmacol* 2002;**57**:915–6). Monitoring levels would seem sensible.

Risperidone + sertraline

See risperidone (4.2.7).

St John's wort + sertraline

See SSRIs + St John's wort (4.3.3.10).

Sumatriptan + sertraline

The literature notes an increased risk of CNS toxicity and recommends avoiding the combination. See also fluoxetine (4.3.2.2).

Sympathomimetics + sertraline

Augmentation of amfetamines is theoretically possible (see sympathomimetics + fluoxetine, 4.3.2.2).

Tolbutamide + sertraline

In a parallel-group study, 200 mg/d sertraline produced a 16% decrease in tolbutamide clearance, possibly via inhibition of CYP2C9 (n = 25, RCT, Tremaine *et al*, *Clin Pharmacokinet* 1997; **31**[Suppl 1]:31–6; n = 25, RCT, Warrington, *Int Clin Psychopharmacol* 1991;**6**[Suppl 2]:11–21).

Tramadol + sertraline

Serotonin syndrome has been reported when a tramadol dose was increased with concomitant sertraline (n = 1, Mason and Blackburn, *Ann Pharmacother* 1997;**31**:175–7).

Tricyclics + sertraline

See SSRIs + tricyclics (4.3.1).

Venlafaxine + sertraline

Acute liver damage possibly related to sertraline and venlafaxine ingestion has been reported (n = 1, Kim *et al*, *Ann Pharmacother* 1999;**3**:381–2).

Warfarin + sertraline

An *in vitro* study indicated that, of the SSRIs, sertraline had the least potent effect on warfarin (Schmider *et al*, *Br J Clin Pharmacol* 1997;**44**:495–8). It may produce only a modest increase in prothrombin time, considered clinically insignificant (n = 12, RCT, 22/7, Apseloff *et al*, *Clin Pharmacokinet* 1997;**32**[Suppl 1]:37–42). However, prothrombin time can be increased by 9% (Wilner *et al*, *Biol Psychiatry* 1991;**29**:354S–355S) and up to a three-point rise in INR has been reported in several patients (mentioned by Askinazi, *Am J Psychiatry* 1996;**153**:135–6).

Zolpidem + sertraline

See SSRIs + zolpidem (4.1.7).

Zotepine + sertraline

See SSRIs + zotepine (4.2.9).

4.3.3 OTHER ANTIDEPRESSANTS

4.3.3.1 AGOMELATINE
Agomelatine is metabolised by CYP1A2 (90%) and CYP9/19 (10%). 2D6 and 3A4 are not involved.

Alcohol + agomelatine
The SPC states that concurrent use is not advisable but there is no kinetic interaction, and only a very minor effect on one of 23 psychometric tests (MI).

Benzodiazepine + agomelatine
Lack of kinetic interaction has been shown (SPC) and there is no interaction between agomelatine 50 mg/d and lorazepam 2.5 mg for seven days (MI).

CIPROFLOXACIN + AGOMELATINE *
This combination is an SPC contraindication.

Fluconazole + agomelatine
Fluconazole does not affect the pharmacokinetics of agomelatine (SPC).

FLUVOXAMINE + AGOMELATINE
Fluvoxamine (a 1A2 and 2C9 inhibitor) may increase agomelatine Cmax and AUC by factors of 47 and 61 respectively, although agomelatine was still well tolerated (SPC).

Lithium + agomelatine
Lack of significant interaction has been shown (SPC), although agomelatine exposure was insignificantly increased.

Paroxetine + agomelatine
Paroxetine does not affect the pharmacokinetics of agomelatine (SPC).

Smoking + agomelatine
Smoking induces 1A2 and reduces agomelatine bioavailability by 33%, considered insignificant (MI).

Theophylline + agomelatine
Lack of interaction has been shown (SPC).

*4.3.3.2 DULOXETINE *
Duloxetine is 95% protein bound and metabolised by 1A2 (but probably does not inhibit it), is a moderate inhibitor and substrate for 2D6 (s = 2, Skinner *et al, Clin Pharmacol Ther* 2003;**73**:170–7) but has no effect on 3A4. Data on interactions is limited but caution is recommended with sedative drugs, e.g. alcohol, benzodiazepines, antipsychotics and sedative antihistamines. Elimination is primarily renal, after extensive metabolism by multiple oxidative pathways, methylation and conjugation (review of kinetics, Wernicke *et al, Expert Opin Drug Saf* 2005;**4**:987–93).

Antacids + duloxetine
Lack of interaction has been shown with a single 40 mg dose of duloxetine (UK SPC).

Beta-blockers + duloxetine
Duloxetine is a 2D6 inhibitor, and can increase metoprolol AUC by 180% (Preskorn *et al, J Clin Psychopharmacol* 2007;**27**:28–34).

CIPROFLOXACIN + DULOXETINE
This combination is a UK SPC contraindication due to the potential for raised duloxetine levels from 1A2 inhibition by ciprofloxacin (UK SPC).

ENOXACINE + DULOXETINE
This combination is a UK SPC contraindication due to the potential for raised duloxetine levels from 1A2 inhibition by enoxacine (UK SPC).

H2-blockers + duloxetine
Lack of interaction has been shown with a single 40 mg dose of duloxetine (UK SPC).

MAOIs + DULOXETINE
This combination is a UK SPC contraindication, due to the risk of serotonin syndrome. Do not use duloxetine within 14 days of stopping an MAOI, or use an MAOI until five days after stopping duloxetine.

Moclobemide + duloxetine
The UK SPC recommends caution, due to the risk of serotonin syndrome, when duloxetine is used with moclobemide.

Olanzapine + duloxetine *
See duloxetine + olanzapine (4.2.5).

Oral contraceptives + duloxetine
There is no reason to suspect an interaction would occur, but there are no formal studies.

Pethidine + duloxetine
Due to the risk of serotonin syndrome, duloxetine should only be used with care with pethidine.

SMOKING + DULOXETINE
Smokers may have duloxetine plasma levels 50% lower than non-smokers (UK SPC).

SSRIs + DULOXETINE
Due to the risk of serotonin syndrome, duloxetine should only be used with care with SSRIs. **Fluvoxamine** may decrease duloxetine's clearance by 77% and increase AUC six-fold, and this combination is a UK SPC contraindication because of the potential for duloxetine toxicity.

St John's wort + duloxetine

The UK SPC recommends caution when duloxetine is used with St John's wort.

Theophylline + duloxetine

Duloxetine had no effect on theophylline in a study in male patients (UK SPC).

Tolterodine + duloxetine

There is no significant interaction (n = 16, RCT, d/b, c/o, 2 x 5/7, Hua et al, Br J Clin Pharmacol 2004;**57**:652–6).

Tramadol + duloxetine

Due to the risk of serotonin syndrome, duloxetine should only be used with care with tramadol.

Tricyclics + duloxetine

Due to the risk of serotonin syndrome, duloxetine should only be used with care with tricyclics.

Triptans + duloxetine

Due to the risk of serotonin syndrome, duloxetine should only be used with care with triptans.

Tryptophan + duloxetine

Due to the risk of serotonin syndrome, duloxetine should only be used with care with tryptophan.

Venlafaxine + duloxetine

Due to the risk of serotonin syndrome, duloxetine should only be used with care with venlafaxine.

Warfarin + duloxetine *

Duloxetine has been shown to have no significant effect on the kinetics of steady-state warfarin (n = 30, 14/7, Chappell et al, J Clin Pharmacol 2009;**49**:1456–66), although there are cases of duloxetine causing severe elevation of INR when combined with warfarin (n = 3, Glueck et al, JAMA 2006;**295**:1517–8).

4.3.3.3 MIANSERIN

ALCOHOL + MIANSERIN

See alcohol (4.7.1).

Benzodiazepines + mianserin

Enhanced sedation may occur.

Carbamazepine + mianserin

Plasma levels of mianserin may be halved by carbamazepine, probably via 3A4 induction (n = 12, Eap et al, Ther Drug Monit 1999;**21**:166–70).

Warfarin + mianserin

There is normally no problem but occasional control difficulties have been reported (Warwick and Mindham, Br J Psychiatry 1983;**143**:308).

4.3.3.4 MIRTAZAPINE

Mirtazapine does not inhibit CYP2D6, 1A2 and 3A and so interactions via these enzymes are unlikely. Mirtazapine is mainly metabolised by CYP2D6 and 1A2 (Montgomery, Int Clin Psychopharmacol 1995;**10**[Suppl 4]:37–45) and if one enzyme is inhibited, the other takes over, so mirtazapine appears less susceptible to P450 interactions. It is 85% protein bound, has linear kinetics from 15–75 mg/d, and 100% is excreted via the urine and faeces.

Review: Clinical pharmacokinetics (Timmer et al, Clin Pharmacokinet 2000;**38**:461–74).

Alcohol + mirtazapine

See alcohol (4.7.1).

Atomoxetine + mirtazapine

See atomoxetine (4.6.4).

Benzodiazepines + mirtazapine

The combination of diazepam and mirtazapine, not surprisingly, produces an additive sedative effect (n = 12, RCT, d/b, c/o, Mattila et al, Pharmacol Toxicol 1989;**65**:81–8) and so anyone on the combination should be warned about driving and other activities.

Carbamazepine + mirtazapine

Mirtazapine has no significant effect on carbamazepine levels but carbamazepine decreases mirtazapine levels by 60%, probably by CYP3A4 induction, and mirtazapine doses may need to be increased (RCT, 4/52, Sitsen et al, Eur J Drug Metab Pharmacokinet 2001;**26**:109–21).

Cimetidine + mirtazapine

Mirtazapine has no effect on cimetidine but mirtazapine levels may be higher (probably by CYP3A4 inhibition), but not enough to require dose reduction (n = 12, d/b, p/c, c/o, Sitsen et al, Eur J Clin Pharmacol 2000;**56**:389–94).

Clozapine + mirtazapine

Lack of significant interaction has been shown (n = 9, 6/52, Zoccali et al, Pharmacol Res 2003; **48**:411–4).

Fluoxetine + mirtazapine *

Fluoxetine 20–40 mg/d caused a clinically insignificant 32% increase in mirtazapine (15 mg/d) plasma levels after an abrupt switch (n = 40, Preskorn et al, Biol Psychiatry 1997;**41**:96S), although mania has been reported with mirtazapine augmentation of fluoxetine (n = 1, Ng, Depress Anxiety 2002;**15**:46–7) and immediately after a switch from fluoxetine, suggesting a combined effect (n = 1, Liu et al, J Psychopharmacol 2009;**23**:220–2).

FLUVOXAMINE + MIRTAZAPINE

Fluvoxamine 50–100 mg/d may increase mirtazapine serum levels 3–4-fold, a significant effect (n = 2, Anttila *et al*, *Ann Pharmacother* 2001;**35**:1221–3) and a serotonin syndrome has been reported with the combination (n = 1, Demers and Malone, *Ann Pharmacother* 2001;**35**:1217–20).

Levodopa + mirtazapine
Psychosis has been reported when mirtazapine was added to a stable levodopa regimen (n = 1, Normann *et al*, *Pharmacopsychiatry* 1997;**30**: 263–5).

Lithium + mirtazapine
No pharmacokinetic interaction has been detected between lithium 600 mg/d and mirtazapine 30 mg (n = 12, 10/7, Sitsen *et al*, *J Clin Psychopharmacol* 2000;**14**:172–6).

MAOIs + mirtazapine
The UK SPC cautiously recommends a two-week gap between stopping an MAOI and starting mirtazapine.

Olanzapine + mirtazapine *
Lack of significant interaction has been shown (n = 7, 6/52, Zoccali *et al*, *Pharmacol Res* 2003; **48**:411–4), although status epilepticus has been reported when olanzapine was added to mirtazapine (n = 1, Spyridi *et al*, *Int J Clin Pharmacol Ther* 2009;**47**:120–3).

Paroxetine + mirtazapine
Mirtazapine had no effect on the kinetics of paroxetine and the combination was better tolerated than either alone, suggesting a lack of clinically relevant interaction (n = 24, RCT, c/o, 6/7 per arm, Ruwe *et al*, *Hum Psychopharmacol* 2001;**16**:449–59).

Phenytoin + mirtazapine
A multiple dose study showed that mirtazapine had no effect on the steady-state kinetics of phenytoin, but that phenytoin reduced mirtazapine levels by a mean of 46%, probably clinically significant (n = 17, RCT, open, Spaans *et al*, *Eur J Clin Pharmacol* 2002;**58**:423–9).

Risperidone + mirtazapine
Mirtazapine 30 mg/d has no effect on risperidone 2–6 mg/d (n = 6, open, 8/52, Loonen *et al*, *Eur Neuropsychopharmacol* 1999;**10**:51–7; see also n = 8, 6/52, Zoccali *et al*, *Pharmacol Res* 2003;**48**: 411–4).

Sertraline + mirtazapine
Hypomania has been reported when mirtazapine 15 mg/d was used to augment sertraline 250 mg/d, which had been only partially effective (n = 1, Soutullo *et al*, *J Clin Psychiatry* 1998;**59**:320).

Smoking + mirtazapine
See mirtazapine + smoking (4.7.4).

Tacrolimus + mirtazapine *
Rapid onset of hypotension with raised tacrolimus levels has been reported when mirtazapine was added (n = 1, Fraile *et al*, *Nephrol Dial Transplant* 2009;**24**:1999–2001).

Tricyclics + mirtazapine
Amitriptyline causes clinically insignificant increases in mirtazapine plasma levels and vice versa (n = 24, Sennef *et al*, *Hum Psychopharmacol* 2003;**38**:91–101).

Venlafaxine + mirtazapine
Serotonin syndrome has been reported during a cross-over (n = 1, Dimellis, *World J Biol Psychiatry* 2002;**3**:167), and when both were also combined with tramadol (n = 1, Houlihan, *Ann Pharmacother* 2004;**38**:411–3). See also 1.14 for rational use of this combination.

Warfarin + mirtazapine
No interaction is known or suspected, but there is insufficient information to confirm this at present (Sayal *et al*, *Acta Psychiatr Scand* 2000;**102**:250–5).

4.3.3.5 MOCLOBEMIDE
Moclobemide is metabolised by CYP2C19, and inhibits 2D6, 2C19 and 1A2.
Review: general (Berlin and Lecrubier, *CNS Drugs* 1996;**5**:403–13).

Alcohol + moclobemide
See alcohol (4.7.1).

Benzodiazepines + moclobemide
No significant interaction occurs (Zimmer *et al*, *Acta Psychiatr Scand* 1990;**360**:84–6).

Bupropion + moclobemide
See MAOIs + bupropion (4.6.6).

Carbamazepine + moclobemide *
Carbamazepine 400 mg/d can reduce moclobemide levels by about 35% (n = 21, open, 4/52, Rakic Ignjatovic *et al*, *Br J Clin Pharmacol* 2009; **67**:199–208).

CIMETIDINE + MOCLOBEMIDE
Cimetidine may reduce the clearance and prolong the half-life of moclobemide, so start with lower doses and monitor closely (n = 8, open, Schoerlin *et al*, *Clin Pharmacol Ther* 1991;**49**:32–8)

Digoxin + moclobemide
Lack of interaction has been reported (Berlin and Lecrubier, *CNS Drugs* 1996;**5**:403–13).

Duloxetine + moclobemide

See duloxetine (4.3.3.2).

Ecstasy/MDMA + moclobemide

Deaths have been reported, with the victims apparently taking moclobemide in an attempt to enhance the effects of MDMA (n = 4, Vuori et al, Addiction 2003;**98**:365–8).

Ibuprofen + moclobemide

Moclobemide is alleged to potentiate the effect of ibuprofen, but lack of interaction has been reported (Berlin and Lecrubier, CNS Drugs 1996; **5**:403–13).

Metoprolol + moclobemide

Concurrent metoprolol and moclobemide results in further lowering of blood pressure, although postural hypotension was not reported (Zimmer et al, Acta Psychiatr Scand 1990;**360**:84–6).

Nifedipine + moclobemide

No significant interaction occurs, apart from some slight reduction in blood pressure (Zimmer et al, Acta Psychiatr Scand 1990;**360**:84–6).

Opiates + moclobemide

Moclobemide is alleged to potentiate the effect of opiates, and dose reductions of morphine and fentanyl may be considered necessary.

Oral contraceptives + moclobemide

No significant interaction has been detected (Zimmer et al, Acta Psychiatr Scand 1990;**360**: 84–6).

Pethidine + moclobemide *

This combination is now SPC contraindication.

SELEGILINE + MOCLOBEMIDE *

Selegiline is an MAO-B inhibitor and if combined with an MAO-A inhibitor, such as moclobemide, could produce full MAO inhibition (albeit reversible). The combination is not recommended but, if the two need to be used together, full MAOI dietary precautions might be required. The combination is now SPC contraindication.

SSRIs + moclobemide

A fatal serotonin syndrome has been reported with moclobemide and **citalopram** (n = 1, Dams et al, J Anal Toxicol 2001;**25**:147–51) but disputed (Isbister et al, J Anal Toxicol 2001;**25**:716–7). Excitation, insomnia and dysphoria have been reported with **fluvoxamine** and moclobemide in refractory depression (n = 36, open, 6/52, Ebert, Psychopharmacology 1995;**119**:342–4), as have headaches and fatigue (review, Dingemanse, Int Clin Psychopharmacol 1993;**7**:167–80). In a study where up to 600mg/d moclobemide was added to established **fluoxetine** therapy, there was no change in the number, intensity or type of adverse events. Fluoxetine markedly inhibited the metabolism of moclobemide but did not lead to excessive accumulation or any indication of development of a serotonin syndrome (n = 18, RCT, open, Dingemanse et al, Clin Pharmacol Ther 1998;**63**:403–13). A serotonin syndrome would also be a possibility with the combination and the UK SPC for moclobemide contraindicates the combination. A fatal case, following overdose of **paroxetine** and moclobemide and subsequent serotonin syndrome, has been reported (Singer and Jones, J Anal Toxicol 1997;**21**:518–20).

Sympathomimetics + moclobemide

The UK SPC recommends avoiding this combination. Phenylephrine may slightly raise blood pressure in people taking high dose (600mg/d) moclobemide (Amrein et al, Psychopharmacology 1992;**106**:S24–S31), but ephedrine produces a greater rise in bp (Dingemanse, Int Clin Psychopharmacol 1993;**7**:167–80). Another study noted no clinically significant interaction, although the pressor effect may be slightly enhanced (review: Zimmer et al, Acta Psychiatr Scand 1990; **360**:84–6).

Tricyclics + moclobemide

The UK SPC contraindicates the combination if the tricyclic (or metabolite) is a serotonin reuptake inhibitor, e.g. clomipramine or imipramine. Serotonin syndrome has been reported with moclobemide and clomipramine, imipramine (Brodribb et al, Lancet 1994;**343**:475–6) and after moclobemide plus either citalopram or clomipramine overdoses (n = 5, fatal, Neuvonen et al, Lancet 1993;**342**:1419), where aggressive therapy may be needed. Lack of interaction has been noted with amitriptyline 150mg/d (e.g. n = 21, Amrein et al, Psychopharmacology 1992; **106**:S24–S31).

Triptans + moclobemide

The literature notes an increased risk of CNS toxicity with **sumatriptan** or **zolmitriptan** and moclobemide (review by Rolan, Cephalalgia 1997;**17**[Suppl 18]:21–7; Morales Asin, Neurologia 1998;**13**[Suppl 2]:25–30), and that lower doses should be used, although a small study suggested combined use with **sumatriptan** was safe with care (n = 14, open, Blier and Bergeron, J Clin Psychopharmacol 1995;**15**:106–9). Moclobemide may significantly potentiate the effects of **rizatriptan** and the combination is not recommended (n = 12, RCT, Van Haarst et al, Br J Clin Pharmacol 1999;**48**:190–6). Moclobemide increases the plasma concentration of **almotriptan** but the combination appears well tolerated (n = 12, RCT, open, c/o, Fleishaker et al, Br J Clin Pharmacol 2001;**51**:437–41) and it may be the triptan of choice.

Tyramine + moclobemide

Moclobemide does not appear to significantly potentiate the pressor effects of tyramine. Dietary restrictions are generally not required, but patients should avoid eating excessive amounts of tyramine-containing foods, especially if they have pre-existing hypertension. Minor pressor effects are not seen until about 100 mg tyramine (Zimmer et al, Acta Psychiatr Scand 1990;**360**:84–6). Even 150 mg tyramine is suggested by some as being safe (Acta Psychiatr Scand 1990;**360**[Suppl]:78–80). The use of this combination has, however, been used to treat severe postural hypotension (e.g. n = 1, Karet et al, Lancet 1994;**344**:1263–5) and in counteracting clozapine-induced hypotension, allowing dose increases to an active therapeutic level (n = 1, Taylor et al, Br J Psychiatry 1995;**167**:409–10).

Venlafaxine + moclobemide

See venlafaxine (4.3.3.9).

Valproate + moclobemide *

Valproate 1 g/d has no effect on moclobemide levels (n = 21, open, 4/52, Rakic Ignjatovic et al, Br J Clin Pharmacol 2009;**67**:199–208).

Warfarin + moclobemide

No interaction has been reported, but moclobemide inhibits CYP1A2 and 2C19 and so the potential for warfarin potentiation exists (Sayal et al, Acta Psychiatr Scand 2000;**102**:250–5).

4.3.3.6 REBOXETINE

Reboxetine is predominantly metabolised in vitro via CYP2D6 and 3A4 (n = 51, Kuhn et al, Int J Clin Pharmacol Ther 2007;**45**:36–46). Reboxetine inhibits both CYP2D6 and CYP3A4 with low binding affinities, but has shown no effect on the in vivo clearance of drugs metabolised by these enzymes. In vitro studies have shown that reboxetine does not inhibit CYP1A2, CYP2C9, CYP2C19, and CYP2E1. Reboxetine should be co-prescribed with caution with potent inhibitors of CYP3A4. Reboxetine is extensively (97%) bound to plasma proteins (particularly the alpha-1 acid glycoprotein fraction) and

may interact with drugs with a high affinity for this fraction, e.g. dipyridamole, propranolol, methadone, imipramine, chlorpromazine (see antipsychotics below) and local anaesthetics.

Alcohol + reboxetine

See alcohol (4.7.1).

Antipsychotics + reboxetine

An interaction is possible (see above). Reboxetine has no effect on **clozapine** or **risperidone** plasma levels (n = 7, Spina et al, Ther Drug Monit 2001;**23**:675–8).

Benzodiazepines + reboxetine

Lack of interaction has been reported, although some mild-to-moderate drowsiness and transient increases in heart rate have been noted.

Carbamazepine + reboxetine

Low serum concentrations of reboxetine have been reported with concurrent carbamazepine (n = 1, Helland and Spigset, J Clin Psychopharmacol 2007;**27**:308–10).

Dipyridamole + reboxetine

An interaction is possible (see introduction).

Disopyramide + reboxetine

The literature advises caution with combination.

Diuretics + reboxetine

There may be an increased risk of hypokalaemia with loop diuretics or thiazides (BNF).

Erythromycin + reboxetine

The literature advises caution with combination.

Flecainide + reboxetine

The literature advises caution with combination.

Fluoxetine + reboxetine

There are no statistically significant effects of reboxetine on fluoxetine or norfluoxetine pharmacokinetics, and a minimal clinical impact is suggested (n = 30, RCT, d/b, p/c, 8/7, Fleishaker et al, Clin Drug Investigat 1999;**18**:141–50), although urinary retention has been reported (n = 1, Benazzi, Can J Psychiatry 2000;**45**:936).

Fluvoxamine + reboxetine

The literature advises caution with combination.

Ketoconazole + reboxetine

Ketoconazole decreases the clearance of the two enantiomers of reboxetine, with no adverse effects, but some caution may be advisable (n = 11, open, Herman et al, Clin Pharmacol Therapeut 1999;**66**:374–9)

Lidocaine + reboxetine

An interaction is possible (see introduction), and with other local anaesthetics. The literature advises caution with the combination.

MAOIs + reboxetine

This has not been evaluated so avoid until further notice, and leave a two-week gap after an MAOI and one week after reboxetine before switching to the other.

Methadone + reboxetine

An interaction is possible (see introduction).

Phenobarbital + reboxetine

Low serum concentrations of reboxetine have been reported with concurrent phenobarbital (n = 1, Helland and Spigset, *J Clin Psychopharmacol* 2007;**27**:308–10).

Potassium-losing diuretics + reboxetine

See diuretics (introduction to 4.3.3.6).

Propafenone + reboxetine

The literature advises caution with combination.

Propranolol + reboxetine

An interaction is possible (see introduction).

Tricyclics + reboxetine

An interaction is possible (see introduction).

Warfarin + reboxetine

No interaction is known or suspected, but there is insufficient information to confirm this at present (Sayal et al, *Acta Psychiatr Scand* 2000; **102**:250–5).

4.3.3.7 TRAZODONE

Trazodone is metabolised by CYP2D6 and inhibits 3A4.

ALCOHOL + TRAZODONE

See alcohol (4.7.1).

Antipsychotics + trazodone

Enhanced hypotension may occur when trazodone was added to either **chlorpromazine** or **trifluoperazine** (n = 2, Asayesh, *Can J Psychiatry* 1986;**31**:857–8).

Buspirone + trazodone

See buspirone (4.1.2).

Carbamazepine + trazodone

See carbamazepine (4.5.1).

Citalopram/escitalopram + trazodone

See citalopram (4.3.2.1).

Clarithromycin + trazodone *

Clarithromycin increases the AUC and half-life of trazodone, enhancing sedative effects (n = 10, c/o, Farkas et al, *Clin Pharmacol Ther* 2009;**85**:644–50).

Cocaine + trazodone

See antidepressants + cocaine (4.7.3).

Digoxin + trazodone

Cases of digoxin toxicity exist with trazodone (n = 2, Rauch and Jenike, *Psychosomatics* 1984;**25**: 334–5).

Fluoxetine + trazodone

See fluoxetine (4.3.2.2).

Gingko biloba + trazodone

Coma has been reported with concomitant use in an Alzheimer's patient (n = 1, Galluzzi et al, *J Neurol Neurosurg Psychiatry* 2000;**68**:679–80).

Interferon alfa + trazodone

See interferon alfa + paroxetine (4.3.2.4).

MAOIs + trazodone

See MAOIs (4.3.4).

Phenytoin + trazodone

See phenytoin (4.5.9).

Venlafaxine + trazodone

See venlafaxine (4.3.3.9).

Warfarin + trazodone

INR and PT can fall when trazodone is added to warfarin, and rise when trazodone is stopped, and so caution is necessary (adjust doses and/ or monitor), especially if trazodone is used as a PRN hypnotic (e.g. n = 1, Small and Giamonna, *Ann Pharmacother* 2000;**34**:734–6; n = 1, Jalili and Dehpour, *Arch Med Res* 2007;**38**:901–4).

4.3.3.8 TRYPTOPHAN

Duloxetine + tryptophan

See duloxetine (4.3.3.2).

Fluoxetine + tryptophan

See fluoxetine (4.3.2.2).

Fluvoxamine + tryptophan

See fluvoxamine (4.3.2.3).

MAOIs + tryptophan

See MAOIs (4.3.4).

4.3.3.9 VENLAFAXINE *

Venlafaxine is metabolised by CYP2D6 to O-desmethylvenlafaxine, a major active metabolite and by CYP3A4 to N-desmethylvenlafaxine. Other, minor, metabolic pathways exist. Venlafaxine has a low potential for CYP2D6 and 3A4 inhibition (Ball et al, *Br J Clin Pharmacol* 1997;**43**:619–26) and does not appear to have a significant effect on other P450 enzymes. 2D6 polymorphism has no effect on desvenlafaxine metabolism, but has significant and predictable effects on venlafaxine (n = 14, open, c/o, Preskorn et al, *J Clin Psychopharmacol* 2009;**29**:39–43). The UK SPC notes that:

- Use of venlafaxine with potent CYP3A4 inhibitors (e.g. ketoconazole, erythromycin) or combinations that inhibit both CYP3A4 and CYP2D6 should be avoided if possible.

Alcohol + venlafaxine

See alcohol (4.7.1).

Anticholinergics + venlafaxine

See anticholinergics (4.6.2).

Antipsychotics + venlafaxine

The UK SPC notes that venlafaxine causes a 70% increase in haloperidol AUC and 88% increase in peak levels, so care is needed as urinary retention has been reported with **haloperidol** (Benazzi, *Pharmacopsychiatry* 1997;**30**:27). Increased **cloza-pine** levels and adverse effects have also been reported, although one study showed that even moderate doses of venlafaxine had no significant effect on clozapine plasma levels (n = 11, Repo–Tiihonen et al, *Neuropsychobiol* 2005;**51**:173–6). Steady-state venlafaxine had no significant effect on the kinetics of a single 1 mg dose of **risperidone**, although some enzyme inhibition led to slightly raised risperidone plasma levels (n = 30, open, Amchin et al, *J Clin Pharmacol* 1999;**39**:297–309).

Atomoxetine + venlafaxine

See atomoxetine (4.6.4).

Benzodiazepines + venlafaxine

A study showed that diazepam 10mg had no significant effect on venlafaxine or metabolite kinetics, but venlafaxine slightly increased diazepam clearance. No clinically significant interaction thus seems likely (n = 17, Troy et al, *J Clin Pharmacol* 1995;**35**:410–9).

Bupropion + venlafaxine

See bupropion (4.6.6).

Carbamazepine + venlafaxine

Carbamazepine 200–400 mg does not appear to effect venlafaxine plasma levels (mean 200mg/d) and metabolite (n = 10, open, 8/52, Ciusani et al, *J Psychopharmacol* 2004;**18**:559–66).

Cimetidine + venlafaxine

A 45% reduction in venlafaxine clearance via reduced first-pass metabolism can result in increased venlafaxine levels and patients should be monitored for dose-related side-effects, e.g. nausea and bp changes. The major metabolite, O-desmethylvenlafaxine, is unaffected.

Co-amoxiclav + venlafaxine

Serotonin syndrome has been reported after single doses of co-amoxiclav during venlafaxine therapy (n = 1, Connor, *J R Soc Med* 2003;**96**:233–4).

Duloxetine + venlafaxine

See duloxetine (4.3.3.2).

ERYTHROMYCIN + VENLAFAXINE *

Potent CYP3A4 inhibitors (e.g. ketoconazole, erythromycin) should only be prescribed with venlafaxine if strictly indicated (UK SPC).

Fluoxetine + venlafaxine

See fluoxetine (4.3.2.2).

INDINAVIR + VENLAFAXINE

A study has shown that venlafaxine reduced indinavir's peak plasma levels by 36% and AUC by 28%, a potentially clinically significant effect (n = 9, Levin et al, *Psychopharmacol Bull* 2001;**35**:62–71).

Ketoconazole + venlafaxine

Ketoconazole increases venlafaxine's AUC and Cmax by about 30% in CYP3A4 extensive metabolisers, but the effect appears erratic in poor metabolisers, variably increasing AUC (0–206%) and Cmax (0–119%), so it's a good job they're relatively rare (n = 21, open, Lindh et al, *Eur J Clin Pharmacol* 2003;**59**:401–6).

Linezolid + venlafaxine

Serotonin syndrome has been reported with the combination (n = 1, Jones et al, *J Antimicrob Chemother* 2004;**54**:289–90; n = 1, Bergeron et al, *Ann Pharmacother* 2005;**39**:956–61).

Lithium + venlafaxine

Venlafaxine has been shown to have no significant effect on lithium kinetics in a single dose study (open, Troy et al, *J Clin Pharmacol* 1996;**36**:175–81), but there are cases of raised lithium levels and of serotonin syndrome (e.g. Mekler and Woggon, *Pharmacopsychiatry* 1997; **30**:272–3; n = 1, Naranjo = probable, *J Clin Pharm Ther* 2006;**31**:397–400). Lithium reduces the renal clearance of venlafaxine but without apparent clinical significance.

MAOIs + VENLAFAXINE

Wyeth state that venlafaxine and MAOIs should not be used together and recommend a 14-day gap after stopping an MAOI before starting venlafaxine, and a seven-day gap after stopping venlafaxine before starting an MAOI. There are many reported cases of severe reactions, e.g. extreme agitation, diaphoresis, rapid respiration and raised CPK levels (n = 1, Phillips and Ringo, *Am J Psychiatry* 1995;**152**:1400–1), hypomania, heavy perspiration, shivering and dilated pupils (n = 1, Klysner et al, Lancet 1995;**346**:1298–9), and serotonin syndrome (e.g. n = 1, Weiner et al, *Pharmacother* 1998;**18**:399–403). Follow the manufacturer's recommendations carefully.

Mirtazapine + venlafaxine
See mirtazapine (4.3.3.4).

Moclobemide + venlafaxine
The UK SPC for venlafaxine states very cautiously that venlafaxine and moclobemide should not be used together and that serious adverse reactions may occur. It recommends a 14-day gap after stopping moclobemide before starting venlafaxine, and a seven-day gap after venlafaxine before moclobemide is used. This seems overcautious, although a serotonin syndrome has been reported (n = 1, Fisher and Davies, *Ann Pharmacother* 2002;**36**:67–71).

Propafenone + venlafaxine
An organic psychosis has been reported, with raised venlafaxine levels (n = 1, Pfeffer and Grube, *Int J Psychiatr Med* 2001;**31**:427–32).

Selegiline + venlafaxine
The UK SPC for venlafaxine states that the combination should not be used and that serious adverse reactions may occur. It recommends a 14-day gap after stopping selegiline before starting venlafaxine, and a seven-day gap after venlafaxine before selegiline is used.

Sertraline + venlafaxine
See sertraline (4.3.2.5).

Sour date nut + venlafaxine
A severe serotonin syndrome with anaphylactic features has been reported with combined sour date nut (jujube) and venlafaxine 37.5 mg/d (n = 1, Stewart, *Am J Psychiatry* 2004; **161**:1129–30).

Trazodone + venlafaxine
A serotonin syndrome has been reported (n = 1, McCue and Joseph, *Am J Psychiatry* 2001; **158**:2088–9).

Tricyclics + venlafaxine
See tricyclics (4.3.1).

Verapamil + venlafaxine
A fatality has been reported (n = 1, Kusman et al, *J Forensic Sci* 2000;**45**:926–8).

Warfarin + venlafaxine
Potentiation of the anticoagulant effects of warfarin has been reported, including increased PT or INR (UK SPC).

4.3.3.10 ST JOHN'S WORT
Although not approved for depression in the UK, this section has been included because concerns about its interactions are frequently raised. Minor serotonin, norepinephrine and dopamine reuptake inhibition activity has been detected from St John's wort (SJW) and might thus potentiate any antidepressants, and so any combinations should in theory be avoided, particularly at high dose. SJW, when taken at recommended doses for depression, is unlikely to inhibit CYP2D6 or 3A4 activity (n = 7, open, Markowitz et al, *Life Sci* 2000;**66**:133–9), but is probably a CYP3A4 and 2C9 inducer (n = 2, Ruschitzka et al, *Lancet* 2000;**355**:548–9). SJW increases the expression of P-glycoprotein, which may have implications for drug interactions (n = 22, Hennessy et al, *Br J Clin Pharmacol* 2002; **53**:75–82). There are reports of serotonin syndrome with SJW and antidepressants in elderly patients (n = 5, Lantz et al, *J Geriatr Psychiatry Neurol* 1999;**12**:7–10). SJW is widely used as self-medication so remember to ask about it (up to 15% have used it recently, and 7% may be taking it at any one time; n = 101, Redvers et al, *Psychiatr Bull* 2001;**25**:254–6).

Reviews: * general interactions (Borrelli and Izzo, *AAPS J* 2009;**11**:710–27, Zhou et al, *J Psychopharmacol* 2004; **18**:262–76; Hammerness et al, *Psychosomatics* 2003;**44**:271–82; Izzo, *Int J Clin Pharmacol Ther* 2004;**42**:139–48; s = 22, Mills et al, *Br Med J* 2004; **329**:27–30).

Alitretinoin + St John's wort
The SPC for alitretinoin states that the combination should not be used with SJW.

Androgens + St John's wort
Short-term administration of SJW does not significantly alter circulating androgen levels in men and women, although 5-alpha-reduced-androgen levels may drop (n = 12, 14/7, Donovan et al, *Phytother Res* 2005;**19**:901–6).

ANTIRETROVIRALS + ST JOHN'S WORT
SJW may induce the metabolism of antiretrovirals, reducing efficacy, and so should not be taken together (CSM warning, 2000). The UK SPC now says **atazanavir** is contraindicated with any products containing SJW, with a similar warning for **maraviroc** (UK SPC). SJW may reduce the levels of **indinavir** (AUC reduced by 57%), reducing efficacy, and so these should not be taken together (n = 8, Piscitelli et al, *Lancet* 2000; **355**:547). The same would probably be true for other protease inhibitors, e.g. ritonavir and saquinavir. Suddenly stopping SJW may require dose adjustment of any anti-HIV drug.

Benzodiazepines + St John's wort
SJW halves **alprazolam's** half-life (n = 12, open,

Markowitz et al, JAMA 2003;**290**:1519–20) but there was no significant interaction between stat doses of alprazolam 1 mg and the Esbericum brand of SJW (n = 28, RCT, p/c, Arold et al, Planta Med 2005;**71**:31–7). SJW significantly reduces **quazepam** plasma levels (n = 13, RCT, p/c, c/o, 14/7, Kawaguchi et al, Br J Clin Pharmacol 2004;**58**:403–10).

Buspirone + St John's wort
See buspirone (4.1.2).

Caffeine + St John's wort
There was no significant interaction between stat doses of caffeine 100 mg and the Esbericum brand of SJW (n = 28, RCT, p/c, Arold et al, Planta Med 2005;**71**:331–7).

Carbamazepine + St John's wort
Carbamazepine reduces hypericum levels by 30%, probably clinically insignificant (n = 33, RCT, p/c, 7/7, Johne et al, Eur J Clin Pharmacol 2004;**60**:617–22). SJW may have no effect on carbamazepine clearance (n = 8, 5/52, Burstein et al, Clin Pharmacol Ther 2000;**68**:605–12), but the CSM has warned that SJW may induce the metabolism of carbamazepine, increasing the risk of seizures, and so should not be taken together (CSM warning, 2000). Suddenly stopping SJW may require dose adjustment of carbamazepine so check levels before and after stopping SJW.

Ciclosporin + St John's wort
SJW causes rapid (within three days) and significant (60%) reduction in ciclosporin plasma levels and may alter the metabolite ratio as well (n = 11, open, 14/7, Bauer et al, Br J Clin Pharmacol 2003;**55**:203–11), so these should not be taken together (CSM warning, 2000; Moschella and Jaber, Am J Kidney Dis 2001;**38**:1105–7). Heart transplant rejection due to SJW has been reported (n = 2, Ruschitzka et al, Lancet 2000;**355**:548).

Cimetidine + St John's wort
Cimetidine produces a 25% increase in hypericum levels, probably clinically insignificant (n = 33, RCT, p/c, 7/7, Johne et al, Eur J Clin Pharmacol 2004;**60**:617–22).

Digoxin + St John's wort
SJW may induce the metabolism of digoxin, reducing AUC by up to 25%, and so these should not be taken together (n = 25, 10/7, s/b, p/c, Johne et al,'Clin Pharmacol Ther 1999;**66**:338–45; Cheng, Arch Intern Med 2000;**160**:2548).

Suddenly stopping SJW may also require dose adjustment of digoxin. There was no significant interaction between stat doses of digoxin and the Esbericum brand of SJW (n = 28, RCT, p/c, Arold et al, Planta Med 2005;**71**:331–7).

Duloxetine + St John's wort
See duloxetine (4.3.3.2).

Fexofenadine + St John's wort
SJW may inhibit the metabolism of fexofenadine (open, c/o, Wang et al, Clin Pharmacol Therapeutics 2002;**71**:414–20).

Ibuprofen + St John's wort
SJW appears to have no significant effect on ibuprofen (n = 8, 21/7, Bell et al, Ann Pharmacother 2007;**41**:229–34).

MAOIs + St John's wort
Minor MAOI activity has been detected from SJW, which might potentiate existing MAOI therapy, and should be avoided, particularly at high dose.

Methadone + St John's wort
SJW induces methadone metabolism, decreasing levels by up to 47% and may precipitate withdrawal symptoms (n = 4, Eich-Hochli et al, Pharmacopsychiatry 2003;**36**:35–7).

Finasteride + St John's wort *
SJW induces the metabolism of finasteride and significantly reduces its AUC and half-life (n = 12, 2/52, Lundahl et al, Eur J Pharm Sci 2009;**36**:433–43).

Lacosamide + St John's wort *
See St John's wort + lacosamide (4.5.4).

Methylphenidate + St John's wort
See St John's wort + methylphenidate (4.6.11).

Omeprazole + St John's wort
SJW may produce 'enormously' decreased omeprazole levels (n = 12, RCT, c/o, Wang et al, Clin Pharmacol Ther 2004;**75**:191–7).

Oral contraceptives + St John's wort
The UK CSM has recommended that since SJW reduces the effectiveness of oral contraceptives, the two should not be taken together (n = 2 pregnancies, Pharm J 2002;**268**:198) and reduced efficacy has been shown (n = 12, open, Hall et al, Clin Pharmacol Ther 2003;**74**:525–35). However, a small study showed no loss of efficacy of Loestrin 1/20® (Galen), with no significant change in serum androgen levels (n = 15, open, Fogle et al, Contraception 2006;**74**:245–8).

Phenobarbital + St John's wort
The CSM has warned that SJW may induce the metabolism of phenobarbital, increasing the risk

of seizures, and so should not be taken together (CSM warning, 2000). Suddenly stopping SJW may require dose adjustment of phenobarbital so check levels before and after stopping SJW.

Phenytoin + St John's wort

The CSM has warned that SJW may induce the metabolism of phenytoin, increasing the risk of seizures, and so should not be taken together (CSM warning, 2000). Suddenly stopping SJW may require dose adjustment of phenytoin so check levels before and after stopping SJW.

Prednisone + St John's wort

Lack of interaction has been shown (n = 8, 28/7, Bell et al, Ann Pharmacother 2007;**41**:1819–24).

SSRIs + St John's wort

Minor serotonin reuptake inhibition activity has been detected from SJW which might potentiate existing SSRI therapy and so should, in theory, be avoided, particularly at high dose.

Statins + St John's wort *

SJW may decrease simvastatin and atorvastatin (but not pravastatin) plasma levels (n = 16, d/b, c/o, 14/7, Fujimura et al, Clin Pharmacol Ther 2002;**71**:63). Reduced (rosuva)statin efficacy has been reported with SJW (n = 1, Gordon et al, Am J Med 2009;**122**:e1–2).

Tacrolimus + St John's wort

SJW induces tacrolimus metabolism via 3A4, which may lead to organ rejection (n = 10, Hebert et al, J Clin Pharmacol 2004;**44**:89–94).

Theophylline + St John's wort

SJW may induce the metabolism of theophylline, reducing efficacy, and so these should not be taken together (CSM warning, 2000), although suddenly stopping SJW may require dose adjustment of theophylline (n = 1, Nebel et al, Ann Pharmacother 1999;**33**:502). Check theophylline levels before and after stopping SJW. One study showed no significant changes from 14 days SJW and a single dose of theophylline (n = 12, open, RCT, c/o, 15/7, Morimoto et al, J Clin Pharmacol 2004;**44**:95–101), so there may be interindividual variation.

Tolbutamide + St. John's wort

There was no significant interaction between stat doses of tolbutamide 500 mg and the Esbericum brand SJW (n = 28, RCT, p/c, Arold et al, Planta Med 2005;**71**:331–7).

Tricyclics + St John's wort

Minor serotonin and norepinephrine reuptake inhibition activity has been detected from SJW, which might thus potentiate existing tricyclic

therapy, and so should, in theory, be avoided, particularly at high dose. Amitriptyline and nortriptyline levels reduced by 22% have been reported (n = 12, Johne et al, J Clin Psychopharmacol 2002;**22**:46–54).

Triptans + St John's wort

The CSM has warned that SJW may increase the serotonergic effects of sumatriptan, naratriptan, rizatriptan and zolmitriptan, with increased adverse effects so avoid the combination.

Tyramine + St John's wort

There is not thought to be an interaction (mentioned by Cupp, Am Fam Physician 1999;**59**: 1239–45).

Verapamil + St John's wort

SJW significantly reduces verapamil bioavailability (AUC 50–60% decreased) via increased first-pass gut metabolism (n = 8, open, Tannergren et al, Clin Pharmacol Ther 2004;**75**:298–309).

Warfarin + St John's wort

SJW may induce the metabolism of warfarin, reducing efficacy, and so these should not be taken together (CSM warning, 2000). Suddenly stopping SJW may require dose adjustment of warfarin so check INR before and after stopping SJW and adjust doses as necessary.

4.3.4 MONOAMINE OXIDASE INHIBITORS (MAOIs)

Review of MAOI interactions; Berlin and Lecrubier, CNS Drugs 1996;**5**:403–13.

Adrenaline + MAOIs

See norepinephrine + MAOIs.

ALCOHOL + MAOIs

See alcohol (4.7.1).

Amantadine + MAOIs

Hypertension occurred in one patient taking amantadine, 48 hours after starting phenelzine (Jack and Daniel, Arch Gen Psychiatry 1984;**41**:726), with one reported case of safe use of both (Greenberg and Meyers, Am J Psychiatry 1985;**142**:273).

AMFETAMINE + MAOIs

See dexamfetamine + MAOIs.

Anaesthetics + MAOIs

With proper monitoring, general and local anaesthesia can be given safely with MAOIs (n = 27, el-Ganzouri et al, Anesth Analg 1985;**64**:592–6), although occasional cases of reactions have been reported (e.g. Sides,

Anesthesia 1987;**42**:633–5). This is generally considered safe, although care with analgesics and sympathomimetics is needed.

Anticholinergics + MAOIs
Enhanced anticholinergic effects have been postulated.

Anticoagulants + MAOIs
An enhanced anticoagulant effect has been shown in animals.

Antipsychotics + MAOIs
Unexplained deaths with levomepromazine exist, but are probably not related to a drug interaction. The combination is a risk factor for NMS and may enhance anticholinergic and EPSEs. Enhanced sedation could occur. There is a case of serotonin syndrome with **phenelzine** and **quetiapine** (n = 1, Kohen *et al, CNS Spectr* 2007;**12**:396–8).

Aspartane + MAOIs
Recurrent headaches following aspartane ingestion have been reported (n = 1, Ferguson, *Am J Psychiatry* 1985;**142**:271).

ATOMOXETINE + MAOIs
See atomoxetine (4.6.4).

Atracurium + MAOIs
A single case report exists of atracurium-induced hypertension (n = 1, Sides, *Anesthesia* 1987;**42**:633).

Barbiturates + MAOIs
Barbiturate sedation may be prolonged. Although little human data exists, be aware of the potential toxicity as one fatality has been reported.

Benzodiazepines + MAOIs

Although there are isolated cases of MAOI toxicity, oedema and hepatotoxicity (e.g. Young and Walpole, *Med J Aust* 1986;**144**:166–7), this is normally considered a safe combination.

Beta-blockers + MAOIs
Propranolol used with MAOIs has caused severe hypertension (Risch *et al, J Clin Psychiatry* 1982;**43**:16) and slight bradycardia (n = 1, Reggev and Vollhardt, *Psychosomatics* 1989;**30**:106–8), although not invariably so (review: Davidson *et al, J Clin Psychiatry* 1984;**45**:81–4). Best to monitor bp carefully, especially in the elderly.

Bretylium + MAOIs
Bretylium may increase the heart rate with MAOIs but it is only dangerous if other sympathomimetics are present. There are no case reports.

Bupropion + MAOIs
See bupropion (4.6.6).

BUSPIRONE + MAOIs
There are four unpublished reports of increased bp and possible CVA, although the combination has been used safely.

Patient information: warning signs of a reaction

If a patient experiences any of the following symptoms, expecially after eating, taking drugs of any type or if unexpected or severe, a reaction should be suspected and appropriate medical attention sought immediately: headache (especially at the back of the head), lightheadedness or dizziness, flushing of the face, pounding of the heart, numbness or stiffness in the neck, photophobia, chest pain or nausea and vomiting. It usually occurs about two hours after the ingestion of the compound.

Treatment for MAOI hypertensive crisis:

- Phenotamine 2–10 mg by slow IV infusion (adults), repeated if necessary.
- If not phentolamine, chlorpromazine 50–100 mg IM can be used, as can diazoxide (50–100 mg by IV injection). Repeat after 10 minutes if necessary.
- Alternative advice might be to bite open a 10 mg capsule of nifedipine, swallow the contents with water (*Am J Psychiatry* 1991;**148**:1616) then go immediately to a hospital casualty department. Due to serious adverse events (stroke, hypotension etc), s/l nifedipine should only be used with care (Marwick, (*JAMA* 1996;**275**:423–4; Grossman et al, *JAMA* 1996;**276**:1328–31). NB: nifedipine is light-sensitive and should not be left in bright light. Safer alternatives include sublingual captopril, clonidine and labetolol (review Matuschka, *J Pharm Tech* 1999;**15**:199–203).
- Cool any fever with external cooling.

Blood pressure should be monitored frequently.

Caffeine + MAOIs

Case reports exist of increased jitteriness with caffeine taken while on MAOIs (Berkowitz et al, Eur J Pharmacol 1971;**16**:315).

Carbamazepine + MAOIs

Carbamazepine is structurally related to the tricyclics and so an interaction has been postulated. There have been case reports of raised carbamazepine levels but a lack of inter-action with **tranylcypromine** (Lydiard et al, J Clin Psychopharmacol 1987;**7**:360) and **phenelzine** (Yatham et al, Am J Psychiatry 1990;**147**:367).

Chloral hydrate + MAOIs

There are two poorly documented case reports of fatal hyperpyrexia and hypertension with chloral hydrate and **phenelzine**. This is not thought to be an important interaction.

Citalopram + MAOIs

There are many reported cases of serotonin syndrome (see 1.32) with other SSRIs and MAOIs and so care is needed if this combination is used (review: Graber et al, Ann Pharmacother 1994;**28**:732–5).

Clozapine + MAOIs

See clozapine (4.2.4).

Cocaine + MAOIs

See cocaine (4.7.3).

Cyproheptadine + MAOIs

An isolated case exists of hallucinations with cyproheptadine and phenelzine (Hahn, Am J Psychiatry 1987;**144**:1242–3).

DEXAMFETAMINE + MAOIs

There is a case report of a death with phenelzine and dexamfetamine (Lloyd and Walker, Br Med J 1965;ii:168–9) and one with amfetamine.

Dextromethorphan + MAOIs

Case reports exist with cough mixtures containing dextromethorphan, but, since all also contained sympathomimetics, these are questionable. Two were fatal so care is advised. Dizziness and muscle spasms with dextromethorphan have been reported (Harrison et al, J Clin Psychiatry 1989;**50**:64–5), as has a serotonin syndrome (Nierenberg et al, Clin Pharmacol Ther 1993; **53**:84–8).

Dextropropoxyphene + MAOIs

Dextropropoxyphene plus **phenelzine** has been reported to produce sedation (n = 1, Garbutt, Am J Psychiatry 1987;**144**:251–2), severe hypotension, ataxia and impaired coordination (n = 1, Zomberg and Hegarty, Am J Psychiatry 1993;**150**:1270).

Disulfiram + MAOIs

See disulfiram (4.6.8).

DOPAMINE/DOXAPRAM + MAOIs

Animal studies show a clear interaction, with side-effects enhanced by MAOIs. The manufacturers recommend that dopamine or doxapram can be used if their initial dose is reduced to one tenth the normal dose and great care is taken.

DULOXETINE + MAOIs

See duloxetine (4.3.3.2).

Ecstasy/MDMA + MAOIs

There is a case of a hypertensive crisis with MDMA/ecstasy and phenelzine (n = 1, Smilkstein et al, J Toxicol Clin Toxicol 1987;**25**:149–59) and two of muscle tension, coma and delirium with raised blood pressure (Kaskey, Am J Psychiatry 1992;**192**:411–2).

Escitalopram + MAOIs

See citalopram + MAOIs.

FLUOXETINE + MAOIs

There are several reported interactions (e.g. Sternbach, Lancet 1988;ii:850–1), including four deaths. A gap must also be left when switching from one to the other (see 2.2.5).

FLUVOXAMINE + MAOIs

There is an SPC recommendation to allow a two-week gap between therapies. There are many reported cases of serotonin syndrome with other SSRIs and MAOIs and so care is needed with this combination.

Ginseng + MAOIs

There are cases of headache, tremor (Shader and Greenblatt, J Clin Psychopharmacol 1985;**5**:65) and mania (Jones and Runikis, J Clin Psychopharmacol 1987;**7**:201–2) with ginseng and phenelzine.

Hypoglycaemics + MAOIs

An enhanced hypoglycaemic effect with insulin and sulphonylureas has been noted.

Indoramin + MAOIs

The SPC for indoramin states this to be a contraindication, as indoramin antagonises alpha-receptors, thus competing with norepinephrine for post-synaptic alpha-receptors, which could cause vasoconstriction and raised blood pressure. No case reports are known.

Isoprenaline + MAOIs

This is a postulated interaction with some evidence that no interaction occurs. No case reports exist.

LEVODOPA + MAOIs

Low dose levodopa with carbidopa or benserazide seems safe but higher doses should be avoided, as should levodopa on its own (*Clin Pharmacol Ther* 1975;**18**:273).

Lithium + MAOIs

Lack of an interaction has been reported (n = 4, Fein *et al*, *Am J Psychiatry* 1988;**145**:249–50).

MAOIs + MAOIs

There is some evidence that different MAOIs may interact with each other, especially if abruptly changed, e.g. isocarboxazid to tranylcypromine (n = 1, Bazire, *Drug Intell Clin Pharm* 1986;**20**: 54–5) and phenelzine to isocarboxazid (Safferman and Masiar, *Ann Pharmacother* 1992;**26**:337–8). Tranylcypromine is metabolised to an amfetamine and an internal autoreaction (i.e. interacts with itself) has been postulated (n = 1, Gunn *et al*, *Br Med J* 1989;**298**:964).

Methadone + MAOIs

Lack of an interaction has been reported (Mendelson, *Med J Aust* 1979;**1**:400).

Methyldopa + MAOIs

There is a single case report of hallucinations with methyldopa and pargyline.

METHYLPHENIDATE + MAOIs

A less severe interaction than with amfetamines would be expected. A single case of headaches and hyperventilation has been reported.

Mirtazapine + MAOIs

See mirtazapine (*4.3.3.4*).

Modafinil + MAOIs

There is a report of successful use of tranyl-cypromine and modafinil for refractory narcolepsy (n = 1, Clemons *et al*, *Sleep Med* 2004; **5**:509–11).

Morphine + MAOIs

This is mainly extrapolation from pethidine. Two cases exist of hypotension and loss of consciousness with IV morphine (Barry, *Anaesth Intens Care* 1979;**7**:194), responsive to naloxone. Low dose morphine and other narcotics, e.g. codeine and fentanyl are probably safe. Methadone may be a suitable alternative. If opiates are used, it is best to start at a third or half the normal dose of opiate and titrate carefully, noting blood pressure and levels of consciousness. See also pethidine.

NEFOPAM + MAOIs

The manufacturers of nefopam recommend avoiding this combination.

Norepinephrine + MAOIs

Although unlikely to cause problems if care is used, norepinephrine is potentially dangerous by injection and/or if other sympathomimetics are present.

Orciprenaline + MAOIs

The manufacturers recommend caution if the two are used together.

Oxcarbazepine + MAOIs

See oxcarbazepine (*4.5.7*).

Oxymetazoline/xylometazoline + MAOIs

There is thought to be little systemic effect when these drugs are used nasally, but use in nose drops and sprays has not been studied.

Paraldehyde + MAOIs

Enhanced CNS sedation and respiratory depression have been suggested.

Paroxetine + MAOIs

Nothing has been reported but see other SSRIs in this MAOI section.

PETHIDINE + MAOIs

This is a well-documented, rapid, severe and potentially fatal interaction, although not inevitable (Evans-Prosser, *Br J Anaesth* 1968;**40**:279–82).

Reboxetine + MAOIs

See reboxetine (*4.3.3.6*).

Salbutamol + MAOIs

No interaction occurs.

SERTRALINE + MAOIs

The manufacturers suggest a one-week washout period after sertraline before an MAOI is used. Several cases of suspected serotonergic syndrome have been reported, so care is essential (e.g. cases and review, Graber *et al*, *Ann Pharmacother* 1994;**28**:732–5).

St John's wort + MAOIs

See St John's wort (*4.3.3.10*).

Sulphonamides + MAOIs

An isolated case exists of adverse effects with sulphafurazole and phenelzine (Boyer and Lake, *Am J Psychiatry* 1983;**140**:264–5).

Suxamethonium + MAOIs

There are three cases of enhancement of suxamethonium by phenelzine (Bodley *et al*, *Br Med J* 1969;**3**:510–2).

SYMPATHOMIMETICS + MAOIs

Hypertension has been reported with many indirectly acting sympathomimetic amines, e.g. ephedrine, metaraminol, pseudoephedrine and phenylpropanolamine. Phenylephrine is found in many OTC cough and cold remedies and can cause a massive rise in blood pressure with MAOIs. Use in nasal sprays and drops is not recommended, although there are no case reports.

Tetrabenazine + MAOIs

Reports exist of a central excitation and hypertension with tetrabenazine.

Trazodone + MAOIs

There are many reported cases of serotonin syndrome with SSRIs and MAOIs and so care is needed with combination (n = 1, Graber et al, Ann Pharmacother 1994;**28**:732–5).

TRICYCLICS + MAOIs

The combination of tranylcypromine and **clomipramine** has caused four deaths and one fatality between tranylcypromine and a single dose of **imipramine** (n = 1, Birkenhager and van den Broek, Eur Psychiatry 2003;**18**:264–5). There are cases of excitation, seizures and hyperpyrexia and a serotonin syndrome after a clomipramine overdose (325–750 mg) with phenelzine (Nierenberg et al, Clin Pharmacol Ther 1993;**53**:84–8).Other MAOI/tricyclic combinations have been used with extreme care (Graham et al, Lancet 1982;ii:440). The dangers could have been exaggerated and the combination may be relatively event-free if the following precautions are taken:

- avoid imipramine, desipramine, clomipramine and tranylcypromine
- prefer amitriptyline
- use oral doses only
- start both drugs simultaneously at low dose, increase slowly and monitor closely.

See also combinations in depression (1.14) for a review of the potentially beneficial effects.

TRIPTANS + MAOIs

The SPCs recommend sumatriptan is not used with MAOIs, or for two weeks after an MAOI has stopped.The UK SPC contraindicates MAOIs with rizatriptan.

Tryptophan + MAOIs

There are cases of hypomania (n = 2, Goff, Am J Psychiatry 1985;**142**:1487–8), behavioural and neurological toxicity with high doses of tryptophan, mostly with tranylcypromine (n = 8, Pope et al, Am J Psychiatry 1985;**142**:491–2), which may respond to propranolol (Guze and Baxter, J Clin Psychopharmacol 1986;**6**:119–20). Potentiation of the therapeutic effect is well known so monitor carefully.

TYRAMINE + MAOIs

Ingestion of dietary tyramine, levodopa or a sympathomimetic drug by a patient on an MAOI can produce a hypertensive crisis, e.g. headache, rapid and prolonged rise in blood pressure, intracranial haemorrhage, acute cardiac failure and death.The effect is probably only seen with slow acetylators, as fast acetylators seem able to handle tyramine and other monoamines better. The effect is hugely variable, but 8 mg tyramine can produce a 30 mmHg rise in bp in about 50% people, and 25 mg and above is potentially dangerous (Blackwell and Mabbitt, Lancet 1965;**1**:938–40). 20–50 mg tyramine produces hypertension with tranylcypromine (Berlin et al, Clin Pharmacol Ther 1989;**46**:344–51). In a normal person, bp rises within 10–20 minutes (range 0–60) of tyramine ingestion, peaking at 20–110 minutes, prolonged if an MAOI is taken. For advice on dietary tyramine, see the following section.

VENLAFAXINE + MAOIs

See venlafaxine (4.3.3.9).

Warfarin + MAOIs

No interaction is known, although tranylcypromine is known to inhibit CYP2C19 and so some minor potential exists (Sayal et al, Acta Psychiatr Scand 2000;**102**:250–5).

Xylometazoline + MAOIs

See oxymetazoline + MAOIs.

FOOD

Compliance with the MAOI diet is often very poor.

Reviews: Cheese and drink tyramine contents (Berlin and Lecrubier, CNS Drugs 1996;**5**:403–13), 'The making of a user–friendly MAOI diet' (Gardner et al, J Clin Psychiatry 1996;**57**:99–104), dietary restrictions (Rapaport, J Clin Psychiatry 2007;**68**[suppl 8]:42–6).

1. General principles

Freshness of food is vital. If there is any sign of spoilage then avoid. Avoid foods that are matured or might be 'spoiling'. Generally, the more 'convenience' the food, the safer it is, e.g. packet soups are generally safe. Although many foods have only small amounts of tyramine, it is possible to have local concentrations, which might give a reaction.

2. Tyramine-containing foods to avoid

The following may be of use as general guidelines:

- Dairy products

Hard cheeses and soft cheeses must be avoided. Special care is needed with salty, bitter tasting, refrigerated cheese. Foods containing cheese (e.g. pizzas and pies, see below) must also be avoided and are a known cause of inadvertent ingestion and death. However, cottage cheese, cream cheeses (e.g. Philadelphia), Ricotta and processed cheese contain only minute amounts of tyramine and large quantities would be needed to produce a reaction.

- **Fruit and vegetables**

Broad bean pods (but not the beans) and banana skins (occasionally cooked as part of whole unripe bananas in a stew) must be avoided. Avocado has been reported to produce a reaction and should be avoided if possible.

- **Game, meat and fish**

Pickled or salted dried herrings and any hung or badly stored game, poultry or other meat that might be 'spoiling' must be avoided. NB. the original reports with pickled herrings may have been due to spoilage in the brine surrounding the fish, and are probably safe.

- **Meat products**

Avoid chicken liver pâté, liver pâté and any other liver that is not fresh. Avoid aged and cured meats (e.g. salami, mortadella, pastrami). Fresh chicken liver, fresh beef liver and fresh pâté should be safe.

- **Pizzas**

Commercially available pizzas from large chain outlets seem safe (analysis by Shulman and Walker, J Clin Psychiatry 1999;**60**:191–3; comment by Feinberg and Holzer, reply by Shulman and Walker, J Clin Psychiatry 2000;**61**:145–6), and even those with double orders of cheese appear safe. Gourmet pizzas from smaller outlets may have higher tyramine contents, especially if mature cheeses are used.

- **Soy and soybean**

Some samples of soy sauce and soybean preparations may have very high tyramine levels. Either avoid entirely or a 10ml maximum is recommended.

> **Soy sauce** (Pearl River, etc) — some have high quantities, ie. up to 3.4mg/15ml, and so double or triple helpings could be well above the threshold for a reaction (Shulman and Walker, J Clin Psychiatry 1999;**60**:191–3)
> **Soybean curd** (e.g. Tofu) — some have high quantities, especially if kept refrigerated for seven days or longer, i.e. up to 5mg per

300mg helping, and so double or triple helpings could well be above the threshold for a reaction (Shulman and Walker, J Clin Psychiatry 1999;**60**:191–3).

- **Yeast and meat extracts**

'Oxo', 'Marmite', 'Bovril' and other meat or yeast extracts must be avoided. Gravy made with 'Bisto' is safe (all contain less than 0.0022mg/g tyramine and a full, half-pint of gravy would contain less than 0.05mg tyramine). Gravy made from juices of the roast or fresh meat should be safe. Brewers yeast (Shulman et al, J Clin Psychopharmacol 1989;**9**:397–402) and bread are safe.

3. Foods known to contain some tyramine where excessive consumption is not advisable, albeit unlikely

Plums, matured pork, sauerkraut, spinach.

4. Foods thought to contain only minute amounts of tyramine

Banana pulp (skins unsafe), chocolate (one anecdotal report of headache), cottage cheese, cream cheese, eggplant, fruit juices, octopus, peanuts, raspberries (minor reports of raised tyramine), sausages, soy milk, tomato, vinegar, yoghurt (commercial), Worcester sauce, eg. Lee and Perrins and others (very low, Shulman and Walker, J Clin Psychiatry 1999;**60**:191–3).

5. Other foods with isolated reports

Chicken nuggets, chapatti, protein dietary supplement, sea kale.

6. Alcoholic drinks

Patient instructions usually state that all alcoholic and some non-alcoholic drinks must be avoided. Real ales may contain up to 110mg/L, with reports of hypertensive crisis after 0.6 pint (79 brand study, Tailor et al, J Clin Psychopharmacol 1994;**14**:5–14). There is some evidence that low or non-alcoholic beers contain significant amounts of tyramine (Murray et al, Lancet 1988;**i**,167–8), shown by three reactions to less than two-thirds of a pint of alcohol-free and 'de-alcoholised' beer (n = 3, Thakore et al, Int Clin Psychopharmacol 1992;**7**:59–60). There is a large variation in other beers, so take in moderation (i.e. 1–2 bottles a day maximum), prefer canned beers from major brewers and take care with de-alcoholised beers. The maximum reported level in Chianti wine is 12mg/L, likely to be dangerous only in overdose. The following may, however, be of use where a particular patient wishes to drink:

> **Avoid:**
> - Chianti
> - Home-made beers and wines
> - Real ales
> - Red wines
>
> **True moderation (e.g. one unit):**
> - White wines
> - Non-alcoholic beers and lagers
>
> **Safest:**
> - Gin, vodka, other clear spirits

Red wines contain phenolic flavanoids, which inhibit the enzymes which metabolise catecholamines, including tyramine (*Br Med J* 1990;**301**:544).

Over-the-counter medicines

Each patient should be warned about the possibility of interactions with over-the-counter medicines. The general advice for patients is:

1. Only buy medicines from a pharmacy

Do not use medicines from supermarket shelves, drug stores or newsagents. Do not take medicines given to you by friends or relatives. Do not take medicines taken before the MAOI was prescribed until advice has been sought.

2. Carry an MAOI card and show it to any doctor, dentist or pharmacist who may treat you.

3. Take special care over any medicines for coughs, colds, 'flu, hay fever, asthma and catarrh.

4.4 LITHIUM

Lithium may interact with other drugs, particularly via changes in renal excretion.

Reviews: interactions with serotonergic agents (may increase prevalence of lithium-induced polyuria; n = 75, 4/12, open, Movig *et al, Br J Psychiatry* 2003;**182**:319–23).

ACE INHIBITORS + LITHIUM

There are many cases of lithium toxicity with ACE inhibitors (n = 9, open, DasGupta *et al, J Clin Psychiatry* 1992;**53**:398–400), especially in the elderly (n = 20, Finley *et al, J Clin Psychopharmacol* 1996;**16**:68–71), so either monitor very carefully (review: Lehmann and Ritz, *Am J Kidney Dis* 1995;**25**:82–7) or use an alternative, e.g. beta-blockers. In a case control study, ACE inhibitors

were most likely to increase lithium toxicity within a month of starting (Juurlink *et al, J Am Geriatr Soc* 2004;**52**:794–8; review by Jacoby, *EBMH* 2004;**7**:120) and there is a case of a five-fold increase in lithium levels after switching from fosinopril to lisinopril, the authors recommending monitoring carefully for four to six weeks after any such change (n = 1, Meyer *et al, Int Clin Psychopharmacol* 2005;**20**:115–8).

Acetazolamide + lithium

Lithium excretion may be increased or, less likely, possibly decreased by acetazolamide (n = 2, Gay *et al, Encephale* 1985;**11**:261–2), probably of minimal importance.

Agomelatine + lithium

See agomelatine (*4.3.3.1*).

Alcohol + lithium

See alcohol (*4.7.1*).

Amfetamines + lithium

Lithium may suppress amfetamine 'highs' (n = 3, Flemenbaum, *Am J Psychiatry* 1974;**131**:820–1).

AMINOPHYLLINE + LITHIUM

See theophylline + lithium.

Amiodarone + lithium

The literature notes an increased risk of hypothyroidism with the combination.

Antacids + lithium

See sodium + lithium.

Antibiotics + lithium

Antibiotics may lead to raised lithium levels (cases within n = 102, Wilting *et al, Bipolar Disord* 2005;**7**:274–80).

Antipsychotics + lithium *

Although generally considered a potentially useful combination, cases of mostly reversible neurotoxicity were reported in the 1980s, particularly with haloperidol (although these may have been undiagnosed NMS), encephalopathy, enhanced EPSE, neurotoxicity or irreversible brain damage. One review suggested that all these symptoms are consistent with lithium toxicity alone, the antipsychotic affecting fluid balance mechanisms and lithium intracellular concentrations (Knorring, *Hum Psychopharmacol* 1990;**5**:287–92). The main risk factors seem to be if high doses of both drugs are used and signs of impending toxicity are ignored.

There are, however, numerous reports for individual drugs. **Chlorpromazine** levels may be lowered by up to 40% by lithium, with enhanced EPSE and rarely neurotoxicity. Combined lithium and **clozapine** appears safe within moderate dose limits and without co-prescription of serotonergic or 1A2-inhibiting drugs (n = 44, Bender et al, Int J Neuropsychopharmacol 2004;**7**:59–63), although there are reports of increased risk of NMS and reversible neurotoxicity (n = 1, Blake et al, J Clin Psychopharmacol 1992;**12**:297–9), including one where lithium levels were below 0.5 mEq/L (n = 1, Lee and Yang, Chung Hua I Hsueh Tsa Chih (Taipei) 1999;**62**:184–7). Cases of diabetic ketoacidosis have also been reported (e. g. n = 1, Peterson and Byrd, Am J Psychiatry 1996;**153**:737–8), and so glucose monitoring might be indicated with this particular combination. While a short study showed a low risk of pharmacokinetic interaction between **risperidone** and lithium (n = 13, open, 9/7, Demling et al, Pharmacopsychiatry 2006;**39**:230–1) there are reports of delirium (n = 1, Chen and Cardasis, Am J Psychiatry 1996;**153**:1233–4), possible NMS (e.g. Bourgeois and Kahn, J Clin Psychopharmacol 2003; **23**:315–7), diabetic ketoacidosis, rabbit syndrome (n = 1, Mendhekar, Can J Psychiatry 2005;**50**:369), encephalopathy (e.g. n = 1, Boora et al, Acta Psychiatr Scand 2008;**117**:394–6) and myocardial infarction (n = 1, Ananth et al, J Clin Psychiatry 2004;**65**:724). Lower **olanzapine** levels were mentioned in one study (Bergemann et al, Pharmacopsychiatry 2004; **37**:63–8), NMS is possible (n = 1, Berry et al, Pharmacother 2003; **23**:55–9) and severe delirium and EPSE occurred in an elderly patient (n = 1, Tuglu et al, J Korean Med Sci 2005; **20**:691–4).

Amisulpride 200 mg/d (n = 24, RCT, d/b, p/c, Canal et al, Int J Neuropsychopharmacol 2003; **6**:103–9), **aripiprazole** (n = 22, 2/52, Citrome et al, J Clin Pharmacol 2005;**45**:89–93) and **quetiapine** have no significant effect on lithium kinetics (n = 10, open, 4/52, Potkin et al, Clin Ther 2002;**24**:1809–23), although slightly increased lithium levels have been reported and increased risk of EPSEs with **sulpiride** (SPC 2009) and rapidly developing delirium when quetiapine was added to lithium (n=1, Miodownik et al, Clin Neuropharmacol 2008;**31**:176–9). Lack of interaction has been shown with **ziprasidone** (n = 25, RCT, Apseloff et al, Br J Clin Pharmacol 2000; **49**[S3]:61–4), although lithium toxicity (n = 2, Miodownik et al, Clin Neuropharmacol 2005; **28**:295–7) and NMS (n = 1, Borovicka et al, Ann Pharmacother 2006;**40**:139–42) have been

reported with the combination.

Baclofen + lithium

Cases of aggravation of movement disorder in Huntington's disease exist (n = 2, Anden et al, Lancet 1973;ii:93).

Benzodiazepines + lithium

There have been several anecdotal reports of reactions, e.g. hypothermia (Naylor et al, Br Med J 1977;**2**:22) and, although a neurotoxic syndrome in combination with lithium has been reported (n = 5, Koczerginski et al, Int Clin Psychopharm 1989;**4**:195–9), routine use of this usually beneficial combination suggests it to be safe.

Beta-blockers + lithium

Bradycardia with propranolol and lithium has been reported (n = 1, Becker, J Clin Psychiatry 1989;**50**:473), although propranolol and nadolol (n = 1, Dave and Langbart, Ann Clin Psychiatry 1994;**6**:51–2) have been used uneventfully for lithium-induced tremor.

Bumetanide + lithium

Although studies have shown a minimal effect, bumetanide may cause lithium toxicity (Kerry et al, Br Med J 1980;**281**:371).

Calcium-channel blockers + lithium

Cases of enhanced effect and toxicity with unchanged plasma levels have been reported with verapamil (Price and Giannini, J Clin Pharmacol 1986;**26**:717–9), as have reduced lithium levels (Weinrauch et al, Am Heart J 1984;**108**:1378–80). Acute EPSE and bradycardia have been reported with diltiazem (n = 1, Binder et al, Arch Intern Med 1991;**151**:373–4).

Candesartan + lithium

There is a case of a patient prescribed 16 mg/d candesartan (an Angiotensin II antagonist) who developed severe lithium toxicity eight weeks later (n = 1, Zwanzger et al, J Clin Psychiatry 2001; **62**:208–9).

Cannabis + lithium

See cannabis (4.7.2).

Carbamazepine + lithium

See carbamazepine (4.5.1), plus 'combinations' in bipolar disorder (1.10) for a review of some beneficial effects.

Cisplatin + lithium

Reports exist of lithium levels decreased by up to 64% (e.g. Vincent et al, Cancer Chemother Pharmacol 1995;**35**:533–4).

Citalopram + lithium

See citalopram (4.3.2.1).

Clonidine + lithium

Lithium may reduce the hypotensive effect of clonidine (Goodnick and Meltzer, *Biol Psychiatry* 1984;**19**:883–9), so monitor carefully.

Cocaine + lithium

See cocaine (4.7.3).

Corticosteroids + lithium

An isolated case exists of lithium reducing the effect of corticosteroids on the kidneys (Stewart et al, *Clin Endocrinol* 1987;**27**:63).

Co-trimoxazole + lithium

Two cases exist of enhanced toxicity with reduced levels (*N Z Med J* 1984;**97**:729–32).

COX-2 inhibitors + lithium

See NSAIDs + lithium.

Dextromethorphan + lithium

Serotonin syndrome has been reported with the combination in a patient also taking fluoxetine (n = 1, Navarro et al, *Gen Hosp Psychiatry* 2006; **28**:78–80).

Digoxin + lithium

Lack of interaction has been shown (n = 6, open, Cooper et al, *Br J Clin Pharmacol* 1984;**18**:21–5).

Dipyridamole + lithium

Lack of interaction has been shown (Wood et al, *Br J Clin Pharmacol* 1989;**27**:749–56).

Disulfiram + lithium

See disulfiram (4.6.8).

Domperidone + lithium

An enhanced risk of EPSE exists.

Escitalopram + lithium

See citalopram/escitalopram (4.3.2.1).

Fluoxetine + lithium

The incidence of problems may be low (n = 110, open, Bauer et al, *J Clin Psychopharmacol* 1996; **16**:130–4) and lack of significant pharma-cokinetic interaction has been shown (n = 10, open, Breuel et al, *Int J Clin Pharmacol Ther* 1995; **33**:415–9). The combination may, however, be poorly tolerated (n = 14, open, Hawley et al, *Int Clin Psychopharmacol* 1994;**9**:31–3), with reports of serotonin syndrome (n = 1, Muly et al, *Am J Psychiatry* 1993;**150**:1565), absence seizures (n = 1, Sacristan et al, *Am J Psychiatry* 1991;**148**:146–7) and acute confusion or lithium toxicity (*Int J Geriatr Psychiatry* 1992;**7**:687–8; review by Levinson et al, DICP *Ann Pharmacother* 1991;**25**:657–61).

Fluvoxamine + lithium

See fluvoxamine (4.3.2.3).

Furosemide + lithium

Studies have shown a minimal effect and furosemide to be the safest diuretic with lithium (e.g. n = 13, RCT, Crabtree et al, *Am J Psychiatry* 1991;**148**:1060–3). In a case control study, loop diuretics most likely to increase lithium toxicity within a month of starting (Juurlink et al, *J Am Geriatr Soc* 2004;**52**:794–8; review by Jacoby, *EBMH* 2004;**7**:120).

Gabapentin + lithium

Although both are exclusively eliminated by renal excretion, a single-dose study showed that the pharmacokinetics of lithium are not altered by gabapentin (n = 13, Frye et al, *J Clin Psychopharmacol* 1998;**18**:461–4).

Herbal diuretics + lithium

A clear case of life-threatening lithium toxicity (4.5 mmol/L) induced by a herbal diuretic preparation has been reported (n = 1, Pyevich and Bogenschutz, *Am J Psychiatry* 2001;**158**:1329).

Hypoglycaemics + lithium

Lithium has been used to improve glucose metabolism and assist the effects of oral hypoglycaemics and insulin (n = 38, Hu et al, *Biol Trace Elem Res* 1997;**60**:131–7).

Iodides + lithium

Enhanced antithyroid and goiter effects of lithium have been reported.

Ispaghula husk + lithium

A single case exists of reduced lithium levels (Perlman, *Lancet* 1990;**335**:416).

Lamotrigine + lithium

Lamotrigine does not cause a significant change in the pharmacokinetics of lithium (n = 20, RCT, 6/7, Chen et al, *Br J Clin Pharmacol* 2000;**50**:193–6).

Levodopa + lithium

Lithium has been used to treat levodopa-induced psychiatric side-effects, e.g. psychosis and mania (n = 1, Braden, *Am J Psychiatry* 1977;**134**:808). Reversible Creutzfeldt-Jakob-like syndrome has also been reported (n = 1, Broussolle et al, *J Neurol Neurosurg Psychiatry* 1989;**52**:686–7).

Levofloxacin + lithium

A case has been reported of severe lithium toxicity (with plasma levels more than doubled) two days after starting levofloxacin in a stable bipolar patient (n = 1, Takahashi et al, *J Clin Psychiatry* 2000;**61**:949–50).

Losartan + lithium

A case has been reported of marked lithium toxicity five weeks after losartan 50 mg/d was added to stable therapy (n = 1, Blanche et al, *Eur J Clin Pharmacol* 1999;**52**:501).

MAOIs + lithium

See MAOIs (*4.3.4*).

METHYLDOPA + LITHIUM

Many cases of rapidly appearing lithium toxicity with normal plasma levels have been reported (e.g. Yassa, *CSAJ* 1986;**134**:141–2).

Metoclopramide + lithium

Enhanced risk of EPSE and of neurotoxicity exists.

Metronidazole + lithium

Cases of toxic lithium levels induced by metronidazole exist (Teicher *et al*, *JAMA* 1987; **257**:3365–6).

Mirtazapine + lithium

See mirtazapine (*4.3.3.4*).

Neuromuscular blocking agents + lithium

A few cases of enhanced blockade have been reported with neostigmine (e.g. Martin and Kramer, *Am J Psychiatry* 1982;**139**:1326–8). Animal studies indicate the possibility of an interaction and so the last dose or two of lithium could be omitted before the use of an NMBA.

NON-STEROIDAL ANTI-INFLAMMATORY DRUGS/COX-2 INHIBITORS + LITHIUM

This is a well-known interaction, probably due to inhibition of renal prostaglandin PGE2 and reduced blood flow. Lithium levels should be monitored frequently if the combination is to be used.

Reviews: NSAIDs (Brouwers and de Smet, *Clin Pharmacokinet* 1994;**27**:462–85), COX-2 (Phelan *et al*, *J Clin Psychiatry* 2003;**64**:1328–34).

Avoid:

- **Indometacin:** lithium levels increased by 61% have been reported (e.g. n = 10, open, Reimann *et al*, *Arch Gen Psychiatry* 1983;**40**:283–6).

Extra care:

- **Ibuprofen:** studies show a variable effect, with a 25% increase in lithium levels possible (e.g. n = 9, open, Ragheb, *J Clin Psychiatry* 1987;**48**:161–3; Bailey *et al*, *South Med J* 1989;**82**:1197). As ibuprofen is available over-the-counter, this interaction should be considered carefully.
- **Diclofenac:** lithium levels may rise by up to 23% (n = 5, Reimann and Frolich, *Clin Pharmacol Ther* 1981;**30**:348–52).
- **Piroxicam:** several cases exist of a slow-onset (e.g. several months) lithium toxicity (e.g. n = 1, Walbridge and Bazire, *Br J Psychiatry* 1985;**147**:206–7).

Care:

- **Azapropazone:** the literature notes the possibility of raised lithium levels.
- **Celecoxib:** several interactions have been reported (e.g. Gunja *et al*, *Intern Med J* 2002; **32**:494), one being life-threatening (Slordal *et al*, *Br J Clin Pharmacol* 2003;**55**: 413–4).
- **Etodolac:** the UK SPC says serum levels of lithium may be increased.
- **Ketoprofen:** raised lithium levels have been reported (n = 1, Singer *et al*, *Therapie* 1981;**36**:323–6).
- **Ketorolac:** lithium levels nearly doubled by ketorolac have been reported (n = 5, Cold *et al*, *J Clin Psychopharmacol* 1998;**18**:33–7).
- **Mefenamic acid:** acute lithium toxicity, possibly with renal damage, has been reported (n = 2, MacDonald and Neale, *Br Med J* 1988;**297**:1339).
- **Meloxicam:** meloxicam 15 mg moderately increases plasma lithium, so plasma levels should be closely monitored (n = 16, Turck *et al*, *Br J Clin Pharmacol* 2000;**50**:197–204).
- **Naproxen:** short-term naproxen has little effect on lithium levels (n = 12, Levin *et al*, *J Clin Psychophamacol* 1998;**18**:237–40), although one study showed some increased lithium levels (n = 7, Ragheb and Powell, *J Clin Psychopharmacol* 1986;**6**:150–4).
- **Phenylbutazone:** doubled lithium levels have been reported (see Ragheb, *J Clin Psychopharmacol* 1990;**10**:49–50).
- **Rofecoxib:** 50 mg/d can increase lithium levels (n = 10, Sajbel *et al*, *Pharmacotherapy* 2001;**21**:380; abstract; n = 1, Lundmark *et al*, *Br J Clin Pharmacol* 2002;**53**:403–4; n = 1, Bravo *et al*, *Ann Pharmacother* 2004;**38**:1189–93).
- **Tiaprofenic acid:** increased serum lithium levels (requiring a dose reduction) occurred in a woman taking fosinopril and lithium to which tiaprofenic acid was added (n = 1, Alderman and Lindsay, *Ann Pharmacother* 1996;**30**:1411–3).

Least risk:

- **Aspirin:** 4 g/d for seven days had no effect on lithium levels in one study (n = 10, open, Reimann *et al*, *Arch Gen Psychiatry* 1983; **40**:283–6), and other studies have only shown a mildly variable effect (e.g. Ragheb, *J Clin Psychiatry* 1987;**48**:425).

- **Sulindac:** reports show either a slightly reduced level of lithium (n = 2, Furnell and Davies, *Drug Intell Clin Pharm* 1986;**19**:374–6), no effect (n = 4, Ragheb and Powell, *J Clin Psychiatry* 1986;**47**:33–4) or raised levels (n = 2, Jones and Stoner, *J Clin Psychiatry* 2000;**61**:527–8).

Oxcarbazepine + lithium
See oxcarbazepine (4.5.6).

Phenytoin + lithium
There are several reports of lithium neurotoxicity, without increased lithium levels (e.g. Raskin, *J Clin Psychopharmacol* 1984;**4**:120).

Potassium iodide + lithium
An additive effect may cause hypothyroidism.

Psyllium + lithium
See Ispaghula husk + lithium.

Quetiapine + lithium
See quetiapine (4.2.6).

Smoking + lithium
See smoking (4.7.4).

Sodium + lithium
Excess sodium (e.g. as bicarbonate in antacids) can reduce lithium levels (e.g. McSwiggan, *Med J Aust* 1978;**1**:38–9) and sodium restriction can lead to lithium intoxication (e.g. Baer et al, *J Psychiatr Res* 1971;**8**:91–105).

Spironolactone + lithium
A rise in lithium levels has been reported (Baer et al, *J Psychiatr Res* 1971;**8**:91–105), as has synergism (see combinations, 1.10).

SSRIs + lithium
See citalopram/escitalopram (4.3.2.1), fluoxetine (4.3.2.2), fluvoxamine (4.3.2.3) and paroxetine (4.3.2.4). No interaction has been seen yet with sertraline.

Tetracyclines + lithium
Cases of lithium intoxication (e.g. McGennis, *Br Med J* 1978;**2**:1183) have been reported so monitor lithium regularly.

THEOPHYLLINE + LITHIUM
Theophylline may reduce lithium levels by 20–30% (Cook et al, *J Clin Psychiatry* 1985;**46**:278–9) as may aminophylline, probably by increased excretion. An increased lithium dose can counteract this so monitoring of levels is essential, especially if theophylline is then stopped. The interaction has been made use of to treat lithium toxicity.

THIAZIDE DIURETICS + LITHIUM
Thiazides reduce the renal clearance of lithium and levels can rise within a few days. Thiazides should only be used where unavoidable and where strict monitoring is used, although it is possible that the effect on lithium is not always dramatic. The combination has occasionally been used in patients where large doses of lithium do not produce therapeutic levels.

- **Bendroflumethiazide** (bendrofluazide): a 24% reduction in lithium excretion has been shown, (Petersen et al, *Br Med J* 1974;**2**:143–5), as has lithium toxicity (n = 1, Vipond et al, *Anesthesia* 1996;**51**:1156–8).
- **Co-amilozide:** single case report (Dorevitch and Baruch, *Am J Psychiatry* 1986;**143**:257–8).
- **Hydrochlorthiazide:** the effect may only be minor (n = 13, RCT, Crabtree et al, *Am J Psychiatry* 1991;**148**:1060–3).
- **Hydroflumethiazide:** one study showed a 24% reduction in lithium excretion (Petersen et al, *Br Med J* 1974;**2**:143–5).
- **Triamterene:** increased lithium clearance may occur (n = 8, open, Wetzels et al, *Nephrol Dial Transplant* 1989;**4**:939–42).

Topiramate + lithium
Elevated and toxic lithium levels have been reported with higher (800 mg/d) doses of topiramate, but not with 500 mg/d (Pinninti and Zelinski, *J Clin Psychopharmacol* 2002;**22**:340; Abraham and Owen, *J Clin Psychopharmacol* 2004;**24**:565–7).

Tricyclics + lithium
See tricyclics (4.3.1).

Trimethoprim + lithium
Lithium toxicity has been reported following addition of trimethoprim (n = 1, de Vries, *Ned Tijdschr Geneeskd* 2001;**145**:539–40).

Triptans + lithium
The literature notes an increased risk of CNS toxicity with sumatriptan.

Valsartan + lithium
There is a report of lithium intoxication with this angiotensin–II antagonist (n = 1, Su et al, *Psychiatry Clin Neurosci* 2007;**61**:204).

Venlafaxine + lithium
See venlafaxine (4.3.3.9).

Warfarin + lithium
No interaction is suspected or reported (mentioned in Sayal et al, *Acta Psychiatr Scand* 2000;**102**:250–5).

Ziprasidone + lithium
See ziprasidone (4.2.8).

4.5 ANTICONVULSANTS

Combining anticonvulsants is a common and essential strategy and so knowledge of interactions is vital, both when adding drugs (or increasing doses) or stopping drugs (or decreasing doses).

Reviews: * detailed review of pharmacokinetic interactions between AEDs (Hachad *et al, Ther Drug Monit* 2002;**24**:91–103), AED–OC interactions (Crawford, *CNS Drugs* 2002; **16**:263–72; concludes that a woman taking carbamazepine, oxcarbazepine, phenobarbital, phenytoin or topiramate, would need an OC with at least 50mcg ethinylestradiol, or Depot Provera given every 10 weeks rather than 12), AEDs and antimicrobials (Desai, *Epilepsia* 2008;49(Suppl 6):47–9), AEDs and chemotherapeutics (Yap *et al, Clin Ther* 2008; **30**:1385–407), P450 interactions with AEDs (Mula, *Curr Drug Metab* 2008;**9**:730–7) and AEDs with other drugs (Díaz *et al, Neurologist* 2008;**14**(6suppl1):S55–65).

4.5.1 CARBAMAZEPINE

Carbamazepine is principally metabolised by CYP3A4 (also CYP2C8), but is also a potent inducer of CYP3A4 and other oxidative mechanisms in the liver. This auto-induction takes up to four weeks to occur, although it is virtually complete after a week. Carbamazepine (CBZ) is metabolised to carbamazepine epoxide (CBZ-E), which may be more toxic than carbamazepine itself and so alteration of the CBZ:CBZ-E ratio by another drug would alter toxicity. Carbamazepine is extensively plasma protein-bound. Major diurnal variations in plasma levels occur, which can be as much as 90% during polytherapy compared to monotherapy (Hoppener *et al, Epilepsia* 1980;**21**:341–50).

Acetazolamide + carbamazepine

CYP3A4 inhibition may raise carbamazepine levels (mentioned in Spina *et al, Clin Pharmacokinet* 1996;**31**:198–214).

Alcohol + carbamazepine

See alcohol (4.7.1).

ANTIPSYCHOTICS + CARBAMAZEPINE *

Antipsychotics lower the seizure threshold, antagonising carbamazepine's anticonvulsant effects and there are also a variety of other well-documented interactions. Carbamazepine reduces **aripiprazole** and metabolite levels by about 70%, probably by CYP3A4 induction, so aripiprazole doses may need to be doubled with carbamazepine, and halved if carbamazepine is discontinued (n=9[c=6], 8/52, Citrome *et al, J Clin Psychopharmacol* 2007;**27**:279–83), although one study did not find a loss of efficacy despite the dramatic level of reductions (n=18, Nakamura *et al, Ther Drug Monit* 2009;**31**:575–8). Lack of interaction has been shown with **asenapine** (US PI). There are cases of **clozapine** levels increasing by up to 100% after carbamazepine was stopped (Raitasuo *et al, Am J Psychiatry* 1993;**150**:169) and of neurotoxicity (n=1, Yerevanian and Hodgman, *Am J Psychiatry* 1985;**142**:785–6). There is also the very real enhanced risk of agranulocytosis (mandatory precaution in SPC), so carbamazepine and clozapine should not be used together (n=1, Gerson, *Lancet* 1991; **338**:262–3). Carbamazepine reduces **haloperidol** levels, with 240mg/d halving haloperidol levels (n=11, Yasui–Furukori *et al, J Clin Psychopharmacol* 2003;**23**:435–40), in a dose-dependent manner, resulting in worsening symptoms and outcome (e.g. n=27, 4/52, Hesslinger *et al, J Clin Psycho–pharmacol* 1999;**19**:310–5). More importantly, a significantly extended QT interval has been shown, probably by increased haloperidol metabolite concentrations. Care is thus needed (n=2, Iwahashi *et al, Am J Psychiatry* 1996;**153**: 135). Carbamazepine increases **olanzapine** clearance by 44% and reduces half-life by 20% (n=47, Linnet and Olesen, *Ther Drug Monit* 2002;**24**:512–7), probably by CYP1A2 induction, but dose adjustment is not needed as olanzapine has a wide therapeutic index (n=11, Lucas *et al, Eur J Clin Pharmacol* 1998; **54**:639–43). Carbamazepine 600–800mg/d may decrease **quetiapine** plasma levels by 80%, presumably by CYP3A4 induction, potentially clinically significant (n=18, Grimm *et al, Br J Clin Pharmacol* 2006;**61**:58–69; n=2, Hasselstrom and Linnet, *Ther Drug Monit* 2004;**26**:486–91), and there is a case of undetectable quetiapine levels with carbamazepine (n=1, Nickl–Jockschat *et al, Clin Neuropharmacol* 2009;**32**:55). Toxic levels of CBZ-E (the toxic CBZ metabolite) raised 3–4-fold have been reported with concurrent quetiapine (n=2, Fitzgerald and Okos, *Pharmacother* 2002; **22**:1500–3). The UK SPC now notes that quetiapine can increase the levels of the metabolite CBZ-epoxide. Carbamazepine may halve plasma levels of **risperidone** and 9-hydroxyrisperidone, probably via 2D6 and 3A4 induction (n = 34, Spina et al, Ther Drug Monit 2000;**22**:481–5; n = 11, Ono et al, Psychopharmacol (Berl) 2002;**162**:50–4), and there are cases of EPSE after carbamazepine was discontinued from a combination with risperidone (n = 2, Takahashi et al, Clin Neuropharmacol 2001;**24**:358–60). Alternatively, risperidone 1 mg/d may increase steady-state carbamazepine levels by 10% over 24 hours and 20% over two weeks (n = 8, Mula and Monaco, Clin Neuropharmacol 2002;**25**:97–100). Carbamazepine causes a substantial reduction in **paliperidone** levels, mostly due to a dose-related increase in renal clearance due to induction of renal P-gp, effect (UK SPC). The Japanese SPC notes that carbamazepine may reduce **zotepine** levels, via CYP3A4 induction. Carbamazepine decreases **ziprasidone** AUC by about 35%, which may require slightly raised doses (n = 25, RCT, 4/52, Miceli et al, Br J Clin Pharmacol 2000;**49**[S3]:65–70).

Antiretrovirals + carbamazepine *

The UK SPC notes the possibility of reduced plasma **indinavir**, **rotinavir** and **saquinavir** levels, probably by 3A4 induction. Carbamazepine toxicity has been reported when **lopinavir/ritonavir** and then **nelfinavir** were added separately to carbamazepine, both increasing CBZ plasma levels by 53%, where reducing CBZ dose by 33% solved the problem (n = 1, Bates and Herman, Ann Pharmacother 2006;**40**:1190–5). Indeed, even a single dose of carbamazepine reduced the half-life of nevirapine (n = 36, open, L'homme et al, J Acquir Immune Defic Syndr 2006;**43**:193–6). Raised carbamazepine levels and toxicity (including hepatic) have been reported with **ritonavir** (n = 1, Kato et al, Pharmacother 2000; **20**:851–4; Antonio et al, Ann Pharmacother 2001;**35**:125–6). **Darunavir** may increase carbamazepine AUC by 45% and carbamazepine a dose reduction of 25–50% is recommended (UK SPC). Carbamazepine significantly reduces **efavirenz** levels and efavirenz significantly reduces carbamazepine (but not CBZ-E) levels (RCT, c/o, open, 6/52, Ji et al, J Clin Pharmacol 2008;**48**:948–56).

Benzodiazepines + carbamazepine

A large study concluded that concomitant clonazepam and carbamazepine results in a 22% increase in clonazepam clearance and a 20% decrease in carbamazepine clearance (n = 183, Yukawa et al, J Clin Psychopharmacol 2001;**21**:588–93), so slightly higher benzodiazepine doses may be needed (Baba et al, Br J Clin Pharmacol 1990;**29**:766–9). Carbamazepine toxicity has occurred after the addition of clobazam (Genton et al, Epilepsia 1998;**39**:1115–8), probably related to progressive increases in norclobazam.

Bupropion + carbamazepine

See bupropion (4.6.6).

Caffeine + carbamazepine

Carbamazepine induces the CYP1A2 metabolism of caffeine (n = 5, Parker et al, Br J Clin Pharmacol 1998;**45**:176–8).

CALCIUM-CHANNEL BLOCKERS + CARBAMAZEPINE

Verapamil increases carbamazepine plasma levels by 50%, via CYP3A4 inhibition (n = 43, open, Bahls et al, Neurology 1991;**41**:740–2). Other evidence, e.g. with **diltiazem** (postoperative ophthalmoplegia and ataxia, n = 1, Wijdicks et al, J Neuroophthalmol 2004;**24**:95) suggests a substantial risk of toxicity. The antihypertensive effect of **nilvadipine** (n = 1, Yasui-Furukori and Tateishi, J Clin Pharmacol 2002;**42**:100–3) and **isradipine** may be reduced. Since no interaction occurs with **nifedipine** (n = 43, open, Bahls et al, Neurology 1991;**41**:740–2), it is the calcium-channel blocker of choice with carbamazepine, although the BNF notes the efficacy of **nifedipine** may be reduced, so care is needed.

Charcoal, activated + carbamazepine

Carbamazepine absorption may be almost completely stopped if activated charcoal is given five minutes after ingestion, with a lesser effect if given after an hour (Neuvonen and Elonen, Eur J Clin Pharmacol 1980;**17**:51–7).

Chinese medicines + carbamazepine

Paeoniae Radix, a traditional Chinese medicine, may increase carbamazepine absorption (in rats, Chen et al, Biol Pharm Bull 2002;**25**:532–5).

CICLOSPORIN + CARBAMAZEPINE

Ciclosporin metabolism is accelerated by carbamazepine, to give reduced plasma levels.

Cisplatin + carbamazepine *

The UK SPC notes that cisplatin might decrease carbamazepine plasma levels.

Citalopram + carbamazepine

See citalopram/escitalopram (4.3.2.1).

Clarithromycin + carbamazepine
See erythromycin + carbamazepine.

Cocaine + carbamazepine
See cocaine (4.7.3).

CORTICOSTEROIDS + CARBAMAZEPINE
Corticosteroid CYP3A4 metabolism is accelerated by carbamazepine, giving a reduced effect (n = 15, open, Bartoszek et al, Clin Pharmacol Ther 1987;**42**:424–32).

DANAZOL + CARBAMAZEPINE
Danazol inhibits carbamazepine metabolism to give an increased effect (n = 6, open, Zielinski et al, Ther Drug Monit 1987;**9**:24–7), so monitor levels and observe for side-effects.

Dantrolene + carbamazepine
Carbamazepine toxicity has been reported when dantrolene and oxybutinin were added to a stable carbamazepine dose (n = 1, Vander et al, Spinal Cord 2005;**43**:252–5).

DEXTROPROPOXYPHENE + CARBAMAZEPINE
Dextropropoxyphene enhances carbamazepine toxicity via CYP3A4 inhibition (e.g. Neurology 1987;**37**[Suppl 1]:87) and levels may rise by 44–77%. In one case, carbamazepine levels increased four-fold over 24 hours and led to cerebellar dysfunction, which resolved over 48 hours (n = 1, Allen, Postgrad Med J 1994;**70**:764). Monitor closely if used together, especially in the elderly (n = 84, open, Bergendal et al, Eur J Clin Pharmacol 1997;**53**:103–6).

Digoxin + carbamazepine
An isolated case exists of bradycardia with digitalis and carbamazepine but not with digoxin.

Disulfiram + carbamazepine
See disulfiram (4.6.8).

Diuretics + carbamazepine
Hyponatraemia may uncommonly occur with furosemide or thiazides (n = 2, Yassa et al, J Clin Psychiatry 1987;**48**:81–3; n = 1, Ranta and Wooten, Epilepsia 2004;**45**:879).

Doxorubicin + carbamazepine *
The UK SPC notes that doxorubicin might decrease carbamazepine plasma levels, and vice versa.

DOXYCYCLINE + CARBAMAZEPINE
Doxycycline metabolism is accelerated by carbamazepine, reducing efficacy and halving half-life (Penttila et al, Br Med J 1974;**2**:470–2). Other tetracyclines appear not to interact.

Enteral feeds + carbamazepine
Carbamazepine suspension absorption has been shown to be slightly slowed and reduced during nasogastric feeding (n = 8, RCT, c/o, Bass et al, Epilepsia 1989;**30**:364–9), so take care with dosing after enteral feeding is stopped.

Escitalopram + carbamazepine
See citalopram/escitalopram (4.3.2.1).

Ethosuximide + carbamazepine
See ethosuximide (4.5.2).

Etretinate + carbamazepine
One girl treated with the combination only responded to etretinate when her carbamazepine was withdrawn (n = 1, Mohammed, Dermatology 1992;**185**:79).

ERYTHROMYCIN + CARBAMAZEPINE
A rapid 100–200% rise in carbamazepine levels has been reported (n = 4, Wroblewski et al, JAMA 1986;**255**:165–7; n = 1, Tatum and Gonzalez, Hosp Pharm 1994;**29**:45) and with IV erythromycin use (Mitsch, Drug Intell Clin Pharm 1989;**23**:878–9), probably via CYP3A4 inhibition. Monitor levels or use an alternative antibiotic. A review of the interaction concluded that the greatest risk is with high doses of both drugs, and least with clarithromycin (Pauwels, Pharmacol Res 2002;**45**:291–8), although clarithromycin can raise CBZ levels significantly, leading to toxicity (n = 10, Gélisse et al, Rev Neurol [Paris] 2007;**163**:1096–9) and hyponatraemia (n = 1, Kanbay et al, South Med J 2007;**100**:222).

Fluconazole + carbamazepine
Fluconazole-induced carbamazepine toxicity has been reported (n = 1, Nair and Morris, Ann Pharmacother 1999;**33**:790–2), with elevated CBZ levels (n = 1, Finch et al, South Med J 2002; **95**:1099–2000; Ulivelli et al, J Neurol 2004;**251**: 622–3).

Fluoxetine + carbamazepine
See fluoxetine (4.3.2.2).

Fluvoxamine + carbamazepine
See fluvoxamine (4.3.2.3).

Gabapentin + carbamazepine
See gabapentin (4.5.3).

Gestrinone + carbamazepine
The UK SPC states that carbamazepine may reduce the activity of gestrinone.

Grapefruit juice + carbamazepine
300 ml grapefruit juice increased carbamazepine levels by 40% and AUC by 41%, probably by CYP3A4 inhibition in the gut wall and liver (n = 10, RCT, Garg et al, Clin Pharmacol Ther 1998; **64**:286–8).

Griseofulvin + carbamazepine

A reduced griseofulvin level by enzyme induction (*Am J Hosp Pharm* 1986;**16**:52) has been postulated.

H2-BLOCKERS + CARBAMAZEPINE

Studies have shown a transient 20% rise in carbamazepine levels with **cimetidine** (n=8, open, 7/7, Dalton et al, *Epilepsia* 1986;**27**:553–8), reduced clearance, prolonged half-life (n=12, open, 8/52, Webster et al, *Eur J Clin Pharmacol* 1984;**27**:341–3) and inhibition of non-renal elimination (n=8, RCT, c/o, Dalton et al, *Epilepsia* 1985;**26**:127–30) via CYP3A4 inhibition. Studies show no interaction with **ranitidine** (e.g. n=8, RCT, Dalton et al, *Drug Intell Clin Pharm* 1985;**19**:941–4), which would thus appear a safer option.

Herbal tea + carbamazepine

For completeness, I thought you'd like to know that rats drinking herbal tea may have raised carbamazepine levels (Thabrew et al, *Drug Metabol Drug Interact* 2003;**19**:177–87).

Honey + carbamazepine

Yes, I was surprised when I saw this too, but you'll be relieved to find there is no interaction (n=10, RCT, c/o, 1/52, Malhotra et al, *Methods Find Exp Clin Pharmacol* 2003;**25**:537–40).

Imatinib + carbamazepine *

Mean trough levels of imatinib are reduced up to 2.9-fold by carbamazepine (n<224, p/c, Pursche et al, *Curr Clin Pharmacol* 2008;**3**:198–203).

Influenza vaccine + carbamazepine

A transient 10% increase in carbamazepine levels occurred in one study (n=55, open, Jann and Fidone, *Clin Pharm* 1986;**5**:817–20), and there is a report of carbamazepine toxicity after influenza vaccination (n=1, Robertson, *Pediatr Neurol* 2002;**26**:61–3).

ISONIAZID + CARBAMAZEPINE

Rapid carbamazepine toxicity may occur via 3A4 inhibition by isoniazid in this potentially serious interaction (Valsalan and Cooper, *Br Med J* 1982;**285**:261–2). It may be potentiated by cimetidine (n=1, Garcia et al, *Ann Pharmacother* 1992;**26**:841–2). Monitor carefully for toxicity.

Isotretinoin + carbamazepine

Isotretinoin may slightly reduce carbamazepine plasma levels and alter the CBZ:CBZ-E ratio (n=1, Marsden et al, *Br J Dermatol* 1988;**119**:403).

Itraconazole + carbamazepine

Sub-therapeutic itraconazole levels may occur with carbamazepine, so monitor for lack of efficacy (n=12, open, Tucker et al, *Clin Infect Dis* 1992;**14**:165–74).

Lacosamide + carbamazepine *

See carbamazepine + lacosamide (*4.5.4*).

Lamotrigine + carbamazepine

See lamotrigine (*4.5.5*).

Lapatinib + carbamazepine *

Carbamazepine decreases lapatinib AUC, Cmax and absorption by 72%, 59% and 28% respectively, probably by CYP3A4 induction, but with no change in half-life (n=24, 20/7, Smith et al, *Br J Clin Pharmacol* 2009;**67**:421–6).

Levetiracetam + carbamazepine

See levetiracetam (*4.5.6*).

Levothyroxine (thyroxine) + carbamazepine

Levothyroxine metabolism is accelerated by carbamazepine, increasing the thyroxine requirements in hypothyroidism.

Lithium + carbamazepine

Although the combination is often used in rapid-cycling bipolar disorder, neurotoxicity may rarely occur without increased plasma levels (Marcoux, *Ann Pharmacother* 1996;**30**:547), and while this is mostly in patients with pre-existing brain damage (n=5, Shukla et al, *Am J Psychiatry* 1984;**141**:1604–6), there is some evidence of minor cognitive impairment with the combination (*Hum Psychopharmacol* 1990;**5**:41–5). An additive anti-thyroid effect can occur, lowering T4 and free T4 levels (n=23, open, Post et al, *Am J Psychiatry* 1990;**147**:615–20) and there is a case of lithium intoxication due to carbamazepine-induced renal failure (n=1, Mayan et al, *Ann Pharmacother* 2001;**35**:560–2). Monitor carefully and regularly for signs of toxicity.

MAOIs + carbamazepine

See MAOIs (*4.3.4*).

Mefloquine + carbamazepine

The SPC states that mefloquine may antagonise the anticonvulsant effect of carbamazepine.

Melatonin + carbamazepine

See melatonin (*4.1.4*).

Methadone + carbamazepine

See methadone (*4.6.10*).

Methylphenidate + carbamazepine

See methylphenidate (*4.6.11*).

Metoclopramide + carbamazepine

There is a report of apparent carbamazepine neurotoxicity occurring after metoclopramide 30 mg/d was added, which resolved when metoclopramide was stopped (n = 1, Sandyk, *Br Med J* 1984;**288**:830).

Metronidazole + carbamazepine

Plasma carbamazepine levels rose by 60% in one case when metronidazole was added, resulting in symptoms of toxicity (n = 1, Patterson, *Ann Pharmacother* 1994;**28**:1304).

Mianserin + carbamazepine

See mianserin (*4.3.3.3*).

Miconazole + carbamazepine

An isolated case report of an adverse response has appeared (n = 1, *Therapie* 1982;**37**:437–41).

Mirtazapine + carbamazepine

See mirtazapine (*4.3.3.4*).

Moclobemide + carbamazepine *

See moclobemide (*4.3.5*).

Modafinil + carbamazepine

See modafinil (*4.6.12*).

Neuromuscular blocking agents + carbamazepine

Studies show reduced responses and recovery times to NMBAs (*Anaesthesiology* 1989;**71**:A784), e.g. vecuronium doses need to be significantly higher in patients on maintenance carbamazepine (n = 8, open, Whalley and Ebrahim, *Br J Anaesth* 1994;**72**:125–6) and recovery times can be 40–60% faster with atracurium and pancuronium (n = 53, open, Tempelhoff et al, *Anesth Analg* 1990;**71**:665–9).

Nicotinamide + carbamazepine *

The UK SPC notes that high-dose nicotinamide can raise CBZ/CBZ-epoxide in adults.

NICOUMALONE + CARBAMAZEPINE

The metabolism of nicoumalone is accelerated by carbamazepine to give a reduced effect.

ORAL CONTRACEPTIVES + CARBAMAZEPINE

The CYP3A4 metabolism of OCs is accelerated by carbamazepine to give a **reduced contraceptive effect** (n = 10, open, Crawford et al, *Br J Clin Pharmacol* 1990;**30**:892–6). Any OC needs to contain at least 50 mcg ethinylestradiol or Depot Provera given every 10 rather than 12 weeks (review by Crawford, *CNS Drugs* 2002; **16**:263–72) or alternative methods used. In the UK, one tablet each of Marvelon® and Mercilon® (Organon), or two tablets of Ovranette® (Wyeth) are often recommended as daily OC.

Orlistat + carbamazepine

A small trial suggested lack of interaction (n = 8, open, 8/52, Hilger et al, *J Clin Psychopharmacol* 2002;**22**:68–70).

Oxcarbazepine + carbamazepine

See oxcarbazepine (*4.5.7*).

Oxybutynin + carbamazepine

See dantrolene + carbamazepine.

Paracetamol + carbamazepine

Co-administration with carbamazepine may reduce the bioavailability of paracetamol (UK SPC) and hepatotoxicity has been reported (n = 1, Parikh et al, *Intern Med J* 2004; **34**:441–2).

Paroxetine + carbamazepine

See paroxetine (*4.3.2.4*).

Phenobarbital + carbamazepine

Phenobarbital induces carbamazepine CYP3A4 metabolism, slightly reducing plasma levels (Christianssen and Dam, *Acta Neurol Scand* 1973;**49**:543–6). Carbamazepine may raise phenobarbital levels but not by a clinically significant amount (d/b, c/o, 4×21/7, Cereghino et al, *Clin Pharmacol Ther* 1975;**18**:733–41).

PHENYTOIN + CARBAMAZEPINE

Phenytoin induces carbamazepine CYP3A4 metabolism, reducing levels, often dramatically (e.g. n = 2, Chapron et al, *Drug Intell Clin Pharm* 1993;**27**:708–11), but with some evidence of increased carbamazepine metabolites in the CSF. Monitoring of CBZ levels is useful, although seizure control may not be affected. Raised carbamazepine levels may result from withdrawal of phenytoin via removal of enzyme induction (n = 2, Chapron et al, *Ann Pharmacother* 1993;**27**:708–11), so carbamazepine levels must be monitored during the de-induction stage to prevent toxicity developing. Raised phenytoin concentrations may occur due to CYP2C19 inhibition (Lakehal et al, *Epilepsy Res* 2002;**52**:79–83) and mean serum levels increase by 35% (some studies by up to 100%), producing neurotoxicity (Browne et al, *Neurology* 1988;**38**:1146–50). The overall clinical effect may be limited but best to monitor the levels of both drugs.

Piperine + carbamazepine *

Piperine (used as a spice and adjuvant in traditional Indian medicines) can significantly raise carbamazepine levels (n = 20, Pattanaik et al, *Phytother Res* 2009;**23**:1281–6).

Pregabalin + carbamazepine

See pregabalin (*4.5.10*).

Primidone + carbamazepine *

The UK SPC notes that primidone can increase the levels of the metabolite CBZ-E.

Probenecid + carbamazepine

Probenecid has a minimal effect on carbamazepine kinetics, but can increase the proportion of CBZ-E via enzyme induction (n = 10, RCT, open, Kim et al, Eur J Clin Pharmacol 2005;**61**:275–80).

Progabide + carbamazepine

Progabide has no effect on carbamazepine levels (n = 24, open, Bianchetti et al, Epilepsia 1987;**28**:68–73), but may slightly increase CBZ-E levels.

PROTON-PUMP INHIBITORS + CARBAMAZEPINE

Carbamazepine induces the CYP3A4 metabolism of omeprazole, but has little or no effect on hydroxylation via CYP2C19 (n = 5, open, Bertilsson et al, Br J Clin Pharmacol 1997;**44**:186–9). Multiple dose omeprazole may decrease carbamazepine clearance by 40% and thus increase levels (Naidu et al, Drug Invest 1994;**7**:8–12). Pantoprazole appears to have no effect on carbamazepine (n = 20, RCT, Huber et al, Int J Clin Pharmacol Ther 1998;**36**:521–4).

Reboxetine + carbamazepine

See reboxetine (4.3.3.6).

RIFAMPICIN + CARBAMAZEPINE

Rapid CYP3A4 induction may lower carbamazepine levels (n = 1, Zolezzi, Am J Psychiatry 2002;**159**:874).

Roxithromycin + carbamazepine

See atorvastatin + carbamazepine.

Rufinamide + carbamazepine

See rufinamide (4.5.11).

Saquinavir + carbamazepine

See protease inhibitors + phenytoin.

Sertraline + carbamazepine

See sertraline (4.3.2.5).

Simethicone + carbamazepine *

There is a report of carbamazepine toxicity after simethicone was started (n = 1, Guneysel et al, J Med Case Reports 2008;**24**:242).

Smoking + carbamazepine

See smoking (4.7.4).

St John's wort + carbamazepine

See St John's wort (4.3.3.10).

Statins + carbamazepine

Transient carbamazepine toxicity has been reported after combination with atorvastatin and roxithromycin (n = 1, Corbin et al, Therapie 2004;**59**:267–9). Carbamazepine reduces the AUC for simvastatin by 75% and the peak by 68%, so increased simvastatin doses would be needed (n = 12, RCT, c/o, Ucar et al, Eur J Clin Pharmacol 2004;**59**:879–82).

Stiripentol + carbamazepine

Stiripentol appears to be a potent inhibitor of CBZ–E formation (n = 14, Tran et al, Clin Pharmacol Ther 2002;**71**:33; Cazali et al, Br J Clin Pharmacol 2003;**56**:526–36).

Tacrolimus + carbamazepine *

Tacrolimus levels have been reduced by 50% (after 11 days) and 70% (after 3/12) by carbamazepine (n = 1, Wada et al, J Heart Lung Transplant 2009;**28**:409–11).

Terfenadine + carbamazepine

There is a case of raised CBZ levels leading to toxicity after starting terfenadine (n = 1, Naranjo = 6, Baath et al, Can J Clin Pharmacol 2006;**13**:228–31).

Theophylline/aminophylline + carbamazepine

Theophylline metabolism is accelerated by carbamazepine to give a reduced effect (Mitchell et al, N Z Med J 1986;**99**:69–70).

Thiazides + carbamazepine

Hyponatremia has been reported with the combination (n = 1, Ranta and Wooten, Epilepsia 2004;**45**:879).

Tiagabine + carbamazepine

See tiagabine (4.5.13).

Tibolone + carbamazepine

The SPC states that carbamazepine may reduce the activity of tibolone.

Topiramate + carbamazepine

See topiramate (4.5.14).

Tramadol + carbamazepine

Carbamazepine may reduce the effectiveness of tramadol.

Trazodone + carbamazepine

Raised carbamazepine levels have been reported with 100mg/d trazodone (n = 1, Romero et al, Ann Pharmacother 1999;**33**:1370).

TRICYCLICS + CARBAMAZEPINE

CBZ may induce the CYP3A4 metabolism of imipramine, doxepin and amitriptyline to give plasma levels reduced by 42–50% (e.g. n = 51, Leinonen et al, J Clin Psychopharmacol 1991;**11**:313–8). This is a common combination and other evidence supports this to be a clinically significant, but not well recognised interaction. However, one study concluded that while the total blood concentration of imipramine drops with carbamazepine, the free fraction remains unchanged, so dose increases may not be necessary (n = 13, Szymura-Oleksiak *et al*, *Psychopharmacology* [Berl] 2001;**154**:38–42).

VALPROATE + CARBAMAZEPINE

Valproate seems to inhibit several carbamazepine metabolic pathways, resulting in raised CBZ-E concentrations (which has led to CBZ-E-induced psychosis, n = 1, McKee *et al*, *Lancet* 1989;**i**:167, and so watch closely for toxicity) but sometimes with unchanged carbamazepine levels (n = 27, Bernus *et al*, *Br J Clin Pharmacol* 1997;**44**:21). In one study, carbamazepine levels fell by about 25% when valproate was added (n = 7, open, Levy *et al*, *Epilepsia* 1984;**25**:338–45). Valproate may also displace carbamazepine from binding sites on plasma proteins (n = 8, open, Macphee, *Br J Clin Pharmacol* 1988;**25**:59–66). Conversely, carbamazepine induces valproate metabolism, reducing plasma levels by about 20% (n = 8, RCT, d/b, c/o, Larkin *et al*, *Br J Clin Pharmacol* 1989;**27**:313–22). This is probably minor but a mean 59% increase in valproate levels can occur on carbamazepine withdrawal (n = 6, open, Jann *et al*, *Epilepsia* 1988;**29**:578–81). Overall, no adjustments in carbamazepine doses are generally necessary, but be aware of the altered metabolite ratio and monitor if clinical symptoms change.

Venlafaxine + carbamazepine

See venlafaxine (*4.3.3.9*).

Vigabatrin + carbamazepine

See vigabatrin (*4.5.15*).

Vincristine + carbamazepine

Carbamazepine significantly increases the clearance of vincristine, probably by CYP3A4 induction (n = 15, open, Villikka *et al*, *Clin Pharmacol Therapeut* 1999;**66**:589–93).

WARFARIN + CARBAMAZEPINE

The metabolism of warfarin is accelerated by carbamazepine, reducing efficacy. Warfarin doses may need to be doubled (n = 5 + 54, Herman *et al*, *Eur J Clin Pharmacol* 2006;**62**:291–6), monitored frequently and reduced carefully if carbamazepine is discontinued (n = 1, Denbow and Fraser, *South Med J* 1990;**83**:981).

Zaleplon + carbamazepine

See zaleplon (*4.1.6*).

Ziprasidone + carbamazepine

See ziprasidone (*4.2.8*).

Zonisamide + carbamazepine

See zonisamide (*4.5.16*).

4.5.2 ETHOSUXIMIDE

Carbamazepine + ethosuximide

Carbamazepine induces ethosuximide's metabolism, reducing plasma levels by about 17% (n = 6, open, 55/7, Warren *et al*, *Clin Pharmacol Ther* 1980;**28**:646–51), although this is probably of minor significance.

Phenytoin + ethosuximide

Phenytoin may reduce ethosuximide plasma levels (n = 198, retrospective, Battion *et al*, *Clin Pharmacokinet* 1982;**7**:176–80).

Sodium oxybate + ethosuximide

See sodium oxybate (*4.6.13*).

Valproate + ethosuximide

Valproate may increase ethosuximide plasma levels by up to 50% via enzyme inhibition, although this may only be a transient effect (n = 6, Pisani *et al*, *Epilepsia* 1984;**25**:229–33), and standard regular monitoring will probably suffice. Adding ethosuximide to valproate may reduce valproate levels by 28% (n = 4) and stopping ethosuximide from an ethosuximide/valproate combination has led to valproate levels rising by 36% (n = 9). The mechanism is unknown (open, Salke–Kellermann *et al*, *Epilepsy Res* 1997;**26**:345–9).

Zotepine + ethosuximide

See anticonvulsants + zotepine (*4.2.9*).

4.5.3 GABAPENTIN

Gabapentin is not metabolised and not protein-bound so there is little chance of an interaction via this mechanism. Excretion is almost completely renal.

Antacids + gabapentin

The antacid 'Maalox' reduces gabapentin levels by 20% when given concurrently. Separating the doses by two hours resulted in only a 5% reduction in levels (Busch *et al*, *Epilepsia* 1993;**34**[Suppl 2]:158), although nothing has been reported with other antacids.

Benzodiazepines + gabapentin

No significant interaction has been noted with clonazepam (n = 127, d/b, p/c, UKGSG, *Lancet* 1990;**335**:1114–7).

Carbamazepine + gabapentin

No significant interaction has been noted (e.g. n = 26, open, Radulovic *et al*, *Epilepsia* 1994; **35**:155–61).

Cimetidine + gabapentin

Cimetidine 1200 mg/d reduces gabapentin clearance by about 10%, which requires no dosage adjustment (Busch *et al*, *Epilepsia* 1993;**34**[Suppl 2]:158).

Levetiracetam + gabapentin

See levetiracetam (*4.5.6*).

Lithium + gabapentin

See lithium (*4.4*).

Oral contraceptives + gabapentin

No change in the kinetics of norethisterone and ethinylestradiol were seen with gabapentin (Busch *et al*, *Epilepsia* 1993;**34**[Suppl 2]:158).

Phenobarbital + gabapentin

One study showed no significant interaction (n = 12, open, 52/7, Hooper *et al*, *Br J Clin Pharmacol* 1991;**31**:171–4).

Phenytoin + gabapentin

Only a slight trend towards an increase in phenytoin levels has been observed (e.g. Graves *et al*, *Pharmacotherapy* 1989;**9**:196), although toxic phenytoin levels have occurred with gabapentin 600 mg/d (e.g. n = 1, Sanchez-Romero *et al*, *Rev Neurol* 2002;**34**:52–3).

Pregabalin + gabapentin

See pregabalin (*4.5.11*).

Valproate + gabapentin

No significant interaction has been noted (n = 127, d/b, p/c, UKGSG, *Lancet* 1990;**335**:1114–7).

Zotepine + gabapentin

See anticonvulsants + zotepine (*4.2.9*).

4.5.4 LACOSAMIDE *

Lacosamide has a low protein binding (< 15%).

Alcohol + lacosamide *

There is no data on the interaction (SPC).

Carbamazepine + lacosamide *

Caution is necessary with this combination as enhanced PR prolongation could occur (SPC). There is no significant pharmacokinetic interaction although lacosamide levels may be reduced by 25% (n = 37, Cawello *et al*, *J Clin Pharmacol* 2010;[in press]).

Class 1 antiarrhythmics + lacosamide *

Caution is necessary with this combination as enhanced PR prolongation can occur (SPC).

Digoxin + lacosamide *

There is no apparent clinically relevant interaction (SPC).

Lamotrigine + lacosamide *

Caution is necessary with this combination as enhanced PR prolongation could occur (SPC).

Metformin + lacosamide *

There is no apparent clinically relevant interaction (SPC).

Omeprazole + lacosamide *

There is no apparent clinically relevant interaction, although lacosamide levels may increase by 19% (SPC).

Oral contraceptives + lacosamide *

There is no apparent clinically relevant interaction (SPC).

Phenobarbital + lacosamide *

There is no significant pharmacokinetic interaction although lacosamide levels may be reduced by 25%.

Phenytoin + lacosamide *

There is no significant pharmacokinetic interaction although lacosamide levels may be reduced by 25%.

Pregabalin + lacosamide *

Caution is necessary with this combination as enhanced PR prolongation can occur (SPC).

Rifampicin + lacosamide *

Rifampicin may induce the metabolism of lacosamide (SPC).

St John's wort + lacosamide *

St John's wort may induce the metabolism of lacosamide (SPC).

Valproate + lacosamide *

There is no significant pharmacokinetic interaction although lacosamide levels may be reduced by 25%.

4.5.5 LAMOTRIGINE

A large naturalistic study showed that lamotrigine levels are lower with co-medication with carbamazepine, ethinylestradiol, fluoxetine, lithium, phenytoin, phenobarbital and topiramate. No other antidepressants or any antipsychotics lowered levels (n = 829, Reimers *et al*, *J Clin Psychopharmacol* 2005;**25**:342–8). Lamotrigine seems to have no effect on P450 enzymes.

Aripiprazole + lamotrigine *

Aripiprazole has no significant effect on lamotrigine (n = 18, open, 2/52, Schieber *et al*, *Hum Psychopharmacol* 2009;**24**:145–52).

Barbiturates + lamotrigine

Lamotrigine has no significant effect on

primidone and phenobarbital (*Epilepsia* 1991;**32** [Suppl 1]:96).

Benzodiazepines + lamotrigine

Lamotrigine has no significant effect on clonazepam (*Epilepsia* 1991;**32**[Suppl 1]:96).

Bupropion + lamotrigine

In a small study, steady–state bupropion 300mg/d had no effect on a single 10mg dose of lamotrigine (n = 12, RCT, Odishaw and Chen, *Pharmacotherapy* 2000;**20**:1448–53).

Carbamazepine + lamotrigine

A higher incidence of CNS side-effects has been noted with the combination (Gilman, *Ann Pharmacother* 1995;**29**:144–51). Toxicity appears more likely to occur when lamotrigine is added to CBZ if the initial CBZ level is high, e.g. greater than 8mg/L, probably via a pharmacodynamic interaction (n = 47, open, Besag *et al, Epilepsia* 1998;**39**:183–7). However, lamotrigine does not seem to raise the levels of CBZ-E and, in fact, may reduce the levels of this active but toxic metabolite (n = 14, open, Eriksson and Boreus, *Ther Drug Monit* 1997;**19**:499–501). Carbamazepine reduces the half-life of lamotrigine from 29 hours to about 15 hours via enzyme induction (n = 23, open, 4/52, Jawad *et al, Epilepsia Res* 1987;**1**:194–201) with clinically important reductions in lamotrigine plasma concentrations reported with carbamazepine (Koch *et al, Eur Psychiatry* 2003;**18**:42). A case of serious lamotrigine rash has been reported after carbamazepine was stopped, presumably as lamotrigine levels increased (n = 1, Surja *et al, J Clin Psychiatry* 2005;**66**:400–1), and there is a case of toxic epidermal necrolysis associated with concomitant use of these two drugs (n = 1, Mansouri *et al, Arch Dermatol* 2005;**141**:788–9).

Citalopram/escitalopram + lamotrigine

See citalopram/escitalopram (*4.3.2.1*).

Clozapine + lamotrigine

See clozapine (*4.2.4*).

Fosphenytoin + lamotrigine

See phenytoin + lamotrigine.

Imatinib + lamotrigine *

Plasma levels of imatinib do not appear to be affected by lamotrigine (n < 224, p/c, Pursche *et al, Curr Clin Pharmacol* 2008;**3**:198–203).

Lacosamide + lamotrigine *

See lamotrigine + lacosamide (*4.5.4*).

Levetiracetam + lamotrigine

See levetiracetam (*4.5.6*).

Lithium + lamotrigine

See lithium (*4.4*).

LOPINAVIR/RITONAVIR (Kaletra®, Abbott) + LAMOTRIGINE

Kaletra® (Abbott) reduced lamotrigine levels by 55%, with a doubling of lamotrigine dose needed to compensate (n = 24, 31/7, van der Lee *et al, Clin Pharmacol Ther* 2006;**80**:159–68).

Olanzapine + lamotrigine

See lamotrigine + olanzapine (*4.2.5*).

ORAL CONTRACEPTIVES + LAMOTRIGINE *

The UK SPC was changed in June 2005 to include advice that lamotrigine reduces the effectiveness of hormonal contraceptives, and OCs may reduce lamotrigine serum levels (52% in AUC and 39% decrease in Cmax for Microgynon 30® [Schering Health]; n = 7, Sabers *et al, Epilepsy Res* 2001;**47**:151–4; see also 33% reduction, n = 24, open, Herzog *et al, Neurology* 2009;**72**:911–4). The advice is:

- In women starting lamotrigine while on OCs, the normal dose escalation should be used.
- In women starting OCs while on lamotrigine, the dose of lamotrigine may need to be increased two-fold (unless taking any drug that induces lamotrigine glucuronidation).
- In women stopping OCs, lamotrigine levels may double, mostly during the first week, a rapid and significant effect (RCT, 2/12, d/b, p/c, c/o, Christensen *et al, Epilepsia* 2007;**48**:484–9), so lamotrigine doses may need to be halved (unless also taking any drug-inducing lamotrigine glucuronidation).

In a controlled study, only the ethinylestradiol component of OCs reduced lamotrigine serum levels, but progestogens did not alter the levels (n = 45, Reimers *et al, Epilepsia* 2005;**46**:1414–7), so advice may need to be considered carefully.

Oxcarbazepine + lamotrigine

See oxcarbazepine (*4.5.7*).

Phenytoin + lamotrigine

Lamotrigine has no effect on phenytoin but phenytoin reduces the half-life of lamotrigine from 29 hours to about 15 hours via enzyme induction (n = 23, open, 4/52, Jawad *et al, Epilepsia Res* 1987;**1**:194–201) by increasing lamotrigine's clearance by 125% (n = 570, chart analysis, Weintraub *et al, Arch Neurol* 2005;**62**:1432–6).

Pregabalin + lamotrigine

See pregabalin (4.5.11).

Risperidone + lamotrigine

See risperidone (4.2.7).

Rufinamide + lamotrigine

See rufinamide (4.5.12).

Sertraline + lamotrigine

Sertraline may increase lamotrigine levels, e.g. sertraline 25mg/d doubled lamotrigine levels in one case and, in another, a 25mg/d dose reduction halved lamotrigine levels, despite a 33% lamotrigine dose increase (n = 2, Kaufman and Gerner, Seizure 1998;**7**:163–5).

Smoking + lamotrigine *

See lamotrigine + smoking (4.7.4).

Topiramate + lamotrigine

Topiramate does not cause a significant change in lamotrigine levels (n = 24, Berry et al, Epilepsia 2002;**43**:818–23) at standard doses (n = 13, open, 22/52, Doose et al, Epilepsia 2003;**44**:917–22).

VALPROATE + LAMOTRIGINE *

Lamotrigine generally has no significant effect on valproate levels (n = 372, open, Mataringa et al, Ther Drug Monit 2002;**24**:631–6) but can potentiate valproate-induced hyper-ammonemic encephalopathy (Fan et al, Prog Neuropsychopharmacol Biol Psychiatry 2008; **32**:1747–8). Valproate inhibits lamotrigine glu-curonidation, doubling plasma levels (n = 38, RCT, Lalic et al, Eur J Drug Metab Pharmacokinet 2009;**34**:92–9), reduced clearance (by 21%), and half-life lengthening from 29 hours to about 59 hours (e.g. n = 570, chart analysis, Weintraub et al, Arch Neurol 2005;**62**:1432–6), probably a dose-dependent (n = 28, open, Kanner and Frey, Neurology 2000;**55**:588–91) rather than concentration-dependent effect (n = 62, open, Gidal et al, Epilepsy Res 2000;**42**:23–31). Lamotrigine should thus start at half the usual dose when used with valproate. The interaction has been used to enhance the effect of both drugs with striking responses in adults and children with intractable epilepsy (Pisani et al, Lancet 1993;**341**:1224). Enhanced ADRs have been reported, e.g. rash (n = 112, open, Faught et al, Epilepsia 1999;**40**:1135–40), disabling postural and action tremor (n = 3, Reutens et al, Lancet 1993;**342**:185–6), lupus (n = 1, Echaniz–Laguna et al, Epilepsia 1999;**40**:1661–3), delirium (n = 1, Mueller and Beeber, Am J Psychiatry 2004;

161:1128–9) and toxic epidermal necrolysis (n = 1, Chang et al, Prog Neuropsychopharmacol Biol Psychiatry 2006;**30**:147–50).

Zonisamide + lamotrigine

See zonisamide (4.5.17).

Zotepine + lamotrigine

See anticonvulsants + zotepine (4.2.9).

4.5.6 LEVETIRACETAM

Levetiracetam has, as yet, no demonstrable drug interactions. It is not bound to plasma proteins, is not extensively metabolised and does not inhibit or induce CYP1A2, 2A6, 2C8/9/10, 2C19, 2D6, 2E1 and 3A4, nor UGT enzymes. A review concluded that there was no need to adjust levetiracetam doses if prescribed with any other AED (n = 590, Perucca et al, Epilepsy Res 2003;**53**:47–56).

Review: Levetiracetam, serum levels and in-fluence of dose and other drugs (n = 297, May et al, Ther Drug Monit 2003;**25**:690–9).

Alcohol + levetiracetam

No data is available.

Carbamazepine + levetiracetam

Lack of pharmacokinetic interaction has been shown, although disabling symptoms consistent with carbamazepine toxicity (but with unchanged levels) have been reported (n = 4, Sisodiya et al, Epilepsy Res 2002;**48**:217–9).

Ciclosporin + levetiracetam

Lack of interaction has been shown in one case (n = 1, Franzoni et al, J Child Neurol 2007; **22**:440–2).

Digoxin + levetiracetam

Lack of pharmacokinetic interaction has been demonstrated (n = 11, RCT, Levy et al, Epilepsy Res 2001;**46**:93–9).

Food + levetiracetam

Levetiracetam absorption is slightly slowed by food, but total absorption remains unchanged.

Gabapentin + levetiracetam

Lack of pharmacokinetic interaction has been demonstrated.

Imatinib + levetiracetam *

Plasma levels of imatinib do not appear to be affected by levetiracetam (n < 224, p/c, Pursche et al, Curr Clin Pharmacol 2008;**3**:198–203).

Lamotrigine + levetiracetam

Lack of pharmacokinetic interaction has been demonstrated.

Oral contraceptives + levetiracetam
Lack of pharmacokinetic interaction has been demonstrated (n = 18, RCT, d/b, c/o, Ragueneau et al, Epilepsia 2002;**43**:697–702).

Phenobarbital + levetiracetam
Lack of pharmacokinetic interaction has been demonstrated.

Phenytoin + levetiracetam
Levetiracetam has no effect on the kinetics of phenytoin (n = 6, open, Browne et al, J Clin Pharmacol 2000;**40**:590–5).

Probenecid + levetiracetam
Probenecid may inhibit the clearance of the primary (inactive) metabolite of levetiracetam, but not of the parent drug.

Valproate + levetiracetam
Lack of pharmacokinetic interaction has been demonstrated (n = 16, open, c/o, Coupez et al, Epilepsia 2003;**44**:171–8).

Warfarin + levetiracetam
Lack of pharmacokinetic interaction has been demonstrated (n = 42, RCT, Ragueneau–Majlessi et al, Epilepsy Res 2001;**47**:55–63).

Zotepine + levetiracetam
See anticonvulsants + zotepine (4.2.9).

4.5.7 OXCARBAZEPINE

Oxcarbazepine and its metabolite MHD inhibit 2C19 and induce 3A4 and 3A5 at higher (n = 4, open, Patsalos et al, Eur J Clin Pharmacol 1990;**39**:187–8), but probably not at lower doses (n = 8, Larkin et al, Br J Clin Pharmacol 1991;**31**:65–71).

Alcohol + oxcarbazepine
Caution should be exercised if alcohol is taken, as additive sedation can occur.

Antipsychotics + oxcarbazepine *
It should be well known that carbamazepine reduces the plasma levels of many antipsychotics. However, as oxcarbazepine seems to have less enzyme-inducing activity when substituted for carbamazepine, it can lead to plasma levels of some antipsychotics (e.g. **haloperidol**, **chlorpromazine** and **clozapine**) increasing by 50–200% over 2–4 weeks (n = 6, Raitasuo et al, Psychopharmacology [Berl] 1994;**16**:115–6). Oxcarbazepine (up to 1200 mg/d), however, may have no effect on **olanzapine** (n = 13) or **risperidone** (n = 12) levels (5/52, Rosaria Muscatello et al, Epilepsia 2005;**46**:771–4). Addition of oxcarbazepine to

amisulpride has been reported to cause NMS (n = 1, Angelopoulos et al, Gen Hosp Psychiatry 2008;**30**:482–4).

Carbamazepine + oxcarbazepine
Addition of oxcarbazepine to carbamazepine has resulted in a 0–22% decrease in carbamazepine levels and a 40% reduction in MHD levels (UK SPC), important perhaps during a switch.

Ciclosporin + oxcarbazepine
Trough ciclosporin levels may fall slightly with oxcarbazepine (n = 1, Rosche et al, Clin Neuropharmacol 2001;**24**:113–6).

Cimetidine + oxcarbazepine
Cimetidine has no effect on the kinetics of oxcarbazepine (n = 8, c/o, Keranen et al, Acta Neurol Scand 1992;**85**:239–42).

Citalopram + oxcarbazepine
Carbamazepine may induce the metabolism and hence reduce plasma levels of citalopram, and when oxcarbazepine is substituted, citalopram plasma levels may rise (n = 2, Leinonen et al, Pharmacopsychiatry 1996;**29**:156–8).

Erythromycin + oxcarbazepine
Erythromycin has no effect on the kinetics of oxcarbazepine (n = 8, c/o, Keranen et al, Acta Neurol Scand 1992;**86**:120–3).

Escitalopram + oxcarbazepine
See citalopram + oxcarbazepine.

Felodipine + oxcarbazepine
Repeated doses of oxcarbazepine reduce felodipine AUC and plasma levels by 28% and 34% respectively, which might slightly reduce its clinical effect (n = 8, open, Zaccara et al, Ther Drug Monit 1993;**15**:39–42).

Fosphenytoin + oxcarbazepine
See phenytoin + oxcarbazepine.

Furosemide + oxcarbazepine
There is a case of acute encephalopathy with this combination (n = 1, Siniscalchi et al, Ann Pharmacother 2004;**38**:509–10).

Imatinib + oxcarbazepine *
Mean trough levels of imatinib are reduced up to 2.9-fold by oxcarbazepine (n < 224, p/c, Pursche et al, Curr Clin Pharmacol 2008;**3**:198–203).

Lamotrigine + oxcarbazepine
There appears to be no significant interaction (n = 47, RCT, s/b, Theis et al, Neuropsychopharmacol 2005;**30**:2269–74), although ADRs may be more common and a retrospective review suggested that lamotrigine plasma levels may fall by 29% and

that reduced lamotrigine doses may be necessary if oxcarbazepine is discontinued (n = 222, May et al, Therap Drug Monit 1999;**21**:175–81).

Lithium + oxcarbazepine

The combination of lithium and oxcarbazepine might theoretically cause enhanced neurotoxicity.

MAOIs + oxcarbazepine

A theoretical risk of interaction exists.

ORAL CONTRACEPTIVES + OXCARBAZEPINE

Oxcarbazepine can produce significant reductions in some OC plasma levels, with some breakthrough bleeding (n = 13, Klosterskov–Jensen et al, Epilepsia 1992;**33**:1149–52; n = 16, RCT, Fattore et al, Epilepsia 1999;**40**:783–7). Any OC needs to contain at least 50 mcg ethinylestradiol, Depot Provera given every 10 rather than 12 weeks (review by Crawford, CNS Drugs 2002;**16**:263–72), or alternative methods used. In the UK, one tablet each of Marvelon® and Mercilon® (Organon), or two tablets of Ovranette® (Wyeth) are often recommended as daily oral contraception.

Phenobarbital + oxcarbazepine

Phenobarbital levels raised by 14% and reduced oxcarbazepine/MHD levels by 30% have been observed with the combination. The clinical significance has not been quantified.

Phenytoin + oxcarbazepine

Doses of oxcarbazepine above 1200 mg/d have been reported to increase phenytoin levels by up to 40% (less than 10% for doses below 1200 mg/d), probably due to CYP2C19 inhibition (Lakehal et al, Epilepsy Res 2002;**52**:79–83) and so close monitoring of phenytoin is essential, especially at higher doses (n = 4, Patsalos et al, Eur J Clin Pharmacol 1990;**39**:187–8).

Propoxyphene + oxcarbazepine

Unlike carbamazepine, propoxyphene has no significant effect on oxcarbazepine kinetics (n = 8, open, Mogensen et al, Acta Neurol Scand 1992;**85**:14–7).

Temozolomide + oxcarbazepine *

Temozolomide does not seem to affect oxcarbazepine pharmacokinetics, although the sample size was small (n = 8, Maschio et al, J Neurooncol 2008;**90**:217–21).

Valproate + oxcarbazepine *

Valproate levels may rise if oxcarbazepine replaces carbamazepine (n = 4, Patsalos et al, Eur J Clin Pharmacol 1990;**39**:187–8), and may need free-valproate levels to detect (n = 1, Xiong

et al, J Clin Psychopharmacol 2008;**28**:472–3). There is also a theoretical increase in the risk of teratogenicity, due to the presence of increased levels of metabolites.

Verapamil + oxcarbazepine

Verapamil can produce a 20% reduction in MHD levels, which could be clinically significant (UK SPC).

Warfarin + oxcarbazepine

Oxcarbazepine does not appear to affect the anticoagulant activity of warfarin (n = 10, 1/52, Kramer et al, Epilepsia 1992;**33**:1145–8).

Zotepine + oxcarbazepine

See anticonvulsants + zotepine (4.2.9).

4.5.8 PHENOBARBITAL AND PRIMIDONE

Alcohol + barbiturates

See alcohol (4.7.1).

ANTICOAGULANTS + BARBITURATES

A well-documented and clinically significant reduction in anticoagulant levels and effects occur with concurrent barbiturates. Doses of the anticoagulant may need to be raised by up to 60% if a barbiturate is started.

ANTIPSYCHOTICS + BARBITURATES

See antipsychotics (4.2.1) and quetiapine (4.2.5).

Benzodiazepines + barbiturates

See benzodiazepines (4.1.1).

Beta-blockers + barbiturates

Plasma levels of **metoprolol** and **propranolol** are reduced by barbiturates (open, Seideman et al, Br J Clin Pharmacol 1987;**23**:267–71), but **timolol** (n = 12, RCT, c/o, Mantyla et al, Eur J Clin Pharmacol 1983;**24**:227–30), **atenolol** and **nadolol** do not appear to be affected.

Bupropion + phenobarbital

See bupropion (4.6.6).

CALCIUM-CHANNEL BLOCKERS + BARBITURATES

Phenobarbital may induce the CYP3A4 metabolism of verapamil (open, Rutledge et al, J Pharmacol Exp Therap 1988;**246**:7–13), diltiazem, isradipine, nicardipine and nifedipine, reducing efficacy and so some care may be needed.

Carbamazepine + phenobarbital

See carbamazepine (4.5.1).

Charcoal, activated + barbiturates

If given within five minutes, activated charcoal can almost completely prevent barbiturate absorption and can be an effective adjunct in overdose treatment (Neuvonen and Elonen, *Eur J Clin Pharmacol* 1980;**17**:51–7).

Chloramphenicol + barbiturates

Chloramphenicol metabolism is accelerated by barbiturates to reduce oral chloramphenicol efficacy (n = 1, Koup *et al*, *Clin Pharmacol Ther* 1978;**24**:571–5).

CICLOSPORIN + PHENOBARBITAL

Even low dose phenobarbital induces the CYP3A4 metabolism of ciclosporin (Carstensen, *et al*, *Br J Clin Pharmacol* 1986;**21**:550–1).

Cimetidine + phenobarbital

Reduced actions of both can occur but this is of very limited significance (n = 8, open, 6/52, Somogyi *et al*, *Eur J Clin Pharmacol* 1981;**19**:343).

Clozapine + phenobarbital

See clozapine (4.2.3).

CORTICOSTEROIDS + PHENOBARBITAL

CYP3A4 induction reduces the effect of some corticosteroids (Brooks *et al*, *NEJM* 1972;**286**:1125–8).

Digoxin + phenobarbital

Digitoxin (but not digoxin) levels can be reduced by up to 50% by phenobarbital, probably via enzyme induction and is of little significance (Kaldor *et al*, *Int J Clin Pharmacol Biopharm* 1975;**12**:403–7).

Disopyramide + phenobarbital

Barbiturates induce the CYP3A4 metabolism of disopyramide, reducing plasma levels (n = 14, open, Kapil *et al*, *Br J Clin Pharmacol* 1987;**24**:781–91).

Doxorubicin + phenobarbital

Indirect results from one study showed that doxorubicin clearance may be increased by barbiturates and so doses may need to be increased (Riggs *et al*, *Clin Pharmacol Ther* 1982;**31**:263).

Doxycycline + phenobarbital

Doxycycline levels are reduced via CYP3A4 induction, reducing its effect, with a halved half-life (Neuvonen and Penttila, *Br Med J* 1974;**2**:535–6). Other tetracyclines appear not to interact.

Ethosuximide + phenobarbital

A possible interaction may lead to reduced phenobarbital effectiveness. A study showed that ethosuximide levels may fall if primidone is used (n = 198, Battino *et al*, *Clin Pharmacokinet* 1982;**7**:176–80).

Fenoprofen + phenobarbital

Phenobarbital may slightly increase fenoprofen metabolism and reduce its efficacy (Helleberg *et al*, *Br J Clin Pharmacol* 1974;**1**:371).

Furosemide + phenobarbital

One study showed no effect of barbiturates on furosemide's diuretic effect (n = 10, open, Lambert *et al*, *Clin Pharmacol Ther* 1983;**34**:170–5).

Gabapentin + phenobarbital

See gabapentin (4.5.3).

Glyceryl trinitrate + phenobarbital

A reduced nitrate effect via enzyme induction may occur.

Griseofulvin + phenobarbital

Cases have been reported of griseofulvin levels reduced by up to 45% by phenobarbital, either by enzyme induction (e.g. *Am J Hosp Pharm* 1986; **16**:52) or reduced absorption.

Indinavir + barbiturates

The plasma levels of indinavir may be reduced by barbiturates via CYP3A4 induction.

Influenza vaccine + phenobarbital

A transient 20% rise in barbiturate levels has been reported (n = 35, open, Jann and Fidone, *Clin Pharm* 1986;**5**:817–20).

Isoniazid + primidone

Steady state primidone levels rose by 80% in a patient given isoniazid 300 mg/d (n = 1, Sutton and Kupferberg, *Neurology* 1975;**25**:1179–81). Blood levels should be monitored.

Ketoconazole + phenobarbital

A case exists of reduced ketoconazole levels in a man taking phenobarbital (n = 1, *Antimicrob Ag Chemother* 1982;**21**:151–8).

Lacosamide + phenobarbital *

See phenobarbital + lacosamide (4.5.4).

Lamotrigine + phenobarbital

See lamotrigine (4.5.5).

Levetiracetam + phenobarbital

See levetiracetam (4.5.6).

Levonorgestrel + phenobarbital

There is a case of a levonorgestrel implant (Norplant) failing twice in a woman also taking phenobarbital (n = 1, Shane–McWhorter *et al*, *Pharmacotherapy* 1998;**18**:1360–4).

Levothyroxine (thyroxine) + barbiturates

Levothyroxine metabolism is accelerated by barbiturates to give a reduced effect and this may increase requirements in hypothyroidism.

Lidocaine + barbiturates

Serum lidocaine levels may be lower in people taking barbiturates (LeLorier, *Toxicol Appl Pharmacol* 1978;**44**:657), via CYP3A4 induction.

MAOIs + phenobarbital

See MAOIs (4.3.4).

Memantine + phenobarbital
See memantine (4.6.9).

Methadone + phenobarbital
See methadone (4.6.10).

Methyldopa + phenobarbital
Methyldopa levels are not reduced by phenobarbital (Kristensen *et al*, *Br Med J* 1973; **1**:49).

Metronidazole + phenobarbital
One study showed metronidazole metabolism to be accelerated by barbiturates, reducing levels by a third (*Clin Pharmacol Ther* 1987;**41**:235).

Modafinil + phenobarbital
See modafinil (4.6.12).

Nicotinamide + primidone
There are reports of reduced conversion from primidone to phenobarbital (n = 1, Bourgeois *et al*, *Neurology* 1982;**32**:1122).

NICOUMALONE + BARBITURATES
Nicoumalone metabolism is accelerated by barbiturates, giving a reduced anticoagulant effect.

ORAL CONTRACEPTIVES + PHENOBARBITAL
Contraceptive failure via CYP3A4 induction is well-established (e.g. n = 5, Back *et al*, *Contraception* 1980;**22**:495–503). Use higher dose OC (equivalent to at least 50 mcg ethinylestradiol), Depot Provera given every 10 rather than 12 weeks (Crawford, *CNS Drugs* 2002;**16**:263–72) and adjust the dose if necessary, or use alternative contraceptive methods. See also levonorgestrel. In the UK, one tablet each of Marvelon® and Mercilon® (Organon) or two tablets of Ovranette® (Abbott) are often recommended as daily oral contraception.

Oxcarbazepine + phenobarbital
See oxcarbazepine (4.5.7).

Paracetamol + phenobarbital
An isolated case of enhanced hepatotoxicity exists (Pirotte, *Ann Int Med* 1984;**101**:403).

Paroxetine + phenobarbital
See paroxetine (4.3.2.4).

Pethidine + phenobarbital
Severe CNS sedation with the combination has been reported (n = 12, open, c/o, Stambaugh *et al*, *J Clin Pharmacol* 1978;**18**:482–90).

Phenylbutazone + phenobarbital
Reduced levels of phenylbutazone may occur (Levi *et al*, *Lancet* 1968;i:1275).

Phenytoin + phenobarbital
See barbiturates + phenytoin (4.5.9).

Pregabalin + phenobarbital
See pregabalin (4.5.11).

Pyridoxine + phenobarbital
Large doses of pyridoxine (e.g. 200 mg/d) can reduce phenobarbital levels by up to 40–50% (Hansson and Sillanpaa, *Lancet* 1976;i:256).

Quetiapine + phenobarbital
See quetiapine (4.2.5).

Quinidine + phenobarbital
CYP3A4 induction may reduce quinidine levels by up to 50% (Rogers and Blackman, *Drug Intell Clin Pharm* 1983;**17**:819–20).

Reboxetine + phenobarbital
See reboxetine (4.3.3.6).

Rifampicin + barbiturates
Rifampicin can induce barbiturate metabolism, so a decreased efficacy might be predicted (for effect on hexobarbital: n = 40, open, See Richter *et al*, *Eur J Clin Pharmacol* 1980;**17**:197–202).

Rufinamide + phenobarbital
See rufinamide (4.5.12)

Smoking + phenobarbital
See smoking (4.7.4).

St John's wort + phenobarbital
See St John's wort (4.3.3.10).

Testosterone + phenobarbital
A reduced steroid effect can occur via CYP3A4 induction.

THEOPHYLLINE + BARBITURATES
Theophylline metabolism is accelerated by barbiturates in premature neonates, giving a reduced effect (n = 24, Kandrokas *et al*, *Ther Drug Monit* 1990;**12**:139–43).

Tiagabine + phenobarbital
See tiagabine (4.5.13).

Topiramate + phenobarbital
See topiramate (4.5.14).

TRICYCLICS + BARBITURATES
See tricyclics (4.3.1).

Tropisetron + phenobarbital
Phenobarbital reduces the plasma levels of tropisetron (BNF).

VALPROATE + PHENOBARBITAL
Valproate may reduce glucuronidation and increase phenobarbital plasma concentrations by up to 25% (mean of 5.87 mg/L, n = 20, Bernus *et al*, *Br J Clin Pharmacol* 1994;**38**:411–6), increasing sedation and other side-effects (e.g. Kapetanovic *et al*, *Clin Pharmacol Ther* 1981;**99**:314), although this may only be transient (review by Keys, *Drug Intell Clin Pharm* 1982;**16**:737–9). Reduce phenobarbital dosage if sedation occurs, and monitor blood levels regularly.

Vigabatrin + phenobarbital
See vigabatrin (4.5.16).
WARFARIN + PHENOBARBITAL
See anticoagulants + barbiturates in this section.
Zaleplon + phenobarbital
See zaleplon (4.1.6).
Zotepine + phenobarbital
See anticonvulsants + zotepine (4.2.9)

4.5.9 PHENYTOIN

Phenytoin has a narrow therapeutic index and is prone to drug–drug interactions via several mechanisms. It is primarily metabolised by 2C9, secondary is 2C19, with genetic polymorphism affecting levels. It is extensively bound to plasma proteins, induces CYP3A4 and has a saturable metabolism. It can be displaced, giving an increased proportion of free active phenytoin, significant where TDM just measures total phenytoin rather than the proportion of free (hence active) phenytoin. Measuring free phenytoin levels may be more appropriate in certain circumstances, e.g. interactions with drugs displacing it from binding sites, as well as hypoalbuminaemia and renal failure, e.g. total plasma levels may be within the alleged therapeutic range. Decreased protein binding produces a decline in total concentration, but no change in free levels (Wilkinson, *Pharmacol Rev* 1987;**39**:1–47).

Thus, low concentrations may appear below the normal therapeutic range, but free (active) levels are appropriate, prompting inappropriately increased doses or discontinuation. More usual concentrations could have toxic (seizure-inducing) free levels, which might provoke an increase in dosage to bring it into the 'optimum' range (see Toler, *Ann Pharmacother* 1994;**28**:808–9).
Review: pharmacokinetic interactions (Nation *et al*, *Clin Pharmacokinet* 1990;**18**:37–60).
Acetazolamide + phenytoin
Case reports indicate that acetazolamide may enhance the osteomalacia secondary to phenytoin use in a few patients (n = 2, Mallette, *Arch Intern Med* 1977;**137**:1013).
ALCOHOL + PHENYTOIN
See alcohol (4.7.1).
Allopurinol + phenytoin
Phenytoin toxicity may occur with repeated high-dose allopurinol (Ogiso *et al*, *J Pharmacobiodyn* 1990;**13**:36–43).

AMIODARONE + PHENYTOIN
Amiodarone reduces phenytoin metabolism, toxicity developing over two weeks (n = 7, open, 8/52, Nolan *et al*, *Am J Cardiol* 1990;**65**:1252–7), so reduce the phenytoin dose by at least 25%.
Anaesthetics + phenytoin
Documentation of an interaction is limited but case reports exist of phenytoin toxicity following halothane (Karlin and Kutt, *J Pediatr* 1970;**76**:941–4) and so caution is needed.
Antacids + phenytoin
Antacids probably reduce phenytoin levels, shown in several studies (e.g. n = 6, McElnay *et al*, *Br J Clin Pharmacol* 1982;**13**:501) and seizure control could be impaired. It is thus best to separate doses by about three hours or use ranitidine (see also cimetidine).
ANTIPSYCHOTICS + PHENYTOIN
See antipsychotics (4.2.1), clozapine (4.2.34), quetiapine (4.2.6), risperidone (4.2.7) and zotepine (4.2.9).
ANTIRETROVIRALS + PHENYTOIN
Phenytoin increases lopinavir clearance, and lopinavir and ritonavir reduce phenytoin levels through 2C9 induction (n = 24, Lim *et al*, *J Acquir Immune Defic Syndr* 2004;**36**:1034–40). A similar effect on reducing levels occurs with **efavirenz** (Spak *et al*, *AIDS* 2008;**22**:164–5), indinavir (BNF) and nevirapine (n = 36, open, L'homme *et al*, *J Acquir Immune Defic Syndr* 2006;**43**:193–6).
Atomoxetine + phenytoin
See atomoxetine (4.6.4).
Ayurvedic herbal mixtures + phenytoin
See shankhapushpi + phenytoin.
Barbiturates + phenytoin
At normal doses it is thought that phenobarbital induces the metabolism of phenytoin, reducing plasma levels, but the clinical effect is probably minimal (n = 6, open, Browne *et al*, *Neurology* 1988;**38**:639–42). Phenytoin serum levels are increased by very high dose barbiturates and the effect may be dose-dependent with a curvilinear relationship (n = 1, Kuranari *et al*, *Ann Pharmacother* 1995;**29**:83–4). Care is also needed if phenobarbital is stopped, as phenytoin levels may change. Phenytoin may raise phenobarbital levels by up to 100%, resulting in increased sedation, probably of minor clinical significance (n = 1, Porro *et al*, *Br J Clin Pharmacol* 1982;**14**:294–7) but regular monitoring should still be done, especially as a case of fatal agranulocytosis has

been reported with the combination (n=1, Laurenson *et al*, *Lancet* 1994;**344**:32–3).

Benzodiazepines + phenytoin

Diazepam, clonazepam and chlordiazepoxide have been reported to potentiate phenytoin leading to possible intoxication (e.g. n=1, Murphy and Wilbur, *Ann Pharmacother* 2003;**37**:659–63), although some studies have not shown this effect. It is best to monitor phenytoin plasma levels regularly. Conversely, phenytoin induces the metabolism of clonazepam, reducing levels by up to 50% (n=27, open, Sjo *et al*, *Eur J Clin Pharmacol* 1975;**8**:249–54).

Bupropion + phenytoin

See bupropion (4.6.6).

Buspirone + phenytoin

See buspirone (4.1.2).

Calcium-channel blockers + phenytoin

High dose diltiazem (720mg/d) increases phenytoin levels, and in one patient a 40% reduction in phenytoin dose was needed to stabilise levels (n=2, Clarke *et al*, *Pharmacotherapy* 1993;**13**:402–5; n=43, Bahls *et al*, *Neurology* 1991;**41**:740–2). Isradipine can raise phenytoin levels, producing toxicity probably by P450 inhibition (n=1, Cachat and Tufro, *Ann Pharmacother* 2002;**36**:1399–402). Lack of interaction between nifedipine and phenytoin has been noted in several studies (e.g. n=8, open, Schellens *et al*, *Br J Clin Pharmacol* 1991;**31**:175–8), although tremor, headache and restlessness with phenytoin levels tripled has been reported, falling to normal after nifedipine was discontinued (n=1, Ahmad *et al*, *J Am Coll Cardiol* 1984;**3**:1581). Verapamil may inhibit phenytoin metabolism (*Neurology* 1991;**41**:740–2). Almost complete lack of verapamil absorption (at up to 400mg/d) has been reported (n=1, Woodcock *et al*, *N Engl J Med* 1991;**325**:1179). The effects of isradipine and nicardipine may be reduced by phenytoin.

CARBAMAZEPINE + PHENYTOIN

See carbamazepine (4.5.1).

Charcoal, activated + phenytoin

Phenytoin absorption is almost completely (98%) prevented if activated charcoal is taken within five minutes and reduced by about 80% if given after one hour (n=6, open, c/o, Neuvonen *et al*, *Eur J Clin Pharmacol* 1978;**13**:213–8). Multiple-dose activated charcoal has been used successfully over several days for phenytoin toxicity

secondary to hepatitis and, extraordinarily, may have some use even up to a week after phenytoin ingestion (n=1, Howard *et al*, *Ann Pharmacother* 1994;**28**:201–3).

Chinese medicines + phenytoin

Phenytoin poisoning after using Chinese proprietary medicines has been reported (n=1, Lau *et al*, *Hum Experimental Toxicol* 2000;**19**:385–6).

Chloral + phenytoin

Dichloralphenazone has been shown to decrease phenytoin levels (n=5, Riddell *et al*, *Br J Clin Pharmacol* 1980;**9**:118P), although whether the chloral part of the molecule was responsible for this is not known.

CHLORAMPHENICOL + PHENYTOIN

Phenytoin toxicity may occur with oral chloramphenicol via enzyme inhibition (*Aust J Hosp Pharm* 1987;**17**:51–3). This is an uncommon combination but a well-documented and serious interaction. Monitor very carefully if the combination has to be used.

Chlorphenamine + phenytoin

Two isolated cases exist of phenytoin intoxication (Pugh *et al*, *Br J Clin Pharmacol* 1975;**2**:173–5) and so care may be needed.

CICLOSPORIN + PHENYTOIN

Ciclosporin levels can be reduced by 80% by phenytoin, via increased metabolism (n=6, Freeman *et al*, *Br J Clin Pharmacol* 1984; **18**: 887–93).

Ciprofloxacin + phenytoin

Raised phenytoin levels have been predicted. Raised phenytoin levels from oral ciprofloxacin have been reported (n=1, Hull, *Ann Pharmacother* 1993;**27**:1283). However, IV ciprofloxacin has led to halved phenytoin levels (n=1, *Int Pharm J* 1992;**6**:109), and resulted in sub-therapeutic levels, seizures and increased phenytoin dose requirements (Dillard *et al*, *Ann Pharmacother* 1992;**26**:263; n=1, Brouwers and de Boer, *Ann Pharmacother* 1997;**31**:498). There is a case of a phenytoin dose increased during ciprofloxacin therapy, only for toxic levels to appear when the antibiotic course was completed (n=1, Pollak and Slayter, *Ann Pharmacother* 1997;**31**:61–4). More frequent phenytoin plasma level monitoring would be wise.

Clinafloxacin + phenytoin

Higher steady state phenytoin levels have been reported with clinafloxacin (Randinitis *et al*, *Drugs* 1999;**58**[Suppl 2]:254–5).

CLOZAPINE + PHENYTOIN

See clozapine (4.2.4).

CORTICOSTEROIDS + PHENYTOIN

Steroid metabolism is accelerated by phenytoin to give a reduced effect (McLelland and Jack, Lancet 1978;i:1096–7) and so higher doses may be needed. Hydrocortisone may be less affected than other steroids. Phenytoin levels may also be changed.

Co-trimoxazole + phenytoin

Raised phenytoin levels have been reported with co-trimoxazole (n = 1, Gillman and Sandyk, Arch Intern Med 1985;**102**:559).

DEXAMETHASONE + PHENYTOIN

Phenytoin levels may be halved by dexamethasone (e.g. n = 1, Lackner, Pharmacother 1991;**11**:344–7; n = 1, Griffiths and Taylor, Can J Hosp Pharm 1999;**52**:96–8) and very high doses of phenytoin may be necessary (e.g. 900mg/d) to maintain levels (case and review by Recueno et al, Ann Pharmacother 1995;**29**:935). Regular and frequent monitoring of phenytoin levels is thus essential.

Dexibuprofen + phenytoin

Phenytoin acute neurological toxicity has been reported with the combination (n = 1, Llinares–Tello et al, Med Clin [Barc] 2007;**128**:239).

Dextropropoxyphene + phenytoin

See propoxyphene + phenytoin.

DIAZOXIDE + PHENYTOIN

Reduced phenytoin levels occur via increased metabolism (Turck et al, Presse Med 1986;**15**:31) so monitor carefully.

DICOUMAROL + PHENYTOIN

Phenytoin levels may rise rapidly by over 100% (Hansen et al, Acta Med Scand 1971;**189**:15–9) via enzyme inhibition. Avoid the combination if at all possible or monitor very carefully.

Digoxin + phenytoin

Phenytoin reduces digoxin half-life by 30% (n = 6, RCT, open, c/o, Rameis et al, Eur J Clin Pharmacol 1985;**29**:49–53) so monitor both carefully.

DISOPYRAMIDE + PHENYTOIN

Phenytoin reduces the plasma levels of disopyramide, possibly to below therapeutic levels (Kessler et al, Clin Pharm 1982;**1**:263–4).

Disulfiram + phenytoin

Phenytoin toxicity and delirium may occur via enzyme inhibition (e.g. n = 1, Brown et al, Ann Emerg Med 1983;**12**:310–3).

Dopamine + phenytoin

Hypotension may occur in patients on dopamine if phenytoin is added (n = 5, Bivins et al, Arch Surg 1978;**113**:245–9), although lack of interaction has been reported in a well studied case (n = 1, Torres et al, Ann Pharmacother 1995;**29**:1300–1).

Doxifluridine + phenytoin

Elevated phenytoin levels have been reported (n = 1, Konishi et al, Ann Pharmacother 2002;**36**:831–4).

DOXYCYCLINE + PHENYTOIN

Doxycycline metabolism is accelerated by phenytoin to give a reduced effect, with a halved half-life (Penttila et al, Br Med J 1974;ii:470). Other tetracyclines appear not to interact, so make dosage adjustments or use an alternative.

Enteral feeds + phenytoin

See nasogastric feeds + phenytoin.

Ethosuximide + phenytoin

See ethosuximide (4.5.2).

FLUCONAZOLE + PHENYTOIN

Oral fluconazole inhibits phenytoin metabolism producing rapid and severe toxicity (Mitchell and Holland, Br Med J 1989;**298**:1315; reviewed by Cadle et al, Ann Pharmacother 1994;**28**:191–5). Continuous phenytoin plasma monitoring is recommended with fluconazole doses of 200mg/d or above (n = 20, RCT, p/c, Blum et al, Clin Pharmacol Ther 1991;**49**:420–5).

Fluorouracil + phenytoin

Cases exist of elevated phenytoin levels 11 weeks after starting fluorouracil and leucovorin, possibly via CYP2C9 inhibition (n = 1, Gilbar and Brodribb, Ann Pharmacother 2001;**35**:1367–70; n = 1, Rosemergy and Findlay, N Z Med J 2002; **115**:U124).

FLUOXETINE + PHENYTOIN

Phenytoin levels raised by 66% have been reported two weeks after fluoxetine was added, with levels falling back to nearly normal within a week of stopping fluoxetine (n = 1, Woods et al, N Z Med J 1994;**107**:19). Conversely, loss of phenytoin efficacy as a result of fluoxetine discontinuation has been reported (n = 1, Shad and Preskorn, J Clin Psychopharmacol 1999;**19**:471).

FLUVOXAMINE + PHENYTOIN

Fluvoxamine may triple phenytoin levels with associated toxicity, probably by 2C9/19 inhibition (n = 1, Mamiya et al, Ther Drug Monit 2001;**23**:75–7).

Folic acid + phenytoin

Serum folate decreases when phenytoin is started and folic acid supplementation is usually used to counteract this folate deficiency. However, folic acid supplementation in folate-deficient patients changes the kinetics of phenytoin and plasma phenytoin levels are then reduced (n=4, open, Berg et al, Ther Drug Monit 1983;**5**:389–99). Folate supplementation should thus be started with phenytoin. If started later, phenytoin levels should be monitored and changes in seizure activity looked for (extensive review by Lewis et al, Ann Pharmacother 1995;**29**:726–35).

Furosemide + phenytoin

The diuretic effect may be reduced by up to 50% by phenytoin (e.g. Bissoli et al, Recenti Prog Med 1996;**87**:227–8), so larger doses may be needed.

Gabapentin + phenytoin

See gabapentin (4.5.3).

Gefitinib + phenytoin *

Phenytoin decreases the anticancer drug gefitinib's levels by about 26% (n=18, RCT, open, c/o, Chhun et al, Br J Clin Pharmacol 2009;**68**:226–37).

Gingko biloba + phenytoin

There is a case of a fatal seizure with the combination, probably due to reduced phenytoin levels via CYP2C19 induction (n=1, Kupiec and Raj, J Anal Toxicol 2005;**29**:755–8).

Glucagon + phenytoin

Patients on phenytoin may get false negatives with glucagon stimulation tests.

Glucocorticoids + phenytoin

A reduced steroid effect via enzyme induction is possible.

Griseofulvin + phenytoin

It is postulated that reduced griseofulvin levels may occur via enzyme induction (Am J Hosp Pharm 1986;**16**:52).

H2-blockers + phenytoin

Phenytoin toxicity has occurred with cimetidine (n=1, Phillips and Hansky, Med J Aus 1984; **141**:602), with a 30% increase in phenytoin levels in other reports (Pharm Int 1985;**6**:223–4; n=9, open, Salem et al, Epilepsia 1983;**24**:284–8) and so toxicity may occur, even with OTC cimetidine (n=9, Rafi et al, Ann Pharmacother 1999;**33**:769–74). The effect is rapid and can occur within two days. An alternative is ranitidine, where lack of interaction has been shown (e.g. Watts et al, Br J Clin Pharmacol 1983;**15**:499–500), although there have been reports of elevated phenytoin levels (e.g. Tse et al, Ann Pharmacother 1993;**27**:1448–51), including one case where oral ranitidine

produced toxic phenytoin levels, which remained high for a week even though the phenytoin was stopped, and only dropped when the ranitidine was also stopped (Tse and Iagmin, Ann Intern Med 1994;**120**:892–3). It is best to monitor phenytoin levels or use an alternative, e.g. famotidine (n=10, RCT, open, c/o, Sambol et al, Br J Clin Pharmacol 1989;**27**:83–7) or nizatidine (Bachmann et al, Br J Clin Pharmacol 1993;**36**:380–2).

Imatinib + phenytoin *

Mean trough levels of imatinib are reduced up to 2.9-fold by phenytoin (n<224, p/c, Pursche et al, Curr Clin Pharmacol 2008;**3**:198–203).

Influenza vaccine + phenytoin

This is reported to reduce total and free phenytoin levels (Smith et al, Clin Pharm 1988;**7**:828–32), although one study showed only a transient 60% increase in levels (Jann and Fidone, Clin Pharm 1986;**5**:817–20).

Irinotecan + phenytoin

Phenytoin appears to decrease plasma levels of irinotecan (Murry et al, J Pediatr Hematol Oncol 2002;**24**:130–3).

ISONIAZID + PHENYTOIN

Phenytoin toxicity may occur via enzyme inhibition (n=1, Witmer and Ritschel, Drug Intell Clin Pharm 1984;**18**:483–6), so observe for toxicity and reduce phenytoin doses if necessary.

KETOCONAZOLE + PHENYTOIN

Phenytoin toxicity may occur via enzyme inhibition. Ketoconazole may also have a reduced effect.

Lacosamide + phenytoin *

See phenytoin + lacosamide (4.5.4).

Lamotrigine + phenytoin

See lamotrigine (4.5.5).

Levetiracetam + phenytoin

See levetiracetam (4.5.6).

Levodopa + phenytoin

Levodopa can be completely antagonised by phenytoin (Mendez et al, Arch Neurol 1975; **32**:44–6), and so increased levodopa doses may be necessary.

Levothyroxine (thyroxine) + phenytoin

Levothyroxine metabolism is accelerated by phenytoin, increasing requirements (Blackshear et al, Ann Int Med 1983;**99**:341–2).

Lidocaine + phenytoin

Phenytoin's central effects may be enhanced if used with lidocaine (Karlsson et al, Eur J Clin Pharmacol 1974;**7**:455–9). Sinoatrial arrest has been reported (Wood, Br Med J 1971;i:645) which was reversed by isoproterenol. The mechanism is probably enhanced cardiac depression.

Lithium + phenytoin
See lithium (4.4).

Losartan + phenytoin
Losartan has no effect on phenytoin, but losartan levels may rise via 2C9 inhibition (n = 16, RCT, c/o, Fischer et al, Clin Pharmacol Ther 2002; **72**:238–46).

Memantine + phenytoin
See memantine (4.6.9).

Methadone + phenytoin
See methadone (4.6.10).

Methotrexate + phenytoin
An increased antifolate effect with phenytoin may occur.

Methylphenidate + phenytoin
See methylphenidate (4.6.11).

METRONIDAZOLE + PHENYTOIN
Mild phenytoin toxicity via enzyme inhibition is possible (Blyden et al, J Clin Pharmacol Ther 1988; **28**:240–5).

MEXILITINE + PHENYTOIN
Mexilitine levels are reduced by up to 50% via enzyme induction so adjust dosage as necessary (n = 6, open, Begg et al, Br J Clin Pharmacol 1982;**14**:219–23).

MICONAZOLE + PHENYTOIN
Phenytoin toxicity via enzyme inhibition has been reported (n = 2, Rolan et al, Br Med J 1983; **287**:1760).

Mirtazapine + phenytoin
See mirtazapine (4.3.3.4).

Modafinil + phenytoin
See modafinil (4.6.12).

Nasogastric feeds + phenytoin
Reduced phenytoin levels have been reported with nasogastric feeds (eg. Osmolite®, Ensure® [Abbott]) and other enteral feeds (Pharm J 1989;**243**:181). One study showed that the AUC of phenytoin was unaffected by enteral feeds but that the absorption patterns were significantly different, with phenytoin sodium more rapidly absorbed (n = 10, RCT, Doak et al, Pharmacother 1998;**18**:637–45). Phenytoin dosage should be spaced to one hour before feeding or two hours after feeding (tube may need to be clamped). Monitor plasma levels frequently (see comment by Au Yeung and Ensom, Ann Pharmacother 2000;**34**:896–905, 32 refs).

Neuromuscular blocking agents + phenytoin
Phenytoin reduces the effects of most NMBAs, e.g. pancuronium (n = 1, Hickey et al, Anesthesia 1988;**43**:757–9; n = 1, Liberman et al, Int J Clin Pharmacol Ther Toxicol 1988;**26**:371–4) and vecuronium, by several mechanisms (n = 22, Wright et al, Anesthesiology 2004;**100**:626–33), although atracurium appears unaffected.

NICOUMALONE + PHENYTOIN
Nicoumalone metabolism is induced by phenytoin, reducing its effect, although enhancement has also been reported.

Nitrofurantoin + phenytoin
There is a report of a stable epileptic developing seizures when nitrofurantoin was added, requiring increased phenytoin dosage (n = 1, Heipertz and Pilz, J Neurol 1978;**218**:297–301).

NSAIDs + phenytoin
One study shows no interaction to occur with ibuprofen (n = 10, open, Bachmann, Br J Clin Pharmacol 1986;**21**:165–9), but toxicity has been reported (n = 1, Sandyk, S Afr Med J 1982;**62**:592). Phenytoin levels may be increased by aspirin via binding displacement (n = 10, open, 11/7, Leonard et al, Clin Pharmacol Ther 1981;**29**:56–60), free levels seeming to remain constant. Transient toxicity may be the only effect and then only at high (900 mg, four-hourly) aspirin doses. Plasma phenytoin levels may be increased by azapropazone via enzyme inhibition (n = 5, open, Geaney et al, Br J Clin Pharmacol 1983;**15**:727–34). Phenytoin toxicity may occur with phenylbutazone via enzyme inhibition and plasma protein displacement (n = 6, open, Neuvonen et al, Eur J Clin Pharmacol 1979;**15**:263–8). Dosage adjustment may be necessary.

ORAL CONTRACEPTIVES + PHENYTOIN
Contraceptive failure via enzyme induction has been reported many times (e.g. JAMA 1986;**256**:238–40). Any OC needs to contain at least 50 mcg ethinylestradiol, Depot Provera given every 10 rather than 12 weeks (Crawford, CNS Drugs 2002;**16**:263–72), or alternative contraceptive methods used. In the UK, one tablet each of Marvelon® and Mercilon® (Organon) or two tablets of Ovranette® (Wyeth) are often recommended as daily oral contraception.

Oxcarbazepine + phenytoin
See oxcarbazepine (4.5.7).

Paroxetine + phenytoin
See paroxetine (4.3.2.4).

Pethidine + phenytoin

Attenuation of pethidine's effect via enzyme induction is possible, with increased metabolite levels (n = 4, open, Pond and Kretschzmar, *Clin Pharmacol Ther* 1981;**29**:273).

Phenindione + phenytoin

No interaction is thought to occur (n = 54, open, Skovsted *et al*, *Acta Med Scand* 1976;**199**:513).

Pregabalin + phenytoin

See pregabalin (*4.5.11*).

PROGABIDE + PHENYTOIN

Phenytoin levels may rise by up to 40% (n = 6, open, Bianchetti, *Epilepsia* 1987;**28**:68–73).

Propoxyphene + phenytoin

Large doses of propoxyphene may raise phenytoin levels (Kutt *et al*, *Ann N Y Acad Sci* 1971;**179**:704), but normal doses have little or no effect (n = 16, open, Hansen *et al*, *Acta Neurol Scand* 1980;**61**:357).

Proton pump inhibitors + phenytoin

A lack of effect of **omeprazole** on phenytoin kinetics has been reported, as has a mild rise in phenytoin levels (n = 10, RCT, d/b, c/o, 9/7, Prichard *et al*, *Br J Clin Pharmacol* 1987;**24**:543–5). The SPC for omeprazole states that there are no significant changes in plasma levels, but patients should be monitored and doses adjusted if necessary. Lack of interaction has been reported with **pantoprazole** (n = 23, RCT, d/b, p/c, c/o, Middle *et al*, *Int J Clin Pharmacol Ther* 1996;**34**:S72–S75).

Pyridoxine + phenytoin

Large doses of pyridoxine (e.g. 200 mg/d) can reduce phenytoin levels by up to 40–50% (Hansson and Sillanpaa, *Lancet* 1976;i:256). Monitoring levels would thus be wise.

Quetiapine + phenytoin

See quetiapine (*4.2.6*).

QUINIDINE + PHENYTOIN

A reduced quinidine effect may occur via enzyme induction (Anon, *N Engl J Med* 1983;**308**:724–5), so monitoring of quinidine levels or effect may be necessary.

RIFAMPICIN + PHENYTOIN

Significant reductions in phenytoin levels may occur via enzyme induction (Abajo, *Br Med J* 1988;**297**:1048).

Rufinamide + phenytoin

See rufinamide (*4.5.12*).

Sertraline + phenytoin

See sertraline (*4.3.2.5*).

Shankhapushpi + phenytoin

It has been recommended to avoid the Ayurvedic herbal mixture shankhapushpi, as decreased plasma phenytoin levels may occur (mentioned by Fugh-Berman, *Lancet* 2000;**355**:134–8).

Sodium oxybate + phenytoin

See sodium oxybate (*4.6.13*).

Statins + phenytoin

Phenytoin can significantly reduce the therapeutic effect of simvastatin and atorvastatin, probably via CYP3A4 induction (n = 1, Murphy and Dominiczak, *Postgrad Med J* 1999;**75**:359–60; n = 1, Khandwala, *South Med J* 2006;**99**:1385–7).

St John's wort + phenytoin

See St John's wort (*4.3.3.10*).

SUCRALFATE + PHENYTOIN

One study showed a small reduction in phenytoin bioavailability (n = 9, open, Hall *et al*, *Drug Intell Clin Pharm* 1986;**20**:607–11) by decreased absorption. This can be avoided by giving phenytoin two hours or more after sucralfate.

Sulphonamides + phenytoin

Phenytoin toxicity is known to be possible via P450 inhibition by co-trimoxazole (Gillman and Sandyk, *Ann Intern Med* 1985;**102**:559) and other sulphonamides, so monitor plasma levels and reduce phenytoin doses if necessary.

Temozolomide + phenytoin

There is a case of delirium probably caused by this combination (n = 1, Levy, *Psychosomatics* 2007;**48**:359–60).

Theophylline + phenytoin

Phenytoin produces a 45% increase in clearance of theophylline, so higher doses may be needed (n = 8, open, Adebayo, *Clin Exp Pharmacol Physiol* 1988;**15**:883–7). Phenytoin absorption may also be reduced (*Int Pharm J* 1989;**3**:98–101). Separating the doses by 1–2 hours may reduce the effect.

Tiagabine + phenytoin

See tiagabine (*4.5.13*).

Ticlopidine + phenytoin

Ticlopidine 500 mg/d inhibits phenytoin clearance so dose adjustment and careful monitoring should be considered (n = 6, Donahue *et al*, *Clin Pharmacol Therapeut* 1999;**66**:563–8; n = 1, Privitera and Welty, *Arch Neurology* 1996; **53**:1191–2), especially since the onset of phenytoin toxicity may be delayed by several weeks (n = 1, Dahm and Brors, *Tidsskr Nor Laegeforen* 2002;**122**:278–80).

Tolbutamide + phenytoin

Mild phenytoin toxicity may occur via increased free levels (n = 18, Tassaneeyakul et al, Br J Clin Pharmacol 1992;**34**:494–8).

Topiramate + phenytoin

See topiramate (4.5.14).

Trazodone + phenytoin

There is a report of phenytoin toxicity developing when relatively high dose trazodone was added (n = 1, Dorn, J Clin Psychiatry 1986;**47**:89).

TRIMETHOPRIM + PHENYTOIN

Plasma phenytoin levels and the antifolate effect may be increased by trimethoprim.

TRICYCLICS + PHENYTOIN

Phenytoin levels may be raised by **imipramine** (Perucca and Richens, Br J Clin Pharmacol 1977; **4**:485–6), but not **nortriptyline** (Houghton and Richens, Int J Clin Pharmacol 1975;**12**:210–6) or **amitriptyline** (Clin Pharmacol Ther 1975;**18**:191–9), probably due to CYP2C19 inhibition (Shin et al, Drug Metab Dispos 2002;**30**:1102–7). Phenytoin levels may need to be monitored frequently. Tricyclics may lower the seizure threshold.

VALPROATE + PHENYTOIN

Valproate inhibits phenytoin metabolism and competes for its binding sites. If enzyme saturation has not occurred then this displacement of phenytoin leads to decreased bound, but increased free phenytoin (n = 12, Lai and Huang, Biopharm Drug Dispos 1993;**14**:365–70). More phenytoin is then metabolised so the net result is reduced total and bound concentrations. The free concentration will remain about the same and lower plasma levels will still contain about the same amount of active/free drug. Thus, beware of raising the dose of phenytoin to bring the total plasma concentration into the 'therapeutic range' as it would then be toxic (Keys, Drug Intell Clin Pharm 1982;**16**:737–9). If the enzyme is saturated, then displacement may lead to a stable total concentration but decreased bound and increased free phenytoin (n = 6, open, Johnson et al, Br J Clin Pharmacol 1989;**27**:843–9). This could lead to toxic effects within the therapeutic range. In practice, phenytoin levels tend to fall initially by up to 50%, then return to normal over about five weeks. Toxicity is possible if levels were higher at the start. Reports of a toxic interaction are not common, but monitoring is essential. Finally, changing valproate from a standard tablet to a slow-release tablet has been shown to result in a

30% rise in phenytoin levels and toxicity (n = 11, Suzuki et al, Eur J Clin Pharmacol 1995;**48**:61–3).

VIGABATRIN + PHENYTOIN

Vigabatrin produces a mean 20–30% reduction in phenytoin levels (n = 8, open, Rimmer and Richens, Br J Clin Pharmacol 1989;**27**:27S–33S) and may compromise seizure control (e.g. n = 89, s/b, Browne et al, Neurology 1987;**37**:184–9).

Vincristine + phenytoin

Phenytoin significantly increases the clearance of vincristine, probably by CYP3A4 induction (n = 15, open, Villikka et al, Clin Pharmacol Therapeut 1999;**66**:589–93).

Voriconazole + phenytoin *

Voriconazole may decrease phenytoin levels dramatically, where even doubling phenytoin dose is insufficient (Alffenaar et al, Br J Clin Pharmacol 2009;**68**:462–3).

WARFARIN + PHENYTOIN

Warfarin metabolism is accelerated by phenytoin, reducing its effect, although enhanced levels of both and deaths have been reported (n = 1, Panegyres and Rischbieth, Postgrad Med J 1991;**67**:98; Meisheri, J Ass Physicians India 1996; **44**:661–2).

Zinc + phenytoin

One case exists of reduced phenytoin levels probably caused by zinc (Am J Hosp Pharm 1988; **18**:297–8).

Zonisamide + phenytoin

See zonisamide (4.5.17).

Zotepine + phenytoin

See anticonvulsants + zotepine (4.2.9).

4.5.10 PIRACETAM

Warfarin + piracetam

Significantly prolonged prothrombin time has been reported with piracetam and warfarin (n = 1, Pan and Ng, Eur J Clin Pharmacol 1983;**24**:711).

4.5.11 PREGABALIN

Pregabalin is excreted by the kidneys, undergoes little metabolism, has no effect on P450 enzymes, and is not bound to plasma proteins so interactions are unlikely. Lack of interaction has also been shown with antidiabetics, diuretics and insulin.

Alcohol + pregabalin

Pregabalin may potentiate the sedative effects of alcohol (SPC).

Benzodiazepines + pregabalin
Pregabalin may potentiate the sedative effects of lorazepam (SPC).

Carbamazepine+ pregabalin
Lack of interaction has been shown (UK SPC).

Gabapentin + pregabalin
Lack of interaction has been shown (UK SPC), but pregabalin displaces gabapentin from receptors.

Lacosamide + pregabalin *
See pregabalin + lacosamide (4.5.4).

Lamotrigine + pregabalin
Lack of interaction has been shown (UK SPC).

Oral contraceptives + pregabalin
Lack of interaction has been shown (UK SPC).

Oxycodone + pregabalin
Pregabalin may enhance the cognitive and motor effects of oxycodone (SPC).

Phenobarbital + pregabalin
Lack of interaction has been shown (UK SPC).

Phenytoin + pregabalin
Lack of interaction has been shown (UK SPC).

Tiagabine + pregabalin
Lack of interaction has been shown (UK SPC).

Topiramate + pregabalin
Lack of interaction has been shown (UK SPC).

Valproate + pregabalin
Lack of interaction has been shown (UK SPC).

4.5.12 RUFINAMIDE

Rufinamide is almost entirely metabolised by hydrolysis to an inactive metabolite but not by any P450 enzyme. It has no effect on 1A2, 2A6, 2C9, 2C19, 2D6, 2E1 but induces 3A4. It is 34% bound to plasma proteins.

Alcohol + rufinamide
No information is available (UK SPC).

Benzodiazepines + rufinamide
No changes in the plasma levels of rufinamide are seen with benzodiazepines but rufinamide induces CYP3A4 and reduces levels of, e.g. triazolam (UK SPC).

Carbamazepine + rufinamide
The plasma levels of rufinamide are reduced by carbamazepine, but carbamazepine is unaffected by rufinamide (UK SPC).

Lamotrigine + rufinamide
No significant interaction has been seen with this combination (UK SPC).

Olanzapine + rufinamide
Rufinamide has no effect on olanzapine kinetics

(UK SPC).

Oral contraceptives + rufinamide
Rufinamide can reduce plasma levels of oral contraceptives by 14–22%, so adequate additional contraceptive measures are recommended (UK SPC).

Phenobarbital + rufinamide
The plasma levels of rufinamide are reduced by phenobarbital but rufinamide has no effect on barbiturates (UK SPC).

Phenytoin + rufinamide
The plasma levels of rufinamide are reduced by phenytoin (UK SPC) and phenytoin clearance is reduced by rufinamide so phenytoin dose reduction may be necessary.

Topiramate + rufinamide
No significant interaction has been seen with this combination (UK SPC).

Valproate + rufinamide
The plasma levels of rufinamide are increased by valproate (UK SPC), especially in people with body weight < 30 kg, so start at 200 mg/d but with a maximum of only 400 mg/d. Rufinamide has no effect on valproate (UK SPC).

Vigabatrin + rufinamide
The plasma levels of rufinamide are reduced by vigabatrin (UK SPC).

4.5.13 TIAGABINE

Tiagabine appears to be metabolised by CYP3A4.

Alcohol + tiagabine
Lack of interaction has been shown (n = 20, RCT, d/b, p/c, c/o, Kastberg et al, Drug Metabol Drug Interact 1998;**14**:259–73), although some caution is still advised.

Benzodiazepines + tiagabine
No interaction with triazolam has been detected (n = 12, RCT, Richens et al, Drug Metabol Drug Interact 1998;**14**:159–77).

Carbamazepine + tiagabine
Tiagabine clearance is 60% greater with carbamazepine, with plasma levels reduced by a factor of 1.5–3, probably by CYP3A4 induction. Tiagabine has no effect on carbamazepine.

Cimetidine + tiagabine
No interaction has been detected.

Digoxin + tiagabine
Lack of interaction has been shown (n = 13, open,

Snel et al, Eur J Clin Pharmacol 1998;**54**:355–7).

Erythromycin + tiagabine

Lack of significant interaction has been shown (n = 13, open, c/o, Thomsen et al, J Clin Pharmacol 1998;**38**:1051–6).

Fosphenytoin + tiagabine

See phenytoin + tiagabine.

Gemfibrozil + tiagabine *

Gemfibrozil increased tiagabine levels by 60–75% in one patient (n = 1, Burstein et al, Ann Pharmacother 2009;**43**:379–82).

Oral contraceptives + tiagabine

No interaction has been detected.

Phenobarbital + tiagabine

Tiagabine clearance is 60% greater in people also taking phenobarbital, with plasma levels reduced by a factor of 1.5–3, probably by CYP3A4 induction. There is no effect on phenobarbital.

Phenytoin + tiagabine

Tiagabine clearance is 60% greater in people also taking phenytoin and plasma levels are reduced by a factor of 1.5–3, probably by CYP3A4 induction. There is no effect on phenytoin.

Pregabalin + tiagabine

See pregabalin (4.5.11).

Theophylline + tiagabine

No interaction has been detected.

Valproate + tiagabine

Tiagabine causes a 10–12% reduction in steady-state valproate levels, while valproate increases free tiagabine levels by about 40% (n = 12, open, Gustavson et al, Am J Ther 1998;**5**:73–9).

Warfarin + tiagabine

No interaction has been detected.

Zotepine + tiagabine

See anticonvulsants + zotepine (4.2.9).

4.5.14 TOPIRAMATE

Topiramate is 13–17% bound to plasma proteins (and thus unlikely to interact with highly bound drugs) and not extensively metabolised. Excretion is mainly via the kidneys. In vitro data suggests that effects on hepatic enzyme metabolism are small and interactions with antipsychotics, tricyclics, antidepressants, caffeine and xanthines are unlikely via this mechanism. Concomitant use with drugs predisposing to nephrolithiasis (renal stone formation) is not recommended, e.g. allopurinol, megadose ascorbic acid, furosemide,

methyldopa, phenolphthalein abuse, steroids and Worcester sauce overdose.

Reviews: Bailer et al, Clin Pharmacokinet 2004; **43**:63–80; Johannessen, Epilepsia 1997; **38**[Suppl 1]:S18–S23.

Acetazolamide + topiramate

There may be an increased risk of renal stone formation in susceptible patients.

Antipsychotics + topiramate

Topiramate up to 200mg/d had no significant effect on the plasma levels of **clozapine** and norclozapine (n = 10), olanzapine (n = 12), **ris–peridone** and **paliperidone** (n = 9), or **quetiapine** (n = 7) and was well tolerated (n = 38, 6/52, Migliardi et al, Clin Neuropharmacol 2007;**30**:107–13).

Barbiturates + topiramate

Topiramate has been shown to have no effect on plasma levels of phenobarbital or primidone (Floren et al, Epilepsia 1989;**30**:646). The effect of the barbiturates on topiramate has not been studied.

Carbamazepine + topiramate

Topiramate has been shown to have no effect on the plasma levels of CBZ or CBZ–E, although there is a suggestion that it may increase CBZ levels (n = 2 + 23, Mack et al, Seizure 2002;**11**:464–7). However, topiramate clearance is increased two-fold by CBZ and half-life reduced (n = 12 open, Britzi et al, Epilepsia 2005;**46**:378–84), and so topiramate doses may need to be lowered if CBZ is reduced or discontinued (n = 12, open, Sachdeo et al, Epilepsia 1996;**37**:774–80).

Citalopram + topiramate *

A case of acute glaucoma has been reported after topiramate was added to stable citalopram (n = 1, Spaccapelo et al, Cases J 2009;**2**:87).

Digoxin + topiramate

Topiramate may decrease the plasma concentration of digoxin, with peak levels reduced by 16%, possibly by reduced bioavailability. Dose reduction or routine digoxin blood levels might be considered.

Fluvoxamine + topiramate *

See topiramate + fluvoxamine (4.3.2.3).

Lamotrigine + topiramate

See lamotrigine (4.5.4).

Lithium + topiramate

See lithium (4.4).

ORAL CONTRACEPTIVES + TOPIRAMATE

Serum estrogen levels are reduced by topiramate

in patients taking combined oestrogen/ progesterone oral contraceptives. An oral contraceptive containing not less than 50mcg of estrogen or Depot Provera given every 10 rather than 12 weeks is recommended, or the use of alternative methods (n = 12, Rosenfeld et al, Epilepsia 1997;**38**:317–23; review by Crawford, CNS Drugs 2002;**16**:263–72). Any changes in bleeding patterns should be reported. There were no contraceptive failures reported in 52 patients in early clinical trials. In the UK, one tablet each of Marvelon® and Mercilon® (Organon) or two tablets of Ovranette® (Wyeth) are often recommended as daily oral contraception.

Phenytoin + topiramate
Decreases in phenytoin clearance may occur in a few patients with topiramate, probably via CYP2C19 inhibition (n = 12, Sachdeo et al, Epilepsia 2002;**43**:691–6). Conversely, topiramate plasma levels are reduced by about 40% by phenytoin, which could be important if phenytoin is withdrawn.

Posaconazole + topiramate *
Posaconazole has been implicated in inducing topiramate toxicity (n = 1, Marriott et al, Ann Intern Med 2009;**151**:143).

Pregabalin + topiramate
See pregabalin (4.5.11).

Rufinamide + topiramate
See rufinamide (4.5.12).

Temozolomide + topiramate *
Temozolomide does not seem to affect topiramate pharmacokinetics (n = 14, Maschio et al, J Neurooncol 2008;**90**:217–21).

Triamterene + topiramate
There may be an increased risk of renal stone formation in susceptible patients.

Valproate + topiramate *
Topiramate has been shown to produce a small but significant increase in valproate clearance, reducing plasma levels, although enhanced valproate side-effects, e.g. apathy, hypothermia and raised LFTs have also been reported (n = 3, Longin et al, Epilepsia 2002:**43**:451–4), as has reversible hepatic failure, which resolved on stopping valproate (n = 1, Bumb et al, Epileptic Disord 2003;**5**:157–9) and hyperammonemic encephalopathy (n = 1, Cheung et al, J Child Neurol 2005;**20**:157–60). Topiramate may enhance the risk and severity of hypothermia from valproate (n = 19, Knudsen et al, J Clin Pharm

Ther 2008;**33**:513–9). Topiramate plasma levels are increased by about 15% by valproate, which could be important if valproate is withdrawn.

Zonisamide + topiramate
See zonisamide (4.5.17).

Zotepine + topiramate
See anticonvulsants + zotepine (4.2.9).

4.5.15 VALPROATE (SODIUM VALPROATE, VALPROIC ACID, DIVALPROEX SODIUM, ETC)

Valproate has a complex metabolism; 50% is metabolised by glucuronidation, 40% by mitochondrial beta-oxidation and 10% by P450 (CYP2C9 and 2C19) enzymes (Sheehan et al, Ann Pharmacother 2006;**40**:147–50).
Review: DeVane, Psychopharmacol Bull 2003; **37**(Suppl 2):25–42.

Antacids + valproate
A slight decrease in valproate absorption with antacids has been noted (n = 7, open, May et al, Clin Pharm 1982;**1**:244–7).

ANTIDEPRESSANTS + VALPROATE
Antidepressants lower the seizure threshold and may antagonise valproate's anticonvulsant effect. Tricyclic levels may be raised by 19% by valproate (n = 15, open, amitriptyline and nortriptyline, Wong et al, Clin Pharmacol Ther 1996;**60**:48–53) and status epilepticus has been reported, with valproate possibly elevating clomipramine to toxic levels (n = 1, DeToledo et al, Ther Drug Monit 1997;**19**:71–3; see also Fehr et al, J Clin Psychopharmacol 2000;**20**:493–4).

Antiretrovirals + valproate
Valproate levels decreased by 48% (resulting in manic relapse) have been reported with lopinavir/ritonavir (Kaletra®, Abbott) probably via glucuronidation-induction (n = 1, Sheehan et al, Ann Pharmacother 2006;**40**:147–50). Valproate produces a dose-dependent inhibition of zidovudine glucuronidation, leading to raised zidovudine levels (Trapnell et al, Antimicrob Agents Chemother 1998;**42**:1592–6), possibly by up to three-fold (n = 1, Akula et al, Am J Med Sci 1997;**31**:244–6), a UK SPC warning, with severe anaemia reported (n = 1, Antoniou et al, Clin Infect Dis 2004;**38**:38–40).

Asenapine + valproate *
See valproate + asenapine (4.2.3).

Aspirin + valproate
Valproate's effect and toxicity may be enhanced

by repeated high-dose aspirin (n = 3, Goulden *et al, Neurology* 1987;**37**:1392–4), and levels may rise by 12–43% (n = 6, open, Orr *et al, Clin Pharmacol Ther* 1982;**31**:642–9).

Benzodiazepines + valproate
See benzodiazepines (*4.1.1*).

BETA-LACTAM ANTIBIOTICS + VALPROATE
Meropenem rapidly decreases valproate levels to potentially sub-therapeutic levels, a serious interaction (n = 3, Nacarkucuk *et al, Pediatr Neurol* 2004;**31**:232–4; n = 1, Coves-Orts *et al, Ann Pharmacother* 2005;**39**:533–7; n = 2, Sala Pinol *et al, Ann Pediatr (Barc)* 2006;**64**:93–5; Clause *et al, Intensive Care Med* 2005;**31**:1293–4) and despite increasing the valproate dose, plasma levels may not return to normal, resulting in the death of several patients (n = 2, Spriet *et al, Am J Health Syst Pharm* 2007;**64**:54–8; see also with **imipenem**, Perea Falomir *et al, Farm Hosp* 2006;**30**:316–7).

Bupropion + valproate
See bupropion (*4.6.6*).

CARBAMAZEPINE + VALPROATE
See carbamazepine (*4.5.1*).

Charcoal, activated + valproate
Activated charcoal reduces the absorption of sodium valproate by 65% (n = 6, Neuvonen *et al, Eur J Clin Pharmacol* 1983;**24**:243–6) but has no effect on valproate elimination (n = 8, Al-Shareef *et al, Br J Clin Pharmacol* 1997;**43**:109–11).

Chitosan + valproate *
Chitosan (a weight-loss product) has caused valproate to drop to almost undetectable levels, with resultant seizures (n = 2, *BMJ* 2009; **339**:b3751).

Clozapine + valproate
See clozapine (*4.2.4*).

Erythromycin + valproate
Valproate levels may rise three-fold when erythromycin is started, resulting in CNS toxicity (n = 1, Redington *et al, Ann Intern Med* 1992;**116**:877–8).

Ethosuximide + valproate
See ethosuximide (*4.5.2*).

Fluoxetine + valproate
See fluoxetine (*4.3.2.2*).

Fluvoxamine + valproate
See fluvoxamine (*4.3.2.3*).

Gabapentin + valproate
See gabapentin (*4.5.3*).

Gingko biloba + valproate
There is a case of a fatal seizure with the combination, probably due to reduced valproate levels via CYP2C19 induction (n = 1, Kupiec and Raj, *J Anal Toxicol* 2005;**29**:755–8).

H2-blockers + valproate
One study showed that cimetidine reduces the clearance and prolongs the half-life of valproate but ranitidine does not interact (n = 12, RCT, Webster *et al, Eur J Clin Pharmacol* 1984;**27**:341–3).

Imatinib + valproate *
Plasma levels of imatinib do not appear to be affected by valproate (n < 224, p/c, Pursche *et al, Curr Clin Pharmacol* 2008;**3**:198–203).

Isoniazid + valproate
Enhanced hepatotoxicity has been reported (n = 1, Dockweiler, *Lancet* 1987;**2**:152).

Lacosamide + valproate *
See valproate + lacosamide (*4.5.4*).

LAMOTRIGINE + VALPROATE
See lamotrigine (*4.5.5*).

Levetiracetam + valproate
See levetiracetam (*4.5.6*).

Meropenem + valproate *
A retrospective analysis shows that meropenem reduces valproate levels by about 82% and remain low for a week after meropenem is stopped, gradually returning to normal over the next week (n = 36, Haroutiunian et al, *J Clin Pharmacol* 2009;**49**:1363–9). Meropenem can produce an unpredictable but rapid decline in valproate levels (Naranjo = 7, n = 1, Gu and Huang, *Am J Geriatr Pharmacother* 2009;**7**:26–33).

Methylphenidate + valproate
See methylphenidate (*4.6.11*).

Moclobemide + valproate *
See valproate + moclobemide (*4.3.3.5*).

Olanzapine + valproate
See valproate + olanzapine (*4.2.5*).

Oral contraceptives + valproate *
A reduced contraceptive effect has not been reported with valproate (Mattson *et al, JAMA* 1986;**256**:238–40; n = 6, Crawford *et al, Contraception* 1986;**33**:23–9), but valproate plasma levels may be higher during drug-free weeks of combined hormonal oral contraceptives than during the 3/52 on it. Indeed, a 23% reduction in valproate levels has been reported when combined with a combined oral contraceptive pill (n = 24, open, Herzog *et al, Neurology* 2009; **72**:911–4). There is a wide inter-individual variation and monitoring valproate may be prudent if adding or discontinuing OCs or

steroids (n = 9, RCT, c/o, Galimberti et al, Epilepsia 2006;**47**:1569–72).

Oxcarbazepine + valproate
See oxcarbazepine (4.5.7).

Paroxetine + valproate
See paroxetine (4.3.2.4).

PHENOBARBITAL + VALPROATE
See phenobarbital (4.5.8).

PHENYTOIN + VALPROATE
See phenytoin (4.5.9).

Pregabalin + valproate
See pregabalin (4.5.11).

Quetiapine + valproate
See quetiapine (4.2.6).

Risperidone + valproate
See valproate + antipsychotics (4.2.1).

Rufinamide + valproate
See rufinamide (4.5.12).

Sodium oxybate + valproate
See sodium oxybate (4.6.13).

Tiagabine + valproate
See tiagabine (4.5.13).

Topiramate + valproate
See topiramate (4.5.14).

Tricyclics + valproate
See antidepressants + valproate.

Vigabatrin + valproate
See vigabatrin (4.5.16).

Warfarin + valproate
Rapidly raised INR (to 3.9) has been reported after a single dose of valproate (Guthrie et al, J Clin Psychopharmacol 1995;**15**:138–9). Care is needed.

Zolpidem + valproate
See zolpidem (4.1.7).

Zonisamide + valproate
See zonisamide (4.5.17).

4.5.16 VIGABATRIN

Vigabatrin is not metabolised, does not induce enzymes and is not protein bound. It is renally excreted.

Carbamazepine + vigabatrin
A 10% rise in carbamazepine levels has been reported with vigabatrin (n = 66, Jedrzejczak et al, Epilepsy Res 2000;**39**:115–20), as has an 18% reduction in steady-state carbamazepine plasma levels (n = 15, Sanchez-Alcaraz et al, J Clin Pharm Ther 2002;**27**:427–30).

Oral contraceptives + vigabatrin
Vigabatrin is unlikely to affect consistently the efficacy of oral contraceptives, although in one study two women showed reduced ethinyloestradiol levels (n = 113, Bartoli et al, Epilepsia 1997;**38**:702–7).

Phenobarbital + vigabatrin
One study reported non-clinically significant 7–11% reductions in barbiturate levels (n=89, s/b, 12/52, Browne et al, Neurology 1987;**37**:184–9).

PHENYTOIN + VIGABATRIN
See phenytoin (4.5.9).

Rufinamide + vigabatrin
See rufinamide (4.5.121).

Valproate + vigabatrin
Lack of interaction has been shown (e.g. McKee et al, Epilepsia 1993;**34**:937–43), but a small rise in levels may occur (Lisart et al, Eur Hosp Pharm 1996;**2**:33–6; disputed by Mumford, Eur Hosp Pharm 1996;**2**:190–1).

Zotepine + vigabatrin
See anticonvulsants + zotepine (4.2.9).

4.5.17 ZONISAMIDE

Zonisamide does not inhibit 1A2 or 2D6, and only weakly inhibits 2A6, 2C9, 2C19 and 2E1. It is partly metabolised by 3A4 and partly by N-acetyltransferases and glucuronidation.

Carbamazepine + zonisamide
Zonisamide does not significantly effect carbamazepine, but 3A4 induction by CBZ reduces zonisamide half-life from 65 to 36 hours (n = 18, Ragueneau-Majlessi et al, Epilepsy Res 2004;**62**:1–11), but an NMS-like state has been reported with the combination (n = 1, Azuma et al, Epilepsia 2007;**48**:1999–2001).

Cimetidine + zonisamide
Lack of interaction has been shown (SPC).

Ketoconazole + zonisamide
Lack of interaction has been shown (SPC).

Lamotrigine + zonisamide
Lack of clinically significant interaction has been shown (n = 20[c = 18], open, Levy et al, Ther Drug Monit 2005;**27**:93–8).

Oral contraceptives + zonisamide
There is apparently no interaction (SPC).

Phenytoin + zonisamide
Lack of clinically relevant interaction has been shown (SPC).

Rifampicin + zonisamide
An interaction is theoretically possible via 3A4 induction (SPC).

Topiramate + zonisamide

The UK SPC recommends caution with the use of zonisamide with carbonic anhydrase inhibitors such as topiramate.

Valproate + zonisamide

Lack of significant interaction has been shown so no dosage adjustments would appear necessary (n = 22 [c = 17], open, Ragueneau-Majlessi et al, Clin Pharmacokinet 2005;**44**:17–23).

4.6 OTHER DRUGS

4.6.1 ACAMPROSATE

Acamprosate is not protein bound, is excreted in the urine and is not significantly metabolised and so probably has a low liability for drug–drug interactions by these mechanisms.

Alcohol + acamprosate

See alcohol (4.7.1).

Benzodiazepines + acamprosate

Lack of interaction with diazepam has been shown.

Disulfiram + acamprosate

Lack of interaction has been shown (n = 118, RCT, p/c, 2 years, Besson et al, Alcohol Clin Exp Res 1998;**22**:573–9).

Food + acamprosate

Food reduces acamprosate's oral absorption.

Naltrexone + acamprosate

Naltrexone significantly increases plasma acamprosate levels, with some increase in ADRs with the combination (n = 23, RCT, d/b, p/c, c/o, 23/7, Johnson et al, J Clin Psychopharmacol 2003;**23**:281–93).

Tricyclics + acamprosate

There is a lack of interaction with imipramine.

4.6.2 ANTICHOLINERGIC OR ANTIMUSCARINIC AGENTS *

The UK SPC now notes that the antimuscarinic effects of orphenadrine can be enhanced by other drugs with antimuscarinic effects, e.g. antihistamines, antispasmodics, tricyclics, phenothiazines, dopaminergic antiparkinsonian agents (e.g. amantadine), and antiarrhythmics (e.g. disopyramide).

Anticholinesterases + anticholinergics

Some antagonism would be expected.

Antipsychotics + anticholinergics

See antipsychotics (4.2.1).

Benzodiazepines + anticholinergics

See benzodiazepines (4.1.1).

Beta-blockers + anticholinergics

Propantheline increases atenolol bioavailability by 36%, increasing its effect (open, Regardh et al, Biopharm Drug Dispos 1981;**2**:79–87) but not that of metoprolol (n = 15, open, Briant et al, Eur J Clin Pharmacol 1983;**25**:353).

Betel nut + anticholinergics

Heavy betel nut consumption has resulted in severe EPSE, possibly by antagonising the effect of procyclidine (n = 1, Deahl, Mov Disord 1989; **4**:330–2).

H2-blockers + anticholinergics

A single–dose study showed possible reduced **cimetidine** absorption (Kanto et al, Br J Clin Pharmacol 1981;**11**:629–31), but not with **ranitidine** (n = 12, open, Donn et al, Pharmacother 1984;**4**:89–92) or **nizatidine** (Knadler et al, Clin Pharmac Ther 1987;**42**:514–20).

Levodopa + anticholinergics

Anticholinergics may reduce the peak blood levels of levodopa and reduce total absorption (Algeri et al, Eur J Pharmacol 1976;**35**:293–9), possibly by slowed gut motility and increased gut metabolism.

MAOIs + anticholinergics

See MAOIs (4.3.4).

Memantine + anticholinergics

See memantine (4.6.9).

Nitrofurantoin + anticholinergics

Nitrofurantoin bioavailability may be increased by anticholinergics (n = 10, Mannisto, Int J Clin Pharmacol Biopharm 1978;**16**:223–8).

Paracetamol + anticholinergics

Propantheline delays the absorption of paracetamol (Nimmo et al, Br Med J 1973;i:587–9).

Procarbazine + anticholinergics

Increased sedation could occur.

SSRIs + anticholinergics

There are several cases of the combination probably causing delirium, e.g. **sertraline** and benzatropine (n = 1, Byerly et al, Am J Psychiatry 1996;**153**:965–6), paroxetine and benzatropine (Armstrong and Schweitzer, Am J Psychiatry 1997;**154**:581–2, where **paroxetine** definitely raised benzatropine levels) and a variety of adverse effects (n = 5, Roth et al, J Clin Psychiatry 1994;**55**:491–5). CYP2D6 inhibition seems the likely mechanism.

Thiazide diuretics + anticholinergics

Thiazide bioavailability may be enhanced (open, Beermann et al, Eur J Clin Pharmacol 1978;**13**: 385–7).

Tricyclics + anticholinergics

See tricyclics (4.3.1).

Venlafaxine + anticholinergics

An acute adverse cutaneous reaction has been reported with venlafaxine and orphenadrine (n = 1, Papadimitriou et al, J Eur Acad Dermatol Venereol 2006;**20**:1019).

Ziprasidone + anticholinergics

See ziprasidone (4.2.8).

Zotepine + anticholinergics

See zotepine (4.2.9).

4.6.3 ANTICHOLINESTERASES

Review: anticholinesterase interactions (Bentue-Ferrer et al, CNS Drugs 2003;**17**:947–63).

4.6.3.1 DONEPEZIL

Donepezil is metabolised slowly by CYP2D6 and 3A4 to multiple metabolites, only one of which appears to be pharmacologically active.

Anticholinergics + donepezil

See anticholinesterases + anticholinergics (4.6.2).

Antipsychotics + donepezil

Donepezil 5 mg/d had no effect on **risperidone** pharmacokinetics in schizophrenia and was well tolerated (n = 31, open, 7/7, Reyes et al, Br J Clin Pharmacol 2004;**58**[Suppl 1]:50–7), although NMS with **bromperidol** (n = 1, Ueki et al, Nippon Ronen Igakkai Zasshi 2001;**38**:822–4) and severe EPSE with risperidone (n = 1, Magnuson et al, Am J Psychiatry 1998;**155**:1459) have been reported.

Cimetidine + donepezil

Lack of significant pharmacokinetic interaction has been reported (n = 19, open, Tiseo et al, Br J Clin Pharmacol 1998;**46**[Suppl 1]:25–9).

Digoxin + donepezil

Lack of significant pharmacokinetic interaction has been reported (n = 12, open, Tiseo et al, Br J Clin Pharmacol 1998;**46**[Suppl 1]:40–4).

Ketoconazole + donepezil

Donepezil levels may rise by around 25% over a week (n = 21, open, Tiseo et al, Br J Clin Pharmacol 1998;**46**[Suppl 1]:30–4).

Memantine + donepezil

See anticholinesterases + memantine (4.6.9).

NMBAs + donepezil

A synergistic effect could be predicted.

NSAIDs + donepezil

The manufacturers of donepezil recommend additional monitoring of patients at risk of developing ulcers, e.g. if taking concomitant NSAIDs.

SSRIs + donepezil

Lack of interaction has been shown between donepezil 5 mg/d and **sertraline** 100 mg/d (n = 19 [c = 16], RCT, open, c/o, Nagy et al, Br J Clin Pharmacol 2004;**58**(Suppl 1):25–33), although case reports exist with **paroxetine** (Carrier, J Am Geriatr Soc 1999;**47**:1037).

Suxamethonium + donepezil

Donepezil is a cholinesterase inhibitor and would be likely to enhance the effect of suxamethonium-type muscle relaxants (n = 1, Crowe and Collins, Anesthiology 2003;**98**:574–5), e.g. during ECT (Walker and Perks, Anesthesia 2002;**57**:1041).

Theophylline + donepezil

Lack of significant pharmacokinetic interaction has been reported (n = 12, open, Tiseo et al, Br J Clin Pharmacol 1998;**46**[Suppl 1]:35–9).

Warfarin + donepezil

Lack of significant pharmacokinetic interaction has been reported (n = 12, open, Tiseo et al, Br J Clin Pharmacol 1998;**46**[Suppl 1]:45–50).

4.6.3.2 GALANTAMINE

Galantamine is 90% bioavailable, has a large VD, low protein binding, and is metabolised by CYP2D6 and 3A4. Galantamine has a minimal effect on P450 enzymes (review by Farlow, Clin Pharmacokinet 2003;**42**:1383–92).

Anticholinergics + galantamine

See anticholinesterases + anticholinergics (4.6.2).

Antipsychotics + galantamine

Lack of interaction has been reported with risperidone (n = 16, RCT, open, c/o, Huang et al, J Clin Pharmacol 2002;**42**:1341–51).

Beta-blockers + galantamine

As galantamine may cause bradycardia, the SPC recommends care with drugs that significantly reduce heart rate, e.g. beta-blockers.

Digoxin + galantamine

As galantamine may cause bradycardia, the SPC recommends care with drugs that significantly reduce heart rate, e.g. digoxin. Galantamine has no effect on the kinetics of digoxin.

Erythromycin + galantamine

A 12% increase in galantamine plasma levels has

been reported, probably by CYP3A4 inhibition.

Ketoconazole + galantamine

A 30% increase in galantamine plasma levels has been reported, probably by CYP3A4 inhibition, and so a reduced maintenance dosage might be appropriate.

Memantine + galantamine

See memantine (4.6.9).

Paroxetine + galantamine

A 40% increase in galantamine plasma levels has been reported, probably by CYP2D6 inhibition, and so a reduced maintenance dosage might be appropriate.

Suxamethonium + galantamine

Galantamine is likely to enhance the effect of suxamethonium-type muscle relaxants.

Warfarin + galantamine

Galantamine has been shown to have no effect on the kinetics of warfarin.

4.6.3.3 RIVASTIGMINE

Rivastigmine has minimal protein binding, a short half-life, is metabolised by esterases (but with little effect on P450 enzymes) and lack of significant interaction has been shown with 22 different therapeutic classes (Grossberg et al, Int J Geriatr Psychiatry 2000;**15**:242–7).

Anticholinergics + rivastigmine

See anticholinesterases + anticholinergics (4.6.2).

Benzodiazepines + rivastigmine

No interaction seen in healthy volunteers.

Digoxin + rivastigmine

No interaction in healthy volunteers has been seen.

Fluoxetine + rivastigmine

No interaction in healthy volunteers has been seen.

Memantine + rivastigmine

See anticholinesterases + memantine (4.6.9).

Suxamethonium + rivastigmine

Rivastigmine may enhance the effect of suxamethonium-type muscle relaxants during anaesthesia.

Warfarin + rivastigmine

No interaction in healthy volunteers has been seen.

4.6.4 ATOMOXETINE

Atomoxetine is metabolised by CYP2D6 and half-life may be longer (five hours vs 21 hours) and peak levels five times higher in poor metabolisers but does not usually need dose reduction, although accumulation can occur (Sauer et al, Clin Pharmacokinet 2005;**44**:571–90). It has no clinically significant effect on CYP1A2, 3A4, 2D6 or 2C9. The UK SPC recommends caution with the potential for potentiation with other noradrenergic drugs, e.g. tricyclics, venlafaxine, reboxetine, mirtazapine, pseudoephedrine or phenylephrine.

Antacids + atomoxetine

Antacids and omeprazole have no effect on atomoxetine bioavailability (UK SPC).

Aspirin + atomoxetine

Lack of interaction has been shown (UK SPC).

Benzodiazepines + atomoxetine

Lack of interaction has been shown with diazepam (UK SPC).

MAOIs + ATOMOXETINE

These should not be used together and a two–week gap is needed after stopping an MAOI before starting atomoxetine (UK SPC).

Methylphenidate + atomoxetine

Lack of additive cardiovascular effects has been shown (UK SPC).

Mirtazapine + atomoxetine

See introduction to 4.6.4.

Phenytoin + atomoxetine

Lack of interaction has been shown (UK SPC).

PPIs + atomoxetine

See antacids + atomoxetine above.

Reboxetine + atomoxetine

See introduction to 4.6.4.

Salbutamol + atomoxetine

Caution is needed with high-dose salbutamol (any route) or other beta-blockers, as the cardiovascular effects of salbutamol can be potentiated (UK SPC).

SSRIs + atomoxetine

Fluoxetine and paroxetine may increase atomoxetine levels via 2D6 inhibition (UK SPC).

Tricyclics + atomoxetine

See introduction to 4.6.4.

Venlafaxine + atomoxetine

There is a case of tic, tremor and speech disturbance with the combination, resolving when atomoxetine was discontinued (n = 1, Bond et al, Clin Toxicol [Phila] 2007;**45**:182–5). See also introduction to 4.6.4.

Warfarin + atomoxetine

Lack of interaction has been shown (UK SPC).

4.6.5 BUPRENORPHINE

Buprenorphine has an extensive first-pass metabolism, but sub-lingual bioavailability is sufficient to allow administration by this route. Half-life can vary widely (3–44 hours). It is highly protein bound (96%), metabolised by CYP2D6 and 3A4. It is a major inhibitor of 2D6 and 3A4, and a weak inhibitor of 1A2, 2B6, 2C9, 2C19 and 2E1, although this is yet to be confirmed in human data (review by Elkader and Sproule, *Clin Pharmacokinet* 2005;**44**:661–80).

Antiretrovirals + buprenorphine *
Ritonavir can produce a significant increase, albeit asymptomatic, in the AUC for buprenorphine, but this does not happen with nelfinavir, lopinavir/ritonavir (n = 10, McCance-Katz et al, *Clin Infect Dis* 2006;**43**[Suppl 4]:S235–46), efavirenz, maraviroc nor delavirdine (n = 10, McCance-Katz et al, *Clin Infect Dis* 2006;**43**[Suppl 4]:S224–34), although there are cases of pharmacokinetic interaction with atazanavir/ritonavir (n = 3, Bruce and Altice, *AIDS* 2006;**20**:783–4), so choose your drugs with care (review by Bruce et al, *Clin Infect Dis* 2006;**43**[Suppl 4]:S216–23; n = 3, Bruce and Altice, *AIDS* 2006;**20**:783–4). Tipranavir/ritonavir have no significant effect on buprenorphine/naloxone levels but tipranavir levels may be substantially reduced, leading to potential loss of efficacy (n=12[c=10], Bruce et al, *Drug Alcohol Depend* 2009;**105**:234–9).

Benzodiazepines + buprenorphine
See benzodiazepines (*4.1.1*).

Cocaine + buprenorphine
No notable interaction has been observed (SPC).

Ketoconazole + buprenorphine
Start with half doses of buprenorphine due to ketoconazole's CYP3A4 inhibition (SPC).

Methadone + buprenorphine
See methadone (*4.6.10*).

Tricyclics + buprenorphine
See tricyclics (*4.3.1*).

4.6.6 BUPROPION

Bupropion is 84% protein bound and primarily metabolised by CYP2B6, with a significant first-pass metabolism, although poor metabolisers may accumulate hydroxybupropion, leading to reduced efficacy (n = 12, Pollock et al, *Ther Drug Monit* 1996;**18**:581–5).
Review: interactions with anticonvulsants (Popli et al, *Ann Clin Psychiatry* 1995;**7**:99–101).

Alcohol + bupropion
There is an increased risk of seizures, so alcohol should be avoided or minimised. Extreme care is needed in overdose, chronic use and in alcohol withdrawal states.

Antipsychotics + bupropion
The CSM recommends caution due to the possible increased risk of seizures.

Antiretrovirals + bupropion
Single doses of bupropion have no effect on lopinavir/ritonavir but lopinavir/ritonavir reduces bupropion levels and may require as much as a 100% bupropion dose increase, probably via 2B6 and UGT induction (n = 12, 4/52, Hogeland et al, *Clin Pharmacol Ther* 2007;**81**:69–75). Ritonavir itself may decrease the metabolism of bupropion, which would increase side-effects.

Baicalin + bupropion *
Baicalin (a Chinese herbal medicine) significantly reduces the plasma levels of bupropion via 2B6 induction (n = 17, Fan et al, *Eur J Clin Pharmacol* 2009;**65**:403–9).

Carbamazepine + bupropion
Carbamazepine induces bupropion metabolism, markedly decreasing bupropion plasma levels (n = 17, RCT, Ketter et al, *J Clin Psychopharmacol* 1995;**15**:327–33).

Ciclosporin + bupropion
A life-threatening decrease in ciclosporin levels has been reported with bupropion (n = 1, Lewis et al, *J Child Adolesc Psychopharmacol* 2001;**11**:193–8).

Cimetidine + bupropion
Cimetidine may inhibit the metabolism of bupropion, and increase adverse effects, although no effect on bupropion SR was seen in one study (n = 24, RCT, open, Kustra et al, *J Clin Pharmacol* 1999;**39**:1184–8).

Clonidine + bupropion
Lack of interaction has been reported (n=8, RCT, d/b, c/o, Cubeddu et al, *Clin Pharmacol Ther* 1984;**35**:576–84).

Clopidogrel + bupropion
A single-dose study showed clopidogrel to significantly inhibit bupropion's 2B6 metabolism, increasing AUC by 60% (n = 12, Turpeinen et al, *Clin Pharmacol Ther* 2005;**77**:553–9).

Fluoxetine + bupropion

Bupropion produces no significant changes in fluoxetine levels (n = 24, open, 8/52, Kennedy et al, J Clin Psychiatry 2002;**63**:181–6) but panic disorder (n = 1, Young, J Clin Psychiatry 1996; **57**:177–8) and delirium (n = 1, Chan et al, J Clin Psychopharmacol 2006;**26**:677–9) have been reported.

Fosphenytoin + bupropion

See phenytoin + bupropion.

Ginkgo biloba + bupropion *

There is no significant interaction, although hydroxybupropion levels may be reduced (n = 14, 2/52, Lei et al, Br J Clin Pharmacol 2009; **68**:201–6).

Guanfacine + bupropion

There is a report of a grand mal seizure with the combination (n = 1, Tilton, J Am Acad Child Adolesc Psychiatry 1998;**37**:682–3).

MAOIs + bupropion

Animal studies have indicated that acute bupropion toxicity might occur, and the combination is contraindicated.

Lamotrigine + bupropion

See lamotrigine (4.5.5).

Levodopa + bupropion

An increased incidence of side-effects has been reported with the combination.

Moclobemide + bupropion

See MAOIs + bupropion.

Paroxetine + bupropion

Bupropion produces no significant changes in paroxetine levels (open, 8/52, Kennedy et al, J Clin Psychiatry 2002;**63**:181–6), but the CSM recommends caution.

Phenobarbital + bupropion

Phenobarbital may induce the metabolism of bupropion, which would reduce its efficacy.

Phenytoin + bupropion

Phenytoin may induce the metabolism of bupropion, which would reduce its efficacy.

Pseudoephedrine + bupropion

There is a report of acute myocardial ischaemia with the combination (n = 1, Pederson et al, Can J Cardiol 2001;**17**:599–601).

Rifampicin + bupropion

Rifampicin may reduce bupropion's half-life by 50%, reducing plasma levels, probably by CYP2B6 induction (n = 18, Loboz et al, Clin Pharmacol Ther 2006;**80**:75–84).

Selegiline + bupropion

See MAOIs + bupropion.

Sertraline + bupropion

A marked adverse reaction has been reported with the combination, where mood appeared to deteriorate and venlafaxine was added, but was later recognised as serotonin syndrome (n = 1, Munhoz, Clin Neuropharmacol 2004;**27**:219–22).

Smoking + bupropion

In a single-dose study, cigarettes had no detectable effect on bupropion kinetics (open, Hsyu et al, J Clin Pharmacol 1997;**37**:737–43).

Ticlopidine + bupropion

A single-dose study showed that ticlopidine significantly inhibited the metabolism of bupropion, increasing AUC by 85% (n = 12, Turpeinen et al, Clin Pharmacol Ther 2005;**77**:553–9).

Tricyclics + bupropion

Bupropion has been reported to increase **imipramine** and **desipramine** levels, through decreased clearance (n = 1, Shad and Preskorn, J Clin Psychopharmacol 1997;**17**:118–9). Also reported with bupropion are seizures with **trimipramine** (n = 1, Enns, J Clin Psychiatry 2001; **62**:476–7), and clomipramine (n = 1, Shin et al, Clin Neuropharmacol 2004;**27**:192–4) and **nortriptyline** toxicity (n = 1, Weintraub, Depress Anxiety 2001;**13**:50–2).

Valproate + bupropion

Valproate does not seem to induce bupropion metabolism, but raised metabolite levels are possible (n = 17, RCT, Ketter et al, J Clin Psychopharmacol 1995;**15**:327–33).

Venlafaxine + bupropion

Bupropion has been shown to produce a significant increase in venlafaxine but decrease O-desmethylvenlafaxine levels (open, 8/52, Kennedy et al, J Clin Psychiatry 2002;**63**:181–6). See also sertraline + bupropion.

Zolpidem + bupropion

There are some reported cases of antidepressants and zolpidem causing short-lived hallucinations (e.g. Elko et al, Clin Toxicol 1998; **36**:195–203).

4.6.7 CLOMETHIAZOLE

Clomethiazole inhibits CYP2E1.

Alcohol + clomethiazole

See alcohol (4.7.1).

Cimetidine + clomethiazole

Cimetidine inhibits the metabolism of clomethiazole, raising plasma levels.

Methadone + clomethiazole
See methadone (4.6.10).

4.6.8 DISULFIRAM

Disulfiram is a potent inhibitor of CYP1A2, 2B6 and 2E1 (the enzyme that metabolises ethanol), but chronic use could affect other enzymes too (n=7, Frye and Branch, *Br J Clin Pharmacol* 2002;**53**:155–62).
Review: disulfiram interactions (*Acta Psychiatr Scand* 1992;**86**[Suppl 369]:59–66).

Acamprosate + disulfiram
See acamprosate (4.6.1).

ALCOHOL + DISULFIRAM
See disulfiram under 'Alcohol abuse and dependence' (1.4) and alcohol (4.7.1).

Antipsychotics + disulfiram
There is a report of psychotic symptoms reappearing when disulfiram was started and an increased first-pass metabolism of perphenazine has been noted (n=1, Hansen *et al*, *Lancet* 1982;**2**:1472).

Benzodiazepines + disulfiram
Disulfiram may inhibit the metabolism of **diaze-pam, chlordiazepoxide** and **temazepam** (n=1, Hardman *et al*, *Lancet* 1994;**344**:1231–2), leading to lengthened half-lives, but not with **oxazepam** (open, MacLeod, *Clin Pharmacol Ther* 1978;**24**:583–9) or **alprazolam** (n=11, 2/52, Diquet *et al*, *Eur J Clin Pharmacol* 1990;**38**:157–60).

Caffeine + disulfiram
Disulfiram may reduce caffeine clearance by 50% (n=21, open, Beach *et al*, *Clin Pharmacol Ther* 1986;**39**:265–70).

Cannabis + disulfiram
See cannabis (4.7.2).

Carbamazepine + disulfiram
Lack of significant interaction has been shown (n=7, open, Krag *et al*, *Acta Neurol* 1981;**63**:395–8).

Cocaine + disulfiram *
There is a case of pronounced paranoia with the combination (n=1, Mutschler *et al*, *J Clin Psychopharmacol* 2009;**29**:99–101).

Colchicine + disulfiram *
A potentially fatal interaction between colchicine and disulfiram has been reported (Chen *et al*, *Prog Neuropsychopharmacol Biol Psychiatry* 2009;**33**:1281).

Isoniazid + disulfiram

CNS toxicity has been reported in patients taking isoniazid who then took disulfiram (Rothstein, *JAMA* 1972;**219**:1216).

Lithium + disulfiram
These appear compatible, with no theoretical or clinical reasons why an interaction should occur.

MAOIs + disulfiram
Delirium has been reported with the combination (n=1, Blansjaar and Egberts, *Am J Psychiatry* 1995;**152**:296; n=1, Circulo, *J Clin Psychopharmacol* 1989;**9**:315–6).

Methadone + disulfiram
See methadone (4.6.10).

Methylphenidate + disulfiram
See methylphenidate (4.6.11).

Metronidazole + disulfiram
Psychotic reactions have been reported (n=2, Hotson and Langston, *Arch Neurol* 1976;**33**:41–2).

NICOUMALONE + DISULFIRAM
An enhanced anticoagulant effect is possible.

Omeprazole + disulfiram
There is a report of confusion, disorientation and catatonia with the combination (n=1, Hajela *et al*, *Can Med Assoc J* 1990;**143**:1207).

Paraldehyde + disulfiram
An enhanced disulfiram reaction is possible (mentioned in Hadden and Metzner, *Am J Med* 1969;**47**:642).

Phenytoin + disulfiram
See phenytoin (4.5.9).

Theophylline + disulfiram
Theophylline levels may be increased via enzyme inhibition. Monitor and reduce the theophylline dose if necessary (n=20, RCT, Loi *et al*, *Clin Pharmacol Ther* 1989;**45**:476–86).

Tricyclics + disulfiram
See tricyclics (4.3.1).

WARFARIN + DISULFIRAM
Prothrombin time can fall by about 10% (Rothstein, *JAMA* 1972;**221**:1051–2), with one study showing a marked effect with reduced warfarin doses sometimes necessary (n=7, open, O'Reilly, *Clin Pharmacol Ther* 1981;**29**:332). The literature notes this to be a significant effect.

4.6.9 MEMANTINE

Memantine is only minimally metabolised, does not inhibit CYP1A2, 2A6, 2C9, 2D6, 2E1 or 3A, or the FMO system, or epoxide hydrolase or sulphation, and so metabolic interactions are unlikely. Raised urinary pH (e.g. infections, diet change, excessive alkalising gastric buffers, etc) may significantly reduce excretion. Plasma protein binding is 45%.

Alcohol + memantine
See alcohol (4.7.1).

Amantadine + memantine
Both are NMDA-antagonists and the combination should be avoided as CNS ADRs may be more frequent. The same may be true with ketamine and dextromethorphan.

Anticholinergics + memantine
The anticholinergic's effects may be enhanced by memantine.

Anticholinesterases + memantine *
Lack of interaction has been shown between memantine and donepezil (n = 19, open, Periclou *et al*, *Ann Pharmacother* 2004;**38**:1389–94) or rivastigmine (n = 16, open, c/o, 7/52, Shua-Haim *et al*, *Clin Drug Investig* 2008;**8**:361–74). A postmarketing survey of patients taking memantine with AChEs suggested that the combination was safe and well-tolerated (n = 158, open, mean 4/52, Hartmann and Mobius, *Int Clin Psychopharmacol* 2003;**18**:81–5).

Antipsychotics + memantine
The antipsychotic effects may be reduced by memantine.

Antispasmodic agents + memantine
The effects may be modified by memantine and dose adjustment may be necessary.

Baclofen + memantine
The effects may be modified by memantine and dose adjustment may be necessary.

Dantrolene + memantine
Dantrolene's effects may be modified by memantine and dose adjustment necessary.

Dextromethorphan + memantine
See amantadine. + memantine

Dopamine agonists + memantine
Dopamine antagonists such as bromocriptine may be enhanced by memantine.

H2–blockers + memantine
A theoretical interaction via competition for cationic transport system exists and there is the potential for increased plasma levels.

Hydrochlorthiazide + memantine
There is a theoretical possibility of reduced diuretic effect.

Ketamine + memantine
See amantadine + memantine.

Levodopa + memantine
The effects of levodopa may be enhanced by memantine.

Phenobarbital + memantine
The barbiturate's effects may be reduced by memantine.

Phenytoin + memantine
There is one case report of interaction.

Procainamide + memantine
A theoretical interaction via competition for cationic transport system exists and there is the potential for increased plasma levels.

Quinidine/quinine + memantine
A theoretical interaction via competition for cationic transport system exists and there is the potential for increased memantine plasma levels.

Smoking + memantine
A theoretical interaction via competition for cationic transport system exists and there is the potential for increased memantine plasma levels.

4.6.10 METHADONE *

Methadone is probably metabolised mainly by CYP3A4 (or not, as the case may be; Kharasch *et al*, *Clin Pharmacol Ther* 2008;**84**:506–12) and partly by 2D6 (but genotype has no apparent effect on clearance; Coller *et al*, *Int J Clin Pharmacol Ther* 2007;**45**:410–7) and 1A2 (and possibly 2B6), and inhibits CYP2D6 and 3A4. Absorption is also variable according to P-glycoprotein status. The (R)-methadone is the active moiety, (S)-methadone being inactive.
Reviews: general (DeMaria, *J Maint Addictions* 2003;**2**:41–57), TDM (Moolchan *et al*, *J Addict Dis* 2001;**20**:55–73).

Alcohol + methadone
See alcohol (4.7.1).

Antipsychotics + methadone *
See methadone + antipsychotics (4.2.1).

Antiretrovirals + methadone *
Although **atazanavir** is a potent CYP3A4 inhibitor, one study showed no clinically relevant interaction with methadone and no dose adjustment needed (n = 16, 2/52, Friedland *et al*, *AIDS* 2005; **19**:1635–41). **Efavirenz** can induce (and inhibit) CYP3A4 and produce withdrawal symptoms from reduced methadone levels (n = 1,

Pinzani et al, Ann Pharmacother 2000;**34**:405–7; n=1, Marzolini et al, AIDS 2000; **14**:1291–2; n=9+52 controls, Esteban et al, Drug Metab Lett 2008;**2**:269–79). Slightly raised methadone levels have been reported with **indinavir**. Reduced methadone levels and AUC by 47% (UK SPC) can occur with **nevirapine** through CYP3A4 induction, precipitating withdrawal (n=5+52 controls, Esteban et al, Drug Metab Lett 2008;**2**:269–79; n=7, Altice et al, AIDS 1999;**13**:957–62). Methadone metabolism and clearance are induced by **nelfinavir** with levels reduced by 40–50%, probably by increasing renal clearance and by altering the S- and R-methadone ratio and despite significant 3A4 inhibition (n=12, Kharasch et al, Drug Alcohol Depend 2009;**101**:158–68). **Ritonavir** may induce the same reduction of 40–50% (Kharasch et al, Clin Pharmacol Ther 2008;**84**:497–505; n=1, Geletko and Erickson, Pharmacother 2000;**20**:93–4), although **ritonavir/saquinavir** has been used without dose adjustment in AIDS patients (n=12, Gerber et al, J AIDS 2001;**27**:153–60). However, although not formally studied, the UK SPC for **maraviroc** states that no interaction is expected. Methadone had no effect on **fosamprenavir-ritonavir**, but methadone levels were reduced AUC by 18%, considered insignificant (n=26, 18/7, Cao et al, Pharmacotherapy 2008;**28**:863–74). Serum levels of **didanosine** can be reduced by about 40% (n=27, open, Rainer et al, J AIDS 2000; **24**:241–8).

Ascorbic acid + methadone
Vitamin C and other urine acidifiers (e.g. ammonium chloride) can decrease methadone plasma levels via increased renal excretion if the pH is less than 6. Methadone's half-life can be halved to around 19–20 hours.

Benzodiazepines + methadone
There is no proven pharmacokinetic interaction but additive sedation can occur (e.g. n=5, RCT, Preston et al, Drug Alc Dep 1986;**18**:195–202).

Buprenorphine + methadone
An antagonistic effect would be predicted and buprenorphine might displace methadone from Mu-opioid receptors, precipitating withdrawal. Enhanced sedation and respiratory depression may occur.

Cannabis + methadone
An interaction would be possible through CYP3A4 induction.

Carbamazepine + methadone
Reduced methadone levels can occur through CYP3A4 induction (Ketter et al, J Clin Psychopharmacol 1991;**11**:198–203; n=43, Bell et al, Clin Pharmacol Ther 1988;**43**:623–9), and methadone-induced respiratory depression has been reported after withdrawal of carbamazepine (n=1, Benitez–Rosario et al, J Pain Symptom Manage 2006;**32**:99–100).

Chloral + methadone
Additive sedation can occur.

Cimetidine + methadone
Raised methadone levels can occur.

Ciprofloxacin + methadone *
A course of ciprofloxacin has caused sudden and profound methadone toxicity (n=1, Herrlin et al, Lancet 2000;**356**:2069–70) and QTc prolongation leading to Torsades de pointes (n=1, Nair et al, Addiction 2008;**103**:2062–4).

Clomethiazole + methadone
Additive sedation can occur.

Cocaine + methadone
Cocaine may accelerate methadone elimination (Moolchan et al, J Addict Dis 2001;**20**:55–73).

Cyclizine + methadone
There are rare reports of hallucinations with the combination.

Dextromethorphan + methadone
Delirium, hypersomnia and confusion has been reported with the combination in an elderly woman (n=1, Lotrich et al, Am J Geriatr Pharmacother 2005;**3**:17–20).

Diphenhydramine + methadone
There are rare reports of additional CNS effects with the combination.

Disulfiram + methadone
Lack of kinetic interaction has been shown (n=7, Tong et al, J Clin Pharmacol 1980;**20**:506–13).

Domperidone + methadone
Increased absorption has been reported.

Erythromycin + methadone
Raised methadone levels could occur through CYP3A4 inhibition.

Fluconazole/ketoconazole + methadone
Methadone levels can rise by a mean of 27% through CYP3A4 inhibition, although one study did not detect any signs of toxicity (n=25, RCT, d/b, p/c, 14/7, Cobb et al, Clin Pharmacol Ther 1998;**63**:655–62).

Fluoxetine + methadone
Lack of significant interaction has been shown

(n = 16, open, 9/52, Batki et al, J Clin Psycho-pharmacol 1993;**13**:243–50).

Fluvoxamine + methadone

Fluvoxamine may inhibit methadone metabolism leading to raised levels (n = 1, DeMaria and Serota, J Addict Dis 1999;**18**:5–12) and severe hypoventilation has been reported (n = 1, Alderman and Frith, Aust N Z J Psychiatry 1999; **33**:99–101).

Fosphenytoin + methadone

See phenytoin.

Grapefruit juice + methadone

Raised methadone levels through CYP3A4 inhibition could theoretically occur.

Hypnotics + methadone

Enhanced sedation can occur.

Lofexidine + methadone

Lofexidine decreases sitting systolic and diastolic bp by 27 and 15 mmHg respectively, and reduced cognitive efficiency compared to placebo when given with methadone, so monitor for cardiovascular and cognitive changes if using the combination (n = 14, d/b, p/c, 11/52, Schroeder et al, Pharmacotherapy 2007;**27**:1111–9).

MAOIs + methadone

See MAOIs (4.3.4).

Metapyrone + methadone

Metapyrone can cause a withdrawal-like syndrome with methadone (n = 15, open, Kennedy et al, Br J Addict 1990;**85**:1133–40).

Naloxone + methadone

This opiate antagonist would block the effect of methadone: this can occur within 5–10 minutes (Tornabene, Ann Intern Med 1974;**81**:349–51).

Naltrexone + methadone

This opiate antagonist would block the effect of methadone.

Paroxetine + methadone

See paroxetine (4.3.2.4).

Phenobarbital + methadone

Enhanced sedation and respiratory depression may occur. Reduced methadone levels have been reported with phenobarbital (e.g. n = 43, Bell et al, Clin Pharmacol Ther 1988;**43**:623–9).

PHENYTOIN + METHADONE

Reduced methadone levels can occur through CYP3A4 induction, with withdrawal symptoms occurring within four days (n = 43, Bell et al, Clin Pharmacol Ther 1988;**43**:623–9). Dosage adjustment may be needed.

Quetiapine + methadone

Quetiapine increases the plasma levels of the active R-methadone enantiomer by about 20%, possibly by CYP2D6 inhibition but this is highly variable and probably not clinically significant, (n = 14, Uehlinger et al, J Clin Psychopharmacol 2007;**27**:273–8).

Reboxetine + methadone

See reboxetine (4.3.3.6).

Rifampicin + methadone

Methadone levels reduce by 30–65% within 4–5 days in 70% patients given rifampicin, through CYP3A4 induction (n = 30, Kreek et al, N Engl J Med 1976;**294**:1104–6).

Risperidone + methadone

There is a report of possible interaction, resulting in irritability and aches (n = 1, Wines and Weiss, J Clin Psychopharmacol 1999:**19**:65–7).

Sodium bicarbonate + methadone

Sodium bicarbonate and other urinary alkalinisers can increase plasma levels via decreased renal excretion.

St John's wort + methadone

See St John's wort (4.3.3.10).

Tricyclics + methadone

Additive sedation might occur. A small study showed desipramine blood levels can double with methadone (n = 5, Maany et al, Am J Psychiatry 1989;**146**:1611–3).

Zidovudine + methadone

Raised zidovudine levels have been reported (AUC increased by 41%) (n = 8, McCance-Katz et al, J Acquir Immune Defic Synd Hum Retrivirol 1998;**18**:435–43).

4.6.11 METHYLPHENIDATE

Atomoxetine + methylphenidate

See atomoxetine (4.6.4).

Carbamazepine + methylphenidate

Carbamazepine has been reported to cause an extreme reduction of methylphenidate levels (n = 1, Behar et al, J Am Acad Child Adolesc Psychiatry 1998;**37**:1128–9).

Ciclosporin + methylphenidate

A rise in ciclosporin levels has been reported with methylphenidate (n = 1, Lewis et al, J Child Adolesc Psychopharmacol 2001;**11**:193–8).

Cocaine + methylphenidate

No pharmacokinetic or physiological interaction seems to occur (n = 7, p/c, Winhusen et al, Pharmacol Biochem Behav 2006;**85**:29–38).

Disulfiram + methylphenidate

There is a case of an acute-onset psychotic episode after a single dose of methylphenidate in a patient taking disulfiram 400mg/d (n = 1, Caci and Baylé, *Am J Psychiatry* 2007;**164**:1759).

Fluoxetine + methylphenidate *

Hallucinations have been reported with the combination (n = 1, Coskun and Zoroglu, *J Clin Psychopharmacol* 2008;**28**:723–5).

Glipizide + methylphenidate

Addition of methylphenidate in a woman also taking glipizide resulted in a 26% reduction in plasma glucose levels, and so an interaction is a possible explanation (n = 1, Gontkovsky et al, *Clin Drug Investig* 2007;**27**:719–25).

MAOIs + methylphenidate

See MAOIs (*4.3.4*).

Modafinil + methylphenidate

See modafinil (*4.6.12*).

Phenytoin + methylphenidate

Phenytoin toxicity has been reported (n = 3, Ghofrani, *Dev Med Child Neurol* 1988;**30**:267–8).

Sertraline + methylphenidate *

Seizures (n = 1, Schertz and Steinberg, *J Child Adolesc Psychopharmacol* 2008;**18**:301–3) and serotonin syndrome (n = 1, Ishii et al, *Psychiatry Clin Neurosci* 2008;**62**:246) have been reported with the combination

St John's wort + methylphenidate

It has been suggested that SJW may reduce the efficacy of methylphenidate in ADHD (Niederhofer, *Med Hypotheses* 2007;**68**:1189).

Tricyclics + methylphenidate

Methylphenidate may inhibit the metabolism of tricyclics producing up to a four-fold increase in levels (e.g. n = 2, Grob and Coyle, *J Dev Behav Pediatrics* 1986;**7**:265–7). Mood and cognitive deterioration has been reported with imipramine and methylphenidate (n = 2, Grob and Coyle, *J Dev Behav Pediatr* 1986;**7**:265–7).

Valproate + methylphenidate

Rapid onset and severe dyskinesia and bruxism has been reported with the combination (n = 2, Gara and Roberts, *J Child Adolesc Psychopharmacol* 2000;**10**:39–43).

4.6.12 MODAFINIL

Modafinil is moderately bound to plasma proteins (62%), essentially to albumin. Renal excretion is the main route of elimination, but is also metabolised by CYP3A4. It inhibits 2C19, 2D6 and a small and concentration-dependent induction of 1A2, 2B6 and 3A4 (Robertson and Hellriegel, *Clin Pharmacokinet* 2003;**42**:123–37). Modafinil is metabolised to two inactive metabolites.

Amfetamines + modafinil

Low dose amfetamines appear to have no significant effects on steady state modafinil (n = 32, RCT, open, Hellriegel et al, *J Clin Pharmacol* 2002;**42**:450–60).

Benzodiazepines + modafinil

Triazolam levels may be significantly reduced by modafinil, probably via 3A4 induction (n = 41, RCT, 4/52, Robertson, *Clin Pharmacol Ther* 2002; **71**:46–56).

Carbamazepine + modafinil

Carbamazepine might reduce plasma modafinil levels (SPC).

Ciclosporin + modafinil

The UK SPC reports a case of a 50% reduction in ciclosporin levels with modafinil.

Cocaine + modafinil

Single doses of IV cocaine have no apparent medical or cardiac interaction with modafinil, although the cocaine euphoria may be significantly blunted (n = 7, open, Dackis et al, *Drug Alcohol Depend* 2003;**70**:29–37; n = 12, Malcolm et al, *Am J Drug Alcohol Abuse* 2006; **32**:577–87).

Dexamfetamine + modafinil

Dexamfetamine has no apparent effect on steady state modafinil levels (n = 32, RCT, open, Hellriegel et al, *J Clin Pharmacol* 2002;**42**:450–60).

Ethinylestradiol + modafinil

Ethinylestradiol levels may be reduced by modafinil, probably via 3A4 induction (n = 41, RCT, 4/52, Robertson, *Clin Pharmacol Ther* 2002;**71**:46–56).

MAOI + modafinil

See MAOIs (*4.3.4*).

Methylphenidate + modafinil

Low-dose methylphenidate does not appear to interact with modafinil (n = 32, RCT, open, Hellriegel et al, *J Clin Pharmacol* 2002;**41**:895–904), although methylphenidate may slightly slow the absorption of modafinil (RCT, Wong et al, *J Clin Pharmacol* 1998;**38**:276–82).

Oral contraceptives + modafinil

Higher dose oral contraceptives containing 50mcg ethinylestradiol should be used.

Phenobarbital + modafinil

Phenobarbital might reduce plasma modafinil levels (SPC).

Phenytoin + modafinil

Phenytoin's clearance might be reduced by modafinil (SPC).

Sodium oxybate + modafinil

See sodium oxybate (4.6.13).

Tricyclics + modafinil

A single dose study showed a clinically important interaction with clomipramine 50mg/d (n=1, Grozinger et al, Clin Neuropharmacol 1998; **21**: 127–9).

Warfarin + modafinil

A single-dose study suggested no interaction (n=28, Robertson et al, J Clin Pharmacol 2002; **42**:205–14) but the UK SPC recommends caution and additional monitoring as warfarin clearance may be reduced.

4.6.13 SODIUM OXYBATE

Sodium oxybate is metabolised by GHB dehydrogenase, eventually to carbon dioxide and water, with no active metabolites. It does not appear to significantly inhibit P450 enzymes 1A2, 2C9, 2C19, 2D6, 2E1, and 3A4 at therapeutic doses.

Alcohol + sodium oxybate

Enhanced CNS depression can occur (SPC).

Benzodiazepines + sodium oxybate

Respiratory depression might be increased and so the combination should be avoided (SPC).

Ethosuximide + sodium oxybate

Ethosuximide inhibits GHB dehydrogenase, which metabolises oxybate, and so an interaction is theoretically possible but there are no human studies or reports (SPC).

Modafinil + sodium oxybate

Lack of interaction has been reported (SPC).

Phenytoin + sodium oxybate

Phenytoin inhibits GHB dehydrogenase, which metabolises oxybate, and so an interaction is theoretically possible but there are no human studies or reports (SPC).

Proton-pump inhibitors + sodium oxybate

Lack of interaction has been reported with omeprazole (SPC).

Tricyclics + sodium oxybate

Lack of interaction has been reported with protriptyline, but adverse effects may be increased with this combination (SPC).

Valproate + sodium oxybate

Valproate inhibits GHB dehydrogenase, which metabolises oxybate, and so an interaction is theoretically possible but there are no human studies or reports (SPC).

Zolpidem + sodium oxybate

Lack of interaction has been reported (SPC).

4.7 NON-PRESCRIBED DRUGS AND 'VICES'

4.7.1 ALCOHOL

Alcohol/ethanol-psychotropic drug interactions can occur frequently and with varied outcome, depending upon:

- alcohol usage (e.g. chronic and/or acute, leading to altered enzymes)
- consumption (amount, time span)
- type of interaction (e.g. additive sedation, antagonism or cross-tolerance)
- what the individual then tries to do (e.g. sleep, drive)
- comorbidity (e.g. asthma).

These variables need to be considered when assessing the effect, or potential effect, of the interaction. Alcohol distribution is wide, with the direct central depressant effect impairing all central functions (e.g. cognition and respiration) which contribute to many of the drug–drug interactions. Alcohol also promotes the action of GABA and may release other amines such as dopamine and endorphins.

Reviews: * general (Jang and Harris, Expert Opin Drug Metab Toxicol 2007;**3**:719–31), in older adults (Moore et al, Am J Geriatr Pharmacother 2007;**5**:64–74).

Acamprosate + alcohol

Continued alcohol consumption may negate the therapeutic effect of acamprosate. There is no detectable pharmacokinetic interaction (review by Nalpas et al, Encephale 1990;**16**:175–9).

Agomelatine + alcohol

See agomelatine (4.3.3.1).

ANTIPSYCHOTICS + ALCOHOL

Enhanced CNS depression is well-documented, resulting in impaired concentration, coordination, judgement, drowsiness and lethargy, as well as hypotension and respiratory depression. Alcohol-related drowsiness is significant with **phenothiazines** and **flupentixol**. EPSE may also be enhanced (Freed, *Med J Aust* 1981;**2**:44–5), as can hepatotoxicity with, eg. **chlorpromazine** (Strubelt, *Biochem Pharmacol* 1980;**29**:1445–9). Single oral doses of **amisulpride** do not seem to enhance the effects of alcohol on the performance and memory of healthy subjects (n = 18, RCT, Mattila *et al*, *Eur J Clin Pharmacol* 1996;**51**:161). No significant difference in performance or gross motor skills has been shown with **aripiprazole**, although 2.5–10 mg/d increases sedation from alcohol (n = 18, p/c, Kranzler *et al*, *Alcohol Clin Exp Res* 2008;**32**:573–9). Enhanced CNS sedation would be expected with **olanzapine**, and raised heart rate and increased postural hypotension have been reported. There is no clear evidence that alcohol reduces antipsychotic efficacy (n = 31, open, Chetty *et al*, *Eur J Clin Pharmacol* 1994;**46**:523–6). Overall, this is a potentially important interaction, especially in the community. Accidental alcohol over-dosage, especially in people with asthma, respiratory depression or chest infections, could prove fatal if combined with antipsychotics.

BARBITURATES + ALCOHOL

Enhanced or prolonged CNS and respiratory depression can occur, seriously impairing concentration and performance. Acute alcohol ingestion may increase barbiturate levels but chronic alcohol use may decrease barbiturate levels (Mezey and Robles, *Gastroenterology* 1974; **66**:248–53). The lethal dose of barbiturates is reported to be up to 50% lower when alcohol is also present (Bogan and Smith, *J Forensic Sci* 1967; **7**:37–45). This is mainly due to additive respiratory depression.

BENZODIAZEPINES + ALCOHOL

Alcohol can enhance the sedation caused by benzodiazepines by 20–30%, a well-established, documented and predictable interaction. Synergistic sedation has been reported with **lorazepam** (d/b, c/o, Lister and File, *J Clin Psychopharmacol* 1983;**3**:66–71), **clorazepate** and **diazepam**. Larger quantities of alcohol may inhibit benzodiazepine metabolism, especially in those with impaired or borderline hepatic function (review by Guthrie and Lane, *Alcoholism* 1986;**10**:686–90). Acute ethanol consumption decreases diazepam clearance by up to 50%, (Laisi *et al*, *Eur J Clin Pharmacol* 1979;**16**:263–70). At low dose, alcohol and **temazepam** appear not

to interact adversely (n = 24, p/c, c/o, Martin and Siddle, *Brain Cogn* 2003;**53**:58–65).

Beta-blockers + alcohol

Alcohol may slightly reduce propranolol absorption and increase clearance (n = 5, open, Grabowski *et al*, *Int J Clin Pharmacol Ther Toxicol* 1980;**18**:317–9; Sotaniemi *et al*, *Clin Pharmacol Ther* 1981;**29**:705–10).

Bupropion + alcohol

See bupropion (4.6.6).

Buspirone + alcohol

A minimal interaction and slightly increased sedation has been reported (n = 24, RCT, Erwin *et al*, *J Clin Psychopharmacol* 1986;**6**:199–209).

Cannabis + alcohol

See cannabis (4.7.2).

Carbamazepine + alcohol

There is virtually nothing published but additive sedation would be expected.

CHLORAL HYDRATE + ALCOHOL

Additive CNS depressant effects occur when alcohol is taken with chloral hydrate. Tachycardia, impaired concentration, disulfiram-like effects and profound vasodilation may also occur (Owen and Taberner, *Br J Pharmacol* 1978; **64**:400).

Clomethiazole + alcohol

Alcohol increases the bioavailability of oral clomethiazole, probably via inhibition of first-pass metabolism (Neuvonen *et al*, *Int J Clin Pharmacol Ther Toxicol* 1981;**19**:552–60).

Citalopram + alcohol

There is little published at present on this. The manufacturers state that citalopram does not enhance the sedation caused by alcohol.

Cocaine + alcohol

See cocaine (4.7.3).

DISULFIRAM + ALCOHOL

Disulfiram inhibits the aldehyde dehydrogenase enzyme, leading to accumulation of acetaldehyde from incomplete alcohol metabolism. The main symptoms of the 'Antabuse reaction' are flushing, sweating, palpitations, hyperventilation, increased pulse, hypotension, nausea and vomiting (often in that order). Arrhythmias and shock can follow. The reaction occurs within 5–15 minutes and can be fatal. Factors affecting the severity of the reaction include the dose of disulfiram, rate and dose of alcohol ingestion, sensitivity, individual aldehyde dehydrogenase activity, concurrent medication (see disulfiram, 4.6.4) and co-existing pulmonary or cardiac disease. Patients should be warned that reactions can occur with disguised sources of alcohol, e.g. 'Listerine' mouthwash, sauces, pharmaceuticals (e.g. cough mixtures) and topical preparations (e.g. shampoo, Stoll and King, *JAMA* 1980;**244**:2045). Delirium has been reported with the combination (Park and Riggio, *Ann Pharmacother* 2001;**35**:32–5).

Escitalopram + alcohol

See citalopram + alcohol.

Fluoxetine + alcohol

Alcohol has no additional significant effect on drowsiness, sedation or task performance tests with fluoxetine 40 mg/d, compared with fluoxetine alone (e.g. Shaw *et al*, *Hum Psychopharmacol* 1989;**4**:113–20).

Fluvoxamine + alcohol

No significant potentiation of the cognitive effects of 40 g IV alcohol by single and multiple doses of 50 mg fluvoxamine occurred in one study (n = 24, van Harten *et al*, *Clin Pharmacol Ther* 1992;**52**:427–35).

Lacosamide + alcohol *

See alcohol + lacosamide (4.5.4).

Levetiracetam + alcohol

See levetiracetam (4.5.6).

Lithium + alcohol

Impaired driving skills have been suggested and alcohol may produce a slight (12%) increase in peak lithium levels (n = 10, RCT, d/b, p/c, c/o, Anton *et al*, *Clin Pharmacol Ther* 1985;**38**:52–5).

MAOIs + ALCOHOL

As well as an interaction occurring with alcoholic and low alcoholic drinks (see MAOIs, 4.3.4), alcohol may increase central catecholamine synthesis and release, and MAOIs may inhibit alcohol dehydrogenase, potentiating alcohol (comprehensive review by Weller *et al*, *Psychosomatics* 1984;**25**:301–9).

Melatonin + alcohol

See melatonin (4.1.4).

Memantine + alcohol

Memantine has no effect on alcohol-induced performance impairment, but may increase some subjective symptoms (n = 18, 3×3/7, d/b, Bisaga and Evans, *Psychopharmacol [Berl]* 2003; **172**:16–24).

Methadone + alcohol

Predictably, increased sedation and respiratory depression may occur with the combination (Bellville *et al*, *Clin Pharmacol Ther* 1971;**12**:607–12), especially in overdose, as could hepatotoxicity.

Chronic high use of alcohol may induce enzymes requiring higher methadone doses and binge drinking may increase methadone excretion via an enhanced diuretic effect.

MIANSERIN + ALCOHOL

Mianserin causes drowsiness, which is enhanced considerably by alcohol (n = 13, RCT, Seppala *et al*, *Eur J Clin Pharmacol* 1984;**27**:181–9).

Mirtazapine + alcohol

Lack of pharmacokinetic interaction has been shown, but additive sedation noted (see Timmer *et al*, *Clin Pharmacokinet* 2000;**38**:461–74).

Moclobemide + alcohol

Some degree of potentiation of the effects of alcohol has been noted, although less than with trazodone and clomipramine (Zimmer *et al*, *Acta Psychiatr Scand* 1990;**360**[Suppl]:84–6). There has also been a case of a fatality with a moclobemide overdose, plus half a bottle of whisky (n = 1, Bleumink *et al*, *Neth J Med* 2003; **61**:88–90).

Oxcarbazepine + alcohol

See oxcarbazepine (4.5.7).

Paraldehyde + alcohol

An enhanced sedative effect can be expected.

Paroxetine + alcohol

Lack of interaction has been shown (review by Boyer and Blumhardt, *J Clin Psychiatry* 1992;**53**[Suppl 2]:132–4).

PHENYTOIN + ALCOHOL

Alcohol has a variable effect on phenytoin so monitor plasma levels regularly. The half-life of phenytoin can be up to 50% shorter in an abstaining alcoholic than in a non-drinker (see also n = 1, Bellibas and Tuglular, *Therapie* 1995; **50**:487–8).

Pregabalin + alcohol

See pregabalin (4.5.11).

Quetiapine + alcohol

Additive sedation would be expected.

Ramelteon + alcohol

See ramelteon (4.1.5).

Reboxetine + alcohol

No potentiation of alcohol's cognitive effects has been reported (UK SPC), and up to 4 mg/d showed no interaction with alcohol in one trial (n = 10, d/b, Kerr *et al*, *Br J Clin Pharmacol* 1996; **42**:239–41).

Rufinamide + alcohol

See rufinamide (4.5.12).

Sertraline + alcohol

There is evidence for a lack of interaction

(review, Warrington, *Int Clin Psychopharmacol* 1991;**6**[Suppl 2]:11–21).

Sodium oxybate + alcohol

See sodium oxybate (*4.6.13*).

Tiagabine + alcohol

See tiagabine (*4.5.13*).

TRAZODONE + ALCOHOL

Additive sedation has been reported (n = 26, d/b, c/o, Warrington *et al*, *Neuropsychobiology* 1986; **15**[Suppl 1]:31–7).

TRICYCLICS + ALCOHOL

Enhanced sedation with most tricyclics is known, but surprisingly little has actually been published and most studies refer to the effect on driving performance. Sedation caused by amitriptyline, maprotiline and doxepin is enhanced by alcohol, but less, or minimally so, with nortriptyline and clomipramine. Both alcohol and tricyclics lower the seizure threshold and care is needed in patients susceptible to seizures. Concurrent alcohol may also increase the oral bioavailability of tricyclics by reducing first-pass metabolism (n = 5, open, Dorian *et al*, *Eur J Clin Pharmacol* 1983;**25**:325–31).

Venlafaxine + alcohol

There appears to be no significant additive effect between alcohol and venlafaxine (n = 16, RCT, d/b, p/c, c/o, Troy *et al*, *J Clin Pharmacol* 1997;**37**: 1073–81).

Zaleplon + alcohol

While zaleplon enhances alcohol performance impairment, the effect appears short-lived and less than triazolam (n = 18, c/o, Roehrs *et al*, *Sleep Med* 2001;**2**:323–32) and zolpidem, albeit less potent on a mg for mg basis (n = 10, RCT, c/o, Drover *et al*, *Clin Ther* 2000;**22**:1443–61).

Zolpidem + alcohol

There is no published information available indicating an interaction.

Zopiclone + alcohol

There appears to be no significant interaction (n = 9, RCT, Hindmarch, *Int Clin Psychopharmacol* 1990;**5**[Suppl 2]:105–13).

Zotepine + alcohol

See zotepine (*4.2.9*).

4.7.2 CANNABIS (TETRAHYDRO-CANNABINOL, SEE ALSO SMOKING)

Cannabis/marijuana is a frequently (and usually secretively) used drug but, with the exception of perhaps tricyclics, has few known important adverse drug interactions.

Alcohol + cannabis

Decreased ethanol metabolism may occur, with enhanced CNS depression (n = 10, RCT, p/c, d/b, c/o, Consroe *et al*, *Psychopharmacol* 1979;**66**:45–50). Cannabis may also reduce peak alcohol levels in modest doses (n = 15, RCT, p/c, Lukas *et al*, *Neuropsychopharmacology* 1992;**7**:77–81).

Antidepressants + cannabis

Mental status changes consistent with delirium and tachycardia and other clinically significant adverse events have been reported following use of marijuana and **tricyclics** (n = 4, Wilens *et al*, *J Am Acad Child Adolesc Psychiatry* 1997; **36**:45–8). Increased heart rate has been reported, e.g. marked sinus tachycardia, possibly via a combined beta–adrenergic effect (e.g. n = 2, Hillard and Vieweg, *Am J Psychiatr* 1983;**140**:626–7). Mania has been reported with **fluoxetine** and cannabis (n = 1, Stoll *et al*, *J Clin Psychiatry* 1991;**52**:280–1).

Antipsychotics + cannabis

Chlorpromazine clearance has been shown to be increased by cannabis smoking, although the clinical significance is not known (n = 31, Chetty *et al*, *Eur J Clin Pharmacol* 1994;**46**:523–6). Cessation of cannabis smoking can lead to **clozapine** intoxication through removal of CYP1A2 induction (n = 1, Zullino *et al*, *Int Clin Psychopharmacol* 2002;**17**:141–3). Additive drowsiness has been reported (review by Benowitz and Jones, *Clin Pharmacol Ther* 1977;**22**:259–68).

Benzodiazepines + cannabis

Additive drowsiness with benzodiazepines and cannabis has been reported (review by Benowitz and Jones, *Clin Pharmacol Ther* 1977;**22**:259–68).

Cocaine + cannabis

See cocaine (*4.7.3*).

CNS depressants + cannabis

The combination has resulted in additive drowsiness (review by Benowitz and Jones, *Clin Pharmacol Ther* 1977;**22**:259–68), e.g. anticholinergics and barbiturates.

Disulfiram + cannabis

There have been two reported reactions; a hypomanic episode in an alcoholic on disulfiram taking marijuana (n = 1, Lacoursiere and Swatek, *Am J Psychiatry* 1983;**140**:242–4) and an acute confusional state (n = 1, Mackie and Clark, *Br J Psychiatry* 1994;**164**:421).

Lithium + cannabis

There is a case of lithium levels raised into the toxic range by secretive use of cannabis (n = 1, Ratey et al, J Clin Psychopharmacol 1981;**1**:32) and additive drowsiness has been reported (review by Benowitz and Jones, Clin Pharmacol Ther 1977;**22**:259–68).

Methadone + cannabis

See methadone (4.6.10).

4.7.3 COCAINE

Review: Ciraulo, J Clin Psychopharmacol 1992;**12**: 49–55 (73 refs).

Alcohol + cocaine

Simultaneous cocaine and alcohol may produce changes in heart rate and blood pressure, increasing the risk of cardiovascular toxicity (Farre et al, J Pharmacol Exp Ther 1993;**166**:1364–73). Combined use has led to enhanced cocaine-induced hepatotoxicity.

Antidepressants + cocaine

In combination with cocaine, desipramine may reduce the effect, fluoxetine has no significant effect (n = 5, Walsh et al, J Clin Psychopharmacol 1994;**14**:396–407), trazodone has minor physiological effects and MAOIs probably augment the pressor effect.

Antipsychotics + cocaine

Flupentixol may reduce cocaine craving and haloperidol may moderate the stimulant effects. Clozapine increases cocaine levels but reduces the cocaine 'high', and some cardiac events (near–syncopal episode) have been reported, so caution is necessary (n = 8, Farren et al, Drug Alcohol Depend 2000;**59**:153–63).

Buprenorphine + cocaine

See buprenorphine (4.6.5).

Cannabis + cocaine

Enhanced cardiotoxicity (e.g. increased heart rate) may occur.

Carbamazepine + cocaine

Cocaine may enhance the cardiac effects of carbamazepine.

Disulfiram + cocaine *

See cocaine + disulfiram (4.6.8).

Lithium + cocaine

Lithium probably has little effect on cocaine.

Methadone + cocaine

See methadone (4.6.10).

Methylphenidate + cocaine

See methylphenidate (4.6.11).

Modafinil + cocaine

See modafinil (4.6.12).

4.7.4 SMOKING

Many people with mental health problems smoke. There are over 3000 different known chemicals in cigarette smoke, but which ones are significant is not fully known. Only a few smoking drug interactions are significant, and only brief details of the more significant psychotropic ones are included here (review by Schein, Ann Pharmacother 1995;**29**:1139–48). The major enzyme metabolising nicotine is probably CYP2A6, with 2B6 and 2D6 playing lesser, but still substantial, roles. Cigarette smoke contains polycyclic aromatic hydrocarbons, which are potent inducers of CYP1A2.

Reviews: general (Zevin and Benowitz, Clin Pharmacokinet 1999;**36**:425–38, 128 refs; Desai et al, CNS Drugs 2001;**15**:469–94, 100 refs).

Agomelatine + smoking

See agomelatine (4.3.3.1).

Antipsychotics + smoking *

Schizophrenics who smoke tend to receive higher doses of antipsychotics than non-smokers (n = 78, open, Goff et al, Am J Psychiatry 1992; **149**:1189–94), possibly via increased hepatic metabolism and renal excretion (n = 90, RCT, d/b, p/c, Salokangas et al, Schizophren Res 1997;**23**:55–60). Plasma levels of **haloperidol** are around 23% lower in smoking than in non-smoking schizophrenic patients (n = 66, open, Shimoda et al, Ther Drug Monit 1999;**21**:293–6; confirmed by another study, n = 63, Pan et al, Ther Drug Monit 1999;**21**:489). **Chlorpromazine** clearance may be increased by cigarette smoking, but the clinical significance is unclear (n = 31, Chetty et al, Eur J Clin Pharmacol 1994;**46**:523–6).

Olanzapine clearance may be higher and half-life 21% shorter in smokers compared to non-smokers, probably via CYP1A2 induction. Smoking cessation can lead to olanzapine intoxication through removal of CYP1A2 induction (n = 1, Zullino et al, Int Clin Psychopharmacol 2002; **17**:141–3). Smoking seems to have no effect on **zotepine** plasma levels (n = 14, Kondo et al, Psychopharmacol [Berl] 1996;**127**:311–4). Lack of interaction has been shown with **amisulpride** levels (n = 85, Bergemann et al, Eur Neuro-

psychopharmacol 2004;**14**:245–50), **ziprasidone** and **aripiprazole**. There is nothing reported with **risperidone**. Many schizophrenics may smoke to relieve subjective distress from the illness and treatment (review, McEvoy, *Curr Opin Psychiatry* 2000;**113**:115–9).

Clozapine levels are lowered by smoking (n = 148, open, Haring *et al*, *Am J Psychiatry* 1990;**147**:1471–5), the 1A2 induction leading to clozapine non-response, but this usually takes two to four weeks to manifest itself (Zullion *et al*, *Int Clin Psychopharmacol* 2002;**17**:141–3). Stopping smoking can be dangerous for someone taking clozapine, e.g. one study showed a mean 72% increase in stable clozapine levels on smoking cessation, with one case so extreme it caused a significant ADR (n = 11, open, Meyer, *J Clin Psychopharmacol* 2001;**21**:569–74). The change in plasma clozapine levels can, in 80% of cases, be predicted by using the formula:

$$\text{Non-smoking level} = 45.3 + (1.474 \times \text{smoking level})$$

Nomograms exist to help predict doses in people on clozapine who smoke, but you'll need a colour copy of the best paper (Rostami–Hodjegan *et al*, *J Clin Psychopharmacol* 2004;**24**:1–9) to make sense of it (review for our Norwegian readers; Molden and Spigset, *Tidsskr Nor Laegeforen* 2009; **129**:623–3).

Valproate has a variable effect on smoking and clozapine (n = 255, Diaz *et al*, *Pharmacopsychiatry* 2008;**41**:81–91):

- Valproate inhibits clozapine metabolism in non-smokers (+16%)
- Valproate induces clozapine metabolism in smokers (−22%)
- Smoking induces clozapine and reduces plasma levels by 20% if not also taking valproate
- Smoking induces clozapine and reduces plasma levels by 46% if taking valproate

Smoking thus induces clozapine metabolism and this induction may be stronger when the patient is taking valproate, and so the effect may be even more marked when stopping smoking.

Benzodiazepines + smoking
Early studies suggested an increased clearance of benzodiazepines in smokers (review by Schein, *Ann Pharmacother* 1995;**29**:1139–48). One re-

view noted increased clearance by smoking of alprazolam, lorazepam, oxazepam and diazepam but not chlordiazepoxide (mentioned in Desai *et al*, *CNS Drugs* 2001;**15**:469–94).

Beta-blockers + smoking
Effects of nicotine on heart rate and blood pressure may negate the effects of beta-blockers.

Bupropion + smoking
See bupropion (4.6.6).

Carbamazepine + smoking
There appears to be no interaction (mentioned in Desai *et al*, *CNS Drugs* 2001;**15**:469–94).

DULOXETINE + SMOKING
See duloxetine (4.3.3.2).

Fluvoxamine + smoking
Fluvoxamine levels are significantly lower in smokers, probably due to CYP1A2 induction (n = 30, open, Yoshimura *et al*, *Neuropsychobiology* 2002;**45**:32–5).

Lamotrigine + smoking *
Lamotrigine levels are about 16% lower in smokers compared to non-smokers, probably via UDPGT2B7 induction (n = 44, Reinsberger *et al*, *Seizure* 2008;**17**:651–3).

Lithium + smoking
Smoking induces CYP1A2 and caffeine is metabolised by CYP1A2. Theoretically, ceasing smoking could raise xanthine levels, which could increase lithium excretion (as with theophylline), lowering levels.

Melatonin + smoking
See melatonin (4.1.4).

Memantine + smoking
See memantine (4.6.9).

Mirtazapine + smoking *
Smokers have mirtazapine levels significantly (25%) lower than non-smokers (n = 95, Lind *et al*, *Clin Pharmacokinet* 2009;**48**:63–70).

Phenobarbital + smoking
Smoking has been shown not to effect the drowsiness caused by phenobarbital (n = 12, d/b, Mirfazaelian *et al*, *Biopharm Drug Dispos* 2001; **22**:403–6).

Propranolol + smoking
Steady-state propranolol levels may be reduced in smokers, via 1A2 induction.

Tricyclics + smoking
Although serum levels of tricyclics fall in smokers, free levels rise, minimising the clinical significance (n = 24, open, Perry *et al*, *Ther Drug Monit* 1986; **8**:279–84).

Valproate + smoking *
See antipsychotics + smoking.
Zolpidem + smoking
See zolpidem (*4.1.7*).

4.8 CYTOCHROME P450 DRUG METABOLISM *

There are currently at least 58 known P450 enzymes, with 388 isoforms described, regulated by 684 genes (Tomaszewski *et al, Acta Pol Pharm* 2008;**65**:319–29). The main recognised P450s are 1A1, 1A2, 2A6, 2B6, 2C8, 2C9, 2C18, 2C19, 2D6, 2E1, 3A3, 3A4, 3A5, 3A6, 3A7, 3A43, 21A2 All have up to 1–70 variations each. These tables (*pp. 401–410*) may be of use in determining actual or potential interactions. There are many discrepancies in the published literature and these tables may inadvertently perpetuate some inaccuracies or incomplete knowledge. The author would be happy to receive any advice on this.

Some points about P450/CYP interactions: *

1. Most have ultrarapid (UM), extensive (EM), intermediate (IM) and poor (PM) metaboliser metabolic variations.
2. Some drugs are metabolised by several enzymes, so if one enzyme is inhibited, another may compensate.
3. A drug may inhibit or induce one enzyme, but be metabolised by another.

4. Onset and offset of inhibition is dependent on the half-life and time to steady state of the inhibitory drug (may be 24 hours to several months) and the drug to be metabolised, but onset is frequently rapid.
5. Onset and offset of induction may take days or several weeks to become apparent, dependent on the inducing drugs half-life, enzyme turnover, age (induction reduces with age) and concurrent liver disease (reduced induction ability).
6. Other enzyme systems are also important. The **UGT** (uridine diphosphate glucuronosyltransferase) enzymes are induced by phenytoin, valproate, phenobarbital and carbamazepine, and lamotrigine is a weak UGT inducer. The Flavin Mono-xygenase (**FMO**) system is also important. Humans have FMO1, FMO3, FM04 and FM05 enzymes in the liver, intestine and kidney. Imipramine, chlorpromazine and orphenadrine are known to be metabolised by this enzyme system.

The general rules for avoiding metabolic interactions are:

1. Avoid reported and predictable interactions.
2. With potential interactions, use reduced doses where possible (start low, go slow).
3. Measure plasma levels of drugs with narrow therapeutic indices.

CYP1A2

Substrates (drugs metabolised by this enzyme)

Agomelatine (90%)	Diazepam	Methadone (minor)
Amiodarone	Duloxetine	Mexiletine (minor)
Anagrelide	Erlotinib (minor)	Mirtazapine (partly)
Asenapine	Erythromycin	Naproxen
Caffeine	Estradiol	Norfloxacin
Carbamazepine (minor)	Flecainide	Olanzapine (partly)
Chlordiazepoxide	Flutamine	Omeprazole
Ciprofloxacin	Fluvoxamine (partly)	Ondansetron
Clarithromycin	Haloperidol (partly)	Oxfloxacin
Clopidogrel (minor)	Lefunomide	Palonosetron (minor)
Clozapine (most)	Lidocaine	Paracetamol
Dextropropoxyphene	Melatonin (partly)	Perphenazine

Substrates (drugs metabolised by this enzyme) continued

Pimozide (possibly)
Promazine
Propafenone
Propranolol
Ramelteon (95% first-pass effect)
Rasagiline (major)
Retinols

Ritonavir
Rofecoxib
Ropinirole
Sibutramine (part)
Tacrine
Tamoxifen
Theophylline
Tizanidine (main)

Tricyclics (tertiary, e.g. amitriptyline, clomipramine, desipramine, trimipramine imipramine)
Verapamil
Warfarin-R (major)
Ziprasidone (minor)
Zotepine

Significant enzyme inducers (decrease levels of substrates)

Cabbage
Caffeine (weak, animal studies)
Carbamazepine?
Charcoal-broiled food

Cigarette smoke (inc. cannabis)
Modafinil (small and dose-dependent)
Omeprazole

Phenobarbital (weak)
Phenytoin (weak)
Rifampin
Ritonavir
Tipranavir (potent)

Significant enzyme inhibitors (increase levels of substrates)

Celery
Cimetidine
Clarithromycin
Diet (low protein/high carbohydrates)
Disulfiram (strong)
Erythromycin
Fluoroquinolones, e.g. ciprofloxacin and

norfloxacin (strong)
Fluvoxamine (potent — other SSRIs only very weak inhibitors)
Grapefruit juice
Griseofulvin?
Isoniazid
Ketoconazole
Mirtazapine (very weak)

Moclobemide
Omeprazole
Parsley
Parsnip
Propafenone (major)
Quercetin (weak)
Sertraline (weak)
Ticlopidone

No effect

Anidulafungin
Asenapine
Bevacizumab
Benzodiazepines
Capecitibane
Cranberry juice
Duloxetine
Emtricitabine
Galantamine
Isotretinoin
Lacosamide
Lanthanum

Lenalidomide
Levetiracetam
Lithium
Memantine
Methylnaltrexone
Mirtazapine
Nelarabine
Olanzapine
Palonosetron
Posaconazole
Pregabalin
Rasagiline

Rufinamide
Sitagliptin
Sulpiride
Sunitinib
Telbivudine
Varenicline
Venlafaxine
Zoledronic acid
Zonisamide
Ziprasidone

CYP1A2 *

1A2 accounts for about 13% of the total liver CYPs, and metabolises 20% of clinically used drugs (Wang and Zhou, *Curr Med Chem* 2009; [in press]) but may also bioactivate a number of biocarcinogens so 1A2 induction can increase carcinogenicity (Zhou et al, *Curr Drug Metab* 2010; [in press]).

CYP2B6

Substrates (drugs metabolised by this enzyme)

Alfentanil	Ifosfamide	Promethazine
Bupropion	Ketamine	Propofol (main)
Carbamazepine	Lidocaine	Rifampicin
Carteolol	S-methadone (major)	Ropivacaine
Clopidogrel	R-methadone (minor)	Selegiline
Cyclophosphamide	Midazolam	Sevoflurane
Dexamethasone	Nevirapine	Tamoxifen
Diazepam	Nicotine	Testosterone
Ecstasy (MDMA)	Orphenadrine	Thiotepa
Efavirenz	Pethidine	Valproic acid
Estrone	Phenobarbital	
Ethinylestradiol	Procainamide	

Significant enzyme inducers (decrease levels of substrates)

Baicalin, (significant)	Modafinil (minor and	Rifampin
Efavirenz	dose-dependent)	

Significant enzyme inhibitors (increase levels of substrates)

Clopidogrel (potent)	Ketoconazole	fluoxetine, fluvoxamine)
Clotrimazole	Memantine	Thiotepa (potent),
Glabridin (a liquorice	OCs (weak)	Ticopidine
extract)	Orphenadine	Tranylcypromine (modest)
HRT (potent)	Raloxifene	Zolpidem (very weak)
Itraconazole	SSRIs (paroxetine,	

No effect *

Anidulafungin	Lithium	Sulpiride
Benzodiazepines	Methylnaltrexone	Sunitinib
Bevacizumab	Nelarabine	Telbivudine
Emtricitabine	Palonosetron	Venlafaxine
Isotretinoin	Posaconazole	Zoledronic acid
Lacosamide	Rasagiline	Zonisamide
Lamotrigine	Rufinamide	Ziprasidone
Levetiracetam	Sertraline	

CYP2B6 *

2B6 accounts for about 2–10% of the total hepatic CYP content and metabolises about 8% clinically used drugs. It is linked to 3A4 and UGT1A1. There are at least 28 known allelic variants, can be 20–250-fold interindividual variation in 2B6 expression and may be some ethnic variations as well (Mo et al, Curr Drug Metab 2010; [in press]; Wang and Tompkins, Curr Drug Metab 2008;**9**:598–610). Probes for 2B6 include bupropion (general reviews by Walsky et al, J Clin Pharmacol 2006;**46**:1426–38, Turpeinen et al, Curr Drug Metab 2006;**7**:705–14) and thioTEPA (Turpeinen et al, Drug Metab Dispos 2004;**32**:626–31).

CYP2C9

Substrates (drugs metabolised by this enzyme)

Agomelatine (10%)
Alosetron
Amiodarone
Amitriptyline
Arachidonic acid
Atorvastatin
Bupropion (8/9)
Carbamazepine (minor)
Celecoxib
Cimetidine
Fluconazole
Fluoxetine
Flurbiprofen

Fluvastatin
Glipizide
Glyburide
Irbesartan
Losartan
Melatonin
Miconazole
NSAIDs (e.g. diclofenac,
  naproxen, piroxicam,
  tenoxicam 8/9)
Phenobarbital
Phenytoin (major)
Retinoids

Rifampicin
Rosiglitazone
Sibutramine
Sildenafil (partly)
Tolbutamide (8/9)
Torasemide
Trimethoprim
Valproate
Valsartan
S-warfarin (major)

Significant enzyme inducers (decrease levels of substrates)

Carbamazepine (weak)
Dexamethasone
Phenobarbital (weak)

Phenytoin (weak)
Rifampin
St John's wort (weak?)

Tipranavir (minor)

Significant enzyme inhibitors (increase levels of substrates)

Amiodarone
Capecitibane
Cimetidine
Cyclizine
Disulfiram
Fluconazole
Fluorouracil
Fluoxetine
Fluvastatin

Fluvoxamine
Gingko biloba (weak)
Ginseng (weak)
Miconazole
Modafinil
Nilotinib (strong)
Omeprazole
Paroxetine (weak)
Phenylbutazone

Promethazine
Sertraline (moderate)
Suprofen
Tamoxifen
Tolcapone (minor)
Topiramate
Tranylcypromine (part)
Valproate
Zafirlukast

No effect *

Anidulafungin
Aripiprazole
Benzodiazepines
Bevacizumab
Cranberry juice
Emtricitabine
Galantamine
Isotretinoin
Lacosamide
Lamotrigine
Lanthanum

Lenalidomide
Lithium
Memantine
Methylnaltrexone
Mirtazapine
Nelarabine
Olanzapine
Palonosetron
Posaconazole
Pregabalin
Rasagiline

Rufinamide
Sitagliptin
Sulpiride
Sunitinib
Telbivudine
Venlafaxine
Varenicline
Ziprasidone
Zoledronic acid
Zonisamide

CYP2C19

Substrates (drugs metabolised by this enzyme) *

Barbiturates
Carisoprodol
Cimetidine
Citalopram (major 60%)
Clobazam
Clopidogrel (needs 2C19
  to be metabolised from
  pro-drug)
Desmethylclobazam
Diazepam (genotype
  important)
Etizolam
Flunitrazepam
Fluoxetine

Fluvoxamine
Indomethacin
Lansoprazole
Melatonin (partly)
Mephenytoin
Midazolam (minor)
Moclobemide (major)
Nelfinavir
Omeprazole (major)
Perphenazine
Pethidine
Phenytoin (minor)
Proguanil
Promazine

Propranolol (part)
Quazepam
Rabeprazole
Ramelteon (minor)
Rifabutin
Rifampicin
Topiramate
Tranylcypromine
Tricyclics (tertiary, e.g.
  amitriptyline, clomipramine,
  imipramine, trimipramine)
R-warfarin (minor)

Significant enzyme inducers (decrease levels of substrates) *

Carbamazepine (weak)
Common sage (dose-
  dependent)

Gingko biloba (low dose,
  weak)
Phenobarbital (weak)

Rifampin
St John's wort (low dose)
Valerian (weak)

Significant enzyme inhibitors (increase levels of substrates) *

Cimetidine
Felbamate
Fluconazole
Fluoxetine (moderate)
Fluvoxamine
Ginkgo biloba (higher dose,
  weak)
Isoniazid (potent)

Ketoconazole
Moclobemide
Modafinil
Nilotinib (strong)
Omeprazole
Oxcarbazepine
Paroxetine (weak)
Phenytoin

Sertraline (weak)
St John's wort (high dose)
Ticlopidine
Tipranavir (potent)
Topiramate
Tranylcypromine (weak)
Tricyclics (e.g. imipramine)
Valproate

No effect *

Anidulafungin
Aripiprazole
Benzodiazepines
Bevacizumab
Cone flower
Emtricitabine
Horse chestnut
Isotretinoin
Lacosamide
Lanthanum
Lenalidomide

Levetiracetam
Lithium
Memantine
Methylnaltrexone
Mirtazapine
Nelarabine
Olanzapine
Palonosetron
Posaconazole
Pregabalin
Rasagiline

Rufinamide
Sitagliptin
Sulpiride
Sunitinib
Telbivudine
Varenicline
Venlafaxine
Ziprasidone
Zoledronic acid
Zonisamide

2C * is a sub-family, containing many closely related enzymes, e.g. 2C9, 2C10, 2C19, etc. About 20% Asians and 3–5% Caucasians are poor CYP2C19 metabolisers. Around 8% population are 2C19 PM (Carlsson *et al, J Anal Toxicol* 2009;**33**:65–76). 2C9 accounts for around 20% total CYP in the liver, and metabolises about 15% of clinical drugs. It has at least 33 variants (Zhou *et al, Toxicology* 2010; [in press]).

CYP2D6

Substrates (drugs metabolised by this enzyme) *

Amfetamines	Duloxetine (partly)	Palonosetron (main)
Amprenavir	Fenfluramine	Paroxetine
Antiarrhythmics type 1c	Fesoterodine (minor)	Phenothiazines
(encainide, flecainide, etc)	Flecainide	(e.g. perphenazine,
Aripiprazole	Fluphenazine	chlorpromazine,
Asenapine (minor)	Fluoxetine (partly)	fluphenazine, thioridazine)
Atomoxetine	Fluvoxamine (partly)	Propafenone
Beta-blockers (especially	Galantamine	Quinidine
lipophilic, metoprolol,	Gefitinib	Risperidone (major)
nebivolol, propranolol,	Haloperidol	Sertindole (partly)
timolol)	Hydrocodone	Tamoxifen (pro-drug,
Buprenorphine	Indoramin	metabolised to active drug)
Carvedilol	Loratadine	Tolcapone (minor)
Chloroquine	Methadone (part)	Tolterodine
Chlorphenamine	Methamfetamine	Tramadol
Cinnarizine	Mexiletine (main)	Trazodone
Ciprofloxacin	Mianserin	Tricyclics — secondary and
Citalopram (minor)	Mirtazapine (minor)	tertiary tricyclics (e.g.
Clozapine (minor, unproven)	Morphine derivatives	nortriptyline, imipramine,
Codeine (to morphine)	Imatinib (minor but can	maprotiline, trimipramine,
Darifenacin (saturable)	be major)	amitriptyline, clomipramine
Debrisoquine	Nefazodone	and desipramine [weak])
Dexfenfluramine	Nicotine (partly)	Venlafaxine (major)
Dextromethorphan	Olanzapine (partly)	Zuclopenthixol
Diazepam	Ondansetron	
Donepezil (partly)	Oxycodone (partly)	

Significant enzyme inducers (decrease levels of substrates)*

Carbamazepine (weak)	Phenobarbital (weak)	Rifampin (weak)
Ginseng (weak)	Phenytoin (weak)	Ritonavir (weak)

Significant enzyme inhibitors (increase levels of substrates)*

Amidarone	Chlorphenamine	Cyclizine
Asenapine (weak)	Chlorpromazine	Dextromethorphan
Buprenorphine (very weak)	Cimetidine	Dextropropoxyphene
Bupropion	Citalopram (very weak/nil)	Diltiazem (weak)
Celecoxib	Clomipramine (moderate)	Diphenhydramine
Chloroquine	Cocaine	Duloxetine

CYP2D6

Significant enzyme inhibitors *continued*

Escitalopram
Fenfluramine?
Flecainide
Fluoxetine (strong)
Fluphenazine
Fluvoxamine (very weak)
Haloperidol (dose-dependent)
Indinavir
Levomepromazine
Methadone (weak?)
Metoclopramide
Metoprolol
Methylnaltrexone (weak)
Mexiletine

Mibefradil
Mirtazapine (very weak/nil)
Moclobemide
Modafinil (small and dose-dependent)
Nefazodone (very weak/nil)
Nicardipine
Nilotinib (strong)
Norfluoxetine (strong)
Paroxetine (strong, dose-related)
Perphenazine
Pindolol
Primaquine
Promethazine

Propafenone
Propanolol
Quinidine
Quinine
Quetiapine
Ritonavir
Sertraline (weak, dose-related, moderate at 150mg/d)
Terbinafine (potent)
Thioridazine
Timolol
Tipranavir (potent)
Tricyclics (all, strong)
Yohimbine

No effect *

Anidulafungin
Aripiprazole
Benzodiazepines
Bevacizumab
Emtricitabine
Galantamine
Isotretinoin
Lacosamide
Lamotrigine
Lanthanum

Lenalidomide
Levetiracetam
Memantine
Mirtazapine
Olanzapine
Palonosetron
Posaconazole
Pregabalin
Rasagiline
Rufinamide

Sitagliptin
Sulpiride
Sunitinib
Telbivudine
Varenicline
Venlafaxine (very weak, nil)
Ziprasidone
Zoledronic acid
Zonisamide

CYP2D6 *

2D6 accounts for only about 2–4% of total liver CYPs but metabolises about 25% of current drugs (Zhou, *Clin Pharmacokinet* 2009;**48**:689–723). Metabolism occurs both in the liver and in the brain. An individual's CYP2D6 status can be determined by giving the probes debrisoquine or dextromethorphan and measuring the ratios of drug and metabolite. Around 5–8% Caucasians, 8.5% African-Americans and 2–10% Asians are slow metabolisers. Up to 29% North Africans and Middle East people (de Leon *et al, Psychosomatics* 2006;**47**:75–85) are ultra-rapid metabolisers (3 or more 2D6 allelles). All CYP2D6 inhibition is probably concentration-dependent and so inclusion in this list only predicts that an interaction could occur, not that it will.

CYP3A3/4

Substrates (drugs metabolised by this enzyme)

Alfentanil
Alitretinoin
Alosetron
Amiodarone (major)
Amprenavir
Androgens
Antihistamines, e.g. astemizole
Aripiprazole
Asenapine (minor)
Benzodiazepines (e.g.
  alprazolam, clonazepam,
  diazepam, flunitrazepam,
  midazolam, temazepam and
  triazolam, but not
  lorazepam)
Bromocriptine
Budesonide
Buprenorphine
Buspirone
Busulfan
Calcium-channel blockers
  (e.g. amlodipine,
  diltiazem, felodipine,
  isradipine, nicardipine,
  nifedipine, verapamil)
Cannabinoids
Carbamazepine
Chloramphenicol
Chloroquine
Ciclosporin
Cimetidine
Ciprofloxacin
Cisapride (restricted in UK)
Citalopram (minor, 30%)
Clindamycin
Clopidrogel
Clotrimazole
Clozapine (partly)
Cocaine
Codeine
Colchicine
Cortisol
Cyclophosphamide
Dapsone
Darifenacin

Dasatinib
Dexamethasone
Dextromethorphan
Digoxin
Disopyramide
Docetaxol
Donepezil (part)
Doxorubicin
Doxycycline
Dutasteride
Efavirez
Ergotamine
Erlotinib (major)
Estradiol and estrogens
Ethosuximide
Ethinylestradiol
Etoposide
Everolimus
Fentanyl
Fesoterodine (main)
Fexofenadine
Fluconazole
Fluoxetine
Flutamine
Fluvoxamine
Fosaprepitant
Galantamine
Gefitinib
Glibenclamide
Glyburide?
Granisetron
Haloperidol
Ifosfamide
Imatinib (major)
Indinavir
Irinotecan
Isoniazid
Isotretinoin
Itraconazole
Ivabradine
Ivermectin
Ketoconazole
Lapatinib
Levonorgestrel
Lidocaine

Lisuride
Lopinavir
Loratadine
Losartan
Macrolides (e.g. erythromycin,
  clarithromycin)
Maravoric
Meloxicam
Methadone (main)
Methylprednisolone
Mianserin
Mibefradil
Miconazole
Mifepristone
Mirtazapine (partly)
Modafinil
Nefazodone
Nelfinavir
Nilotinib
Ondansetron
Orphenadrine
Oxycodone (prob minor)
Paclitaxel
Paracetamol
Paricalcitol (?)
Perphenazine
Pethidine
Phenobarbital
Phenytoin
Pimozide (mostly)
Prednisone
Progesterone
Proguanil
Propafenone
Promazine
Protein-pump inhibitors
  (lansoprazole [weak],
  omeprazole, rabeprazole)
Quetiapine (mostly)
Quinidine
Quinine
Ramelteon (minor)
Reboxetine
Rifampin
Rimonabant

CYP3A3/4

Substrates, i.e. drugs metabolised by this enzyme *continued*

Risperidone (partly)
Ritonavir
Saquinavir
Sertindole (partly)
Sertraline
Sibutramine (main)
Sildenafil (partly)
Sirolimus
Sitagliptin (limited except in
   renal failure)
Sodium fusidate
Sorafenib
Statins (e.g. atorvastatin,
   cerivastatin, lovastatin,
   pravastin, simvastatin)
Steroids (e.g.

dexamethasone)
St John's wort
Sunitinib
Tacrolimus
Tamoxifen
Temsirolimus
Testosterone
Theophylline
Tiagabine
Tipranavir
Tolcapone (minor)
Tolterodine
Tolvaptan
Topiramate (possibly)
Trabectedin
Tricyclics — tertiary (e.g.

imipramine, amitrip-
   tyline, clomipramine)
Valproate
Vardenafil
Venlafaxine
Vinblastine
Vincristine
Vinorelbine (major)
R-warfarin (minor)
Zaleplon (secondary route)
Ziprasidone (most)
Zolpidem (mainly)
Zonisamide (part)
Zopiclone (mostly)
Zotepine

Significant enzyme inducers (decrease levels of substrates)

Barbiturates (all)
Carbamazepine (induces
   3A4 about 46% more than
   oxcarbazepine)
Cortisol
Dexamethasone
Efavirez
Ethosuximide
Flucloxacillin

Modafinil (small and dose-
   dependent)
Nevirapine (?)
Omeprazole
Oxcarbazepine
Phenobarbital
Phenytoin
Pioglitazone
Prednisone

Primidone
Rifampin (rapid)
Rufinamide (moderate
   effect)
St John's wort (moderate)
Topiramate (dose-
   dependent, especially
   at high doses)
Troglitazone

Significant enzyme inhibitors (increase levels of substrates)

Acetazolamide
Amiodarone
Atazaivir (moderate)
Buprenorphine (weak/
   moderate)
Cannabinoids
Cimetidine (moderate)
Citalopram (weak)
Clotrimazole
Danazol
Dextropropoxyphene
Diltiazem (weaker)
Echinacea purpurea (weak)
Erlotinib
Fluconazole (strong)
Fluoxetine (weak)

Fluvoxamine (moderate)
Fosaprepitant (minor)
Gestodene
Gingko biloba
Grapefruit juice (weak)
Imatinib
Indinavir (moderate)
Isoniazid (potent)
Itraconazole (strong)
Ivabradine (very weak)
Ketoconazole (strong)
Lopinavir
Macrolides (some, e.g. clarith-
   romycin, erythromycin,
   strong)
Methadone (weak?)

Metronidazole
Mibefradil
Miconazole (strong)
Mifepristone
Nefazodone (strong)
Nelfinavir
Nilotinib (strong)
Norfluoxetine (moderate)
Orange juice (weak)
Paroxetine (weak)
Posaconazole (potent)
Quinine
Ritonavir (moderate)
Saquinavir
Sertindole (weak)
Sertraline (minor)

Significant enzyme inhibitors (increase levels of substrates) *continued*		
Statins (atorvastatin, fluvastatin)	Trazodone	Verapamil (weak)
Stiripentol (variable)	Tricyclics (moderate)	Zafirlukast
Terbinafine	Troleandomycin (strong)	
	Venlafaxine (very weak)	

No effect *		
Aliskiren	Ivabradine	Pioglitazone
Anidulafungin	Lamotrigine	Pregabalin
Aripiprazole	Lanthanum	Rasagiline
Asenapine	Lenalidomide	Rosaconazole
Benzodiazepines	Levetiracetam	Sitagliptin
Bevacizumab	Lithium	Sunitinib
Capecitibane	Memantine	Telbivudine
Cranberry juice	Methylnaltrexone	Varenicline
Duloxetine	Mirtazapine	Zoledronic acid
Emtricitabine	Nelarabine	Zonisamide
Galantamine	Olanzapine	Ziprasidone
Isotretinoin	Palonosetron	

CYP3A3/4 * (very similar structures, and are often grouped together). CYP3A4 is an important P450 enzyme, metabolising at least 50% of all marketed medications (Zhou, *Curr Drug Metab* 2008;**9**:310-22), and may account for up to 50–60% of the total liver P450. There is little generic polymorphism so little inter-individual variation exits. CYP3A4 occurs in the liver, gut and, possibly, the brain. Ultra-rapid metabolisers have not yet been identified. Debrisoquine is a probe. Midazolam is more reliable, although simvastatin, lovastatin and buspirone are alternatives (s=113, Ohno *et al*, *Clin Pharmacokinet* 2007;**46**:681–96).

5 DRUG-INDUCED PSYCHIATRIC DISORDERS

The drugs listed in each section have been reported to cause that condition in some context (e.g. standard dose, high dose, prolonged courses, etc). The main references next to the drug should be consulted to ascertain the circumstances of reports. The references are offered without qualification and no indication of frequency or status of reports can be given as this information is not really available, except where a side–effect is well recognised, BNF, listed. For completeness, drugs not available in every country are also listed.

Sub–divisions are based on the UK BNF, chapters: (although many drugs appear in several sections)

- CNS: anxiolytics and hypnotics (including BDZs)
- CNS: antipsychotics (including lithium)
- CNS: antidepressants (including bupropion)
- CNS: analgesics
- CNS: anticonvulsants
- CNS: antiparkinsonian drugs
- CNS: others
- Gastrointestinal drugs
- Cardiovascular drugs
- Respiratory drugs
- Anti–infection drugs
- Endocrine system drugs
- Malignancy and immunosuppressant drugs
- Musculoskeletal and analgesics
- Others

The BNF side–effect categories generally mean:

- Very common = more than one in 10 people get this side–effect
- Common one in 10 to one in 100 (1–10%)
- Uncommon or less common = 1 one in 100 to one in 1,000 (0.1–1%)
- Rare = one in 1,000 to one in 10,000 (0.01–0.1%)
- Very rare = less than one in 10,000 (≤0.01%).

Each side–effect may be dose–related (the higher the dose, the more likely you are to get it, especially a higher starting dose) and may abate with time.

5.1 ANXIETY, AGITATION AND NERVOUSNESS

- CNS — anxiolytics and hypnotics *
Benzodiazepine withdrawal (n = 43, d/b, p/c, 7/52, abrupt is much worse than gradual withdrawal, e.g. Am J Psychiatry 1984;**141**:848–52)
Clomethiazole
Sodium oxybate (BNF common)
Temazepam
Zopiclone (n = 1, Ir Med J 2007;**100**:511; n=1, Prog Neurol Psychiatry 2009;**13**:20–4)

- CNS — antipsychotics *
Aripiprazole initiation (n = 2, J Clin Psychiatry 2004;**65**:132–3; n = 3, Pharmacother 2007; **27**:1339–42; after clozapine discontinuation, n=1, J Clin Psychiatry 2009;**70**:141–3)
~ high–dose (n = 1, J Neuropsychiatry Clin Neurosci 2007;**19**: 481–2)
~ after clozapine discontinuation (n=1, J Clin Psychiatry 2009;**70**:141–3)
Olanzapine (Can J Psychiatry 1998;**43**:1054)
Risperidone (n = 1, Am J Psychiatry 1995;**152**:1096–7; n=1, Psychiatry Clin Neurosci 1999;**53**:682)
Zotepine (BNF, common)

- CNS — antidepressants *
Early worsening of anxiety and agitation with antidepressants is well–known but very poorly researched (Br J Psychiatry 2009;**194**:483–90).
Mianserin abrupt withdrawal (n = 1, panic anxiety, Jpn J Psychiatry Neurol 1989;**43**:155–9)
Moclobemide (incidence 5–10%, J Neural Transm 1989;**28** [Suppl]:S77–S89)
Reboxetine (BNF, rare)
SSRIs (BNF, common)
→ citalopram (cases in Eur J Clin Pharmacol 1986;**31**:18–22)
→ fluoxetine (incidence 9%? e.g. J Clin Psychiatry 1985;**46**(3 Pt 2):32–7)
→ paroxetine (incidence 11%? Acta Psychiatr Scand 1989;**80**[Suppl 350]:117–37)

→ paroxetine withdrawal (rebound anxiety, review, *Can J Clin Pharmacol* 2006;**13**: 69–74)
→ SSRI withdrawal (BNF)
Tricyclics (e.g. amitriptyline, lofepramine at < 2%, review in *Drugs* 1989;**37**: 123–40)

• CNS — analgesics *
Buprenorphine (BNF, common)
Fentanyl (BNF, common)
Frovatriptan (BNF, less common)
Morphine
Nefopam
Oxycodone (BNF, common)
Pentazocine (e.g. *Br Med J* 1974;**2**:224)
Pizotifen (BNF, rare)
Sumatriptan in people with panic disorder (n = 15, RCT, d/b, p/c, *Eur Neuropsychopharmacol* 2005;**15**:279–82)

• CNS — anticonvulsants *
Carbamazepine (*J Am Acad Child Adolesc Psychiatry* 1988;**27**:500–3)
Clonazepam
Ethosuximide
Gabapentin (BNF, common)
Gabapentin withdrawal (n = 1, *J Clin Psychiatry* 1998;**59**:131)
Lamotrigine
Levetiracetam (BNF, common)
Phenobarbital and other barbiturates
Piracetam (BNF, uncommon)
Rufinamide (BNF, common; 1–10% incidence, UK SPC)
Topiramate (BNF, common)
Valproate (n = 1, *J Neuropsychiatry Clin Neurosci* 2001;**13**:528–30)
Vigabatrin
Zonisamide (SPC)

• CNS — antiparkinsonian drugs *
Amantadine
Anticholinergics (BNF, common)
Baclofen (used in Parkinson's Disease, UK SPC change 2009)
Bromocriptine
Levodopa (BNF, common)
Rotigotine (BNF, less common)

• CNS — others *
Alcohol (review, n = 285, *Aggress Behav*

2007;**33**:327–38)
Anticholinesterases (n = 4, *J Neuropsychiatry Clin Neurosci* 1992;**4**:189–94) e.g.:
→ donepezil (n = 1, *Int J Geriatr Psychiatry* 2003;**18**:657–8)
→ rivastigmine (incidence <5%, inc transdermal patches; UK SPC, common)
Aprepitant (BNF, less common)
Atomoxetine (BNF, common; n = 1, *Pediatrics* 2004;**114**:895–6)
Botulinum toxin A injection (BNF, less common; *South Med J* 1999;**92**:738)
Bupropion (incidence 9.7%; BNF, common)
Caffeine (n = 22 children, d/b, p/c, c/o, *J Am Acad Child Adolesc Psychiatry* 1994;**33**:407–15)
Cannabis (n = 79, no association, *Psychiatry Res* 2003;**118**:1–8)
Dexamfetamine
Flumazenil (BNF, common)
Gamma–Hydroxybutyrate (GHB) intoxication (n = 66 with toxicity, 60% incidence, *Am J Emerg Med* 2005;**23**:316–20)
Ginseng (reported, inc. abuse, see *Arch Gen Psychiatry* 1998;**55**:1033–44)
Granisetron (unconfirmed, e.g. *Eur J Cancer* 1990;**26**[Supp 1]:S19–23)
Heroin withdrawal (*Int J Addict* 1992;**27**:25–35)
LSD (n = 16, responds to clonazepam, *Int Clin Psychopharmacol* 2003;**18**:101–5)
Memantine (n = 3, *J Neurol Neurosurg Psychiatry* 2007;**78**:546)
Memantine abrupt discontinuation (n = 2, *Geriatr Gerontol Int* 2009;**9**:202–5)
Metoclopramide (n = 1, *Psychiatry Clin Neurosci* 2007;**61**:193–5)
Modafinil (BNF, common, n = 2, *J Clin Psychopharmacol* 2005;**25**:628–9)
Naltrexone (BNF, common)
Orlistat (BNF, common)
Palonosetron (BNF, less common)
Rimonabant (BNF, common; see SPC, *Lancet* 2007;**370**:1671–2)
Sibutramine (BNF, common)
Sodium oxybate (BNF, common)

• Gastrointestinal drugs *
Bismuth intoxication (*Postgrad Med J* 1988;**64**:308–10)
H2 blockers (BNF, rare) e.g.:
→ cimetidine (*Adv Psychiatric Treat* 2005;**11**:68)

→ famotidine (mentioned in *Digestion*
1985;**32** [Suppl 1]:24–31)
Misoprostol
Omeprazole

• Cardiovascular drugs *
Adrenaline/epinephrine (BNF, common)
Atenolol withdrawal (n = 1, *Am J Psychiatry*
1994;**151**:1840)
Cilostazol (BNF, less common)
Doxazosin (incidence 2.4%)
Epoprostenol (BNF, common)
Fondaparinux sodium (BNF, rare)
Hydralazine (BNF, rare)
Isoproterenol (*Psychopharmacol Bull*
1985;**21**:424–7)
Methoxamine
Methyldopa (rare)
Moexipril (BNF, common)
Nicardipine (rare)
Nifedipine (*An Med Interna* 1992;**9**:362)
Ramipril (BNF, less common)
Sodium nitroprusside (BNF, common)
Streptokinase (see *Drugs* 1973;**5**:357)
Telmisartan (BNF, less common)

• Respiratory drugs *
Aminophylline
Ephedrine (BNF, common)
Mizolastine (BNF, common)
Montelukast (SPC, FDA warning 2009)
Phenylpropanolamine OD (*Lancet*
1979;**314**:1367–8)
Pseudoephedrine (n = 1, *Eur J Clin Pharmacol*
1978;**14**:253–9)
Salbutamol
Theophylline (*Med Clin (Barc)* 1987;**88**:549–50)

• Anti–infection drugs *
Atazanavir (BNF, less common)
Azithromycin (BNF, rare)
Chloroquine and mefloquine (*Adv Psychiatr Treat*
2005;**11**:66)
Clarithromycin (BNF, very rare)
Co–trimoxazole (n = 1, *J Clin Psychopharmacol*
1991;**11**:144–5)
Daptomycin (BNF, less common)
Darunavir (BNF, common)
Efavirenz (BNF, common)
Enfuvirtide (BNF, common)
Ertapenem (BNF, rare)

Ganciclovir (BNF, common; *N Engl J Med*
1990;**322**:933–4; *Adv Psychiatr Treat*
2005;**11**:66)
Isoniazid (*Lancet* 1989;**334**:735–6)
Levamisole (rare, *N Engl J Med*
1990;**322**:352–8)
Lopinavir with ritonavir (BNF, less common)
Mefloquine (BNF, less common; *Pharm J*
1989;**243**:561)
Penicillins (*Adv Psychiatr Treat* 2005;**11**:66)
Piperazine (see *Trans R Soc Trop Med Hyg*
1976;**70**:358)
Quinine (*Adv Psychiatr Treat* 2005;**11**:66)
Quinupristin with dalfopristin (BNF, less
common)
Ribavirin (BNF, common)
Ritonavir (BNF, common)
Stavudine (BNF, less common)
Voriconazole (BNF, common)
Zidovudine (BNF, common)

• Endocrine system drugs *
Corticosteroids (BNF, less common; *Adv
Psychiatr Treat* 2005;**11**:68; incidence may be
as high as 5–6% in adults, usually emerges
within a few days or weeks, risk may be
higher with higher doses, *MHRA Drug Safety
Update* 2007;1–9)
    → dexamethasone — overall risks:
        • dose–related (but not time, duration
        or severity)
        • female gender
        • PMH (but only weak association)
        (see *Arch Gen Psychiatry* 1981;**38**:471–7)
    → methyltestosterone
    → prednisone (especially in children, cases
    in *Clin Paediatr* 1990;**29**:382–8)
Danazol (BNF, common)
Levothyroxine
Testosterone and esters (BNF, common)
Zoledronic acid (BNF, less common)

• Malignancy and immunosuppressant drugs *
Buserelin (BNF, less common)
Ciclosporin (*Adv Psychiatr Treat* 2005;**11**:68)
Clofarabine (BNF, common)
Glatiramer acetate (BNF, common)
Imatinib (BNF, less common)
Interferons, e.g.:
    → interferon alfa (responds to
    benzodiazepines, n = 2, *J Psychopharmacol*

2004;**18**:41–6)
→ peginterferon alfa 2a + ribavirin (n = 176, incidence < 36%, *Aliment Pharmacol Ther* 2008;**27**:257–65)
Letrozole (BNF, less common)
Octreotide
Trastuzumab (BNF, less common)
Tretinoin (BNF, common)

- Musculoskeletal and analgesics *

Abatacept (BNF, less common)
Baclofen (BNF, common; n = 2, *Lancet* 1977;**2**:44)
Etoricoxib (BNF, less common)
Leflunomide (BNF, common)
Methocarbamol (BNF, less common)
NSAIDs (*Adv Psychiatric Treat* 2005;**11**:68), e.g.:
→ ibuprofen (overdose, *Am J Emerg Med* 1998;**16**: 549–50)
→ indometacin (n = 1, *South Med J* 1983;**76**:679–80)
→ mefenamic acid
→ naproxen
→ naproxen + chloroquine (*Ann Pharmacother* 1993;**27**: 1058–9)

- Others *

Atropine eye drops (n = 1, *J Ped Ophthalmol Strabis* 1985;**22**: 38–9)
Cyclopentolate eye drops (n = 1, *Nervenarzt* 2009;**80**:967–9)
Deferasirox (BNF, less common)
Flunisolide
Isotretinoin (BNF, rare; n = 45 [c = 23], no association with anxiety, *J Dermatolog Treat* 2004;**15**:153–7)
Ketamine (BNF, common)
Lidocaine (n = 15, incidence 73%, *Am J Psychiatry* 1987;**144**:159–63)
Neostigmine (cases in *Dtsch Med Wochenschr* 1966;**91**:699)
Organic solvents (n = 77, up to 36% can develop anxiety clusters, *Psychosom Med* 2000;**62**:746–50)
Phenylephrine (rare)
Pyridostigmine (rare)
Ropivacaine (BNF, less common; n = 3 after nerve block, *Reg Anesth Pain Med* 1999;**24**:175–8)
Sevoflurane (n = 169, common, reduced by clonidine, *Anesth Analg* 2005;**101**:1619–22)

Sildenafil (BNF common)
Tacrolimus (BNF, rare; *Adv Psychiatr Treat* 2005;**11**:68)
Vardenafil (BNF, rare)
Yohimbine (mentioned in *Arch Gen Psychiatry* 1998;**55**: 1033–44)
Zafirlukast (FDA warning 2009)

5.2 AGGRESSION, INCLUDING HOSTILITY AND VIOLENCE

Review: Shaw and Fletcher, *Adv Drug React Toxicolog Rev* 2000;**19**: 35–45, 64 refs.

- CNS *

Alcohol (review, n = 285, *Aggress Behav* 2007;**33**:327–38)
Alcohol withdrawal
Amantadine (cases in *Br Med J* 1972;**3**:50)
Amfetamine withdrawal
Anticholinesterases (n = 4, *J Neuropsychiatry Clin Neurosci* 1992;**4**:189–94)
→ donepezil (e.g. n = 1, *Am J Psychiatry* 1998;**155**:1632–3; n=1, *Int J Geriatr Psychiatry* 2003;**18**:657–8)
Atomoxetine (*Pediatrics* 2004;**114**:895–6)
Barbiturate withdrawal
Benzodiazepines (incidence < 1%, *J Clin Psychiatry* 1988;**49**:184–8; during prolonged benzodiazepine use: *Can J Psychiatry* 2000; **45**:89–90; aggressogenic effect from diazepam, n = 60 male, *Addict Behav* 2002;**27**: 167–77; review *CNS Drugs* 1998;**9**:41–57), e.g.:
→ alprazolam (greater response to provocation, n = 23, RCT, p/c, 8/52, *J Affect Disord* 1995;**35**:117–23)
Carbamazepine
Gabapentin (n = 1, *J Neuropsychiatry Clin Neurosci* 2001;**13**:424; n = 2, *Epilepsia* 1996;**37**:501–2)
Lamotrigine (survey, n = 19, *Epilepsia* 1998;**39**:280–2)
Levetiracetam (SPC)
Modafinil (n = 2, *J Clin Psychopharmacol* 2005; **25**:628–9)
Naloxone IV (n = 2, *Ann Pharmacother* 1992; **26**:196–8)
Olanzapine (*Can J Psychiatry* 1998;**43**: 1054)
Paroxetine withdrawal (*Lancet* 1995;**346**:57)
Tricyclics (rare)
Venlafaxine (n = 1, *J Am Acad Child Adolesc Psychiatry* 2003;**42**: 383–4)

Vigabatrin (e.g. *Drugs* 1991;**41**:889–926)

● **Others** *
Anabolic steroids, e.g. oxandrolone
Anabolic steroid withdrawal
Cyproheptadine (n = 1, *J Am Acad Child Adolesc Psychiatry* 1998;**37**:668–70)
Omeprazole
Sildenafil (review, n = 274, *Ann Pharmacother* 2002;**36**:1129–34)
Steroids high dose (*Lancet* 1987;**2**:750–1)
Testosterone (highly variable, n = 56 men, RCT, p/c, c/o, 3×6/52, *Arch Gen Psychiatry* 2000;**57**:133–40)

5.3 BEHAVIOURAL CHANGES

● **CNS** *
Barbiturates
Benzodiazepines:
→ clonazepam (*Dev Med Child Neurol* 1991; **33**:362–5)
Carbamazepine (*J Paediatrics* 1982;**101**:785–7)
Donepezil (e.g. n = 7, *Am J Psychiatry* 1998;**155**: 1632–3)
Gamma–Hydroxybutyrate (GHB) intoxication (n = 66 with toxicity, 60% incidence, *Am J Emerg Med* 2005;**23**:316–20)
Levetiracetam (n = 553, incidence 7%, *Neurology* 2003; **61**:1218–21)
Levodopa
Levodopa + carbidopa
Lithium + antipsychotics

● **Others**
Anabolic steroids (n = 1, bizarre after brief exposure to low potency, *Am J Psychiatry* 1992;**149**:271–2)
Bismuth (*Acta Neurologica Belgica* 1979;**79**:73)
Methyldopa + haloperidol
Prazosin (n = 1, bizarre behaviour, *Am J Psychiatry* 2008;**165**:744–5)
Prednisone withdrawal (*JAMA* 1989;**261**:1731)
Theophylline (disputed — not in children, *JAMA* 1992;**267**:2621–4)

5.4 DELIRIUM (ACUTE ORGANIC PSYCHOSIS) AND CONFUSION

Drug-induced delirium is usually an acute reaction and always with fluctuating levels of awareness of self and environment. It is most frequent in frail or dementing elderly, drug abusers and with pre-existing organic brain disease, and is strongly associated with anticholinergic activity:
● high risk drug groups are tricyclics and typical antipsychotics
● medium risk drugs include benzodiazepines, sedatives, dopamine-activating drugs, anticonvulsants, histamine H2 receptor blockers, digoxin, beta-blockers and analgesics. Most of these do not have direct anticholinergic effects but *in vitro* have been shown to bind to muscarinic receptors.

Reviews: * drug-induced delirium and management (Brown, *Semin Clin Neuropsychiatry* 2000;**5**: 113–24), in elderly (Moore and O'Keeffe, *Drugs Aging* 1999;**15**:15–28; Inouye, *Dement Geriatr Cogn Disord* 1999;**10**:393–400), management and causes (Attard et al, *CNS Drugs* 2008;**22**:631–44), drugs with anticholinergic properties (Cancelli et al, *Neurol Sci* 2009;**30**:87–92).

● **CNS — anxiolytics and hypnotics** *
Benzodiazepine withdrawal
Benzodiazepines, e.g.:
→ alprazolam (n = 1, *Clin Neuropharmacol* 1998;**21**:201–3)
→ diazepam as pre-med (n = 1, *Indian J Ophthalmol* 1989;**37**:35–6)
Chloral and derivatives
Clomethiazole
Clomethiazole withdrawal
Zolpidem (several cases, e.g. n = 1, *Ann Pharmacother* 2001;**35**:1562–4; n = 1, elderly, *Psychosomatics* 2004;**45**:88–9)
Zopiclone withdrawal (n = 1, *Age Ageing* 2005; **34**:526–7)

● **CNS — antipsychotics** *
Aripiprazole high-dose (n = 1, *J Neuropsychiatry Clin Neurosci* 2007;**19**:481–2)
Butyrophenones
Clozapine (may occur in 10%, especially in older people also taking other anticholinergics; n = 139, *Pharmacopsychiatry* 2003;**36**:156–60)
Clozapine withdrawal (n = 3, *J Clin Psychiatry* 1997;**58**:252–5)
Lithium (e.g. n = 1, *Am J Psychiatry* 1983; **140**:1612; n = 1, *Psychiatr Prax* 2000; **27**:296–7; n = 1, *Practitioner* 2009; **253**:28–30)
Olanzapine (n = 1[elderly], *J Clin Psychiatry*

2004;**65**;582–3; n = 1, *Ann Pharmacother* 2006;**40**:135–8)

Olanzapine + opioid (n = 2, *J Pain Symptom Manage* 2005;**29**:330–2)

Phenothiazines (esp. sedative ones)

Quetiapine toxicity (n = 1, *Aust N Z J Psychiatry* 2009;**43**:781)

Quetiapine + lithium (n = 1, *Clin Neuropharmacol* 2008;**31**:176–9)

Risperidone (n = 1, *Can J Psychiatry* 1998;**43**: 194; n = 1, *J Child Adolesc Psychopharmacol* 2005; **15**:520–5)

• CNS — antidepressants *
Bupropion (cases, e.g. *J Clin Psychiatry* 1990;**51**: 307–8)

Bupropion + fluoxetine (n = 1, *J Clin Psychopharmacol* 2006;**26**:677–9)

MAOIs, e.g.:
→ phenelzine (*J Clin Psychiatry* 1987;**48**: 340–1)
→ tranylcypromine (*J Clin Psychopharmacol* 1997;**17**:430–2)
→ tranylcypromine abuse (*J Clin Psychopharmacol* 2000;**20**:270–1)

Mianserin (n = 1, *Br Med J* 1988;**296**: 137; n = 5, *Eur Neuropsychopharmacol* 1995;**5**:147–9)

Mirtazapine (n = 3, *Int Clin Psychopharmacol* 2000;**15**:239–43)

SSRIs, e.g.:
→ fluoxetine (n = 1, *Am J Psychiatry* 1995; **152**:295–6)
→ paroxetine (n = 1, *Pharmacopsychiatry* 2007;**40**:199–200)
→ paroxetine withdrawal (n = 1, *J Neuropsych Clin Neurosci* 2004;**16**: 119–20)
→ paroxetine and benzatropine (n = 1, *Am J Psychiatry* 1997;**154**:581–2)

Trazodone (n = 3, *Int Clin Psychopharmacol* 1998;**13**:225–8)

Tricyclics (*J Clin Psychiatry* 1983;**44**: 173–6), e.g.:
→ imipramine (n = 1, *Am J Psychiatry* 1983;**140**:1517–8)

Venlafaxine (n = 1, *Can J Psychiatry* 2003;**48**: 129)

• CNS — analgesics *
Dextropropoxyphene withdrawal

Ergotamine + caffeine (n = 1, *Pharmacother* 2002;**22**:126–9)

Fentanyl (*Anesthesiology* 1995;**83**:869–71)

Methadone (during switch from fentanyl, *J Pain Symptom Manage* 2001;**21**:177–8)

Nalbuphine

Narcotics

Opioids (n = 1, *J Pain Symptom Manage* 2004; **27**:268–73)

Papaveretum

Tramadol (n = 11, *Curr Problems* 1995;**21**:2; n = 1, *Pharmacopsychiatry* 2006;**39**:194–9)

• CNS — anticonvulsants *
Barbiturate withdrawal

Barbiturates (dose–related)

Benzodiazepines (common cause, see anxiolytics)
→ clonazepam (*Mil Med* 1997;**162**:3)
→ midazolam (alone and with propofol, n = 1, *Anesth Prog* 2006;**53**:95–7)

Carbamazepine (especially early in therapy; as part of SIADH, *Psychiatr Prax* 2001;**28**:48–9)

Ethosuximide

Gabapentin abuse (n = 1, *J Psychiatr Pract* 2009;**15**:314–9)

Lacosamide (common, SPC)

Phenytoin (dose–related)

Pregabalin (SPC; *Clin Neuropharmacol* 2009;**32**:236–7)

Primidone

Phenytoin + temozolomide (n = 1, *Psychosomatics* 2007;**48**:359–60)

Topiramate (reversible dementia, n = 1, *Clin Neuropharmacol* 2008;**31**:62; n = 1, *Bipolar Disord* 2001;**3**:211–2)

Valproate (n=272, usually in first 2/52, can be serious, more common in elderly, *Pharmacopsychiatry* 2009;**42**:61–5)

Valproic acid loading dose (n=1, *J Clin Psychiatry* 2005;**66**:801–2)

Valproate + lamotrigine (n = 1, *Am J Psychiatry* 2004;**161**:1128–9)

Zonisamide (*J Clin Psychopharmacol* 2004; **4**:110–1; SPC)

• CNS — antiparkinsonian drugs
Amantadine (n=1, *Am J Psychiatry* 1980;**137**:240–2)

Amantadine withdrawal (n=3, *Neurology* 1998;**50**:1456–8)

Anticholinergic drugs (particular association, *J Am Geriatr Soc* 1988;**36**:525; n = 278, *Arch Internal Med* 2001;**161**: 1099–105)

Bromocriptine

Levodopa (*Lancet* 1973;**ii**:929)

Lisuride

Pergolide withdrawal (*Clin Neuropharmacology* 1988;**11**:545–8)

Ropinirole (common, SPC)

Selegiline

• CNS — others *

Alcohol + disulfiram (n = 1, *Ann Pharmacother* 2001;**35**:32–5)

Alcohol withdrawal (n=1, persistent after heavy use, *Am J Psychiatry* 1997;**154**:846–51)

Amfetamines

Anticholinesterases, e.g.:
  → donepezil (n = 1, *J Clin Psychiatry* 2002;**63**: 250–1)
  → rivastigmine (incidence <5%)
  → rivastigmine transdermal patches (UK SPC, common)

Baclofen (used in Parkinson's Disease, UK SPC change 2009)

Betahistine (n = 1, *Ned Tijdschr Geneeskd* 2004;**148**:2338–41)

Caffeine (n=1, overdose and physical stress, *Am J Psychiatry* 1978;**135**:855–6)

Cannabis (in cookies, n = 1, *CNS Spectr* 2006;**11**:262)

Cocaine (*Am J Emerg Med* 1996;**14**:425–8; n=333, *Am J Forensic Med Pathol* 1999;**20**:120–7; n = 3 deaths, *Ned Tijdschr Geneeskd* 2009;**153**:1014–7)

Disulfiram (n = 5, *Am J Psychiatry* 1974;**131**:1281; n = 1, *Nihon Arukoru Yakubutsu Igakkai Zasshi* 2006;**41**:535–40)

Disulfiram + alcohol (n = 1, *Ann Pharmacother* 2001;**35**:32–5)

Disulfiram + tranylcypromine (n = 1, *Am J Psychiatry* 1995;**152**:296)

Ergotamine–caffeine (n = 1, *Pharmacother* 2002;**22**;126–9)

Gamma–butyrolactone (GBL) withdrawal (n = 1, *Pharmacopsychiatry* 2009;**42**:202–3)

Gamma–hydroxy butyrate (GHB) (n = 1, *Gen Hosp Psychiatry* 2000;**22**:213–5)

Hyoscine, transdermal (n = 1, *JAMA* 1988;**260**:478)

MDMA/ecstasy (n = 3, *J Psychoactive Drugs* 1999;**31**:167–70)

Metoclopramide (*J Clin Psychopharmacol* 1987;**7**:281–2; overdose SPC)

Nabilone

Naltrexone (*Presse Med* 1999;**28**:1361–2)

Nicotine (*J Pain Symptom Manage* 1998;**16**:76–7)

Nicotine withdrawal (*J Pain Symptom Manage* 1998;**15**:S18; n = 5, *Neurology* 2001;**57**:551–3)

Psilocybin in wild mushrooms (n = 1, *Lakartidningen* 1995;**92**:3779–80)

Sodium oxybate (SPC)

Solvent intoxication

• Gastrointestinal drugs *

H2 receptor antagonists (*Adv Psychiatr Treat* 2005;11:68), e.g.:
  → cimetidine (e.g. *Ann Intern Med* 1992;**115**:658–9)
  → famotidine (n = 1, after switch from cimetidine; *Ann Pharmacother* 2001;**35**:1045–8; n = 6, *Psychosomatics* 1996;**37**:349–55)
  → nizatidine (n = 1, *J Clin Psychiatry* 1997;**58**:327)
  → ranitidine (*Ann Intern Med* 1992;**115**:658–9; n=1, IV, *Br Med J* 1987;**294**:1616)

Loperamide (*J Pediatr* 1990;**117**:467–71; *ibid* 1991;**118**:656–7)

Methixene

Misoprostol (n = 1, *Drug Intell Clin Pharm* 1991;**25**:133–4)

Omeprazole (*J Neurol* 2000;**247**:56–7; n = 1, *Am J Emerg Med* 2008;**26**:519)

Sulfasalazine (*Adv Psychiatr Treat* 2005;11:68)

• Cardiovascular drugs *

Alpha–adrenoceptor blockers e.g. doxazosin, prazosin (*Adv Psychiatr Treat* 2005;11:66)

Amiloride

Amiodarone (n = 1, *Am J Psychiatry* 1999;**156**:1119; *Am J Geriatr Psychiatry* 2003;11:696–7)

Beta-blockers (e.g. *Postgrad Med J* 1990;**66**:1050–2;)
  → atenolol (n = 1, *Br Med J* 1988;**297**:1048)
  → metoprolol (n = 24, *Cardiovasc Drugs Ther* 2002;**16**:161–5; n = 1, *Ned Tijdschr Geneeskd* 2005;**149**:2183–6)
  → propranolol (*Can J Psychiatry* 2004;**49**:645; n = 3, *Gaoxiong Yi Xue Ke Xue Za Zhi* 1994;**10**:40–7)

Calcium-channel blockers (*Adv Psychiatr Treat*

2005;**11**:66), e.g.:
→ verapamil (n = 1, *Am J Psychiatry* 1987;
144:248)

Clonidine (n = 7, *Int J Cardiol* 2006;**113**:276–8)

Digitalis (n = 1, *Clin Cardiol* 1995;**18**:351–2)

Digoxin (*Am Heart J* 1983;**106**:419; *J Clin Pharmacol* 1979;**19**:747)

Disopyramide (*Adv Psychiatr Treat* 2005;**11**:66)

Diuretics (via severe K + loss)

Flecainide toxicity (n = 1, *Ann Pharmacother* 2009;**43**:1366–9)

Hydralazine

Lidocaine

Methyldopa (*Adv Psychiatr Treat* 2005;**11**:66)

Mexilitine

Nitrates (*Adv Psychiatr Treat* 2005;**11**:66)

Procainamide

Sodium nitroprusside (*Psychosomatics* 1995;
36:83–5)

Spironolactone

Statins (MHRA warning, *Drug Safety Update* 2008;**1**:10)

Sulphonamide diuretics (*Adv Psychiatr Treat* 2005;
11:66)

• **Respiratory drugs** *

Aminophylline

Antihistamines, sedating (*Adv Psychiatr Treat* 2005;**11**:68)

Dextromethorphan (n = 1, *Am J Geriatr Pharmacother* 2005;**3**:17–20)

Diphenhydramine (*Psychosomatics* 1994;
35:399–402)

Diphenhydramine + linezolid (n = 1, *Ann Pharmacother* 2004;**38**:62–5)

Doxapram

Mentholatum (n = 1, *Am J Psychiatry* 2000;**157**:
483–4)

Phenylpropanolamine O/D (*Br Heart J* 1982;
47:51–4)

Promethazine + cyproheptadine overdose
(n = 1, *Australas Psychiatry* 2007;**99**:242–4)

• **Anti-infection drugs** *

These may indirectly cause delirium if inducing diarrhoea and dehydration.

Aciclovir (e.g. n = 1, *Nervenarzt* 1998;**69**:1015–8;
n = 1, *Clin Infect Dis* 1995;**21**:435–6)

Amphotericin B (*Adv Psych Treat* 2005;**11**:66;
Psychosomatics 1984;**25**:706)

Azithromycin (*Can J Psychiatry* 2002;**47**:585–6;

n = 1, *Med Clin (Barc)* 2006;**126**:439; n = 2,
Surg Neurol 2003;**59**:509–11)

Cefazolin (n = 1, *Br Med J* 1989;**299**:393)

Cephalexin (n = 1, *J Adolesc Health* 2006;
39:782–3)

Chloramphenicol (*Clin Pharmacol Ther* 1970;
11:194)

Chloroquine

Ciprofloxacin (e.g. n = 1, *Ann Pharmacother* 1997;**31**:252)

Clarithromycin (n = 1, *Ned Tijdschr Geneeskd* 2001;**145**:225–8; n = 1, *Eur Respir J* 2006;**28**:
671–2; *J Antimicrob Chemother* 2007;**59**:331)

Co-trimoxazole (n = 1, *Hum Exp Toxicol* 2000;
19:149–51)

Cycloserine

Fluconazole (*Gen Hosp Psychiatry* 2003;**25**:297–8)

Foscarnet sodium (*Adv Psych Treat* 2005;**11**:66)

Gancyclovir (*N Engl J Med* 1990;**322**:933–4)

Gatifloxacin (*Psychosomatics* 2003;**44**:85–6;
n = 1, *J Am Geriatr Soc* 2006;**54**:871)

Isoniazid (*Br Med J* 1969;i:461)

Itraconazole (*Psychosomatics* 2003;**44**:260–1)

Levofloxacin (*Clin Neurol Neurosurg* 2005;
107:998–9; n = 1, *Gen Hosp Psychiatry* 2008;**30**:381–3)

Mefloquine (*Pharm J* 989;**243**:561;*Lancet* 1993;
341:632)

Ofloxacin (*J Clin Psychiatry* 1992;**53**:137–8)

Oseltamivir (n = 1, *Int J Geriatr Psychiatry* 2007;
22:935–6)

Penicillin

Piperacillin + tazobactam (n = 1, *Nephrol Dial Transplant* 2004;**19**:1341)

Piperazine

Quinine (*Adv Psych Treat* 2005;**11**:66)

Rifampicin

Streptomycin

Sulfadiazine

Sulphonamides

Tobramycin (*JAMA* 1982;**248**:1971–2)

• **Endocrine system drugs**

Adrenocorticotropin

Clomifene (n = 1, *Psychosomatics* 2007;**48**:65–6)

Corticosteroids (n = 1, *Gen Hosp Psychiatry* 1996;**18**:196–202)

Hypoglycaemics (oral)

Methylprednisolone

Triamcinolone

• **Malignancy and immunosuppressant drugs** *

Acytokine
Ciclosporin (*Adv Psychiatr Treat* 2005;**11**:68)
Interferon alfa (*Arch Intern Med* 1987;**147**:1557–80; n = 1, *Am J Psychiatry* 2000;**157**:1705–7)
Interleukin–2 + interferon alfa (n = 1, *Anticancer Res* 2001;**21**:3699–700)
Nelarabine (common, SPC)
Tamoxifen (n = 273, no adverse effect on cognition, *J Clin Oncol* 2009;**27**:5144–52)

• **Musculoskeletal and analgesics** *
Aspirin toxicity (*Lancet* 1971;**2**:242)
Baclofen
Baclofen withdrawal (n = 1, elderly man, *Br Med J* 2001;**323**:870; n = 23, review, *Psychosomatics* 2005;**46**:503–7)
Corticosteroids (incidence may be as high as 5–6% in adults, usually emerges within a few days or weeks, risk may be higher with higher doses, *MHRA Drug Safety Update* 2007;1–9)
COX–2 inhibitors:
→ celecoxib (*J Neuropsychiatry Clin Neurosci* 2001;**13**:305–6)
→ rofecoxib (*J Neuropsychiatry Clin Neurosci* 2001;**13**:305–6; *Psychosomatics* 2004;**45**:361–3)
Etodolac (SPC)
Hydroxychloroquine
Methotrexate (*Adv Psychiatr Treat* 2005;**11**:68)
NSAIDs (*Adv Psychiatr Treat* 2005;**11**:68), e.g.:
→ fenoprofen
→ ibuprofen (*Arthritis Rheum* 1982;**25**:1013)
→ ibuprofen + tacrine (n = 1, *Am J Psychiatry* 1996;**153**:842)
→ indometacin, inc. OD (*Drugs* 1980;**19**:220–42)
→ ketoprofen (*J Clin Psychopharmacol* 1999;**19**:95–6)
→ naproxen (cases)
→ salicylates? (*Psychosomatics* 1987;**28**:344)
→ sulindac (*JAMA* 1980;**243**:1630)
→ tiaprofenic acid (*CMAJ* 1987;**137**:1022–3)

• **Others** *
Anesthetic agents (incidence 56%, *Br J Psychiatry* 2001;**178**:360–6)
Atropine and homatropine eye drops
Cyclopentolate eye drops (n = 1, *Nervenarzt* 2009;**80**:967–9)
Herbal medicines (*Psychiatr Serv* 1999;**50**:969–70)
Homatropin eye drops (n = 1, *Clin Neurol Neurosurg* 1987;**89**:53–4)
Iodoform gauze (n = 1, *Lancet* 1997;**350**:1294)
Mercury intoxication (n = 1, *Appl Neuropsychol* 2008;**15**:79–91)
Mouthwash containing alcohol (n = 1, *Mil Med* 2009;**174**:828–31)
Nitrous oxide abuse (n = 1, *Arch Neurol* 1983;**40**:446–7)
Propofol (n = 1, *Can J Anaesth* 1996;**43**:877)
Sevoflurane (*Anesth Analg* 1999;**88**:1308–10; *Minerva Anestesiol* 2002;**68**:402–5)
Tacrolimus (*Adv Psychiatr Treat* 2005;**11**:68)
Tolterodine + anticholinesterases (*J Am Geriatr Soc* 2002;**50**:1165–6)
Typewriter correction fluid (n = 1, *Psychosomatics* 1986;**27**:665–6)
Valerian root withdrawal (*JAMA* 1998;**280**:9966–7)

5.5 DEPRESSION (SEE ALSO SUICIDAL IDEATION)

Occurs mainly in patients with a history of depression.
Review: * general (Patten and Barbui, *Psychother Psychosom* 2004;**73**:207–99).

• **CNS — anxiolytics and hypnotics** *
Benzodiazepines (BNF, common, especially resistant depression):
→ alprazolam (n = 15, incidence 33% at 3–10 mg/d, *Am J Psychiatry* 1987;**144**:664–5; n = 2, *J Clin Psychiatry* 1993;**54**(Suppl):78–84)
→ clobazam (n = 1, *Br Med J* 1983;**286**:1246–7)
→ clonazepam
→ clorazepate
→ lorazepam (n = 8, incidence 27%, *Am J Psychiatry* 1989;**146**:1230–1)
Benzodiazepine withdrawal (n = 3, *Can J Psychiatry* 1988;**33**:626–7; n = 4, *Psychol Med* 1984;**14**:937–40; diazepam abuse discontinuation, n = 1, *DICP* 1989;**23**:989–90)
Buspirone (incidence 3%? *J Clin Psychiatry* 1982;**43** [sect 2]:100–2)
Hypnotics (n = 5535 + 2318, increased incidence with hypnotic use, 2% vs 0.9%, *BMC Psychiatry* 2007;**21**:42)

Sodium oxybate (BNF, less common)
Zaleplon (BNF, less common)
Zopiclone (BNF, rare)

- CNS — antipsychotics *
Aripiprazole (BNF, less common)
Clozapine (n = 1, managed successfully by SSRIs, *Eur Neuropsychopharmacol* 1998;**8**:239–40)
Fluphenazine depot (n = 1, *Br Med J* 1969;**3**:564–7)
Pimozide (n = 4, *J Clin Psychiatry* 1997;**58**:433–6)
Quetiapine (n = 1, *Clin Neuropharmacol* 2005; **28**:133–5)
Risperidone (BNF, common; n = 17, incidence 29%, *J Clin Psychiatry* 2002;**63**:1040–4)
Ziprasidone (n = 3, *Clin Neuropharmacol* 2007;**30**:357–61)
Zotepine (BNF, common)
Zuclopenthixol

- CNS — antidepressants *
Bupropion (BNF, less common)
Duloxetine (induction of ultra-rapid cycling, n = 1, *J Clin Psychopharmacol* 2007;**27**:115–6; n = 2, *Clin Pract Epidemol Ment Health* 2008; **4**:18)
Tricyclics
  → nortriptyline (n = 2, *Br Med J* 1964;**2**:1593)

- CNS — analgesics *
Codeine — long-term use (n = 339, community survey, *J Clin Psychopharmacol* 1999;**19**:373–6)
Eletriptan (BNF, less common)
Fentanyl (transdermal)
Frovatriptan (BNF, less common)
Pentazocine (*South Med J* 1975;**68**:808)
Sumatriptan (n = 1, *J Clin Psychopharmacol* 1995; **15**:81–2)
Tramadol (n = 1, *Am J Psychiatry* 1996;**153**: 843–4)

- CNS — anticonvulsants *
Barbiturates (BNF, less common)
Carbamazepine (BNF, less common)
Ethosuximide (BNF, less common)
Felbamate (FDA warning 2008)
Gabapentin (BNF, uncommon; FDA warning 2008)
Lacosamide (common, SPC)
Lamotrigine (rare, *Epilepsia* 1991;**32**[Suppl

2]:S17–21; n = 1, *J Clin Psychiatry* 2006; **67**:1159–60)
Levetiracetam (BNF, common; n = 1, *J Clin Psychiatry* 2006; **67**:1159–60)
Oxcarbazepine (BNF, uncommon)
Phenobarbital (*Pediatrics* 1990;**85**:1086–91)
Phenytoin (n = 2, *Arch Phys Med Rehab* 1990; **71**:422–3; n = 1, *Harefuah* 1993;**124**:762–4)
Piracetam (BNF, less common)
Pregabalin (BNF, uncommon)
Primidone (n = 241, incidence 42%, *Epilepsy Behav* 2005;**6**:413–6)
Tiagabine (BNF, rare)
Topiramate (BNF, common; n = 70, risk factors, *Epilepsia* 2003;**44**:1573–7; n = 1, *Am J Psychiatry* 2001;**158**:1736)
Vigabatrin (BNF, common; incidence < 10%, *Neurology* 1991;**41**:363–4; n = 10, *J Neurol Neurosurg Psychiatry* 1993;**56**:925–8)
Zonisamide (BNF, common; *J Clin Psychopharmacol* 2004;**24**:110–1)

- CNS — antiparkinsonian drugs *
Amantadine (*JAMA* 1972;**222**:792–5)
Anticholinergics, e.g.:
  → benzatropine (BNF, less common)
Botulinum toxin A (n = 1, *South Med J* 1999; **92**:738)
Levodopa (BNF, common, review in *N Engl J Med* 1976;**295**:814–8)
Rasagiline (BNF, common)
Tetrabenazine (BNF, common; n = 1, *J Neurol Neurosurg Psychiatry* 1999;**67**:550)

- CNS — others *
Amfetamine withdrawal (*Br J Hosp Med* 1993; **49**:361–3)
Anticholinesterases, e.g.:
  → galantamine (BNF, common)
  → rivastigmine (BNF, less common)
Atomoxetine (BNF, common)
Botulinum toxin A injection (*South Med J* 1999; **92**:738)
Bupropion (during smoking cessation, rare, *J Clin Psychiatry* 1999;**60**:436–41)
Caffeine withdrawal (review in *N Engl J Med* 1992;**327**:1160–1)
Dexamfetamine withdrawal (BNF, uncommon)
Disulfiram (BNF, rare; case in *Arch Neurol* 1976;**33**:141)
Ergotamine (BNF, very rare)

Flumazenil (incidence < 1%)

Heroin withdrawal (*Int J Addict* 1992;**27**:25–35)

LSD (n = 1, responded to reboxetine, *Isr J Psychiatry Relat Sci* 2002;**39**:100–3)

MDMA/Ecstasy (*Lancet* 1996;**347**:833; former chronic users report higher levels of depression than matched controls — n = 29, *J Psychopharmacol* 2001;**15**:181–6; *J Psychopharmacol* 2006;**20**:411–6; review, *J Psychoactive Drugs* 2007;**39**:31–9; n = 402, suggestion it does not lead to long-term depression, *J Psychopharmacol* 2008;**22**: 47–54)

Memantine (BNF, very rare)

Methylphenidate (BNF, common)

Modafinil (BNF, common)

Nabilone (BNF, less common)

Nalbuphine

Naltrexone (probably not a cause, n = 80, *J Psychiatry Neurosci* 2006;**31**:38–45)

Nicotine dependence and withdrawal (incidence 4%, *Addict Behav* 2003;**28**:461–70)

Ondansetron (n = 1, *Am J Psychiatry* 1995;**152**: 1101; n = 1, *S Afr Med J* 1997;**87**:1013–4)

Orlistat (n = 1, *Can J Psychiatry* 2000;**45**:87)

Oxetorone (n = 1, *Cephalalgia* 1996;**16**:560–1)

Pizotifen (BNF, rare)

Rimonabant (BNF, common; *Lancet* 2007;**370**: 1671–2)

Sibutramine (BNF, common)

Smoking (roughly doubles chance of risk of depression in women; n=971, *Br J Psychiatry* 2008;**193**:322–6)

Smoking cessation, especially if previous MDD (n = 304, *Am J Psychiatry* 2000;**157**:368–74; n = 100 with history of MDD, *Lancet* 2001;**357**:1929–32; see also *Lancet* 2001; **357**:1900–1)

Sodium oxybate (SPC)

Tetrabenazine

- Gastrointestinal drugs *

Diphenoxylate

H2-blockers: (BNF, rare), e.g.:
  → cimetidine (several cases, e.g. *Can J Psychiatry* 1981;**26**:260–1)
  → famotidine (rare reports)
  → ranitidine (n = 3, *Am J Psychiatry* 1986;**143**:915–6; n = 3, *Aust NZ J Psychiatry* 1991;**25**:4199–8)

Metoclopramide (BNF, less common; n = 1,

Am J Geriatr Psychiatry 1997;**5**:79–82; n = 1, *Psychopharmacol Bull* 2002;**36**:82–93)

Proton pump inhibitors (BNF, rare), e.g.:
  → omeprazole (unproven reports)

Sulfasalazine (BNF, less common)

- Cardiovascular drugs *

See also suicidal ideation.

ACE inhibitors, e.g.:
  → enalapril (BNF, less common; n = 1, *South Med J* 1989;**82**:402–3)
  → imidapril (BNF, less common)
  → lisinopril (rare)
  → quinapril (BNF, less common; n = 1, *Am J Psychiatry* 1999;**156**:1114–5)
  → ramipril (BNF, less common)

Alpha-blockers (BNF, common; case–control study concluding no association, *Pharmacoepidemiol Drug Saf* 2002;**11**:55–61)

Amiodarone (n = 1, *Br J Psychiatry* 1999;**174**:366–7)

Beta-blockers (n = 381, concludes no increase in depression in first year, *J Am Coll Cardiol* 2006;**48**:2209–14), e.g.:
  → acebutol (mentioned in *Am J Med* 1987; **83**:223–6)
  → atenolol (*J Hum Hypertens* 1987;**1**:87–93; n = 1, *Actas Esp Psiquiatr* 2006;**34**:352–4)
  → celiprolol (BNF, less common)
  → metoprolol (incidence 5%? review in *Drugs* 1977;**14**:321–48)
  → nadolol (*Lancet* 1982;i:1286; no different to placebo, d/b, p/c, *J Neuropsychiatry* 1992;**4**:187–9)
  → nebivolol (BNF, less common)
  → propranolol (n = 1, resolved with switch to atenolol, *Am J Psychiatry* 1982; **139**:1187–8)
  → sotalol (*Ann Pharmacother* 2004;**38**: 1321–2)
  → timolol

Calcium-channel blockers, e.g.:
  → diltiazem (BNF, less common; *Br Med J* 1989;**299**:796)
  → felodipine (*Br Heart J* 1987;**58**:122–8)
  → isradipine (BNF, rare)
  → nicardipine (BNF, uncommon; cases mentioned in *Br J Clin Pharmacol* 1985;**20**[Suppl]:178–86; n = 2, *J Assoc Physicians India* 2002;**50**:1432–4)
  → nifedipine (n = 1, *Br J Psychiatry*

1991;**159**:447–8; n = 1, *Br J Psychiatry* 1990;**158**;889)

Clonidine (BNF, common; 1% incidence, case study in *Postgrad Med J* 1993;**69**: 327–8; when used for ADHD; *J Clin Psychopharmacol* 2008;**28**:725–6)

Cyclopenthiazide (BNF, rare)

Digoxin (BNF, less common)

Digoxin intoxication (*Psychosomatics* 2001; **42**:369–70)

Doxazosin (BNF, common)

Flecainide (BNF, rare)

Furosemide (BNF, caution in depression)

Hydralazine

Indoramin (BNF, less common)

Losartan (*Ugeskr Laeger* 1997;**159**:2106–8)

Methyldopa (BNF, common; review in *Am J Psychiatry* 1983;**140**:534–8)

Moxonidine (BNF, C/I)

Prazosin (BNF, uncommon)

Procainamide (BNF, common)

Statins (BNF, less common; n = 2813, no association with depression or suicide and probably lowers incidence [*Arch Intern Med* 2003;**163**:1926–32]. See also suicidal ideation C5.15)

Streptokinase (cases, e.g. *Drugs* 1973;**5**: 357–445)

Telmisartan (BNF, rare)

Valsartan + hydrochlorothiazide overdose (n = 1, *Dtsch Med Wochenschr* 2003;**128**;2534–6)

Verapamil (*Can J Psychiatry* 1993;**38**:299–300)

• Respiratory drugs *

Alimemazine

Antihistamines (BNF, rare)

Astemizole (debatable, *Drugs* 1984;**28**:38–61)

Cinnarizine (*Br Med J* 1988;**297**:722; n = 1, *Rev Neurol* 1999;**28**:876–8)

Doxapram (BNF, C/I in depression)

Ephedrine (as part of a psychosis, *Br Med J* 1968;**2**:60)

Hydroxyzine (some reports)

Montelukast (BNF, rare)

Phenylpropanolamine (n = 1, persistent, *Am J Psychiatry* 1990;**147**:367–8; n = 1, *Milit Med* 1986;**151**:387–8)

Pulmicort Turbohaler (n = 1, *Lakartidningen* 1996;**93**:2083)

Theophylline (n = 2, *Br Med J* 1980;**281**: 1322)

Zafirlukast (FDA warning 2009)

• Anti-infection drugs *

Amprenavir (BNF, less common)

Antituberculous drugs (*Lancet* 1989;**ii**:735–6)

Atazanavir (BNF, less common)

Cefradine (n = 1, *Med J Aus* 1973;**2**:742)

Chloramphenicol (BNF, less common; rare mild cases)

Chloroquine and mefloquine (*Adv Psychiatr Treat* 2005;**11**:66)

Clofazimine (*Adv Psychiatr Treat* 2005;**11**:66)

Clotrimazole — oral (review in *Drugs* 1975; **9**:424)

Co-trimoxazole (BNF, very rare but severe cases, e.g. *Drug Intell Clin Pharm* 1988; **22**:267)

Cycloserine (BNF, less common; *Adv Psychiatr Treat* 2005;**11**:66)

Dapsone (n = 1, *Br Med J* 1989;**298**:1524)

Efavirenz (BNF, common; n = 355, no higher risk than placebo, *Clin Infect Dis* 2006;**42**:1790–9)

Ertapenem (BNF, rare)

Ethionamide (*Adv Psychiatr Treat* 2005;**11**:66)

Ganciclovir (BNF, common)

Griseofulvin (as part of psychosis, n = 1, *JAMA* 1974;**229**:1420)

Linezolid (BNF, common)

Lopinavir with ritonavir (BNF, less common)

Mefloquine (BNF, less common; n = 1, *Pharmacopsychiatry* 2002;**5**:200–2; n = 1, *J Clin Psychopharmacol* 2005;**25**:399–400; CSM warning, *Curr Prob Pharmacovig* 1999;**25**: 15)

Metronidazole (n = 1, *Am J Psychiatry* 1977;**134**:329–30)

Peginterferon alfa and ribavirin (n = 162, moderate to severe depressive symptoms seem to be common, especially with higher doses of ribavirin; *J Clin Psychiatry* 2005;**66**:41–8)

Piperazine (cases, e.g. *J Indian Med Assoc* 1976; **66**:33)

Posaconazole (BNF, rare)

Primaquine (n = 1, *Ann Int Med* 1980;**92**:435)

Quinolones (BNF, less common)
→ ciprofloxacin (very rare)

Ribavirin (BNF, less common)

Stavudine (BNF, less common)

Sulphonamides

Trimethoprim (*Adv Psychiatr Treat* 2005;**11**:66)

Voriconazole (BNF, common)

Zidovudine (BNF, uncommon)

- **Endocrine system drugs** *
Buserelin (BNF, uncommon)
Cabergoline (BNF, less common)
Choriogonadotropin alfa (BNF, less common)
Clomifene (BNF, common)
Corticosteroids (BNF, rare but incidence may
be as high as 5–6% in adults, usually emerges
within a few days or weeks, risk may be
higher with higher doses, MHRA *Drug
Safety Update* 2007; 1–9; *Adv Psychiatr Treat*
2005;**11**:68)
→ deflazacort (SPC)
→ dexamethasone (up to 40% incidence,
Arch Gen Psychiatry 1981;**38**:471–7)
→ methyltestosterone (rare)
→ prednisolone (*J Assoc Physicians India* 1973;
21:909)
→ prednisone (review in *Clin Paediatr* 1990;
29:382–8)
Cyproterone acetate (BNF, C/I in depression)
Danazol (rare cases, *Am J Obstet* 1977;**27**:130)
Depo-Provera (unlikely to cause, n = 495,
Contraception 1998;**57**:237–40)
Estrogens for HRT (BNF, less common)
Finasteride (n = 19, *J Dermatol* 2002;**29**:665–9;
n = 128, *BMC Clin Pharmacol* 2006;**7**:7)
Gestrinone (BNF, common)
Iodine long–term (BNF, common)
Mecasermin (rare, UK SPC)
Norplant implant (unlikely to cause or
exacerbate, n = 910, *Contraception*
1998;**57**:241–5)
Oestrogens for HRT (BNF, uncommon)
Oral contraceptives, combined (BNF, rare;
n = 1238, concludes that synthetic
estrogen and progestogens may have
lower depressive symptoms than placebo,
Psychoneuroendocrinology 2007;**32**:843–53;
opposite conclusion from pilot study in
Expert Opin Drug Saf 2007;**6**:371–4)
Progestogens (BNF, caution in depression; *Drug
Treatment Psychiatry* 1982;**12**:234–5)
Progestogen-only oral contraceptives (BNF,
common)
Teriparatide (BNF, common)
Testosterone and esters (BNF, common)
Testosterone abuse cessation (n = 1, *Can J
Psychiatry* 1994;**39**:317–8)
Tibolone (BNF, rare)

- **Malignancy and immunosuppressant drugs** *
Reviews: Cytokine-induced depression (Wichers
and Maes,*Int J Neuropsychopharmacol* 2002;**5**:375–
88; Schiepers *et al, Prog Neuropsychopharmacol
Biol Psychiatry* 2005;**29**:201–17).

Bicalutamide (BNF, less common)
Bortezomib (BNF, common)
Ciclosporin (n = 1, *Lijec Vjesn* 2007;**129**:74–6; *Adv
Psychiatric Treat* 2005;**11**:68)
Cyproterone (BNF, caution in depression)
Dasatinib (BNF, common)
Erlotinib (BNF, less common)
Exemestane (BNF, common)
Glatiramer (BNF, less common)
Gonadorelin agonist therapy for ovarian
suppression (treated with sertraline, d/b, p/c,
Fertil Steril 2000;**74**:984–6; *Depress Anxiety*
1998;**7**:171–7)
Gonadorelin analogues (BNF, rare)
Goserelin (n = 1, *Psychosomatics* 2006;**47**:360–1)
Imatinib (BNF, less common)
Interferons (prevalence and management,
n = 185 and review, Scalori *et al, Dig
Liver Dis* 2005;**37**:102–7; Asnis *et al, Prog
Neuropsychopharmacol Biol Psychiatry* 2005;
29:808–18; *Prog Neuropsychopharmacol Biol
Psychiatry* 2005;**29**:201–17), e.g.:
→ aldesleukin
→ interferon + ribavirin (*Psychosomatics*
2006;**47**:254–6)
→ interferon alfa (BNF, uncommon; n = 44,
can cause or exacerbate, *Psychiatr
Pol* 2006;**40**:799–808; n = 1, *J ECT*
2007;**23**:291–2; review, *Int J Methods
Psychiatr Res* 2007;**16**:186–201; but
appears relatively common with
hepatitis C; n = 39, incidence 33%,
Mol Psychiatry 2002;**7**:942–7; can be
treated with paroxetine [*N Engl J Med*
2001;**344**:961–6], sertraline [*Med J Aus*
2000;**173**:359–61] or methylphenidate
[n = 1, *J Psychopharmacol* 2006; **20**:687–9];
review of mechanisms and management,
Br J Hosp Med (Lond) 2007;**68**:307–10)
→ interferon beta (BNF, caution in
depression)
Letrozole (BNF, common; n = 1, *Bipolar Disord*
2006;**8**:516–8)
Leuprolide/leuprorelin (n = 1, *J Clin Psychiatry*
2003;**64**:341–3)

→ leuprolide acetate (BNF, common)

Mesna (BNF, common)

Mithramycin

Mycophenolate mofetil (n = 1, *Pharmacother* 2008;**28**:136–9)

Nilotinib (BNF, less common)

Nilutamide (n = 1, *Therapie* 1997;**52**:79–81)

Octreotide (rare)

Sorafenib (BNF, common)

Tacrolimus (BNF, common)

Tamoxifen (two large studies show no increased risk [n = 2943, *Psychosomatics* 2007;**48**:205–10; n = 11064, *J Natl Cancer Inst* 2001;**93**:1615–23], n = 1, prevented by venlafaxine, *Psychosomatics* 2009;**50**:162–5)

Toremifene (BNF, less common)

Trastuzumab (BNF, common)

Tretinoin (BNF, common)

Triamcinolone (incidence up to 8%, see *Br Med J* 1969;**i**:682)

- Musculoskeletal and analgesics

Baclofen (BNF, less common; rare cases, e.g. *Arch Intern Med* 1985;**145**:1717–8; psychotic, n = 1, *J Clin Psychiatry* 1992;**53**:211–2)

Cytokine modulators

   → abatacept (BNF, uncommon)

   → adalimumab (BNF, uncommon)

   → etanercept (BNF, uncommon)

   → infliximab (BNF, uncommon)

   → rituximab (BNF, uncommon)

Dantrolene (BNF, common)

Etodolac (SPC, rare)

Nabilone

NSAIDs (BNF, uncommon)

   → diflunisal (< 1% incidence)

   → flurbiprofen (> 1% incidence?)

   → ibuprofen (uncommon, *Arthritis Rheum* 1982;**25**:1013)

   → indometacin (BNF, rare; incidence 4%? *Br Med J* 1972;**4**:398)

   → indometacin withdrawal (*Br J Rheumatol* 1992;**31**:211)

   → naproxen (rare)

   → sulindac

- Others *

Acetazolamide (BNF, common)

Acitretin (*J Drugs Dermatol* 2005;**4**:690–6)

Allopurinol

Anagrelide (BNF, less common)

Anesthetic agents (in elderly, n = 140, *Br J Psychiatry* 2001;**178**:360–6)

Apraclonidine (BNF, common)

Betaine (BNF, less common)

Betaxolol eye drops (n = 2, *Aust NZ J Psychiatry* 2001;**35**:569–71)

Brimonidine (BNF, common)

Brinzolamide (BNF, common)

Carbaryl (psychotic, n = 1, *Am J Psychiatry* 1995;**152**:646–7)

Dianette (SPC)

Dorzolamide eye–drops (*Can J Ophthalmol* 1999;**34**:93–4)

Etretinate (*Br Med J* 1989;**298**:964)

Flunisolide (inhaled, incidence 1–3%)

Isotretinoin (BNF, rare; one review noted a incidence 1–11%, *Semin Cutan Med Surg* 2007;**26**:210–20; and a larger one showed a statistically significant association, n = 30496, *J Clin Psychiatry* 2008;**69**:526–32; although it may abate over 6/12, n = 100, *Psychol Rep* 2006;**99**:897–906; n = 10, incidence 90% in bipolar patients, *J Affect Disord* 2009;**424** [*in press*])

Inositol (n = 3, *Am J Psychiatry* 1996;**153**:839)

Medroxyprogesterone acetate (Depo-Provera; n = 457, three years, 12% increase cf. non-users, *Contraception* 2000;**61**:385–90)

Mercaptamine (BNF, common)

Nitrous oxide (risk factor? *J Clin Psychopharmacol* 2007;**27**:238–9)

Oral contraceptives combined (incidence 16–56%, review in *J Adolescent Health Care* 1981;**2**:53–64)

Organophosphate pesticides (related to cumulative lifetime exposure, n = 29074, *J Occup Environ Med* 2006;**48**:1005–13; n = 761, *Ann Epidemiol* 2002;**12**:389–94)

Pegaptanib (BNF, less common)

Sodium phenylbutyrate (BNF, less common)

Tacrolimus (*Adv Psychiatric Treat* 2005;**11**:68)

Vitamin A intoxication (*Psychosomatics* 1992; **33**:117–8)

Xylometazoline (n=1, child, *JAMA* 1970; **211**:123–4)

5.6 HALLUCINATIONS (INCLUDING VISUAL DISTURBANCES, SEE ALSO PSYCHOSIS)

- CNS — anxiolytics and hypnotics *

Benzodiazepines (n = 1, musical, *Can J Psychiatry* 1991;**36**:609–11), e.g.:

→ lorazepam overdose (n = 65, *Ann Pediatr (Paris)* 1984;**31**:286–9)

→ midazolam IV (*Drug Intell Clin Pharm* 1989; **23**:671–2)

→ temazepam (n = 1, visual, *J Am Geriatr Soc* 2006;**54**:1627–8)

→ triazolam (n = 1 in dental surgery, *Anesth Prog* 2005;**52**:17–20)

Benzodiazepine withdrawal (n = 1, visual, *Psychiatr Prax* 1997;**24**:309–10)

Zaleplon (BNF, uncommon; n = 1, dose-related, *Clin Toxicol (Phila)* 2008;**46**:344–5)

Zolpidem (n = 5, *J Toxicol Clin Toxicol* 1998;**36**:195–203; distorted perception, n = 1, *Ann Pharmacother* 2003;**37**:683–6)

Zolpidem + fluvoxamine (n = 1, *Int Psychogeriatr* 2006;**18**:749–51)

Zopiclone (BNF, rare; *Pharm J* 1990;**245**:210)

• CNS — antipsychotics *

Lithium (n = 1, visual and auditory, *Nervenartz* 1993;**64**:747–9)

Olanzapine (BNF, common; n = 1, hypnopompic hallucinations, *Can J Psychiatry* 2004;**49**:496–7)

• CNS — antidepressants *

Review: factors associated with visual hallucinations with antidepressants (*Hum Psychopharmacol* 2004;**19**:577–84).

Bupropion (BNF, very rare; tactile, n = 2, *J Clin Psychiatry* 2006;**67**:1820–1)

Bupropion + valproate (n = 1, visual and auditory, *Can J Psychiatry* 2000;**45**:198–9)

Duloxetine (BNF, v rare)

MAOIs, e.g.:

→ phenelzine (BNF, rare; n = 1, *Am J Psychiatry* 1994;**151**:450)

→ tranylcypromine (n = 1, *Psychiatr Prax* 1993;**20**:116)

Moclobemide (pseudohallucinations, n = 1, *Pharmacopsychiatry* 2005;**38**:179–81)

Reboxetine (BNF, very rare)

SSRIs (BNF, uncommon), e.g.

→ citalopram (n = 1, complex visual, *Prog Neuropsychopharmacol Biol Psychiatry* 2009;**33**:575–6)

→ fluoxetine (n = 1, *Am J Psychiatry* 1993; **150**:1750)

→ fluoxetine + zolpidem (n = 1, *J Forensic Sci* 2004;**49**: 392–3)

→ fluoxetine + dextromethorphan (n = 1, *Am J Psychiatry* 1992;**149**:1406)

→ paroxetine, excessive use (n = 1, *Psychiatry Clin Neurosci* 2003;**57**:548–9)

→ paroxetine OD (*Psychiatr Clin Neurosci* 2003;**57**:548–9)

→ sertraline (n = 1, *J Clin Psychiatry* 2004;**65**:446–7)

Tricyclics (musical, *Biol Psychiatry* 1996;**40**:309–10), e.g.:

→ amitriptyline low dose (visual, *J Clin Psychopharmacol* 1988;**8**:75–6)

→ clomipramine (n = 1, visual, *Acta Psychiatr Scand* 1999;**99**:388–90; n = 1, musical, *Br J Psychiatry* 1991;**159**:888–9)

→ doxepin (n = 1, visual, *Aust NZ J Psychiatry* 1982;**16**:295–6)

→ imipramine

→ maprotiline (n = 1, *Acta Psychiatr Scand* 2000;**101**:476–7)

Venlafaxine (BNF, uncommon, n = 1, *J Clin Psychiatry* 2009;**70**:601–3)

• CNS — analgesics *

Buprenorphine (rare, incidence < 1%, *Br Med J* 1988;**296**:214)

Buprenorphine–epidural (n = 5, *Br Med J* 1989; **298**:928–9)

Methadone (*J Am Acad Child Adolesc Psychiatry* 1999;**38**: 355–6)

Morphine (n = 1, but not with oxycodone, *Lancet* 1988;**2**:912)

Morphine SR and methadone (*Lancet* 1987;**2**: 392)

Nefopam (BNF, uncommon; *Curr Probl* 1989; **1**:89)

Oxycodone (n = 1, musical, *Am J Geriatr Psychiatry* 2003;**11**:470)

Oxycodone + sertraline (n = 1, *J Clin Pharmacol* 2001;**41**:224)

Pentazocine

Tramadol (n = 6, *Curr Probl* 1995;**21**:2; n = 1, visual and auditory, *Ann Med Interna* 2003; **20**:493; n = 1, visual, *Acta Clin Belg* 1996;**51**:184–6)

• CNS — anticonvulsants *

Carbamazepine hypersensitivity (n = 1, *Pharmacopsychiatry* 2006;**39**:192–3)

Gabapentin (BNF, rare)

Lamotrigine (BNF, common; n = 1, *Am J*

Psychiatry 2006;**163**:749–50)
Levetiracetam (BNF, uncommon)
Midazolam (BNF, common; n = 1, visual, *Ann Pharmacother* 1989;**23**:671–2; oral n = 1, visual, *Rev Esp Anestesiol Reanim* 1995; **42**:76–7)
Phenobarbital (BNF, common)
Phenytoin (n = 1, *Drug Intell Clin Pharm* 1988;**22**:1003–4; n = 1, *Epilepsy Behav* 1990;**71**:422–3)
Pregabalin (BNF, uncommon)
Primidone (n = 241, incidence 43%; *Epilepsy Behav* 2005;**6**:413–6)
Sodium valproate (BNF, rare)
Topiramate (n = 1, auditory, *J Clin Psychiatry* 2001;**62**:653; *Epileptic Disord* 2008;**10**:240)
Vigabatrin (BNF, visual disturbance common)
Zonisamide (BNF, very rare; n = 3, *Pharmacotherapy* 2003;**23**:93–6)

- **CNS — antiparkinsonian drugs** *
Amantadine (BNF, common; n = 1, *Med J Aus* 1973;**1**: 444)
Amantadine overdose (n = 1, *Pediatr Emerg Care* 1991;**7**:89–92)
Anticholinergics, e.g.:
   → trihexyphenidyl (n = 1, tactile, *Rinsho Shinkeigaku* 2005;**45**:125–7; abuse, *Med Clin (Barc)* 1991;**97**:239)
Dopamine agonists:
   → apomorphine (BNF, common)
   → bromocriptine (BNF, common; incidence < 1%, *Ann Int Med* 1984;**101**: 149)
   → pergolide (BNF, common; in up to 13%, e.g. *Neurology* 1982;**32**:1181–4)
   → pergolide withdrawal (*Clin Neuropharmacology* 1988;**11**:545–8)
   → pramipexole (BNF, common)
   → ropinirole (BNF, common; n = 1, transient, *Prog Neuropharmacol Biol Psychiatry* 2008; **32**:1087–8)
   → rotigotine (BNF, common)
Entacapone (BNF, common)
Levodopa (BNF, common; incidence < 26% in elderly, e.g. *Postgrad Med J* 1989;**65**: 358–61)
Levodopa-carbidopa + paroxetine (n = 1, *Ned Tijdschr Geneeskd* 2002;**146**:1056–7)
Rasagaline (BNF, common)
Riluzole added to memantine/bupropion (n = 1, *J Clin Psychopharmacol* 2006;**26**:218–20)
Selegiline (BNF, common; esp. combined with

levodopa and/or dopamine agonists, n = 94, *Parkinsonism Relat Disord* 2004;**10**:235–42)
Tolcapone (BNF, common)

- **CNS — others** *
Alcohol
Amfetamines (*Biol Psychiatry* 1980;**15**: 749)
Anticholinesterases, e.g.:
   → donepezil (BNF, common; n = 1, hypnopompic, *J Psychopharmacol* 2000; **14**:303–4)
   → galantamine (BNF, rare)
   → rivastigmine (BNF, very rare)
Atomoxetine (MHRA warning 2009)
Ginseng (n = 1, *Acta Psychiatr Scand* 2002; **105**:76–8)
Guanfacine (n = 1, *J Am Acad Child Adolesc Psychiatry* 2003;**42**:1387)
Hyoscine patch (n = 1, *Lakartidningen* 1995;**92**:638)
Khat (n = 3, hypnagogic, *Acta Psychiatr Scand* 1988;**78**:458–61; n = 4, *Br J Hosp Med* 1995; **54**:322–6)
LSD (*J Nerv Mental Dis* 1991;**179**:173–4)
Meclizine + metaxalone (n=1, *Ann Pharmacother* 2004;**38**:1968–9)
Memantine (BNF, uncommon; n = 3, *J Neurol Neurosurg Psychiatry* 2007;**78**:546; exacerbation, n = 3, *Neurology* 2005;**65**:481–2)
Methylphenidate (*Neurology* 2004;**63**:753–4; US FDA warning in children; low-dose n = 1, *J Child Neurol* 2009;**24**:1005–7)
Methylphenidate + fluoxetine (n = 1, *J Clin Psychopharmacol* 2008;**28**:723–5)
Metoclopramide OD (SPC)
Modafinil (n = 1, *J Clin Psychopharmacol* 2009; **29**:408)
Nabilone (BNF, uncommon)
Naltrexone (BNF, very rare)
Prolintane + diphenhydramine (n = 1, visual, *Pharmacopsychiatry* 2002;**35**:24–5)
Sodium oxybate (SPC)
Varenicline (UK SPC; n = 1, *J Med Case Reports* 2009;**3**:7560)
Varenicline withdrawal (n = 1, *Am J Psychiatry* 2009;**166**:619–20)

- **Gastrointestinal drugs** *
Bismuth toxicity (n = 1, *Actas Luso Esp Neurol Psiquiatr Cienc Afines* 1984;**12**:427–33)

H2-antagonists (BNF, rare)
  → cimetidine (n = 3, *Gen Hosp Psychiatry* 1980;**2**:233–6; *Arch Intern Med* 1983; **98**:677)
  → famotidine (n = 1, *Pharmacother* 1998;**18**:404–7)
  → ranitidine (n = 1, *Eur J Clin Pharmacol* 1985;**29**:375–6)
Proton-pump inhibitors (omeprazole, lansoprazole etc; BNF, very rare)
Sulfasalazine (BNF, uncommon)

• Cardiovascular drugs
ACE inhibitors (*Postgrad Med J* 1993;**69**:240), e.g.
  → quinapril (*NZ Med J* 1999;**112**:83)
Beta-blockers, e.g.:
  → metoprolol (visual, *Psychosomatics* 2006; **47**:537–8)
  → pindolol (n = 1, visual, *Harefuah* 1983; **104**:226–7)
  → propranolol (n = 1, musical, *J Nerv Ment Dis* 1998;**186**:192–4; n = 1, *Intensive Care Med* 1999;**25**:336–7)
  → timolol (*JAMA* 1980;**244**:768)
Calcium-channel blockers, e.g.:
  → diltiazem (n = 1, *Psychiatr Prax* 1998; **25**:91–2)
Clonidine (n = 3, *Ann Int Med* 1980;**93**:456–7; n = 1, *Clin Ter* 2000;**991**:45–7)
Clopidogrel (BNF, very rare)
Digoxin (*Arch Neurol* 1983;**40**:386; *Ann Int Med* 1979;**91**:865)
Disopyramide
Flecainide (BNF, rare; n = 1, visual, *Postgrad Med J* 1986;**62**:61–2)
Flunarizine (n = 1, *Rev Neurol* 2006;**42**:399–7)
Isosorbide dinitrate (n = 1, visual, *Psychosomatics* 1987;**28**:555–6)
Pentoxifylline (musical, *Neurology* 1993;**43**: 1621–2)
Prazosin (auditory, *J Clin Psychopharmacol* 1988; **8**:228)
Procainamide
Streptokinase (reported in *Drugs* 1973;**5**:357–445)

• Respiratory drugs *
Decongestants (containing pseudoephedrine and triprolidine; n = 4, *Br Med J* 1984; **288**:1688; n = 3, *Br Med J* 1984;**288**:1369)
Desloratadine (BNF, very rare)

Dextromethorphan (n = 1, *Psychosomatics* 1996; **37**:71–4)
Doxapram (BNF, common post-op)
Montelukast (BNF, very rare; FDA warning 2009)
Phenylpropanolamine (*JAMA* 1981;**245**:601–2)
Promethazine (*Acta Paediatrica Scand* 1989; **78**: 131–2)
Pseudoephedrine (BNF, rare)
Salbutamol (nebulised) (*Br Med J* 1986; **292**:1430; n = 1, probably due to fluorocarbon propellant, *Pediatr Emerg Care* 1994;**10**:87–8)
Zafirlukast (FDA warning 2009)

• Anti-infection drugs *
Aciclovir (BNF, very rare)
Amoxicillin (n = 1, *Br J Clin Pract* 1996;**50**:279; *Practitioner* 1985;**229**:301–2)
Cefalosporins and other beta-lactams (*Adv Psychiatr Treat* 2005;**11**:66)
  → cefaclor (BNF, rare)
  → ceftazidime (*BMJ* 1998;**297**:858)
  → ertapenem (BNF, very rare)
Chloroquine (*Adv Psychiatr Treat* 2005;**11**:66)
Ciclosporin (visual, *Neurology* 1991;**41**:1996; *Transplantation* 1987;**43**:768–9)
Clarithromycin (n = 1, *Farm Hosp* 2007;**31**: 321–3; n = 1, visual, *Int J Clin Pharmacol Ther* 2002;**40**:20–2; n = 1, visual, *Am J Kidney Dis* 1996;**27**:143–6)
Co-trimoxazole (BNF, rare)
Efavirenz (significantly reduced with stepped dose increase, n = 114, RCT, d/b, *Ann Intern Med* 2009; [*in press*])
Erythromycin + nitrazepam/triazolam (n = 1, *Psychiatry Clin Neurosci* 1996;**50**:337–9)
Famciclovir (BNF, very rare)
Flucytosine (BNF, common)
Gatifloxacin (n = 1, *Psychosomatics* 2006;**47**:360)
Gentamicin (*JAMA* 1977;**238**:53)
Isoniazid (n = 1, *Presse Med* 2006;**35**:425–6; *Psychosomatics* 1993;**34**:537–9)
Itraconazole, oral (n = 1, *Clin Infect Dis* 1995; **21**:456)
Maraviroc (uncommon, UK SPC)
Mefloquine (BNF, uncommon; n = 1, psychotic, *Psychiatr Prax* 1999;**26**:252–4; *Adv Psychiatr Treat* 2005;**11**:66; *N Engl J Med* 1990;**322**:1752–3)
Osteltamivir (SPC, < 1% incidence)
Quinolones (BNF, uncommon; review, esp in

elderly, *Prescrire Int* 2008;**17**:20), e.g.:
  → ciprofloxacin (*Arch Intern Med* 1989;**110**:170–1; n = 1, visual, *Arch Soc Esp Oftalmol* 2007;**82**:299–301)
  → levofloxacin (n = 2, visual, *Nippon Ronen Igakkai Zasshi* 1999;**36**:213–7)
  → nalidixic acid (*Nouv Presse Med* 1980;**9**:455)
  → norfloxacin (n = 1, *J Assoc Physicians India* 1996;**44**:504)
Voriconazole (BNF, common; n = 1, *Rev Clin Esp* 2005;**205**:632–3; n = 1, musical, *Infection* 2004;**32**:293–5; n = 12, *Clin Infect Dis* 2008; **47**:7–10)

* Endocrine system drugs *
Alendronic acid (n = 1, auditory and visual, *Pharmacotherapy* 2004;**24**:799–802)
Cabergoline (BNF, common)
Corticosteroids (incidence may be as high as 5–6% in adults, usually emerges within a few days or weeks, risk may be higher with higher doses, *MHRA Drug Safety Update* 2007;1–9)
Disodium pamidronate (BNF, rare, *Ann Rheum Dis* 1992;**51**:927–8)
Estrogen (n = 1, visual, *Am J Ophthalmol* 2000; **129**:407)

* Malignancy and immunosuppressant drugs*
Bevacizumab (n = 1, visual, *Am J Ophthalmol* 2007;**143**:169–70)
Chlorambucil (n = 1, *Ir Med J* 1984;**77**:288–9)
Ifosfamide (n = 6, visual, *Cancer* 1994;**73**:1509–14; n = 5, *Drugs Aging* 2007;**24**:967–73)
Hydroxycarbamide
Vincristine (n = 2, visual, *Clin Lab Haematol* 1994; **16**:355–7)

* Musculoskeletal and analgesics *
Baclofen (BNF, common; used in Parkinson's Disease, UK SPC change 2009)
COX–2 inhibitors:
  → celecoxib (auditory n = 1, *Am J Psychiatry* 2000;**157**:1022–3)
  → etoricoxib (BNF, very rare)
Hydrochloroquine (n = 1, *Ann Dermatol Venereol* 2004;**131**:471–3)
NSAIDs, e.g.:
  → fenbufen (*Br Med J* 1985;**290**:822)
  → flurbiprofen (BNF, uncommon)
  → indometacin (rare, e.g. n = 1, visual, *Int Clin Psychopharmacol* 1986;1:263–6; n = 32,

Can J Anaesth 2003;**50**:586–8)
  → piroxicam (visual, *Presse Med* 1995; **24**:504)
  → salicylates
  → sulindac (auditory and visual, *Psychosomatics* 1990;**31**:461–2)
Tizanidine (BNF, common)

* Others *
Anagrelide (n = 1, visual, *Eur J Haematol* 2004; **73**:223–4)
Atropine toxicity (n = 1, visual, *Can J Neurol Sci* 1991;**18**:18–27)
Benzydamine (as in Difflam, n = 78, 50% incidence, *Rev Bras Psiquiatr* 2009;**31**:208–12)
Erythropoietin (visual, *Psychosomatics* 1998; **39**:83–5; n = 5, *N Engl J Med* 1991;**325**:285; *J Neurol* 1999;**246**:614–6)
Isoflurane withdrawal (n = 1, *Acta Paediatr* 1993; **82**:885–6)
Ketamine (BNF, very common; *Minerva Anestesiol* 1983;**49**:299–8; *Anaesthesia* 1990;**45**:422)
Mercaptamine (BNF, rare)
Nitrous oxide (*J Am Dent Assoc* 1980;**101**: 595–7)
Phenylephrine (*JAMA* 1982;**247**:1859)
Propofol (n = 1, *Acta Anaesthesiol Scand* 1998; **42**:739–41; n = 1, erotic, *Rev Esp Anestesiol Reanim* 2000;**47**:90–2)
Radiographic contrast media (n = 2, review, *Br J Clin Pharmacol* 1999;**47**:226–7)
Tolterodine (n = 1, *BJU Int* 1999;**84**:1109)

5.7 MANIA, HYPOMANIA OR EUPHORIA

Antidepressant-induced mania may be a marker for increased vulnerability to antidepressant-induced cycle acceleration. The most common symptoms of drug-induced mania are increased activity, rapid speech, elevated mood and insomnia. The main risk factors are prior history, family history or concurrent mood disorder. Steroids, levodopa, triazolobenzodiazepines and hallucinogens are most commonly associated. A sudden switch to mania or hypomania may be indicative of the diagnosis of 'bipolar III'.

* CNS — anxiolytics and hypnotics
Benzodiazepines:
  → alprazolam (*J Clin Psychiatry*

1987;**48**:117–8)

→ clorazepate (n = 5, *Ann Med Psychol (Paris)* 1987;**145**:855–60)

→ midazolam (euphoria possible)

Benzodiazepine withdrawal (n = 1, abrupt, *Acta Psychiatr Scand* 1989;**79**:406–7)

Buspirone (n = 1, *Br J Psychiatry* 1991;**158**: 136–7)

Lorazepam withdrawal (n = 2, *J Affect Disord* 1989;**17**:93–5)

● CNS — antipsychotics *

Review: mania has been reported to be induced by olanzapine, risperidone, quetiapine and ziprasidone, but not (or only very rarely) with clozapine or typicals, including amisulpride (Rachid *et al, J Clin Psychiatry* 2004;**11**:1537–45).

Amisulpride (n = 1, *Prog Neuropsychopharmacol Biol Psychiatry* 2009;**13**:1572–3)

Aripiprazole (n = 1, *Am J Psychiatry* 2007;**164**:172–3; n = 1, *Pharmacopsychiatry* 2007;**40**:37–8)

Lithium toxicity (n=3, *Drug Intell Clin Pharm* 1987;**21**:979–81)

Lithium + imipramine (n=1, *Br J Psychiatry* 1988;**153**:828–30)

Olanzapine (review, concludes half of reports are poorly documented but, in the others, mood–elevating effects were prominent, n = 26, *J Clin Psychiatry* 2000;**61**:649–55; Lilly post-hoc analysis of two RCTs failed to show evidence of olanzapine–induced mania; n = 254, Baker *et al, J Affect Disord* 2003;**73**:147–53)

Olanzapine/fluoxetine combination (no greater risk than olanzapine or placebo over 8/52, n = 833, *J Clin Psychiatry* 2005;**66**:611–6)

Quetiapine (e.g. n = 1, *Eur Neuropsycho-pharmacol* 2003;**13**:135–6; n = 1, *Can J Psychiatry* 2003;**48**:349–50; n = 1, *Rev Bras Psiquitr* 2009: **31**:286–7)

Risperidone (review concludes that half of the reports are poorly documented but, in the others, mood–elevating effects were prominent, n = 26, *J Clin Psychiatry* 2000;**61**:649–55; e.g. *Ann Pharmacother* 1999;**33**:380–1)

Risperidone withdrawal (n = 1, *J Clin Psychiatry* 1998;**59**:620–1)

Ziprasidone (n = 14 worldwide, reviewed in *Clin Neuropharmacol* 2005;**28**:83–6; n = 1,

CNS Spectr 2007;**12**:578–9; n = 1, *J Clin Psychopharmacol* 2008;**28**:711–3)

Ziprasidone + SSRI (n = 1, *J Clin Psychiatry* 2003; **64**:1393–4)

● CNS — antidepressants

Antidepressant–induced mania is well known (especially in bipolar III), as is the spontaneous swing from depression to hypomania in bipolars. Depressed bipolar II patients may be less vulnerable than in bipolar I to switch to mania/hypomania when treated with an antidepressant and an adjunctive mood stabiliser (n = 184, 10/52, Altshuler *et al, Am J Psychiatry* 2006;**163**:313–5). Risk factors include:

● increased number of antidepressant trials
● history of substance misuse (n = 53, Goldberg and Whiteside, *J Clin Psychiatry* 2002;**62**:792–5; n=98, *J Clin Psychiatry* 2006; **67**:1341–5)
● in bipolar depression, during acute and maintenance. Venlafaxine appears worst, sertraline medium and bupropion lowest risk (n = 159, RCT, 10/52, Leverich *et al, Am J Psychiatry* 2006;**163**:232–9)
● Higher doses — SSRI–induced hypomania may be dose-related (n = 2, Ramasubbu, *Acta Psychiatr Scand* 2001;**104**:236–9)

Switching can be reduced by using adjunctive lithium (n = 44, review by Henry *et al, J Clin Psychiatry* 2001;**62**:249–55).

Reviews: general (Benazzi, *J Affect Disord* 1997; **46**:73–7), avoiding drug–induced switching in bipolar depression (Henry *et al, Drug Saf* 2003; **26**:337–51; Andrade, *J Clin Psychiatry* 2004;**65**: 987–93).

Bupropion (rare, *Am J Psychiatry* 1991;**148**:541; n = 1, within a week, *Bipolar Disord* 2001;**3**:159–60)

Bupropion discontinuation (n = 1, *J Clin Psychiatry* 2004;**65**:277)

Duloxetine (rare in unipolar depression; *J Affect Disord* 2005;**87**:115–9; n = 1, *J Psychopharmacol* 2009;**23**:592–6)

Flupentixol (n = 6, *Eur Psychiatry* 2002;**17**: 349–52)

MAOIs, e.g.

→ isocarboxazid (n = 3, *J Clin Psychiatry* 1986; **47**:40–1)

→ isocarboxazid withdrawal (n = 2, *J Clin*

Psychopharmacol 1985;**5**: 340–2)
→ phenelzine (e.g. *Biol Psychiatry* 1985;**20**: 1009–14)

Mianserin

Mirtazapine (n = 1, *Br J Psychiatry* 1999;**175**: 390; n = 1 + review, *Int Clin Psychopharmacol* 2002;**17**:319–22; n = 1 after switch from fluoxetine, *J Psychopharmacol* 2009;**23**:220–2; n = 1, *Aust N Z J Psychiatry* 2008;**42**:1070–1)

Mirtazapine withdrawal (n = 1, *Br J Psychiatry* 1999;**175**: 390)

Mirtazapine + fluoxetine (n = 1, *Depress Anxiety* 2002;**15**:46–7)

Mirtazapine + sertraline (n = 1, *J Clin Psychiatry* 1998;**59**: 320)

Reboxetine (n = 3, *J Clin Psychiatry* 2001;**62**: 655–6)

SSRIs, e.g.:
→ citalopram (n = 1, *Aust NZ J Psychiatry* 2003; **37**:776–7; n = 1, *Gen Hosp Psychiatry* 2007;**29**:374–6; n = 1, *Psychosomatics* 2008; **49**:362–3)
→ citalopram + silbutramine (n = 1, *J Clin Psychiatry* 2002;**63**: 165)
→ escitalopram (n = 1, *Eur Psychiatry* 2004; **19**:455–6; n = 1, *Mil Med* 2003;**168**:2; n = 2, *Psychopharmacol Bull* 2009;**42**:89–91)
→ fluoxetine (e.g. n = 1, *Am J Psychiatry* 1991;**148**: 1403–4; n = 3, *J Child Adolesc Psychopharmacol* 1998;**8**:73–80)
→ fluvoxamine (case series in *Ann Pharmacother* 1993;**27**:1455–7; n = 1, *World J Biol Psychiatry* 2001;**2**:201–4; n = 1, *J Psychiatry Neurosci* 2003;**28**: 134–5)
→ paroxetine (n = 1, psychotic mania, *Am J Psychiatry* 1995;**152**: 1399–440; n = 79, incidence 8.9%; *Hum Psychopharmacol* 2003;**18**:565–8)
→ sertraline (n = 1, *Acta Psychiatr Scand* 2003;**108**:70–4)
→ sertraline withdrawal (*Can J Psychiatry* 2002;**47**:584–5)

St John's wort (n = 12, review in *Int J Clin Pharmacol Ther* 2004;**2**:473–80)

Trazodone (n = 3, *Br J Psychiatry* 1991; **158**:275–8; n = 2, *Am J Psychiatry* 1985; **142**:386; n = 1, *Br J Psychiatry* 1987;**151**:274)

Tricyclics, e.g.:
→ amitriptyline (*Br Med J* 1991;**303**:331–2, 720, 1200; *Neurology* 1989;**39**: 305)
→ amitriptyline withdrawal (n = 1, *J Clin Psychiatry* 1980;**41**:33–4)

→ clomipramine (n = 25, RCT, incidence 24%, *Arch Gen Psychiatry* 1979; **36**: 560–5; inc. abuse n = 3, *Addiction* 2007;**102**:1166–7)
→ desipramine (n = 2, both also manic with trazodone, *Am J Psychiatry* 1985;**142**:386)
→ desipramine withdrawal (n = 2, *Am J Psychiatry* 1983;**140**: 624–5)
→ dosulepin abuse (n = 3, *Addiction* 2007; **102**:1166–7)
→ imipramine (n = 25, RCT, incidence 4%, *Arch Gen Psychiatry* 1979;**36**: 560–5)
→ imipramine withdrawal (n = 1, *Am J Psychiatry* 1986;**143**:260)

Tryptophan + MAOI (n = 2, *Am J Psychiatry* 1985;**142**: 1487–8)

Venlafaxine (n = 1, *Can J Psychiatry* 2004;**49**: 496; n = 1, *Can J Psychiatry* 2004;**49**:786–7)

Venlafaxine withdrawal (n = 1, *Int J Neuropsychopharmacol* 2003;**6**:89–90; n = 1, *Ann Pharmacother* 2007;**41**:359–60)

Venlafaxine + lithium + valproate (n = 1, *Therapie* 2006;**61**:531–3)

- CNS — analgesics

Buprenorphine (n = 1, *Aust N Z J Psychiatry* 2004;**38**: 560–1; incidence up to 1%, *Br J Clin Pract* 1980; **34**: 144–6)

Codeine + paracetamol (n = 1, *Aust N Z J Psychiatry* 1998;**32**:586–8)

Frovatriptan (n = 1, *J Neuropsychiatry Clin Neurosci* 2005;**17**:430–1)

Nefopam IM (euphoria, *Br J Anaesth* 1979;**51**:691–5)

Pentazocine (*South Med J* 1975;**68**: 808)

Tramadol (n = 1, *Am J Psychiatry* 1997;**154**: 1624)

- CNS — anticonvulsants *

Carbamazepine (*J Clin Psychiatry* 1984;**45**:272–4)

Carbamazepine withdrawal (n = 1, *Br J Psychiatry* 1995;**167**:698)

Clonazepam (*Drug Intell Clin Pharm* 1991;**25**: 938–9)

Ethosuximide

Gabapentin (n = 1, *Br J Psychiatry* 1995;**166**:679–80; comment in *Br J Psychiatry* 1995;**167**:549; n = 1, *Br J Psychiatry* 1999;**175**:291)

Lamotrigine (e.g. n = 3, *Am J Psychiatry* 2006 **163**:159–60; n = 1, *Aust N Z J Psychiatry* 2006; **40**:718; no increase in switch to mania in Bipolar I, n = 1258, 6/12, open, p/c, *J Clin*

Psychiatry 2009;**70**:1273–80; possible n=1, *J Clin Psychopharmacol* 2009;**29**:508–9)

Phenobarbital (*Pediatrics* 1984;**74**: 1133)

Pregabalin (SPC)

Topiramate (n=1, *J Neurol Neurosurg Psychiatry* 2002;**73**: 208–9; *J Clin Psychopharmacol* 2005; **25**: 196–7)

Vigabatrin (n=1, *Lancet* 1994;**343**: 606–7)

Zonisamide (*J Clin Psychopharmacol* 2004; **24**: 110–1; n=1, *J Clin Psychopharmacol* 2006; **26**:439–40)

- CNS — antiparkinsonian drugs

Amantadine (n=1, *J Clin Psychiatry* 1989; **50**: 143–4)

Bromocriptine (n=600, incidence 1.3%, *Br Med J* 1984;**289**: 1101–3; postpartum mania, n=1, *J Gynecol Obstet Biol Reprod* [Paris] 2006;**35**:79–81; n=1, *Am J Psychiatry* 1981;**138**:980–2)

Levodopa (e.g. *N Engl J Med* 1971;**285**: 1326)

Levodopa + carbidopa (*J Clin Psychopharmacol* 1985;**5**: 338–9)

Pramipexole (n=1, *Am J Psychiatry* 2007;**164**:351)

Procyclidine abuse (e.g. n=1 and review, *Br J Psychiatry* 1982;**141**:81–4)

- CNS — others *

Amfetamine withdrawal (*J Clin Psychiatry* 1980;**41**: 33–4)

Atomoxetine (MHRA warning 2009; n=1, *J Clin Psychopharmacol* 2004;**24**: 567–8; n=1, *Pediatrics* 2004;**114**:895–6)

Bromide (n=1, *Am J Psychiatry* 1976;**133**:228–9)

Bupropion (n=1, *Aust N Z J Psychiatry* 2008; **42**:746)

Caffeine (*Gen Hosp Psychiatry* 2003;**25**: 138–9)

Cannabis (n=4815, dose–related increased risk, *J Affect Disord* 2006;**95**:103–10; comment by Skosnik, *EBMH* 2007;**10**:61; regular use increases illness severity, n=3459, *J Nerv Ment Dis* 2009;**197**:35–40)

Cyclizine

Dexamfetamine (n=1 and review, *Am J Psychiatry* 1976;**133**:1177–80)

Disulfiram (*J Clin Psychopharmacol* 1986;**6**: 178–80; *J Am Acad Child Adolesc Psychiatry* 1988;**27**: 500–3; high dose n=1, *J Clin Psychopharmacol* 2007;**27**:224–5)

Fenfluramine (e.g. *Med J Aus* 1976;**2**:537; *Am J*

Psychiatry 1997;**154**:711)

Ginseng (n=1, *Acta Psychiatr Scand* 2002;**105**: 76–8)

LSD (n=1, *Am J Psychiatry* 1981;**138**:1508–9)

Methylphenidate (n=1, *J Clin Psychiatry* 1986;**47**:566–7; see also n=137, *Psychopharmacol Bull* 2008;**41**:37–47)

Modafinil (n=1, *Am J Psychiatry* 2005;**162**:813–4; n=1, *J Clin Psychopharmacol* 2006;**67**:1817 see also n=137, *Psychopharmacol Bull* 2008;**41**:37–47)

Nicotine withdrawal (n=1, *Am J Psychiatry* 1992;**149**:708; n=1, *Am J Psychiatry* 1990; **147**:1254–5)

Sibutramine (n=1, *Int J Neuropsychopharmacol* 2002;**5**:283–4)

Silbutramine + citalopram (n=1, *J Clin Psychiatry* 2002;**63**:165)

Stimulants (methylphenidate, amfetamine, modafinil)

Varenicline (n=1, relapse of pre–existing bipolar, *J Clin Psychiatry* 2007;**68**:1269–70; n=1, bipolar patient, *Clin Neuropharmacol* 2009; **32**:117–8)

- Gastrointestinal drugs *

H2 blockers, e.g.:

→ cimetidine (n=2, *J Clin Psychiatry* 1983; **44**:267–8)

→ famotidine (n=1, *Pharmacopsychiatry* 2002;**35**:992–4)

→ ranitidine oral (n=1, after 2/7, *Am J Psychiatry* 1988;**145**:271)

→ ranitidine IV (case in *South Med J* 1987; **80**: 1467)

Metoclopramide (n=1, *J Clin Psychiatry* 1984; **45**:180–1)

- Cardiovascular drugs *

ACE inhibitors e.g.:

→ captopril (n=1, *Am J Psychiatry* 1985; **142**:759–60; n=1, *Am J Psychiatry* 1993;**150**: 1429–30)

→ lisinopril (n=1, *Psychosomatics* 1995; **36**:508–9)

Beta–blockers, e.g.:

→ propranolol (*South Med J* 1984;**77**: 1603)

→ propranolol withdrawal (n=1, *Am J Psychiatry* 1986;**143**: 1633)

Calcium–channel blockers, e.g.:

→ diltiazem (*Clin Cardiology* 1984;**7**:611–2; n=1, *Clin Cardiol* 1986;**9**:39)

Clonidine (n=1, *Am J Psychiatry* 1982;**139**: 1083)

Clonidine withdrawal (*J Clin Psychopharmacol* 1981;1: 93–5; n = 1, *Am J Psychiatry* 1984; 141:993)

Digoxin (*Med J Rec* 1929;130: 381–2)

Hydralazine

Isosorbides (*Adv Psych Treat* 2005;11:66)

Methyldopa withdrawal (n = 1, *Am J Psychiatry* 1989;146:1075–6)

Omega-3 fatty acids (n = 1, *Arch Gen Psychiatry* 2000;57:715–6)

Procainamide (n = 1, *Am J Psychiatry* 1988;145: 129–30)

• Respiratory drugs *

Alimemazine (rare cases)

Aminophylline

Beclomethasone aerosol (n = 1, in stable bipolar person, *Am J Psychiatry* 1989;146: 1076–7)

Beclomethasone nasal spray (n = 1, *Br J Psychiatry* 1989;155:871–2)

Cyproheptadine (rare, e.g. *Am J Psychiatry* 1980; 137:378–9)

Dextromethorphan (*Psychosomatics* 1996; 37:71–4; *Psychosomatics* 1996;37; 571–3)

Dextromethorphan abuse (cases in *Br Med J* 1986;293:597; *Br Med J* 1993;306:896)

Ephedrine (*J Clin Psychopharmacol* 1983;3:97–100; and in a herbal diet supplement, n = 1, *Am J Psychiatry* 1995;152:647)

Phenylephrine (*Am J Psychiatry* 1981;138:837–8)

Phenylpropanolamine (n = 3, *Am J Psychiatry* 1981;138:392)

Pseudoephedrine (n = 1, *Tijdschr Psychiatr* 2007; 49:125–9; n = 1, *NZ Med J* 2002;199:86; *Psychiatr J Uni Ott* 1987 12:47–8)

Salbutamol

• Anti-infection drugs *

Generally low risk, most commonly with (in decreasing order) clarithromycin, ciprofloxacin, ofloxacin, then co-trimoxazole, metronidazole and erythromycin. It can be enduring in a very few people.

Reviews: short review, *Prescrire Int* 2003;12:183; n = 103, Abouesh *et al, J Clin Psychopharmacol* 2002;22:71–81.

Antituberculous drugs (*Lancet* 1989;ii: 735–6)

Chloroquine (n = 1, *Br J Psychiatry* 1991; 159: 164–5 + 735; n = 6, *Int J Psychiatry Med* 1993;23:349–56)

Ciprofloxacin (*Psychosomatics* 2007;48:363)

Clarithromycin (n = 1, *Am J Psychiatry* 1998; 155: 1626; n = 1, *Int J Neuropsychopharmacol* 2004;7:99–100)

Dapsone (n = 1, *Br Med J* 1989;298: 1524)

Efavirenz overdose (n = 1, *Clin Infect Dis* 2001; 33:270–1)

Ethambutol (n = 1, *Med J Aust* 1996;164:445–6)

Foscarnet sodium (*Adv Psychiatr Treat* 2005; 11:66)

Isoniazid (n = 5, *Br Med J* 1957;ii:743–6)

Isoniazid (aka isonicotinic acid hydrazine) and pyridoxine (*Can J Psychiatry* 1988;33:675–6)

Ketoconazole (*Adv Psychiatr Treat* 2005;11:66)

Mefloquine (n = 1, *Singapore Med J* 2006;47: 549–50; n = 1, *South Med J* 2008;101:550–1; n = 1, child, *J Child Neurol* 2009;24:1008–9)

Mepacrine (*Mayo Clin Proc* 1989;64: 129)

Quinacrine (n = 1, *Mayo Clin Proc* 1989;64: 129–30)

Tetracyclines (*Adv Psychiatr Treat* 2005;11:66)

Valaciclovir (n = 1, *Psychosomatics* 2009;50: 293–6)

Zidovudine (*JAMA* 1988;259: 3406; n = 2, *Med J Aust* 1989;150:339–41)

• Endocrine system drugs *

Review: steroid–induced mania (risk factors; *Can J Clin Pharmacol* 2001;8:109–12)

Adrenocorticotropin (*Psychosomatic Med* 1953;15: 280–91)

Androgens (*J Clin Psychiatry* 1985;46:354–5)

Clomifene (n = 1, *Psychosomatics* 2007;48:65–6)

Corticosteroids (n = 1, *Cephalagia* 2001; 21:852–4; *Clin Pharm* 1987;6: 186; n = 1, *Anesthesiology* 1996;85: 1194–6; incidence may be as high as 5–6% in adults, usually emerges within a few days or weeks, risk may be higher with higher doses, *MHRA Drug Safety Update* 2007;1–9; may respond to quetiapine, *Can J Psychiatry* 2005;50:77–8):

→ cortisone (*Psychosomat Med* 1953;15: 589–97)

→ deflazacort (SPC)

→ dexamethasone (incidence up to 31%, *Arch Gen Psychiatry* 1981;38:471–7; *J Adolesc Health* 1994;99:345–7)

→ hydrocortisone (*J Nerv Ment Dis* 1979; 167: 229–36; n = 1, *Postgrad Med J* 1992; 68: 41–3)

→ prednisolone + clarithromycin (n = 1, *Can J Psychiatry* 1997;42:778)

→ prednisone + bromocriptine (n = 1, *Gen*

Hosp Psychiatry 1991;**13**:345–6)

→ prednisone (*J Affect Disord* 1983;**5**: 319–24)

→ triamcinolone (rare cases)

Dehydroepiandrosterone DHEA (dehydroepiandrosterone, prasterone) (n = 1, *Encephale* 2002;**28**:563–6; n = 1, *Ann Pharmacother* 2000;**34**:1419–22; n = 1, *Am J Psychiatry* 1999;**156**:971; *Biol Psychiatry* 1999; **45**:241–2)

HRT (n = 1, *Am J Geriatr Psychiatry* 1997;**5**: 179–81)

Levothyroxine (n = 1, *J Am Acad Child Adolesc Psychiatry* 2005;**44**:211)

Quinagolide (n = 1, *Gen Hosp Psychiatry* 2007; **29**:464)

Testosterone patches (n = 1, *Am J Psychiatry* 1999;**156**:969)

Triiodothyronine (*J Clin Psychiatry* 1986;**47**:521–32)

- Malignancy and immunosuppressant drugs *

Anastrozole (n = 1, *Bipolar Disord* 2006;**8**:516–8)

Ciclosporin (*Biol Psychiatry* 1984;**19**:1161–2)

Interferons (*J Postgrad Med* 2007;**53**:990; *Can J Psychiatry* 2004;**49**:867–8), e.g.:

→ interferon alfa (n = 1, *J Postgrad Med* 2006; **52**:207–9; n = 4, *Cancer* 2000;**89**:356–62; n = 1, *Ir J Med Sci* 2007;**176**:137–9; *Hosp Med* 1999;**60**:381–2; n = 93, incidence 16%, *J Clin Psychiatry* 2005;**66**:1050–7)

→ interferon alfa withdrawal (n = 1, *Psychiatry Clin Neurosci* 2002;**56**:647–8; n = 44, incidence 5%, *Arch Gen Psychiatry* 1998;**55**:88–9)

→ peginterferon + ribavirin (n = 1, *Am J Psychiatry* 2004;**161**:429)

Letrozole (n = 1, *Bipolar Disord* 2006;**8**:516–8)

Leuprolide (n = 1, *Biol Psychiatry* 1999;**45**: 243–4)

Procarbazine (*Br Med J* 1982;**284**:82)

Triptorelin (n = 1, *Br J Psychiatry* 1999:**175**;290–1)

- Musculoskeletal and analgesics

Baclofen (e.g. *Biol Psychiatry* 1982;**17**:757–9; inc high-dose, e.g. n = 1, *J Clin Psychopharmacol* 1992;**12**:299–7)

Baclofen withdrawal (n = 1, *Am J Psychiatry* 1980; **137**:1466–7)

Indometacin (*J Clin Psychopharmacol* 1987;**7**: 203–4)

- Others *

Aspartame high–dose (n = 1, *Psychosomatics* 1986;**27**:218–20)

Calcium IV (*J Nerv Ment Dis* 1980;**168**: 562–3)

Decongestants

Energy drink containing caffeine, taurine and inositol (*Can J Psychiatry* 2001;**46**:454–5)

Herbal remedies (n = 1, *Am J Psychiatry*1998; I**55**:1627)

Horny Goat weed (n = 1, *Psychosomatics* 2004;**45**:536–7)

Inositol (n = 3, *Am J Psychiatry* 1996;**153**:839)

Ma-hung (a herb in weight–loss supplements n = 1, *Pharmacotherapy* 2003;**23**:380–3)

Metrizamide (*N C Med J* 1984;**45**:759)

Sildenafil (relapse, n = 1, *Int J Neuro–psychopharmacol* 2004;**7**:525)

Yohimbine? (see *Arch Gen Psychiatry* 1998; **55**:1033–44)

5.8 MOVEMENT DISORDERS, EXTRA-PYRAMIDAL DISORDERS

Four distinct types of drug–induced extra–pyramidal or movement disorders are common, especially with antipsychotics. These are dystonias, akathisias, pseudoparkinsonism and dyskinesias. All can occur acutely or be delayed (tardive). Acute reactions are usually at the start of treatment or after a dose increase and are usually reversible. The tardive forms are not invariably reversible on discontinuation of the drug or on dose reduction and can be aggravated by anticholinergics.

Reviews: causes (Thanvi and Treadwell, *Postgrad Med J* 2009;**85**:322–6; Susatia and Fernandez, *Curr Treat Options Neurol* 2009;**11**:162–9).

5.8.1 PSEUDOPARKINSONISM

Pseudoparkinsonism is characterised by akinesia, tremor and rigidity, and generally occurs within a month of the start of treatment.

Reviews: * postural induced-tremor in psychiatry (Arbaizar *et al*, *Psychiatry Clin Neurosci* 2008; **62**: 638–45), extensive (Mena and de Yébenes, *Expert Opin Drug Saf* 2006;**5**:759–71), in the elderly (Esper and Factor, *Mov Disord* 2008; **23**: 401–4).

- CNS — antipsychotics *

Review: antipsychotic drug–induced movement disorders (Blanchet, *Can J Neurol Sci* 2003; **30**

[Suppl 1]:S101–7)

Aripiprazole (many cases, e.g. n = 1, *Am J Psychiatry* 2006;**163**:160–1; n = 1, *Aust N Z J Psychiatry* 2006;**40**:194–5; n = 1, *Int Clin Psychopharmacol* 2006;**21**:127–9; *J Psychopharmacol* 2008; **28**:352–3; n=2, *J Med Case Reports* 2009; **3**:6448)

Chlorpromazine (n = 1, *Psychiatr Pol* 2007;**41**: 495–501)

Clozapine (n = 1, *Ann Pharmacother* 2000;**34**: 615–8)

Lithium
→ short-term (*J Neurol Sci* 2000; **176**: 78–9)
→ long-term (e.g. n = 2, *Br J Psychiatry* 1980;**136**:191; n = 2, *Tijdschr Psychiatr* 2009; **51**:123–7)
→ toxicity (n = 1, *Acta Neurol Taiwan* 2007; **16**;231–3)

Olanzapine overdose (n = 1, *Am J Psychiatry* 1998;**155**:1630–1)

Risperidone (n = 1, 2 mg/d, *Lancet* 1995; **346**:226; n = 1, possible, *Am J Psychiatry* 1996;**153**:843)

Ziprasidone IM (n = 1, *Am J Psychiatry* 2005; **23**:92–3)

- CNS — antidepressants *

Bupropion (n = 1, *J Clin Psychiatry* 1992;**53**:157–9; *Mov Disord* 2007;**22**:1830–1)

MAOIs

Mirtazapine (*J Pain Symptom Manage* 2008;**36**: 5–6)

SSRIs (annual incidence may be around 0.1– 0.2%; Gerber and Lynd, *Ann Pharmacother* 1998;**32**:692–8):
→ fluoxetine (n = 21, *Parkinsonism Relat Disord* 2002;**8**:325–7; mean latency for tremor 54 days, mild and remitted in 50% over a mean of 35 days after discontinuation; n = 2, *Am J Psychiatry* 1989;**146**:1352–3)
→ fluoxetine withdrawal (n = 1, *Am J Psychiatry* 1991;**148**:1263)
→ paroxetine (cases reported in *Current Problems* 1993;**19**:1; incidence as with other SSRIs, *Lancet* 1993;**341**:624)
→ sertraline (n = 1, *Am J Psychiatry* 1994; **151**:288)
→ sertraline and oxycodone (n = 1, *J Clin Pharmacol* 2001;**41**:224)

Trazodone (*Clin Neuropharmacol* 1988;**11**:180–2; n = 1, *Nephron* 2002;**90**:222–3)

Tricyclics

- CNS — analgesics
Nabilone
Pethidine and other opioids

- CNS — anticonvulsants *
Carbamazepine (incidence of tremor may be 22%, *NEJM* 1992;**327**:765–71)
Lacosamide (common, SPC)
Lamotrigine (n = 1, *Mov Disord* 2006;**21**:2269–70)
Levetiracetam (n = 1, *Clin Neuropharmacol* 2005;**28**:188–90; n = 1, *Clin Neuropharmacol* 2006;**29**:303–4)
Oxcarbazepine (n = 1, *Parkinsonism Relat Disord* 2009;[in press])
Phenytoin (n = 1, *Singapore Med J* 2006;**47**:981–3)
Rufinamide (incidence 1–10%, UK SPC)
Topiramate + fluvoxamine (n = 1, *Clin Neuropharmacol* 2008;**31**:366–7)
Valproate (incidence 5–10%, especially if > 3 years, *Mov Disord* 2007;**22**:130–3; mechanism unclear as usually unresponsive to l-dopa; *Parkinsonism Relat Disord* 1999;**5**:67–8; n = 10, *Pharmacopsychiatry* 2006;**39**:9–12; *Prog Neuropsychopharmacol Biol Psychiatry* 2008;**32**:1351–2)
Zonisamide (SPC)

- CNS — antiparkinsonian drugs
Bromocriptine
Levodopa

- CNS — others *
Anticholinesterases:
→ donepezil (n = 1, *Ann Pharmacother* 1998; **32**:610–1)
→ rivastigmine
Atomoxetine + venlafaxine (n = 1, *Clin Toxicol* [Phila] 2007;**45**:182–5)
Cocaine abuse (*Arch Internal Med* 1997; **157**:241; as a risk factor; review, n = 106, *Psychopharmacol Bull* 2008;**41**:5–10)
Cyclizine
Dexamfetamine
Metoclopramide (n = 1, *J Perianesth Nurs* 2008; **23**:292–9)
Ondansetron (*Ann Pharmacother* 1994; **28**:280; *Ann Pharmacother* 1996;**30**:196)
Tetrabenazine

- Gastrointestinal drugs

Cimetidine (n = 1, possible, *Postgrad Med J* 1982;**58**:527–8)

Domperidone (rare, case in *Helv Paediatr Acta* 1984;**39**:285–8)

Metoclopramide (incidence 2–30%, cases in, e.g. *Ann Int Med* 1989;**149**:2486–92)

Prochlorperazine (common, e.g. *Lancet* 1984; **2**:1082–3)

- **Cardiovascular drugs** *

Review: calcium-channel blockers as cause of EPS (*Ann Pharmacother* 1995;**29**:73–5)

Amiodarone (*Ann Neurol* 1989;**25**:630–2)

Diazoxide (n = 6, *Br Med J* 1973;**3**:474–5)

Diltiazem (*Am J Med* 1989;**87**:95–6)

Flunarizine (*Arq Neuropsiquiatr* 2004;**62**:784–8)

Methyldopa (*Can Med Assoc J* 1966; **95**:928)

Metirosine

Mexilitine

Nifedipine (*Br Med J* 1978;i:1619)

Tocainide

Trimetazidine (8% incidence, n = 258, *Therapie* 2005;**60**:419–22)

- **Respiratory drugs** *

Antihistamines:
> → brompheniramine (*NEJM* 1975;**293**:486)
> → cinnarizine (*Arq Neuropsiquiatr* 2004;**62**:784–8; *Lancet* 1987;i:1324; n = 1, *Rev Neurol* 1999;**28**:876–8)
> → diphenhydramine (*NEJM* 1977;**296**:111)

Montelukast (FDA warning 2009)

Orciprenaline

Promethazine (*Clin Pharm* 1984;**3**:83)

Salbutamol

Terbutaline

Zafirlukast (FDA warning 2009)

- **Anti-infection drugs**

Aciclovir

Cephaloridine

Chloroquine

- **Endocrine system drugs**

Mecasermin (rare, UK SPC)

Medroxyprogesterone

Prednisolone (increases incidence with neuroleptics, review in *JAMA* 1973;**224**:889)

- **Malignancy and immunosuppressant drugs** *

Ciclosporin (n = 1, *Transplant Proc* 2008; **40**:2823–4; 13% point prevalence, n = 60, *Arq Neuropsiquiatr* 2005;**63**:592–6)

Interferons
> → peginterferon–IFN–α 2a (n = 1, *Arq Neuro Psiquiatr* 2009;**67**:715–6)

Nelarabine (very common, SPC)

Octreotide high-dose (n = 1, *Neurology* 2008; **70**:2345–6)

- **Musculoskeletal and analgesics**

Etodolac (SPC)

Fenoprofen

Flurbiprofen (*Br Med J* 1990;**300**:549)

Ibuprofen (n = 1, *Postgrad Med J* 1987;**63**:593–4)

Indometacin

Mefenamic acid (n = 1, *J Roy Soc Med* 1983;**76**:35)

Sulindac (n = 1, *Ann Neurol* 1985;**17**:104–5)

- **Others** *

Distigmine bromide (n = 1, *Rinsho Shinkeigaku* 2005;**45**:600–2)

Ethylene glycol + methanol (n = 2, *Clin Pharmacol Ther* 2007;**81**:114–21)

Manganese intoxication (*Chang Gung Med J* 2007;**30**:385–95; review *Neurotoxicology* 2006;**27**:340–6)

Organophosphates (chlorpyrifos overdose; n = 1, *Clin Toxicol (Phila)* 2005;**43**:877–9)

5.8.2 AKATHISIA

Characterised by motor restlessness, with an inability to stay still. Onset is around 6–60 days and has been implicated with all antipsychotics, but especially with the high potency ones.

Review: symptoms, classification, general (Gattera et al, *Aus J Hosp Pharm* 1994; **24**:480–9).

- **CNS — anxiolytics and hypnotics** *

Alprazolam

Buspirone (n = 1, *J Clin Psychopharmacol* 1988;**8**:296–7; n = 1, *Ann Intern Med* 1983; **99**:94–5)

Lorazepam (n = 1, *Oncology* 1990;**47**:415–7)

Melatonin withdrawal (*Mov Disord* 1999; **14**:381–2)

- **CNS — antipsychotics** *

Review: * akathisia is observed with all antipsychotics, but is more common in bipolar than schizophrenia (s = 77, Kane et al, J Clin Psychiatry 2009;**70**:627–43).

Aripiprazole (n = 1, J Clin Psychiatry 2007;**68**: 1814–5)

Clozapine (incidence 6% claimed: Psychopharmacology 1995;**118**:52–6; but may be rarer, see Biol Psychiatry 1991;**29**:1215–9; acute nocturnal, n = 1, J Clin Psychopharmacol 2007;**27**:205)

Haloperidol (review in Psychopharmacol 1985; **21**:69–72)

Lithium (n = 1, J Neurol Sci 2000;**176**:78–9)

Olanzapine (incidence 6%)

Pipotiazine (study in Curr Ther Res 1981;**29**: 903–14)

Prochlorperazine (n = 140, incidence 44% with IV, Ann Emerg Med 1999;**34**:469–75)

Promazine

Quetiapine (n = 1, Mov Disord 2003;**18**:712–3; n = 1, Aust N Z J Psychiatry 2006;**40**:607–8; n = 2, Psychosomatics 2005;**46**:291–301)

Risperidone (Neurology 1995;**45**:14–9)

Risperidone withdrawal (n = 1, Am J Psychiatry 1997;**154**:437–8; n = 2, Actas Esp Psiquiatr 2002;**30**:195–7)

Risperidone + levomepromazine (n = 1, Eur Psychiatry 2002;**17**:294–5)

Sulpiride (n = 1, Clin Neuropharmacol 1994; **17**:481–3)

Ziprasidone dose reduction (n = 5, Am J Psychiatry 2006;**163**:546)

Zuclopenthixol (study in Pharmatherapeutica 1989;**5**:380–6)

- CNS — antidepressants *

Review: SSRI–induced akathisia (Koliscak and Makela, J Am Pharm Assoc (2003) 2009;**49**:e28–36).

Mianserin (n = 3, Br J Psychiatry 1989;**155**:415–7)

Mirtazapine (Med J Aust 2002;**176**:242; n = 1, J Clin Psychopharmacol 2008;**28**:467)

SSRIs, e.g.:

→ citalopram (n = 1, J Clin Psychiatry 1988; **49**[Suppl]:18–22)

→ fluoxetine (e.g. J Clin Psychiatry 1991; **52**:491–3; n = 1, dose dependent, J Psychopharmacol 2003;**17**:451–2)

→ paroxetine (n = 3, Compr Psychiatry 1996;**37**:122–4; Can J Psychiatry 2000;

45:398)

→ sertraline (n = 1, Am J Psychiatry 1993;**150**:986–7; mistaken for panic attack, n = 1, Psychiatr Serv 2002;**53**:1477–8)

Tricyclics (Br Med J 1986;**292**:1529), e.g.:

→ imipramine (n = 1, J Clin Psychopharmacol 1987;**7**:254–7)

→ nortriptyline (Am Fam Physician 1993; **48**:1024–6)

→ tricyclics and conjugated estrogens (n = 3, Am J Psychiatry 1984;**141**:696–7)

Venlafaxine withdrawal (n = 1, Am Fam Physician 1997;**56**:455–62)

Venlafaxine + methimazole (n = 1, Gen Hosp Psychiatry 2009;**31**:388–90)

- CNS — analgesics *

Sumatriptan (n = 1, J Neurol 1997;**244**:131–2)

- CNS — anticonvulsants *

Carbamazepine (n = 1, Am J Psychiatry 1986; **143**:1190–1; NZ Med J 1992;**105**:182)

Ethosuximide (n = 1, Am J Dis Child 1978; **132**:527–8)

- CNS — antiparkinsonian drugs

Levodopa (review in Neurology 1990; **40**:340–5)

- CNS — others *

Alcohol (as trigger factor, JAMA 1976; **236**:2422–3)

Antiemetics, e.g. metoclopramide and prochlorperazine (many cases, e.g. n = 3, Gan To Kagaku Ryoho 2006;**33**:267–9; n = 56, Acad Emerg Med 2007;**14**:799–21)

Cocaine (recent use is a risk factor for antipsychotic-induced, n = 106, Psychopharmacol Bull 2008;**41**:5–10)

Methysergide (n = 1, Clin Neuropharmacol 1988;**11**:87–9)

Metoclopramide (n = 1, Milit Med 1987; **152**:585–6)

Ondansetron (n = 1, Cancer 1992;**69**:1275)

- Cardiovascular drugs *

Atenolol (n = 1, J Clin Psychopharmacol 1986; **6**:390)

Diltiazem (n = 1, Ann Intern Med 1983;**99**:794)

Flunarizine (n = 1, Rev Clin Esp 1991;**188**:384)

Midodrine + promethazine (n = 1, JAMA

2006;**295**:2000–1)

Trimetazidine (n = 1, *Therapie* 2005;**60**:603–5)

Verapamil (*Lancet* 1991;**338**:893)

- Respiratory drugs *

Alimemazine

Cinnarizine (n = 1, *Rev Neurol* 1999;**28**:876–8)

Promethazine + midodrine (n = 1, *JAMA* 2006; **295**:2000–1)

- Malignancy and immunosuppressant drugs

Interferon alfa (*Gen Hosp Psychiatry* 1999; **21**:134–5)

5.8.3 DYSTONIAS

Dystonias includes oculogyric crisis, trismus and torticollis. They may occur within 72 hours of start of therapy and occur more frequently with high-potency antipsychotics, where the incidence may be as high as 10% (*Applied Therapeutics*, Koda-Kimble, 2004).

Review: general (van Harten *et al*, *Br Med J* 1999;**319**: 623–6, 34 refs).

- CNS — anxiolytics and hypnotics *

Benzodiazepines, e.g.:

→ bromazepam (n = 1, *Biomed Pharmacother* 1992;**46**:375–6)

→ diazepam (n = 2, *J Emerg Med* 1988;**6**: 491–3)

→ midazolam (*Br Med J* 1990;**300**:614)

Buspirone (n = 1, *Neurology* 1990;**40**:1904; discussion in *Neurology* 1991;**41**:1850)

- CNS — antipsychotics *

Review: n = 43, *Int J Neuropsychopharmacol* 2001; **4**:393–7.

Amisulpride (n = 1, *J Clin Psychopharmacol* 2008;**28**:573–4; *Aust NZ J Psychiatry* 2008;**42**:430–1; low dose n = 1, *J Clin Psychopharmacol* 2008;**28**:573–4)

Aripiprazole (many cases, e.g. n = 1, *Ann Pharmacother* 2006;**40**:775–7; n = 1, *J Am Acad Child Adolesc Psychiatry* 2007;**46**:306–7; n = 1, *J Neuropsychiatry Clin Neurosci* 2007; **19**:89–90; n = 1, after single dose, *Am J Addict* 2007;**16**:244; *J Clin Psychopharmacol* 2008;**28**:245–7; n = 1, *Tijdschr Psychiatr* 2009; **51**:761–5)

Clozapine (rare, n = 1, *Am J Psychiatry*

1995;**152**:647–8; n = 1, *Am J Psychiatry* 1994;**151**:1096; occulygyric crisis, n = 3, *Clin Drug Investig* 2007;**27**:861–4)

Clozapine withdrawal, abrupt (cases, *J Clin Psychiatry* 1998;**59**:472–7)

Flupentixol decanoate (n = 1, *Br Med J* 1981; **282**:1756)

Fluspirilene (n = 1, *Nervenarzt* 1994;**65**:647)

Haloperidol (n = 62, incidence 37%, in first episode, *Am J Psychiatry* 1994;**151**:1819–21; *Rev Esp Anaetesiol Reanim* 2004;**51**:229–31)

Lithium (n = 1, *Neurol India* 2002;**50**:473–5)

Loxapine

Olanzapine (n = 1, *Am J Psychiatry* 1999; **156**:1662; tardive n = 1, *Neurol Sci* 2001; **22**:331–2; n = 1, *J Clin Psychopharmacol* 2006;**26**:431; *J Clin Psychiatry* 1998;**59**:384)

Olanzapine overdose (n = 1, *J Emerg Med* 2006; **30**:311–7)

Pimozide (low–dose n = 1, *J Am Acad Child Adolesc Psychiatry* 1993;**32**:640–2; n = 1, delayed by 12 hours in child, *J Toxicol Clin Toxicol* 2004;**42**:977–81)

Prochlorperazine

Quetiapine (e.g. n = 1, *Ann Pharmacother* 2004; **38**:719–20; n = 1, *Aust N Z J Psychiatry* 2006;**40**:607–8; n=1, *J Am Geriatr Soc* 2009;**57**:918–9)

Risperidone (e.g. n = 1, *Am J Psychiatry* 1996; **153**:577; n = 1, *Lancet* 1999;**353**:981; persistent, n = 1, *Psychiatr Danub* 2008; **20**:329–31)

Sulpiride (n = 1, *Clin Neuropharmacol* 1991; **14**:463–4)

Ziprasidone (e.g. 240 mg/d, n = 1, *Prog Neuropsychopharmacol Biol Psychiatry* 2007;**31**:546–7; n = 2, *J Clin Psychiatry* 2006;**67**:326–7; n = 1, *Am J Psychiatry* 2005; **162**:2191)

Zuclopenthixol (study in *Acta Psychiatr Scand* 1991;**84**:14–6)

- CNS — antidepressants *

Bupropion (BNF, rare; n = 1, *J Clin Psychiatry* 1997;**58**:218; n = 1, *Ann Pharmacother* 2002; **36**:251–4; *Aten Primaria* 2001;**28**:507–8)

Bupropion abrupt withdrawal (n = 1, *Prog Neuropsychopharmacol Biol Psychiatry* 2007; **31**:766–8)

MAOIs, e.g.:

→ phenelzine (n = 1, *J Clin Psychopharmacol* 1990;**10**:144–5)

→ tranylcypromine (n = 1, *J Clin Psychopharmacol* 1989;**9**:229–30)

Mirtazapine (n = 1, *J Clin Psychiatry* 2002; **63**:452–3; n=1, *Tijdschr Psychiatr* 2006: **48**:153–7; *Tijdschr Psychiatr* 2006;**48**:993–7)

SSRIs, e.g.:

→ citalopram (dystonic rabbit syndrome; n = 2, *Clin Neuropharmacol* 2005;**28**:289–91)

→ escitalopram (*Clin Neuropharmacol* 2007; **30**:124–6; n = 1, *Int Arch Allergy Immunol* 2006;**140**:27–9)

→ fluoxetine (e.g. n = 1, *Mov Disorder* 2001;**16**:767–9; n = 1, *Rev Neurol* 2004; **38**:99; n = 1, persistent, *Intern Med J* 2008; **38**:672–4)

→ fluvoxamine (*J Clin Psychopharmacol* 1993; **13**:220–1)

→ paroxetine (cases reviewed in *Curr Prob* 1993;**19**:1; n = 1, *J Psychopharmacol* 2002; **16**:395–7)

→ paroxetine withdrawal (n = 1, *Rev Neurol* 2008;**46**:253–4)

→ sertraline (n = 1, *J Clin Psychopharmacol* 1999;**19**:98–100; mistaken for panic attack, n = 1, *Psychiatr Serv* 2002;**53**:1477–8)

Tricyclics, e.g.:

→ amitriptyline (*J Neurol Neurosurg Psychiatry* 1992;**55**:414)

→ amitriptyline and doxepin (n = 1, *Am J Psychiatry* 1988;**145**:649)

→ clomipramine withdrawal (*Aust NZ J Psychiatry* 2001;**35**;696)

Venlafaxine

● CNS — analgesics *

Ergotamine (*Mov Disord* 1991;**6**:263–4; *Mov Disord* 1992;**7**:188–9)

Sumatriptan (BNF, very rare; n = 1, *Ann Pharmacother* 1994;**28**:1199; n = 1, *Cephalagia* 1998;**18**:360–1; *J Neurol* 1997; **244**:131–2)

● CNS — anticonvulsants *

Carbamazepine (n = 1, *N Z Med J* 1994;**107**: 360–1; n = 1, *Gen Hosp Psychiatry* 2002; **24**:114–5; n = 1, oculogyric crisis, *J Neurosurg* 2008;**109**:944–5)

Gabapentin (n = 1, *Ann Pharmacother* 2005;

39:380–2; n = 1, possible case, *Br J Anaesth* 2007;**99**:218–20)

Midazolam (n = 1, *BMJ* 1990;**300**:614)

Phenobarbital (n = 1, *Clin Pediatr (Phila)* 1992;**31**:252)

Phenytoin (n = 1, *Dev Med Child Neurol* 1984; **26**:677–8)

Tiagabine (n = 3, *Epilepsia* 2001;**42**:944–6)

● CNS — antiparkinsonian drugs *

Benzatropine (n = 1, child, *Ann Emerg Med* 1986;**15**:594–6)

Bromocriptine (n = 5, *Neurology* 1993;**43**: 2319–22)

Entacapone (BNF, common)

Levodopa (BNF, common)

Rotigotine (BNF, less common)

Tetrabenazine (n = 4, *Ann Neurol* 1985;**17**: 200–2)

Tolcapone (BNF, common)

Trihexyphenidyl withdrawal (n = 1, *Mov Disord* 1989;**4**:349–53)

● CNS — others *

Amfetamine (risk factor with aripiprazole, *Prog Neuropsychopharmacol* 2008;**32**:1756–7)

Amfetamine + haloperidol (n = 2, *Br J Psychiatry* 1994;**165**:276)

Betahistine (n = 1, *Neurologia* 2000;**99**:417)

Clebopride (*Rev Neurol* 1997;**25**:2060)

Cocaine (including crack) in its own right or as a risk factor with dopamine–blocking drugs (n = 2, *Am J Emerg Med* 1997;**99**:513–5; n = 1, *South Med J* 1997;**90**:1050–2; n = 29, two years, *J Clin Psychiatry* 1998;**59**:128–30)

Cocaine withdrawal (*Neurology* 1989;**39**:996–7; *Neurology* 1990;**40**:863–4)

Cyclizine (*Anaesthesia* 2004;**59**:413–4; *Anaesthesia* 2003;**58**:928; n = 1, *Anaesthesia* 2003;**58**:257–60)

Disulfiram (n = 1, *Mov Disord* 1991;**6**:166–70)

Domperidone (n = 1, *Mov Disord* 1991;**6**:79–81)

MDMA/ecstasy (*Mov Disord* 2004;**19**:1386–7; n = 1, *Mov Disord* 1995;**10**:353)

Methamphetamine (n = 1, *Psychiatry Clin Neurosci* 2007;**61**:691–4)

Methylphenidate (n = 1, *J Child Neurol* 1994;**9**: 45–6)

Metoclopramide (BNF, less common; n = 2, *Tidsskr Nor Laegeforen* 2001;**121**:2162–3; incidence 3%, see *NEJM* 1983;**309**:433; cases in, e.g. *Ann Intern Med* 1989;**149**:2486–92)

Prochlorperazine (controlled by hyoscine patch
n = 1, *J Emerg Med* 2006;**30**:299–301; n = 1,
Am J Phys Med Rehabil 1993;**72**:97–8; n = 1, *Ir
J Med Sci* 2007;**176**:53–4)

Rivastigmine (n = 1, *Am J Health Syst Pharm*
2007;**64**:2468–70)

- **Gastrointestinal drugs** *

Cimetidine (n = 1, *Ann Emerg Med* 1987; **16**:
1162–4; n = 1, *J Emerg Med* 2001; **21**:27–9)

Ranitidine (e.g. n = 1, *J La State Med Soc* 1997;
149:36–8; n = 1, *Am J Emerg* 1999;**17**:258–60)

- **Cardiovascular drugs** *

Amiodarone (isolated case in *Lancet* 1979;**1**:81–2)

Flecainide (n = 1, *Mov Disord* 1992;**7**:62–3)

Midodrine + perphenazine (n = 1, *J Neurol* 2008;
255:767–8)

Midodrine + risperidone (n = 1, *J Neuropsychiatry Clin Neurosci* 2000;**12**:285–6)

Nifedipine (*Ann Intern Med* 1985;**104**:125)

Propranolol (n = 1, *Arch Neurol* 2000;**57**:570–1)

Verapamil (n = 1, *J Clin Pharmacy Ther* 1998;**23**:
79–80)

- **Respiratory drugs** *

Alimemazine

Cetirizine (*Neurology* 2006;**66**:143–4; n = 1,
Pediatr Emerg Care 2008;**24**:627–8)

Cinnarizine (n = 101, *Mov Disord* 1989;**4**:139–46)

Dextromethorphan (*J Toxicol Clin Toxicol* 1996;
34:351–2)

Diphenhydramine:

   → oral (*Ann Intern Med* 1989;**111**:92–3; *Clin
Pharm* 1989;**8**:471; n = 1, *Pharmacotherapy*
1994;**14**:491–6)

   → IV (*Ann Intern Med* 1989;**111**:92–3)

Flunarizine (n = 101, *Mov Disord* 1989;**4**:139–46)

Phenylpropanolamine (*Clin Pediatr (Phila)* 1997;
36:57–8)

Promethazine (n = 1, *Clin Pharm* 1984;**3**:83–5;
n = 1, *Pediatr Emerg Care* 1987;**3**:91–2)

- **Anti-infection drugs** *

Chloroquine (with metronidazole; n = 1, *Drug
Intell Clin Pharm* 1988;**22**:308–10)

Erythromycin (n = 1, *Am J Emerg Med* 1992;
10:616)

Foscarnet (n = 1, *Am J Ther* 2008;**99**:184–6)

Lamivudine (n = 2, *Clin Neuropharmacol* 2005;

28:193–4)

Quinine (*An Med Interna* 2003;**20**:650–1)

Spiramycin (n = 1, *Can J Psychiatry* 1997;**42**: 665–6)

- **Malignancy and immunosuppressant drugs** *

Capecitabine (n = 1, *Acta Oncol* 2008;**47**:1161–5)

Etoposide (n = 1, *Drug Intell Clin Pharm* 1988;
22:41–2)

Peginterferon alfa (*Mov Disord* 2007;**22**:747–8)

- **Musculoskeletal and analgesics**

Azapropazone (n = 1, *J Neurol Neurosurg
Psychiatry* 1988;**51**:731–2)

Indometacin (n = 1, *J Neurol Neurosurg Psychiatry*
1988;**51**:731–2)

Penicillamine (review, *Arch Neurol* 1987;**44**:490–3)

- **Others** *

Acetazolamide (n = 1, *Eur J Neurol* 2000;**7**:
237–40)

Alfentanil (n = 1, *Anesth Analg* 1991;**72**:557–8)

Contrast Media (n = 1, *J Emerg Med* 2001;
21:499–7)

Copper (n = 1, *Lancet* 1990;**335**:410)

Cyanide (n = 1, *J Neurol Neurosurg Psychiatry*
1992;**55**:198–9)

Insecticides (cholinesterase inhibitors, n = 1, *Drug
Intell Clin Pharm* 1988;**22**:311–2)

Ketamine abuse (*Ann Emerg Med* 1982;
11:673–5)

Permethrin (n = 1, *Pharmacotherapy* 2005;**25**:
448–50)

Propofol (BNF, very rare; n = 45, *Anesth Analg*
2002;**94**:1237–40; n = 1, *Paediatr Anaesth*
2005;**99**:597–601)

Propofol + fentanyl (n = 1, *Br J Anaesth* 2000;**84**:
828–9)

Sevoflurane (*Anaesthesiology* 1999;**90**:1299–6)

5.8.4 DYSKINESIAS

If (tardive) dyskinesia (TD) is of late onset, it
can be a potentially irreversible movement
disorder with possible relationship to drug, dose
and duration (see *6.7*). The risk of developing
definitive TD is half with the use of atypicals
(risperidone, olanzapine or quetiapine) than
with conventional antipsychotics (haloperidol or
thioridazine), even among patients at high risk
of the condition (n = 240, Dolder and Jeste, *Biol
Psychiatry* 2003;**53**:142–5).

Review: * non-therapeutic risk factors (s = 8, Tenback et al, Mov Disord 2009;[in press]).

- CNS — anxiolytics and hypnotics

Buspirone (n = 1, J Clin Psychopharmacol 1988;**8**:296–7; n = 1, J Clin Psychiatry 1988; **49**:322–3; n = 2, Mov Disord 1993;**8**:331–4)

Midazolam (Palliat Med 2000;**14**:435–6)

- CNS — antipsychotics *

Amisulpride (n = 1, Prog Neuropsychopharmacol Biol Psychiatry 2007;**31**:586–7; n = 1, Schizophr Res 2006;**88**:232–4; n = 1, J Neuropsychiatry Clin Neurosci 2009;**21**:104–5)

Aripiprazole (n = 1, after 18/12 for refractory depression, CNS Spect 2006;**11**:435–9; n = 1, Brain Inj 2008;**22**:99–102; n = 2, Prog Neuropsychopharmacol Biol Psychiatry 2009;**33**:743–4; n = 1, J Psychopharmacol 2009;**23**:214–5; n = 2, J Clin Psychopharmacol 2009;**29**:185–6)

Aripiprazole + tamoxifen (n = 1, Am J Psychiatry 2007;**164**:1436–7)

Clozapine (n = 1, J Clin Psychiatry 2002;**63**:167–8; n = 3, Eur Psychiatry 2003;**18**:260–1; n = 1, after 10 years, Am J Psychiatry 2003;**160**:588; n = 1, Prog Neuropsychopharmacol Biol Psychiatry 2005;**29**:633–5)

Clozapine withdrawal, abrupt (n = 4, J Clin Psychiatry 1998;**59**:472–7)

Flupentixol decanoate (Psychopharmacol 1983; **81**:359–62)

Haloperidol (many cases)

Lithium (n = 130, incidence 9%, J Clin Psychiatry 1996;**57**:22–8; n = 1, J Neurol Sci 2000;**176**:78–9)

Lithium + carbamazepine (n = 1, J Clin Psychopharmacol 1994;**14**:146–7)

Lithium + neuroleptics (n = 1, persistent, Pharmacopsychiatry 1998;**31**:201–4)

Loxapine

Olanzapine (e.g. n = 1, J Clin Psychiatry 1999; **60**:870; J Neuropsychiatry Clin Neurosci 2006;**18**:132; n = 1, Psychiatry Clin Neurosci 2003;**57**;605–6)

Pimozide (incidence 35% reported, probably rarer, Neurology 1982;**32**:335–6)

Quetiapine (e.g. n = 1, Am J Psychiatry 2001;**158**:1737; n = 1, oropharyngeal and facial dyskinesia, J Clin Psychopharmacol 2008;**28**:705–6; n = 1, World J Biol Psychiatry

2009;**10**:54–7)

Risperidone (many cases, e.g. n = 1, Ann Pharmacother 2000;**34**:1487–8; n = 1, J Clin Psychiatry 1999;**60**:485–7; although a lower incidence has been reported in the elderly with low–dose, n = 330, RCT, open, 12/52, Am J Psychiatry 2000;**157**:1150–5; n = 1, Neurol India 2009;**57**:94–5)

Risperidone/citalopram abrupt withdrawal (n = 1, Ann Pharmacother 2000;**34**:269)

Sulpiride (Clin Neuropharmacol 1990;**13**:248–52)

Ziprasidone (n = 1, Natl Med J India 2007;**20**: 271–2; n = 1, Am J Psychiatry 2002;**159**:1436; n = 1, Am J Psychiatry 2004; **161**:175–6; Can J Psychiatry 2005;**50**:567–8)

- CNS — antidepressants *

Bupropion (J Clin Psychiatry 1997;**58**:218)

Duloxetine (n = 1, Pharmacopsychiatry 2006;**39**:237–8)

Mirtazapine (n = 1, Mov Disord 2005;**20**:771)

SSRIs (review of movement disorders caused by SSRIs; Leo, J Clin Psychiatry 1996;**57**:449–54):
  - → citalopram (n = 1, J Clin Psychiatry 2007; **68**:803)
  - → escitalopram + itopride (a D2 antagonist antinauseant, n = 1, Prog Neuropsychopharmacol Biol Psychiatry 2009;**33**:380–1)
  - → fluoxetine (e.g. n = 5555, incidence 0.2%, Am J Psychiatry 1991;**148**:1403; n = 1, Mov Disord 1996;**11**:324–6; n = 3, Psychiatr Serv 1996;**47**:991–3)
  - → fluoxetine + low dose haloperidol (n = 1, Am J Psychiatry 1991;**148**:683)
  - → fluvoxamine (n = 1, J Clin Psychopharmacol 1993;**13**:365–6)
  - → paroxetine (J Clin Psychopharmacol 1996; **16**:258–9)
  - → paroxetine + sumatriptan (n = 1, persistent, Biol Psychiatry 1997;**42**:144–6)
  - → sertraline (n = 1, J Clin Psychopharmacol 1997;**17**:138–9)

Tricyclics, e.g.:
  - → clomipramine (n = 9, Am J Psychiatry 1993;**150**:165–6)
  - → doxepin (10% incidence in study in J Clin Psychopharmacol 1987;**7**:243–6)

Venlafaxine

- CNS — analgesics *

Fentanyl (Mov Disorder 1995;**10**:679–80)

- CNS — anticonvulsants *

Review: Zaatreh, *Expert Opin Drug Saf* 2003;**2**: 385–93.

Carbamazepine (n = 2, *Cleve Clin J Med* 1990; **57**:367–72)

Gabapentin (n = 1, *J Clin Psychopharmacol* 2001; **21**:623–4; n = 1, *Mov Disorder* 2007; **22**:288–9)

Lamotrigine overdose (n = 1, *J Child Neurol* 2008; **23**:243)

Midazolam (*Palliat Med* 2000;**14**:435–6)

Phenytoin (n = 1, *Arq Neuropsiquiatr* 1999;**57**: 356–60; *Indian Pediatr* 1998;**35**:274–6)

- CNS – antiparkinsonian drugs *

Apomorphine abuse (n = 1, *Mov Disord* 2005; **20**:105–8)

Bromocriptine (n = 1, low–dose, *Acta Med Port* 1992;**5**:347)

Levodopa (common)

Trihexyphenidyl (n = 1, *Mov Disord* 1993;**8**:512–4)

- CNS — others *

Atomoxetine (n = 2, with other drugs, *Clin Toxicol (Phila)* 2007;**45**:182–5)

Benzatropine (study showed worsening TD — *Neuropsychobiology* 1980;**6**:109)

Cannabis (n = 51, *Schizophr Res* 1993;**11**:3–8)

Cocaine (recent use is a risk factor for antipsychotic–induced, n = 106, *Psychopharmacol Bull* 2008;**41**:5–10; n = 1, *Neurology* 2001;**56**:964–5; 1525)

Donepezil (*Ann Pharmacother* 2000;**34**:1347)

Diphenhydramine (n = 1, *Can J Psychiatry* 1985; **30**:370–1)

Methylphenidate (n = 1, *Prim Care Companion J Clin Psychiatry* 2002;**4**:158–9; n = 1, seven-year-old boy, *Pediatr Neurol* 2007;**37**:287–8; n = 1, short-lived in six-year-old boy, *J Child Adolesc Psychopharmacol* 2007;**17**:378–81)

Metoclopramide (BNF, FDA warning, directly related to total doses taken; many cases, e.g. *Neurology* 1984;**34**:238–9; *J Clin Pharmacol* 2008;**48**:379–84; n = 1, *Mov Disord* 2005; **20**:86–9)

Norpseudoephedrine (n = 2, *J Neurol* 1994;**241**: 167–9)

Prochlorperazine long-term (n = 1, *South Med J* 1996;**89**:989–91)

Stimulants in ADHD (n = 127, incidence 9% , *Arch Pediatr Adolesc Med* 1994;**148**: 859–61)

- Gastrointestinal drugs *

Tiemonium (n = 1, *Fundam Clin Pharmacol* 2007; **21**:657–8)

- Respiratory drugs *

Aminophylline (*Pediatr Neurol* 1992;**8**:997)

- Anti-infection drugs *

Ciprofloxacin (n = 1, *Hosp Med* 2000;**61**:142–3; n = 1, *J Neurol* 1996;**243**:616–7)

Ofloxacin (n = 1, *Mov Disord* 2004;**19**:731–2)

- Musculoskeletal and analgesics *

Baclofen (n = 1, *Arch Phys Med Rehabil* 1993; **74**:766–7)

- Others *

Phenylalanine (exacerbates TD, n = 18, d/b, p/c, *Neuropsychopharmacology* 1997;**16**:136–46)

Propofol (*Anesth Analg* 1996;**83**:420–2)

5.8.5 OTHER MOVEMENT DISORDERS

5.8.5.1 CATATONIA

Review: in young people (*J Am Acad Child Adolesc Psychiatry* 1999;**38**:1040–6), general (Duggal and Singh, *Drugs Today* [Barc] 2005;**41**:599–607).

- CNS — general *

Alcohol withdrawal (n = 1, *Med Sci Monit* 2009; **15**:129–31)

Amfetamine (pseudocatatonia, *Postgrad Med* 1977;**61**:275–7)

Aripiprazole (possible case, *J Clin Psychopharmacol* 2009;**29**:503–4)

Benzodiazepine withdrawal (n = 5, *J Clin Psychopharmacol* 1996;**16**:315–9; *Pharmacopsychiatry* 2001;**34**:41–2)

Bupropion (n = 1, *J Clin Psychiatry* 1992;**53**:210)

Clonazepam withdrawal (n = 1, *Psychosomatics* 2009;**50**:289–92)

Clozapine (*Can J Psychiatry* 2001;**46**:458)

Clozapine withdrawal (e.g. n = 1, *Clin Neuropharmacol* 2004;**27**:216–8; *Aust N Z J Psychiatry* 2009;**43**:283–4)

Cocaine (n = 1, *Am J Psychiatry* 1998;**155**:1629)

Disulfiram (n = 1, *Arch Neurol* 1989;**46**:798–804; n = 1, *Am J Psychiatry* 1992;**149**:1279–80)

Donepezil (n = 1, *No To Shinkei* 2004;**56**:881–4)

Fluphenazine (n = 1, *Br J Psychiatry* 1973;**122**:240)

Gabapentin (n = 1, *Am J Ger Pharmacother* 2009;

7:220–4)

Hydroxyzine (n = 1, *No To Shinkei* 2005;**57**: 45–9)

Levetiracetam (n = 1, *Epilepsy Behav* 2006;**8**: 303–7)

Lithium (n = 1, *J Clin Psychopharmacol* 2007;**27**: 410–2)

Loxapine (n = 1, *J Clin Psychiatry* 1983;**44**:10–2)

LSD (n = 1, *Aust N Z J Psychiatry* 1995;**29**:324–7; ibid 696–7)

MDMA/ecstasy (*BMJ* 1994;**308**:717–8; n = 1, *J Am Acad Child Adolesc Psychiatry* 2002;**41**:892)

Morphine epidural (n = 1, *Lancet* 1980;**2**:984; n = 1, *Acta Anaesthesiol Scand* 1981;**25**:445–6)

Phenelzine + haloperidol (n = 1, *Can J Psychiatry* 1988;**33**:633–4)

Pipotiazine (n = 1, *Br J Psychiatry* 1988;**152**: 865–6)

Prochlorperazine (n = 1, *Postgrad Med* 1976; **60**:171–3)

Risperidone (n = 1, *Acta Psychiatr Scand* 1999;**99**:223–6)

Tramadol + pethidine (n = 1, *J Formos Med Assoc* 2007;**106**:323–6)

Valproate + risperidone (n = 1, *Neuropsychiatry Neuropsychol Behav Neurol* 1998;**11**:997–63)

Zotepine (n = 1, *Pharmacotherapy* 2005;**25**: 1156–9)

- **Others** *

Allopurinol (n = 1, *Br Med J* 1991;**302**:970)

Azithromycin (n = 1, *J Clin Psychiatry* 2006;**67**: 492–3)

Baclofen (*J Clin Psychopharmacol* 1986;**6**: 387–8; cases, *Clin Neuropharmacol* 1992; **15**:56–62)

Ciprofloxacin (*J Clin Psychiatry* 1993;**54**: 199–6)

Cycloserine

Efavirenz (*AIDS* 2002;**16**:1841–2)

Omeprazole + disulfiram (n = 1, *CMAJ* 1990; **143**:1207–8)

Oral contraceptive (n = 1, *Mov Disord* 2009; **24**:2166–7)

Phenylpropanolamine overdose (n = 1, *J Clin Psychiatry* 1985;**46**:288–9)

Piperazine (mentioned in *Trans Roy Soc Trop Med Hyg* 1976;**70**:358)

Prednisone (n = 1, *J Geriatr Psychiatry Neurol* 1989;**2**:41–4)

Sibutramine (n = 1, *J Psychosom Res* 2008; **64**:107–9)

Steroids (n = 1, *Br J Psychiatry* 1991;**158**:125–7;

Br J Psychiatry 1991;**159**:445)

5.8.5.2 CATAPLEXY

Cataplexy is a rare transient sudden loss of muscle tone, often triggered by emotions.

Clozapine (*J Neuropsychiatry Clin Neurosci* 2007;**19**:87–8)

Clomipramine withdrawal (n = 3, *Neurologia* 2002;**17**:113–6)

Fluoxetine withdrawal (n = 1, *Neurology* 2005; **65**:967–8)

Prazosin (n = 1, *Sleep* 1989;**12**:254–6)

Venlafaxine withdrawal (n = 1, *J Sleep Res* 2005;**14**:207–8)

5.8.5.3 CHOREAS

- **CNS** — antipsychotics *

Chlorpromazine (n = 1, *Postgrad Med J* 1970; **540**: 633–4)

Haloperidol (many cases)

Lithium toxicity (n = 1, *Eur J Neurol* 2003;**10**: 743–4; n = 1, *Seishin Shinkeigaku Zasshi* 2003; **105**:1206–12; *Rev Neurol* 1998;**26**:841; n = 1, *Mov Disord* 1996;**11**:733–7)

Quetiapine withdrawal (n = 1, *Rev Neurol* 2004; **38**;1094)

Risperidone (n = 1, *J Clin Psychiatry* 1999;**60**:85–7)

Sulpiride (n = 1, *J Psychopharmacol* 1993;**7**:290–2; n = 6, *Clin Neuropharmacol* 1990;**13**:248–52)

- **CNS** — antidepressants

Fluoxetine (n = 1, *J Clin Psychiatry* 1999; **60**: 868–9; n = 1, *Neurology* 1996; **46**; 853)

Mianserin (n = 1, *Br J Psychiatry* 1989;**154**:13–4)

Paroxetine (n = 1, after a single dose, *Br J Psychiatry* 1997;**170**:193–4)

Trazodone low dose (n = 1, *Eur Neurol* 2006; **55**:101–2)

- **CNS** — anticonvulsants

Anticonvulsants (review of choreas and possible interactions as cause; Zaatreh *et al*, *Seizure* 2001;**10**:596–9).

Carbamazepine (*J Neurol Neurosurg Psychiatry* 1982;**45**:560)

Carbamazepine overdose (n = 4, *Neurology* 1988;**38**;755–9)

Gabapentin (n= 1, *Clin Rheumatol* 2008;**27**:389–90; n = 2, *Arch Neurol* 1997;**54**:910–2; *Neurology* 1996;**46**:851–2)

Lamotrigine (n = 1, *J Child Neurol* 2003;**18**:479–80; *J Child Neurol* 2006;**21**:357–8)

Lamotrigine + phenytoin (n = 3, *Seizure* 2001;**10**: 596–9)

Lamotrigine overdose (n = 1, *J Child Neurol* 2008; **23**:243)

Phenytoin (e.g. n = 3, *Neuropediatrics* 2001; **32**:231–5; *Postgrad Med J* 1990;**66**:1089; n = 1, *S Afr Med J* 1981;**60**:627–8)

Valproate (n = 1, *Pediatr Neurol* 2006;**35**:356–8; n = 3, *Arch Neurol* 1994;**51**:702–4; n = 1, *Seizure* 2002;**11**:205–6)

- **CNS — antiparkinsonian drugs**

Anticholinergics (n = 1, *Med J Aust* 1979;**1**:465):
→ trihexyphenidyl (n = 1, *Nippon Ronen Igakkai Zasshi* 1992l;**29**:686–9)

Levodopa (BNF)

- **CNS — others**

Amfetamines (review, *Emerg Med Australas* 2005;**17**:277–80; n = 1, *Mov Disord* 2004;**19**;840–2; chronic abuse, e.g. *J Clin Psychopharmacol* 1988;**8**:146)

Cocaine (cases in *Am J Emerg Med* 1991;**9**: 618–20; including crack (*Med Clin (Barc)* 2006;**126**:555; n = 9, *Biol Psychiatry* 1999; **45**:1630–5)

Donepezil (n = 1, *Ann Pharmacother* 2000;**34**: 1347; *J Neurol* 2007;**254**:1752–3)

Methadone (n = 1, *J Pain Symptom Manage* 2003; **26**:688–91; n = 1, *Clin J Pain* 2001;**17**:375–7; n = 1, *Pharmacopsychiatry* 1998;**31**:143–5)

Methamphetamine (*Ann Intern Med* 1994;**121**: 986)

Methylphenidate (n = 1, *Neurology* 1978;**28**: 1041–4)

Modafinil + tranylcypromine (n= 1, *Am J Psychiatry* 2007;**164**:684)

- **Gastrointestinal drugs**

H2–blockers, e.g.:
→ cimetidine (n = 1, *Ann Intern Med* 1982; **96**:126; n = 1, *Ann Intern Med* 1982;**96**:531)
→ ranitidine (n = 1, *Lancet* 1988;**2**:158)

Metoclopramide (n = 1, *Am J Ther* 2006;**13**: 543–4; *South Med J* 1986;**79**:1465)

Sulfasalazine (n = 1, *BMJ* 1991;**302**:1025)

- **Anti-infection drugs**

Ciprofloxacin (*Mov Disord* 2005;**20**:513–4)

Trimethoprim-sulfamethoxazole (n = 1, *Paediatr Infect Dis J* 2005;**24**:934–5)

Valacyclovir + famciclovir (n = 1, *South Med J* 2001;**94**:655)

- **Others** *

Anabolic steroids (*Br Med J (Clin Res Ed)* 1981; **283**:349–50)

Baclofen (*Ann Neurol* 1990;**28**;839)

Ciclosporin (n = 1, *Ann Neurol* 1993;**33**:108–9)

Cyclizine (n = 1, *J Neurol Sci* 1977;**31**:237–44)

Cyproheptadine (n = 1, *Mov Disord* 1989;**4**:81–4)

Dienoestrol/dienestrol

Digoxin toxicity (n = 1, *J Neurol Neurosurg Psychiatry* 1984;**47**:419; n = 1, *Mov Disord* 1999;**14**:877–9)

Diphenhydramine (n = 2, *Chudoku Kenkyu* 2007; **20**:1299–9)

Estrogen as topical vaginal cream (n = 1, *Mov Disord* 1991;**6**:355–7)

HRT (n = 1, *BMJ* 1991;**302**:762)

Interferons:
→ interferon alfa (*Neurology* 2002;**58**:328–30; n = 1, *Nippon Naika Gakkai Zasshi* 1997; **86**:1036–8)

Levofloxacin (n = 1, *Nippon Ronen Igakkai Zasshi* 1999;**36**:213–7)

Luteinizing hormone–releasing hormone analog (n = 1, *J Neurol* 2008;**255**:1264–5)

Oral contraceptives (BNF, rare; n = 1, *J Neurol Neurosurg Psychiatry* 2004;**75**:327–8; n = 2, *Rev Med Chil* 1999;**127**:468–71)

Propofol (n = 1, *Anesth Analg* 1996;**82**:670)

Trimetazidine (*Rev Med Intern* 2008;**29**:512–5)

5.8.5.4 TICS (including exacerbation of Tourette's syndrome)

- **CNS — general** *

Amisulpride (n = 1, *Clin Neuropharmacol* 2006; **29**:163–4)

Atomoxetine (n = 1, *J Child Adolesc Psychopharmacol* 2005;**15**:331–3; n = 1, *CNS Spectr* 2008;**13**:301–3; n = 2, *Int J Psychiatry Med* 2007;**37**:499–24)

Atomoxetine + venlafaxine (n = 1, *Clin Toxicol* [Phila] 2007;**45**:182–5)

Caffeine (n = 2, *Pediatrics* 1998;**101**:E4)

Carbamazepine (*Clin Neuropharmacol* 1989;**12**:298–302; n = 1, *Epileptic Disord*

2000;**2**:39–40; n = 3, *Epilepsia* 1993;**34**: 965–8)

Clozapine (n = 1, *Am J Psychiatry* 1995;**152**:649; n = 1, *Aust NZ J Psychiatry* 2005;**39**:202; n = 1, exacerbation, *Aust N Z J Psychiatry* 2008; **42**:1068–70)

Cocaine (several e.g. *NEJM* 1986;**315**:398; n = 1, *Am J Psychiatry* 1996;**153**:965)

Escitalopram (n = 1, *Int Clin Psychopharmacol* 2005;**20**:177–8)

Fluoxetine (cases in *Ann Pharmacother* 1993; **27**:725–6; n = 1, Tourette's, *Am J Psychiatry* 1994;**151**:946–7)

Haloperidol (n = 2, tics, *Am J Psychiatry* 1986; **143**:1176–7)

Lamotrigine (n = 3, *Neurology* 1999;**52**:1191–4; n = 5, *Epilepsia* 2000;**41**:862–7; n = 1, vocal and motor tics, *Am J Psychiatry* 2006; **163**:159)

Quetiapine (n = 1, *J Clin Psychiatry* 2002;**63**: 1184–5)

Risperidone withdrawal (n = 1, *J Am Acad Child Adolesc Psychiatry* 1997;**36**:162–3)

Sertraline (n = 1, *Int Clin Psychopharmacol* 2005;**20**:177–8; n = 1, *Pharmacopsychiatry* 2007;**40**:289–90; n = 1, *Mov Disord* 1995; **10**:682–4)

Stimulants (frequent cause, especially in children treated for ADHD, incidence may be about 8% with methylphenidate, 6% with dexamfetamine; n = 555, chart review, Varley et al, *Compr Psychiatry* 2001;**42**:228–33):
→ amfetamines (*JAMA* 1982;**247**:1729–31, n = 1, *Mov Disord* 2004;**19**:840–2)
→ dexamfetamine (see amfetamines)
→ methylphenidate (*JAMA* 1982;**247**:1729–31)

Sulpiride (review of n = 17, *Seishin Shinkeigaku Zasshi* 2006;**108**:459–65)

● Others *
Anabolic steroids (e.g. methandrostenolone, testosterone; *NEJM* 1990;**322**:1674)

Clonidine (n = 1, *J Child Neurol* 2001;**16**:380–1; n = 1, *J Am Acad Child Adolesc Psychiatry* 1989; **28**:583–6)

Growth hormone (human, n = 1, *Eur Neurol* 2007;**57**:116–7)

Mercury poisoning (n = 1, *Arch Dis Child* 2000; **83**:174–5)

Ofloxacin (n = 1, *Ann Pharmacother* 1996;**30**: 138–41)

Sibutramine (BNF, may exacerbate)

Prednisolone (n = 2, *Nervenarzt* 1998;**69**:1111–4)

5.9 NEUROLEPTIC MALIGNANT SYNDROME

NMS is mostly related to the use of therapeutic or high doses of neuroleptics, particularly pheno-thiazines and high potency drugs. It frequently occurs within 4–11 days of initiation, or alteration of dosages of neuroleptic therapy. NMS may be due to a sudden and profound reduction in dopaminergic function, caused by dopamine blocking drugs. See *6.8*.

Reviews: * atypicals as causes (*Expert Opin Drug Saf* 2003;**2**:21–35; Trollor et al, *CNS Drugs* 2009; **23**:477–92).

● CNS — antipsychotics *
Be aware that NMS with atypicals might actually be serotonin toxicity via 5HT1A partial agonism (Odagaki, *Curr Drug Saf* 2009;**4**:84–93).

Amisulpride (n = 1, *Clin Neuropharmacol* 2007; **30**:245–6; n = 1, *J Neuropsychiatry Clin Neurosci* 2007;**19**:488–9)

Amisulpride + oxcarbazepine (n = 1, *Gen Hosp Psychiatry* 2008;**30**:482–4)

Aripiprazole (e.g. n = 1, *J Clin Psychopharmacol* 2006;**26**:534; n = 1 without fever, *J Okla State Med Assoc* 2006;**99**:435–8; n = 1, Naranjo high probability, *Clin Neuropharmacol* 2007;**30**:47–51; low dose, *J Psychiatr Pract* 2007;**13**:117–9)

Aripiprazole + fluoxetine (n = 1, possible, *Am J Psychiatry* 2005;**162**:397–8)

Aripiprazole + lithium (n=1, *J Clin Psychopharmacol* 2006;**26**:434–6)

Bromperidol + donepezil (n = 1, *Nippon Ronen Igakkai Zasshi* 2001;**38**:822–4)

Chlorpromazine (e.g. n = 2, *Biol Psychiatry* 1983; **18**:1441–6; n = 1, *Trop Doct* 1992;**22**:92–3)

Clozapine (rare, but cases exist, e.g. n = 2 and review, *Ann Pharmacother* 1999;**33**:623–30; long-term n = 1, *Chang Gung Med J* 2001;**24**: 522–5; n = 1, *Ann Intern Med* 2002;**137**:374; after 30 years uneventful treatment; n = 1, *Anasthesiol Intensivmed Notfallmed Schmerzther* 2006;**41**:125–7; n = 1, *J Am Acad Child Adolesc Psychiatry* 2005;**44**:1101–2; after 10 years, n = 1, *Crit Care Resusc* 2007; **9**:338–40)

Clozapine + paroxetine (n = 1, *Aging Clin Exp Res* 2006;**18**:266–70)

Clozapine + risperidone (n = 1, *Prog Neuropsychopharmacol Biol Psychiatry* 2002;**26**:407–9)

Clozapine + venlafaxine (n = 1, *Can J Psychiatry* 2004;**49**:497–8)

Flupentixol (SPC, n = 1, possible, *Br J Psychiatry* 1988;**152**:558–9)

Fluphenazine (reviewed in *Compr Psychiatry* 1985;**26**:63–70)

Fluphenazine decanoate (n = 1, *Ann Pharmacother* 2005;**39**:1131–5)

Haloperidol (many cases, e.g. *J Trauma* 1989;**29**: 1595–7; in pregnancy, n = 1, *Obstet Gynecol* 2001;**98**:906–8; following clozapine discontinuation, n = 1, *Aust NZ J Psychiatry* 2005;**39**:947–8)

Haloperidol + olanzapine (n = 1, *Am J Psychiatry* 2001;**158**:650–1)

Lithium (possible cases in *J Clin Psychopharmacol* 1987;**7**:339–41)

Lithium + amitriptyline (n = 1, *J Psychiatry Neurosci* 1995;**20**:305–6)

Lithium + risperidone (possible case in *Am J Psychiatry* 1995;**152**:1096)

Lithium + ziprasidone (n = 1, *Ann Pharmacother* 2006;**40**:139–42)

Loxapine (n = 1, *Br J Psychiatry* 1991;**159**:572–3)

Olanzapine (atypical syndrome, n = 1, *Pharmacotherapy* 2002;**22**:641–4; n = 1, with severe hypernatraemia, *Hum Psychopharmacol* 2001; **16**:279–81; 2.5 mg/d, n = 1, *Am J Psychiatry* 2003;**160**:796; n = 1, atypical with normal CK, *Acta Psychiatr Scand* 2005;**112**:238–40; *Actas Esp Psiquiatr* 2006;**34**:144–5; n = 1, *Pharmacotherapy* 2006;**26**:1180–2)

Olanzapine + chlorpromazine overdose (n = 1, *J Med Toxicol* 2009;**5**:27–31)

Olanzapine + fluphenazine (n = 1, *J Clin Psycho-pharmacol* 2003;**23**:672–4)

Olanzapine + levomepromazine (n = 1, *Acta Psychiatr Scand* 2000;**102**:231–3)

Olanzapine + lithium (n = 1, *Pharmacother* 2003;**23**:255–9)

Olanzapine + rivastigmine (n = 1, *Pharmacotherapy* 2008;**28**:403–5)

Paliperidone (n = 1, *J Neuropsychiatry Clin Neurosci* 2007;**19**:477–8)

Paroxetine + alprazolam (n = 1, Naranjo = 6,

Neuropsychopharmacol Biol Psychiatry 2006;**30**:1176–8)

Perphenazine (n = 1, *Otolaryngol Head Neck Surg* 1992;**106**:206–8; n = 1, *Pharmacol Toxicol* 1987;**60**:221–3)

Promazine

Quetiapine (atypical n = 1, *J Clin Psychopharmacol* 2009;**29**:497–9; n = 1 after no dose changes and review of n = 13, *Ann Pharmacother* 2009;**43**:785–91; n = 1, Stanley and Hunter, *Br J Psychiatry* 2000;**176**:497; n = 1, *J Neuropsych Clin Neurosci* 2002;**14**:87; n = 1, *Am J Psychiatry* 2002;**159**:149–50)

Quetiapine + fluvoxamine (n = 1, *Am J Psychiatry* 2005;**162**:812)

Risperidone (many cases, e.g. n = 1, *J Child Adolesc Psychopharmacol* 2005;**15**:844–5; n = 1, *Curr Drug Saf* 2009;**4**:119–20; n = 1, *J Natl Med Assoc* 2009;**101**:273–5)

Risperidone + haloperidol (during switch, n = 1, *Ann Pharmacother* 2001;**35**:698–701)

Risperidone + lithium (*J Clin Psychopharmacol* 2003;**23**:315–7; n = 1, *J Clin Psychiatry* 2004; **65**:724)

Risperidone + ritonavir + indinavir (n = 1, *Psychosomatics* 2000;**41**:453–4)

Sulpiride + maprotiline withdrawal (n = 1, *Jpn J Med* 1991;**30**:387–91)

Ziprasidone (*J Clin Psychopharmacol* 2002;**22**: 624–6; n = 1, adolescent, *Clin Ther* 2004;**26**: 1105–8; n = 1, on second day, *World J Biol Psychiatry* 2007;**8**:42–4)

Zotepine (n = 1, *Pharmacotherapy* 2005;**25**: 1156–9)

Zotepine + valproate + benzodiazepine (n = 2, *Psychiatr Clin Neurosci* 2003;**57**:369–71)

Zuclopenthixol (n = 1, *Br J Psychiatry* 1989;**154**: 562–3)

- CNS — antidepressants *

Review: n = 23, Assion *et al*, *Eur Arch Psychiatry Clin Neurosci* 1998;**248**:231–9.

Amoxapine + lithium (n = 1, *Ann Clin Psychiatry* 2000;**12**:107–9)

SSRIs:

→ citalopram overdose (n = 1, *Can J Psychiatry* 2000;**45**:941–2)

→ fluoxetine monotherapy (n = 1, *Biol Psychiatry* 1990;**28**:518–21)

→ paroxetine monotherapy (n = 1, *Rinsho Shinkeigaku* 2006;**46**:575–8; n = 1, *Seishin*

Shinkeigaku Zasshi 2004;**106**:723–6)
→ paroxetine + olanzapine (n = 1, *J Clin Psychopharmacol* 2003;**23**:671–2)
→ paroxetine + promethazine (n = 1, *Nervenartz* 1997;**68**:664–6)
→ sertraline withdrawal (n = 1, *J Clin Psychopharmacol* 2009;**29**:300–1)

Tricyclics:
→ clomipramine (n = 1, *Br Med J* 2004; **329**:1333–5)
→ desipramine (n = 1, *Neurology* 1990; **40**:1797–8)
→ imipramine withdrawal (n = 1, *J Clin Psychopharmacol* 1987;**7**:53–4)
→ nortriptyline (n = 1, *Am J Emerg Med* 1999; **17**:736–7)
→ trimipramine (n = 1, *J Clin Psychiatry* 1989;**50**:144–5)
→ overdose (*J Assoc Physicians India* 2002; **50**:614)

Phenelzine (many cases, e.g. *Can Med Assoc J* 1991;**145**:817–9)

Venlafaxine (n = 1, *J Formos Med Assoc* 2006;**105**: 90–3; n = 1, *Lancet* 2000;**355**:2164–5)

Venlafaxine + trifluoperazine (n = 1, *Lancet* 2000;**354**:289–90)

- **CNS — anticonvulsants** *

Carbamazepine (may also complicate symptoms, n = 1, *Br J Psychiatry* 1990;**157**:437–8; n = 1, *Br J Psychiatry* 1994;**164**:270; n = 1, *South Med J* 1991;**84**:1378–80)

Carbamazepine withdrawal (n = 1, *Am J Psychiatry* 1990;**147**:1687)

Oxcarbazepine + amisulpride (n = 1, *Gen Hosp Psychiatry* 2008;**30**:482–4)

Phenytoin toxicity (*S Afr Med J* 1988;**73**:620–1)

Tiapride (n = 1, *Clin Neuropharmacol* 1996;**19**: 539–40; n = 1, *Rev Rhum Ed Fr* 1994; **61**:362)

Zonisamide + carbamazepine (n=1, *Epilepsia* 2007;**48**:1999–2001)

- **CNS — antiparkinsonian drugs** *

Amantadine (SPC)

Amantadine withdrawal (n = 1, *Am J Psychiatry* 1994;**151**:451–2; n=1, *Eur J Pediatr* 2001; **160**:401; *Neurology* 1991;**41**:942–3)

Anticholinergic withdrawal (n = 1, *Int Clin Psychopharmacol* 1996;**11**:207–9)

Bromocriptine to pergolide (rapid switch, n = 1, *Parkinsonism Relat Disord* 2002;**9**:116)

Fava bean abrupt withdrawal (n = 1, *Mov Disord* 2005;**20**:630–1; NB Fava beans contain appreciable amounts of levodopa)

Levodopa (n = 1, *Intern Med* 1992;**31**:1298–302)

Levodopa withdrawal (n = 1, *Med J Aust* 1991; **155**:53–4; n = 1, *J Clin Anesth* 1995;**7**:652–6; n = 3, *JAMA* 1985;**254**:2792–5)

Levodopa and bromocriptine withdrawal (n = 1, *Singapore Med J* 2001;**42**:85–8)

Tetrabenazine long–term (n=1, *Mov Disord* 1997;**12**:246–8; *Mov Disord* 1996;**11**:95)

Tolcapone withdrawal (n = 1, *Am J Med* 2000; **108**:517–8)

- **CNS — others** *

Anticholinesterases (n = 1, *Int J Geriatr Psychiatry* 2006;**21**:193–4), e.g.:
→ donepezil (n = 1, *Int J Neuropsychopharmacol* 2004;**7**:101–3)
→ donepezil + maprotiline (n = 1, *Neurology* 2003;**60**:1050–1)
→ donepezil + olanzapine (n = 1, *Nat Clin Pract Neurol* 2008;**4**:170–4)

Cocaine (review, *Am J Emerg Med* 1996;**14**: 425–8; n = 1, *Tijdschr Psychiatr* 2006;**48**; 399–404)

Cocaine + amfetamine overdose (fatal, n = 1, *Med Clin (Barc)* 1996;**106**:717–8)

Domperidone (n = 1, *Dig Dis Sci* 1992;**37**:946–8)

LSD (n = 1, fatal, *J Neurol Neurosurg Psychiatry* 1991;**54**:741–3)

LSD + alcohol (n = 1, *Br J Addict* 1990;**85**:990–1)

Methylphenidate (n = 1, *Pediatr Neurol* 1998;**19**: 299–301; n = 1, *Prim Care Companion J Clin Psychiatry* 2006;**8**:47)

Metoclopramide (several cases, e.g. *Arch Intern Med* 1987;**147**:1495–7; *Ann Pharmacother* 1999;**33**:644–5; n = 1, *J Burn Care Res* 2006; **27**:237–41)

Metoclopramide withdrawal (n = 1, *Aust N Z J Med* 1995;**25**:261)

Prochlorperazine (n = 1, *J Emerg Med* 1996;**14**: 727–9)

- **Others** *

Alimemazine (n = 1, *Eur J Pediatr* 2002;**161**:259–61)

Baclofen abrupt withdrawal (n = 1, *J Psychopharmacol* 2001;**99**:61–3; n = 1, *Med Clin (Barc)* 2006;**127**:79)

Compulsive water drinking (*Med J Aust* 1989; **150**:457–8)

Diphenhydramine (n = 1, *Vet Hum Toxicol* 1988; **30**:58–9)

Diphenhydramine + diprophyllin overdose (n = 1, *J Neurol Sci* 1999;**162**:108–9)

Ganciclovir (n = 1, *Pharmacother* 2000;**20**: 479–83)

Iron (low levels? *Lancet* 1987;**i**:1234–6)

Oral contraceptives (n = 1, *Drug Intell Clin Pharm* 1989;**23**:811)

Organophosphate poisoning (n = 1, *Can J Anesth* 1995;**42**:1027–30)

Promethazine (n = 1, *Aust N Z J Psychiatry* 2005; **39**:113–4)

Promethazine + lorazepam (n = 1, *Aust N Z J Psychiatry* 2001;**35**:250–1)

Rifampicin + chlorpromazine (n = 1, *J Korean Med Sci* 2008;**23**:734–6)

5.10 OBSESSIVE-COMPULSIVE SYMPTOMS

Reviews: typical antipsychotic–induced OCD (*Prog Neuropsychopharmacol Biol Psychiatry* 2003: **27**;333–46).There is a 3% incidence with clozapine, olanzapine and risperidone in Asians, although in this study no cases were reported with quetiapine (Mahendran *et al, J Clin Psychiatry* 2007;**68**:542–5).

• CNS — anxiolytics and hypnotics *
Benzodiazepine withdrawal (n = 1, *Br J Psychiatry* 1987;**150**:272; n = 1, *J Nerv Ment Dis* 1988; **176**:688–91)

• CNS — antipsychotics *
Reviews: antipsychotics (review of drug–induced OCD and treatment; Sareen *et al, J Affect Disord* 2004;**82**:167–74). For risperidone and olanzapine, there are no differences in incidence but severity is associated with longer duration of olanzapine treatment (n = 113, *J Clin Psychiatry* 2002;**63**:104–7; n = 6, *J Clin Psychopharmacol* 2002; **22**:461–7; n = 2, *J Child Adolesc Psychopharmacol* 2003;**13** Suppl 1:S89–92).

Clozapine (e.g. n = 40, 20% incidence, *Compr Psychiatry* 2009;**50**:437–42; n = 59 on clozapine, 24% had OCD; Mukhopadhaya *et al, J Psychopharmacol* 2009;**23**:6–13; especially early in schizophrenia, n = 121, *J Clin Psychiatry* 1999;**60**:364–5; n = 1, *Psychiatr Clin Neurosci* 2005;**59**:219–22; although one study showed it might be of

some use for OCD symptoms in people with schizophrenia; n = 15, Reznik *et al, Pharmacopsychiatry* 2004;**37**:52–6; n = 1, *Aust NZ J Psychiatry* 2007;**41**:293–4; n = 7, *Clin Neuropharmacol* 2009;**32**:227–9)

Haloperidol (n = 20, 10% incidence, *Compr Psychiatry* 2009;**50**:437–42)

Olanzapine (n = 2, *Am J Psychiatry* 1999;**156**: 799–800; severity associated with duration of treatment: n = 113, *J Clin Psychiatry* 2002; **63**:104–7; review, n = 9, *Int Clin Neuropsychopharmacol* 2004;**7**:375–7)

Quetiapine (n = 1, *Prog Neuropsychopharmacol Biol Psychiatry* 2006;**30**:724–7; n = 5, *J Clin Psychopharmacol* 2006;**26**:396–400)

Risperidone (dose dependent case, *Aust N Z J Psychiatry* 1998;**32**:299–301; n = 1, *Br J Psychiatry* 1999;**174**:559; n = 2, children, *J Child Adolesc Psychopharmacol* 2003;**13**[Suppl 1]:S89–92)

• CNS — antidepressants *
Fluoxetine (n = 3, *Am J Psychiatry* 1991;**148**: 1262–3)

• CNS — analgesics *
Codeine abuse (n = 2, *Acta Psychiatr Scand* 1989; **79**:619–20)

• CNS — anticonvulsants
Gabapentin withdrawal (n = 1, *J Clin Psychiatry* 1998;**59**:131)

Topiramate (n = 1, *Psychiatry Clin Neurosci* 2006; **60**:394)

• CNS — others *
Methamphetamine (*J Clin Psychiatry* 1999;**60**: 337–8; n = 1, *J Am Acad Child Adolesc Psychiatry* 1998;**37**:135)

Methylphenidate (*J Am Acad Child Adolesc Psychiatry* 1998;**37**:135; n = 1, *Can J Psychiatry* 2001;**46**:89; n = 1, *CNS Spectr* 2003;**8**:612–3)

Modafinil (n = 2, exacerbation of symptoms, *Prim Care Companion J Clin Psychiatry* 2008; **10**:164–5)

Stimulants (n = 1, *Biol Psychiatry* 1985;**20**:1332–7)

• Anti-infection drugs *
Isoniazid (*J Clin Psychiatry* 1990;**51**:387)

• Endocrine system drugs *
Corticosteroids (may respond to fluvoxamine,

Clin Neuropharmacol 2009;**32**:176–7):
  → cortisone (n=1, *Pharmacopsychiatry* 2002;
    35:72–4)

- **Malignancy and immunosuppressant drugs** *
Interferons (*Gen Hosp Psychiatry* 2006;**28**:
  357–8)

5.11 PANIC ATTACKS

- **CNS — anxiolytics and hypnotics** *
Benzodiazepines:
  → alprazolam (*J Am Board Fam Pract* 2002;**15**:
    69–72)
  → clobazam withdrawal (n=2, *Br Med J* 1981;
    282:1931–2)
  → diazepam discontinuation after long-term
    abuse (n=1, *Drug Intell Clin Pharmacy* 1989;
    23:989–90)
Buspirone (case + correspondence in *Lancet*
  1989;**2**:46–7, 615, 682–3)

- **CNS — antipsychotics** *
Review: long-term (n=45, incidence 20%,
Psychiatry Clin Neurosci 1999;**53**:91–4).

Clozapine (n=1, *Am J Psychiatry* 2000;**157**:2056)
Olanzapine (e.g. hyperventilation, n=1, *J Psych
  Neurosci* 2002;**27**:360–3)
Risperidone (in people with post-LSD visual
  disorder, n=3, *J Clin Psychopharmacol* 1996;
  16:238–41)

- **CNS — antidepressants** *
Amitriptyline abrupt discontinuation (n=1, *Am J
  Psychiatry* 1981;**138**:117–8)
Mianserin discontinuation (n=1, *Jpn J Psychiatry
  Neurol* 1989;**43**:995–9)
Mirtazapine discontinuation (*Can J Psychiatry*
  2000;**45**:570–1)
SSRIs:
  → citalopram (n=1, *South Med J* 2002;**95**:
    1088–9)
  → fluoxetine (unless initial doses kept very
    low, e.g. *J Clin Psychopharmacol* 1987;
    7:329–32; n=1, *J Neuropsychiatry Clin
    Neurosci* 1989;**1**: 219–20)
  → fluoxetine + bupropion (*J Clin Psychiatry*
    1996;**57**:177–8)
  → sertraline (n=1, *Clin Neuropharmacol*
    2000;**23**:164–8)

Trazodone

- **CNS — analgesics** *
Opiate blockade (*J Clin Psychopharmacol*
  1987;**7**:361–2)
Sumatriptan (n=125, incidence 7.2%, *Am J
  Psychiatry* 1996;**153**:1505; single dose n=15,
  RCT, d/b, p/c, *Eur Neuropsychopharmacol*
  2005;**15**:279–82)

- **CNS — anticonvulsants** *
Pregabalin (BNF, less common)
Topiramate (n=1, *J Clin Psychopharmacol*
  2001;**21**:461–2; n=1, *J Clin Psychiatry* 2006;
  67:326–7; *Pharmacopsychiatry* 2008;**41**:79)

- **CNS — antiparkinsonian drugs** *
Amantadine (n=1, *J Clin Psychiatry* 1996;**57**:374)
Levodopa (n=31, *Acta Neurol Scand* 1993;**87**:
  14–8)
Pramipexole (*Eur J Neurol* 2007;**14**:e1)

- **CNS — others** *
Amfetamines (n=3, *Biol Psychiatry* 1992;**32**:91–5;
  n=1, *J Clin Psychopharmacol* 1998;**18**:95–6;
  methamphetamine n=1, *J Anxiety Disord*
  1997;**11**:113–6)
Caffeine hyperreactivity (n=98, RCT, d/b, 1/52,
  Psychiatry Res 2009;**169**:149–53; *J Nerv Ment
  Dis* 1993;**181**:327–30)
Cannabis (n=1, *Acta Psychiatr Scand* 1998;**98**:
  254–5; *J Am Acad Child Adolesc Psychiatry*
  2000;**39**:1467)
Cocaine (*Biol Psychiatry* 1991;**29**:403–6; reviews:
  Am J Drug Alcohol Abuse 1992;**18**:57–62;
  Biol Psychiatry 1996;**40**:938–40; *J Addict Dis*
  1992;**11**:47–58)
Fenfluramine (n=1, *Braz J Med Biol Res* 1997;
  30:887–90)
MDMA/Ecstasy (n=3, *Biol Psychiatry* 1992;**32**:
  91–5)
Metoclopramide (n=1, *Psychopharmacol Bull*
  2002;**36**:82–93)
Naltrexone (n=1, *Am J Psychiatry* 1998;**155**: 447)
Sibutramine (n=1, *Am J Psychiatry* 2002;**159**:
  1793–4)
Smoking cessation (n=2, *J Clin Psychiatry* 2002;
  63:594–5)
Sumatriptan (n=125, incidence 7%, panic
  being interpretation of side-effects such as
  chest pain, palpitations, etc, *Am J Psychiatry*

1996;**153**:1505)
Varenicline (BNF, less common)

- **Gastrointestinal drugs** *
Pentagastrin (laboratory probe, n = 14,
incidence 86% in people with OCD,
p/c, *Psychopharmacology (Berl)* 1996;**126**:
339–44; n = 25, RCT, p/c, d/b, c/o, *Psychoneuroendocrinology* 2002;**27**:417–29)

- **Cardiovascular drugs** *
Carvedilol (n = 1, *Ann Pharmacother* 2002;**36**:
1736–40)
Isoproterenol (n = 131, incidence 66%, p/c, d/b,
Biol Psychiatry 1988;**24**:891–902)
Pentoxifylline (n = 1, *Am J Psychiatry* 1994;**151**:
290)

- **Respiratory drugs** *
Doxapram (*Biol Psychiatry* 1993;**33**:295–7;
n = 10, s/b, *Psychiatry Res* 2005;**133**:253–61)
Epinephrine/adrenaline (n = 25, incidence 67%,
d/b, p/c, *J Affect Disord* 1996;**39**:133–40;
n = 50, incidence 68%, RCT, d/b, *Biol
Psychiatry* 1998;**44**:1017–26)
Salbutamol (n = 1, *Eur Neuropsychopharmacol*
1997;**7**:241–2)
Theophylline (n = 1, *An Med Interna* 1990;**7**:53;
n = 1, *Rev Clin Esp* 1988;**183**:280)

- **Anti-infection drugs** *
Chloroquine and mefloquine (*Adv Psychiatr Treat*
2005;**11**:66)
Co-trimoxazole (n = 1, *J Clin Psychopharmacol*
1991;**11**:144–5)
Mefloquine (BNF, less common; incidence 0.3%,
n = 35,370, *Drug Saf* 2004;**27**:203–13)
Metronidazole (*South Med J* 1985;**78**:627)
Rifampicin (n = 1, *Pharmacotherapy* 2005;**25**:
435–7)

- **Endocrine system drugs** *
Dexamethasone (*J Adolesc Health* 1994;**99**:
345–7; n = 1, *Am J Psychiatry* 1984;**141**:1647;
J Psychiatry Neurosci 1997;**22**:346–7)
Estrogen (n = 1, *Am J Psychiatry* 1994;**151**:1246;
Psychosomatics 1988;**29**:433–5)
Levonorgestrel implant (n = 2, *J Clin Psychiatry*
1994;**55**:478–80)
Oral contraceptive, combined (n = 2, *J Clin
Psychiatry* 1992;**53**:163–5; n = 1, *Acta Obstet

Gynecol Scand 1992;**71**:87–90)
TRH (thyrotropin releasing hormone) (n = 99,
Depress Anxiety 2003;**17**:78–87)

- **Malignancy and immunosuppressant drugs** *
Interferons (n = 1, *Gen Hosp Psychiatry* 2005;**27**:
329–37)

- **Musculoskeletal and analgesics** *
Infliximab (n = 1, *Dig Dis Sci* 2006;**51**:1056)
Oxaprozin (n = 1, *Am J Psychiatry* 1995;**152**:149)

- **Others** *
Aspartame (n = 1, unproven, high dose, *Lancet*
1986;**12**:631)
Carbon dioxide (mentioned in *Am J Psychiatry*
1994;**151**:292–3)
Flumazenil (n = 36, incidence 9%, d/b, *J
Psychopharmacol* 1998;**12**:146–50; n = 1,
given as part of ECT, *J ECT* 2009;**25**:145)
Isotretinoin (n = 1, *Rev Med Chil* 2006;**134**:
1565–7)
Lactate oral (e.g. in calcium lactate tablets, case
in *Ann Pharmacother* 1995;**29**:539–40)
Organic solvents (n = 3, *Am J Psychiatry* 1987;
144:1056–8)
Oxymetazoline (n = 1, *J Clin Psychiatry* 1987;**48**:
293)
Oxymetazoline withdrawal (n = 1, *J Clin
Psychiatry* 1987;**48**:293)
Phenylephrine (n = 1, *Br J Psychiatry* 1980;**136**:
297–9)
Procaine (in Penicillin G, n = 3, *Am J Psychiatry*
1988;**145**:1317)
Sodium lactate (study in *Arch Gen Psychiatry*
1989;**46**:135–40)
Tyramine (*J S C Med Assoc* 2002;**98**:187–92)
Yohimbine (see *Arch Gen Psychiatry* 1998;**55**:
1033–44; n = 16, p/c, *Psychiatry Res* 1993;**48**:
119–33)

5.12 PARANOID OR SCHIZOPHRENIC-LIKE PSYCHOSES (SEE ALSO HALLUCINATIONS 5.6)

This is characterised by paranoid delusions and
hallucinations in a person with little clouding of
consciousness. The literature on drug-induced
psychosis is extensive but mainly case reports
and short uncontrolled studies. A classification
has been proposed:

- Intoxication mimicking functional: (e.g.

drug-induced), e.g. stimulants and cannabis. Persists for several days until the drug has cleared.

- **Psychoactive drugs altering the clinical presentation of an existing psychosis:** e.g. cannabis or amfetamines, etc. creating a more aggressive and disturbed schizophrenic patient (Davison and Roth, *Br J Psychiatry* 1996;**168**:651).
- **Chronic hallucinations induced by substance abuse:** insight usually present, no clouding of consciousness, continue despite long-term abstinence, e.g. alcoholic hallucinosis, LSD or cannabis flashbacks.
- **Drug-induced relapse of functional psychosis:** e.g. schizophrenia.
- **Withdrawal states:** e.g. delirium tremens, benzodiazepine or barbiturate withdrawal.
- **Others:** acute intoxication/confusion with clouding of consciousness, post-intoxication depression, e.g. post-amfetamine crash, panic/anxiety attacks, e.g. from hallucinogens such as LSD.
- **True drug-induced psychosis:** any psychotic symptoms which occur with drug intoxication and then persist after elimination of the causing drug, e.g. one to two drug-free weeks.

Review: substance-induced psychosis (Mathias *et al, J Clin Psychiatry* 2008;**69**:358–67).

- **CNS — hallucinogens, etc (major cause)**

Cannabis (acute onset, usually resolves in 2–7 days, *Acta Psychiatr Scand* 1991;**83**:34–6). At higher doses, cannabis is a risk factor for the development or relapse of schizophrenia, e.g. there is a two-fold increase in relative risk for later schizophrenia. Cannabis itself, however, is neither a sufficient nor necessary cause for psychosis but should be discouraged in vulnerable youths (Arseneault *et al, Br J Psychiatry* 2004;**184**:110–7; review by Macleod, *Adv Psychiatr Treat* 2007;**13**:400–11; systematic review, s = 35, *Lancet* 2007; **370**: 319–28).

Dimethoxy-methylamfetamine (DOM)
LSD
Khat chewing (n = 4, *Br J Hosp Med* 1995;**54**: 322–6)
Mescaline
MDE/Eve (n = 1, *Arch Gen Psychiatry* 1993;**50**:75)
MDMA/Ecstasy (n = 1, *Br J Psychiatry* 1991;**159**: 713–5)
Petrol (n = 2, *Am J Psychiatry* 1964;**120**:757–61)
Phencyclidine (angel dust)
Psilocybin (magic mushrooms) (n = 3, *Br J Psychiatry* 1978;**132**:602)

- **CNS — stimulants (major cause)** *
Review: systematic (s = 54, Curran *et al, Br J Psychiatry* 2004;**185**:196–204).

Adderall® (n = 1, *J Am Board Fam Pract* 2002; **99**:498–500)
Amfetamines (e.g. treatment/review in *Topic Emerg Med* 1985;**7**:18–32; *Gen Hosp Psychiatry* 1996;**18**:117–20)
Cocaine (n = 50, incidence 68%, *Am J Psychiatry*, 1991;**148**:495–8)
Diethylpropion (n = 1, *Int Clin Psychopharmacol* 1993;**8**:67–70; n = 5, *Clin Neuropharmacol* 1988;**11**:183–8)
Ephedrine (review in *Br J Psychiatry* 1987;**150**: 252–5)
Methamfetamine (n = 1, *Am J Psychiatry* 1999;**4**:662; *Australas Psychiatry* 2006;**14**:86–9)
Phencyclidine (n = 10, *South Med J* 1988;**81**:565–7)
Phentermine (n = 1, *Zhonghua Yi Xue Za Zhi* [Taipei] 1998;**61**:44–7)
Phenylephrine (e.g. *JAMA* 1982;**247**:1859–60)
Phenylpropanolamine (*Am J Psychiatry* 1990;**147**:367–8; n = 1, *Am J Psychiatry* 2000; **157**:1021–2)
Pseudoephedrine (many cases, e.g. *South Med J* 1990;**83**:64–5)
Solvents (review, *Nihon Arukoru Yakubutsu Igakkai Zasshi* 2005;**40**:471–84; *Br J Psychiatry* 1989; **155**:132; n = 1, *Nihon Arukoru Yakubutsu Igakkai Zasshi* 1996;**31**:475–82)

- **CNS — anxiolytics and hypnotics** *
Benzodiazepines:
  → alprazolam
  → lorazepam (*Br J Psychiatry* 1985:**147**:211; *Br J Psychiatry* 1986;**148**:344; pre-operative, n = 1, *Anaesthesia* 2003;**58**:1036)
  → lormetazepam (n = 1, *Pharmacopsychiatry* 1993;**26**:102–3)
  → midazolam (possible case in *Drug Intell Clin Pharm* 1989;**23**:671–2)
  → nitrazepam (BNF, C/I in psychosis)

→ nitrazepam normal-dose withdrawal
(n = 2, J *UOEH* 1988;**10**:337–40)

→ triazolam (e.g. *Pharmacopsychiatry*1989;**22**:115–9)

→ triazolam withdrawal (J *Clin Psychiatry*
1987;**48**:168–9)

Benzodiazepine withdrawal (*Int J Geriatr
Psychiatry* 1995;**10**:901–2; *Psychosomatics*
1997;**38**:160–1)

Buspirone (n = 1, *Am J Psychiatry* 1991;**148**:1606;
J *Psychopharmacol* 1993;**7**:295–300; n = 1,
Psychosomatics 1992;**33**:332–5)

Chloral

Melatonin (n = 1, *Ann Pharmacother* 1997;**31**:1408)

Oxybate (BNF, less common)

Zolpidem (*Lancet* 1992;**339**:813; n = 2, *Ann Clin
Psychiatry* 1996;**8**:89–91; n = 1, J *Am Geriatr
Soc* 1997;**45**:533–4)

Zolpidem withdrawal (n = 2, *Ugeskr Laeger*
1993;**155**:2711–3)

Zopiclone (some cases reported — *WHO Drug
Information* 1990;**4**:179)

- CNS — antipsychotics *

Antipsychotic withdrawal (rebound psychosis
as opposed to relapse; n = 1, *Can J Psychiatry*
1989;**34**:227–9; in Tourette's; *Biol Psychiatry*
1993;**34**:341–2)

Aripiprazole (n = 1, J *Clin Psychiatry* 2005;**66**:
1339; n = 4, *Int Clin Psychopharmacol* 2004;
19:45–8; as both add-on and during tapered
crossover; and as adjunct to risperidone,
n = 1, J *Clin Psychiatry* 2007;**68**:1445–6)

Chlorpromazine (n = 1, *Can Med Assoc J* 1970:
102:642; n = 1, *Brain Inj* 1993;**7**:77–83)

Clozapine withdrawal (e.g. rebound psychosis,
study in *Psychopharmacol* 1988;**24**:260–3;
n = 3, J *Clin Psychiatry* 1997;**58**:252–5)

Haloperidol (*Drug Intell Clin Pharm* 1981;**15**:209)

Olanzapine (psychotic mania, *Eur Psychiatry*
1999;**14**:410–1)

Risperidone (n = 1, J *Child Adolesc Psychopharmacol* 2005;**15**:520–5)

- CNS — antidepressants *

Antidepressants may account for 8% admissions
due to drug-induced psychosis or mania (n = 533,
J *Clin Psychiatry* 2001;**62**:30–3)

Bupropion (many cases, e.g. n = 1, *Pharmacopsychiatry* 2002;**35**:247–8; J *Psychiatr Pract*
2007;**13**:336–8; n = 1, J *Am Board Fam*

Med 2008;**21**:244–5; overdose n = 1, *Prog
Neuropsychopharmacol Biol Psychiatry* 2005;
29:149–51)

Mirtazapine (BNF, may aggravate psychotic
states; added to levodopa, n = 1, *Pharmacopsychiatry* 1997;**30**: 263–5)

Phenelzine (BNF, rare; e.g. n = 1, *Br J Psychiatry*
1991;**159**:716–7)

SSRIs, e.g.:

→ fluoxetine (J *Nerv Mental Dis* 1990;
178:55–8; n = 1, J *Am Acad Child Adolesc
Psychiatry* 2007;**46**:944–5)

→ fluvoxamine (n = 2, *Schizophr Res*
1995;**16**:77–9; n = 1, *Can J Psychiatry* 2000;
45:762; n = 1, *Hum Psychopharmacol*
2003;**18**:477–8)

→ paroxetine (case of psychotic mania, *Am J
Psychiatry* 1995;**152**:1399–440)

→ sertraline (n = 4, *Ann Clin Psychiatry* 1997;
9:99–7)

St John's wort (n = 1, *Hum Psychopharmacol*
2004;**19**:275–6; review, n = 17, possible
association, *Int J Clin Pharmacol Ther* 2004;
42:473–80)

Trazodone (n = 1, J *Neuropsych Clin Neurosci*
2005;**17**:253–4)

Tricyclics (BNF, may aggravate psychosis; review,
concludes any psychosis is temporary and
rare, s = 20, n = 177, J *Affect Disord* 2008;
106:279–84)

Venlafaxine + propafenone (*Int J Psychiatr Med*
2001;**31**:427–32)

- CNS — analgesics *

Anticholinergic toxicity from antidiarrhoeal
preparation (n = 1, *Br J Psychiatry*
1990;**157**:758–9)

Buprenorphine (BNF, less common)

Buprenorphine withdrawal (n = 1, *Am J
Psychiatry* 2008;**165**:399–400)

Butorphanol (J *Neuropsychiatry Clin Neurosci*
1998;**10**:236–7)

Codeine OD (n = 1, *Neurobehavioral Toxicol
Teratol* 1985;**7**:93–4)

Diamorphine (BNF, caution in psychosis)

Dipipanone (BNF, uncommon)

Fentanyl (BNF, v rare)

Methadone withdrawal (e.g. n = 2, J *Clin
Psychiatry* 1995;**56**:73–6)

Morphine intrathecal (*Anesth Analg* 1993;**77**:
1298–9)

Naltrexone (after heroin detox, n = 1, *Am J Addict* 2005;**14**:486–7)

Oxycodone (BNF, caution in psychosis)

Paracetamol overdose (*Gen Hosp Psychiatry* 1997;**19**;149–50)

Pentazocine (esp. hallucinations, e.g. *Br Med J* 1974;**2**:224)

- CNS — anticonvulsants *

Psychosis induced by anticonvulsants may be the result of 'forced normalisation'. Risk factors include temporal lobe epilepsy (TLE), treatment resistance, past history of psychosis or affective disorder, and becoming suddenly seizure-free (best to do this gradually). Drug regimens should be changed gradually and compliance should be maintained to prevent epileptic psychoses (n = 44, Matsuura, *J Neurol Neurosurg Psychiatry* 1999;**67**:231–3).

Carbamazepine (BNF, rare)

Carbamazepine toxicity (*Lancet* 1989;i:167)

Carbamazepine withdrawal (n = 1, *Br J Clin Pract* 1996;**50**:350–1)

Clonazepam (n = 1, *J Nerv Ment Dis* 1982;**170**: 117)

Clonazepam withdrawal (*J Clin Psychopharmacol* 1986;**6**:193)

Ethosuximide (BNF, rare)

Gabapentin (exacerbation of psychosis in schizophrenic, n = 1, *Can J Psychiatry* 2002;**47**:975–6)

Lamotrigine (*Epilepsy Behav* 2007;**11**:476; n = 4, incidence 0.2%, *Epilepsy Behav* 2007;**11**:133–9)

Levetiracetam (BNF, less common; cases within n = 517, *Neurology* 2003;**61**:704–6; n = 1, long-term, *Can J Psychiatry* 2004;**49**:868; *Can J Psychiatry* 2005;**50**:948; n = 1, *Med Clin* [Barc] 2007;**129**:278)

Oxcarbazepine (n = 1, *Epilepsy Behav* 2008; **12**:492–3)

Phenytoin toxicity (*Drug Intell Clin Pharm* 1988; **22**:1003–4; n = 1 for trigeminal neuralgia, *Epilepsy Behav* 2003;**4**:771–2; *Clin Pediatr* [Phila] 1993;**32**:107–10)

Pregabalin (n = 1, *Seizure* 2006;**15**:208–10)

Tiagabine (BNF, rare; RCT shows no significant risk; n = 554, *Epilepsia* 2002;**43**:394–8; n = 1, *Neuropsychiatr* 2007;**21**:59–61; n = 596, 1.5% incidence, esp. with previous episodes, *Epilepsy Behav* 2003;**4**:548–52)

Topiramate (n = 596, 1.5% incidence, esp. with previous episodes, *Epilepsy Behav* 2003; **4**:548–52; discussion in *J Clin Psychiatry* 2004;**65**:145–6; n = 2, *Expert Opin Drug Saf* 2006;**5**:741–2; n = 1, >400mg/d, *Am J Psychiatry* 2005;**162**:1542; n = 2, *Clin Neuropharmacol* 2006;**29**:168–9)

Valproate (isolated cases, e.g. *Clin Electro-encephalography* 1982;**13**:50–3)

Vigabatrin (BNF, less common; n = 1, *Acta Med Port* 2000;**13**:111–4; review, *Acta Neurol Scand* 1996;**93**:1–8; n = 14, *J Neurol Neurosurg Psychiatry* 1991;**54**:435–9)

Vigabatrin withdrawal (*Med J Aust* 1992;**156**:291; letter in *Lancet* 1990;**335**:1279)

Zonisamide (BNF, less common; n = 74, incidence 13–18%, *Seizure* 2000;**9**:65–70; n = 1, *Am J Psychiatry* 2007;**164**:682)

- CNS — antiparkinsonian drugs *

The incidence with Parkinsonian treatments may be as high as 20–30%.

Review: Kuzuhara, *J Neurol* 2001;**248**(Suppl 3): 28–31.

Amantadine (n = 2, exacerbation of schizophrenia, *Am J Psychiatry* 1986;**143**: 1170–1; overdose, n = 1, *Ann Emerg Med* 1990;**19**:668–70)

Anticholinergics (in people with Alzheimer's Disease, n = 230, *Clin Pharmacol Ther* 2008; **84**:63–8):
→ biperidin (*Med Clin (Barc)* 1992;**99**:79)
→ trihexyphenidyl

Barbiturates

Cabergoline (BNF, caution in psychosis; n = 2, exacerbation of schizophrenia when used as adjunct, *Gen Hosp Psychiatry* 2008;**30**:378–80)

Dopamine agonists:
→ bromocriptine (BNF, rare; *An Med Interna* 2003;**20**:50–1; n = 1, *J Natl Med Assoc* 1993;**85**:700–1; low–dose n = 1, *Acta Obstet Gynecol Scand* 1991;**70**:375–6; n = 2, *Harefuah* 1990;**118**:203–4)
→ bromocriptine + pseudoephedrine (n = 1, *J Fam Pract* 1997;**45**:164–6)
→ pergolide (BNF, caution in psychosis; esp. hallucinations, incidence ≤13%, e.g. *Neurology* 1982;**32**:1181–4)
→ pramipexole (BNF, *Psychiatry Clin Neurosci* 2008;**62**:245)

→ ropinirole (BNF, less common; n = 95, 14% incidence, *Ann Pharmacother* 2009;**43**:1426–32; n = 1, *Prog Neuro-psychopharmacol Biol Psychiatry* 2008;**32**:1087–8; n = 1, *Am J Psychiatry* 2006;**163**:457–8)

→ rotigotine (BNF, less common)

Levodopa (esp. hallucinations — *Arch Neurol* 1970;**23**:193–200)

Lisuride (a few cases, e.g. *Lancet* 1986;**2**:510)

Selegiline (a few cases, e.g. *Neurology* 1981;**31**: 19–23)

- **CNS — others** *

Review: drug-induced symptoms in Parkinson's Disease (Kuzuhara, *J Neurol* 2001;**248**(Suppl 3): 28–31).

Adderall® (n = 1, *J Am Board Fam Pract* 2002; **99**:498–500)

Alcohol

Alcohol, caffeine and 'vigueur fit' (n = 1, *Med Sci Law* 2001;**41**:331–6)

Amfetamine (*Gen Hosp Psychiatry* 1996;**18**:117–20; treatment for this, review *Cochrane Database Syst Rev* 2009;**1**:CD003026)

Atomoxetine (n = 1, transient, *J Child Adolesc Psychopharmacol* 2009;**19**:319–20)

Bupropion (n = 1, *Indian J Psychiatry* 2009;**51**: 53–4; n = 2, *Pharm World Sci* 2009;**31**:238–40)

Caffeine (n = 1, *CNS Spectr* 2009;**14**:127–9)

Cannabis (regular use increases illness severity, n = 3459, *J Nerv Ment Dis* 2009;**197**:35–40; review of mechanisms, *Curr Opin Psychiatry* 2007;**20**:116–20; earlier onset of use might be associated with greater risk of developing psychosis, n = 472, *Acta Psychiatr Scand* 2008;**118**:209–13; may also reduce brain volume over five years; *Am J Psychiatry* 2008; **165**;490–6)

Cocaine (review of risk factors, e.g. low BMI, n = 69, *Isr J Psychiatry Relat Sci* 2005;**42**:45–50)

Cocaine + OTC cold cure (*J Clin Psychiatry* 1989;**50**:147)

Dexamfetamine (BNF, less common; *Pediatrics* 2004;**113**:1466)

Dexfenfluramine (*Am J Psychiatry* 1997;**154**: 1624–5)

Diethylpropion (n = 1, *Int Clin Psychopharmacol* 1993;**8**:67–70; n = 5, *Clin Neuropharmacol* 1988;**11**:183–8)

Disulfiram (BNF, rare; C/I in psychosis; n = 1, *Ned Tijdschr Geneeskd* 2002;**146**:571–3; n = 1, *Br Med J* 1992;**305**:763; n = 1, *Ned Tijdschr Geneeskd* 2002;**146**:965):

→ high-dose (n = 1, *J Clin Psychopharmacol* 2007;**27**:224–5)

→ low-dose (n = 1, *Prog Neuro-psychopharmacol Biol Psychiatry* 2008; **32**:311–2)

Ephedra alkaloids (in 'vigueur fit' tablets; n = 1, *Med Sci Law* 2001;**41**:331–6; n = 7, *South Med J* 2003;**96**:718–20)

Gamma-hydroxybutyrate (GHB) withdrawal (n = 8, *Ann Emerg Med* 2001;**37**:147–53)

Hyoscine (n = 4 plus review, *Fortschr Neurol Psychiatr* 1998;**66**:289–95)

Hyoscine transdermal patches (n = 1, *Nervenarzt* 1997;**68**:77–9; Transderm®, *Neurology* 2000; **54**:1877; *Postgrad Med* 1988;**84**:73–6; n = 3, *Can J Hosp Pharm* 1994;**47**:67–9)

Khat (n = 1, *Tijdschr Psychiatr* 2007;**49**:763–7; review of association in Somalia, n = 4854, *BMC Med* 2005;**3**:5; n = 1, *Ethiop Med J* 1997; **35**:137–9)

Khat + mushrooms (n = 4, *World J Biol Psychiatry* 2004;**5**:49–53)

MDMA/ecstasy (n = 1, *Lijec Vjesn* 2000;**122**:27–30; n = 1, persistent after single dose, *Psychosomatics* 2001;**42**:525–7; n = 1, very persistent, *Psychol Rep* 2004;**95**:192–6; n = 32, *Eur Addict Res* 2002;**8**:133–40)

Memantine (BNF, less common; *Lancet* 1991;**338**:1022–3; n = 1, *J Clin Psychiatry* 2005; **66**:658–9; n = 3, *Neurology* 2005;**65**:481–2)

Methamphetamine (n = 21, 6/12 follow-up, *Zhonghua Yi Xue Za Zhi [Taipei]* 2001; **64**:388–94; n = 309, incidence 13%, McKetin et al, *Addiction* 2006;**101**:1473–8; n = 39, *Psychiatry Res* 2008;**157**:273–7)

Methylphenidate (BNF, v rare)

Methysergide (n = 1, *Neuropsychobiology* 1989; **22**:125–7)

Metoclopramide (n = 2, *Ann Pharmacother* 2002; **36**:1387–90)

Modafinil (may exacerbate: n = 1, *Arch Gen Psychiatry* 2002;**59**:292–3; n = 1, *Am J Psychiatry* 2005;**162**:1983; n = 1, *Intern Med J* 2008;**38**:677–8)

Nabilone (BNF, common)

Naltrexone (after heroin detox, n = 1, *Am J Addict* 2005;**14**:486–7)

Nandrolone (n = 1, *Psychiatr Prax* 2003;**30**(Suppl 3):S73–4)

Nicotine, abrupt withdrawal (n = 1, *Am J Psychiatry* 1994;**151**:452)

Promethazine (rare but possible, e.g. *NEJM* 1960; **263**:747)

Silbutramine (n = 1, *Am J Psychiatry* 2000; **157**:2057–8; *J Clin Psychopharmacol* 2007;**27**:399–7; n = 1, *J Psychosom Res* 2008;**64**:107–9; *J Clin Psychopharmacol* 2007; **27**:726–7)

Sodium oxybate (SPC)

Varenicline (n = 1, relapse of pre-existing schizophrenia, *J Clin Psychiatry* 2007;**68**:1269; n = 1, *CNS Spectr* 2008;**13**:511–4; n = 1, *Pharmacotherapy* 2009;**29**:852–7)

- **Gastrointestinal drugs** *

Antidiarrheals (OTC) (n = 1, *Br J Psychiatry* 1990; **157**:758–9)

Bismuth toxicity (*Am Fam Physician* 1988;**38**: 244–6)

Cimetidine (*Indian Pediatr* 1989;**26**:1061–2; n = 1, *Am J Psychiatry* 1980;**137**:1112–3)

Dicycloverine

- **Cardiovascular drugs** *

ACE inhibitors, e.g.:
  → lisinopril (*Psychiatr Prax* 1998;**25**:204)

Amyl nitrate (Martindale, 1993)

Beta–blockers (see under depression for differentials), e.g.:
  → atenolol (rare, n = 1, *Am J Psychiatry* 1983; **140**:1382)
  → propranolol (well known, e.g. *Biol Psychiatry* 1989;**25**: 351–4; n = 1, *Am J Emerg Med* 1995;**13**:536–7)
  → propranolol withdrawal (*Biol Psychiatry* 1989;**25**:351–4)

Calcium–channel blockers, e.g.:
  → diltiazem (n = 1, *Arch Intern Med* 1991; **151**:373–4; *J R Soc Med* 1988;**81**:296–7)
  → enalapril (n = 1, *Drug Intell Clin Pharm* 1991; **25**:558–9)
  → nifedipine (possible case in *J Am Geriatr Soc* 1984;**32**:408; *Am J Med* 1987;**83**:389; n = 1, *Am J Med* 1986;**81**:705–6)
  → quinapril (n = 1, *J Am Geriatr Soc* 2000;**48**: 9933)

Clonidine (n = 1, *Prog Neuropsychopharmacol* 1980;**4**:21)

Clonidine withdrawal (n = 3, *Am J Psychiatry* 1982;**139**: 110–2)

Digoxin toxicity (BNF, v rare; *J Nerv Mental Dis* 1978;**166**:817; *Lijec Vjesn* 1991;**113**:417–9)

Disopyramide (BNF, very rare; e.g. *Lancet* 1978;**1**: 858 + 1152)

Dopamine infusion (*Biol Psychiatry* 1992;**31**: 1225–7)

Doxazosin (n = 1, *Br Med J* 1997;**314**:1869)

Hydralazine

Lidocaine IV (n = 6, *Ann Intern Med* 1982;**97**: 149–50)

Losartan (*Cardiology* 1996;**87**:569–70)

Methyldopa (BNF, mild psychosis is common; *Adv Psych Treat* 2005;**11**:66)

Mexilitine (n = 1, *Am Heart J* 1984;**107**:1091–8)

Nitrates, e.g. isosorbides (*Adv Psychiatr Treat* 2005;**11**:66)

Pentoxifylline (*J Assoc Physicians India* 1992;**40**: 479)

Procainamide (BNF, uncommon; *Crit Care Nurse* 1993;**13**:70–2)

Quinidine (n = 1, *Med J Aust* 1990;**153**:47–9)

Simvastatin (n = 3, *Ned Tijdschr Geneeskd* 1993; **137**:1312–5)

Tocainide (*Br Med J* 1984;**288**:606–7)

- **Respiratory drugs** *

Betamethasone (n = 1, *No To Shinkei* 1992;**44**: 913–6)

Chlorphenamine OD (n = 1, *Med J Aust* 1973; **1**:382–6)

Coricidin cold medicine (*Ann Pharmacother* 2005;**39**:9977–8)

Cyproheptadine (*Indian J Pediatr* 1989;**56**:521–3; n = 1, *Pediatr Emerg Care* 1986;**2**:183–5)

Dextromethorphan (review, *Addict Biol* 2005;**10**:325–7; n = 1, *Am J Psychiatry* 2000; **157**:304)

Diphenhydramine (e.g. *Am J Emerg Med* 1997;**99**: 548–9; n = 1, *Am J Emerg Med* 1986;**4**:369–71; n = 2, *Chudoku Kenkyu* 2007;**20**:125–9)

Diphenhydramine overdose (n = 1, *Dtsch Med Wochenschr* 1988;**113**:180–3)

Ephedrine (n = 1, *Harefuah* 1994;**127**:166–8;299)

Phenylpropanolamine (with caffeine, *Biol Psychiatry* 1991;**30**:401–4; n = 1, *Gen Hosp Psychiatry* 1994;**16**:358–60; n = 1, *Am J Psychiatry* 2000;**157**:1021–2)

Phenylpropanolamine + amantadine (n = 1, *Gen*

Hosp Psychiatry 1995;**17**:457–8)

Promethazine (n = 1, *Psychosomatics* 2004;**45**: 89–90)

Salbutamol (*Biol Psychiatry* 1989;**26**:631–3)

Salbutamol inhaler (n = 1, *J Clin Psychopharmacol* 1995;**99**:446–7)

Theophylline (n = 1, *J Clin Psychopharmacol* 1989; **9**:65–6)

- Anti-infection drugs *

Aciclovir (BNF, rare; *Adv Psych Treat* 2005;**11**:66)

Amoxicillin + clarithromycin (n = 1, *Paediatr Anaesth* 2005;**99**:703–5)

Antifungals, e.g.:
  → amphotericin B IV (n = 1, *Ariz Med* 1972; **29**:322)
  → griseofulvin (*Adv Psychiatr Treat* 2005;**11**: 66)
  → posaconazole (BNF, common)

Antimalarials, e.g.:
  → chloroquine (n = 1, *Am J Ther* 2007;**14**: 406–7; n = 1, recurrent, *Indian J Med Sci* 1996;**50**:302–4; n = 1, *Presse Med* 2003; **32**:117; *Lancet* 1985;**2**:37)
  → lariam (severe is extremely low, e.g. one in 6000, *Pharm J* 1996;**256**:184)
  → mefloquine (BNF, less common; n = 1, *PNG Med J* 2002;**45**:219–21; n = 179, more common in females and first-time users; *Eur J Clin Pharmacol* 2002;**58**:441–5; n = 1, after single therapeutic dose, responded to quetiapine, *Malar J* 2006;**5**:74)
  → quinine (*Br J Psychiatry* 1988;**153**:575–6)

Antiretrovirals, e.g.:
  → efavirenz (BNF, less common; e.g. n = 1, *Clin Infect Dis* 2007;**45**:128–30; n = 1, *Clin Infect Dis* 2005;**40**:22–3)

Antituberculous drugs (*Lancet* 1989;ii:105; 735–6):
  → cycloserine (BNF, common; *Adv Psychiatr Treat* 2005;**11**:66)
  → ethambutol toxicity (n = 1, *Int J STD AIDS* 2007;**18**:287–8)
  → isoniazid (BNF, common; caution in psychosis; *Adv Psychiatr Treat* 2005;**11**:66; *Gen Hosp Psychiatry* 2007;**29**:85–6; n = 1, *Ann Pharmacother* 1998;**32**:889–91; n = 1, *Mil Med* 1996;**161**:707; n = 1, *Pediatr Emerg Care* 2002;**18**:25–7)
  → rifampicin (*Indian J Lepr* 1992;**64**:537–9)

Carbaryl (n = 1, *Am J Psychiatry* 1995;**152**:466–7)

Cephalosporins (*Aust NZ J Psychiatry* 2003;**37**: 627–8), e.g.:

→ cefuroxime (*Lancet* 1984;i:965)
→ cephalexin (n = 1, *Med J Aust* 1973;i:497)
→ cephalothin (*Drug Intell Clin Pharm* 1974;**8**: 71)

Ciclosporin (n = 1, *Lijec Vjesn* 2007;**129**:75–6)

Colistin (BNF, rare)

Co-trimoxazole (e.g. n = 1, *Pediatrics* 2005;**199**: 739–41; n = 1, *Pharmacopsychiatry* 2006;**39**: 236–7)

Dapsone (BNF, uncommon at low doses; *J Indian Med Assoc* 1989;**87**:120–1; *Indian J Pediatr* 1988;**55**:993–4; n = 1, *J Trop Med Hyg* 1993;**96**:274–6; *Br Med J* 1989;**299**:324)

Ethionamide (*Adv Psychiatr Treat* 2005;**11**:66)

Foscarnet (BNF, common; *Adv Psychiatr Treat* 2005;**11**:66)

Ganciclovir (BNF, less common; n = 1, *Pharmacother* 2000;**20**:479–83; *N Eng J Med* 1996;**335**:1397)

Gatifloxacin (*Am J Geriatr Psychiatry* 2003; **11**:470–1; n = 1, *J Am Geriatr Soc* 2006;**54**: 871; *Psychosomatics* 2007;**48**:87)

Ketoconazole (n = 1, idiosyncratic and v rare, *Am J Psychiatry* 1990;**147**:677)

Levamisole (*Ann Pharmacother* 1998;**32**:134–5)

Macrolides, e.g.:
  → clarithromycin (BNF, v rare; *Med J Malaysia* 2006;**61**:263; *Eur J Clin Microbiol Infect Dis* 1999;**18**:70–1; n = 1, *Psychiatr Bull* 2004;**28**: 98–9)
  → erythromycin (n = 2, *Arch Internal Med* 1986;**146**:897–9)
  → erythromycin + bromocriptine (n = 1, *Neurologia* 1997;**12**:429)
  → nalidixic acid (many cases, e.g. *Br Med J* 1965;**2**:590)

Mefloquine (n = 1, child, *J Child Neurol* 2009;**24**: 1008–9)

Mepacrine (BNF, rare, transient)

Metronidazole (BNF, v rare; *J Fam Pract* 1988;**27**: 323–5; n = 1, *Am J Psychiatry* 1997;**154**:1170–1)

Nitrofurantoin (*Adv Psychiatr Treat* 2005;**11**:66)

Penicillin (several cases, e.g. *Br J Psychiatry* 1990; **156**:554)

Primaquine (n = 1, *Ann Intern Med* 1980;**92**:435)

Quinacrine (e.g. n = 1, *Hum Psychopharmacol* 2002;**17**:357–9; n = 1, *J Fam Pract* 1991;**32**: 526–8)

Quinolones (*Adv Psychiatr Treat* 2005;**11**:66), e.g.:
  → ciprofloxacin (n = 1, *Ann Pharmacother* 1992;**26**: 930–1; n = 1, *Postgrad Med J*

1998;**74**:189–90; n = 1, *Eur Psychiatry* 2003;**18**:262–3; n = 1, *Psychosomatics* 2007;**48**:269; n = 1, *Arch Ophthalmol* 2002; **120**:665–6)

→ levofloxacin (rare but can be serious, SPC, n = 1, *Gen Hosp Psychiatry* 2008;**30**:381–3)

→ nalidixic acid (BNF, less common; injection n = 1, *J Forensic Sci* 1986;**31**:1145–9)

→ norfloxacin (*J Assoc Physicians India* 1994;**42**: 844)

→ ofloxacin (*Psychiatr Prax* 1996;**23**:251; n = 2, *Int J STD AIDS* 2003;**14**:636–7)

→ pefloxacin (n = 1, *Prog Neuropsychopharmacol Biol Psychiatry* 1996;**20**:343–7)

Sulfadiazine (n = 2, *Clin Infect Dis* 1992;**99**:556–7)

Tobramycin (a few cases, e.g. *Pediatr Pulmonol* 1988;**4**:201–4)

Trimethoprim (*Adv Psychiatr Treat* 2005;**11**:66)

Triple therapy for H Pylori (*J Am Board Fam Pract* 2002;**99**:66–8)

Valaciclovir (n = 1, *Psychosomatics* 2009;**50**: 293–6)

- **Endocrine system drugs** *

Adrenocorticotropin

Carbimazole

Clomifene (n = 1, *Hum Reprod* 1997;**12**:706–7; n = 2, *Am J Psychiatry* 1997; **154**:1169–70)

Corticosteroids (aggravation of schizophrenia, incidence may be as high as 5–6% in adults, usually emerges within a few days or weeks, risk may be higher with higher doses, *MHRA Drug Safety Update* 2007;1–9; review, *Gen Hosp Psychiatry* 2003;**25**:27–33; n = 6, *J Clin Psychiatry* 2000;**61**:261–7; review in *Drug Saf* 2000;**22**:111–22):

→ corticosteroid withdrawal (*J Pain Symptom Manage* 2007;**34**:118–9)

→ deflazacort (aggravation of symptoms, SPC)

→ dexamethasone withdrawal (*Lijec Vjesn* 1988;**110**:94–6)

→ prednisone (usually >40mg/d, e.g. *J Clin Psychiatry* 1982;**43**:75–6 inc. brief overview; case and discussion in *Br J Psychiatry* 1993;**162**:549–53; low dose n = 1, *Endocr J* 2006;**53**:255–8)

→ prednisolone + clarithromycin (n = 1, *Gen Hosp Psychiatry* 1998;**20**:325–6)

→ triamcinolone (SPC, dose–related; nasal spray n = 1, *Prog Neurol Psychiatry* 2007;**11**:31–2)

Desmopressin (n = 1, *Lancet* 1981;**2**:808)

Estrogen withdrawal (review, n = 26, *J Acta Psychiatr Scand* 2001;**104**:323)

Iodine, radioactive (n = 1, *Am J Psychiatry* 2009; **166**:1067–8)

Insulin abuse (*Br Med J* 1971;**4**:792–3)

Methyltestosterone (*Lancet* 1987;i:863)

Quinagolide (BNF, v rare)

- **Malignancy and immunosuppressant drugs** *

Ciclosporin (*Psychosomatics* 1993;**34**:101–2)

Gonadorelin (*Br J Psychiatry* 1999;**175**:290–1)

Ifosfamide (BNF, common; e.g. n = 1, *Farm Hosp* 2006;**30**:399–6; n = 1, *Psychooncology* 2007;**16**:956–60)

Interferons e.g.:

→ interferon alfa (e.g. n = 1, psychotic depression, *J Psychopharmacol* 2005;**19**: 102–5; n = 1, *Pharmacopsychiatry* 2007;**40**:146–8; n = 1, persistent, *J Clin Psychopharmacol* 2006;**26**:446–7)

→ peginterferon alfa 2b + ribavirin (n = 1, *Int Clin Psychopharmacol* 2005;**20**:289–90; n = 1, *Braz J Infect Dis* 2006;**10**:406–7)

Leuprorelin acetate (n = 1, *Nervenarzt* 2007;**78**: 691–5)

Tacrolimus (BNF, rare; n = 1, *Int J Neuropsychopharmacol* 2006;**9**:493–4)

- **Musculoskeletal and analgesics** *

Allopurinol (n = 1, causing relapse, *Schizophr Res* 2007;**93**:409)

Aspirin (*JAMA* 1965;**193**:555–8)

Baclofen (e.g. n = 1, *Ann Pharmacother* 2006; **40**:2071–3; psychotic depression, n = 1, *J Clin Psychiatry* 1992;**53**:211–2; intoxication, n = 18, *Przegl Lek* 2004;**61**:389–91)

Carisoprodol withdrawal (n = 1, *Ann Clin Psychiatry* 2008;**20**:173–4)

Chloroquine (BNF, rare)

Hydroxychloroquine (BNF, rare)

Indometacin (rare, e.g. cases within n = 32, *Can J Anaesth* 2003;**50**:586–8; n = 1, *Postgrad Med J* 2000;**76**:736–7)

Indometacin + ciprofloxacin (n = 1, *Rev Clin Esp* 1992;**191**:401)

Pyridostigmine (n = 1, *Deutsch Med Wschr* 1966; **9**:699)

Sulindac (*JAMA* 1980;**243**:1420)

- **Others** *

Atropine (oral, IV, eye drops, e.g. *DICP Ann*

Pharmacother 1990;**24**:708–9; n = 4
plus review, *Fortschr Neurol Psychiatr*
1998;**66**:289–95; *J Assoc Physicians India* 1990;
38:444–5)

Brimonidine eye drops (*Arch Ophthalmol* 2000;
118:1132–3)

Butane (n = 1, *Psychiatry Clin Neurosci* 2001;**55**:
163)

Colubrina — see Mabi bark

Cyanide (*Arch Environ Health* 1997;**52**:245–6)

Cyclobenzaprine (n = 1, *Can J Psychiatry* 2000;**45**:
763–4)

Cyclopentolate eye drops (e.g. n = 1, *J Cataract
Refract Surg* 2003;**29**:1026–30; n = 1, *Klin
Monatsbl Augenheilkd* 1989;**194**:458–61)

Distigmine bromide (n = 1, *Eur Psychiatry* 2003;
18:318–9)

Flumazenil (*Lancet* 1992;**339**:488–9)

Herbal preparations and supplements (n = 1, *Int
J Psychiatry Med* 2007;**37**:279–82; n = 1, *S D
Med* 2008;**61**:173–7)

Inhalants (n = 40, responds to carbamazepine,
Psychiatr Serv 1998;**49**:812–5)

Insect repellant (*Psychosomatics* 2001;**42**:78–80;
n = 1, after 2/52 topical application of DEET,
Am J Psychiatry 1987;**144**:1103–4)

Iohexol (n = 1, *Neuroradiology* 1994;**36**:141)

Isotretinoin (no evidence for increase in
psychosis or any other psychiatric disorder,
n = 21911, *Arch Dermatol* 2000;**136**:1231–6;
possible case, *J Clin Psychiatry* 1999; **60**:
407–8; n = 5, *Int Clin Psychopharmacol*
2005;**20**:39–41)

Ketamine (discussion, *Am J Psychiatry* 1997;**154**:
805–11)

Ketorolac (BNF, less common)

Lactate oral (e.g. in calcium lactate tablets, case
in *Ann Pharmacother* 1995;**29**:539–40)

Mabi bark tea (n = 1, *Br J Psychiatry* 1992;**161**:
404–7; hotly disputed, *Br J Psychiatry* 1993;
162:275)

Methazolamide (n = 1, *Pharmacotherapy* 1997;
17:387–9)

Metrizamide (n = 1, prolonged, *Psychosomatics*
1986;**27**:373–5)

Mouthwash containing alcohol (n = 1, *Mil Med*
2009;**174**:828–31)

Nitrous oxide abuse (n = 1, *J Med Toxicol* 2006;
2:71–4)

Nutmeg (*J R Soc Med* 1993;**86**:179–80; *Br J
Psychiatry* 1993;**162**:131)

Oral contraceptive, combined (n = 1, *Gynecol
Endocrinol* 2007;**23**:361–2)

Organic solvents (n = 2, *Nihon Arukoru Yakubutsu
Igakkai Zasshi* 2007;**42**:76–81)

Oxybutynin (n = 2, *Clin Drug Investig* 2006;**26**:
603–6)

Oxymetazoline nasal spray (*CMAJ* 1994;**150**:
375–6; several cases, e.g. *Scott Med J* 1982;
27:175–6)

Peyote plant (n = 1, *J Clin Psychiatry* 2004;**65**:
1433–4)

Phenylephrine (*JAMA* 1982;**247**:1859)

Pilocarpine (*Psychosomatics* 2005;**46**:88)

Procaine penicillin (n = 1, *Int J Dermatol* 1995;
34:627–9)

Salvia divinorum (n = 1, *Am J Psychiatry* 2009;
166:832)

Styrene exposure (n = 1, *J Clin Exp Neuropsychol*
1990;**12**:798–806)

Thallium poisoning (n = 1, *J Assoc Physicians India*
2006;**54**:53–5)

Timolol eye drops (n = 163 from National
Registry reports, *J Clin Psychopharmacol* 1987;
7:264–7)

Toluene (*Br J Psychiatry* 1991;**158**:578)

Trichloroethylene abuse (n = 1, *Arch Neurobiol
(Madr)* 1989;**52**:198–202)

Yohimbine (unproven, see *Arch Gen Psychiatry*
1998;**55**:1033–44)

5.13 SEROTONIN SYNDROME

Serotonin syndrome (SS) has been reported
with a variety of antidepressants, buspirone,
carbamazepine, pethidine, dextromethorphan
and levodopa, usually in combination but can
be monotherapy or in overdose. There was an
FDA alert on SS with SSRIs/SNRIs and triptans,
but other data suggests SS is rare and the
combination should not be prohibited (n = 29,
MedGenMed 2007;**9**:48). There were 7349
reported cases of SS and 93 deaths in USA in
2002 (Bush *et al*, *J Palliat Med* 2006;**9**:1257–9).
It is not idiopathic, but a predictable adverse
consequence of excess serotonergic agonism.

Reviews: * general (Dvir and Smallwood, *Gen
Hosp Psychiatry* 2008;**30**:284–7), misdiagnosis
(n = 7, Attar–Herzberg *et al*, *Isr Med Assoc J* 2009;
11:367–70).

- Monotherapy *

Amantadine (n = 1, *Am J Emerg Med* 2008; **26**:5–6)

Chlorphenamine? (*Singapore Med J* 2006;**47**: 1014)

Dexfenfluramine (n = 1, *JAMA* 1996;**276**:1220–1)

Duloxetine (n = 1, *Aust N Z J Psychiatry* 2009; **43**:581–2)

MDMA/ecstasy (*JAMA* 1993;**269**:869–70; review of risks; *Aust N Z J Psychiatry* 2007; **41**:649–55; see also *Pharmacol Biochem Behav* 2002;**71**:837–44)

Methadone (n=1, *J Palliat Med* 2006;**9**: 1257–9)

Mirtazapine (n = 1, *Ann Pharmacother* 2002;**36**: 641–3; n = 1, *Clin Neuropharmacol* 2003;**26**: 54–7)

Pethidine (n = 1, *Br J Anaesth* 2009;**103**:369–70)

SSRIs, e.g.:

→ citalopram (n = 1, *Kaohsiung J Med Sci* 2005;**21**:326–8; at low dose *J Clin Psychopharmacol* 2000;**20**:713–4; n = 1, after a first–time low dose, *Neurotoxicology* 2007;**28**:1272–4; n = 1, misdiagnosed as fibromyalgia, *Phys Ther* 2008;**88**:757–65)

→ fluoxetine (n = 1, *Psychiatr Pol* 1995;**29**:529–38; = 1, *Psychopharmacol Bull* 2008;**41**:76–9)

→ fluvoxamine (e.g. after single dose n = 1, *Ann Emerg Med* 1999; **34**:806–7; mild syndrome may occur in 43% on fluvoxamine alone, n = 37, *Int J Neurosci* 2001;**109**:165–72)

→ paroxetine (*Am J Emerg Med* 1995;**13**:606–7; at standard dose in 80-year-old, n = 1, *Am J Ther* 2006;**13**:550–2; delayed effect, n = 1, *Consult Pharm* 2009; **24**:64–8)

→ sertraline low dose (*J Clin Psychopharmacol* 2000;**20**:713–4; single 50 mg dose in nine-year-old, *Clin Toxicol (Phila)* 2008;**46**:845–9)

→ sertraline overdose (n = 1, *Arch Pediatr Adolesc Med* 1997;**151**:1064–7)

Sibutramine overdose (n = 1, child, *Clin Toxicol [Phila]* 2009;**47**:598–601)

Suanzaorentang (*J Clin Psychopharmacol* 2008; **28**:113–4)

Tandospirone (n = 1, *Rinsho Shinkeigaku* 2002; **42**:892–4)

Trazodone (*Int J Geriatr Psychiatry* 1997; **12**:129–30)

Tricyclics e.g.:

→ amitriptyline (n = 1, *Postgrad Med J* 2000;**76**: 254–6)

→ clomipramine (*J Clin Psychopharmacol* 1999;**19**:285–7; possible case after withdrawal of clozapine: *Ann Pharmacother* 2001;**35**:180–2)

→ dosulepin overdose (n = 1, *J Child Adolesc Psychopharmacol* 1998;**8**:201–4)

Venlafaxine (e.g. n = 1, *Postgrad Med J* 2000; **76**:254–6; n = 1, *Psychiatry Clin Neurosci* 2006;**60**:121–2; 37.5 mg/d, n = 1, *Ann Pharmacother* 2003;**37**:209–11)

- **Combinations, including SSRIs** *

Citalopram + buspirone (n = 1, *Int Clin Psychopharmacol* 1997;**12**:61–3)

Citalopram + fluconazole (n = 2, Levin *et al*, *Gen Hosp Psychiatry* 2008;**30**:372–7)

Citalopram/trazodone + linezolid (n = 1, *Ann Pharmacother* 2005;**39**:956–61)

Citalopram + linezolid (n = 1, *J Am Med Dir Assoc* 2004;**5**:111–3)

Citalopram + linezolid + mirtazapine (n = 1, *J Intensive Care Med* 2005;**20**:351–3)

Citalopram + methylene blue + (n = 1, *Med J Aust* 2008;**189**:534–5)

Citalopram + moclobemide (*Med Clin [Barc]* 1999;**113**:677–8)

Citalopram overdose + moclobemide (*Lancet* 1993;**342**:1419; fatal, n = 1, *Anaesthetist* 2006;**55**:1189–96; n = 1, fatal, *J Anal Toxicol* 2001;**25**:147–51)

Citalopram + pethidine (n = 1, *Psychosomatics* 2007;**48**:361–3)

Citalopram + quetiapine (n = 1, *N Z Med J* 2006;**119**:2058)

Citalopram + St John's wort (*Pharm J* 2007; **278**:487)

Citalopram + tramadol (n = 1, *Am J Psychiatry* 2004;**161**:1129)

Citalopram + trazodone + linezolid (n = 1, *Ann Pharmacother* 2005;**39**:956–61)

Dextromethorphan + SSRIs (evidence that supra-therapeutic dextromethorphan doses are needed with an SSRI to create SS (n = 2, *Clin Toxicol (Phila)* 2008;**46**:771–3)

Escitalopram + cyclobenzaprine (a tricyclic muscle-relaxant, n = 1, *Am J Emerg Med* 2008; **26**:1069)

Fluoxetine/moclobemide/clomipramine

overdose (fatal case in *Anaesth Intensive Care* 1995;**23**:499–502)

Fluoxetine + buspirone (*Ann Pharmacother* 2000;**34**:871–4)

Fluoxetine + carbamazepine (n = 1, *Lancet* 1993; **42**:442–3)

Fluoxetine + dextromethorphan (n = 1, *Gen Hosp Psychiatry* 2006;**28**:78–80)

Fluoxetine + hydromorphone (n = 1, *Prescrire Int* 2004;**13**:57)

Fluoxetine + olanzapine (n = 1, *World J Biol Psychiatry* 2004;**5**:114–5)

Fluoxetine + lithium (n = 1, *Ugeskrift for Laeger* 1995;**157**:1204–5)

Fluoxetine + mirtazapine (*Int J Geriatr Psychiatry* 1998;**13**:495–6; n = 1, *Ann Pharmacother* 2001;**35**:1217–20)

Fluoxetine + moclobemide (e.g. *Pharmaco-psychiatry* 1996;**29**:162; n = 1, *Can J Anaesth* 2000;**47**:246–50)

Fluoxetine + nefazodone (n = 1, *J Clin Psychiatry* 2000;**61**:146)

Fluoxetine + paroxetine (n = 1, *Am Fam Physician* 1995;**52**:1475–82)

Fluoxetine + Parstelin (n = 1, *Anaesthesia* 1991; **46**:507–8)

Fluoxetine + pethidine (n = 1, *Anesthesiology* 2003;**98**:9911–2)

Fluoxetine + sertraline (n = 1, *Clin Pharmacol Ther* 1993;**1**:84–8)

Fluoxetine + tramadol (n = 1, *J Royal Soc Med* 1999;**92**:474–5)

Fluoxetine + trazodone (*Biol Psychiatry* 1996; **39**:384–5)

Fluoxetine + venlafaxine (*Ann Pharmacother* 1998;**32**:432–6)

Fluvoxamine + oxycodone (n = 1, *Ann Pharmacother* 2006;**40**:155–7)

Paroxetine + lithium (n = 1, *Pharmaopsychiatry* 1997;**30**:106–7)

Paroxetine + methylene blue (n = 1, *Can J Anaesth* 2008;**55**:36–41)

Paroxetine + moclobemide (n = 1, fatal, *J Anal Toxicol* 1997;**21**:518–20; *J Accid Emerg Med* 1999;**16**:293–5)

Paroxetine + moclobemide + selegiline (all low dose, n = 1, *J Chin Med Assoc* 2009;**72**:446–9)

Paroxetine + nefazodone (n = 1, *Ann Emerg Med* 1997;**29**:113–9)

Paroxetine + OTC cold remedy (*Am J Emerg Med* 1994;**12**:642–4)

Paroxetine + risperidone (*J Clin Psycho-pharmacol* 2000;**20**:103–5)

Paroxetine + tramadol (n = 11, *Int Clin Psychopharmacol* 1997;**12**:181–2)

Paroxetine + trazodone (*Psychosomatics* 1995; **36**:159–60)

Sertraline + amitriptyline (*Ann Pharmacother* 1996;**30**:1499–500)

Sertraline + bupropion + venlafaxine (n = 1, *Clin Neuropharmacol* 2004; **27**:219–22)

Sertraline + buspirone + loxapine (n = 1, *Therapie* 1999;**54**:269–71)

Sertraline + clomipramine (n = 1, *J Med Assoc Thai* 2005;**88**:993–6)

Sertraline + dolasetron (n = 1, *J Psychopharmacol* 2002;**16**:191)

Sertraline + erythromycin (n = 1, *Pharmacotherapy* 1999;**19**:894–6)

Sertraline + linezolid (n = 1, *Clin Infect Dis* 2002;**34**:1651–2; n = 1, *Pharmacotherapy* 2006;**26**:269–76)

Sertraline + metoclopramide (n = 1, *Ann Pharmacother* 2002;**36**:67–71)

Sertraline + phenelzine (n = 1, *Ann Pharmacother* 1994;**28**:732–5)

Sertraline + risperidone + trazodone (n = 1, *CNS Spectr* 2007;**12**:396–8)

Sertraline + tramadol (n = 1, *Ann Pharmacother* 1997;**31**:175–7; n = 1, *Aust Pres* 2002;**25**:19; n = 1, *Clin Neuropharmacol* 2004;**27**:150–1)

Sertraline + tranylcypromine (n = 1, *Clin Pharm* 1993;**12**:222–5)

SSRIs + risperidone (n = 2 [one fatal], *Ann Pharmacother* 2003;**37**:388–91)

- **Combinations, including MAOIs/ moclobemide (see also above)** *

Moclobemide + clomipramine overdose (*Intensive Care Med* 1997;**23**:122–4; *J Toxicol Clin Toxicol* 1998;**36**:31–2)

Moclobemide + clomipramine (n = 1, *Br Med J* 1993;**306**:248)

Moclobemide + pethidine (possible case, *Med J Aust* 1995;**162**:554)

Moclobemide + venlafaxine overdose (n = 1, *Forensic Sci Int* 2009; [in press])

Phenelzine + clomipramine (n = 1, *Clin Pharmacol Therap* 1993;**53**:84–8)

Phenelzine + cyclobenzaprine (n = 1, *Anesth Analg* 2006;**103**:1466–8)

Phenelzine + dextromethorphan (n = 1, *Clin*

Pharmacol Therap 1993;**53**:84–8)

Phenelzine + quetiapine (n = 1, *CNS Spectr*
2007;**12**:396–8)

Tranylcypromine + modafinil? (n = 1, *Am J*
Psychiatry 2007;**164**:684),

Tranylcypromine + venlafaxine (cases in *Vet*
Hum Toxicol 1996;**38**:358–61; *Hum Exp*
Toxicol 1997;**16**:14–7)

- Other combinations (see also above) *

Buprenorphine + naloxone (Suboxone single
dose, n = 1, *Am J Emerg Med* 2008;**26**:840)

Clomipramine + olanzapine (n = 1, *Minerva*
Anestesiol 2008;**74**:41–5)

Dextromethorphan + chlorphenamine (n = 1,
Pediatr Emerg Care 2007;**23**:829–31)

Duloxetine + cyclobenzaprine (n = 1, *Anesth*
Analg 2006;**103**:1466–8)

Fentanyl + 5HT3 antagonist (n = 1,
Psychosomatics 2001;**42**:258–60)

Herbal detox cocktail (*Am J Emerg Med* 2004;
22:625–6)

Linezolid + duloxetine (n = 1, *J Clin*
Psychopharmacol 2006;**26**:681–3)

Linezolid (review of cases, *Pharmacotherapy*
2006;**26**:1784–93)

Linezolid (shortly after stopping paroxetine,
n = 1, *Clin Infect Dis* 2002;**34**:1651–2)

Linezolid + pethidine (n = 1, *Clin Infect Dis* 2008;
46:264–5)

Linezolid + tryptophan + metoclopramide
(n = 1, *Med Intensiva* 2009;**33**:360–1)

Methylene blue (when added to an
antidepressant, n = 1, *Neurocrit Care*
2009;**11**:88–93; paroxetine, n = 1, *J*
Psychopharmacol 2010;[in press])

Mirtazapine + tramadol + olanzapine (n = 1, *Am*
J Psychiatry 2002;**159**:672–3)

Nortriptyline + selegiline (n = 1, *J Neurol* 2000;
247:811)

St John's wort + buspirone (n = 1, *J Psycho-*
pharmacol 2002;**16**:401)

Tramadol + venlafaxine + mirtazapine (n = 1,
Ann Pharmacother 2004;**38**:411–3)

Tramadol abuse added to sertraline +
trazodone (n = 1, *Indian J Psychiatry* 2009;
51:68)

Trazodone + amitriptyline (n = 1, *Int Clin*
Psychopharmacol 1996;**11**:289–90)

Trazodone + nefazodone (n = 1, *Am J Psychiatry*
2000;**157**:1022)

Venlafaxine + amitriptyline (n = 1, *Postgrad Med J*
2000;**76**:254–6)

Venlafaxine + co–amoxiclav (n = 1, *J R Soc Med*
2003;**96**:233–4)

Venlafaxine + dexamfetamine (n = 1, *Med J Aust*
2002;**176**:240–1)

Venlafaxine + linezolid (n = 1, *J Antimicrob*
Chemother 2004;**54**:289–90; n = 1, *Ann*
Pharmacother 2005;**39**:956–61)

Venlafaxine + lithium + valproate (n = 1,
Therapie 2006;**61**:531–3)

Venlafaxine + maprotiline + reboxetine (n = 1,
Eur Psychiatry 2004;**19**:456–7)

Venlafaxine + metoclopramide (n = 1, *Ann*
Pharmacother 2002;**36**:67–71)

Venlafaxine + mirtazapine (n = 1, *World J Biol*
Psychiatry 2002;**3**:167)

Venlafaxine + selegiline (n = 1, *J Clin*
Psychopharmacol 1997;**17**:66–7)

Venlafaxine + sour date nut (n = 1, *Am J*
Psychiatry 2004;**161**:1129–30)

Venlafaxine + St John's wort? (*Presse Med* 2000;
29:1285–6)

Venlafaxine + trazodone (n = 1, *Am J Psychiatry*
2001;**158**:2088–9)

5.14 SLEEP PROBLEMS

5.14.1 SLEEP DISTURBANCES

Review of non-psychotropic causes: Novak and
Shapiro, *Drug Safety* 1997;**16**:133–49.

- CNS — anxiolytics and hypnotics

Lorazepam

Zolpidem (hypnagogic, on temporary
withdrawal, n = 1, *J Toxicol Clin Toxicol* 2003;
41:869–72)

- CNS — antipsychotics

Benperidol

Chlorpromazine

Clozapine abrupt withdrawal (n = 1, *Eur Arch*
Psychiatry Clin Neurosci 1996;**246**:79–82)

Fluspirilene

Olanzapine (somnambulism, n = 2, *Am J*
Psychiatry 2001;**158**:1158)

Risperidone (sleep-related eating disorder, n = 1,
J Clin Psychiatry 2004;**65**:273–4)

Sulpiride

- CNS — antidepressants *

Bupropion (incidence 11%)

Duloxetine (insomnia, BNF common)

MAOIs (hypersomnia, mainly tranylcypromine and phenelzine, *Am J Psychiatry* 1989; **146**:1078; n = 8, dose-related, *Am J Psychiatry* 1988;**145**:1552–6)

Mirtazapine (n = 1, *Br J Clin Pharmacol* 2009;**67**: 135–6)

SSRIs (all SSRIs can disrupt sleep architecture so are best taken in the morning, RCT, n = 14, *J Clin Psychiatry* 2001;**62**:642–52; somnambulism, n = 1, *J Pharm Tech* 1999; **15**:204–7):

→ fluoxetine

→ paroxetine (somnambulism, n = 1, *J Clin Psychiatry* 2003;**64**:483)

Trazodone

Tricyclics

● **CNS — analgesics**

Nefopam

● **CNS — anticonvulsants**

Lamotrigine (n = 109, incidence 6%, dose-related, *Epilepsia* 1999;**40**:322–5)

Levetiracetam (hypersomnia, n = 1, *Epilepsia* 2005;**46**:588–9)

Phenytoin

Rufinamide (insomnia, incidence 1–10%, UK SPC)

● **CNS — antiparkinsonian drugs** *

Amantadine (4% incidence, *J Clin Psychiatry* 1981;**42**:9; *Rev Neurol* 1997;**25**:2062)

Biperiden withdrawal (n = 2, *Int Clin Psychopharmacol* 2000;**15**:357–9)

Bromocriptine

Pramipexole (n = 6, *Mov Disord* 2000;**15**:658–63; n = 40, 52% incidence of somnolence, *Mov Disord* 2000;**99**:658–63)

Ropinirole and/or pramipexole (n = 2, *Pharmacother* 2000;**20**:724–6)

● **CNS — others** *

Anticholinesterases:

→ donepezil (n = 2, *J Am Geriatr Soc* 1998; **46**:119–20)

→ rivastigmine (incidence < 5%)

Ginseng (common, *Drugs Exp Clin Res* 1996; **22**:65–72)

Methylphenidate

Methysergide

Modafinil (UK SPC)

Nicotine (n = 252, *J Clin Psychiatry* 2001;**62**: 319–24)

Raltegravir (n = 2, *AIDS Patient Care STDS* 2009; **23**:689–90)

Sibutramine

Sodium oxybate (SPC)

● **Gastrointestinal drugs**

Bismuth toxicity (*Postgrad Med J* 1988;**64**: 308–10)

Propantheline

Ranitidine (see *Adv Psychiatr Treat* 1999;**5**:30–8)

Sulfasalazine

● **Cardiovascular drugs** *

Amiodarone (frequent, e.g. *Am J Cardiol* 1983; **52**:975–9)

Beta-blockers:

→ atenolol (very common, *Adv Psychiatr Treat* 1999;**5**:30–8)

→ carvedilol (n = 1, *Ann Pharmacother* 2002; **36**:1736–40)

→ propranolol (very common, *Adv Psychiatr Treat* 1999;**5**:30–8)

Calcium-channel blockers:

→ diltiazem (see *Adv Psychiatr Treat* 1999; **5**:30–8)

→ isradipine (up to 3%, *Am J Med* 1989; **86**[Suppl 4A]:98–102)

→ nifedipine (see *Adv Psychiatr Treat* 1999; **5**:30–8)

Clonidine for ADHD (*J Clin Psychopharmacol* 2008;**28**:725–6)

Digoxin (see *Adv Psychiatr Treat* 1999;**5**:30–8)

Statins (MHRA warning, *Drug Safety Update* 2008;**1**:10; *Drug Saf* 2008;**31**:1115–23), e.g.:

→ lovastatin (*Lancet* 1994;**343**:973)

● **Respiratory drugs** *

Aminophylline

Brompheniramine

Montelukast (FDA warning 2009)

Pseudoephedrine

Theophylline

Zafirlukast (FDA warning 2009)

● **Anti-infection drugs**

Cefalosporins (*Adv Psychiatr Treat* 2005;**11**:66)

Chloroquine (*Presse Med* 1991;**20**:659)

Cinoxacin

Ciprofloxacin (n = 1, *Lancet* 1986; **1**:819–22)

Efavirenz (dose-related, *J Acquir Immune Defic Syndr* 2001; **28**:399–400)

Fleroxacin (n = 2, *Int Clin Psychopharmacol* 1994; **9**:295–6)

Ganciclovir (*Adv Psychiatr Treat* 2005; **11**:66)

Griseofulvin (*Adv Psychiatr Treat* 2005; **11**:66)

Maraviroc (insomnia, common, UK SPC)

Nitrofurantoin (*Adv Psychiatr Treat* 2005; **11**:66)

Quinolones (*Adv Psychiatr Treat* 2005; **11**:66)

- **Endocrine system drugs**

Clomifene

Corticosteroids (incidence may be as high as 5–6% in adults, usually emerges within a few days or weeks, risk may be higher with higher doses, *MHRA Drug Safety Update* 2007; 1–9)
  → deflazacort (SPC)
  → triamcinolone

Tolazamide

- **Malignancy and immunosuppressant drugs**

Thalidomide cessation (n = 1, *Gastroenterology* 2001; **120**:1567–8)

Trabectedin (insomnia, common, UK SPC)

- **Musculoskeletal and analgesics**

Diclofenac

Diflunisal

Etodolac (insomnia, SPC)

Fenoprofen

Indometacin

Naproxen (*Eur J Rheumatol Inflamm* 1981; **4**:87–92)

Sulindac

- **Others**

Eculizumab (insomnia, uncommon, SPC)

Mercury poisoning (n = 99, *Arq Neuropsiquiatr* 2000; **58**:32–8)

Sarin toxicity (n = 161, *Percept Mot Skills* 2005; **100**:1121–6)

5.14.2 VIVID DREAMS AND NIGHTMARES *

Nightmares — a review noted that drugs affecting serotonin, noradrenaline and dopamine are clearly associated with reports of nightmares, and that immunological drugs and those affecting GABA, histamine and acetylcholine are also possible causative agents (Pagel and Helfter, *Hum Psychopharmacol* 2003; **18**:59–67).

Baclofen

Beta-blockers:
  → atenolol (*Clin Pharm Ther* 1979; **25**:8)
  → propranolol (*Adv Drug React Bull* 1983; **99**:364)

Clonidine (*Adv Drug React Bull* 1983; **99**:364)

Digoxin toxicity (*Ann Intern Med* 1980; **93**:639)

Famotidine (n = 1, *Pharmacother* 1998; **18**:404–7)

Galantamine (n = 1, nightmares, *J Am Geriatr Soc* 2009; **57**:565)

Indometacin (rare, n = 202, 2.5 years, incidence 0.5%, *Br Med J* 1965; **2**:1281–4)

Mirtazapine (SPC at < 1 in 10 000)

Nalbumetone (*Pharm J* 1990; **244**:764)

Nicotine patches (*Pharm J* 1992; **249**:384)

Pergolide (e.g. *Clin Neuropharmacol* 1986; **9**:160–4)

SSRI withdrawal

Verapamil (*NEJM* 1988; **318**:929–30)

Withdrawal from barbiturates, benzodiazepines, narcotics, etc

5.15 SUICIDAL IDEATION (SEE ALSO DEPRESSION) *

Although suicidal ideation is not the same as actual suicide, more suicidal ideation is associated with more suicide attempts and completions (1,404,470 reports on 832 drugs, Robertson and Allison, *PloS One* 2009; **4**:e7312). In men, suicide risk is strongly inversely related to BMI, but not height or physical activity (n = 1829, Mukamal et al, *Arch Intern Med* 2007; **167**:468–75), except in extreme obesity where attempted suicide increases (Dong et al, *Int J Obes (Lond)* 2006; **30**:388–90).

- **CNS — anxiolytics and hypnotics** *

Benzodiazepines (n = 1, *Br J Gen Pract* 2007; **57**: 407–9):
  → alprazolam (caution in SPC)
  → chlordiazepoxide (SPC)

Sodium oxybate (SPC; BNF less common)
Zaleplon (BNF caution)
Zolpidem (SPC)

- CNS — antipsychotics (including lithium)*

Antipsychotics can cause akathisia, with the risk of suicide (review, CNS Spectr 2007;**12**(9 Suppl 14):1–13).

Aripiprazole (BNF very rare, SPC now says that there is no increased risk of suicidality in bipolar disorder)

Flupentixol (SPC; BNF)

- CNS — antidepressants (including bupropion) *

Suicidal ideation has been reported for many decades with antidepressants. However, suicidal ideation is not necessarily the same as actual suicide or suicide attempt, e.g. up to 8.8% of 10–24-year-olds had considered or attempted suicide in 2002, whereas the actual rate was 0.0028%, suggesting a different phenomenon (Seemüller et al, Acta Psychiatr Scand 2009;**119**:166–7, reply by Castelpietra).

In profound depression, suicidal ideation may be related to increasing motivation, to short-term akathisia, misdiagnosis of bipolar depression in younger adults and many other factors (n = 1090, Zisook et al, J Affect Disord 2009;**117**:63–73). If depression improves, suicidal ideation reduces (n = 1693, Olfson and Marcus, J Clin Psychiatry 2008;**69**:425–32).

Risk factors for treatment-emergent suicidal ideation or worsening in adults (n = 1909, Zisook et al, J Affect Disord 2009;**117**:63–73):

- drug abuse
- severe depression
- melancholic features
- age.

A number of studies have now shown that the risk of suicidality with antidepressants is greater in younger people (e.g. s = 372, n = 99231, Stone et al, BMJ 2009;**339**:b2880). A WHO systematic review also concluded that the risk with SSRIs is increased in adolescents, reduced in adults and much reduced in older adults (s = 8, n > 200000, Barbui et al, CMAJ 2009;**180**:291–7). Finally, a major FDA analysis has shown:

Age	Suicidal behaviour	Suicidal ideation
<25	Increased (OR 2.3)	Increased (OR 1.6)
25–64	No significant change (OR 0.87)	Possibly reduced (OR 0.79)
>64	Decreased (OR 0.06)	Decreased (OR 0.37)

This increase in younger people may be because bipolar disorder is often (as yet) undiagnosed in younger people, and antidepressants may be harmful in bipolar by promoting a mixed state, particularly difficult in younger people. Reduction in antidepressant use from 2003 does not seem to have been associated with an increase or decrease in suicide behaviour in young people to 2005 (Wheeler et al, BMJ 2008;**336**:542–5).

In adolescents with SSRI-resistant depression (n=334, Brent et al, Am J Psychiatry 2009;**166**:418–26):

- median time to suicidal event was 3/52, predicted by high baseline suicidal ideation, family conflict, and drug and alcohol use
- median time to non-suicidal event was 2/52, predicted by previous history of non-suicidal self-injury
- venlafaxine associated with slightly higher rate of self-harm.

Duloxetine (SPC; BNF rare; case series, J Clin Psychopharmacol 2008;**28**:101–2; n = 2, Clin Pract Epidemol Ment Health 2008;**4**:18)

MAOIs:

→ isocarboxazid (SPC; BNF in susceptible persons)

→ phenelzine (SPC; BNF in susceptible persons)

Mirtazapine (SPC; BNF rare; associated with statistically significant lower suicidal risk than placebo; s = 15, RCT, d/b, p/c, World J Biol Psychiatry 2007;**26**:1–6)

Moclobemide (SPC)

SSRIs (no association with risk of suicide: Curr Problems 2000;**26**:11–2):

→ citalopram (SPC: may be genetic linkage; n = 1447, incidence 8.6%, Arch Gen Psychiatry 2007;**64**:689–97; n = 1915, incidence 6%, 14/12, *Am J Psychiatry* 2007; **164**:1530–8)

→ escitalopram (SPC; lower than with nortriptyline, n = 811, RCT, open, 12/52, *BMC Med* 2009;**7**:60)

→ fluoxetine (SPC; two Lilly analyses of the FDA databases on suicide show no increase in the risk of treatment-emergent suicide with use of fluoxetine for MDD [s = 18, n = 3751, Beasley *et al, J Clin Psychopharmacol* 2007;**27**:682–6], nor for non-MDD conditions [s = 53, n = 11448, d/b, p/c, *Psychol Med* 2007;**37**:1585–93], although older data suggested a possible problem [*Am J Psychiatry* 1990;**147**:1570–2; disproven in s = 17, n = 3065, d/b, *Br Med J* 1991;**303**:685–92])

→ fluvoxamine (n = 1, akathisia resulting in suicide attempt, *J Clin Psychiatry* 1999;**60**:869)

→ paroxetine (SPC, may be higher than formally reported, *BMC Psychiatry* 2006; **6**:55)

→ paroxetine withdrawal (n = 4, *J Psychopharmacol* 2008;**22**:330–2; overall incidence of definite suicidal behaviour with paroxetine is the same as placebo but is higher in adults < 30 years old (s = 57, n = 14911, p/c, *J Affect Disord* 2009;[in press])

→ sertraline (SPC, but a meta-analysis showed that the 0.04% incidence of suicides with sertraline [n = 4 from n = 10917] was similar to 0.03% with placebo [n = 3 from n = 9006], s = 126, n = 19923, d/b, p/c, *J Clin Psychiatry* 2009; **70**:674–83)

Reboxetine (SPC; BNF rare)
Trazodone (SPC)
Tricyclics:
  → clomipramine (SPC)
  → lofepramine (SPC)
  → nortriptyline (SPC)
  → trimipramine (SPC)
Tryptophan (SPC; BNF)
Venlafaxine (SPC; BNF very rare; has higher suicide rate than citalopram, fluoxetine and dosulepin but there may be confounding factors, e.g. use in more severe MDD might explain this; n = 219,088, *BMJ* 2007;**334**:242)

- **CNS — analgesics** *
Dihydrocodeine (SPC)
Paracetamol
Ziconotide (SPC, uncommon)

- **CNS — anticonvulsants** *
A meta-analysis has shown that 32.5% of all deaths of people with epilepsy are due to suicide and 13.5% of all registered suicides are committed by epileptics so suicide in epilepsy is disturbingly frequent (s = 30, n = 51216, Pompili *et al, Epilepsy Behav* 2006;**9**:641–8). AEDs are associated with a small increase in risk of suicidal thoughts and behaviour, sometimes as soon as one week after starting (BNF) and this must be taken seriously. However, consistent taking of anticonvulsants in Denmark is associated with substantial reduction in risk of SI, similar to lithium (n = 16645, Smith *et al, J Affect Disord* 2009;**117**:162–7).

Barbiturates (BNF uncommon)
Benzodiazepines, e.g.:
  → clobazam (SPC, especially in elderly or children)
  → clonazepam, diazepam, flurazepam, loprazolam, lorazepam, midazolam, nitrazepam, temazepam (SPC; BNF rare)
Carbamazepine (suicidality, FDA warning 2008)
Ethosuximide (SPC)
Felbamate (suicidality, FDA warning 2008)
Gabapentin (BNF, uncommon; suicidality, FDA warning 2008)
Lacosamide (SPC)
Lamotrigine (suicidality, FDA warning 2008)
Levetiracetam (suicidality, FDA warning 2008; SPC; BNF rare)
Oxcarbazepine (SPC, FDA warning 2008)
Phenytoin (SPC)
Pregabalin (suicidality, FDA warning 2008; reports, SPC addition)
Tiagabine (suicidality, FDA warning 2008; SPC)
Topiramate (SPC; BNF less common, FDA warning 2008)
Valproate (reports, SPC addition, FDA warning 2008)
Vigabatrin (BNF rare)
Zonisamide (SPC; BNF less common, FDA warning 2008)

- **CNS — antiparkinsonian drugs**
Levodopa (SPC; BNF very rare)

- CNS — others *

Acamprosate (mentioned SPC)

Alcohol (risk of suicide is primarily associated with the quantity of alcohol consumed per drinking day, but not with drinking frequency nor overall alcohol consumption; n = 47,654, *Soc Psychiatry Psychiatr Epidemiol* 2007;**42**:153–60)

Atomoxetine (SPC; BNF less common, n = 1, *J Paediatr Child Health* 2008;**44**:596–8)

Bupropion (SPC, rare)

Caffeine (in bipolars, high coffee consumption is significantly associated [OR 1.79] with suicidal acts; n = 352, *Bipolar Disorder* 2009; **11**:494–503)

Cannabis (young users may possibly be more at risk, n = 2033, *Acta Psychiatr Scand* 2008; **118**:395–403; n = 1, *Case Report Med* 2009; [in press])

Disulfiram (SPC)

Galantamine (SPC, very rare)

Memantine (association, SPC; BNF very rare)

Methylphenidate (SPC; BNF less common)

Modafinil (SPC; BNF rare)

Naltrexone (BNF rare)

Nicotine (high nicotine consumption is significantly associated [OR 2.42] with suicidal acts in bipolar people [n = 352, *Bipolar Disorder* 2009;**11**:494–503] and in adolescent females [OR 4.7, n = 508, *Compr Psychiatry* 2009;**50**:293–8])

Sibutramine (SPC)

Varenicline (SPC; BNF less common, no association, n = 80,660, *BMJ* 2009;**339**:b3805; n = 1, *Am J Psychiatry* 2008;**165**:774; n = 1, *J Anal Toxicol* 2009;**33**:118–20)

- Cardiovascular drugs

ACE inhibitors (a review has shown that there is no greater risk of suicidal ideation with ACE inhibitors, n = 58 529, *Br J Clin Pharmacol* 2001;**52**:313–8; n = 743, *Eur J Clin Pharmacol* 2007;**63**:591–6)

Beta-blockers (one review has shown that users of medium and high lipid–soluble beta–blockers may be associated with an increased risk of suicide, n = 58 529, *Br J Clin Pharmacol* 2001;**52**:313–8; but another sudy showed no increased risk; n = 743, *Eur J Clin Pharmacol* 2007;**63**:591–6)

Calcium-channel blockers (reviews have shown

no greater risk of suicidal ideation with calcium-channel blockers, n = 58 529, *Br J Clin Pharmacol* 2001;**52**:313–8; n = 743, *Eur J Clin Pharmacol* 2007;**63**:591–6; n = 153 458, *Br Med J* 2000;**320**:1251)

Omega-3 fatty acids (low plasma levels may be a risk factor for suicide or depression: *Am J Psychiatry* 2006;**163**:1100–2)

Statins — there is insufficient evidence that low cholesterol is associated with increased risk of suicidal ideation and might actually be lower (n = 2813, *Arch Intern Med* 2003;**163**:1926–32; see also n = 930, *J Clin Psychiatry* 2008;**69**:1920–7), but increased dietary intake may reduce impulsive and aggressive behaviours (*Pharmacopsychiatry* 2002;**35**:1–5). Other data had suggested a higher incidence of low cholesterol in parasuicide [n = 100, *Br J Psychiatry* 2000;**177**:77–83] and suicide [n = 783, *Acta Psych Scand* 2001;**104**:37–41]; but high risk of violent suicide with high cholesterol, n = 37 635, *Am J Psychiatry* 2000;**157**:648–50). Statins are implicated (MHRA warning, *Drug Safety Update* 2008;**1**:10), e.g.

  → atorvastatin (very low-density lipoprotein cholesterol levels are not associated with increased suicide, n = 10001, *Am J Cardiol* 2007;**100**:747–52)

  → simvastatin (*Curr Problems* 1992;33: n = 4, *Lancet* 1993;**341**:14)

- Respiratory drugs

Montelukast (FDA change 2009; SPC, rare; BNF very rare; but a review concluded there was no association, *Expert Opin Drug Saf* 2009;**8**:273–82)

- Anti-infection drugs

Antiretrovirals — multiple switching of agents is associated with higher distress and suicide than single or non-switchers in ART therapy (n = 779, *Int J STD AIDS* 2007;**18**:700–4):

  → disoproxil (SPC; BNF less common)

  → emtricitabine (SPC; BNF less common)

  → efavirenz (SPC; BNF less common; not associated with increased suicide risk, n = 355, 48/52, *Clin Infect Dis* 2006; **42**: 1790–9)

  → tenofovir (SPC; BNF less common)

Cycloserine (SPC, psychosis with suicidal

tendencies)

Levofloxacin (SPC, very rare)

Ofloxacin (SPC, very rare)

Mefloquine (SPC, rare; BNF rare; n = 1, *Presse Med* 2006;**35**:789–92)

Ribavirin (SPC; BNF oral, more common in children)

- **Endocrine system drugs**

Systemic corticosteroids (SPC; BNF especially high doses and during withdrawal):

→ beclomethasone (SPC, BNF as above)

→ cortisone (SPC, BNF as above)

→ deflazacort (SPC, BNF as above)

→ dexamethasone (SPC, BNF as above)

→ fludrocortisone (SPC, BNF as above)

→ hydrocortisone (SPC, BNF as above)

→ methylprednisolone (SPC, BNF as above)

→ prednisolone (SPC, BNF as above)

→ triamcinolone (SPC, BNF as above)

- **Malignancy and immunosuppressant drugs**

Aldesleukin (suicide, n = 1, *J Am Osteopath Assoc* 1993;**93**:799–800)

Interferons:

→ interferon alfa

→ interferon beta-1a and 1b

→ peginterferon alfa (SPC; BNF uncommon, contraindication for some in severe depression or suicidal ideation)

- **Others** *

Alitretinoin (SPC, very rare)

Baclofen (SPC)

Isotretinoin (SPC; BNF rare; review, *Int J Dermatol* 2006;**45**:789–99; review, *Psychol Rep* 2007;**100**:1312–4; incidence 1–11%, *Semin Cutan Med Surg* 2007;**26**:210–20; n = 30496, statistically significant association, *J Clin Psychiatry* 2008;**69**:526–32; n = 100, showed reduced depressive symptoms over 6/12, *Psychol Rep* 2006;**99**:897–906; and in 2006, the UK MHRA concluded that there is no firm evidence of an association between isotretinoin and suicidal ideation, although there are reported cases; n = 10, incidence 30% in bipolar patients, *J Affect Disord* 2009; [in press])

Zafirlukast (FDA warning 2009)

6 MANAGEMENT OF SIDE-EFFECTS

Without wishing to state the blindingly obvious, we know that all drugs have side-effects. These may range from being mild and transient to being intolerable or life-threatening. If switching or discontinuing the causative agent is not clinically possible (e.g. patient preference, clinical response), managing undesirable adverse effects may allow continued treatment, improve compliance and lead to better outcomes.

STANDARD STRATEGIES TO TRY FIRST INCLUDE:

- Drug — alter formulation (i.e. SR/MR, liquid, injection).

- Dose — adjust total daily dose (increasing rarely works, but a systematic and gradual decrease should be tried to determine the minimum effective dose).

- Dose — manipulate frequency and timings (e.g. split, or load to one particular time).

- Dose — consider drug holiday (e.g. omitting doses on particular days, although this is likely only to be helpful for some specific ADRs).

- Dose — consider slower dose escalation (including stopping and restarting more gently), particularly with buspirone, many tricyclics and SSRIs.

- Monitor plasma levels to optimise the dose if possible, e.g. tricyclic ADRs are clearly correlated with plasma levels (review for our Polish readers by Grzesiak et al, Psychiatr Pol 2003;**37**:825–37).

- Switch to a drug from a different chemical group.

- Discontinue completely.

- Discontinue any concurrent drugs that might be interacting.

- Wait for the side-effect to wear off, or at least to get more tolerable.

- Initiate adjunctive therapies (additional drugs, physical management strategies).

All of these routine strategies may be of some importance and relevance for each side-effect. This chapter comments on some of the above, along with additional strategies. Data in this area of therapy is notably sparse, and the author would be grateful for any additional ideas.

Disclaimers:
- Some drug doses are quoted as total daily doses but many will need to be given as divided doses.
- Drugs and strategies are not in any particular order within each section, and are in alphabetical order where possible.

Review:
Haddad, Dursun and Deakin (2005) *Adverse Syndromes and Psychiatric Drugs*. Oxford University Press, Oxford (ISBN 0-19-852748-9)

6.1 Anticholinergic and related side-effects

Anticholinergic, blurred vision

Antidepressants **Switch** to an antidepressant with less anticholinergic side-effects (see *2.1.2*).
Beware of glaucoma developing (see *3.6*).
Bethanechol 30–90 mg/d may be effective but often poorly tolerated.
Pilocarpine 1% drops QDS may restore pupilary responsiveness and have been used if desipramine-induced (Salah and Cameron, *Am J Psychiatry* 1996;**153**:579).

Anticholinergic, constipation

Antidepressants Ensure adequate fluid intake.
(usually tricyclics) Usually requires bran or a bulking or lubricating laxative, e.g. lactulose, docusate.
Bethanechol 30–90 mg/d may be effective but often poorly tolerated.

Clozapine * As for tricyclics, but it is important to take this seriously as it may lead on to potentially fatal paralytic ileus, with or without previous abdominal symptoms (there are over 30 cases of fatal clozapine-induced constipation, e.g. n = 2, Hibbard et al, *Psychosomatics* 2009;**50**:416–9; review, n = 102, Palmer et al, *J Clin Psychiatry* 2008;**69**:759–68).
Risk factors for clozapine-induced constipation:

* Recently starting clozapine
* High clozapine dose or plasma level
* Use of concomitant anticholinergics
* Intercurrent illness

Additional actions:

* Regular physical monitoring, especially during higher risk times
* Appropriate and timely use of laxatives
* Ensure adequate fluid intake
* Early referral before life-threatening pathological changes start

Once resolved, preventative measures (high-fibre diet, adequate fluid intake, stool softeners and exercise) must be used to allow clozapine to continue safely (n = 1, Pelizza et al, *Acta Biomed* 2007;**78**:144–8).

Anticholinergic, dry mouth (xerostomia)

General advice

* **Stimulate salivary flow** — sugarless gum and other confectionary (e.g. wine gums) stimulate salivary flow (avoid those with sugar as this can promote dental caries and weight gain).
* Artificial **saliva sprays** (most contain methylcellulose or glycerin, e.g. Glandosane® [Fresenius Kabi]).
* Ensure adequate **hydration**.
* **Distigmine** bromide, but this has its own notable adverse effects, e.g. digestive, urinary and dermatological (n = 25, open, Wolpert et al, *Fortschr Neurol Psychiatr Grenzgeb* 1980;**48**:224–33).
* **Pilocarpine** 10–30 mg/d, as 2–3 times a day, may resolve the problem within a day if caused by clozapine, olanzapine, benzatropine, tricyclics or mirtazapine, with no significant side-effects (naturalistic overview, Masters, *Am J Psychiatry* 2005;**162**:1023).

Review: dietary and dental advice to avoid dental consequences (Boyd et al, *Nutr Rev* 1997;**55**:362–8).

SSRIs **Switching** to fluvoxamine may be effective if paroxetine-induced (n = 1, Arima et al, *Ann Pharmacother* 2005;**39**:567–71).
Stop olanzapine, which may enhance the effect (n = 1, Hori et al, *Prog Neuropsychopharmacol Biol Psychiatry* 2006;**30**:758–60).

Tricyclics **Coffee** — chewing 15 g cappuccino coffee for five minutes may help (n = 10, open, Chodorowski, *Przegl Lek* 2002;**59**:392–3).
Pilocarpine (peripheral cholinergic) may not be effective but **bethanechol** has been used at 5–10 mg at night, or up to 60 mg/d sublingually to promote

salivation (titrate dose slowly upwards, may be poorly tolerated).
Yohimbine 4mg/d may be effective for 3–4 hours (Bagheri et al, Br J Clin Pharmacol 1994;**37**:93–6).

Anticholinergic, urinary retention

Tricyclics
Once other physical causes have been excluded, the best course of action is probably to discontinue and/or switch. It can be a medical emergency (Tueth, Am J Emerg Med 1994;**12**:212–6) so must be taken seriously.
Bethanechol 30–90mg/d may be effective, albeit poorly tolerated (Hermesh et al, Drug Intell Clin Pharm 1987;**21**:877–9).

Antipsychotics
Aripiprazole 10mg/d has been successful as an alternative antipsychotic for urinary retention caused by haloperidol, olanzapine and risperidone (n = 1, Sahoo, Isr J Psychiatry Relat Sci 2007;**44**:74–5).

Urinary hesitancy (see also anticholinergic effects)

Reboxetine
Doxazosin 1mg/d (n = 1, Szabadi, Br J Psychiatry 1998;**173**:441–2).
Tamsulosin 0.4mg/d may be rapidly successful (within 20 minutes) and well tolerated (n = 8 males, Kasper and Wolf, Eur Neuropsychopharmacol 2002;**12**:119–22; n = 1, Kasper, Psychopharmacol 2002;**159**:445–6).

Urinary incontinence

Venlafaxine
Sertraline, switch to (n = 1, Polimeni et al, Clin Neuropharmacol 2005;**28**:247–8).
Duloxetine might be an alternative if stress-related.

6.2 Blood disorders

Review: * Haematological toxicity from psychotropics and how to treat (Flanagan and Dunk, Hum Psychopharmacol 2008;**23**:27–41).

Bleeding

SSRIs
Discontinue, or switch to a non-SSRI may be the best option.
Stop any NSAIDs (inc. aspirin), prescribe a less gastrotoxic NSAID or co-prescribe gastroprotective drugs (Dalton et al, CNS Drugs 2006;**20**:143–51; Mort et al, Pharmacotherapy 2006;**26**:1307–13).
Vitamin C 500mg/d has been used (n = 1, Tielens, Am J Psychiatry 1997;**153**:883; Rasker, Ned Tijdschr Genneesk 1993;**137**:618).

Blood dyscrasias
Neutropenia, agranulocytosis

Clozapine *
'Red result' — immediate cessation mandatory
Even a major **dose reduction** is unlikely to help in the short-term.
***GCSF/filgrastim** may be effective and logical (e.g. n = 1, Schuld et al, Acta Psychiatr Scand 2000;**102**:153–5; Sperner-Unterweger et al, Br J Psychiatry 1998;**173**:82–4; n = 3, Lamberti et al, J Clin Psychiatry 1995;**56**:256–9), and may shorten the duration of hospitalisation (n = 11, Chengappa et al, Psychopharmacol Bull 1996;**32**:111–21). It can also be used long term (11–48/12, n = 3, Hagg et al, Int Clin Psychopharmacol 2003;**18**:173–4). Doses above 0.3mg/wk may be more successful, although any rechallenge still needs extreme care (n = 5, Joffe et al, Am J Psychiatry 2009;**166**:236).
'Amber result' — advice on management
Exclude any interacting or contributing drugs, e.g. carbamazepine (case reports, Imbarlina et al, Eur Psychiatry 2004;**19**:506–9; see Chapter 4.2.3), antibiotics, etc.
Take the blood sample in the afternoon: neutrophil levels have a diurnal variation and a transient and harmless neutropenia (not requiring discontinuation) may occur in the morning (morning pseudoneutropenia,

n = 1, Esposito et al, World J Biol Psychiatry 2003;**4**:192–4).

Exercising before a sample, **B12** and oral **folate** have also been used.

Lithium (n = 2, Papetti et al, Encephale 2004;**30**:578–82; n = 1, Brunoni et al, Prog Neuropsychopharmacol Biol Psychiatry 2008;**32**:2006–7) has been used to prevent a patient going red by reversing a low wbc, e.g. during an 'amber' phase or raising baseline wbc where a low count exists, allowing clozapine to start. Although lithium protects against neutropenia (e.g. Silverstone, J Clin Psychopharmacol 1998;**18**:86–8), it does not protect against neutropenia progressing to agranulocytosis (Paton and Esop, Psychiatr Bull 2005;**29**:186–8). Plasma levels of 0.4 mmol/l have been used.

After care and re-exposure:

In 53 patients rechallenged with clozapine after leucopenia or neutropenia, 38% had a further dyscrasia and, in most, it was more severe, longer-lasting and occurred more quickly (incidence peaks at 5.5 weeks), but 55% of these 53 were rechallenged successfully and remained in treatment (n = 53, Dunk et al, Br J Psychiatry 2006;**188**:255–63).

Reviews: * management (Esposito et al, Eur J Clin Pharmacol 2005;**60**:759–64), rechallenge (n = 1 and extensive review, Ghaznavi et al, Am J Psychiatry 2008;**165**:813–8).

Eosinophilia
Clozapine

Clozapine-induced eosinophilia has an incidence of 13%, and resolves in nearly all without intervention (n = 160, Chatterton, Aust N Z J Psychiatry 1997;**31**:874–6) and probably is not a predictor of neutropenia (n = 70, Ames et al, J Clin Psychiatry 1996;**57**:579–81), but monitor carefully anyway, especially in women (n = 118, > 3/52, Banov et al, J Clin Psychiatry 1993;**54**:466–9).

Switching to quetiapine can be a successful alternative (n = 1, Zipris et al, Isr J Psychiatry Relat Sci 2007;**44**:54–6).

6.3 Cardiac effects

Hypertension
Antipsychotics

Beta-blockers and other general strategies are often adequate, e.g. **propranolol** has been used if the hypertension is aripiprazole-induced (n = 1, Borras et al, Am J Psychiatry 2005;**162**:2392). **Pindolol** 5 mg BD has been used when clozapine-induced (where nifedipine was ineffective; n = 1, Shiwach, Clin Neuropharmacol 1998;**21**:139–40; see also review of 82 cases with clozapine; Henderson et al, J Clin Psychiatry 2004;**65**:686–9).

Clozapine

Hypertension is usually transient over the first month, so reduce the dose or rate of upward titration.

Antihypertensives may be necessary if persistent or severe (n = 82, retrospective chart, Henderson et al, J Clin Psychiatry 2004;**65**:686–9).

Review: management (Shiwach, Clin Neuropharmacol 1998;**21**:139–40).

MAOIs

For hypertensive crisis, refer to a specialist unit immediately for specialist care, e.g. using British Hypertension Society guidelines for malignant hypertension (see also Elliot, J Clin Hypertens [Greenwich] 2004;**6**:587–92).

Hypotension
MAOIs

Hypotension occurs in about 10% people on MAOIs (n = 61, Remnick et al, Prog Neuropsychopharmacol Biol Psychiatry 1989;**13**:497–504) and usually needs specialist medical care.

Metoclopramide (Patterson, J Clin Psychopharmacol 1987;**7**:112–3).

Plasma expansion, e.g. salt tablets or fludrocortisone (review by Cockhill and Remick, *Can J Psychiatry* 1987;**32**:803–8).

Postural (orthostatic) hypotension
General strategies:
- Self-care (e.g. if lying down, dangle legs for a minute before rising slowly and attempting to stand).
- Use support stockings.
- Slower dose titration.
- Plasma volume expansion, e.g. fluid and increased sodium chloride intake.
- Desmopressin, indomethacin and erythropoietin can be used in extreme cases.
- Midodrine, an alpha-adrenergic agonist, is licensed and available in some countries (review by McClellan *et al*, *Drugs Aging* 1998;**12**:76–86), e.g. for tricyclics (n = 1, Maskall and Lam, *J Psychiatry Neurosci* 1993;**18**:276–7).

Review: general (Freeman, *Semin Neurol* 2003;**23**:435–42).

Additional strategies:

Tricyclics	**Fludrocortisone** has been used but obviously has long-term side-effects (Chobanian *et al*, *N Engl J Med* 1979;**301**:68–73).
	Yohimbine 12 mg/d (n = 12, d/b, c/o, p/c, Lacomblez *et al*, *Clin Pharmacol Ther* 1989;**45**:241–51).
MAOIs	**Brewed coffee** (Pollack and Rosenbaum, *J Clin Psychiatry* 1987;**48**:3–8).
	Fludrocortisone (Simonson, *Am J Psychiatry* 1964;**120**:1118–9).
	Levothyroxine or liothyronine has been suggested (see review, Whybrow and Prange, *Arch Gen Psychiatry* 1981;**38**:106–13).
	Methylphenidate 10–15 mg (case series, Feighner *et al*, *J Clin Psychiatry* 1985;**46**:206–9; mentioned in Pollack and Rosenbaum, *J Clin Psychiatry* 1987;**48**:3–8), but beware of ADRs.
	Salt tablets 600–1800 mg BD (n = 1, Munjack, *J Clin Psychiatry* 1984;**45**:89–90; mentioned in Pollack and Rosenbaum, *J Clin Psychiatry* 1987;**48**:3–8).
	Review: general (Cockhill and Remick, *Can J Psychiatry* 1987;**32**:803–8).
Antipsychotics	The effect is probably alpha-adrenergic-related so slower dose titration and lower doses are logical. Tolerance usually develops.
Clozapine	**Bovril and moclobemide** has been used for severe clozapine-induced postural hypotension (n = 1, Taylor *et al*, *Br J Psychiatry* 1995;**167**:409–10).
	Fludrocortisone (n = 1, Testani, *J Clin Psychiatry* 1994;**55**:497–8).

QTc prolongation
General strategies (see *Chapter 3.2* for risk factors and short review)
- **Switching** drugs is usually essential. If not possible, use the lowest doses in simple drug regimens.
- Avoiding metabolic interactions minimises the impact.
- **Magnesium** ion (Mg^{++}) orally at a mean dose of magnesium oxide 15 mg/kg/d shortens QTc, and can be given long term with appropriate monitoring. **Magnesium** sulphate by IV injection has been used and recommended by the American Heart Association (n = 24, Bachman, *J Clin Psychiatry* 2003;**64**:733–4).
- **Beta-blockers** are often ineffective (mentioned by Bachman, *J Clin Psychiatry* 2003;**64**:733–4).

Reviews: antipsychotics and QTc prolongation (Vieweg, *Prim Care Companion J Clin Psychiatry* 2003; **5**:205–15; Taylor, *Acta Psychiatr Scand* 2003;**107**:85–95; Zareba and Lin, *Psychiatr Q* 2003;**74**:291–306).

Tachycardia

Antipsychotics *	Amisulpride may be slightly safer than olanzapine for tachycardia (n = 33, Wang *et al*, *Neuropsychobiology* 2008;**57**:200–5).
Clozapine *	Tachycardia is common (up to 67%) early in treatment, but usually resolves over 4–6 weeks (n = 100, Marinkovic *et al*, *Prog Neuropsychopharmacol Biol Psychiatry* 1994;**18**:537–44). However, it may be the first, or only, presenting symptom of (often fatal) cardiomyopathy (e.g. n = 26, Hagg *et al*, *J Clin*

Psychopharmacol 2001;**21**:382–8), and so this must be fully excluded first. If the tachycardia is persistent and/or associated with chest pain, this may also indicate myocarditis (review of n = 26 where it was fatal in 46% of cases, Hagg *et al*, *J Clin Psychopharmacol* 2001;**21**:382–8). Myocarditis is most common (80%) in the first month (n = 25, Hill and Harrison-Woolrych, *N Z Med J* 2008;**121**:68–75), but can occur at any time, e.g. even after six years therapy (n = 1, Tanner and Culling, *Postgrad Med J* 2003;**79**:312–3) where discontinuation would be essential.

Slower dose escalation may help.

Manage nicotine and caffeine intake.

Discontinuation usually results in rapid resolution (e.g. n = 1, Stampfer and Swanepoel, *Australas Psychiatry* 2005;**13**:80–2).

Beta-blockers may help if the tachycardia is anticholinergic/noradrenergic-related, although the literature on this is minimal. Metoprolol is often used first-line as it has a short half-life, and can be converted to atenolol. A young male with hypokinetic cardiomyopathy, who needed to continue clozapine, had the cardiac effects managed successfully over five years with carvedilol and captopril (n = 1, Rostagno *et al*, *Gen Hosp Psychiatry* 2008;**30**:280–3).

6.4 Central adverse effects

Abnormal dreams and nightmares

Antidepressants	**Alter time** of the dose from night to morning if appropriate.
	Discontinue or switch drugs may be the only option.
	Discontinue tramadol (n = 1, Devulder *et al*, *Acta Clin Belg* 1996;**51**:184–6) and possibly other similar drugs that may exacerbate the effect.

Anorexia

Valproate	Could be a sign of impending hepatic failure. Investigate immediately and discontinue if necessary.

Ataxia

Lithium	This is usually a sign of lithium toxicity and neurotoxicity, and requires immediate action, e.g. discontinuation or dose reduction. If acute, dialysis may be needed. Consider also the global clinical picture, as ataxia may occur with 'normal' therapeutic lithium plasma levels.
	Discontinue any exacerbating drugs, e.g. clozapine (Lee and Yang, *Zhonghua Yi Xue Za Zhi [Taipei]* 1999;**62**:184–7).
	Buspirone (high-dose) has been used for ataxia due to lithium toxicity (n = 1, Megna and O'Dell, *Arch Phys Med Rehabil* 2001;**82**:1145–8).

Delirium *

- Discontinue any causative agent (see 5.4).
- There is very limited evidence (no p/c studies) for the use of antipsychotics to treat delirium (s = 14, Seitz *et al*, *J Clin Psychiatry* 2007;**68**:11–21; atypicals for delirium, Peritogiannis *et al*, *Psychiatry Clin Neurosci* 2009;**63**:623–31).

Review: * systematic review (Campbell *et al*, *J Gen Intern Med* 2009;**24**:848–53).

Antidepressants	**Donepezil** may help if tricyclic overdose-induced (rapidly effective in n = 1, Noyan *et al*, *Prog Neuropsychopharmacol Biol Psychiatry* 2003;**27**:885–7).
Antipsychotics	**Reduce** any concurrent anticholinergics.
	Switch to an antipsychotic with low anticholinergic effects (*Table 2.1.4*) or discontinue if no clear indication. **Quetiapine** has been used if risperidone-induced (n = 1, Kato *et al*, *Psychosomatics* 2005;**46**:374–5) and **haloperidol** used if clozapine-induced (Spisla and Bunter, *Psychiatr Prax* 1997;**24**:308).

Reduce dose, e.g. clozapine-induced delirium appears to be dose-related (n = 139, Centorrino et al, *Pharmacopsychiatry* 2003;**36**:156–60).

Propofol has been used successfully for post-ictal delirium with clozapine-ECT therapy (n = 1, Sienaert et al, *J ECT* 2004;**20**:254–7).

Depression
Tetrabenazine   Discontinue, or use antidepressants.

Reboxetine (n = 1, Schreiber et al, *J Neurol Neurosurg Psychiatry* 1999;**67**:550)

Drowsiness or sedation (see also fatigue)
Antipsychotics *   Wait, as tolerance often partly develops.

Adjust dose, e.g. lower dose, bias full dose to night or early evening or spread out throughout the day.

Avoid other concurrent CNS depressants.

Methylphenidate 20–40 mg/d has been used if clozapine-induced (with great care; Miller, *Am J Psychiatry* 1996;**153**:1231–2).

*Modafinil 200 mg/d has been used if sedation is induced by clozapine (n = 3, Makela et al, *J Clin Psychiatry* 2003;**64**:485–6), risperidone or olanzapine, with no exacerbation of psychosis. However, a pilot study was unable to show a significant effect from modafinil for clozapine-induced sedation (n = 35, d/b, p/c, 8/52, Freudenreich et al, *J Clin Psychiatry* 2009;**70**:1674-80) and a critical review concludes that the evidence is fairly poor but it may work (s = 6, Saavedra-Velez et al, *J Clin Psychiatry* 2009;**70**:104–12).

Levetiracetam   Can be minimised by starting at a lower dose.

MAOIs *   For phenelzine-induced daytime somnolence, triazolam (or presumably another short-acting hypnotic) can help sleep and reduced daytime somnolence (n = 3, Gray, *Am J Psychiatry* 1989;**146**:1078).

Mirtazapine   Start at higher dose: 30 mg/d may produce less drowsiness than 15 mg/d (mirtazapine is a highly potent H1 receptor blocker, and at 30 mg/d the noradrenergic enhancement may counteract some of the histamine blockade).

SSRIs   Modafinil, used adjunctively to SSRIs at the start of treatment, may enhance the onset of action in people with MDD and fatigue (n = 29, open, 6/52, Ninan et al, *J Clin Psychiatry* 2004;**65**:414–20, MS; n = 16, 3/52, open, Schwartz et al, *J Clin Psychiatry* 2004;**65**:1223–7).

Topiramate   Modafinil (Berigan, *Prim Care Companion J Clin Psychiatry* 2002;**4**:249–50).

Valproate   Investigate immediately and discontinue if necessary. May be indicative of impending hepatic failure or encephalopathy.

Modafinil (Berigan, *Can J Psychiatry* 2004;**49**:72–3).

Dysphoria
Antipsychotics   Procyclidine may be effective (n = 51, King et al, *Br J Psychiatry* 1995;**167**:480–2).

Review: Voruganti and Awad, *Can J Psychiatry* 2004;**49**:285–9.

Fatigue (see also drowsiness or sedation)
Antipsychotics   Adjust dose or spread the doses out throughout the day.

Modafinil has limited efficacy. A small study failed to show any differences vs placebo on fatigue, attention, working memory and executive functioning (n = 24 [c = 20], 8/52, d/b, p/c, Sevy et al, *J Clin Psychiatry* 2005;**66**:839–43), although a smaller study showed it may be effective in some people (n = 11, open, 4/52, Rosenthal and Bryant, *Clin Neuropharmacol* 2004;**27**:38–43).

Topiramate   Modafinil (Berigan, *Prim Care Companion J Clin Psychiatry* 2002;**4**:249–50).

Hypomania
Antidepressants   Mania from antidepressants is restricted to people with bipolar disorder

(review by Chun and Dunner, *Bipolar Disord* 2004;**6**:32–42). Beware of inducing rapid-cycling with antidepressants, which may be more prevalent in people given multiple antidepressant trials (see C5).

Discontinuation is the absolute priority, with short-term management of the manic episode.

May be dose-related with SSRIs (n = 1, Ramasubbu, *Acta Psychiatr Scand* 2001;**104**:236–8), but may only be transient with trazodone (n = 3, Jabeen and Fisher, *Br J Psychiatry* 1991;**158**:275–8).

Switch antidepressants once resolved; venlafaxine appears to have the highest risk of inducing mania, sertraline has an intermediate risk and bupropion the lowest (n = 159, RCT, 10/52, Leverich *et al*, *Am J Psychiatry* 2006;**163**:232–9).

Adjunctive mood stabilisers, e.g. lithium, may be protective.

Review: Goldberg and Truman, *Bipolar Disord* 2003;**5**:407–20.

Insomnia

Antidepressants * (SSRIs, bupropion, venlafaxine)	**Standard hypnotic therapy** (time-limited) may be adequate, e.g. zolpidem 5–10 mg/d if SSRI-induced (n = 190, RCT, d/b, 5/52, Asnis *et al*, *J Clin Psychiatry* 1999;**60**:668–76). * **Adjust time of doses**, e.g. prefer morning doses, as all (esp. SSRIs) can disrupt sleep architecture. **Quetiapine** 50 mg/d was effective for phenelzine-induced insomnia non-responsive to BDZs, Zs and antihistamines (n = 1, Sokolski and Brown, *Ann Pharmacother* 2006;**40**:567–70). **Trazodone** 50–75 mg may be effective in patients on MAOIs (e.g. n = 21, open, Jacobsen, *J Clin Psychiatry* 1990;**51**:298–302). It was also highly effective at 100 mg at night for insomnia induced by SSRIs (n = 12, d/b, p/c, c/o, 2×7/7, Kaynak *et al*, *Sleep Med* 2004;**5**:15–20), bupropion (67% improved, n = 17, RCT, p/c, d/b, c/o, Nierenberg *et al*, *Am J Psychiatry* 1994;**151**:1069–72) and venlafaxine (especially in people with increased inner tension; n = 50 [c = 42], open, 4/52, Bertschy *et al*, *Pharmacol Res* 2005;**51**:79–84).
Antidepressants * (MAOIs)	**Adjust time of doses**, e.g. take last dose of the day in the evening rather than (MAOIs) late at night. For MAOIs, the last dose should be before 3.00 PM. **Switch** to isocarboxazid. **Hypnotics** may help sleep but have no effect on daytime somnolence (n = 8, Teicher *et al*, *Am J Psychiatry* 1988;**145**:1552–6).
Aripiprazole *	Add a hypnotic agent during the first days of treatment, administer in the morning or divide the dose of aripiprazole into two daily half doses (AM and PM — review, Cassano *et al*, *Clin Drug Invest* 2007;**27**:1–13; Aitchison *et al*, *J Psychopharmacol* 2009;**23**:231–40).
Lamotrigine	Insomnia is probably dose-related so reduce dose, switch (n = 109, Sadler, *Epilepsia* 1999;**40**:322–5) or use hypnotics.
Methylphenidate	**Mirtazapine** can be used (chart review, Adler *et al*, *Curr Psychiatry Rep* 2006;**8**:409–15).

Irritability, jitteriness or agitation

SSRIs	**Slower dose titration** (or restarting more slowly) usually helps. **Valproate** has been used for fluoxetine-induced irritability in autism (Anagnostou *et al*, *J Clin Psychopharmacol* 2006;**26**:444–6).
Tricyclics	**Slower dose titration** (or restarting more slowly) usually helps. **Iron supplements** to resolve any low serum iron (Yeragani *et al*, *Neuropsychobiology* 1992;**25**:8–10).

Aripiprazole *	Perphenazine was used twice (n = 2, Pohl et al, J Clin Psychiatry 1986;**47**:427). Agitation is common when switching to aripiprazole and must be managed. Benzodiazepines (esp. lorazepam) during switch-over period (Aitchison et al, J Psychopharmacol 2009;**23**:231–40). Anticholinergic drugs. Antihistaminic drugs (e.g. diphenhydramine; Aitchison et al, J Psychopharmacol 2009;**23**:231–40). Valproic acid. Gabapentin. **Review:** Cassano et al, Clin Drug Invest 2007;**27**:1–13.

Nausea

Antidepressants	**Slower dose increases** help initially. See Table 2.1.2 for advice on anti-depressants with a lower incidence of nausea. Short-term antinauseants may have a role. **Cisapride** has been used (n = 6, Russell, J Clin Psychopharmacol 1996;**16**:35–7), so presumably similar antiemetics may be effective. **Slow-release** tablets/capsules reduce the peak plasma level effect, as would splitting doses throughout the day. **Gorei-san** (TJ-17), a Japanese herbal medicine may help if SSRI-induced (n = 3, open, Yamada et al, Psychiatr Clin Neurosci 1999;**53**:681). **Mirtazapine** may help if the nausea is SSRI-induced (Pedersen and Klysner, Int Clin Psychopharmacol 1997;**12**:59–60) and 15 mg at night may be effective within four days (n = 1, Caldis and Gair, Can J Psychiatry 2004;**49**:707; n = 3, Pedersen et al, Int Clin Psychopharmacol 1997;**12**:59–60). **Milnacipran and olanzapine** have been used for severe antidepressant-induced nausea (n = 1, Yoshida et al, Pharmacopsychiatry 2007;**40**:84–5).
Antipsychotics	**Antiemetics**, e.g. ondansetron may be effective but **avoid** metoclopramide or prochlorperazine for the first 1–2 months, or if there is a history of EPSE. **Prochlorperazine** has been effective for quetiapine-withdrawal nausea, where ondansetron had failed (n = 1, Kim and Staab, Am J Psychiatry 2005;**162**:1020), but see warning above.
Aripiprazole *	Nausea is usually transient so administer aripiprazole with or after food, reduce the dose or add an antiemetic if other measures fail (review, Cassano et al, Clin Drug Invest 2007;**27**:1–13), e.g. domperidone (Aitchison et al, J Psychopharmacol 2009;**23**:231–40)

Nocturnal enuresis (see also urinary incontinence)

Clozapine	**Avoid or reduce fluids** at night or after 6.00 PM, have planned night awakenings, enuresis alarms, and voiding before going to bed. **Adjust dose** and bias towards morning if possible. **Desmopressin** can be used intranasally at 10 mcg in each nostril at bedtime (n = 1, Aronowitz et al, Am J Psychiatry 1995;**152**:472; Steingard, J Clin Psychiatry 1994;**55**:315–6), although hyponatraemia can occur (n = 1, Sarma et al, Aust N Z J Psychiatry 2005;**39**:949). **Oxybutinin** (mentioned in Lurie and Hosmer, J Clin Psychiatry 1997;**58**:404). **Tolterodine** (there is one case where it did **not** work, whereas desmopressin did: n = 1, English et al, Ann Pharmacother 2001;**35**:867–9). **Trihexyphenidyl** 5 mg/d at bedtime (n = 2, Poyurovsky et al, Int Clin Psychopharmacol 1996;**11**:61–3).

Obsessive-compulsive symptoms

Antipsychotics *	**Standard treatments** may be adequate, e.g. **fluoxetine** if quetiapine-induced (n = 1, Ozer et al, Prog Neuropsychopharmacol Biol Psychiatry 2006;**30**:724–7).

Valproate has been used for augmentation in clozapine-induced OCD (n = 1, Zink et al, *Pharmacopsychiatry* 2007;**40**:202–3).
Aripiprazole 20 mg/d adjunctively has been effective for clozapine-induced OCD (n = 7, Englisch et al, *Clin Neuropharmacol* 2009;**32**:227–9)
Reduced dose — clozapine-induced OCD symptoms may be related to high clozapine/norclozapine plasma levels, so try reducing the dose or measuring plasma levels (n = 39, Lin et al, *Ther Drug Monit* 2006;**28**:303–7).

Benzodiazepines * Pregabalin has been successful if BDZ-induced (Oulis et al, *Prog Neuropsychopharmacol Biol Psychiatry* 2008;**32**:2000–1).

Panic

SSRIs Discontinue if panic symptoms are citalopram-induced (n = 1, Brauer et al, *South Med J* 2002;**95**:1088–9).

Sedation (see drowsiness)

Seizures

Clozapine * Clozapine-induced seizures are usually dose-related, so reduce the dose or rate of increase, or stop and restart if seizures occur. The incidence rises markedly above 600 mg/d.

Discontinue any other drugs likely to reduce the seizure threshold.
Carry out an **EEG** to test for ictal activity, as abnormal EEGs are not uncommon with clozapine or olanzapine (n = 323, Centorrino et al, *Am J Psychiatry* 2002;**159**:109–15).

* **Valproate** is standard management (case of successful concurrent valproate at low-dose clozapine 125 mg/d; n = 1, Foster and Olajide, *J Psychopharmacol* 2005;**19**:93–6), but the literature is remarkably sparce on this. It may be underused as only 24% patients on clozapine at risk of seizures may receive prophylactic valproate (n = 81, Sparshatt et al, *Psychiatric Bull* 2008;**32**:262–5).
Other anticonvulsants include gabapentin (up to 2100 mg/d, n = 1, Usiskin et al, *Am J Psychiatry* 2000;**157**:482–3; Landry, *Am J Psychiatry* 2001;**158**:1930–1) and **topiramate** (Navarro et al, *Am J Psychiatry* 2001;**158**:968–9).
Review: * management (Wong et al, *Can J Psychiatry* 2007;**52**:457–63).

6.5 Dermatological effects

Lithium is a major cause of cutaneous reactions, often characterised by pathological findings of neutrophilic infiltration (can cause or make worse). The general advice with lithium is:

- Check personal and family history of skin diseases before prescribing; the incidence is also higher in males (n = 108, Chan et al, *J Affect Disord* 2000;**57**:107–13; review by Yeung and Chan, *Am J Clin Dermatol* 2004;**5**:3–8).
- Mild or moderate dermatoses — use specific or systemic therapy.
- Severe or persistent dermatoses — use specific or systemic therapy; try dose reduction or discontinuation or rechallenge at lower dose.
- Most reactions seem to be dose-related, usually not too serious and may resolve on continuation, so dose reduction and discontinuation (if dose reduction does not help) are options.
- Exclude other factors, e.g. infections, other medication changes.

Review: cutaneous reactions from lithium (Yeung and Chan, *Am J Clin Dermatol* 2004;**5**:3–8)

Acne

Lithium **Systemic antibiotics** (avoid tetracycline because of interaction, see Malt, *Br Med J* 1978;**2**:502)
Topical retinoids (tretinoin; Remmer and Falk, *J Clin Psychiatry* 1986;**47**:48).
Reduce dose or discontinue.
Wait (may spontaneously resolve even with continued treatment, n = 2,

Kusumi, *Dis Nerv Sys* 1971;**32**:853–4).

Alopecia

- Check trace minerals, as low plasma levels of copper and zinc may predispose to hair loss, so oral supplementation may be effective (Ftemi and Calabrese, *Ann Pharmacother* 1995;**29**:1302;Tasaki et al, *J Dermatol* 1993;**20**:21–4).
- Other standard management includes hair care techniques and minoxidil.

Review: McKinney et al, *Ann Clin Psychiatry* 1996;**8**:183–5.

Carbamazepine	May occur in 6% and resolve after withdrawal, but can take several months.
Lithium	May occur in 12–19% patients (Mercke et al, *Ann Clin Psychiatry* 2000;**12**:35-42), either de novo or exacerbated. May occur in the first 6/12 treatments, and is more common in women.
	Alopecia may resolve with continued treatment (Ghadirian et al, *J Clin Psychiatry* 1986;**47**:212–3) or withdrawal (but might take several months).
	Exclude hypothyroidism as a causative factor (9%, Mortimer and Dawber, *Int J Dermatol* 1984;**23**:603–4) and other causes, e.g. stress, other drugs.
SSRIs	Occurs more in women and there may be an association with sertraline so switch if appropriate, e.g. to paroxetine or trazodone (may help if sertraline-induced; n = 1, Gautam, *Ann Pharmacother* 1999;**33**:631–7).
	Review: Hedenmalm et al, *Pharmacoepidemiol Drug Safety* 2006;**15**:719–25.
Valproate *	The incidence is 5–6% (range 2.6–15%). It is usually transient and slight and often resolves without alteration of dose, although may take 6/12 to regrow.
	* **Dose reduction** may help as alopecia is considered to be dose-dependent (28% incidence at high dose, 5% at low dose) so dose reduction may help (Mercke et al, *Ann Clin Psychiatry* 2000;**12**:35–42).
	Check copper and zinc levels as low levels may predispose to hair loss with valproate (Ftemi and Calabrese, *Ann Pharmacother* 1995;**29**:1302;Tasaki et al, *J Dermatol* 1993;**20**:21–4).

Darier's disease

Lithium	Topical retinoids.

Exfoliative dermatitis

Lithium	**Discontinue** — although rare (e.g. Sarantidis and Waters, *Br J Psychiatry* 1983;**143**:42–50) it is serious and discontinuation is usually the only option.

Folliculitis

Lithium	**Observation** (as it is often transient, starting several months after commencing lithium and resolving spontaneously), keep lithium levels stable. **Topical antibiotics and corticosteroids.**

Hair loss

Venlafaxine	**Discontinue or switch**, and it may resolve within a month (Pitchot and Ansseau, *Am J Psychiatry* 2001;**158**:1159–60).

Maculopapular eruption

Lithium	Usually occurs within three weeks of starting treatment. **Topical corticosteroids.** **Oral antihistamines.** **Reduce dose or discontinue** (can recur on rechallenge).

Photosensitivity

Antipsychotics	**Exclude other causes**, e.g. SLE and porphyria. **Avoid direct sunlight** or sun-lamps. **Use a high factor** sun-block cream. **Reduce** doses or **switch** drugs (there is no reliable comparative information but chlorpromazine is almost certainly the worst). **Reviews:** antipsychotics (Warnock and Morris, *Am J Clin Dermatol* 2002;

3:629–36), antipsychotics, antidepressants and anxiolytics (Harth and Rapoport, *Drug Saf* 1996;**14**:252–9).

Phenytoin

Can be the presenting symptom of serious reactions (review by Scheinfeld, *Expert Opin Drug Saf* 2004;**3**:655–65).

If mild, can reintroduce cautiously but discontinue immediately if it recurs.

Pigmentation
Imipramine

Blue-grey pigmentation, often facial, is probably due to melanin deposits. **Laser** (Q-switched alexandrite and ruby) treatment may be effective, better with higher doses (n = 1, Atkin and Fitzpatrick, *J Am Acad Dermatol* 2000;**43**:77–80).

Switch to an SSRI (e.g. sertraline, n = 1, Metelitsa et al, *J Cutan Med Surg* 2005;**9**:341–5).

Chlorpromazine

Withdrawal — chlorpromazine-pigmentation is almost completely reversible on withdrawal. CPZ lenticular pigmentation may persist whereas corneal changes may resolve slowly over several years on discontinuation.

Switch drugs, e.g. levomepromazine (n = 4), trifluoperazine (n = 1), combination (n = 5) (Bloom et al, *Acta Psychiatr Scand* 1993;**87**:223–4) can help. Other data supports a switch to haloperidol (n = 4, Thompson et al, *Acta Psychiatr Scand* 1988;**78**:763–5).

Psoriasis
Lithium

Lithium takes about a month to exacerbate psoriasis (but this is not inevitable: Skoven and Thormann, *Arch Dermatol* 1979;**115**:1185–7) and 10 months to induce it *de novo*.

Conventional topical therapy (e.g. topical corticosteroids and calcipotriol). **Oral retinoids.**

Reduce dose (as it is apparently dose-dependent) or discontinue (rarely necessary and takes many weeks to resolve on discontinuation).

Rash
Review: * ACHSS (anticonvulsant hypersensitivity syndrome; n = 32, Newell et al, *Pediatr Dermatol* 2009;**26**:536–46).

Anticonvulsants *
(general)

Switch AED * Skin rash with one AED seems to increase risk of rash with another, especially combinations involving carbamazepine or phenytoin. Specific cross-sensitivity rates may be useful for AED selection and counselling of patients (n = 1875, Hirsch et al, *Neurology* 2008;**71**:1527–34).

Rash with first AED	Second AED	Chance of rash with second AED
Carbamazepine	Lamotrigine	20% (n = 50)
Carbamazepine	Oxcarbazepine	33% (n = 15)
Carbamazepine	Phenobarbital	26.7% (n = 30)
Carbamazepine	Phenytoin	57.6% (n = 59)
Lamotrigine	Carbamazepine	26.3% (n = 38)
Lamotrigine	Oxcarbazepine	20% (n = 15)
Lamotrigine	Phenytoin	38.9% (n = 36)
Oxcarbazepine	Carbamazepine	71.4% (n = 7)
Oxcarbazepine	Lamotrigine	37.5% (n = 8)
Phenobarbital	Carbamazepine	66.7% (n = 12)
Phenobarbital	Phenytoin	53.3% (n = 15)
Phenytoin	Carbamazepine	42% (n = 81)
Phenytoin	Lamotrigine	18.9% (n = 74)
Phenytoin	Phenobarbital	19.5% (n = 41)

Oral corticosteroids (n = 1, Verrotti et al, *Int J Immunopathol Pharmacol* 2000;**13**:49–53).

Antihistamines, topical corticosteroids and H2-blockers have also been used.

Avoid paracetamol — adverse cutaneous reactions with carbamazepine and valproate (e.g. EM, SJS and TEN) can be enhanced by paracetamol (n = 72, Gau et al, *J Clin Psychopharmacol* 2008;**28**:509–17).

Carbamazepine *

Occurs in about 10–13% of people and there may be a genetic susceptibility (Hung et al, *Pharmacogenet Genomics* 2006;**16**:297–306), e.g. in Chinese (n = 24, Miller, *Epilepsy Curr* 2008;**8**:120–1).

If treating the rash rather than discontinuing, full laboratory test monitoring (including LFTs, FBC, U&E) must be carried out frequently to exclude agranulocytosis, aplastic anaemia (n = 10, Cates and Powers, *Ann Pharmacother* 1998;**32**:884–7) or internal organ involvement, which may occur in rare cases and be potentially fatal.

Slow increments (syrup 0.1 mg/d, doubling alternate days over 4/52) has been successful in preventing recurrence of rash (n = 1, Boyle and Lawlor, *Am J Psychiatry* 1996;**153**:1234; see also n = 1, Eames, *Lancet* 1989;**1**:509–10).

Oral corticosteroids, e.g. prednisone (n = 20, only four had to discontinue, Murphy et al, *Neurology* 1991;**41**:144–5).

Lamotrigine *

Take seriously: although relatively rare, rash may be the first sign of a potentially fatal Stevens-Johnson syndrome (n = 1175, RCT, Ketter et al, *J Clin Psychiatry* 2006;**67**:400–6) or toxic epidermal necrolysis (where the skin takes a red appearance and peels off) and so **must** be taken very seriously (review: Antai-Otong, *Perspect Psychiatr Care* 2005;**41**:193–6).

Prevention:

Risk factors: It is more common in females (relative risk of 1.8; Wong et al, *Ann Pharmacother* 1999;**33**:1037–42), people with a previous anticonvulsant rash and in the under 13s (n = 988, Hirsch et al, *Epilepsia* 2006;**47**:318–22).

Slow dose titration — the risk of rash is almost abolished by following the manufacturer's recommended titration schedule (n = 254, Huang et al, *Kaohsiung J Med Sci* 2002;**18**:66–72), especially the initial dose (n = 1955, Calabrese et al, *J Clin Psychiatry* 2002;**63**:1012–9). The starting dose in adults should be 25 mg/d for two weeks, then 50 mg/d for two weeks, then increasing every 1–2 weeks, halved if added to valproate (where rash is also more likely to occur) or if allergic to trimethoprim, and doubled if combined with concurrent enzyme-inducing drugs, e.g. phenytoin, carbamazepine, etc.

Preventative dermatological advice should be given, e.g. avoid other new medicines, foods, cosmetics, deodorants, detergents and fabric softeners, and avoid sunburn or exposure to poison ivy/oak (n = 100, Ketter et al, *J Clin Psychiatry* 2005;**66**:642–5). This may be effective in minimising the danger of this serious adverse reaction.

Valproate may not necessarily be an additional risk factor (n = 52, P-Codrea Tigaran et al, *Acta Neurol Scand* 2005;**111**:191–4). Lamotrigine can be added to valproate without increased risk of rash if started at very low initial doses (n = 108, Faught et al, *Epilepsia* 1999;**40**:1135–40), but the risk is 3–4 times more common with the combination (n = 103, Li et al, *Arq Neuropsiquiatr* 1996;**54**:47–9).

Management:

Corticosteroids for mild non-progressive types.

* **IV immunoglobulins and corticosteroids** are essential in specialist care

settings for more severe reactions. **Toxic epidermal necrolysis** caused by lamotrigine has responded to intravenous immunoglobulin and amniotic membranes (n = 1, Schwartz et al, Arch Dermatol 2008; **144**:724–6).
Switching may be the best option in epilepsy (long-term follow up, n = 2, Feliciani et al, Int J Immunopathol Pharmacol 2003; **16**:89–93).
Aftercare:
*****Very careful rechallenge** may be possible in some patients with a much slower dose escalation (n = 52, P-Codrea Tigaran et al, Acta Neurol Scand 2005; **111**:191–4). Leave a gap of 1–2 months, then restart at 0.1 mg/d (n = 7, Besag et al, Seizure 2000; **9**:2820–6), then 2.5–5 mg/d for 2/52, increasing by 5 mg/d every 2/52 to 25 mg/d, then as per SPC (n = 52, P-Codrea Tigaran et al, Acta Neurol Scand 20055; **111**:191–4). In one trial, 88% re-exposures were successful, with a very slow titration rate crucial in reducing recurrence (n = 44, Lorberg et al, Int J Neuropsychopharmacol 2009; **12**:257–65).

Phenytoin

Rash can be the presenting symptom of serious reactions (review by Scheinfeld, Expert Opin Drug Saf 2004; **3**:655–65).
If mild, can re-introduce cautiously but discontinue immediately if it recurs.

Antipsychotics
Antidepressants

Clozapine — see Fong et al, J Psychopharmacol 2005; **19**:107.
Fluoxetine — care needed, as rash can develop into more serious Stevens-Johnson syndrome or toxic epidermal necrolysis (Lyell syndrome).
Switching may not be effective as there can be cross-reactivity with other SSRIs (n = 2, Beauquier and Fahs, Encephale 1998; **24**:62–4; n = 1, Sannicandro et al, Pharmacotherapy 2002; **22**:516–8; paroxetine and sertraline n = 1, Warnock and Azadian, Ann Pharmacother 2002; **36**:631–3).
Avoid chocolate, which might be a precipitant (n = 1, Cederberg et al, BMC Psychiatry 2004; **4**:36), although this could be a tough call.
Antihistamine and topical steroids are widely mentioned in the literature as effective where rash is mild and self-limiting, e.g. fluoxetine and paroxetine rash has responded to oral diphenhydramine and topical hydrocortisone cream (n=1, Sannicandro et al, Pharmacotherapy 2002; **22**:516–8).

Rivastigmine *

Rash and itchiness with rivastigmine patches is a well recognised ADR, is mild in about 20% of patients but is common with all transdermal preps. There are two mechanisms: allergic dermatitis (tends to spread out from patch) and irritant dermatitis (just the patch area itself). Management includes:
Varying the site — best areas compared to the back are the upper arm and chest, with the lower back better than the upper back. Do not apply to excessively hairy, broken, burned, cut or irritated skin. The patch application site should be moved daily and do not use the exact same site for at least 14 days.
Skin care: If cleaning the skin before patch application, gently wash with water and dab dry with a cloth or towel.
- Avoid shaving, vigorous rubbing or use of alcohol-based cleansers or gels on the area as they may damage the integrity of the stratum corneum, the thin outer layer of skin.
- Gently clean the skin and apply moisturisers after every patch removal to reduce irritation and promote healthy skin.
- Remove the patch carefully to avoid surface damage to frail skin.
- Any irritant dermatitis (localised to the patch) should be left to resolve spontaneously, which is usually within several days without any intervention.

Treat any allergic dermatitis (hypersensitivity to patch adhesive or rivastigmine, presenting as localised redness that can spread beyond the edge of the patch) should be left to resolve spontaneously, usually within two weeks once the patch is removed. However, once allergic, patients will continue to experience skin reactions with subsequent use.

- **Use moisturising creams** and lotions for skin irritation (dryness, scaling, fissures or cracks).
- **Antihistamines and calamine lotion** can help itchiness but have no effect on irritant or allergic dermatitis.
- **Potent topical corticosteroids** may help severe allergic dermatitis, with referral to a dermatologist and discontinuation considered.

Seborrheic dermatitis

Lithium — Ketoconazole shampoo. Topical or systemic antifungal agents.

Sweating

Antidepressants * — Discontinuation or dose-reduction usually improves this rapidly.

Adjunctive therapies

Sweating can be a significantly irritating ADR for patients, especially those on tricyclics. Drugs tried include:

- * **Aripiprazole** 10–20 mg/d has been used for SSRI/duloxetine-induced sweating in women (Lu et al, J Clin Psychopharmacol 2008;**28**:710–1).
- **Beta-blockers** (propranolol, atenolol, labetalol) probably make sweating worse and should be excluded before other therapies are tried (n=1, Butt, J Clin Psychiatry 1989;**50**:146–7).
- **Benzatropine** 0.5–1 mg/d if venlafaxine-induced (Pierre and Guze, J Clin Psychopharmacol 2000;**20**:269).
- **Clonidine** 0.2 mg/d may help dramatically within 24 hours, (n=1, Feder, J Clin Psychiatry 1995;**56**:35; and for nortriptyline and paroxetine-induced; n=1, Mago and Monti, J Clin Psychiatry 2007;**68**:639–40), although stopping it sometimes helps (Leeman, J Clin Psychiatry 1990;**51**:258–9).
- **Cyproheptadine** 4 mg either BD or at night (n=5, open, Ashton and Weinstein, Am J Psychiatry 2002;**159**:874–5).
- **Mirtazapine** has been successful for 'hot flushes' in women (n=22[c=16], Perez et al, J Support Oncol 2004;**2**:50–6), although sedation was a tolerance problem (n=27[c=20], open, 12/52, Biglia et al, Breast J 2007;**13**:490–5). It may be dose-dependent, perhaps via 5-HT2/3 antagonism and influence on regulation of body temperature and diaphoresis (n=1, Buecking et al, Eur J Clin Pharmacol 2005;**61**:543–4).
- **Terazosin** 2 mg/d (n=1, Leeman, J Clin Psychiatry 1990;**51**:258–9; very effective for venlafaxine or sertraline-induced, n=1, Mago and Monti, J Clin Psychiatry 2007;**68**:639–40).

Reviews: case and brief review (Marcy and Britton, Ann Pharmacother 2005; **39**:748–52), general (Butt, J Clin Psychiatry 1989;**50**:146–7), pathophysiology of tricyclic-induced (Leeman, J Clin Psychiatry 1990;**51**:258–9).

6.6 Endocrine effects *

Metabolic syndrome is a term used to describe a series of endocrine disturbances such as weight gain, hypertriglyceridemia and increased insulin, glucose, and low-density lipoprotein cholesterol levels. These are associated with antipsychotic use and raise the risk of diabetes and cardiac problems.
Reviews: * Hert et al, World Psychiatry 2009;**8**:15–22; Meyer and Stahl, Acta Psychiatr Scand 2009;**119**: 4–14.

Diabetes:
Diabetes insipidus
Diabetes insipidus (not related to diabetes mellitus) is caused by poor kidney function or inadequate antidiuretic hormone production and is commonly reported with lithium and clozapine. It is becoming more common anyway, and often underdiagnosed and so screening before prescribing helps exclude pre-existing diabetes, for which any medication would obviously get the blame.

- Discontinuing the causative drug if possible is the obvious strategy.
- If urine volumes exceed 4 L/day, use thiazides and/or amiloride.
- NSAIDs (e.g. indometacin) may help in severe cases.

Diabetes mellitus

Type 1: person is unable to produce any insulin (previously known as insulin-dependent diabetes).

Type 2: person is unable to produce enough insulin or the insulin fails to work (insulin resistance, formerly non-insulin dependent diabetes mellitus [NIDDM], mature-onset diabetes).

- May be caused by decreased insulin sensitivity and weight gain.
- Monitor carefully if there is a family history or risk factors exist.

General management includes:

- The most potent strategies are to adjust lifestyle changes, e.g. manage obesity, smoking, exercise and diet.
- Oral hypoglycaemics, e.g. metformin (increases utilisation of insulin not increases production, n = 40, RCT, d/b, 14/52, Baptista *et al*, *Can J Psychiatry* 2006;**1**:192–6) or insulin can be considered.

Review: diabetes and atypicals (Clarke and Burge, *Diabetes Technol Ther* 2003;**5**:669–83).

Clozapine | **Discontinue** (although it may not always resolve, n = 2, Tovey *et al*, *J Psychopharmacol* 2005;**19**:207–10).

Orlistat has been used (Pavlovic, *Eur Psychiatry* 2005;**20**:520).

Reviews: Haupt and Newcomer, *J Clin Psychiatry* 2001;**62**(Suppl 27):15–26; Henderson, *CNS Drugs* 2002;**16**:77–89.

Olanzapine | **Discontinue** drug (may not always resolve, see Koller and Doraiswamy, *Pharmacotherapy* 2002;**22**:841–52).

Reduced dosage may help (n = 237, Koller and Doraiswamy, *Pharmacotherapy* 2002;**22**:841–52).

Switch to an alternative antipsychotic, e.g. quetiapine (n = 6 and review, Ashim *et al*, *J Psychopharmacol* 2004;**18**:128–32), risperidone (n = 1, Wu *et al*, *Psychiatry Clin Neurosci* 2006;**60**:115–6), aripiprazole (De Hert *et al*, *Diabetes Care* 2006;**29**:2329–30) or ziprasidone (Spivak *et al*, *Am J Psychiatry* 2002;**159**:1606; mean −14 mg/dL reduction in serum glucose, n = 84, Montes *et al*, *Prog Neuropsychopharmacol Biol Psychiatry* 2007;**31**:383–8).

* **Rosiglitazone** — 4–8 mg/d improved glycaemic control in olanzapine metabolic disturbance but not Hb1c or lipids (n = 30, RCT, d/b, p/c, 12/52, Baptista *et al*, *Pharmacopsychiatry* 2009;**42**:14–9) and 4 mg/d non-significantly improved glucose utilisation and insulin sensitivity and reduced LDL in clozapine metabolic disturbance (n = 18, RCT, d/b, p/c. 8/52, Henderson *et al*, *Acta Psychiatr Scand* 2009;**119**:457–65).

Hepatotoxicity
Valproate | **Early discontinuation** and supportive therapy is usually vital (Konig *et al*, *Epilepsia* 1999;**40**:1036–40)

Dose reduction may be possible if monitored with extreme care (n = 1, Lackmann, *Pharmacology* 2004;**70**:57–8).

L-carnitine can help, especially if given IV and within the first five days (n = 92, Bohan *et al*, *Neurology* 2001;**56**:1405–9; n = 1, Romero-Falcon *et al*, *Eur J Intern Med* 2003;**14**:338–40), and it can also be given prophylactically (review of evidence by Leheureux *et al*, *Crit Care* 2005;**9**:431–40).

Garlic organosulfur and **gingko biloba** use has been postulated (Sabayan *et al, Med Hypotheses* 2007;**68**:512–4).

Hyperammonaemia
Valproate

Discontinuation, as this is usually rapidly reversible (n = 2, Carlson *et al, J Am Acad Child Adolesc Psychiatry* 2007;**46**:356–61; n = 2, Panda and Radhakrishnon, *J Assoc Physicians India* 2004;**52**:746–8) but can lead to coma.
Reduce dose, as it may be plasma level related (n = 2, Wadzinski *et al, J Am Board Fam Med* 2007;**20**:499–502).
Stop other drugs that may exacerbate, e.g. phenobarbital, topiramate (Segura-Bruna *et al, Acta Neurol Scand* 2006;**114**:1–7) and pivmecillinam (n = 1, Lokrantz *et al, Acta Neurol Scand* 2004;**109**:297–301).
L-carnitine can correct carnitine deficiency (Segura-Bruna *et al, Acta Neurol Scand* 2006;**114**:1–7) and be well tolerated (n = 19, LoVecchio *et al, Am J Emerg Med* 2005;**23**:321–2).
Review: Stewart, *J Am Geriatr Soc* 2005;**53**:1080.

Hypercalcemia (hyperparathyroidism) *
Lithium *

Although very rare, hypercalcemia/hyperparathyroidism is a recognised ADR (review, Saunders *et al, World J Surg* 2009;**33**:2314–23):
Surgery (bilateral or unilateral parathyroidectomy).
Calcimimetic therapy (a potential alternative to parathyroidectomy).

Hypercholesterolaemia
Antipsychotics

Standard treatments for reducing cholesterol, e.g. statins are effective (n = 28, Ojala *et al, J Psychopharmacol* 2008;**22**:33–8).
Switch drugs, e.g. aripiprazole (significant decrease, n = 15 olanzapine, n = 9 others, Spurling *et al, J Clin Psychiatry* 2007;**68**:406–9) or ziprasidone (mean –24.1 mg/dL total cholesterol, n = 84, Montes *et al, Prog Neuropsychopharmacol Biol Psychiatry* 2007;**31**:383–8).
Discontinue any beta-blockers, which may enhance clozapine's effect on cholesterol (n = 50, Batmiller *et al, Schizophr Res* 2003;**59**:49–57).

Hyperglycaemia
Clozapine

Standard hypoglycaemic therapies
Orlistat has been used (Pavlovic, *Eur Psychiatry* 2005;**20**:520).
Amisulpride has a lower hyperglycaemic effect compared to clozapine (n = 22, 12–16/52, Rettenbacher *et al, J Psychopharmacol* 2007;**21**:400–4), although unlikely to be therapeutically equivalent.
Reviews: Haupt and Newcomer, *J Clin Psychiatry* 2001;**62**(Suppl 27):15–26; Henderson, *CNS Drugs* 2002;**16**:77–89.

Hyperlipidaemia
Antipsychotics *

Hyperlipidaemia has been reported with all antipsychotics (decreasing incidence from clozapine, olanzapine, risperidone, quetiapine, ziprasidone to first generation) except aripiprazole.
Manage risk factors, such as weight gain, dietary changes and glucose intolerance (Koro and Meyer, *Essent Psychopharmacol* 2005;**6**:148–57).
Discontinue any beta-blockers which may enhance the effects on lipids (n = 50, Batmiller *et al, Schizophr Res* 2003;**59**:49–57).
Lipid-lowering therapy, e.g. rosuvastatin (n = 100, 3/12, De Hert *et al, J Clin Psychiatry* 2006;**67**:1889–96).
Switch drugs:
- **Amisulpride or ziprasidone** (Rettenbacher *et al, Int Clin Psychopharmacol* 2006;**21**:369–72) and **risperidone** (n = 15, Su *et al, Psychopharmacology* [Berl] 2005;**183**:383–6) may be alternatives if olanzapine or clozapine-induced.

- * **Aripiprazole** has resolved clozapine (n = 1, Ball et al, Ann Pharmacother 2005;**39**:1570–2) and olanzapine (s = 3, n=546, RCT, Newcomer et al, Schizophr Res 2008;**106**:300–7) induced hyperlipidaemia and may be the best option (n = 13,133 vs 17,240, Olfson et al, Am J Psychiatry 2006;**163**:1821–5; mean –6.2 mg/dL in triglycerides, n = 84, Montes et al, Prog Neuropsychopharmacol Biol Psychiatry 2007;**31**:383–8), although raised lipids and triglycerides have been linked with improved PANSS scores (n = 55, RCT, p/c, d/b, 8/52, Procyshyn et al, J Psychiatry Neurosci 2007;**32**:31–8).
- **Fluvoxamine** 50 mg/d has been used for clozapine-induced hyperlipidaemia, partly by altering the clozapine:norclozapine ratio and possibly partly by facilitating a reduced clozapine dose via CYP1A2 inhibition (n = 68, RCT, 12/52, Lu et al, J Clin Psychiatry 2004;**65**:766–71; see also Chapter 4.2.3).

Hyperprolactinaemia

Hyperprolactinaemia is more common in bipolar disorder and schizophrenia (Bushe and Shaw, J Psychopharmacol 2007;**21**:768–73) and is linked to longer-term clinical sequelae, such as osteoporosis, hip fractures and possibly breast cancer.

Reviews: * general (Bostwick et al, Pharmacotherapy 2009;**29**:64–73), drug causes (review, Torre and Falorni, Ther Clin Risk Manag 2007;**3**:929–51)

Antidepressants	**Switch** — occurs in 22% women and 4.5% men with fluoxetine (n = 87, open, 12/52, Papakostas et al, J Clin Psychiatry 2006;**67**:952–7).
Antipsychotics *	**Reducing the dose** of the causative agent may help.

Check clinical relevance or importance (remembering the potential long-term effects of raised prolactin), especially if it is resulting in amenorrhoea in women or testosterone deficiency in men.

Test for a lesion by stopping the drug temporarily (or switching to a prolactin-sparing antipsychotic) to see if prolactin returns to normal, and/or performing a CT scan (Molitch, Mayo Clin Proc 2005;**80**:1050–7).

HRT/combined oral contraceptive in women and exogenous testosterone in men (see Molitch, Mayo Clin Proc 2005;**80**:1050–7) may help, and avoid the need to switch drugs (Miller, CNS Spectr 2004;**9**[8 Suppl 7]:28–32).

***Switch drugs: ***

Switching to a prolactin sparing drug (Table 2.1.4) is first-line strategy: A comparison of the prolactin-raising effect of antipsychotics in children and adolescents, concludes that quetiapine, ziprasidone and clozapine are best, amisulpride and risperidone worst, but there is insufficient data on the rest (s = 29, Roke et al, J Child Adolesc Psychopharmacol 2009;**19**:403–14).

- * **Aripiprazole** may be an alternative as it can reduce prolactin in its own right, but is not always successful (Paulzen and Grunder, Int J Neuropsychopharmacol 2006;**10**:149–51). In a switching study, augmenting with aripiprazole or switching (either abruptly or cross-over) to aripiprazole, significantly reduced prolactin levels within a week, maintained for eight weeks (n=269, 8/52, Byerly et al, Schizophr Res 2009;**107**:218–22; see also n = 23 [n = 20], Lu et al, Prog Neuropsychopharmacol Biol Psychiatry 2008;**32**:1978–81; n = 555, RCT, open, 26/52, Hanssens et al, BMC Psychiatry 2008;**22**:95; MS).
- **Olanzapine** has been used if risperidone-induced (n = 17, c/o, Lin et al, J Clin Psychiatry 2006;**67**:1470–1).
- **Quetiapine** has a low incidence of hyperprolactinaemia (20%; n = 70, Stevens et al, J Child Adolesc Psychopharmacol 2005;**15**:893–900) and

switching to quetiapine from typicals may be successful in about 65% of cases (n = 69, Nakajima et al, Pharmacopsychiatry 2005;**38**:17–9).

- **Risperidone** — switching patients from oral to RLAI may reduce prolactin levels, possibly by reducing surges in 9-OH-risperidone levels (35% reduction, n = 25, open, 12/52, Bai et al, J Clin Psychopharmacol 2007;**27**:306–8).

Adjunctive therapies: *

- **Aripiprazole** augmentation may be successful (15 mg/d for risperidone depot, Wahl and Ostroff, Am J Psychiatry 2005;**162**:1542–3; n = 1, Rainka et al, J Clin Pharm Ther 2009;**34**:595–8), e.g. with haloperidol, aripiprazole 15–30 mg/d significantly reduced prolactin levels, with 88% normal after 8/52 compared to 4% with placebo, and reversal of symptoms in most (n = 56, p/c, 8/52, Shim et al, Am J Psychiatry 2007;**164**:1404–10), but it may exacerbate hallucinations in a few patients (n = 7, Lee et al, Prog Neuropsychopharmacol Biol Psychiatry 2006;**30**:714–7).

Dopamine agonists should generally be avoided as they may precipitate psychosis, but with careful monitoring and dose adjustment may be successful in selected cases where other strategies have failed (review of bromocriptine and cabergoline; Colao et al, Nat Clin Pract Endocrinol Metab 2006;**2** 200–10). There may be significant differences in tolerability of dopamine agonists, with cabergoline probably the best (review by Chanson et al, Ann Endocrinol [Paris] 2007;**68**:113–7).

- **Amantadine** has been successful on all measures of hyperprolactinaemia in 90% patients (n = 10, open, 7/52, Correa et al, J Clin Psychopharmacol 1987;**7**:91–5).
- **Bromocriptine** may reverse the hyperprolactinaemia and galactorrhoea from olanzapine (n = 1, Miller and Sebastian, J Clin Psychiatry 2005;**66**:269–70) and amisulpride (n = 1, Bliesener et al, Pharmacopsychiatry 2004;**37**:189–91).
- ***Cabergoline** is longer-acting, better tolerated and may be superior to bromocriptine in efficacy (Biller et al, J Reprod Med 1999;**44** [12Suppl]: 1075–84). Cabergoline 0.125–0.25 mg/d has been used if risperidone-induced (58% had a statistically significant reduction, with no adverse affects and no deterioration in psychosis; n = 19, 8/52, Cavallaro et al, J Clin Psychiatry 2004;**65**:187–90; n = 4, mean dose 0.3 mg/d, Cohen and Biederman, J Child Adolesc Psychopharmacol 2001;**11**:435–40). Use a lower dose as the standard starting dose of 0.5mg/d or higher might cause psychosis (n = 2, Chang et al, Gen Hosp Psychiatry 2008;**30**:378–80).
- **Pergolide** – mentioned in some reviews (see below).
- ***Peony-glycyrrhiza decoction** (PGD, a herbal medicine) 45 g/d was as effective as bromocriptine 5 mg/d at reducing risperidone-induced hyperprolactinaemia in women with schizophrenia, and also improved symptoms of raised prolactin (n = 20, RCT, c/o, 3x4/52, Yuan et al, J Clin Psychopharmacol 2008;**28**:264–70).

Reviews: management of antipsychotic-induced hyperprolactinaemia (Haddad and Wieck, Drugs 2004;**64**:2291–314; Miller, CNS Spectr 2004;**9**[8 Suppl 7]:28–32; see also Gillam et al, Pediatr Endocrinol Rev 2004;**2**[Suppl 1]:108–14), general (Verhelst and Abs, Treat Endocrin 2003;**2**:23–32; Bankowski and Zacur, Clin Obstet Gynecol 2003;**46**:349–62).

Hyperthyroidism
Lithium *

Lithium can raise TSH levels, which have been linked strongly with an increased risk of depression, so monitor regularly and manage (s = 2, n = 32, RCT, d/b, p/c, 18/12, Frye et al, Acta Psychiatr Scand 2009;**120**:10–3).

Carbimazole (n = 9 and review, Barclay et al, Clin Endocrinol [Oxf] 1994; **40**:759–64).

Radioactive iodine (n = 3, Dwarakanathan, Endocr Pract 1998;**4**:201–3).

Hyponatraemia

Risk factors for hyponatraemia include older age, female gender, low body weight, concurrent drugs (e.g. diuretics, NSAIDs, carbamazepine, cancer chemotherapy), reduced renal function, comorbidity (e.g. hypothyroidism, diabetes, COPD), and hotter weather (review Jacob and Spinler, Ann Pharmacother 2006;**40**:1618–22), so monitor serum sodium over several weeks in higher risk patients. Rapid correction is extremely hazardous.

- On drug withdrawal, sodium usually returns to normal within two weeks.
- Smoking may exacerbate hyponatraemia.
- Rechallenge may be possible without recurrence (review, Kirby and Ames, Int J Geriatr Psychiatry 2001;**16**:484–93). If necessary, restart at low dose, increase slowly and monitor carefully.
- If sodium > 125 mmol/l, monitor daily until above 135 mmol/L. If < 125 mmol/L, refer for urgent specialist medical care.
- Loop diuretics have been used (Jacob and Spinler, Ann Pharmacother 2006;**40**:1618–22).
- Restrict fluid intake.

Review: * Management (Munger, Am J Health Syst Pharm 2007;**64**:253–65).

Antidepressants *   May be due to inappropriate antidiuretic hormone secretion.

Use a lower risk antidepressant. According to CSM data to 2005, the risks are as follows (although there is doubtless under-reporting for all drugs):

- Highest risk (> 1% incidence): citalopram, escitalopram, fluoxetine, sertraline.
- Medium risk (0.5–1% incidence): amitriptyline, clomipramine, dosulepin, doxepin, imipramine, lofepramine, moclobemide, paroxetine, venlafaxine.
- Lowest risk (< 0.5% incidence): nortriptyline, trazodone, phenelzine, tranylcypromine, mirtazapine, reboxetine.

* **Mirtazapine** appears, overall, to have the lowest risk based on current evidence and the level of reported problems (cases have been reported, e.g. profound hyponatraemia; n = 2, Cheah et al, Am J Geriatr Pharmacother 2008;**6**:91–5), although all antidepressants have reported associations.

If it recurs on rechallenge and antidepressants are essential, consider water restriction and/or careful use of demeclocycline.

Demeclocycline use is controversial and some texts recommend avoiding it with antidepressants.

Reviews: Spigset and Hedenmalm, Drug Saf 1995;**12**:209–25; Cawley, Ann Pharmacother 2007;**41**:840–50.

Antipsychotics   Can be caused by water intoxication, SIADH or severe hyperlipidaemia and/or hyperglycaemia.

If caused by water intoxication (serum and urine osmolality both low):

- **Fluid restriction** (refer to DGH if sodium < 125 mmol/L).
- **Switch drugs**, e.g. clozapine (may reverse hyponatraemia/hypoosmolemia; n = 8, 18–24/52, open, Canuso and Goldman, J Neuropsychiatry Clin Neurosci 1999;**11**:86–90), olanzapine, risperidone or quetiapine.
- There is no evidence that altering doses is effective.

If caused by SIADH (high urine but low serum osmolality):

- **Fluid restriction** (refer to DGH if sodium < 125 mmol/L).
- **Switch** antipsychotic as soon as possible. A low incidence has been reported with aripiprazole (n = 1, Bachu et al, Am J Ther 2006;**13**:370–2).

- **Consider demeclocycline** (probably directly blocks the renal tubule effect of antidiuretic homone; usual dose range is 0.9–1.2 g daily, reduced to 600–900 mg/d for maintenance, see standard texts).
- **Discontinue any concurrent desmopressin** (n = 1, Sarma et al, *Aust N Z J Psychiatry* 2005;**39**:1726–31).
- **Lithium** has been used (mentioned in Madhusoodanan et al, *Adverse Drug React Toxicol Rev* 2002;**21**:17–29).

Review: Spigset and Hedenmalm, *Drug Saf* 1995;**12**:209–25.

Hypothyroidism

Lithium

Lithium inhibits thyroid release but compensatory mechanisms normally operate in most patients. It is more common in people with circulating thyroid antibodies (n = 150, Bocchetta et al, *J Endocrinol Invest* 2007;**30**:363–6). Refer to an endocrinologist if TSH levels are repeatedly abnormal.

Lithium withdrawal tends to resolve euthyroid or hypothyroid goitres

Supplementary thyroxine therapy is indicated for overt hypothyroidism. Treatment with thyroxine for subclinical hypothyroidism is controversial.

Manage weight, especially during the first year, which can be highly predictive of hypothyroidism (Henry, *J Psychiatry Neurosci* 2002;**27**;104–7).

Reviews: general (Fagiolini et al, *Epidemiol Psichiatr Soc* 2006;**15**:123–7), mechanisms (Bocchetta and Loviselli, *Clin Pract Epidemol Ment Health* 2006;**12**:23; Johnson and Eagles, *Br J Psychiatry* 1999;**175**:336–9).

Polyuria and renal impairment (often a symptom of diabetes insipidus)

Lithium

About 20% of people on lithium develop decreased renal function and polyuria, but this is probably only progressive in a few, with a change in therapy only recommended if serum creatinine concentration rises above 200 micromol/l (van Gerven and Boer, *Ned Tijdschr Geneeskd* 2006;**150**:1715–8). It may be due to lithium's effect on vasopressin at a hypothalamic level and a decrease in GFR. The main strategies are:

- **Reduce dose** to the lowest possible, making it once daily (if not already) although there is little data to support this.
- **Switch** to an alternative drug if possible (e.g. valproate has been used; n = 7, Stoll et al, *J Clin Psychiatry* 1996;**57**:356–9).
- **Discontinue** any other drugs that might be contributing.
- **Stop any serotonergic antidepressants** that may enhance polyuria (n = 75, Movig et al, *Br J Psychiatry* 2003;**182**:319–23).
- **Diuretics** such as amiloride have been used (n = 1, Finch et al, *Pharmacotherapy* 2003;**23**:546–50), but great care is needed with interactions, see *Chapter 4.4* (mentioned in van Gerven and Boer, *Ned Tijdschr Geneeskd* 2006;**150**:1705–9).
- **NSAIDs** such as ketoprofen 100 mg IV have been effective in acute lithium toxicity presenting as severe nephrogenic diabetes mellitus (n = 1, Tran-Van et al, *Presse Med* 2005;**34**:1137–40), as has indomethacin 150 mg (rapidly effective, within 36 hours; n = 1, Lam and Kjellstrand, *Ren Fail* 1997;**19**:183–8; 50 mg TDS, n = 1, Martinez et al, *South Med J* 1993;**86**:971–3), probably by blocking lithium's prostaglandin-inducing activity. Adequate hydration is essential.
- **Refer** to renal specialists for advice (although they are likely to recommend discontinuation).

Reviews: effect of lithium on renal function (n = 20, Turan et al, *Prog Neuropsychopharmacol Biol Psychiatry* 2002;**26**:561–5), avoiding lithium toxicity based on renal clearance (Thomsen and

Schou, *Pharmacopsychiatry* 1999;**32**:83–6), general (van Gerven and Boer, *Ned Tijdschr Geneeskd* 2006;**150**:1705–9), risk factors (n = 75, Movig et al, *Br J Psychiatry* 2003;**182**:319–23).

Weight gain *

Numerous mechanisms for drug-induced weight gain have been proposed, including:

- Sedation — leading to decreased activity.
- Thirst — anticholinergic dry mouth may lead to an increased intake of fluids and calories.
- Reduced metabolism — fat and carbohydrate oxidation.
- Increased food intake via neurotransmitter-mediated increase in appetite, e.g. via blockade of receptors such as 5-HT2A, 5-HT2C (n = 123, Reynolds et al, *Lancet* 2002;**359**:2086–7), H1 or H2 (n = 92, males, retrospective, Wirshing et al, *J Clin Psychiatry* 1999;**60**:358–63) and perhaps D2, and polypeptides such as CCK. 5-HT2C polymorphism appears to determine circulating leptin levels so might explain the mechanism (e.g. n = 30, RCT, d/b, Kluge et al, *J Clin Psychopharmacol* 2007;**27**:662–6).
- * Changes in levels of leptin (Baptista and Beaulieu, *Can J Psychiatry* 2002;**47**:742–9; Gorobets, *Bull Exp Biol Med* 2008;**146**:348–50), a multifunctional polypeptide produced by fat cells to reduce appetite (by signalling the size of the adipose tissue to the brain) and to increase energy expenditure. Weight gain induced by clozapine, olanzapine and other antipsychotics may be related to an increase in leptin levels via hypothalamic neurons that mediate the effects leptin on the control of food intake (Reynolds et al, *J Psychopharmacol* 2006;**20**[4 Suppl]:15–8).
- Other polypeptides may also be implicated, e.g. reductin and cytokines, mainly tumour necrosis factor alpha (TNF-alpha) and ghrelin (a fast-acting hormone which plays a role in meal initiation; clozapine, olanzapine, risperidone, amisulpride all cause raised ghrelin but quetiapine does not; n = 112, Esen-Danaci et al, *Prog Neuropsychopharmacol Biol Psychiatry* 2008;**32**:1434–8).
- Induction of abdominal fat deposition, combined with a dysfunction of the normal leptin control of weight (n = 46, 10/52, Zhang et al, *Br J Psychiatry* 2004;**184**:58–62).
- Fluid retention — via peripheral oedema, a minor effect.
- Endocrine effects — increased prolactin levels (which may promote adiposity and is related to weight gain in men; open, p/c, Baptista et al, *Pharmacopsychiatry* 1997;**30**:250–5), variation in cortisol or altered insulin secretion.

Reviews: * general (s = 248, Gentile, *Obes Rev* 2009;**10**:527–42; Faulkner and Cohn, *Can J Psychiatry* 2006;**51**:502–11; Ness-Abramof and Apovian, *Drugs Today (Barc)* 2005;**41**:547–55; Ruetsch et al, *Encephale* 2005;**31**:507–16), aetiological factors (Virk et al, *Obes Rev* 2004;**5**:167–70), review of non-pharmacological interventions (Alvarez-Jiménez et al, *Br J Psychiatry* 2008;**193**:101–7), therapeutic options (Cordes et al, *Fortschr Neurol Psychiatr* 2008;**76**:703–14), in bipolar (review, Torrent et al, *Acta Psychiatr Scand* 2008;**118**:4–18).

Antidepressants *	**Switch** antidepressants. SSRIs have the lowest short-term weight gain potential, although there is a tendency for weight gain after 6–12 months. **Tricyclics** should be **avoided** as they cause carbohydrate craving (Paykel, *Br J Psychiatry* 1973;**123**:501–7) and a decreased metabolic rate (Fernstein et al, *Biol Psychiatry* 1985;**20**:688–92), a double whammy. **Bupropion** for SSRI-induced weight gain (see review by Demyttenaere and Jaspers, *J Psychopharmacol* 2008;**22**:792–804). **Naltrexone** can produce a reduction in continuous hunger and a small weight loss at eight weeks for tricyclic-induced weight gain (open, Zimmermann et al, *Biol Psychiatry* 1997;**41**:47–9).
Antipsychotics	**Education**; WWW (**w**arn, **w**eigh, **w**atch): **Warn:** counsel patients with a higher risk of weight gain, e.g. female, prone to overeating under stress, narcissistic personality traits, family or personal history of obesity and a greater than 6.5 kg difference between adult maximum and minimum weights. **Weigh:** take a baseline weight, warn of the unpredictable nature of

weight gain, that the effect plateaus after several months, and the need to optimise calorie intake.

Watch: most weight is gained in the first few months, so ensure the patient seeks advice from a dietician early, since it is easier to prevent weight gain than lose it once it has happened. Moderate physical exercise may be helpful and excessive intake of high calorie fluids should be avoided. Weight management includes all possible variations on 'eat less, move more' (see Sharpe *et al, J Clin Psychiatry* 2005;**66**:951–2 for explanation of 'move more' but not mentioning the "Keep Fit Calypso").

* **Manage more carefully where risk factors exist:**
- Increased parents' BMI
- Patient's pre-morbid BMI (higher predicts 12.5% of gain with olanzapine)
- Female gender
- Schizophrenia spectrum disorder (trend)
- Age (negative correlation, more common in younger, gain is reduced by 0.6kg for every extra 10 years of age)
- High cumulative olanzapine dose

(n = 118; 12/52, Smith *et al, Int Clin Psychopharmacol* 2008;**23**:130–7; n = 65, Gebhardt *et al, J Psychiatr Res* 2009;**43**:620–6; n = 164, < 24/52, Ujike *et al, J Clin Psychiatry* 2008;**69**:1416–22).

Cochrane concludes that modest weight loss can be achieved with selected pharmacological and non-drug therapies but that the data is limited by small sample sizes, duration and intervention variety (s = 23, Faulkner *et al, Cochrane Database Syst Rev* 2007;**1**:CD005148).

Behavioural interventions:

Dietary interventions and nutritional education may be effective, e.g.
- Regular dietician visits and self-directed dieting with weight loss as a treatment goal (n = 35 [c = 29], 15/12, Kalarchian *et al, J Clin Psychiatry* 2005;**66**:1058–63; n = 70, RCT, 4/12, Littrell *et al, J Nurs Scholar* 2003; **35**:237–41).
- Individual nutritional education for 3–6/12 after starting olanzapine may be successful, although studies are small and excluded obese people (Evans *et al, Aust N Z J Psychiatry* 2005;**39**:479–86; critical review by Isaacs, *EBMH* 2006;**9**:11; programme focused on nutrition, exercise and motivation; n = 31 [c = 21], 12/12, Menza *et al, J Clin Psychiatry* 2004;**65**:471–7).
- Weight management programmes may be effective (e.g. n = 48 [c = 36], RCT, 12/52, Kwon *et al, J Clin Psychiatry* 2006;**67**:547–53). Attending group sessions regularly over a year also helps (n = 93, Pendlebury *et al, Acta Psychiatr Scand* 2007;**115**:286–94).

Exercise may help. Those doing light jogging for 30 minutes three times a week plus reducing food intake by 500kcal/d gained 2kg less than those just receiving olanzapine 10–20mg/d for mania (n=28, RCT, 8/52, Milano *et al, Adv Ther* 2007;**24**:123–34).

Lifestyle intervention and metformin were both superior for antipsychotic-induced weight gain on all measures, with the combination being the most effective (n = 128, RCT, p/c, 12/52, Wu *et al, JAMA* 2008;**299**:185–93).

Medication interventions: *

Reduce dose, as there is preliminary evidence that weight gain with clozapine and olanzapine is related to **plasma** levels, but not dose, but there is insufficient evidence on other 2nd generation antipsychotics (Simon *et al, J Clin Psychiatry* 2009;**70**:1041–50).

Slower introduction has been postulated to lead to a lower final weight gain. Intermittent antipsychotic use is not recommended but has been suggested (Buchanan and Carpenter, *CNS Drugs* 1996;**5**:240–5).

Switch drugs: * (see *2.1.3* and CATIE for a table of the relative risks)

* **Aripiprazole** (see also adjunctive) has been used if olanzapine-induced (n = 53 [c = 29], open, 12/12, Schorr et al, *Acta Psychiatr Scand* 2008;**118**:246–50; significant decrease, n = 15 olanzapine, n = 9 others, Spurling et al, *J Clin Psychiatry* 2007;**68**:406–9) as has **risperidone** (n = 15, Su et al, *Psychopharmacology(Berl)* 2005;**183**:383–6; n = 121, Meyer et al, *Clin Ther* 2005;**27**:1930–41), although when switched to aripiprazole in a small study, a third deteriorated mentally, and in the remainder who improved, there was no alteration in weight or metabolic outcomes (n = 15, open, 4/12, Kim et al, *J Clin Psychopharmacol* 2007;**27**:365–8).

* **Quetiapine** — in olanzapine-induced weight gain, a Lilly study showed that switching to quetiapine led to increased relapses and no significant weight improvements (n = 133, 13/52, Deberdt et al, *Ther Clin Risk Manag* 2008;**4**:713–20).

Adjunctive therapies: *

Few, if any, adjunctive therapies have been shown to have any sustained or robust effect. The following, in alphabetical order, are the best of the bunch:

* **Acetazolamide** has been used as an alternative to topiramate (n = 1, Schneiderhan and Marvin, *Am J Ther* 2007;**14**:581–4).

* **Amantadine** 100–300 mg/d may be well-tolerated and attenuated weight gain or modestly promoted weight loss in some patients who had already gained weight with olanzapine 5–20 mg/d (n = 125, RCT, d/b, p/c, 16/52, Deberdt et al, *Eur Neuropsychopharmacol* 2005;**15**:13–21) but not in all studies (n = 25, Bahk et al, *Psychiatr Clin Neurosci* 2004;**58**:163–7).

* * **Aripiprazole** 15 mg/d significantly reduced weight and BMI from olanzapine, but had no effect on overall cholesterol, although serum triglycerides, VLDC and VLDL all decreased significantly (d/b, p/c, c/o, 10/52, Henderson et al, *J Clin Psychopharmacol* 2009;**29**:165–9).

* * **Bofu-tsusho-san** (an Oriental herbal medicine) can attenuate weight gain from olanzapine (Yamamoto and Inada, *Psychiatry Clin Neurosci* 2008;**62**:747).

* **Bupropion** 150–300 mg/d as an adjunct to olanzapine (mean duration 26/12) produced modest weight loss, with 50% losing > 3% (n = 8 [c = 7], open, 24/52, Gadde et al, *J Clin Psychopharmacol* 2006;**6**:409–13; review by Gadde and Xiong, *Expert Rev Neurother* 2007;**7**:17–24).

* * **Modafinil** 200 mg/d reduced the weight gained with olanzapine by 50% (from 0.89 to 0.47 kg/m2; n = 50 [c = 40], RCT, d/b, p/c, 3/52, Roerig et al, *Biol Psychiatry* 2009;**65**:607–13), the effect being maintained for three years in a patient on clozapine, possibly by reducing clozapine-induced fatigue, reversed on discontinuation (n = 1, Henderson et al, *Ann Clin Psychiatry* 2005;**17**:95–7).

* **Orlistat** has a modest effect that may only be seen in men (n = 71 [c = 63], RCT, d/b, p/c, 16/52, Joffe et al, *J Clin Psychiatry* 2008;**69**:706–11), although is poorly tolerated and requires good compliance with a low-fat diet.

* **Quetiapine** has been used as an adjunct to clozapine; after six months' therapy patients had 25% of their dose converted to quetiapine (using ratio 1 mg clozapine:2 mg quetiapine) for 10 months. Average weight

loss was 0.22–10.5 kg after one month, and maintained, with 100% user satisfaction reported (n = 65, open, 10/12, Reinstein et al, Clin Drug Invest 1999;**18**:99–104; review by Werneke et al, Int Clin Psychopharmacol 2002;**17**:145–60).

- **Reboxetine** co-prescribed when starting olanzapine may help (n = 26 [c = 20], RCT, p/c, d/b, 6/52, Poyurovsky et al, Am J Psychiatry 2003;**160**:297–302).
- * **Switching to orodispersible olanzapine** — a recent RCT failed to show any loss of weight with orodispersible tablets compared to plain tablets (RCT, d/b, p/c, 16/52, Karagianis et al, Schizophr Res 2009;**113**:41–8; MS) although there are continued reports, e.g. a mean weight loss 6.6 kg; n = 17, open, 16/52, de Haan et al, Psychopharmacol 2004;**175**:389–90; n = 2, weight loss 15 kg maintained for 12/12, Kozumplik et al, Psychiatr Danub 2009;**21**:71–4).
- **Topiramate** 200 mg/d may be effective (100 mg/d is ineffective; n = 66, RCT, d/b, p/c, 12/52, Ko et al, Clin Neuropharmacol 2005;**28**:169–75) and has helped with olanzapine-induced weight gain (n = 1, Levy et al, J Clin Psychiatry 2002;**63**:1045; n = 3, Lin et al, Psychiatr Clin Neurosci 2005;**59**:613–5), with reduced adiposity in women (n = 43, RCT, d/b, p/c, 10/52, Nickel et al, J Clin Psychopharmacol 2005;**25**:211–7; n = 26 [c = 13], open, 12/12, Vieta et al, J Clin Psychopharmacol 2004;**24**:374–8). Adjunctive topiramate (mean 200 mg/d) in overweight schizophrenics has produced continued weight loss over 6/12 (n = 10, Lévy et al, Can J Clin Pharmacol 2007;**14**:234–9) and improved mood (both depressive and manic) and dropped BMI by two points at 12/52 in refractory obese bipolar patients (n = 30, open, 12/52, Gabr iel, Eat Weight Disord 2007;**12**:48–53).

Less useful strategies:

Other drugs have been tried but those listed below are either of no use or are theoretical prospects only:

- **Appetite suppressants** may exacerbate psychosis or fail to work.
- **Estrogen** shows a possible preventative role in animal studies (see Baptista, Acta Psychiatr Scand 1999;**100**:3–16).
- **Fluoxetine** is ineffective if olanzapine-induced (n = 30, RCT, d/b, 8/52, Poyurovsky et al, Am J Psychiatry 2002;**159**:1058–60; n = 31, RCT, d/b, Bustillo et al, Neuropsychopharm 2003;**28**:527–9).
- **Fluvoxamine** (50 mg/d) may allegedly attenuate weight gain and metabolic disturbances from clozapine, perhaps by allowing lower doses to be used, although the interaction can be dramatic and dangerous (n = 68, RCT, 12/52, Lu et al, J Clin Psychiatry 2004;**65**:766–71).
- **H2-antagonists** such as famotidine (n = 14, d/b, p/c, 6/52, Poyurovsky et al, Eur Neuropsychopharmacol 2004;**14**:332–6) and nizatidine are ineffective for olanzapine-induced weight gain (n = 175, d/b, p/c, 16/52, Cavazzoni et al, Eur Neuropsychopharmacol 2003;**13**:81–5) but may have some effect (n = 59, RCT, d/b, 8/52, Atamaca et al, Hum Psychopharmacol 2003;**18**:457–61). Ranitidine reduced the weight gain from olanzapine in 60% cases (RCT, open, Lopez-Mato et al, Vertex 2003;**14**:85–96) and may stop weight gain with quetiapine although not reduce any weight already gained (n = 47, RCT, Atmaca et al, Hum Psychopharmacol 2004;**19**:37–40).
- **Melatonin** augmentation helps in rats, but human data is currently unavailable (Raskind et al, Neuropsychopharmacol 2007;**32**:284–8).

- **Memantine** augmentation had a significant effect for clozapine-induced weight gain (n = 1, Scharfer *et al, Pharmacopsychiatry* 2007;**40**:149–51).

- * **Metformin** does not aid loss of olanzapine-induced weight gain (n = 40, RCT, d/b, p/c, 14/52, Baptista *et al, Can J Psychiatry* 2006;**51**:192–6), but has been shown to help attenuate weight gain from olanzapine in drug-naive first-episode schizophrenics (n = 40 [c = 37], RCT, d/b, 12/52, Wu *et al, Am J Psychiatry* 2008;**165**:352–8). It has been shown to prevent weight gain when started with a range of atypicals (n = 39, RCT, d/b, p/c, Klein *et al, Am J Psychiatry* 2006;**163**:2072–9) but not in adolescents taking risperidone (n = 49 [c = 32], RCT, d/b, p/c, 12/52, Arman *et al, Saudi Med J* 2008;**29**:1130–4). In patients stable on clozapine, addition of metformin 500–1000 mg/d has resulted in a mean weight loss of 1.87 kg (n = 61 [c = 56], RCT, d/b, p/c, 14/52, Carrizo *et al, Schizophr Res* 2009;**113**:19–26). Metformin only increases utilisation of insulin not the production, so can be safe long-term but not without the risk of, e.g. lactic acidosis.

- **Phenylpropanolamine** is ineffective for clozapine-induced weight gain (n = 16, RCT, d/b, 12/52, Borovicka *et al, J Clin Psychiatry* 2002; **63**:345–8).

- **Sibutramine** 15 mg/d significantly reduced olanzapine-induced weight gain (8 lb *vs* 2 lb) but increased bp and disturbed sleep in some patients (n = 37, RCT, d/b, p/c, 12/52, Henderson *et al, Am J Psychiatry* 2005;**162**:954–62). However, it was ineffective for clozapine-induced weight gain (n = 21, RCT, d/b, p/c, 12/52, Henderson *et al, Acta Psychiatr Scand* 2007;**115**:101–5). Addition of sibutramine (10–20 mg/d) to metformin (850–1700 mg/d) was no more effective than metformin alone for reducing olanzapine-induced weight gain (n = 28, d/b, p/c, 12/52, Baptista *et al, Psychiatry Res* 2008;**159**:250–3). It is contraindicated in 'psychiatric illness' so should not be used with another serotonergic drug.

Reviews: general (Faulkner and Cohn, *Can J Psychiatry* 2006;**51**:502–11; Gentile, *Drug Saf* 2006;**29**:303–19; Faulkner *et al, Acta Psychiatr Scand* 2003;**108**:324–32; Ananth *et al, Ann Clin Psychiatry* 2004;**16**:75–85), genetics (Muller and Kennedy, *Pharmacogenomics* 2006;**7**:863–87).

Lithium

Weight gain occurs predominantly during the first 1–2 years of treatment, occurs more often in people already overweight and may be more common in women than men.

Manage thirst, as increased thirst has been noted in 89% and strongly correlates with weight gain. Increased hunger/food intake has not been directly shown (*J Psychopharmacol* 1990;**4**:303) and so the predominant mechanism may be increased intake of high-calorie drinks.

Thyroid status should also be assessed as a possible contributory cause.

Counselling, e.g. use of plain/low-calorie beverages, along with normal sodium intake, dietary advice and monitoring, particularly during the first year, may be adequate (general review by Baptista *et al, Pharmacopsychiatry* 1995;**28**:35–44).

Lamotrigine may be an alternative as it is associated with weight loss, there being no significant differences in non-obese patients (n =554, s = 2, d/b, p/c, 12/12, Bowden *et al, Am J Psychiatry* 2006;**163**:1199–201).

Topiramate can safely be added to lithium or valproate in bipolar I manic or mixed episodes to significantly reduce weight (n = 287, RCT, d/b, p/c, 12/52, Chengappa *et al, J Clin Psychiatry* 2006;**67**:1698–1706; MS).

Mirtazapine	Weight gain is difficult to manage, switching may be the only option. **Ranitidine** at night is probably of no use.
SSRIs	Weight gain tends to occur later in the first year of therapy. **Topiramate** up to 250mg/d has produced a mean 4kg loss of weight (n = 15, open, 10/52, Van Ameringen et al, J Clin Psychiatry 2002;**63**:981–4).
Valproate	Valproate-induced weight gain may have a variety of mechanisms, but seems more common in people with normal or below normal weight before starting (n = 70, Corman et al, Can J Neurol Sci 1997;**24**:240–4) and so warning people in advance may be advantageous. **Get a new set of genes** (n = 5 twin pairs, Klein et al, Obes Res 2005;**13**:1330–4). OK, it's not realistic, but may help to explain to some people that weight gain with valproate isn't all their 'fault'. **Lamotrigine** may be an alternative (n = 222, open, Morrell et al, Epilepsy Res 2003;**54**:189–99), but carbamazepine may not be suitable (n = 211, Easter et al, Seizure 1997;**6**:121–5).
Zonisamide	**Bupropion** augmentation of zonisamide may help weight loss in the short-term in obese women (n = 18, RCT, open, 12/52, Gadde et al, J Clin Psychiatry 2007;**68**:1226–9).

6.7 Movement disorders

Blepharospasm (see also tardive dystonia)
Blepharospasm is a sustained, forced, involuntary closing of the eyelids, often a presenting symptom of tardive dystonia.

Antipsychotics	Switching antipsychotics is usually the main effective strategy, e.g. to **clozapine**, (n = 4, Levin and Reddy, J Clin Psychiatry 2000;**61**:140–3) or **quetiapine** (n = 1, Reeves and Liberto, Mov Disord 2003;**18**:1072–3). **ECT** has been used (n = 1, Sienaert and Peuskens, J ECT 2005;**21**:132–4).

Bruxism (teeth grinding)
Bruxism is defined as grinding, clenching and forceful teeth or jaw movements, usually during sleep. Almost everyone bruxes, but bruxism is where it is severe enough to cause damage or distress.
General review: (Lobbezoo et al, J Oral Rehabil 2006;**33**:293–300).

Antidepressants *	* **Dose reduction** usually leads to resolution (n = 4, Ellison and Stanziani, J Clin Psychiatry 1993;**54**:432–4) but can take several months to resolve (n = 1, Alonso-Navarro et al, Clin Neuropharmacol 2009;**32**:111–2). * **Buspirone** has been used if bruxism is induced by venlafaxine (40mg/d, significantly effective over 4/52: Pavlovic, Int J Neuropsychopharmacol 2004;**7**:523–4; Jaffee and Bostwick, Psychosomatics 2000;**41**:535–6; n = 1, Kuloglu et al, J Psychopharmacol 2010; [in press]) or SSRIs (n = 4, Bostwick and Jaffee, J Clin Psychiatry 1999;**60**:857–60), e.g. fluoxetine (n = 1, Sabuncuoglu et al, Spec Care Dentist 2009;**29**:215–7). **Gabapentin**, if venlafaxine-induced (n = 1, Brown and Hong, J Am Dent Assoc 1999;**130**:1467–9). **ECT**, if fluvoxamine-induced (n = 1, Miyaoka et al, J ECT 2003;**19**:170–2).
Antipsychotics *	**Dose reduction** usually leads to resolution. * **Switch** to low-dose clozapine (n = 1, 16/52, Mendhekar and Andrade, J Neuropsychiatry Clin Neurosci 2009;**21**:105–6). **Propranolol** (case where concurrent akathisia also improved; n = 2, Amir et al, Clin Neuropharmacol 1997;**20**:86–9). **Lamotrigine** has been used successfully (n = 1, McMeekin, J S C Med Assoc 2007;**103**:69–73).

Dysphagia

Difficulty in swallowing or painful swallowing has been reported with many antipsychotics.

Reviews: drug-induced (Bulling, *Aust N Z J Med* 1999;**29**:748) and neuroleptic dysphagia (Sokoloff and Pavlakovic, *Dysphagia* 1997;**12**:177–9).

Antipsychotics	Dysphagia generally responds rapidly to discontinuation (e.g. n = 1, Stewart, *Dysphagia* 2003;**18**:274–5). In life-threatening dysphagia, **benzodiazepines** (clonazepam) or oral **anticholinergics** may be effective (trihexyphenidyl, n = 2, Hayashi *et al*, *Clin Neuropharmacol* 1997;**20**:77–81; benzatropine, n = 1, Nair *et al*, *Gen Hosp Psychiatry* 2001;**23**:231–2), although if used regularly, anticholinergics may be a causative or exacerbating factor.

EPSE, akathisia

Neuroleptic-induced akathisia (NIA) is a subjective unpleasant feeling of inner restlessness and the urge to move, with rocking while standing or sitting, lifting feet as if marching on the spot, and crossing and uncrossing legs while sitting. NIA has been associated with suicidal behaviour (s = 83, Hansen, *Hum Psychopharmacol* 2001;**16**:495–505) and subjective cognitive dysfunction and so needs treating (n = 67, Kim and Byun, *J Clin Pharm Ther* 2007;**32**:461–7). It is probably an imbalance of cortical and nigrostriatal dopaminergic innervation and has been reported with other drugs.

Reviews: general (Miller and Fleischhacker, *Drug Saf* 2000;**22**:73–81;71 refs), effect on clinical outcome (n = 34, Luthra *et al*, *Gen Hosp Psychiatry* 2000;**22**:276–80), use of serotonin-based drugs (Poyurovsky and Weizman, *Br J Psychiatry* 2001;**179**:4–8; including an algorithm), NIA and violence (Leong and Silva, *J Forensic Sci* 2003;**48**:187–9).

Antidepressants	**Reduce** the dose, as it is dose-related at least for fluoxetine (n = 1, Hansen, *J Psychopharmacol* 2003;**17**:451–2). **Switch** antidepressants, e.g. **paroxetine** for fluoxetine-induced (n = 1, Bauer *et al*, *J Clin Psychiatry* 1996;**57**:593–4) or **mianserin** 15 mg/d (n = 1, Poyurovsky *et al*, *Int Clin Psychopharmacol* 1995;**10**:111–4). **Propranolol** has also been used if fluoxetine-induced (Fleischhacker, *Biol Psychiatry* 1991;**30**:531–2). **Review:** SSRI-induced akathisia (Koliscak and Makela, *J Am Pharm Assoc* 2009;**49**:28–36).
Antipsychotics *	**Reducing the dose or switching** antipsychotics is the main strategy. * For **aripiprazole**, reduce dose, use benzodiazepines, adrenoceptor antagonists (propranolol), gabapentin or anticholinergic agents (review, Cassano *et al*, *Clin Drug Invest* 2007;**27**:1–13; Aitchison *et al*, *J Psychopharmacol* 2009;**23**:231–4).

Adjunctive therapies:

The following drugs may be useful in the short or long-term if the dose or drug cannot be changed:

- **Anticholinergics** may have some efficacy if the akathisia forms part of an EPSE but are generally considered less useful. Biperiden 5 mg iv may be rapidly effective (within 10 minutes) for severe akathisia (n = 23, open, Hirose and Ashby, *Int J Psychiatry Med* 2000;**30**:185–94). Cochrane concludes that there is no reliable evidence to support or refute the use of anticholinergics in acute NIA (Lima *et al*, *CDSR* 2006;**4**:CD003727).
- **Benzodiazepines**, e.g. clonazepam 0.5–3 mg/d (mean 1.7 mg/d) have been used and 81% patients in one study improved, with the effect prominent in two days (n = 21, open, *Acta Psychiatr Scand* 1989;**80**:106–7). Diazepam 10–17 mg IV (at 5 mg/30sec) has also provided rapid relief of acute NIA (n = 18, open, Hirose and Ashby, *J Clin Psychiatry* 2002;**63**:524–7).
- **Beta-blockers**, e.g. propranolol 30–80 mg/d can produce a dramatic and

persistent improvement (especially if not part of an EPSE), but may take up to three months to act in chronic cases (d/b, p/c, Kramer *et al, Biol Psychiatry* 1988;**24**:823–7). Other lipophilic beta-blockers, e.g. metoprolol (RCT, Adler *et al, Biol Psychiatry* 1990;**27**:673–5) and betaxolol (n = 19, RCT, p/c, c/o, *Am J Psychiatry* 1992;**149**:647–50) may be effective for olanzapine-induced akathisia (n = 1, Kurzthaler *et al, Am J Psychiatry* 1997;**154**:1316). Nadolol, sotalol and atenolol are probably ineffective.

- **Cyproheptadine** 16 mg/d may be effective, supported by a robust trial (n = 30, RCT, d/b, 7/7, Fischel *et al, J Clin Psychopharmacol* 2001;**21**:612–5).
- **Diphenhydramine** IV may rapidly (over 30 minutes) reduce the symptoms of acute NIA from IV prochlorperazine (n = 87, open, Vinson, *J Emerg Med* 2004;**26**:265–70).
- **Gabapentin**, where a dose-related response has been reported (n = 1, Pfeffer *et al, Int Clin Psychopharmacol* 2005;**20**:179–81).
- **Mianserin** 5 mg/d may produce a significant improvement in NIA and dysphoria (n = 15, RCT, 5/7, Poyurovsky *et al, Br J Psychiatry* 1999;**174**:238–42; n = 1, Stryjer *et al, Eur Psychiatry* 2004;**19**:237–8).
- * **Mirtazapine** has a 53% response rate (cf placebo 8%) in NIA (s = 5, n=125, Hieber *et al, Ann Pharmacother* 2008;**42**:841–6), probably via 5HT2A/2C antagonism.
- **Ropinirole** 18 mg/d has helped aripiprazole-induced tardive akathisia (n = 1, Hettema and Ross, *J Clin Psychiatry* 2007;**68**:1814–5).
- **Thiamine** (vitamin B1) high-dose (1.2 g/d) may be useful for acute NIA (n = 20, RCT, p/c, d/b, 5/7, Lerner *et al, J Clin Psychiatry* 2004;**65**:1550–4).
- **Trazodone** 100 mg/d may produce a marked improvement (n = 9, 5/7, Stryjer *et al, Clin Neuropharmacol* 2003;**26**:137–41).
- **Zolmitriptan** (a selective 5HT1D inhibitor) 7.5 mg/d can produce a significant and rapid improvement in NIA, even in chronic and resistant cases, warranting further trials (n = 8, open, 3/7, Gross-Isseroff *et al, Int Clin Psychopharmacol* 2005;**20**:23–5).

Less use:

Other drugs tried, usually without success, include:

- **Amantadine** (n = 4, Zubenko *et al, J Clin Psychopharmacol* 1984;**4**:218–20).
- **Apomorphine** low dose may reduce objective (movement) effects but not subjective distress (Karstaedt and Pincus, *Neurology* 1993;**43**:611–3).
- **Buspirone** has only a minor effect, with only 20% showing any effect (n = 10, Poyurovsky and Weizman, *Int Clin Psychopharmacol* 1997;**12**:263–8).
- **Granisetron** is ineffective (n = 10, 4/7, Poyurovsky and Weizman, *Int Clin Psychopharmacol* 1999;**14**:357–60).
- * **Iron supplements** — although there is no relationship between plasma iron and chronic akathisia (Barnes *et al, Br J Psychiatry* 1992;**161**:791–6), IV iron has been used successfully in iron-deficient akathisia (n = 1, Cotter and O'Keeffe, *J Neurol Neurosurg Psychiatry* 2007;**78**:548).
- **Moclobemide** (n = 1, Ebert and Demling, *Pharmacopsychiatry* 1991;**24**: 29–31).
- **Tryptophan** (n = 6, open, *Biol Psychiatry* 1990;**27**:671–2).
- **Lorazepam** (Yassa and Grouix, *J Clin Psychopharmacol* 1989;**9**:70–1)
- **Mianserin** (n = 1, Poyurovsky *et al, Int Clin Psychopharmacol* 1995;**10**:261–3).

Lithium *

EPSE, dyskinesias (acute or tardive)

Tardive dyskinesia (TD) is an involuntary hyperkinesia, which increases with anxiety, goes away during sleep and in some cases may be irreversible. Symptoms include choreas, tics, dystonias and orolingual dyskinesias, but not tremor. It is generally seen as repetitive, involuntary and purposeless movements of, e.g. the tongue, neck and jaw. It may be a late symptom of schizophrenia and antipsychotics might in fact just bring such symptoms forward (rather than cause them), e.g. brain structures are similar (n=93, McCreadie et al, Arch Gen Psychiatry 2002;**59**:332–6) and TD fluctuates with time (n=37, McCreadie et al, Br J Psychiatry 2002;**181**:135–7).

Risk factors include the length of exposure to antipsychotics in the elderly, alcohol consumption, advancing age, being male, previous head injury, presence of organic brain disease, structural brain damage, earlier drug-induced Parkinsonism, akathisia or dystonias, being left-handed, being diabetic, concurrent affective or negative symptoms and having a parent with schizophrenia who themselves has or had a dyskinesia.

Reviews: * general (Correll and Schenk, Curr Opin Psychiatry 2008;**21**:151–6; Soares-Weiser and Fernandez, Semin Neurol 2007;**27**:159–69; Remington, Curr Opin Psychiatry 2007;**20**:131–7), in children (Correll and Kane, J Child Adolesc Psychopharmacol 2007;**17**:647–56), 'miscellaneous' treatments (Soares-Weiser and Joy, Cochrane Database Syst Rev 2003 2:CD000208).

Antidepressants	**Mirtazapine** has been used for bupropion-induced TD (n=1, Kohen and Sarcevic, Movement Disord 2006;**21**:584–5).
Antipsychotics *	**Withdrawal** or **dose reduction** are the usual strategies, although the risk of relapse may be high.

Drug **'holidays'** seem detrimental.

Transient dose increases may help occasionally, but only in the short-term. **Withdraw** or reduce any anticholinergic drugs if possible, as these can provoke or exacerbate TD, although are not a risk factor as such (Soares and McGrath, CDSR 2000;**2**:CD000204). Indeed, trihexyphenidyl is now contraindicated for use in TD.

Switching antipsychotics: *

Switching to an atypical is usually considered the main strategy, including:

- * **Aripiprazole** may be effective if induced by quetiapine (n=1, Rizos et al, World J Biol Psychiatry 2009;**10**:54–7), risperidone (Caykoylu et al, Prog Neuropsychopharmacol Biol Psychiatry 2009;**33**:571–2) or haloperidol (n=3, Osorio et al, Neurotox Res 2010; [in press]).
- **Clozapine** may improve TD, especially with dystonic features, e.g. >50% reduction in symptoms has been seen (n=7, open, Bassitt et al, Eur Arch Psychiatr Clin Neurosci 1998;**248**:209–11) and may also be effective over the longer term (n=7, open, five years, Louza and Bassitt, J Clin Psychopharmacol 2005;**25**:180–2).
- **Olanzapine**, where there are case reports of a marked reduction in pre-existing symptoms of TD (n=2, Soutullo et al, J Clin Psychopharmacol 1999;**19**:100–1; n=2, Agarwal and Kumar, J Clin Psychiatry 2001;**62**:298–9).
- **Quetiapine** where, in a switch study, it maintained psychotic symptom control but reduced TD compared to haloperidol (n=45, RCT, 12/12, s/b, Emsley et al, J Clin Psychiatry 2004;**65**:696–701; see also n=3, Alptekin and Kivircik, Int Clin Psychopharmacol 2002;**17**:263–4). Adjunctive quetiapine has been used for risperidone-induced TD (n=1, Nelson et al, Clin Neuropharmacol 2003;**26**:297–8).
- **Risperidone**, where the response may occur in a few weeks and then be maintained (n=40, 48/52, Bai et al, Int Clin Psychopharmacol 2005;**20**:79–85; n=49, RCT, d/b, p/c, 16/52, Bai et al, J Clin Psychiatry 2003;**64**:1342–8; MS; review by Tandon, EBMH 2004;**7**:83).

Adjunctive therapies: *

Adjunctive therapies are usually considered to be of low efficacy, although tetrabenazine is licensed:

- **Tetrabenazine** is licensed in the UK, with a starting dose of 12.5 mg, titrated to 25–75 mg/d (maximum 200 mg/d). In refractory TD, tetrabenazine (mean 58 mg/d) has significantly improved AIMS scores (n = 20, 20/52, Ondo et al, Am J Psychiatry 1999;**156**:1279–81; see informal follow-up of 400 patients: n = 526, Jankovic and Beach, Neurology 1997;**48**:358–62). It may have long-term efficacy (n=448, mean 2.3 years, Kenney et al, Mov Disord 2007;**22**:193–7).
- **Amantadine** was superior to placebo in one study (d/b, c/o, p/c, 18/52, Angus et al, J Clin Psychopharmacol 1997;**17**:88–91).
- **Buspirone** at up to 180 mg/d may be useful (n = 8, open, 12/52, Moss et al, J Clin Psychopharmacol 1993;**13**:204–9).
- **Cyproheptadine** at 8–24 mg/d has significantly improved haloperidol-induced TD (n = 10, open, Lee et al, J Serotonin Res 1994;**1**:91–5).
- **Donepezil**, where a pilot study indicated that 5–10 mg/d might suppress symptoms of TD (n = 10, open, 8/52, Caroff et al, J Clin Psychiatry 2001;**62**:772–5).
- **Gabapentin** has improved long-term TD, with an average improvement of 47.5% (n = 25, open, 12/12, Hardoy et al, J Affect Disord 2003;**75**:125–30).
- **Galantamine** 8–24 mg/d as an adjunct to stable antipsychotic doses has reduced AIMS-rated scores, but not statistically significant, although there was a statistically significant deterioration on discontinuation (n = 35, RCT, d/b, p/c, c/o, 2 × 12/52, Caroff et al, J Clin Psychiatry 2007;**68**:410–5; MS).
- **Levetiracetam** (500–3000 mg/d) was well tolerated and significantly reduced AIMS scores (43% vs 19%) compared to placebo (n = 50, RCT, d/b, p/c, 12/52, Woods et al, J Clin Psychiatry 2008;**69**:546–54; see also n = 16, open, 3/12, Meco et al, Clin Neuropharmacol 2006;**29**:265–8).
- **Melatonin** 10 mg/d has been shown to decrease AIMS scores in TD (n = 22, d/b, p/c, c/o, 6/52, Shamir et al, Arch Gen Psychiatry 2001;**58**:1049–52).
- **Naltrexone** plus clonazepam have reduced TD scores compared with each drug individually (n = 23, RCT, d/b, p/c, Wonodi et al, J Clin Psychopharmacol 2004;**24**:441–5).
- **Ondansetron** (a 5-HT3 antagonist) 12 mg/d has been used successfully (n = 12, open, 12/52, Sirota et al, Am J Psychiatry 2000;**157**:287–9; although this could have been an interaction).
- **Piracetam** (mean 4800 mg/d) appears to be effective for TD symptoms (n = 40, RCT, d/b, p/c, c/o, 2 × 4/52, Libov et al, J Clin Psychiatry 2007;**68**:1031–7).
- **Pyridoxine** (Vitamin B6) 200 mg/d has produced a rapid and sustained reduction in TD symptoms (e.g. n = 1, Lerner and Liberman, J Clin Psychiatry 1998;**59**:623–4) and 1200 mg/d was clearly superior to placebo for reducing the symptoms of TD (n = 50, RCT, d/b, p/c, c/o, 26/52, Lerner et al, J Clin Psychiatry 2007;**68**:1648–54).
- * **Sodium oxybate** resolved olanzapine-induced TD, with a 2/52 latency of onset (n = 1, Berner, J Clin Psychiatry 2008;**69**:862).
- **Thiamine** was effective in one small but careful study (n = 15, RCT, d/b, p/c, 4/52, Lerner et al, Am J Psychiatry 2001;**158**:1511–4).
- * **Yi-gan san**, Japanese herbal medicine (n = 22, open, 12/52, Miyaoka et al, Prog Neuropsychopharmacol Biol Psychiatry 2008;**32**:761–4).
- * **Zopiclone** has been used (n = 1, Sugawara et al, Prog Neuropsychopharmacol Biol Psychiatry 2009;**33**:727–8).

Less useful:

Many adjunctive therapies have been tried but few have any real use. The following are not in the useful group:

- **Baclofen**, see GABA agonists.
- **Benzodiazepines** have been used but Cochrane concludes that they have no proven advantage over placebo (Bhoopathi and Soares-Weiser, *Cochrane Database Syst Rev* 2000;**2**:CD000205).
- **Calcium-channel blocker** use is not supported by any robust studies (s = 0, n = 0, Soares-Weiser and Rathbone, *Cochrane Database Syst Rev* 2004;**1**:CD000206), although older reviews were more positive (review by Cates *et al*, *Ann Pharmacother* 1993;**27**:191–6, 14 refs).
- **Cholinergic drugs** (e.g. choline, lecithin, ACEIs) are probably ineffective (see systematic review; s = 11, n = 261, RCTs, Tammenmaa *et al*, *Prog Neuropsychopharmacol Biol Psychiatry* 2004;**28**:1099–107).
- **Citalopram** was ineffective in one study (n = 13, Korsgaard *et al*, *Clin Neuropharmacol* 1986;**9**:52–7).
- **GABA agonists/enhancers** such as baclofen and valproate. Cochrane concludes from the eight small, short-term studies that the evidence is inconclusive and unconvincing (s=8, n=547, Soares *et al*, *Cochrane Database Syst Rev* 2004;**4**:CD000203).
- **Insulin** (low-dose) has been suggested as superior to placebo (see McGrath and Soares, *Cochrane Database Syst Rev* 2000;**2**:CD000208).
- **Lithium** has no consistent positive effect (e.g. Yassa *et al*, *Can J Psychiatry* 1984;**29**:36–7) and may even be detrimental.
- **Valproate**, see GABA agonists.
- **Vitamin E** probably has no significant effect (up to 1600 iu/d; n = 40, RCT, 20/52, Dorevitch *et al*, *Biol Psychiatry* 1997;**41**:114; n = 158, RCT, up to two years, Adler *et al*, *Arch Gen Psychiatry* 1999;**56**:836–41; Soares and McGrath, *CDSR* 2000;**2**:CD000209), but may perhaps be effective in a small subgroup of patients (s = 18, Boomershine *et al*, *Ann Pharmacother* 1999;**33**:1195–202).

EPSE, Parkinsonism

Pseudoparkinsonism or Parkinsonian side-effects include akinesia, rigidity, bradykinesia and coarse tremor at rest. They are usually associated with antipsychotics but can occur with many drugs (*Chapter 5.8*).

Antidepressants, (especially tricyclics)	**Switch drugs** or treat as per antipsychotics. **Benzodiazepines**, e.g. diazepam (mentioned in Pollack and Rosenbaum, *J Clin Psychiatry* 1987;**48**:3–8). **Propranolol** 40–120 mg/d has been used (mentioned in Pollack and Rosenbaum, *J Clin Psychiatry* 1987;**48**:3–8). **Review:** Gill *et al*, *J Clin Psychopharmacol* 1997;**17**:377–89.
Antipsychotics	**Dose reduction** of any antipsychotic. **Switch** to an antipsychotic with lower EPS, e.g. quetiapine, olanzapine or aripiprazole. **Anticholinergics** (antimuscarinics) are first-line treatments. They include **benzatropine** (also has antihistaminic properties and a long half-life of up to 24 hours), **orphenadrine** (which is probably more toxic: Slørdal and Gjerden, *Br J Psychiatry* 1999;**174**:275–6), **procyclidine** (with a disputed abuse potential) and **trihexyphenidyl** (benzhexol; with a reported abuse and dependence potential; Frauger *et al*, *Therapie* 2003;**58**:541–7). They may improve survival (n = 88, 10-year prospective study, Waddington *et*

al, Br J Psychiatry 1998;**173**:325–9) and compliance, and may actually only be detrimental to positive symptoms during acute phases (when excess dopaminergic activity is thought to occur) but not during stable phases (Tandon and Dequardo, *Am J Psychiatry* 1995;**152**:814–5). Anticholinergics may adversely effect memory, exacerbate TD, and abrupt withdrawal can produce rebound EPS and cholinergic rebound. They are best prescribed only for overt symptoms and discontinued gradually after three months, reinstated only if symptoms reappear. If, however, they aid long-term compliance that may be a benefit that outweighs the risks.

Review: managing antipsychotic-induced parkinsonism (Mamo *et al*, *Drug Saf* 1999;**20**:269–75).

Adjunctive therapies:

* **Diphenhydramine** 25–300 mg (oral or parenteral) may rapidly be effective (within minutes) and maintenance doses of 25–50 mg TDS have been widely used (n = 5, RCT, Granana *et al*, *Medicina* [B Aires] 1999;**59**:38–42).
* **Donepezil** may have some use in treating EPSE in the elderly (n = 7, open, Bergman *et al*, *J Clin Psychiatry* 2005;**66**:107–10).
* **Estrogen** at high plasma levels has been reported to reduce hyperkinetic symptoms of EPSE in women with psychosis (n = 25, RCT, Thompson *et al*, *Acta Psychiatr Scand* 2000;**101**:130–4).
* **Iron supplementation** may help EPSE if associated with iron-deficient anaemia (n = 1, Yoshida *et al*, *Nihon Shinkei Seishin Yakurigaku Zasshi* 2004;**24**:29–31).
* **Kava special extract** WS1490 has been claimed to significantly improve EPSE (n = 42, open, Boerner and Klement, *Wien Med Wochenschr* 2004; **154**:508–10).
* **Zolpidem** 5 mg QDS has been used successfully to treat persistent and unresponsive EPSE (n = 1, Farver and Khan, *Ann Pharmacother* 2001; **35**:435–7).

Less use:

Some drugs that have been tried but failed include:

* **Amantadine** is not recommended for EPSE but may be effective (d/b, c/o, Silver *et al*, *J Clin Psychiatry* 1995;**56**:167–70) and better tolerated than anticholinergics in elderly patients (review by Mamo *et al*, *Drug Saf* 1999; **20**:269–75).
* **Calcium** orally.
* **Mianserin** is ineffective (Korsgaard and Friis, *Psychopharmacol* [Berl] 1986;**88**:109–11).
* **Quinine**.

EPSE, dystonia (including oculogyric crisis)

Dystonia is a syndrome of sustained or slow involuntary muscular contractions, resulting in twisting of the neck, limbs, trunk or face. Acute dystonia from antipsychotics is more likely to occur in younger and more severely ill people, especially if antipsychotic-naïve. It can present as an oculogyric crisis (review by Abe, *World J Biol Psychiatry* 2006;**7**:70–4).

Review: general (Balash and Giladi, *Eur J Neurol* 2004;**11**:361–70).

Antidepressants	**Switching drugs** is the main strategy.
	Epinephrine 0.3 mg has been used for escitalopram-induced oculogyric dystonia (n = 1, Patel and Simon, *Int Arch Allergy Immunol* 2006;**140**:27–9).
	Mianserin has been used at low dose for fluoxetine-induced dystonia (Poyurovsky *et al*, *Mov Disord* 1997;**12**:1102–5).

Antipsychotics **Acute dystonia:**
- **Anticholinergics** are usually effective for acute dystonias (e.g. laryngeal dystonia: Christodoulou and Kalaitzi, *J Psychopharmacol* 2005;**19**:307–11) and **procyclidine** is the standard UK treatment.
- **Diphenhydramine** (oral or parenteral) can be used and has been reported to produce rapid reversal of dystonic reactions, e.g. oculogyric crisis (Leigh *et al*, *Ann Neurol* 1987;**22**:3–17).

Tardive dystonia:
Switching antipsychotic is the first choice strategy:
- **Clozapine** may improve severe and persistent (e.g. Sieche and Giedke, *J Clin Psychiatry* 2000;**61**:949).
- **Olanzapine** may have some role (n = 4, s/b, Lucetti *et al*, *Clin Neuropharmacol* 2002;**25**:71–4).
- **Quetiapine** has been used if the dystonia is induced by risperidone, olanzapine (n = 2, Gourzis *et al*, *Clin Neuropharmacol* 2005;**28**:195–6; n = 1, Sasaki *et al*, *J Clin Psychiatry* 2004;**65**:583–4) or amisulpride (n = 1, Fountoulakis *et al*, *Schizophr Res* 2006;**88**:232–4).

Others:
In resistant cases, other strategies may be worth trying:
- **Benzodiazepines** — a multiple drug-resistant disabling dystonia responded partly to clozapine and virtually completely when clonazepam was added (n = 1, Shapleske *et al*, *Br J Psychiatry* 1996;**168**:516–8).
- **Botulinum toxin** may possibly relieve the pain and symptoms of dystonia (n = 34, open, Tarsy *et al*, *Clin Neuropharmacol* 1997;**20**:90–3).
- **Levodopa** combined with an anticholinergic has been used (n = 1, Looper and Chouinard, *Can J Psychiatry* 1998;**43**:646–7).
- **Levetiracetam** has helped generalised dystonia (n = 1, 20/52, Sullivan *et al*, *Parkinsonism Relat Disord* 2005;**11**:469–71).
- **Tetrabenazine** has been used for olanzapine-induced tardive dystonia (n = 1, Rauchverger *et al*, *J Neuropsychiatry Clin Neurosci* 2007;**19**:484–5).

Less useful:
- **Anticholinergics** are less effective in tardive dystonia (e.g. n = 32, Wojcik *et al*, *Am J Psychiatry* 1991;**148**:1055–9).
- **Carbamazepine** is ineffective (*Psychopharmacol Bull* 1985;**21**;345–6). Other drugs tried include baclofen and bromocriptine.

Laryngospasm (see also dystonia)
Benzodiazepines **Flumazenil** may be effective in 25 minutes if laryngospasm is midazolam-induced (n = 1, Davis *et al*, *Ann Emerg Med* 1998;**32**:263–5).

Myoclonus
Myoclonus presents as shock-like, involuntary movements. It can also be caused by CNS infections, systemic metabolic disorders or neurodegenerative disorders. General management includes:
- **Discontinuation, switching** or **dose reduction** usually resolves myoclonus.
- It can be a symptom of serotonin syndrome and akathisia, so exclude these first.
- **Discontinue** any other causative drugs, e.g. levodopa, tricyclics, lamotrigine (n = 1, Rosenhagen *et al*, *J Clin Psychopharmacol* 2006;**26**:346–7) and bismuth salts (including OTC products).

Review: Jimenez-Jimenez, *CNS Drugs* 2004;**18**:93–104.

Other strategies:
Antidepressants **Valproate**, if sertraline-induced (n = 1, Ghaziuddin *et al*, *J Child Adolesc Psychopharmacol* 2001;**11**:199–202).
Antipsychotics **Carbamazepine**, if clozapine-induced, but beware of the potential interaction (n = 5, Bak *et al*, *J Clin Psychiatry* 1995;**56**:418–22).

Haloperidol may be an alternative if olanzapine-induced (n = 1, Camacho *et al, Clin Neuropharmacol* 2005;**28**:145–7).

Valproate, if clozapine-induced (n = 1, Meltzer and Ranjan, *Am J Psychiatry* 1994;**151**:1246–7).

Pisa syndrome (antipsychotic-induced pleurothonus)

Persistent dystonia of the trunk is a rare ADR from long-term antipsychotics.

Review: Suzuki and Matsuzaka, *CNS Drugs* 2002;**16**:165–74.

Antipsychotics	**Switching** to olanzapine has worked if risperidone-induced (n = 1, Nishimura *et al, J Neuropsychiatry Clin Neurosci* 2007;**19**:202–3).
	Switching to clozapine has worked if olanzapine-induced, with psychotic symptoms improved and Pisa syndrome declined over six weeks (n = 1, Arora *et al, Ann Pharmacother* 2006;**40**:2273–5).
	Anticholinergics help about 40% (n = 1, Bhattacharya *et al, Mov Disord* 2000;**15**:1285–7; Suzuki *et al, J Clin Psychopharmacol* 1999;**19**:277–80).
Galantamine *	**Memantine** has been used as an alternative (Chen *et al, Int J Geriatr Psychiatry* 2008;**23**:660–1).

Restless legs (may also be akathisia)

Antidepressants *	Although there are anecdotal reports, there is no clear association between antidepressants and restless legs (n = 200, Brown *et al, Sleep Med* 2005;**6**:443–50).
	Re-exposure may be possible without recurrence with **mirtazapine** (n = 1, Pae *et al, Psychiatr Clin Neurosci* 2004;**58**:669–70).
	* **Exclude other drugs**, e.g. D2 receptor antagonists such as domperidone (n = 1, Chang *et al, Prog Neuropsychopharmacol Biol Psychiatry* 2006;**30**:316–8), tramadol and dopamine-blockers, plus possibly antihistamines and non-opioid analgesics (n = 14, Kim *et al, Hum Psychopharmacol* 2008;**23**:615–20).
	Bupropion may be a therapy in its own right (n = 3, Kim *et al, Clin Neuropharmacol* 2005;**28**:298–301).
Antipsychotics *	**Benzodiazepines, e.g. clonazepam** have been used (n = 1, Horiguchi *et al, Int Clin Psychopharmacol* 1999;**14**:33–6).
	* **Ropinirole** — has been used if caused by olanzapine (n = 5, Kang *et al, J Psychopharmacol* 2009;**23**:597–601) or quetiapine (n = 2, Urbano and Ware, *J Clin Psychopharmacol* 2008;**28**:704–5).

Tremor (see EPSE, Parkinsonism and under 'others')

6.8 Neuroleptic malignant syndrome (NMS)

NMS is a rare and potentially fatal idiosyncratic dose-independent ADR resulting in a sudden loss in control of body temperature. The main symptoms are hyperthermia or fever and severe muscle rigidity, with two or more of: diaphoresis, dysphagia, tremor, incontinence, altered consciousness, tachycardia, altered blood pressure, leucocytosis and raised creatinine phosphokinase concentration. Body temperature rises rapidly and can be fatal in 1–3 days, although death rates are reducing due to increased awareness, early intervention, and the use of newer antipsychotics (n = 68, Ananth *et al, J Clin Psychiatry* 2004;**65**:464–70). It is probably caused by a sudden over-blockade of dopaminergic function, resulting in a disruption to the thermoregulatory centre.

Risk factors include: *

- **History** (previous NMS, known cerebral compromise, previous ECT).
- **Mental state** (agitation, overactive and/or in need of restraint or seclusion, catatonia, affective disorder [Berardi *et al, Hum Psychopharmacol* 2002;**17**:99–102], mental retardation).
- **Physical state** (dehydration, postpartum, Parkinson's disease, young and male, high serum creatinine phosphokinase [n = 32, Hermesh *et al, J Clin Psychopharmacol* 2002;**22**:252–6]).

- **Drugs** (see *Chapter 5.9*, e.g. high potency antipsychotics, IM therapy, high doses over short periods, abrupt or recent changes, rapid neuroleptisation, and concurrent MAOIs and carbamazepine).
- **Genetic** vulnerability (n = 2 siblings, Ziegenbein *et al, Ann Pharmacother* 2006;**40**:574–5)
- **Catatonia**, also a prodromal state (n = 17, White and Robins, *CNS Spectr* 2000;**5**:58–65).

Neuroleptic rechallenge:
Rechallenge with antipsychotics may show a high rate of recurrence, although most people may be able to tolerate antipsychotics again if monitored carefully and a two-week recovery period is allowed (n = 15, Rosebush *et al, J Clin Psychiatry* 1989;**50**:295–8). Rechallenge with clozapine has been successful (Weller and Kornhuber, *Br J Psychiatry* 1992;**161**:855–6). Depots are contraindicated.

Reviews: risk factors (Gupta *et al, Int J Psychiatry* 2003;**45**:30–5; n = 20, Berardi *et al, Hum Psychopharmacol* 2002;**17**:99–102; n = 15, controls n = 45, Viejo *et al, Acta Psychiatr Scand* 2003;**107**:45–9), general (*Prescriber* 2006;**17**:18–23; Strawn *et al, Am J Psychiatry* 2007;**164**:870–6).

Antipsychotics	**Immediate management** is essential.

Withdraw any antipsychotics, lithium and antidepressants.

Correct any dehydration and hyperpyrexia, e.g. using ice packs, re-hydration, and sedation with benzodiazepines if necessary.

Measure WCC, U&E, LFT and CPK to assess diagnosis, cause and response.

Manage acute symptoms, initially using a first-line agent below:

First line strategies:

- **Dantrolene** IV (a skeletal muscle relaxant used for malignant hyperthermia) is usually the treatment of choice. It reduces the duration and mortality of NMS (n = 9, Nisijima and Ishiguro, *Biol Psychiatry* 1993;**33**:45–8) and reduces body temperature in 2–24 hours. There are some views that it might prolong the course of symptoms compared to supportive therapy (Rosebush *et al, Br J Psychiatry* 1991;**148**:709–12).
- **Bromocriptine** 7.5–60 mg/d reduces the duration and mortality of NMS (Sakkas *et al, Psychopharmacol Bull* 1991;**27**:381–4). There are some views that it might sometimes prolong the course of symptoms compared to supportive therapy (Rosebush *et al, Br J Psychiatry* 1991;**148**:709–12).
- **Amantadine** 100 mg BD may be the third-line choice (mentioned by Waldorf, *AANA J* 2003;**71**:389–94).

Other strategies:

- **Anaesthetics** have been used for emergency treatment in a person recovering from NMS (Parke and Wheatley, *Anesthesia* 1992;**47**:908–9).
- **Anticoagulants** used to provide complete anticoagulation have been suggested as adjunctive therapy to reduce death as a result of pulmonary embolism (van Harten and van Agtmael, *Am J Psychiatry* 1995;**152**:1103).
- **Apomorphine** s/c 2 mg three-hourly for three days then 2 mg QD for two days can improve NMS significantly (n = 1, Lattanzi *et al, Am J Psychiatry* 2006;**163**:1450–1), and as rapidly as monotherapy (n = 1, Wang and Hsieh, *Movement Disord* 2001;**16**:765–7; n = 1, Gambassi *et al, Aging Clin Exp Res* 2006;**18**:266–70).
- **Benzodiazepines** (IV lorazepam or diazepam) can be used if dantrolene and bromocriptine have failed. Predominantly, catatonic symptoms may rapidly respond to diazepam, including via continuous IV administration (Miyaoka *et al, Am J Psychiatry* 1997;**153**:882), although its longer half-life may complicate recovery (Velamoor, *Br J Psychiatry* 1992;**160**:135–6).
- **ECT** has been used for low-dose quetiapine-induced NMS (n = 1, Bora *et al, Eur Psychiatry* 2003;**18**:323).
- **Levodopa** IV may be an effective alternative to dantrolene (Nisijima *et al,*

Biol Psychiatry 1997;**41**:913–4), as may carbidopa/levodopa (Shoop and Cernek, *Ann Pharmacother* 1997;**31**:119).

- **Nifedipine** 25 mg s/l has been used (Talley and Taylor, *Psychosomatics* 1994;**35**:168–70).

Aftercare:

1. Review NMS symptoms to confirm diagnosis.
2. Review psychiatric diagnosis and the need for further antipsychotics.
3. Consider alternative management strategies.
4. Leave as long a gap as possible before restarting antipsychotics (e.g. 14 days), considering also the risks of untreated psychosis.
5. Choose an antipsychotic from a different group to the causative agent, particularly of low potency or any previously used without problem. Start low and go slow. Contraindicate depots.
6. Perform alternate day CPK monitoring, interpreted in the context of the global clinical picture.
7. Perform daily temperature, pulse and muscle tone measures, weekly wbcs and ensure adequate hydration and nutrition.
8. Obtain an informal or formal second opinion, as informed consent for re-exposure may not be possible. Inform family and carers of the decisions and risks (and document this).
9. Educate patients, carers and care team of the symptoms of early NMS and of the appropriate action to take, ie. seek urgent medical advice.

Review: guidelines for the re-introduction of antipsychotics following NMS (Williams and MacPherson, *Irish J Psychiatr Med* 1997;**14**:147–8).

6.9 Serotonin syndrome

This potentially dangerous adverse reaction is attributed to a toxic hyperserotonergic state from hyper-stimulation of the brain stem and spinal chord 5HT1A and 5HT2 receptors. Onset is usually within a few hours of drug or dose changes, usually resolves in about 24 hours and can be fatal.

Sternbach's diagnostic criteria

1. At least three of the following: mental state changes (e.g. confusion), agitation/restlessness, sweating, diarrhoea, fever, hyperreflexia, tachycardia, myoclonus, lack of co-ordination, shivering, and tremor. Other symptoms can include nausea, vomiting, tachycardia, myoclonus, hypertension, convulsions and multiple organ failure.
2. Other causes ruled out, e.g. infection, metabolic disturbances, substance abuse or withdrawal.
3. No concurrent antipsychotic dose changes.

The Hunter Serotonin Toxicity Criteria (Dunkley et al, *QJM* 2003;**96**:635–42) may be more specific and an alternative to Sternbach's criteria.

Reviews: general (Isbister et al, *Med J Aust* 2007;**187**:361–5; Boyer and Shannon, *N Engl J Med* 2005;**352**:1112–20; Gillman, *Biol Psychiatry* 2006;**59**:1046–51), Serotonin Syndrome Rating Scale to aid diagnosis (Hegerl et al, *Eur Arch Psych Clin Neurosci* 1998;**248**:96–103).

All drugs [*]   **Discontinue** all serotonergic drugs (see *Chapter 5.14*), including over-the-counter sympathomimetics (usually adequate management in mild cases).

Symptomatic support, e.g. cooling blankets and fans.

Benzodiazepines, e.g. lorazepam (1–2 mg by slow IV injection every 30 minutes until excessive sedation occurs) may be superior to clonazepam, which has a lower affinity for peripheral benzodiazepine receptors (e.g. Nierenberg and Semprebon, *Clin Pharmacol Ther* 1993;**53**:84–8).

Chlorpromazine has been used for its sedative effect (n = 1, Graham, *Med J Aust* 1997;**166**:166–7).

* **Cyproheptadine** (a non-specific 5-HT blocker) at 4–8 mg orally (but perhaps as high as 10–20 mg), repeated every 2–4 hours up to 0.5 mg kg/d maximum (beware of urinary retention) has been claimed to be the best antiserotonergic drug strategy, with case reports of rapid success (n = 3, McDaniel, *Ann Pharmacother* 2001;**35**:870–3; Baigel, *Eur J Anaesthiol* 2003;**20**:586–8; n=2, Levin *et al*, *Gen Hosp Psychiatry* 2008;**30**:372–7).
Mirtazapine blocks 5-HT2 and 5-HT3 receptors and may reduce serotonergic toxicity (Hoes, *Pharmacopsychiatry* 1996;**29**:81).
* **Nitroglycerin** (2 mg/kg/min) has been reported to be rapidly successful in severe SS (n = 1, Brown and Skop, *Ann Pharmacother* 1996;**30**:191; n = 1, Brown, *Am J Emerg Med* 2004;**22**:510).
Propranolol (1–3 mg every five minutes, up to 0.1 mg/kg) may be useful, as it blocks 5-HT1A and 5-HT2 receptors (Guze and Baxter, *J Clin Psychopharmacol* 1986;**6**:119–20).

6.10 Sexual side-effects

General
The main stages of sexual activity that can be affected by psychotropics (as well as, of course, the conditions they may be treating) are libido, arousal/lubrication, erectile issues and orgasmic disorders. Many studies do not differentiate between these stages and refer to generic 'sexual dysfunction'. This section includes general advice and then stage-specific strategies to improve sexual problems.
Review: female sexual dysfunction (Clayton, *J Clin Psychiatry* 2006;**67**:991–2).

General sexual dysfunction
Anticonvulsants *   Switching drugs:
* * **Lamotrigine** improves sexual function, testosterone levels and gonadal efficiency compared to carbamazepine and phenytoin (n = 85, Herzog *et al*, *Neurology* 2005;**65**:1016–20). It improves most measures of sexual function, especially in women, including people both starting on lamotrigine as a first anticonvulsant (n = 79) and those switching (n = 62) on to it (n = 141, open, 8/12, Gil-Nagel *et al*, *Seizure* 2006;**15**:142–9).
* * **Levetiracetam** has no apparent adverse sexual or endocrine effects in men or women (n = 136, p/c, Svalheim *et al*, *Epilepsy Behav* 2009;**16**:281–7).
* * **Oxcarbazepine** — in 228 males with epilepsy and pre-existing sexual dysfunction, 79% showed improvement when switched to oxcarbazepine and 10% had no problems at the trial end with the effect more marked if they had previously been on an enzyme-inducing AED (n=673, 12/52, Luef *et al*, *Acta Neurol Scand* 2009;**119**:94–9). Carbamazepine significantly reduces testosterone levels and androgen levels in men and women, which will adversely effect sexual function (n = 160, RCT, d/b, 12/12, Lossius *et al*, *Epilepsia* 2007;**48**:1875–82), so don't switch to it.
Exogenous testosterone and **aromatase inhibitors** (to reduce testosterone's metabolism) have been tried for male sexual dysfunction.
Reviews: general (Stimmel and Gutierrez, *CNS Spectr* 2006;**11**[8 Suppl 9]:31–7; Montouris *et al*, *Epilepsy Behav* 2005;**7** Suppl 2:S7–14).
Antidepressants *   * **General interventions** include behavioural strategies, psychotherapy, delaying drug intake until after sexual activity, reduction in dosage, drug holidays, adjuvants and switching. Sexual side-effects from SSRIs do not seem to abate with time (n = 119, Landén *et al*, *J Clin Psychiatry* 2005;**66**:100–6).

Untreated MDD symptoms may have a greater impact on global sexual functioning than actual antidepressant ADRs (n = 114, RCT, d/b, p/c, 8/52, Clayton et al, J Sex Med 2007;**4**:917–29; n=70, RCT, d/b, 8/52, Lanza di Scalea et al, J Clin Psychiatry 2009;**70**:423–8).

Switch drugs:

* * Switching antidepressants is often the main strategy. The adverse effect in decreasing order of impact is sertraline, venlafaxine, citalopram, paroxetine, fluoxetine, imipramine, phenelzine, duloxetine, escitalopram, and fluvoxamine, with no difference from placebo shown with agomelatine, amineptine, bupropion, moclobemide and mirtazapine (meta-analysis by Serretti and Chiesa, J Clin Psychopharmacol 2009;**29**:259–66).

- * Agomelatine has minimal effect compared to paroxetine (n = 92 healthy males, RCT, p/c, d/b, 8/52, Montejo et al, J Psychopharmacol 2010;**24**:111–20) and venlafaxine (n = 276 (n = 193 sexually active; n = 111 remitted], d/b, 12/52, Kennedy et al, J Clin Psychopharmacol 2008;**28**:329–33).

- * Bupropion has placebo-level sexual ADRs (s = 7, n = 1463, RCT, d/b, Thase et al, J Clin Psychiatry 2005;**66**:974–81), but is probably not effective as an adjunct in SSRI-induced sexual dysfunction (s = 3, RCTs, review by Demyttenaere and Jaspers, J Psychopharmacol 2008;**22**:792–804).

- Escitalopram has been claimed to have less sexual ADRs than similar antidepressants (Ashton et al, J Sex Marital Ther 2005;**31**:257–62).

- Mirtazapine has lower sexual ADRs than other antidepressants, apart from the potentially counter-productive sedation (n = 78, open, 6/12, Saiz-Ruiz et al, Hum Psychopharmacol 2005;**20**:435–40; n = 102, open, 6/12, Osvath et al, Neuropsychopharmacol Hung 2005;**7**:177–86).

- Moclobemide may have lower sexual ADRs (n = 5, open, Ramasubbu, J Psychiatr Neurosci 1999;**224**:45–50).

- * Pregabalin has reversed citalopram-induced sexual dysfunction within 3/7 in GAD in males suffering from poor libido, arousal and orgasmic satisfaction (n=2, Oulis et al, J Clin Psychopharmacol 2008;**28**:362–3).

- Reboxetine lacks serotonin-related sexual ADRs (n = 450, RCT, d/b, 8/52, Clayton et al, Int Clin Psychopharmacol 2003;**18**:151–6; 6% incidence vs 39% with citalopram in women; n = 357, RCT, d/b, 24/52, Langworth et al, J Clin Psychopharmacol 2006;**26**:121–7).

Adjunctive therapies:

- Ephedrine 50mg was shown to be effective for SSRI-induced sexual dysfunction but, then again, so was placebo (n = 19 women, RCT, p/c, c/o, 8/52, Meston, J Sex Marital Ther 2004;**30**:57–68).

- Gingko biloba (some spectacular individual responses have been noted but no statistically significant differences; n = 24 [c = 11], RCT, t/b, p/c, 12/52, Wheatley, Hum Psychopharmacol 2004;**19**:545–8).

- * Methylphenidate OROS was ineffective in improving antidepressant-induced sexual dysfunction but at least it did not exacerbate the dysfunction (Pae et al, Clin Neuropharmacol 2009;**32**:85–8).

- Ropinirole up to 2–4mg/d was effective in 54% (n = 13 [3F, 10M], open, 4/52, Worthington et al, Int Clin Psychopharmacol 2002; **17**:307–10).

- * Sildenafil 50–100mg may help all domains of sexual function in women (n = 49, RCT, d/b, p/c, 8/52, Nurnberg et al, JAMA 2008;**300**:395–404).

- * Trazodone, a 5HT2A antagonist, has been associated with improvement in sexual function as an adjunct in people with SSRI-induced sexual dysfunction in all four domains (n = 20 [c = 15], Stryjer et al, Clin Neuropharmacol 2009;**32**:82–4).

No efficacy:
- **Granisetron** (n = 12, RCT, d/b, p/c, 14/7, Jespersen et al, Int Clin Psychopharmacol 2004;**19**:161–4).

Reviews: * managing antidepressant-induced sexual dysfunction (Taylor, Curr Psychiatry Rep 2006;**8**:431–6; Rudkin et al, Cochrane Database Syst Rev 2004;**4**:CD003382; Tayor et al, J Affect Disord 2005;**88**:241–54; Balon and Segraves, J Sex Marital Ther 2008;**34**:353–65), sexual ADRs of newer antidepressants (Schweitzer et al, Aust N Z J Psychiatry 2009;**43**:795–808).

Antipsychotics

* Sexual dysfunction occurs at higher rates in schizophrenia (86–96%) than in the general population (n = 179, MacDonald et al, Br J Psychiatry 2003;**182**:50–6). 40–60% feel that psychotropics cause their sexual problems and 42% men and 15% women have admitted that they had stopped their medication at some point due to this side-effect (n = 51, Rosenberg et al, J Sex Marital Ther 2003;**29**:289–96). Sexual dysfunction may occur in 45% people on typicals, with hyperprolactinaemia the predominant cause (n = 101, Smith et al, Br J Psychiatry 2002;**181**:49–55). However, raised prolactin may not necessarily be the only cause as in first episodes sexual dysfunction may occur despite normal prolactin levels (n = 74, open, van Bruggen et al, Psychoneuroendocrinology 2009;**34**:989–95).

General principles:

Normalise prolactin, e.g. by switching to a prolactin-sparing antipsychotic such as olanzapine (Ahl et al, Ann N Y Acad Sci 2004;**1032**:289–90) or quetiapine (cf risperidone and fluphenazine; n = 27, RCT, d/b, Kelly and Conley, Psychoneuroendocrinology 2006;**31**:340–6). **Aripiprazole** has helped either as an alternative (45%) or adjunct (55%) to another antipsychotic, with prolactin significantly reduced, improvement in libido, reduced erectile and ejaculation and reduced menstrual dysfunction, established from 12/52 and maintained for 6/12 (n = 27 [c = 22], 26/52, open, Mir et al, J Psychopharmacol 2008;**22**:244–53; see also (n = 555, RCT, open, 26/52, Hanssens et al, BMC Psychiatry 2008;**8**:95). Although olanzapine might be suitable in the short-term, prolactin levels may be little different to haloperidol at 9/12 (n = 63, RCT, 9/12, Costa et al, J Psychopharmacol 2007;**21**:165–70).

Reviews: in men (Khawaja, J Ayub Med Coll Abbottabad 2005;**17**:73–5) and in women (Smith, J Clin Psychopharmacol 2003;**23**[3 Suppl 1]:S27–32).

Libido (see also general advice section)

Libido and desire is controlled by the mesolimbic dopamine reward pathway and facilitated by NA and 5-HT. Testosterone is essential for male and estrogen and progesterone for female sexual behaviour. It is unclear to what extent psychotropics effect libido specifically.

Antidepressants   Switch drugs to, e.g. **moclobemide** (n = 5, open, Ramasubbu, J Psychiatr Neurosci 1999;**224**:45–50), **bupropion** or **mirtazapine**.

Antipsychotics   **Raised prolactin** may be the predominant cause, so check and, if raised, see the hyperprolactinaemia section for options, as bromocriptine may be of use (review, Zeitlin and Rajfer, Rev Urol 2000;**2**:39–42).

Arousal (lubrication and erection) — (see also general advice section)

Arousal mechanisms involve acetylcholine (facilitates erection/lubrication), adrenergic fibres (cause detumescence), cAMP (smooth muscle relaxation), dopamine (stimulates sexual arousal in females) and nitric oxide (activates the production of cGMP).

Review: options for oral pharmacotherapy in ED (Vitezic and Pelcic, Int J Clin Pharmacol Ther 2002;**40**;393–403).

Antidepressants	**Switching drugs** is the main strategy, e.g. to:

- **Bupropion** (n = 18 ethnic minority women, open, 10/52, Dobkin et al, *J Clin Psychopharmacol* 2006;**26**:21–6).
- **Moclobemide** (n = 5, open, Ramasubbu, *J Psychiatr Neurosci* 1999;**224**: 45–50).
- **Mirtazapine**.

Adjunctive therapies:
- * **PDE-5 inhibitors**, e.g. sildenafil are effective for drug-induced erectile dysfunction (s = 15, n = 904, Taylor et al, *J Affect Disord* 2005;**88**:241–54), including men with ED at the time of diagnosis of MDD that then persists, despite the resolution of the depressive symptoms (RCT, 12/52, Tignol et al, *Int Clin Psychopharmacol* 2004;**19**:191–9). Vardenafil 10mg is also well-tolerated and effective for ED in chronic schizophrenia, and independent of ED severity or prolactin levels (n = 25 [c = 21], open, 12/52, Mitsonis et al, *J Clin Psychiatry* 2008;**69**:206–12).
- **Pentoxifylline** may improve ED caused by borderline arterial insufficiency (n = 36, Peskircioglu et al, *Br J Urol* 1996;**77**:563–5).
- **Yohimbine** given 1–2 hours pre-intercourse has been shown to improve antidepressant-induced ED (review by Labbate et al, *J Clin Psychiatry* 2003; **64**[Suppl 10]:11–9).

Antipsychotics	**Switching drugs** is the main strategy, e.g. to:

- **Olanzapine**, if haloperidol-induced (n = 1, Tsai and Hong, *Gen Hosp Psychiatry* 2000;**20**:391–2; n = 570, Bitter et al, *Int Clin Psychopharmacol* 2005;**20**:19–21; part of SOHO study).
- **Quetiapine** (n = 28) may improve erectile function and lubrication compared to other antipsychotics (n = 86, 6/12, open, Montejo-Gonzalez et al, *J Clin Psychopharmacol* 2005;**25**:533–8).

Adjunctive therapies:
- **Amantadine** 100mg/d may help (n = 6, open, 6/52, Valevski et al, *Clin Neuropharmacol* 1998;**21**:355–7).
- **PDE-5 inhibitors**, e.g. sildenafil can be effective if ED is induced by olanzapine (n = 10, 4/52, Atmaca et al, *Int J Impot Res* 2002;**14**:547–9) or risperidone (n = 32 [c = 31], RCT, d/b, p/c, c/o, Gopalakrishnan et al, *Am J Psychiatry* 2006;**163**:494–9; n = 12, open, Aviv et al, *J Clin Psychiatry* 2004;**65**:97–103). Cochrane concludes that sildenafil may be useful but the data is very limited (Berner et al, *Cochrane Database Syst Rev* 2007;1:CD003546).

Carbamazepine	**Oxcarbazepine**, switch to (n = 4, Sachdeo and Sathyan, *Curr Med Res Opin* 2005;**21**:1065–8).

Anorgasmia (see also general advice section)

Noradrenaline exerts an excitatory or facilitatory action on orgasm. Serotonin 5HT2A receptor agonism is inhibitory on orgasm.

Antidepressants *	Anorgasmia from antidepressants is a common phenomenon. A minor effect can be advantageous in some men (by delaying ejaculation), but almost invariably considered disadvantageous in women.

Dose adjustment:
- reduce dose
- omit selected doses (e.g. at weekends)
- use a single daily dose, e.g. one taken at night will give trough levels the next evening, useful if that is when sexual activity occurs
- partial drug holiday (i.e. missing specific days, although as David Baldwin once said, you'd need a sabbatical for fluoxetine, due to its long half-life).

Wait for spontaneous resolution (occurs in less than a third).
Withdraw drug — anorgasmia is rapidly reversible on drug withdrawal.
Switch drugs:
Switching drugs may often be the main choice, but frequently a major problem if the patient has responded to the causative agent:

- **Bupropion** (probably fairly useful as it has a low serotoninergic effects). Switching to bupropion SR may be successful for escitalopram-induced anorgasmia (s = 2, n = 830, RCT, d/b, p/c, 8/52, Clayton *et al*, *J Clin Psychiatry* 2006;**67**:736–46).
- **Duloxetine** is alleged to have a lower anorgasmic effect (s = 4, RCT, d/b, p/c, n = 1466, Delgado *et al*, *J Clin Psychiatry* 2005;**66**:686–92).
- **Escitalopram** (better than paroxetine: Bielski *et al*, *Ann Clin Psychiatry* 2005;**17**:65–9).
- **Mirtazapine** has placebo-level effects on orgasmic capacity. This is probably because although it increases serotonin, it blocks serotonin's anorgasmic effect on 5HT2A receptors.
- **Trazodone** (if you can stay awake long enough) 50–200 mg/d may help men with psychogenic ED (s = 6, n = 396 men, RCTs, > 1/52, Fink *et al*, *BJU Int* 2003;**92**:441–6), although an earlier study found no effect (n = 34, RCT, p/c,4/52, Enzlin *et al*, *Int J Impot Res* 2000;**12**:223–8).
- **Venlafaxine** 75 mg daily had no effect on premature ejaculation and therefore might be better than an SSRI at not causing it (n = 31, p/c, s/b, c/o, Kilic *et al*, *Int J Androl* 2005;**28**:47–52).

Adjunctive therapies:
Many adjunctive therapies have been tried and may work for some individuals. These are purely in alphabetical order as there is no robust way of assessing their relative efficacies:

- **Bethanechol** taken 1–2 hours before intercourse has been claimed to relieve tricyclic-induced anorgasmia, but may only occasionally be successful.
- **Bupropion** was effective in 46% of women and 75% of men, most improvement occurring in the first two weeks (open, n = 24, 7/52, Gitlin *et al*, *J Sex Marital Ther* 2002;**28**:131–8), but an RCT failed to show an effect in SSRI-induced anorgasmia (n = 30, RCT, p/c, Masand *et al*, *Am J Psychiatry* 2001;**158**:805–7).
- **Buspirone** 20–60 mg/d has improved 58% people with SSRI-induced sexual problems (cf. 30% on placebo; n = 117, p/c, > 4/52, Landen *et al*, *J Clin Psychopharmacol* 1999;**19**: 268–71).
- **Cyproheptadine** 2–4 mg 30–60 minutes before sex (provided one can then stay awake) may help if SSRI-induced, although relapse of depression has been reported (see 4.3.2.2). 4 mg (but not 2 mg) the day before intercourse has been used for anorgasmia induced by citalopram (being referred to by the male patient as 'the catapult pills' Lauerma, *Acta Psychiatr Scand* 1996;**93**:69–70), fluvoxamine (n = 1, Arnott and Nutt, *Br J Psychiatry* 1994;**164**:838–9) and MAOIs (Decastro, *Am J Psychiatry* 1985;**142**:783).
- **Dronabinol**, a synthetic cannabinol, one hour before sex has increased libido, arousal, lubrication, orgasm and overall quality, but beware of people wandering around with grins on their faces in case they get drug-tested (n = 1, Salerian, *J Clin Psychiatry* 2004;**665**:1146–7).
- **Loratadine** 15 mg/d may rapidly reverse SSRI-induced anorgasmia in men and women (n = 10, case series, Brubaker, *J Clin Psychiatry* 2002;**63**:534).

- **Methylphenidate** (Roeloffs et al, J Clin Psychiatry 1996;**57**:548) and dextroamfetamine (15–20 mg/d) have been used successfully for SSRI-induced anorgasmia (n = 5, Bartlik, J Sex Marital Ther 1995;**21**:264–71).
- **Mianserin** 7.5–15 mg/d as add-on for SSRI-induced 'sexual dysfunction' may be successful in 65% within 1–2 weeks, with no adverse effects (n = 16, open, 3/52, Aizenberg et al, Clin Neuropharmacol 1999;**22**:347–50; n = 17, open, 3/12, Dolberg et al, Psychopharmacol [Berl] 2002;**161**:404–7), although the only RCT showed no significant difference in women (n = 75, RCT, d/b, p/c, 4/52, Michelson et al, J Psychiatr Res 2002;**36**:147–52).
- **Mirtazapine** improved function in premenopausal females with SSRI-induced sexual side-effects (n = 148, RCT, p/c, 6/52, Michelson et al, J Psychiatr Res 2002;**36**:147–52). Stimulation of the 5HT2A receptor inhibits orgasm, but mirtazapine blocks 5HT2A receptors, reversing the anorgasmic effect, and this may happen at relatively low doses, e.g. 7.5–15 mg/d.
- * **PDE-5** inhibitors such as **sildenafil** 50–100 mg, taken 30–60 minutes pre-sex, may help SSRI-induced anorgasmia in men (n = 90, RCT, p/c, 6/52, Nurnberg et al, JAMA 2003;**289**:56–64) and in women (n = 98 [c = 89], RCT, d/b, p/c, 8/52, Nurnberg et al, JAMA 2008;**300**:395–404), but high doses may be needed (50–200 mg/d) to overcome the problem (n = 21, open Seidman et al, J Clin Psychiatry 2003;**64**:721–5).
- **Yohimbine** 5.4–10.8 mg has been used if SSRI-induced and a retrospective chart review and survey showed it to be more effective than amantadine and cyproheptadine (n = 596, Keller Ashton et al, J Sex Marital Ther 1997;**23**:165–75), although it was no better than placebo in the main RCT (n = 148, RCT, p/c, 6/52, Michelson et al, J Psychiatr Res 2002;**36**:147–52). Yohimbine can cause insomnia, so rolling over and going to sleep afterwards may be trickier.

Less useful:

- **Amantadine** 200–300 mg/d was ineffective in the main study (n = 57, RCT, p/c, 8/52, Michelson et al, Am J Psychiatry 2000;**157**:239–43), but there are cases of use in SSRI-induced anorgasmia (n = 596, Keller Ashton et al, J Sex Marital Ther 1997;**23**:165–75).
- **Ginkgo biloba** has failed to show any significant reversal of SSRI-induced sexual dysfunction (n = 37, RCT, p/c, 2/12, Kang et al, Hum Psychopharmacol 2002;**17**:279–84).
- **Granisitron** (5-HT3 antagonist) has been used to treat fluoxetine-induced anorgasmia, but 1–2 mg was ineffective in one study, although a significant placebo response was noted (n = 20, p/c, c/o, Nelson et al, J Clin Psychiatry 2001;**62**:469–73).

Antipsychotics

Switch drugs:

- **Quetiapine** has a lower incidence of problems than risperidone and fluphenazine (n = 27, RCT, d/b, Kelly and Conley, Psychoneuroendocrinology 2006;**31**:340–6).

Adjunctive therapies:

- **Amantadine** 100 mg/d did not help in one study (n = 6, open, 6/52, Valevski et al, Clin Neuropharmacol 1998;**21**:355–7).

Opiates

Buprenorphine probably has less sexual ADRs than methadone as it causes suppression of plasma testosterone (n = 105, Bliesener et al, J Clin Endocrinol Metab 2005;**90**:203–6).

Methadone produces a dose-dependent inhibition of orgasm (n = 92, Brown et al, J Addict Disord 2005;**24**:91–106), so dose reduction may help.

| Anticonvulsants | Topiramate-induced anorgasmia responds to dose reduction or discontinuation (n = 7, Sun et al, Headache 2006;**46**:1450–3). |

Ejaculation problems (see also general advice section)

| All drugs | **Discontinue or reduce dose**, e.g. if tricyclic-induced (Aizenberg et al, J Clin Psychiatry 1991;**52**:461–3). Retrograde ejaculation from risperidone 8 mg/d promptly responds to dose reduction (n = 1, Loh et al, Int Clin Psychopharmacol 2004;**19**:111–2). Discontinuation generally works for clozapine (n = 3, Talmon et al, Harefuah 1994;**126**:509–10). Trazodone ejaculatory inhibition resolves within 48 hours of stopping (n = 1, Kaufman et al, J Sex Marital Ther 2007;**33**:225–30).
Switch drugs, e.g. ED and inappropriate ejaculation with reboxetine resolved when switched sertraline (n = 1, Sivrioglu et al, Prog Neuropsychopharmacol Biol Psychiatry 2007;**31**:548–50).
Tamsulosin has been used for reboxetine-induced painful ejaculation (n = 2, Demyttenaere and Huygens, Eur Neuropsychopharmacol 2002;**12**:337–41), and intermittent use may help with other causes (n = 405, Goktas et al, J Urol 2006;**175**:650–2). |

Priapism

Early treatment (within 4–6 hours, before local hypoxemia) reduces morbidity, the need for invasive procedures and impotence, and may prevent or minimise long-term complications.

* Immediate short-term treatment includes conservative measures, e.g. pain control, vigorous hydration, and cold compress before urology consultation.
* Active treatments include cavernosal penile aspiration, irrigation, instillation of vasoactive agents, intracavernosal injection of phenylephrine (n = 1, Davol and Rukstalis, Urology 2005;**66**:880) and, if necessary, shunting procedures.

> **Terbutaline** orally may be effective for about 40% (cf. 15% with placebo), so may be worth a try (n = 68, RCT, p/c, Priyadarshi, Int J Impot Res 2004;**16**:424–6; n = 75, RCT, p/c, Lowe and Jarow, Urology 1993;**42**:51–4).
> **Switching** — if antipsychotic related, switch to one with a lower propensity to cause priapism (highest with chlorpromazine, and risperidone; see review by Compton and Miller, J Clin Psychiatry 2001;**62**:362–6). With risperidone, priapism has occurred with a switch from oral to IM so try to switch back (n = 1, Kirshner and Davis, J Clin Psychopharmacol 2006;**26**:626–8).

Reviews: general (Wang et al, Int Clin Psychopharmacol 2006;**21**:245–8; Kalsi et al, Hosp Med 2002; **63**:224–5), antipsychotics (Sood et al, Int Clin Psychopharmacol 2008;**23**:9–17).

6.11 Others, side-effects

Gastric irritation or nausea

| Valproate | Take with or after food.
Slow-release or enteric-coated tablets may help.
Avoid fizzy drinks with the liquid or soluble tablets. |
| Galantamine * | **Switching** to the XL preparation has a disappointingly low impact on reducing nausea (n = 965, RCT, d/b, p/c, 6/12, Dunbar et al, Clin Ther 2006;**28**:365–72, MS). Rivastigmine patches might be an alternative (see C2). |

Glaucoma

| Topiramate | **Discontinuation** usually quickly leads to reversal (Anon, Prescrire Int 2003;**12**:61).
Methylprednisolone and mannitol may be rapidly effective if acute (n = 1, Rhee et al, Am J Ophthalmol 2006;**141**:1133–4). |

Laser surgery or peripheral iridectomy may be longer-term options (n = 83, Fraunfelder *et al*, *Ophthalmology* 2004;**111**:109–11).

Hypersalivation (see also sialorhoea)

Lithium **Propantheline** may give some symptomatic relief (n = 1, Donaldson, *Am J Psychiatry* 1982;**139**:1350–1).

Incontinence (see also noctural enuresis)

Clozapine This may be due to alpha-adrenergic antagonism and usually resolves spontaneously within 3/12 in nearly all cases (n = 16, Warner *et al*, *Int Clin Psychopharmacol* 1994;**9**:207–9).

Reducing fluid intake during the evening may help.

Alpha-adrenergic agonists; ephedrine was rapidly effective at 150 mg at night in 16 patients with the problem, with response maintained over 12/12 (n = 57, Fuller *et al*, *J Clin Psychiatry* 1996;**57**:514–8).

DDAVP® (Ferring)/Desmopressin intranasally has been used symptomatically (n = 1, English *et al*, *Ann Pharmacother* 2001;**35**:867–9).

Oxybutinin has been used (Lurie and Hosmer, *J Clin Psychiatry* 1997; **58**:404).

Tolterodine has been used, albeit unsuccessfully (n = 1, English *et al*, *Ann Pharmacother* 2001;**35**:867–9).

Review and case series: Warner *et al*, *Int Clin Psychopharmacol* 1994;**9**:207–9.

Jaundice (see also hepatotoxicity)

Valproate Could be impending hepatic failure. Investigate immediately and discontinue if necessary.

Mastalgia (see also hyperprolactinaemia)

Venlafaxine **Check prolactin** and take appropriate action.

Bromocriptine 5 mg/d has been used for mastalgia occurring in weeks 5–13 of therapy, with no recurrence on discontinuation (n = 1, Bhatia *et al*, *J Clin Psychopharmacol* 2000;**20**:590–1).

Megaloblastic anaemia

Anticonvulsants Folic acid may be used if caused by, e.g. phenytoin or phenobarbital.

Oedema

Lithium **Reduce dose**, as this common effect may be dose-related.

Diuretics may be useful but see *Chapter 4.4* for interactions.

Trazodone **Reduction** in dose or **discontinuation** may be rapidly successful (n = 10, Barrnett *et al*, *J Clin Psychopharmacol* 1985;**5**:161–4).

Valproate * **Discontinuation** — usually occurs after long-term treatment (but can be after short-term use), can have fluctuating presentation and rapidly improves when valproate is stopped (n = 2, Lin *et al*, *Int J Neuropsychopharmacol* 2010; [in press]).

Nausea (see gastric irritation)

Osteopenia (see also osteoporosis and hyperprolactinaemia)

Antipsychotics **Correct** any raised prolactin abnormalities.

Standard therapies, e.g. alendronic acid 5 mg/d has improved spine and hip T-scores by 7% and 9% respectively over a year (n = 1, Howes and Smith, *Am J Psychiatry* 2004;**161**:756).

Osteoporosis (see also osteopenia) *

General * **Beer drinking** — I couldn't resist mentioning that quantitative bone ultrasound values for women (pre-, peri- and post-menopausal) are greater in beer drinkers (in moderation of course) compared to non-beer or non-wine drinkers, possibly due to the phytoestrogen content (n = 1697, Pedrera-Zamorano *et al*, *Nutrition* 2009;**25**:1057–63).

Pain at site of injection

Depots   **Warm baths** and regular exercise can help.

Change site or systematically alternate injection sides.

Check injection technique, as Z-tracking technique may not always be meticulously followed (Belanger-Annable, *Canadian Nurse* 1985;**81**:1–3).

Raised LFTs

Valproate   Raised LFTs are not uncommon but usually transient, so monitor LFTs (including prothrombin time) until it returns to normal.

Discontinue if the prothrombin time is abnormally prolonged.

Salicylates (inc. OTC) may exacerbate so should be discontinued.

Sialorhoea (hypersalivation)

Clozapine *   Hypersalivation may be a lack of the swallowing reflex (rather than excess saliva production; n = 17, Rabinowitz *et al*, *Biol Psychiatry* 1996;**40**:1132–4) or due to clozapine's pharmacology, e.g. M4 activation or alpha-2 blockade, so hypersalivation may be an inaccurate term for this side-effect.

Review: * Cochrane concludes there is insufficient evidence for any treatment (s = 15, Syed *et al*, *Cochrane Database Syst Rev* 2008;**3**:CD005579; comment by Sockalingham and Remington, *EBMH* 2009;**12**:12).

Physical strategies:
- Propping pillows up at night helps a little in some people.
- Reduce caffeine intake (n = 1, Odom-White and de Leon, *J Clin Psychiatry* 1996;**57**:175–6).

Adjunctive therapies:

Adjunctive therapies are usually the only realistic option for this unpleasant and common, but not life-threatening ADR. The following are probably in descending order of efficacy:
- **Atropine** 1% eye drops, one drop given orally at bedtime may be rapidly effective (n = 3, Antonello and Tessier, *J Psychiatry Neurosci* 1999;**24**:250; Comley *et al*, *Aust N Z J Psychiatry* 2000;**34**:1033–4).
- **Hyoscine** hydrobromide 300 mcg sucked and swallowed up to TDS.
- * **Moclobemide** 150–300 mg/d showed a beneficial effect in 66% patients (n = 14, 2/52, Kreinin *et al*, *Clin Neuropharmacol* 2009;**32**:151–3).
- **Pirenzapine (**M1/M4 blocker) 25–100 mg/d is frequently used (n = 29, Schneider *et al*, *Pharmacopsychiatry* 2004;**37**:43–5) and has no interaction with clozapine, although it may not always be useful (n = 20, RCT, d/b, c/o, p/c, Bai *et al*, *J Clin Psychopharmacol* 2001;**21**:608–11).
- **Quetiapine**, through allowing reduced clozapine dosage.
- **Sulpiride** (150–300 mg/d) may have some efficacy (n = 18, open, 3/52, Kreinin *et al*, *Isr J Psych Relat Sci* 2005;**42**:61–3), as may amisulpride ('strong ameliorating effect'; n = 20, RCT, d/b, p/c, c/o, Kreinin *et al*, *Int Clin Psychopharmacol* 2006;**21**:99–103).
- **Tricyclics** (e.g. amitriptyline; Praharaj and Arora, *Br J Clin Pharmacol* 2006;**63**:128–9) can be useful, predominantly for their anticholinergic effect (Copp *et al*, *Br J Psychiatry* 1991;**159**:166).

Less use:
- * **Amisulpride** has been used for clozapine-induced sialorrhea (Praharaj *et al*, *J Clin Psychopharmacol* 2009;**29**:189–90)
- **Anticholinergics** or antimuscarinics are generally ineffective, although **trihexyphenidyl** 5–15 mg/d at bedtime reduced secretions by 44% in one study (n = 14, open, Spivak *et al*, *Int Clin Psychopharmacol* 1997;**12**:213–5). Trihexyphenidyl plus terazosin 2 mg/d (Reinstein *et al*, *Clin Drug Invest*

1999;**17**:97–102) may be better than either drug alone. **Biperiden** 6 mg/d has been effective in a case resistant to propranolol and clonidine (n = 1, Richardson et al, Am J Psychiatry 2001;**158**:1329–30).

- * **Botulinum toxin** (injected into the parotid gland) has been used successfully (n = 9, p/c, 16/52, Steinlechner et al, Psychopharmacology (Berl) 2010;**207**:593–7; n = 1 and review, Kahl et al, Nervenarzt 2005;**76**:205–8) although the evidence is weak (s = 6, Lim et al, Clin Otolaryngology 2006;**31**:267–72).
- * **Bupropion** has helped (n = 1, Stern et al, Prog Neuropsychopharmacol Biol Psychiatry 2009;**33**:1578–80).
- **Chewing gum** has been used to stimulate salivation and swallowing.
- **Clonidine** 50–100 mcg/d increases adrenergic tone and reduces patient-reported hypersalivation (wet area on pillow) without adverse effects (n = 12, open, 4/52, Parharaj et al, J Psychopharmacol 2005;**19**:426–8), although it might exacerbate depression and psychosis. Clonidine patches (0.1 mg/week) have been used.
- **Guanfacine** (Webber et al, J Clin Psychopharmacol 2004;**24**:675–6).
- * **Ipratropium** (sublingually or intranasal spray) has limited efficacy (Freudenreich et al, J Clin Psychopharmacol 2004;**24**:98–100; n = 10, Calderon et al, Int Clin Psychopharmacol 2000;**15**:49–52) and the only RCT showed no sublingually efficacy compared to placebo (n = 20, RCT, d/b, p/c, 6/52, Sockalingam et al, J Clin Psychiatry 2009;**70**:1114–9).
- **Lofexidine** 0.2 mg BD has been used as an alpha-2 agonist in the short-term (testing the theory that hypersalivation is due to clozapine's alpha-2 antagonism; n = 1, 1/12, Corrigan et al, Br J Psychiatry 1995;**167**:412; rebuttal of theory by Szabadi, Br J Psychiatry 1996;**169**:380–1).
- **Propantheline** 7.5 mg/d has been used.
- **Scopolamine** patches (Gaftanyuk and Trestman, Psychiatr Serv 2004; **55**:318).
- **Septoplasty** was dramatically successful in one patient with a deviated septum causing him to breathe through his mouth (n = 1, Conry et al, Am J Psychiatry 1996;**153**:444).

Reviews: general (Praharaj et al, Psychopharmacol [Berl] 2006;**185**:265–73; Davydov and Botts, Ann Pharmacother 2000;**34**:662–5; Freudenreich, Drugs Today [Barc] 2005;**41**:411–8).

Tremor (see also EPSE, Parkinsonism)

Lithium *
Dose reduction is appropriate since tremor is dose/plasma level related. **Beta-blockers** are standard therapy, e.g. **propranolol** 30–40 mg/d (n = 5, Lapierre, Can Med Assoc J 1976;**114**:619–20), **metoprolol** (comparison with propranolol, Zubenko et al, Psychiatry Res 1984;**11**:163–4), **atenolol** and **nadolol** (for a hepatically-compromised patient; n = 1, Dave and Langbart, Ann Clin Psychiatry 1994;**6**:51–2).

* **Pregabalin** (n = 1, Marks et al, Int J Neuropsychopharmacol 2008;**11**:879–81). **Vitamin B6** 900–1200 mg/d was completely effective in 80% patients (open, n = 5, Miodownik et al, Int J Psychiatr Med 2002;**32**:103–8). **Linoleic acid** is ineffective (Schou, Prostaglandins Med 1980;**5**:343–4; Anton, Prostaglandins Med 1980;**5**:321–2).

Review: Gelenberg and Jefferson, J Clin Psychiatry 1995;**56**:283–7.

Vomiting

Valproate
Could be impending hepatic failure. Investigate immediately and discontinue if necessary.

PSYCHOTROPIC DRUGS

This section details currently and formerly available psychotropic drugs in the UK. The dates are rarely definitive. A drug may be licensed but not launched, it may be different in different countries, may be launched but not promoted, different salts or presentations may exist; medicines may be discontinued but not withdrawn, or may be much stock left so continues to be used. Patents may exist for the drug, manufacturing process, different salts, presentation/formulation appearance, packaging, license/ use, patent extension or protection may be gained, the ten-year rule may apply for new chemical entities. The author would be grateful for any clarifications and corrections.

NAME	UK LAUNCH	UK PATENT EXPIRY	UK STATUS	COMMENTS
Acamprosate	1996	Expired 2002	Available	
Acetazolamide	1953	Expired	Available	
Agomelatine (Valdoxan®)	2009	-	Available	
Alprazolam	1983	Expired c1992	Available	Black list in UK
Amisulpride	1997	Expired 2001	Available	
Amitriptyline	1961 SR caps 1971	Expired	Available	SR caps discontinued 2000
Amobarbital (amylobarbital, amylo-barbitone, Amytal®)	c1923	Expired	Tablets discontinued 2006 Injection 2000	Commercial reasons
Amoxapine (Asendis®)	1989	Expired	Discontinued 2006	Commercial reasons
Asenapine	TBA	-	License applied	Available USA 2009
Aripiprazole	2004 IM inj 2008	2014	Available	
Atomoxetine	2004	Expires 2016	Available	Patent extension in some countries
Beclamide (Nydrane®)	c1956	Expired	Discontinued 1987	Commercial reasons
Benperidol	1973	Expired	Available	
Benzatropine Benztropine	1950s	Expired	Discontinued 2008	Injection available only, as import
Benzoctamine (Tacitin®)	1971	Expired	Discontinued 1983	Commercial reasons
Biperiden (Akineton®)	c1957	Expired	Discontinued 2003	Commercial reasons
Buprenorphine	1980 (USA 2003) 1999 for SM	Expired 2006	Available	Suboxone 2007 (with naloxone)

NAME	UK LAUNCH	UK PATENT EXPIRY	UK STATUS	COMMENTS
Bupropion	2000 (US 1985 for depression)	Expired in most countries	Available	
Buspirone	1987	Expired 2000	Available	
Butobarbitone (Sonergan®)	1931	Expired	Available	
Butriptyline (Evadyne®)	1975	Expired	Discontinued 1993	Commercial reasons
Carbamazepine	1962 (1965 for epilepsy), SR tabs 1989 Suppositories 1994	Expired	Available	
Chloral Hydrate	1870s	Expired	Available	First synthesis 1832, first medical use 1869. Noctec capsules discontinued 1996
Chlordiazepoxide	1960	Expired	Available	Injection discontinued 1988
Chlormethiazole Clomethiazole	First patent 1938 First used for DTs in 1959 Syrup 1972	Expired	Available	Infusion discontinued 2000
Chlormezanone (Trancopal®)	c1961	Expired	Withdrawn 1996 worldwide	Toxic epidermal necrolysis
Chlorpromazine	1954	Expired	Available	
Chlorprothixene (Taractan®)	1959	Expired	Discontinued 1987	Commercial reasons
Citalopram	1995 Drops 2000	Expired 2002	Available	
Citrated calcium carbimide (Abstem®)	1977	Expired	Discontinued 1984	Commercial reasons
Clobazam	1979	Expired 1997	Available	
Clomipramine	1970	Expired	Available	Injection discontinued 2002, syrup 2001
Clonazepam	1974	Expired c1995	Available	
Clorazepate Dipotassium (Tranxene®)	1973	Expired c1988	Discontinued 2005	Lack of use after black-listing
Clozapine	1990	Expired	Available	
Cyclobarbitone (Rapidal®, Phanodorm®)	c1920s	Expired	Discontinued 1988	Lack of use and toxicity

Name	UK LAUNCH	UK PATENT EXPIRY	UK STATUS	Comments
Deprol® (meprobamate and benactyzine)	1965	Expired	Discontinued 1970s	Commercial reasons
Desipramine (Pertofran®)	1963	Expired c1988	Discontinued 1977	Commercial reasons/ toxicity
Dexamphetamine (dexamfetamine, dextroamphetamine)	1937	Expired	Available	First synthesised 1887. Marketed 1932 for nasal congestion, as stimulant 1935 and Dexadrine® launched 1937
Diazepam	1963	Expired	Available	
Dibenzepine (Noveril®)	1970	Expired	Discontinued 1981	Commercial reasons
Dichloralphena-zone (Welldorm®)	1940s?	Expired	Discontinued 1992 (converted to chloral betaine)	Production problems
Disulfiram	1949 (1951 in USA)	Expired	Available	First synthesised 1881
Donepezil	1997	Expires Feb 2012	Available	
Dosulepin/dothiepin	1969	Expired	Available	
Doxepin	1969	Expired	Available	
Droperidol (Droleptan®)	c1980	Expired	Withdrawn 2001	Due to QTc issues.
Duloxetine	2005 for depression (2004 for stress incontinence)	Unclear due to patent extensions, c2009	Available	Basic US patent expires 2008
Escitalopram	2002	Expires 2014	Available	
Eslicarbazepine	2009		Available	
Ethosuximide	1982ish	Expired	Available	
Ethotoin (Peganone®)	1957	Expired	Discontinued 1985	Commercial reasons
Fencamfamin (Reactivan®)	c1965	Expired	Withdrawn 1986	Abuse and dependency
Fenfluramine (Ponderax®)	1968	Expired	Withdrawn 1997	Toxicity (deaths) and abuse
Flumazenil	1988	Expired 2002	Available	
Flunitrazepam (Rohypnol®)	1982	Expired	Withdrawn 1986	Abuse
Fluoxetine	1989, Liquid 1992	Expired 2000	Available	

NAME	UK LAUNCH	UK PATENT EXPIRY	UK STATUS	COMMENTS
Flupentixol	1965	Expired	Available	
Flupentixol Decanoate	1972 Low vol 1992	Expired	Available	
Fluphenazine Decanoate (Modecate®)	1968	Expired	Available	
Fluphenazine Enanthate (Moditen®)	1966	Expired	Discontinued 1991	Commercial reasons
Fluphenazine HCI (Moditen®)	c1967	Expired	Discontinued 2008	Commercial reasons
Flurazepam	1973	Expired	Available	
Fluspirilene (Redeptin®)	1975	Expired	Discontinued 1995	Commercial reasons, import in UK
Fluvoxamine	1987	Expired 1996	Available	
Fosphenytoin	1998	Expired US 2007	Available	
Gabapentin	1993	Expired 2000	Available	
Galantamine	2000 Syrup 2003 XL 2008?	Expires Jan 2012	Available	
Glutethimide (Doriden®)	1954	Expired	Discontinued 1983	Commercial reasons
Haloperidol	1959	Expired	Available	
Haloperidol decanoate	1982	Expired 2000	Available	
Heptabarbitone (Medomin®)	1950s?	Expired	Discontinued 1985	
Hexobarbital	c1940	Expired	Discontinued1960s	
Hydergine® (codergocrine)	c1975	Expired	Discontinued 2005	Commercial reasons
Hydroxyzine	c1958	Expired	Available	
Imipramine	1959	Expired	Available	
Iprindole (Prondol®)	c1972	Expired	Discontinued 1995	Commercial reasons
Iproniazid (Marsilid®)	1958	Expired	Discontinued 1987	Commercial reasons
Isocarboxazid	1959–60	Expired	Available	
Ketazolam (Anxon®)	1980	Expired	Discontinued 1990	Commercial reasons
Lacosamide	2008		Available	
Lamotrigine	1991 Dispersible tablets 1994	Expired 2005	Available	

Name	UK LAUNCH	UK PATENT EXPIRY	UK STATUS	Comments
Levetiracetam	2000 syrup 2005	Expires 2010	Available	
Levomepromazine	c1950s	Expired	Available	
Limbitrol® (amitriptyline and chlordiazepoxide)	c1966	Expired	Discontinued 1994	Commercial reasons
Lithium carbonate	c1955? (first mania license in USA in 1970) Priadel 1968 Liskonum 1980	Expired	Available	
Lithium citrate tablets (Litarex®)	1982	Expired	Discontinued 2001	Commercial reasons
Lofepramine	1983	Expired	Available	
Lofexidine	1992	Expired 2003	Available	
Loprazolam	1983	Expired 1995	Available	
Lorazepam	1971	1982	Available	
Lormetazepam	1980	Expired	Available	
Loxapine (Loxapac®)	1989	Expired 1996	Discontinued 2003	Commercial reasons
Maprotiline (Ludiomil®)	1975	Expired c1989	Discontinued 2005/6	Commercial reasons
Mazindol (Teronac®)	1960s (1973 USA)	Expired	Discontinued 1992	Commercial reasons
Meclofenoxate (Lucidril®)	1966	Expired	Discontinued 1982	Commercial reasons
Medazepam (Nobrium®)	1968	Expired	Discontinued 1994	Lack of use after black-listing
Memantine	2002	Expires 2014	Available	
Meprobamate (Equanil®)	1955	Expired	Discontinued 2002	Commercial reasons
Methadone	c1947 (as analgesic)	Expired	Available	First synthesised 1937
Methixene (Tremonil®)	1970s	Expired	Discontinued 1994	Commercial reasons
Methohexitone (Brietal®)	c1957	Expired	Discontinued 1999	Commercial reasons
Methoin (Mesontoin®)	1940s	Expired	Discontinued 1981	Commercial reasons
Methylphenidate	1954 (for fatigue and depression) Equasym 2000 Concerta 2002 Medikinet 2007	Expired	Available	First synthesised 1944, off market in mid-1980s, reintroduced 1995

Name	UK LAUNCH	UK PATENT EXPIRY	UK STATUS	Comments
Methylpheno-barbitone®	1935	Expired	Discontinued 2001	Commercial reasons
Methyprylon(e) (Noludar®)	c1958	Expired	Discontinued 1989	Adverse effects and commercial reasons
Mianserin	1976	Expired	Available	
Midazolam	1982	Expired 1995	Available	
Mirtazapine	1997	Expired 2005	Available	
Moclobemide	1993	Expired 2002	Available	
Modafinil	1998	Unclear, 2003 or 2009	Available	
Motipress® (fluphenazine 1.5mg and nortriptyline 30mg)	1976	Expired	Discontinued 2003	Commercial reasons
Motival® (fluphenazine 0.5mg and nortriptyline 10mg)	1973	Expired	Discontinued 2006	Commercial reasons
Naltrexone	1988	Expired 2007	Available	
Nefazodone (Dutonin®)	1995	Expired 2007	Withdrawn 2002	Hepatic ADRs
Nialamide	1950s	Expired	Discontinued 1970s	
Nitrazepam	1965	Expired	Available	
Nomifensine (Merital®)	1977	Expired	Withdrawn worldwide 1986	Haemolytic anaemia
Nortriptyline	1963	Expired c1988	Available	
Olanzapine	1996 Velotabs 2001 IM injection Depot 2010	Expires Sept 2011	Available	Patent challenge may change patent expiry
Opipramol (Insidon®)	1970s	Expired	Discontinued 1981	Available in Germany
Orphenadrine	c1951	Expired	Available	Injection discontinued 1990
Oxazepam	c1965	Expired c1987	Available	
Oxcarbazepine	2000	Expired 2000	Available	
Oxprenolol	c1968 1983 for anxiety	Expired	Available	
Oxypertine (Integrin®)	c1950s	Expired	Discontinued 2002	Commercial reasons
Paliperidone	2007		Available	
Paraldehyde	First used as AED in 1882	Expired	Available	

Name	UK LAUNCH	UK PATENT EXPIRY	UK STATUS	Comments
Paramethadione (Paradione®)	1970s?	Expired	Discontinued UK 1984	Commercial reasons
Paroxetine	1991 (liquid 1997)	Expired 2006	Available	
Parstelin® (tranylcypromine 10mg, trifluoperazine 1mg)	<1964	Expired	Discontinued 1999	Commercial reasons
Pemoline (Volital®, Kethamed®, Ronyl®)	1975 in USA	Expired	Withdrawn 1997	Withdrawn worldwide 2005 due to liver toxicity
Pentobarbitone Sodium (Nembutal®)	c1919	Expired	Discontinued 1986	Commercial reasons
Pericyazine	1966	Expired	Available	
Perphenazine	1957	Expired 1987	Available	Injection discontinued 1990
Phenelzine	1959–60	Expired	Available	
Phenobarbitone sodium (Gardenal®)	1912	Expired	Available	
Phenytoin	1938	Expired	Available	
Pimozide	1971	Expired	Available	
Pipothiazine	1983	Expired	Available	
Piracetam	1992	Expired	Available	
Pramindole®	1968	Expired	Discontinued 1981	Commercial reasons
Prazepam®	1982	Expired c1988 in US	Discontinued 1988	Lack of use after black-listing
Pregabalin	2004 (epilepsy) 2007 (GAD)	Expires 2018	Available	
Primidone	1952	Expired	Available	Suspension discontinued 2000
Prochlorperazine	1950s	Expired	Available	
Procyclidine	1951 UK	Expired	Available	
Promazine	1955	Expired	Available	
Promethazine	c1951 (USA)	Expired	Available	OTC in UK from 1985
Propranolol	1965 1973 (anxiety)	Expired	Available	
Protriptyline (Concordin®)	1967	Expired	Discontinued 2000	Commercial reasons
Quetiapine	1997, 2009 (bipolar) 2009 XL	Expires 2012	Available	

NAME	UK LAUNCH	UK PATENT EXPIRY	UK STATUS	COMMENTS
Reboxetine	1997	Expired 2004	Available	
Remoxipride (Roxiam®)	1990	Expired	Suspended 1993, withdrawn 1994	Aplastic anaemia
Risperidone	1993 Quicklets 2003 Consta 2002	Expired 2007	Available	
Rivastigmine	1998, liquid 2001	July 2012	Available	
Secobarbital (Seconal sodium)	1934	Expired	Available	Was quinalbarbitone
Sertindole (Serdolect®)	1996	Expires 2011	Available on named-patient basis only (see *Chapter 1.23*)	Voluntarily withdrawn 1998, reintroduced 2003 on named-patient basis only
Sertraline	1991	Expired 2005	Available	
Sodium oxybate	2006		Available	
Sodium valproate	1977 1988 Injection 1993 Convulex 1994 Chrono	Expired	Available	
Sulpiride	1983	Expired	Available	
Sulthiame (Ospolot®)	c1965	Expired	Discontinued 1986	Commercial reasons
Tacrine (Cognex®)	Licensed 1997 in UK	Expired	Never marketed	
Temazepam	1969	Expired	Available	
Tetrabenazine	1950s	Expired	Available	
Thiopropazate (Dartalan®)	c1950s	Expired	Discontinued 1984	Commercial reasons
Thioproperazine (Majeptil®)	1950s	Expired	Discontinued 1981	Commercial reasons
Thioridazine (Melleril®)	1958	Expired	Voluntary withdrawn 2005 (liquids 2004)	Restricted due to QTc prolongation. Import from Victoria International, Switzerland
Thiothixene (Navane®)	1967	Expired	Discontinued c1980	Commercial reasons
Tiagabine	1998	Expires 2011	Available	
Topiramate	1995	Expired 2009	Available	
Tranylcypromine	1959–60	Expired	Available	
Trazodone	1980 SR tabs 1992	Expired	Available	

NAME	UK LAUNCH	UK PATENT EXPIRY	UK STATUS	COMMENTS
Triazolam (Halcion®)	1978	Expired	License revoked 1993	Adverse effects
Triclofos sodium	1962	Expired	Available as syrup	
Trifluoperazine	1958 Spansules 1967	Expired	Available	Injection discontinued 1995
Trifluperidol	1967	Expired	Discontinued 1981, reintroduced c1986	Commercial reasons
Trihexyphenidyl	c1955	Expired	Available	Was benzhexol
Trimipramine	1966	Expired c1988	Available	
Triptafen® preps (perphenazine + amitriptyline	1970s	Expired	Available	
Troxidone (Triodone®)	1960s	Expired	Withdrawn 1985	Toxicity (especially teratogenicity) and commercial reasons
Tryptophan	Available as food supplement Licensed for depression Optimax® 1971, Pacitron® 1976	Expired	Available	Discontinued 1990 after reports of Eosinophilia Myalgia Syndrome. Reintroduced 1994
Tybamate	1966	Expired	Discontinued 1970s	
Valproate semisodium	2000	Expired 2008	Available	
Valproic acid	1993	Expired	Available	
Venlafaxine	1995	Expires 2008 XL expiry 2012	Available	
Vigabatrin	1989	Expired 1996	Available but restricted	
Viloxazine (Vivalan®)	1974	Expired	Discontinued 2000	Commercial reasons and toxicity
Zaleplon (Sonata®)	2000	Expires 2011	Available	
Zimelidine (Zelmid®)	1982	Expired	Withdrawn 1983	Guillaine-Barré syndrome
Ziprasidone (Zeldox®, Geodon®)	Licensed but never launched		Never launched	SPC restrictions made non-viable
Zolpidem	1994	Expired 2002	Available	
Zonisamide	2005		Available	
Zopiclone	1999	Expired	Available	

Name	UK LAUNCH	UK PATENT EXPIRY	UK STATUS	Comments
Zotepine	1998	Expired	Available	Japan since 1982
Zuclopenthixol acetate	1990	Expired	Available	Clopenthixol until 1985
Zuclopenthixol decanoate	1978	Expired	Available	Clopenthixol until 1985
Zuclopenthixol oral	1982	Expired	Available	Clopenthixol until 1985

NEW DRUGS EXPECTED

Name, trade name and manufacturer	Details
Amibegron (Sanofi-Aventis)	Selective beta-3 adrenoceptor agonist antidepressant (beta-3 adrenoceptors are activated by noradrenaline)
Armodafinil (Nuvigil®, Cephalon)	Armodafinil is the r-enantiomer of modafinil, presumably with similar effects but a longer half-life (12–15 hours)
Asenapine (Zydis®, Organon/ Pfizer) *	A 5HT2 antagonist and D2 partial agonist licensed in USA for schizophrenia and mania (see Chapter 1). Oral melt form of 'fragile wafer'. Asenapine 10mg/d is as effective as risperidone and superior to placebo in acute schizophrenia, (n = 174, RCT, p/c, 6/52, Potkin et al, J Clin Psychiatry 2007;**68**:1492–1500; MS)
Bifeprunox (Wyeth, Solvay/ Lundbeck) *	Bifeprunox is a partial D2 and 5-HT1A antagonist. Although 20mg/d is effective in acute schizophrenia (n = 589, RCT, d/b, p/c, 6/52, Casey et al, Psychopharmacol [Berl] 2008;**200**:317–31; Bishara and Taylor, Drugs 2008;**68**:2269–92). Development was discontinued in 2009
Blonanserin (Lonasen®, Dainippon) *	Blonanserin is a D2 and 5HT antagonist antipsychotic and has been compared successfully to haloperidol (n = 307, d/b, p/c, RCT, 6/52, Garcia et al, CNS Drugs 2009;**23**:615–25), but appears to have little significant potential
Brivaracetam (Rikelta®, UCB)	In phase III for partial-onset seizures and myoclonic seizures, and is related to levetiracetam **Review:** Malawska and Kulig, Expert Opin Investig Drugs 2008;**17**:361–9
Carisbamate (J&J)	In phase III for epilepsy (2008), and is a novel neuromodulator (Kulig and Malawska, Idrugs 2007;**10**:720–7; safe in elderly; n = 48, RCT, d/b, p/c, Levy et al, Epilepsy Res 2008;**79**:22–30)
Desvenlafaxine (Pristiqs®, Wyeth) *	Metabolite of venlafaxine, for depression, anxiety and non-hormonal vasomotor symptoms associated with menopause. No reported adverse cardiac effects. Effective for depression (n = 461, RCT, d/b, p/c, 8/52, DeMartinis et al, J Clin Psychiatry 2007;**68**:677–88; MS). Launched USA in 2008 for depression, see Chapter 1 (depression, unlicensed)
Dimebolin (Dimebon, Pfizer and Medivation) *	Dimebolin (also known as latrepirdine) is a neuroprotective for Alzheimer's and Huntington's diseases. It is also an antihistamine, but seems to work via mitochondria. UK license expected 2011. It is effective for mild-to-moderate Alzheimer's (n = 183, RCT, d/b, p/c, 26/52, Doody et al, Lancet 2008;**372**:207–15; review as novel neuroprotector and cognitive enhancer (n = 14, open, Bachurin et al, Ann N Y Acad Sci 2001;**939**:425–35)

NAME, TRADE NAME AND MANUFACTURER	DETAILS
Docosahexaenoic acid	An omega-3 fatty acid supplement, in phase III for Alzheimer's (2008)
Eplivanserin (Sanofi-Aventis, 2010?) *	5HT2A antagonist, to be known as an ASTAR (antagonists of serotonin two A receptors), for chronic insomnia characterised by difficulty staying asleep. License applied for possible 2010 launch. Four phase III studies have been completed, shows rapid hypnotic effect with no hangover. EMEA license application withdrawn December 2009
Esmirtazapine (Organon)	5-HT2 blocker in phase III trials for insomnia and hormonal flushes
Eszopiclone (Lunesta, GSK/ Sepracor) *	An analogue of zopiclone, this is licensed in the USA with no limit to the time of treatment and with enhanced quality of life and improved work performance (n = 830, RCT, d/b, p/c, Walsh et al, Sleep 2007;**30**:959–68). Eszopiclone 2–3mg appears to have no discontinuation, tolerance or rebound effects (n = 308, RCT, p/c, 7/52, Zemmit et al, Curr Med Res Opin 2004;**20**:1979–91; p/c, s/b, 8/52, Krystal et al, J Clin Sleep Med 2007;**3**:48–55) and was effective cf. placebo and zolpidem (n = 65, RCT, d/b, p/c, Erman et al, J Clin Sleep Med 2008;**4**:229–34). License declined in Europe in May 2009 as eszopiclone was not considered a separate molecule and so patent protection would not apply, and marketing would be unviable **Reviews:** * Wilson and Nutt, J Psychopharmacol 2008;**22**:703–6; Hair et al, CNS Drugs 2008;**22**:975–8
Guanfacine (Tenex®, Shire)	An alpha-2-adrenoceptor agonist for ADHD, submitted for approval in USA, already marketed for hypertension
Iloperidone (Zomaril®, Vanda) *	Iloperidone is an antagonist of NA-alpha2C, D2, D3, 5HT1A and 5HT6 receptors now approved in USA for schizophrenia (May 2009). Its high alpha(1)-adrenoceptors affinity can lead to haemodynamic adverse effects (Bishara and Taylor, Drugs 2008;**68**:2269–92). A monthly depot being investigated. It is effective for schizophrenia (s = 3, n = 1943, RCT, d/b, p/c, 6/52, J Clin Psychopharmacol 2008;**28**[Suppl 1]:S4–11; Citrome, Int J Clin Pract 2009;**63**:1237–48; s = 3, n = 1644 [c = 1326], RCT, d/b, Kane et al, J Clin Psychopharmacol 2008;**28**[2 Suppl 1]:S29–35; s = 3, n = 1943, RCT, d/b, p/c, 6/52, Potkin et al, J Clin Psychopharmacol 2008;**28**[2 Suppl 1]:S4–1)
Indiplon MR® (Neurocrine Biosciences/Pfizer)	Quick-acting GABA-A modulator for transient sleep disorders. Approvable in USA subject to more trials (2008). Has been used for post-bedtime dosing in people with difficulty maintaining sleep (n = 264, RCT, d/b, p/c, 4/52, Roth et al, Sleep 2007;**30**:1731–8) and in the elderly (n = 358, RCT, d/b, p/c, 2/52, Walsh et al, Sleep Med 2007;**8**:753–9)
Leuprolide acetate or leuprorelin (Lupron®, Eligard®, Wyeth)	Licensed for prostate cancer but now in phase III for Alzheimer's disease (2008), although ADRs are a problem **Review:** Wilson et al, Expert Opin Investig Drugs 2007;**16**:1851–63
Lisdexamfetamine dimesylate (Vyvance®, Shire) *	Vyvance is lisdexamphetamine, which is dexamfetamine bound to the amino acid, l-lysine and is a long-acting pro-drug of d-amfetamine. It is inactive until metabolised in the GI tract, releasing d-amphetamine, reducing the abuse potential. It is licensed in USA and Canada for ADHD, including adults. It may have a lower abuse potential than d-amfetamine in people with a history of stimulant abuse (n = 36, Jasinski and Krishnan, J Psychopharmacol 2009;**23**:419–27) **Reviews:** Weber and Siddiqui, CNS Drugs 2009;**23**:419–25; Cowles, Ann Pharmacother 2009;**43**:669–76; Najib, Clin Ther 2009;**31**:142–76

NAME, TRADE NAME AND MANUFACTURER	DETAILS
Lurasidone (Dianippon) *	Lurasidone blocks D2, 5HT7, 5HT2A, 5HT1A and alpha2C recptors. It may be useful for memory impairment in schizophrenia. Phase III studies (e.g. PEARL 2) in schizophrenia have been positive and an FDA application is expected in Q2 2010. The dose is 40-120mg/d and appears weight neutral **Review:** Meyer et al, Expert Opin Investig Drugs 2009;**18**:1715–26
Methylphenidate (Daytrana®, Shire) *	Daytrana® is a daily patch with a nine-hour duration. Shire are doing another study to confirm efficacy. It appears as effective as oral methylphenidate (n = 282, RCT, d/b, p/c, 7/52, Findling et al, J Clin Psychiatry 2008;**69**:149–59)
Mifepristone (Corlux®, Mifegyne®, Exelgym)	A glucocorticoid type-II receptor (GRII) antagonist and progesterone receptor antagonist for depression and psychosis, approval awaited in USA
Naltrexone depot (Vivitrol®, Alkermes)	Naltrexone extended-release depot suspension, licensed in USA as long-term relapse prevention in alcohol dependence. UK license delayed **Review:** Swainston Harrison et al, CNS Drugs 2007;**21**:83–7
Nalmefene (Revex®?, Lundbeck) 2011? *	Nalmefene is an opioid antagonist related to naltrexone, being investigated for alcohol dependence. Targeted use may be viable (n = 403, RCT, d/b, p/c, 28/52, Karhuvaara et al, Alcohol Clin Exp Res 2007;**31**:1179–87)
Nemonapride	Nemonapride is essentially a typical antipsychotic drug, similar in structure to sulpiride, which has been available for some time in Japan. It has efficacy against positive symptoms and has shown some antidepressant and anxiolytic properties, although efficacy data for it are somewhat limited (Bishara and Taylor, Drugs 2008;**68**:2269–92)
Nicergoline (Sermion®, Farmitalia)	In phase III studies for Alzheimer's disease, and may help protect cells against beta-amyloid toxicity (Caraci et al, Brain Res 2005;**1047**:30–7)
Paliperidone palmitate (Invega®, Janssen-Cilag) 2010-1?	Paliperidone palmitate (Invega Sustenna®) was approved in USA in 2009. It is the palmitate ester of paliperidone, the major metabolite of risperidone, formulated as a long-acting injection for IM use (see paliperidone in C1). Efficacy studies have shown positive results, with low potential for anticholinergic adverse effects, including cognitive dysfunction. EPSE and postural hypotension appear greater than with placebo. (Bishara and Taylor, Drugs 2008;**68**:2269–92; n = 1795, Samtani et al, Clin Pharmacokinet 2009;**48**:585–600)
Ramelteon (Rozerem®, Takeda)	Ramelteon is an MT1, MT2 and MT3 receptor agonist for insomnia, with no abuse potential in previous sedative abusers, even at massive doses (n = 14, d/b, p/c, c/o, 18/7, Johnson et al, Arch Gen Psychiatry 2006;**63**:1149–57), and no clinically meaningful change in sleep architecture, residual effects or withdrawal or rebound (n = 405, RCT, d/b, p/c, 5/52, Zammit, J Clin Sleep Med 2007;**3**:495–504; n=451, RCT, d/b, p/c, 6/12, Mayer et al, Sleep 2009;**32**:351–60) and a sustained effect over one year (n = 1213, open, one year, Richardson et al, J Clin Psychiatry 2009;**70**:467–76). In older adults (> 65 years) there was no middle-of-the-night balance, mobility or memory issues with ramelteon (n = 33, RCT, d/b, p/c, c/o, Zammit et al, J Clin Sleep Med 2009;**5**:34–40). It is available in USA, was due to be launched UK 2010 **Reviews:** Pandi-Perumal et al, Nat Clin Pract Neurol 2007;**3**:221–8; Borja and Daniel, Clin Ther 2006;**28**:1540–55

Name, trade name and manufacturer	Details
Retigabine (GSK/Valeant) *	Retigabine is a neuronal KCNQ/Kv7 potassium channel opener, license application 2010 in the EU and the US, as adjunctive therapy to treat adult epilepsy patients with partial-onset seizures (failed neuropathic pain trials) and may be licensed for adjunctive therapy (n = 399[c=279], RCT, d/b, 16/52, Porter et al, Neurology 2007;**68**:1197–204)
Rosiglitazone (Avandamet®, GSK)	This thiazolidinedione is in phase III trials for a potential for delaying cognitive decline (n = 30, RCT, d/b, p/c, 6/12, Watson et al, Am J Geriatr Psychiatry 2005;**13**:950–8)
Saredutant (Sanofi-Aventis)	Saredutant is an antagonist at the neurokinin-2 receptor, which works by blocking the effects of the tachykinin neurokinin A at the NK-2 receptor and has an antidepressant and anxiolytic effect
Selegiline Transdermal System (Emsam®, BMS)	Selegiline Transdermal System (6–12 mg/24 hours) is licensed in USA for depression, with insomnia and application-site reactions the main adverse effects (n = 265, RCT, d/b, p/c, 8/52, Feiger et al, J Clin Psychiatry 2006;**67**:1354–61) and relapse prevention over a year in responders (n = 322, d/b, p/c, 52/52, Amsterdam and Bodkin, J Clin Psychopharmacol 2006;**26**:579–86) **Reviews:** Goodnick, Expert Opin Pharmacother 2007;**8**:59–64; Frampton and Plosker, Drugs 2007;**67**:257–67; Robinson and Amsterdam, J Affect Disord 2008;**105**:15–23)
Talnetant (GSK)	Talnetant is an orally active NK3 antagonist, under phase II/III trials for schizophrenia
Tarenflurbil (Flurizan®)	R-flurbiprofen is in phase III for mild Alzheimer's disease
Tasimelteon (Vanda) *	Tasimelteon is a melatonin agonist (VEC-162) acting on M1 and M2 receptors. Phase II and III studies have been successful (s = 2, n = 450, RCT, d/b, p/c, Rajaratnam et al, Lancet 2009;**373**:482–91) **Review:** (Hardeland, Curr Opin Investig Drugs 2009;**10**:691–701)
Tramiprosate (Alzhemed®, Neurochem)	In phase III trials for Alzheimer's as an anti-amyloid protein agent **Review:** Wright, Drugs Today [Barc] 2006;**42**:291–8; see Santa-Maria et al, Mol Neurodegener 2007;**2**:17
Volinanserin (Sanofi-Aventis, 2011?)	In phase III trials for insomnia (2008)
Xaliproden (Xaprila®, Sanofi-Aventis)	Xaliproden is a non-peptide compound that activates the synthesis of endogenous neurotropins, in phase III trials for Alzheimer's disease
Zolpidem CR (Sanofi-Aventis)	A two-layered tablet giving quick release and slower release with no residual effects from 6.26–12.5 mg/d in the elderly (n = 24, RCT, d/b, p/c, c/o, Hindmarsh et al, Br J Clin Pharmacol 2006;**62**:538–45; n = 205 [c = 198]. RCT, d/b, p/c, 3/52, Walsh et al, Am J Geriatr Psychiatry 2008;**16**:44–57; review by Barkin, Am J Ther 2007;**14**:299–305)

INDEX

All the main psychotropic drugs are indexed according to their BNF or other main indications in *Chapter 1*, but obviously may appear elsewhere. In order to keep the index down to a manageable size, you are then referred to the index listing for that drug's chemical or therapeutic group. Individual drugs should be looked up under their drug group.

527

Abbreviations

FOR DETAILS OF STUDIES:

n = number of patients

RCT = randomised controlled trial

d/b = double-blind

c/o = cross-over

o/p = out-patient

s/b = single blind (trial)

p/c = placebo-controlled

MS = manufacturer's study

OTHER ABBREVIATIONS:

AAPCD = American Academy of Pediatrics Committee on Drugs

ACh = acetylcholine

ACEI = ACE inhibitors

AD = Alzheimer's disease

ADHD = attention deficit hyperactivity disorder

ADD = attention deficit disorder

ADL = activities of daily living

ADME = absorption, distribution, metabolism and excretion

ADR = adverse drug reaction

AED = anti-epileptic drug

AFP = alpha-fetoprotein

AIMS = abnormal involuntary movement scale

AN = anorexia nervosa

APE = acute psychiatric emergency

APA = American Psychiatric Association

AWS = alcohol withdrawal syndrome

BAP = British Association for Psychopharmacology

BD = twice a day

BDD = body dysmorphic disorder

BDI = Beck Depression Inventory

BDZ = benzodiazepine(s)

BED = binge-eating disorder

BMA = British Medical Association

BMI = body mass index

BN = bulimia nervosa

BNF = British National Formulary

BPD = borderline psychiatric disorder

BPRS = Brief Psychiatric Rating scale

BPSD/BPSSD = behavioural and psychological (signs and) symptoms of dementia

bp = blood pressure

BP = British Pharmacopoeia

CBT = cognitive behavioural therapy

CBZ = carbamazepine

CBZ-E = carbamazepine-epoxide

CCK = cholecystokinin

CGI = clinical global impression

ChEIs = cholinesterase inhibitors

CHD = coronary heart disease

CNS = central nervous system

CPK = creatinine phosphokinase

CSE = convulsive status epilepticus

CSM = Committee on the Safety of Medicines

CVAE = cerebrovascular adverse events

D1 = dopamine-1 (receptor)

D2 = dopamine-2 (receptor)

DA = dopamine

DDD = defined daily dose

DSM-IV = Diagnostic Statistical Manual IV

DT = delirium tremens

e/c = enteric-coated

ECG = electrocardiogram

ECT = electroconvulsive therapy

EBMH = *Evidence-Based Mental Health* (journal)

EEG = electro-encephalogram

EPO = evening primrose oil

EPSE = extra-pyramidal side-effects

FBC = full blood count

FDA = federal Drug Agency

GABA = gamma-aminobutyric acid

GAD = generalised anxiety disorder

GB = Ginkgo Biloba

GFR = glomerular filtration rate

GTC = generalised tonic-clonic (seizure)

HAL-PRO = haloperidol + promethazine

5-HT = 5-hydroxytryptamine

HF = heart failure

IED = intermittent explosive disorder

IV = intravenous

IM = intramuscular

INR = international normalised ratio

IPT = interpersonal therapy

ISE = ion-selective electrode

ITT = intention to treat

KP = Korsakoff's psychosis

L/A = long-acting

LD = low dose

LFT = liver function tests

LTG = lamotrigine

MAOI = mono-amine oxidase inhibitor

MCM = major congenital malformations

MDD = major depressive disorder

MHA = Mental Health Act (1983)

MHRA = Medicines and Healthcare products Regulatory Agency (was CSM/MCA)

MI = manufacturers' information

MMSE = mini-mental state examination

MS = mood stabiliser

NA = noradrenaline

NCSE = non-convulsive status epilepticus

NE = norepinephrine

NICE = National Institute for Clinical Excellence

N/K = not known

NMDA = N-methyl-D-aspartate receptor

NMS = neuroleptic malignant syndrome

NPI = Neuropsychiatric Inventory

NNH = numbers needed to harm

NNT = numbers needed to treat

NPSA = National Patient Safety Agency (UK)

NSAIDs = non-steroidal anti-inflammatory drugs

OCD = obsessive-compulsive disorder

O/C = oral contraceptive

OD = overdose

OFC = olanzapine-fluoxetine combination

OTC = over-the-counter (medicine)

PD = personality disorder; pro-drug

PMH = previous medical history

PMS = pre-menstrual syndrome

PPHN = persistent pulmonary hypertension in the newborn

PT = prothrombin time

PTSD = post-traumtic stress disorder

PUFA = polyunsaturated fatty acid

QoLS = Quality of Life scale

QTc = corrected QT interval

REM = rapid eye movement

RIMA = reversible inhibitor of monoamine-A

RPSGB = Royal Pharmaceutical Society of Great Britain

RT = rapid tranquillisation

SA = short-acting

SAD = seasonal affective disorder

s/c = subcutaneous

SDS = Severity of Dependence scale

SF = sugar-free

SFQ = sexual functioning questionnaire

SIB = self-injurious behaviour

SIDS = sudden infant death syndrome

SJW = St John's wort

SPC = summary of product characteristics

SSRI = serotonin-selective reuptake inhibitor

STEP-BD = systematic treatment enhancement program for bipolar disorder

SUD = substance use disorders

t½ = half life

TAU = treatment as usual

TCA = tricyclic antidepressant

TD = tardive dyskinesia

TDM = therapeutic drug monitoring

TEAEs = treatment emergent adverse events

THC = tetrahydrocannabinol

TIA = transient ischaemic attack

TRS = treatment-resistant schizophrenia

U&E = urea and electrolytes

USP = United States Pharmacopoeia

VaD = vascular dementia

YMRS = Young Mania Rating scale